Contents

Games and audio pronunciations are available on the student Evolve website.

Acknowledgments

A teacher's greatest joy is learning that students found they were a step ahead because of having taken their class. Fresh ideas, sometimes a hint that makes a difficult term easier or an exercise that challenges one to think differently not only stimulates the brain but also makes learning more fun!

Each edition of *Building a Medical Vocabulary* results from collective hard work and dedication to accuracy.

Suggestions from instructors, students, and reviewers have been incorporated, and production would not be possible without the producers, editors, proofreaders, and all whose expertise has produced an outstanding book. I am blessed to have worked with Linda Woodard, Kelly Skelton, and Carolyn Kruse to produce a book that is "tried and true".

Peggy Leonard, MT, MEd

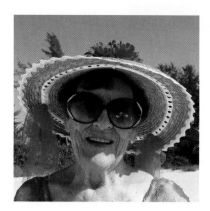

Peggy C. Leonard, at home in Florida

Dedicated to the instructors and students
whose enthusiasm and influence
have helped shape this book and to my
family who support me in so many ways.

BUILDING A MEDICAL VOCABULARY

with Spanish Translations

10th EDITION

PEGGY C. LEONARD, MT, MEd
Fort Myers, Florida

ELSEVIER

ELSEVIER

3251 Riverport Lane
St. Louis, Missouri 63043

BUILDING A MEDICAL VOCABULARY WITH SPANISH TRANSLATIONS,   ISBN: 978-0-323-42794-4
TENTH EDITION

Notices

Previous editions copyrighted 2015, 2012, 2009, 2005, 2001, 1997, 1993, 1988, 1983.

International Standard Book Number: 978-0-323-42794-4

Senior Content Strategist: Linda Woodard
Content Development Manager: Luke Held
Content Development Specialist: Kelly Skelton
Publishing Services Manager: Julie Eddy
Project Manager: Abigail Bradberry
Design Direction: Ashley Miner
Artist: Jeanne Robertson

Printed in Canada

Last digit is the print number: 9   8   7   6   5   4   3   2

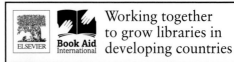

Reviewers

Tammy S. Clossen, RDH, PhD
Assistant Professor of Dental Hygiene
Pennsylvania College of Technology
Williamsport, Pennsylvania

Rita R. Courier, MA, CCA
Adjunct Instructor
North Central Michigan College
Petoskey, Michigan

Coleen Dent Jones, MS Edu
Professor and Program Director for Office and Medical
Office Technology
Valencia College—Osceola Campus
Kissimmee, Florida

Barbara Emert-Strouse, RDH Med
Assistant Professor
Pennsylvania College of Technology
Williamsport, Pennsylvania

Sandra Hertkorn, Director
Director of Operations
All Inclusive Medical Services Ambulatory Clinic
Carmichael, California

Carolyn M. Kruse, DC
Instructional Consultant
Kruisin Editorial & Voice
O'Fallon, Missouri

Jennifer A. Mai, PT, DPT, PhD, MHS, NCS
Associate Professor of Physical Therapy
Clarke University
Dubuque, Iowa

Sean F. Peck, MEd, EMT-P
Associate Faculty
Arizona Western College
Yuma, Arizona

Susan E. Saullo, RN, MS, MT (ASCP)
Adjunct Instructor
ITT Technical Institute
Lake Mary, Florida

Brian S. Spence, MSRS (Ed), RT(R)
Radiologic Technology Program Director
Tarrant County College
Fort Worth, Texas

Charles Kent Williston BA, MS, CPC
Instructor
Traviss Career Center
Lakeland, Florida

Contributors

Erinn Kao, RPh, PharmD, PRS
Pharmacist
St. Charles, Missouri

Brian S. Spence, MSRS (Ed), RT(R)
Radiologic Technology Program Director
Tarrant County College
Fort Worth, Texas

How to Use this Book

The tenth edition of *Building a Medical Vocabulary* is now even more interactive! It can be used in a medical terminology course or as self-paced material for anyone pursuing a career in the health professions.

THE MOST INTERACTIVE TEXT ON THE MARKET!

After learning the meaning of word parts and how they are combined using a logical, step-by-step learning method, you begin recognizing and writing new terms in the first chapter! *Immediate involvement and feedback* within the programmed method provide motivation not found in other systems.

TEXT ORGANIZATION

Strong Foundation: Chapters 1 through 3
Chapters 1 through 3 provide a foundation for chapters about the body systems. Be sure to study the first three chapters *in sequence,* because each chapter builds on the material learned in the previous chapter.

Body Systems (Chapters 4 through 13) Can Be Studied in Any Sequence
Because you can easily change the sequence of the body systems chapters, the book adapts well for use in conjunction with anatomy, physiology, or introductory medical science courses. *The organization of systems chapter material reflects the medical process: anatomy and physiology, diagnostic tests and procedures, pathologies, and surgical and therapeutic interventions.*

New! Chapter 14 on Oncology
Oncology applies to all body systems. Oncology can be studied before or after any systems chapter, to coordinate with your program.

Review: Comprehensive Review and Comprehensive Glossary/Index
Use the Index/Glossary to review terms for the big exams. To prepare for the final, complete the Self-Test after Chapter 14; it reviews the entire text!

Appendices
Appendices include abbreviations, word parts, Spanish translations, and exercise answers.

CHAPTER FEATURES

New! More Health Care Reports!
Now even more practice with real-life documents helps you gain confidence.

New! Dedicated Pharmacology!
Now every chapter introduces relevant drug classes and includes updated generic and trade names! The understanding of drug classes integrates easily into medical terminology and brings learning about body systems full circle to medical treatment of pathologies.

PHARMACOLOGY

Many of the agents in this chapter may be found together in combination drugs to treat multiple facets of a disease at once.

Drug Class: Effects and Uses

Antianginal Drugs: Relax blood vessels of the heart to treat and prevent angina
isosorbide dinitrate (Isordil)   nitroglycerin (Nitrostat)
isosorbide mononitrate (Imdur)   ranolazine (Ranexa)

Key Point Boxes

Key points help you focus on the most important material.

> 🔑 **KEY** POINT **Two important types of circulation occur each time the heart beats:**
> - **Systemic circulation:** The general circulation that carries oxygenated blood from the heart to the tissues of the body and returns the blood with much of its oxygen exchanged for carbon dioxide back to the heart
> - **Pulmonary circulation:** The circuit that the blood makes from the heart to the lungs for the purpose of ridding the body of carbon dioxide and picking up oxygen

Beyond the Blueprint

Information beyond the usual realm helps anchor word memory.

> ➤ **BEYOND** THE BLUEPRINT Occasionally you will encounter a word that doesn't seem to fit the rules because it isn't composed of word roots that make sense to you. For example, a cataract, which is an eye condition characterized by loss of transparency of the lens, is named for a Greek word that means waterfall. Perhaps the first physician who observed a cataract thought it resembled looking through a waterfall.

Look at .... ted word .... ing

Caution: Students at Work

Caution boxes help you distinguish between terms and word parts that look alike but have different meanings.

> **Be Careful With These!**
>
> -*ase* (enzyme) vs. -*ose* (sugar)
> *diagnosis* (identification of disease) vs. *prognosis* (predicted outcome)
> -*gram* (a record) vs. -*graph* (an instrument) vs. -*graphy* (a process)
> -*ia* (condition) vs. -*iac* (one who suffers)
> *iatrogenic* (unfavorable response to medical treatment) vs. *idiopathic* (disease without an apparent or known cause)
>
> *incision* (cutting into) vs. *excision* (cutting out, removal)
> -*lysin* (that which destroys) vs. -*lytic* (capable of destroying)
> -*phagia* (eating, swallowing) vs. -*phasia* (speech)
> -*plasia* (formation, development) vs. -*plasty* (surgical repair)
>
> -*rrhage* (excessive bleeding) vs. -*rrhea* (discharge) vs. -*rrhexis* (rupture)
> *sign* (objective) vs. *symptom* (subjective)
> -*tome* (cutting instrument) vs. -*tomy* (cutting into)
> -*tomy* (cutting into) vs. -*stomy* (formation of an opening)

More, More, More Exercises

Know if you understand a section before moving ahead. "Chunking" exercises chop material into manageable pieces.

FIND IT!
EXERCISE 14

Draw a slash between the combining forms and the suffixes in the following list of adjectives, all meaning "pertaining to" different structures or conditions. Then find the meanings of the word parts within the definitions. You may be wondering how you know which suffix to use, but this exercise will help you remember by visualizing the terms. (Draw the slash, and then perform the remainder of the activity as a mental exercise.) Think!

1. **blepharal** pertaining to the eyelids
2. **cancerous** pertaining to cancer
3. **cerebral** pertaining to the brain or the cerebrum
4. **mammary** pertaining to the breast
5. **tracheal** pertaining to the trachea (windpipe)

ANALYZE IT!
EXERCISE 15

Break these words into their component parts. Then write the meaning of each term.

1. lactase _____
2. lactose _____
3. pyromania _____
4. pyromaniac _____
5. neural _____

Making Connections, Finetuning Terms, Opting for Opposites
Compare-and-contrast exercises improve your ability to communicate in the specialized language of health care.

NEW! Expanded Art Program Has Even More Full-Color Illustrations and Photos
Full-color art and photos enhance learning and make difficult concepts easier to understand.

Mini-Glossaries
Rapid-fire recall of word parts in condensed "bytes" change the pace plus reinforce earlier learning.

Learn the following terms for various surgical procedures:

cryosurgery Destruction of small growths, such as warts, by application of extreme cold; **cryotherapy**

débridement The removal of foreign material and dead or damaged tissue, especially from a wound. To **débride** is to remove by dissection.

electrodessication Destruction of superficial skin growths by burning with an electric spark

escharotomy Surgical incision of constricting necrotic tissue resulting from a severe burn, done to relieve pressure from severe swelling and restore blood flow

incision and drainage (I&D) Opening of an infected wound and withdrawal of its fluids and discharges

onychectomy Excision of a nail; declawing of an animal

Expanded Index/Glossary
Now with more terms than ever, the Index/Glossary serves as a concise dictionary of medical terms. It is a superb study tool for a final exam and an excellent reference once you have completed the text.

New Chapter on Oncology!
An entire chapter devoted to this timely topic, Chapter 14 on Oncology applies to all body systems and can be taught in or out of sequence with body systems.

Medical Process
Orientation to the medical process is your reality check on how terms fit into patient presentation, diagnostics, and care, involving you in the center of the medical arena by understanding its world of terms. Recognizing terms that fit into each part of the medical process helps you make the connections between medicine and its terminology.

Career Highlights
What medical profession will you choose? Possible health career options and related website resources are included.

A Career as a Radiologic Technologist

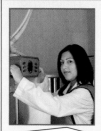

Radiologic technologists (RTs) play a vital role in diagnosis. They perform diagnostic imaging examinations, creating the images that radiologists evaluate. RTs work with many types of imaging, including plain x-ray examinations, magnetic resonance imaging (MRI), computed tomography (CT), mammography, sonography, and fluoroscopy. RTs can also be trained to administer radiation therapy treatments. Meet Jeanne Jones, an RT who works at a community hospital. She is positioning a patient for an x-ray examination of the abdomen. Jeanne loves her work, because she knows that radiologists, as well as patients, count on her to provide the best diagnostic tools possible. To learn more, visit the website *www.asrt.org.*

Boldfaced Terms and Pronunciations
Boldfaced terms are listed at the end of each chapter with their pronunciations; these lists coordinate with the audio files on the student Evolve web site, so you master pronunciation.

Spanish Terms

Every chapter presents related Spanish terms, and Appendix II summarizes all the Spanish terms presented in the text.

End-of-Chapter Self-Tests

Complete the end-of-chapter self-test, and check your answers in Appendix IV to ensure that you understand the material.

STUDENT EVOLVE WEBSITE FEATURES

Games help you rehearse and rapidly recall word parts and term meanings. Additional exercises offer practice.

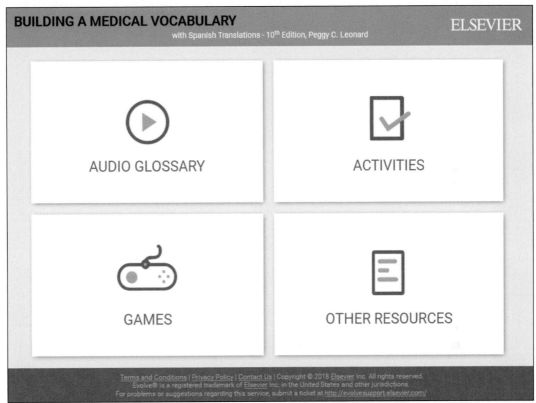

BUILDING A MEDICAL VOCABULARY
with Spanish Translations - 10th Edition, Peggy C. Leonard — ELSEVIER

AUDIO GLOSSARY   ACTIVITIES

GAMES   OTHER RESOURCES

Terms and Conditions | Privacy Policy | Contact Us | Copyright © 2018 Elsevier Inc. All rights reserved.
Evolve® is a registered trademark of Elsevier Inc. in the United States and other jurisdictions.
For problems or suggestions regarding this service, submit a ticket at http://evolvesupport.elsevier.com/

The student Evolve website also includes mobile-ready flashcards and quizzes, animations, audio glossary, anatomy coloring book, and career videos.

INSTRUCTOR EVOLVE WEBSITE FEATURES

TEACH Instructor Resources

The instructor resources on the Evolve website include a Test Bank, image collection, and the TEACH Instructor Resources: lesson plans, PowerPoint slides, and classroom handouts.

Building Medical Terms Starting With Medical Specialties

You'll find a career highlight in every chapter, introducing you to professions in which medical terminology is commonly used.

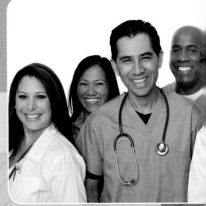

CONTENTS

LEARNING OUTCOMES

Basic Understanding

In this chapter you will learn to do the following:

1. Identify the roles of word roots, prefixes, suffixes, and combining forms.
2. Identify examples of combining forms, prefixes, suffixes, and word roots, and recognize them in medical terms.
3. Demonstrate correct usage of the combining vowel by correctly joining word parts to write medical terms.
4. Use the rules in this chapter to write singular and plural forms and to identify eponyms, acronyms, and abbreviations.
5. Use the rules in this chapter to pronounce medical terms correctly.
6. Write the meanings of selected word parts and use them to build and analyze terms.
7. Match the terms for medical specialists with the areas in which they specialize, or write the medical specialties when given the area of expertise.
8. Identify the specialty associated with various medical conditions.
9. List five categories for classifying medical terms that are used in this book.

Greater Comprehension

10. Spell medical terms accurately.
11. Write the meanings of terms and abbreviations, including those in a health report presented in this chapter.
12. Recognize the meanings of general pharmacological terms from this chapter as well as the drug classes and their uses.
13. Identify terms as a medical specialty, a specialist, another type of noun, or an adjective.
14. Pronounce terms correctly.

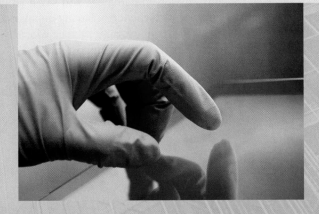

FUNCTION FIRST

The material in this chapter provides a blueprint for learning medical vocabulary. Using medical specialties (many of which you already recognize) as a foundation, you begin building new terms.

It is important to study material in the order in which it is presented within a chapter. It is also important to study Chapters 1 through 3 in sequential order, because these early chapters form the foundation for learning material about the body systems in Chapters 4 through 13. A blueprint is a photographic print of plans or something intended as a guide (Fig. 1.1). Be sure to work all of the exercises, because this helps you retain the material and often provides greater understanding.

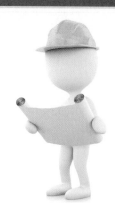

Figure 1.1 **This book provides a blueprint for learning medical terminology.** First, build the Foundation: Chapters 1–3. Then study Chapters 4–14.

Use this functional study guide as you work through each chapter.
1. Read each page in the chapter, writing answers in the blanks.
2. You'll see that variety keeps your mind engaged and you'll quickly begin writing medical terms you haven't seen before!
3. Pay attention to the visuals, reading the material that accompanies them.
4. Working every exercise and checking your answers will assure that you haven't missed important concepts and terms.
5. Work through all the Self-Test before checking the answers. This prepares you for a written test over the material in the chapter.
6. You'll be amazed at how quickly you'll begin building a medical vocabulary!

LEARNING MEDICAL TERMINOLOGY

1-1 This book provides an excellent guide to learning medical terminology, also called medical vocabulary. You've probably noticed that medicine has a language of its own.

1-2 In this book, you will use programmed learning, which consists of blocks of information (such as the one you're reading), often containing blanks in which you will write answers. After writing an answer, you will check to see if it is correct by comparing your answer with that in the left column, called the *answer column*.

🔑 **KEY** POINT **Cover the answer column while you are filling in the blanks.** To do this, position the bookmark so that it covers only the answer column. After writing your answer in a blank, check it by sliding the bookmark down just enough to see the answer. (Most are just one word.) When you are not using the bookmark to cover the answer column, use it to mark your place in the book.

frame

1-3 You have just read two frames. Information contained in frames throughout this book will help you learn medical terms. A block of information with a number is called a _____.

Write the answer in the preceding blank, and check it immediately. It is important to write your answer, because writing it will help you to remember it better than if you just think of the answer (Fig. 1.2). Always check your answer immediately, and say it aloud if possible. This is especially helpful when you are not familiar with the term. Saying an answer aloud helps you remember it. If you make an error, look back at previous frames to see where you went wrong. Otherwise, you may repeat the error without realizing why it is incorrect.

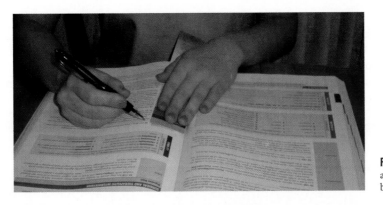

Figure 1.2 Write your answer. It is always important to write your answer because that helps you remember it.

1-4 This text provides frequent exercises to reinforce what you are learning. Answers are located in Appendix IV. If you are uncertain about pronunciation, check the BMV List at the end of the chapter. When you've completed the material in the chapter, a Self-Test helps integrate what you've learned. (Those answers are also found in Appendix IV.)

Be sure to complete all of the exercises! If you can't complete a blank, you'll see the correct response when you check your answers.

BUILDING WORDS

1-5 Word building is a system of learning the meaning of various word parts to understand and write new words. Because it is impractical to memorize the medical dictionary, you will use a system of word _____ to learn medical terms.

building

1-6 Pay close attention to spelling. For example, cyt(o) means cell, but cyst(o) means a bladder or sac; incision means to cut into, but excision means to cut out or remove. (When using a computer, be careful with Spell Check, because many medical terms aren't included in its program.) If you mistakenly say, "I sent an electrocardiograph to Dr. Gomez," you are saying that you sent a machine rather than a heart tracing (an electrocardiogram).

🔑 **KEY** POINT **A change of only one letter can result in a different term.** Be careful when writing a term. Example: the ilium is a pelvic bone, and the ileum is part of the small intestine; hydr(o) means water, and hidr(o) means perspiration.

CONSTRUCTED TERMS

1-7 Many medical terms are constructed terms (words that are made up of multiple word parts, which have meanings). You need only to learn the English translation of Greek or Latin word parts used in medical terms, and you already know some of them (for example, tonsillitis, dentist, anatomy, and appendectomy).

🔑 **KEY** POINT **In a constructed term, the word parts are key in decoding a term.** Word roots, combining forms, prefixes, and suffixes are word parts. Learning the meaning of these word parts eliminates the necessity of memorizing each new term you encounter. It is important to learn to recognize combining forms, prefixes, and suffixes in terms and how to combine them to write medical terms.

parts

Word roots, combining forms, prefixes, and suffixes are called word _____.

Word Roots

root

1-8 Most words, even ordinary words, have a word root (or stem). The word root is the foundation of the word. It is usually accompanied by a prefix or suffix or both. Word roots are the building blocks for many terms related to anatomy, diagnosis, and medical procedures. You see by reading this information that most words have a word _____.

 TOOL TIP!   *Beyond the Blueprint features give extra information to help you anchor your learning with interesting tidbits.*

➤ **BEYOND** THE BLUEPRINT Occasionally you will encounter a word that doesn't seem to fit the rules because it isn't composed of word roots that make sense to you. For example, a cataract, which is an eye condition characterized by loss of transparency of the lens, is named for a Greek word that means waterfall. Perhaps the first physician who observed a cataract thought it resembled looking through a waterfall.

WORD ORIGIN
Watch for this clue to tell you the origin of words.
D. German (Deutsch)
G. Greek
I. Italian
L. Latin

Look at the Greek and Latin words and their associated word roots in Table 1.1. By adding prefixes and suffixes, you will soon begin writing medical terms. (Don't be concerned about learning the meaning of the word parts in the early part of Chapter 1 just yet; however, you're expected to remember the word parts beginning with those on page 13. (Don't worry. You'll be reminded!)

1-9 You will sometimes learn two word roots that have the same meaning. Table 1.1 shows both the Greek word root *nephr* for kidney and the Latin word root *ren* for kidney. As a general rule, Latin roots are used to write words naming and describing structures of the body, whereas Greek roots are used to write words naming and describing diseases, conditions, diagnosis, and treatment.

Use this as a guideline only, because you will quickly learn exceptions. For example, both dermal and cutaneous mean *pertaining to the skin.* Likewise, both nephric and renal mean *pertaining to the kidney.*

Latin

When two medical terms have the same meaning but look very different, it is probably because the origins of the word roots are from two different languages, Greek and _____.

Table 1.1	Origin of Word Roots	
Word Root	**Greek or Latin Origin**	**Use in a Word**
nephr	*nephros* (G., kidney)	nephritis
psych	*psyche* (G., mind)	psychology
caud	*cauda* (L., tail)	caudal
or	*oris* (L., mouth)	oral
ren	*renes* (L., kidney)	renal
pharmac	*pharmakon* (G. drug)	pharmacist

Combining Forms

form

1-10 A vowel (usually "o") is often inserted between word roots to make the word easier to pronounce and to connect word parts. This vowel is called a *combining vowel.* A word root with a vowel attached is called a *combining form* and looks like this: speed(o).

🔑 **KEY** POINT Combining forms are the foundation of words and will be recognized in this book as word parts that end in an enclosed vowel. In thermometer, the combining form therm(o) is joined with another part of the word, meter. The parentheses are not included when the combining form joins other word parts. In cardiology and gastrology, cardi(o) and gastr(o) are the combining forms.

Study Table 1.2 and observe that a combining vowel is added to a word root to write a combining _____.

cephal(o)

1-11 Some compound words are composed of two word roots or words. The term *cephalometer* is composed of a word root and a word, cephal and meter. Write the combining form for cephal: _____.

Table 1.2 Examples of Word Roots and Combining Forms			
Word Root	**Combining Form**	**Meaning**	**Use in a Word**
blephar	blephar(o)	eyelid	blepharospasm
cephal	cephal(o)	head	cephalometry
fung	fung(i)	fungus	fungicide
or	or(o)	mouth	oropharynx
path	path(o)	disease	pathology

Collarbone and eyelid are examples of two words joined to form a new term.

You will learn the combining form for word roots, because word roots are often combined with other word parts. Combining forms act as the foundation for most terms. There are combining forms for all body structures and other nouns.

WRITE IT!
EXERCISE 1

Combining forms for six body structures are shown. Write the word root for each body structure that is labeled. (Number 1 is done as an example.)

1. ophthalm(o) _____*ophthalm*_____

2. nas(o) _____, rhin(o) _____

3. thorac(o) _____

4. spondyl(o) _____, vertebr(o) _____

5. abdomin(o) _____

(Use Appendix IV to check your answers.)

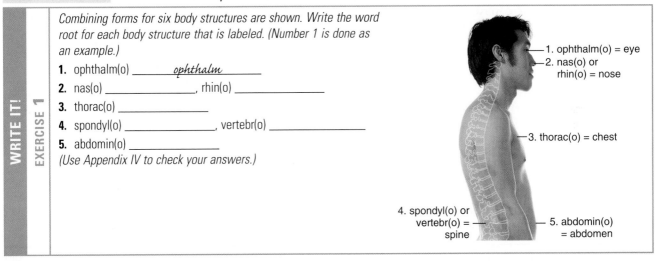

1. ophthalm(o) = eye
2. nas(o) or rhin(o) = nose
3. thorac(o) = chest
4. spondyl(o) or vertebr(o) = spine
5. abdomin(o) = abdomen

SELECT IT!
EXERCISE 2

Write either combining form *or* word root *after each of the following word parts: (Number 1 is done as an example.)*

1. aden(o) _____*combining form*_____

2. bil(i) _____

3. cyan _____

4. derm(a) _____

5. duoden _____

6. electr _____

7. gloss(o) _____

8. hemat _____

(Use Appendix IV to check your answers.)

Prefixes

1-12 A prefix is a word part that is placed before a word root to modify its meaning.

🔑 **KEY** POINT **A prefix written alone is usually followed by a hyphen. An-, anti-, and peri- are examples of prefixes.**

hyphen

When written alone, a prefix is usually followed by a _____.

water

1-13 In anhydrous, hydrous refers to water, and the prefix an- means without. Combining the two meanings, anhydrous means without _____.

sub-

1-14 In subnormal, sub- means below. In subnormal, which part of the word is the prefix? _____

below

Normal is a familiar word that we use to mean agreeing with the regular and established type. Its meaning is changed when a prefix is added. Subnormal means _____ normal.

Suffixes

1-15 A suffix is attached to the end of a word or word part to modify its meaning. Suffixes are joined to combining forms to write nouns (names; the subject of the sentence), adjectives (descriptive words), and verbs (action words). So, suffixes categorize the term by placing it in a group.

 KEY POINT **A suffix written alone is usually preceded by a hyphen.** The hyphen placed before a suffix indicates that another part precedes it. In the term *tonsillitis,* -itis means inflammation.

suffix

Blepharitis means inflammation of the eyelid. The word part blephar refers to the eyelid and is the word root. The word part -itis means inflammation and is being used as what part of the word?

_____

TOOL TIP! *Write your answer in the blank; then check it right away to be sure you understand. Check your spelling, too!*

dyspnea

1-16 Occasionally a word is composed of only a prefix and a suffix. Join dys- and -pnea to write a new word: _____. The prefix dys- means bad, painful, or difficult, and -pnea means breathing. Dyspnea means difficult breathing.

Visualize the relationship of prefixes, combining forms, and suffixes as you study Fig. 1.3.

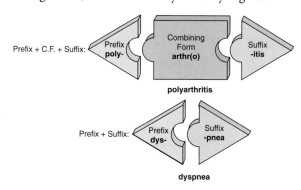

Figure 1.3 **The relationship of prefixes, combining forms, and suffixes.**

SELECT IT! EXERCISE 3

Write combining form, prefix, *or* suffix *for each of the following word parts:*

1. brady- _____
2. -cele _____
3. eu- _____
4. -graphy _____
5. hydr(o) _____
6. -iasis _____
7. mal- _____
8. phon(o) _____

SELECT IT! EXERCISE 4

A prefix or suffix is underlined in each of the following terms. Identify each underlined part as a prefix or a suffix.

1. <u>ad</u>hesion _____
2. adeno<u>pathy</u> _____
3. bili<u>ary</u> _____
4. der<u>mal</u> _____
5. <u>endo</u>cardial _____
6. hemato<u>logy</u> _____
7. <u>hypo</u>glossal _____
8. <u>micro</u>scope _____

(Use Appendix IV to check your answers.)

Using Word Parts to Write Terms

1-17 You have learned that medical terms are composed of word roots, combining forms, prefixes, and suffixes. You will now learn to combine these word parts to write medical terms.

 KEY POINT **You don't always need the combining vowel, so here's the rule: Use the combining vowel before suffixes that begin with a consonant and before another word root.**

consonant

(There are exceptions to the rule, and you will learn the exceptions as you progress through the material. For now, remember to drop the vowel before a suffix that begins with a vowel.) The rule for using the combining vowel shows us that the combining vowel is used in two cases. In one case, the combining vowel is used before a suffix that begins with a _____.

BUILD IT! EXERCISE 5

Use the rule you just learned to build terms, knowing that ot(o) means ear.

Combining Form + Suffixes	Term and Meaning
1. ot(o) + -ic =	_____, pertaining to the ear
2. ot(o) + -itis =	_____, inflammation of the ear
3. ot(o) + -logy =	_____, study of the ear
4. ot(o) + -plasty =	_____, plastic surgery of the ear
5. ot(o) + -rrhea =	_____, discharge from the ear
6. ot(o) + -tomy =	_____, incision of the ear

gastroenterology

1-18 The combining vowel is also used to join two combining forms. When combining gastr(o), meaning stomach, and enter(o), meaning intestine, gastroentero results. (Of course, this is not a complete word, because it needs a suffix.) Combine gastr(o) + enter(o) + -logy to write a term that means the study of the stomach, intestines, and related structures: _____.

carpal

1-19 The wrist is also called the *carpus*. Write a word that means pertaining to the wrist by combining carp(o), meaning wrist, and -al, meaning pertaining to: _____.

aortitis

1-20 The combining form aort(o) means aorta, and -itis means inflammation. Join the two word parts to write a term that means inflammation of the aorta: _____. (Check your spelling carefully.)

BUILD IT! EXERCISE 6

Combine the word parts to write medical terms.

1. tonsill(o) + -itis _____
2. ur(o) + -emia _____
3. cardi(o) + aortitis _____
4. ur(o) + genital _____
5. enter(o) + -itis _____
6. enter(o) + cyst _____
(Use Appendix IV to check your answers.)

1-21 The word-building rules are summarized in Table 1.3.

🔑 **KEY** POINT **In general, most prefixes require no change before they are joined with other word parts.** Notice that prefixes are not included in the rule concerning use of the combining vowel. (A few exceptions will be noted later.)

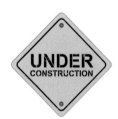

Table 1.3   Word-Building Rules
Joining Combining Forms
The combining vowel is usually retained between two combining forms.
Example: gastr(o) + enterology = gastroenterology
Joining Combining Forms and Suffixes
The combining vowel is usually retained when a combining form is joined with a suffix that begins with a consonant.
Example: enter(o) + -logy = enterology
The combining vowel is usually omitted when a combining form is joined with a suffix that begins with a vowel.
Example: enter(o) + -ic = enteric
Joining Other Word Parts and Prefixes
Most prefixes require no change when they are joined with other word parts.
Examples: peri- + appendicitis = periappendicitis; dys- + -pnea = dyspnea

BUILD IT! EXERCISE 7

Combine the word parts to write terms.

1. peri- + appendicitis _____
2. uni- + lateral _____
3. anti- + septic _____
4. an- + -emia _____
(Use Appendix IV to check your answers.)

1-22 If you correctly answered Exercises 6 and 7, you have learned the rules for using word parts to write medical terms. In this program, you will be using combining forms, prefixes, and suffixes to build many new words.

> 🔑 **KEY** POINT **Remember these simple rules for recognizing word parts:**
> - A combining form will be recognized as a word part that has a vowel enclosed in parentheses as its ending; example: appendic(o).
> - Prefixes will be designated by placing a hyphen after the word part (example: peri-).
> - Suffixes will be designated by placing a hyphen before the word part (example: -itis).

BUILD IT!   EXERCISE 8

Combine the following word parts to write medical terms.

1. acid(o) + -osis   _____
2. acr(o) + -megaly   _____
3. anti- + -emesis   _____
4. bronch(o) + -scopy   _____
5. dys- + -phagia   _____

6. hypo- + thyroid(o) + -ism   _____
7. leuk(o) + cyt(o) + -osis   _____
8. mal- + absorption   _____
9. my(o) + metr(o) + -ium   _____
10. thromb(o) + phleb(o) + -itis _____

(Use Appendix IV to check your answers.)

Breaking Apart Constructed Terms

1-23 You will also learn to recognize word parts as components of other words. To help you distinguish the component parts of medical terms, the words will often be divided by a diagonal line between the component parts.

two
For example, how many component parts are there in the word aden/oma? _____

three
How many component parts does peri/ophthalm/itis have? _____

> 🔑 **KEY** POINT **When looking at a new word, begin by looking at the suffix (Fig. 1.4).** Recognizing suffixes will help you identify the word as a noun, a verb, or an adjective. You will know the meaning of many suffixes after studying Chapters 2 and 3. After deciding the meaning of the suffix, go to the beginning of the word, and read across from left to right, interpreting the remaining elements to develop the full sense of the term.

When you use the suggested method, the interpretation of word parts in peri/ophthalm/itis is inflammation, around, eye. The full sense of the term is inflammation of tissues around the eye. See Fig. 1.5 to summarize what you have learned about writing and interpreting medical terms.

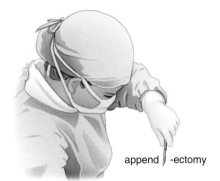

append | -ectomy

Figure 1.4 Dissect words into component parts. Look for a suffix first; then look for other word parts you recognize.

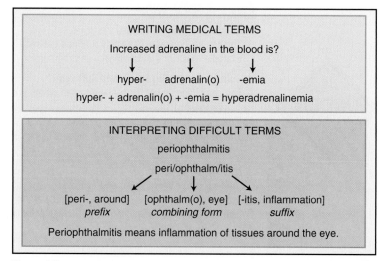

WRITING MEDICAL TERMS

Increased adrenaline in the blood is?

↓   ↓   ↓
hyper-   adrenalin(o)   -emia

hyper- + adrenalin(o) + -emia = hyperadrenalinemia

INTERPRETING DIFFICULT TERMS

periophthalmitis

peri/ophthalm/itis

[peri-, around]   [ophthalm(o), eye]   [-itis, inflammation]
prefix   *combining form*   *suffix*

Periophthalmitis means inflammation of tissues around the eye.

Figure 1.5 Examples of using prefixes, suffixes, and combining forms to write and interpret medical terms.

1-24 Now that you have learned about word parts and how to analyze terms, you need to be aware that some terms do not follow the rules you have learned. In other cases, two spellings are accepted. Whenever you are in doubt, check a medical dictionary. Two spellings of the same term usually come about through popular use (for example, both thoracentesis and thoracocentesis mean surgical puncture of the chest wall). As we progress through the material, such exceptions are noted.

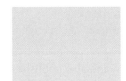

NONCONSTRUCTED TERMS AND VOCABULARY AIDS

Acronyms and Eponyms

acronyms

1-25 Nonconstructed terms are not formed from a combination of word parts, and sometimes include a person's name (for example, Parkinson) or acronyms, words formed from initials that are pronounceable (for example, CABG, pronounced as "cabbage"). Word building will not be as helpful when analyzing nonconstructed terms. Words formed from initials that are pronounceable, such as "cabbage" for CABG are _____.

🔑 **KEY** POINT **Eponyms are names of diseases, organs, procedures, or body functions that are derived from the name of a person.** A cesarean section, a surgical procedure in which the abdomen and uterus are incised to deliver an infant, is an eponym and named after the manner in which Julius Caesar was supposedly born. Parkinson disease and Alzheimer disease are also eponyms. Eponyms are usually capitalized; however some eponyms used to write adjectives are written in lowercase (for example, cesarean section).

CIRCLE IT! **EXERCISE 9**

Circle the eponyms in the following list.
1. Alzheimer disease vs. wasting disease
2. Beckman thermometer vs. oral thermometer
3. cesarean section vs. frozen section
4. cardiac catheter vs. Foley catheter
5. electronic fetal monitor vs. Holter monitor

Abbreviations

1-26 Abbreviations are shortened forms of words or phrases. Abbreviations include the following:
- Letters (The abbreviation for complete blood cell count is CBC.) Remember that some abbreviations, acronyms such as TURP (meaning transurethral resection of the prostate), are pronounced as words.
- Shortened words (The abbreviation stat. is short for *statim,* which is Latin for at once or immediately.)

Abbreviations and symbols save time but can be confusing, because some have more than one meaning. The abbreviation C means canine tooth, carbon, and Celsius, among others. Also, some uppercase abbreviations have different meanings than the lowercase equivalents (CC means chief complaint, and cc means cubic centimeter).

abbreviations

Shortened words or phrases are called _____.

🔑 **KEY** POINT **Using abbreviations and symbols can be dangerous.** The Institute for Safe Medication Practices publishes lists of what are considered dangerous abbreviations and recommends that certain terms be written in full, because they are easily mistaken for one with another meaning (for example, qn, meaning nightly or at bedtime, is misinterpreted as qh, which means every hour). In addition, use only abbreviations that are approved by your employer (generally consistent with those of your professional organization).

1-27 Abbreviations are presented in this book because many are still commonly used, but particular caution must be taken in both using and reading abbreviations. If a common abbreviation is missing, you may wish to check to see if its use is discouraged by the Institute for Safe Medication Practices. The Institute's website address is *www.ismp.org.*

TOOL TIP!   *Use abbreviations sparingly and with caution!*

Commission

The Joint Commission (TJC) is recognized nationwide as a symbol of quality, and also publishes an official "Do Not Use" List of Abbreviations and Symbols. The Joint Commission is an independent, not-for-profit organization that accredits and certifies subscriber hospitals and other health care organizations. Look for their "Do Not Use" list of abbreviations under the "Topics" tab, then choose "Patient Safety" at *www.jointcommission.org* and in Table 1.7 of this chapter. If you are unsure if an abbreviation should be used, check the website for The Joint _____.

MATCH IT! EXERCISE 10

Match the examples in the left columns with the type of term in the right column.

_____ **1.** CPR   _____ **5.** lig.   **A.** abbreviation

_____ **2.** D&C   _____ **6.** PFT   **B.** eponym

_____ **3.** Gram stain   _____ **7.** Raynaud disease

_____ **4.** Foley catheter _____ **8.** stat.

Plurals

abrasions; cysts

1-28 When you see a noun in its singular form, you will learn to write a plural for that term, but be aware that sometimes more than one plural is acceptable. Although plurals of many medical terms are formed using rules you may already know, it is important to learn rules that apply when terms have special endings.

Many plurals are formed by simply adding an "s" to the singular term. Write plurals by adding an "s" to these singular terms:

abrasion _____; cyst _____

branches, brushes
sinuses

1-29 Many nouns that end in "s," "ch," or "sh" form their plurals by adding "es." The plural of abscess is abscesses. Write plurals by adding "es" to these terms:

branch _____; brush _____;
sinus _____

capillaries; ovaries
extremities

1-30 Singular nouns that end in "y" preceded by a consonant form their plurals by changing the "y" to "i" and adding "es." For example, the plural of allergy is allergies. Change the "y" to "i" and add "es" to write plurals of these nouns:

capillary _____; ovary _____;
extremity _____

1-31 Use Table 1.4 to learn the rules for forming other plurals of medical terms, but be aware that there are a few exceptions and that only major rules are included. Many dictionaries show the plural forms of nouns and can be used as references. Also notice that some terms have more than one acceptable plural. Get more practice with plurals at *http://evolve.elsevier.com/Leonard/building*.

WRITE IT! EXERCISE 11

Write the plural form for each of the following singular nouns.

1. capsule _____   **6.** meninx _____

2. cataract _____   **7.** neurosis _____

3. calculus _____   **8.** protozoon _____

4. cortex _____   **9.** vertex _____

5. diagnosis _____   **10.** virus _____

Table 1.4 Forming Plurals of Nouns With Special Endings

If the Singular Ending Is	The Plural Ending Is	Examples (Singular)	Examples (Plural)
is ——————→ es		diagnosis, prognosis, psychosis	diagnoses, prognoses, psychoses
(Some words ending in is *form plurals by dropping the* is *and adding* ides, *as in epididymis and epididymides.)*			
um ——————→ a		atrium, ileum, septum, bacterium	atria, ilea, septa, bacteria
us ——————→ i		alveolus, bacillus, bronchus	alveoli, bacilli, bronchi
(Some singular terms ending in us *form plurals by dropping the* us *and adding either* era *or* ora, *for example, viscus and viscera and corpus and corpora. Others form plurals by simply adding* es; *for example, virus becomes viruses.)*			
a ——————→ ae		vertebra, patella, petechia	vertebrae, patellae, petechiae
ix ——————→ ices		appendix, varix, cervix	appendices, varices, cervices
(Through common use, appendixes and cervixes have become acceptable plural forms.)			
ex ——————→ ices		cortex	cortices
ax ——————→ aces		thorax	thoraces (thoraxes is also acceptable)
ma ——————→ s or mata		carcinoma, sarcoma	carcinomas or carcinomata, sarcomas or sarcomata
on ——————→ a		protozoon, spermatozoon	protozoa, spermatozoa
(Some singular forms ending in on *form plurals by adding* s; *for example, chorion becomes chorions.)*			
nx ——————→ nges		phalanx, larynx	phalanges, larynges

WRITE IT!
EXERCISE 12

Write the singular form of each of the following plural nouns.

1. appendices _____
2. fungi _____
3. larynges _____
4. prognoses _____

5. sarcomata _____
6. spermatozoa _____
7. syndromes _____
8. thrombi _____

(Use Appendix IV to check your answers.)

Pronunciation of Medical Terms

dren
ī
short

1-32 A medical term is easier to remember when you know how to pronounce it. Be aware that there are different ways to pronounce some medical terms. If you have not already done so, study the rules for pronunciation that are found at the back of this book. Do this before proceeding to the remaining frames of this chapter.

In the term adrenaline (uh-**dren**-uh-lin), which syllable has the primary accent? _____

In adrenalitis (uh-drē-nul-**ī**-tis), which syllable has the primary accent? _____

Is the "a" in angiectomy (an-jē-**ek**-tuh-mē) pronounced as a long or short "a"? _____

Some letter combinations are unusual (Table 1.5).

Table 1.5 Pronunciation of Unusual Letter Combinations

Spelling	Pronounced as	Example
eu	ū	euphoria
ph	f	pharmacy
pn	n	pneumonia
ps	s	psychology
pt	t	ptosis
rh	r	rheumatic

lō
short

1-33 In ankylosis (ang-kuh-**lō**-sis), which is the primary accented syllable? _____
Is the vowel in the sis syllable pronounced as a long or short "i"? _____

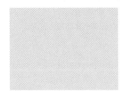 **KEY** POINT **There are three ways to learn pronunciation:**
- Terms in boldface type are shown with their pronunciations in the BMV List at the end of each chapter.
- Use the Evolve website to listen to the pronunciations.
- Use end-of-chapter exercises, "Categorizing Terms and Practicing Pronunciation," and be prepared to pronounce terms in class.

While looking at the terms at the end of each chapter (for example Chapter 1, pages 34 and 35, listen to the pronunciations on the Evolve website. Look closely at the spelling, and be sure that you know its meaning. If you can't recall its meaning, reread the frames that pertain to the term. (The Glossary Index in the back of the book may also help.) Once you've mastered the chapter, use the audio files on the Evolve website to test your recognition and spelling of terms.

WRITE IT!
EXERCISE 13

Write answers in the blanks to review your understanding of the rules of pronunciation used in this book. Use the pronunciation shown in question 1 to answer 2, 3, and 4.

1. How many syllables does the term hypercalcemia (hī-pur-kal-**sē**-mē-uh) have? _____
2. Is the e in the syllable sē long or short? _____
3. Which syllable receives the primary accent? _____
4. List all vowels that are pronounced as long vowels: _____

 MEDICINE AND ITS SPECIALTIES

prefix

1-34 You have learned that prefixes, suffixes, and combining forms are word parts that are used to write medical terms. Which word part is placed before a word root to modify its meaning? _____

combining

1-35 Some word parts end in an enclosed vowel—for example, psych(o). You recognize this type of word part as a _____ form.
This chapter introduces several combining forms associated with the medical specialties. You will also learn a few prefixes and suffixes that are used in naming both the specialties and the specialists.

TOOL TIP! *Note! You will learn many word parts as you study each chapter. Beginning now, you are expected to remember the meanings of word parts and terms that are introduced.*

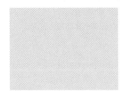 **KEY** POINT **Essential terms are included in the BMV List that follows each chapter's Self Test.** You need to remember their meanings and correct spellings.

suffix

1-36 Which word part is attached to the end of a word or word part to modify its meaning? _____
Suffixes are added to other word parts (mainly combining forms) to write terms.
The American Medical Association (AMA) is made up of the largest group of physicians and medical students in the United States, which includes recognized medical specialties, as well as general care physicians. Study these suffixes that pertain to the studies or the physicians.

TOOL TIP! *Make flash cards for word parts and their meanings whenever you see the flash card symbol!*

Word Parts: Suffixes Used in Writing Medical Specialists and Their Specialties

Suffix	Meaning	Suffix	Meaning
Terms About Specialists		**Terms About Specialties**	
-er, -ist	one who	-ac, -al, -ar, -ic, -ical	pertaining to
-iatrician	practitioner	-iatrics, -iatry	medical profession or treatment
-logist	one who studies; specialist	-logic, -logical	pertaining to the science or study of
		-logy	study or science of

Use the electronic flash cards on the Evolve website or make your own set of flash cards using the above list. Select the word parts just presented, and study them until you know their meanings. Do this each time a set of word parts is presented.

---

one

1-37 The suffixes -er and -ist mean _____ who.

You know many terms that contain these suffixes—for example, practitioner (one who practices) and specialist (one who is devoted to a special field or occupation). In medicine, a specialist is a person who has advanced education and training in one area of practice, such as internal medicine, dermato/logy, or cardio/logy.

study

1-38 The suffix -logy means the _____ or science of, and the suffix -logist means one who studies or a specialist.

Also notice that several suffixes in the list, including -ic and -ical, mean pertaining to.

profession

1-39 The suffixes that are mentioned in the last two frames are not used exclusively in writing medical terms. You will be able to think of many words that use these word parts. The suffixes -iatrics and -iatry are more specific for medicine and mean the medical _____ or a medical treatment.

MATCH IT! **EXERCISE 14**

Match the suffixes in the left columns with their meaning in the right column. Some choices will be used more than once.

_____ **1.** -ac   _____ **5.** -ic

_____ **2.** -er   _____ **6.** -ist

_____ **3.** -iatrician _____ **7.** -logist

_____ **4.** -iatry   _____ **8.** -logy

A. medical profession or treatment
B. one who
C. one who studies; specialist
D. practitioner
E. pertaining to
F. study or science of

1-40 The term *medicine* has several meanings, including a drug or a remedy for illness. A second meaning of medicine is the art and science of diagnosis, treatment, and prevention of disease. Medicine recognizes that a person is a composite of physical, social, spiritual, emotional, and intellectual needs (holistic needs, Fig. 1.6).

WORD ORIGIN
holistic *(G.)*
holos, whole

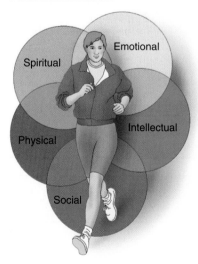

Figure 1.6 Holistic health needs. This viewpoint recognizes the integrated aspects of a person's physical, emotional, intellectual, social, and spiritual needs.

🔑 **KEY** POINT **The holistic viewpoint considers the person as a functioning whole.** **Holistic health** views the individual as an integrated system in which the separate parts interact and influence one another. (Reminder: boldface terms are included in the BMV List, which is an alphabetical list at the end of each chapter.)

holistic
Recognizing that a person is a composite of physical, social, emotional, spiritual, and intellectual needs is a _____ viewpoint. Read about alternative medicine on the Evolve website (*http://evolve.elsevier.com/Leonard/building*).

1-41 **Family practice** is a medical specialty that encompasses several branches of medicine and coordinates health care for all members of a family. A family practice physician often acts as the **primary health care provider,** referring complex disorders to other specialists. The family practice physician has largely replaced the concept of a general practitioner (GP).

1-42 **Internal medicine** is a clinical (nonsurgical) specialty of medicine that deals specifically with the diagnosis and treatment of diseases of the internal structures of the body. The specialist is called an **internist.**

🔑 **KEY** POINT **Don't confuse an** *internist* **with the term** *intern.* An intern in many clinical programs is any immediate postgraduate trainee. A physician intern is in postgraduate training, learning medical practice under supervision before being licensed as a physician. An internist, however, is a licensed medical specialist.

internist
A physician who specializes in internal medicine is an _____.
Study the following combining forms associated with the medical specialties and remember the names of the medical specialties.

Word Parts: Combining Forms: Selected Medical Specialties

Combining Form(s)	Meaning	Medical Specialty	Medical Specialist
cardi(o)	heart	**cardiology**	**cardiologist**
crin(o)	to secrete	**endocrinology**	**endocrinologist**
dermat(o)	skin	**dermatology**	**dermatologist**
esthesi(o)	feeling or sensation	**anesthesiology**	**anesthesiologist**
gastr(o), enter(o)	stomach, intestines*	**gastroenterology**	**gastroenterologist**
ger(a), ger(o), geront(o)	elderly or aged	**geriatrics**	**geriatrician**
gynec(o)	female	**gynecology**	**gynecologist**
immun(o)	immune	**immunology**	**immunologist**
ne(o), nat(o)	new, birth	**neonatology**	**neonatologist**
neur(o)	nerve	**neurology**	**neurologist**
obstetr(o)	midwife	**obstetrics**	**obstetrician**
onc(o)	tumor	**oncology**	**oncologist**
ophthalm(o)	eye	**ophthalmology**	**ophthalmologist**
orth(o), ped(o)	orth(o) means straight, ped(o) means child (sometimes, foot)	**orthopedics**	**orthopedist (orthopedic surgeon)**
ot(o), laryng(o)	ear, larynx	**otolaryngology**	**otolaryngologist**
path(o)	disease	**pathology**	**pathologist**
ped(o)	child (sometimes, foot)	**pediatrics**	**pediatrician**
psych(o)	mind	**psychiatry**	**psychiatrist**
radi(o)	radiant energy, radiation (sometimes, radius)	**radiology**	**radiologist**
rheumat(o)	rheumatism	**rheumatology**	**rheumatologist**
rhin(o)	nose	**rhinology**	**rhinologist**
ur(o)	urinary tract (sometimes, urine)	**urology**	**urologist**

*Enter(o) sometimes refers specifically to the small intestine.

 Audio files for boldfaced terms are found on the student Evolve website!

WRITE IT! EXERCISE 15

Write meanings for these combining forms.

1. crin(o) _____
2. esthesi(o) _____
3. gastr(o) _____
4. geront(o) _____
5. gynec(o) _____

6. laryng(o) _____
7. nat(o) _____
8. ne(o) _____
9. orth(o) _____
10. rhin(o) _____

WRITE IT! EXERCISE 16

Write the combining form you just learned for the following meanings.

1. child _____
2. ear _____
3. eye _____
4. foot _____
5. heart _____

6. immune _____
7. mind _____
8. nerve _____
9. skin _____
10. urinary tract _____

FIND IT! EXERCISE 17

Draw a slash before the suffixes in the following list of new adjectives (descriptive terms). Then, find the meanings of the word parts within the definition. Draw the slash, and then perform the remainder of the activity as a mental exercise. This is one way to begin recognizing unfamiliar words. Think! (The first one is done as an example.) When you are working in your chosen profession, you may need to use a medical dictionary to know the full meaning of a term.

1. **dermatologic, dermatological** pertaining to dermatology (skin specialty)
   dermato/logic, dermato/logical: dermat(o), skin; -logic or -logical, pertaining to the study of.
2. **cardiologic** pertaining to cardiology (heart specialty)
3. **cardiac** pertaining to the heart
4. **gastric** pertaining to the stomach
5. **neurologic, neurological** pertaining to neurology or the nervous system

6. **ophthalmologic, ophthalmological** pertaining to ophthalmology (eye specialty)
7. **ophthalmic** pertaining to the eye
8. **otic** pertaining to the ear
9. **pediatric** pertaining to pediatrics or the health of children
10. **pathologic, pathological** pertaining to pathology or caused by a diseased condition

WRITE IT! EXERCISE 18

Write the medical specialty associated with the following new terms:

1. **geriatric** _____
2. **immunologic** _____
3. **obstetric, obstetrical** _____

4. **orthopedic** _____
5. **radiologic** or **radiological** _____

dermal

1-43 One's preference determines the use of dermatologic or dermatological, and either term means pertaining to dermatology or pertaining to the skin. Many adjectives are written either way. Combine derm(o) and -al to write another term that means pertaining to the skin: _____.

pathologist

1-44 Pathology is the general study of the characteristics, causes, and effects of disease. The specialist in pathology is a _____. A pathologist collaborates with most of the other medical specialties.

Pathology has many specialties and subspecialties.

A pathologist is certified in **clinical** or **anatomic pathology** or both. A **clinical pathologist** is a physician who is certified in the laboratory study of disease, and there are many subspecialties. An **anatomic pathologist** is certified in the study of the effects of disease on the structure of the body. Subspecialties include surgical pathologists and those who specialize in autopsies. When surgical specimens are obtained, a surgical pathologist studies the appearance of the tissue, a technician specially trained in this area prepares thin slices of the tissue, and then the tissue is examined microscopically. During a surgery the surgical pathologist sometimes performs a frozen section method to determine how the operation should be modified or completed.

obstetrician

1-45 Many gynecologists also specialize in obstetrics. **Obstetrics** (OB) deals with pregnancy, labor, delivery, and immediate care after childbirth; however, obstetr(o) means midwife. Midwives assisted women during childbirth before obstetrics developed as a medical specialty.

Write the name of the physician who specializes in obstetrics: _____.

Nurse midwives manage normal pregnancies, labor, and childbirth. A nurse midwife is a registered nurse with advanced education and clinical experience in obstetrics and care of newborns. Nurse midwives work with women having normal pregnancies and uncomplicated deliveries.

neonatologist

1-46 **Neo/nato/logy** is the branch of medicine that specializes in the care of newborns, infants from birth to 28 days of age. A physician who specializes in neonatology is a _____.

> **BEYOND** THE BLUEPRINT Neonatal refers to the period of time covering the first 28 days of life. Newborns are given a physical examination (PE) soon after birth (Fig. 1.7). In general, weight triples and height increases by 50% in the first year of a healthy infant's life. Head circumference is also measured, and subsequent measurements are taken for the first few years. A rapidly rising head circumference suggests increased pressure inside the skull, and an unusually small head may indicate underdevelopment of the brain.

pediatrics

1-47 The word root for child is ped(o). **Ped/iatrics** is devoted to the study of children's diseases. Because diseases of children are often quite different from diseases encountered later in life, most parents prefer to take their children to a physician who specializes in _____.

The suffix -iatrician, which means practitioner, is used to write the name of the physician who specializes in pediatrics. A **ped/iatrician** specializes in the development and care of infants and children and in the treatment of their diseases (Fig. 1.8).

endocrinologist

1-48 The science of the endocrine glands and the hormones they produce is **endocrinology.** A specialist in endocrinology is called an _____.

Glands are organs that secrete material not related to ordinary metabolism. Those that secrete hormones into the bloodstream are endocrine glands. One example of an endocrine gland is the adrenal gland, which secretes adrenaline (epinephrine) into the bloodstream.

The **endo/crine** glands secrete chemical messengers called *hormones* into the bloodstream. These hormones play an important role in regulating the body's metabolism. The prefix endo- means inside. The suffix -crine, from the combining form crin(o), means to secrete. A gland is an organ with specialized cells that secrete material not related to their ordinary metabolism.

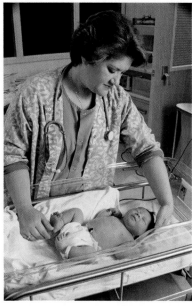

Figure 1.7 Nurse caring for a newborn in the neonatal unit.

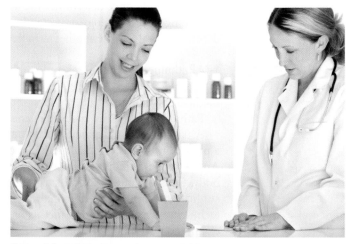

Figure 1.8 Pediatrician with young child. Skill levels and much information are gained while watching and talking to a child at play.

geriatrician

1-49 Three combining forms—ger(a), ger(o), and geront(o)—mean old age or the aged. The scientific study of all aspects of the aging process and issues encountered by older persons is **geronto/logy.** The branch of medicine that deals with the problems of aging and the diseases of older persons is geriatrics. A physician who specializes in gerontology is a _____.

The selection of the correct combining form may be confusing. Common usage determines which term is proper. Practice will help you to remember.

> **BEYOND** THE BLUEPRINT The older adult population is growing faster than the rest of the population. Gerontologic nursing is the care of older adults based on specialty knowledge of gerontology. Subcategories of older adults include living independently, physically active, cognitively impaired, and chronically ill. The usual teaching method of demonstration and return demonstration increases the possibility of successful learning by the patient, especially an older person.

otolaryngologist

1-50 An **otologist** specializes in **otology,** the study of the ear, including the diagnosis and treatment of its diseases and disorders. Physicians who specialize in ear, nose, and throat disorders are ear, nose, and throat (ENT) specialists, or otolaryngologists. The combining form ot(o) means ear and laryng(o) means **larynx,** or the voice box. **Oto/laryngo/logy** commonly refers to the branch of medicine dealing with diseases and disorders of the ears, nose, throat, and nearby structures (Fig. 1.9). An _____ is a physician who practices otolaryngology.

Ophthalmology (ophth) specializes in the diagnosis and treatment of disorders of the eye, including the performance of certain eye surgeries (Fig. 1.10).

anesthesiologist

1-51 An/esthesio/logy is the branch of medicine concerned with the administration of anesthetics and with their effects. The physician who administers anesthetics during surgery is an _____. An **an/esthetist** is a nurse or other person trained in administering anesthetics.

🔑 **KEY** POINT An **anesthetic** is a drug or agent that is capable of producing a complete or total loss of feeling. The prefix an- means no, not, or without. The literal interpretation of anesthesiology is the study of no feeling, but you need to remember that it is the branch of medicine concerned with the administration of drugs that produce a loss of feeling. Written alone, the term *anesthetic* means producing or characterized by anesthesia.

anesthetic

The postanesthesia care unit (PACU) is an area adjoining surgery or other areas where anesthesia is administered. Patients are assessed and cared for while recovering from anesthesia. The drug or agent that produces partial or total anesthesia is an _____.

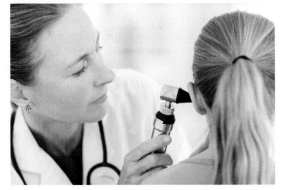

Figure 1.9 Otolaryngology. An otolaryngologist specializes in ear, nose, and throat disorders.

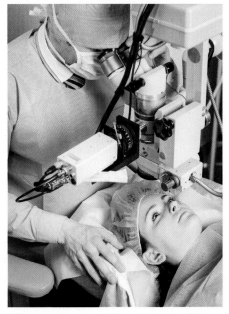

Figure 1.10 Surgeon using a video microscope for eye surgery.

BUILD IT!

EXERCISE 19

Build medical terms for the following definitions by using the word parts you have learned. The first question is done as an example.

1. obstetrician's specialty   _____*obstetr*/*ics*_____

2. endocrine gland specialist   _____/_____/_____

3. female specialty   _____/_____

4. otolaryngology specialist   _____/_____/_____

5. specialty of a pediatrician   _____/_____

6. specialist in the general study of disease   _____/_____

7. specialty of an anesthesiologist   _____/_____/_____

8. specialty of caring for newborns   _____/_____/_____

1-52 The rapidly changing specialty, **onco/logy,** is concerned with the study of malignancy. The combining form onc(o) means tumor. Tumor can sometimes mean a swelling but as used here means an uncontrolled growth of tissue. Not all tumors are malignant (become worse and threatening to cause death) (Table 1.6).

Table 1.6 Tumors	
Not Malignant	**Malignant**
Slow growing	Rapidly growing
Does not invade	Invades surrounding tissue

1-53 The combining form radi(o) means radiation or radiant energy. (Sometimes radi[o] is used to mean radius, a bone of the forearm, but usually it refers to radiant energy.) **Radio/logy** is the use of various forms of radiant energy (such as x-rays) in the diagnosis and treatment of disease. The physician who studies and interprets radiographs (x-ray examinations) is a

radiologist

_____. **Roentgenology** is a branch of radiology dealing with the use of roentgen rays (x-rays).

➤ **BEYOND** THE BLUEPRINT Sometimes radiology is called *roentgenology*, which is named after its discoverer, Wilhelm Conrad Röntgen (with the unusual "o" as already shown). Radiology includes the use of other forms of radiant energy for diagnostic and therapeutic purposes.

1-54 Radiology deals with radioactive substances and radiant energy in the diagnosis and treatment of disease. X-rays pass through some substances and expose radiographic film or digital image receptors to create an image, which enables the radiologist to view internal structures of the body.

1-55 The combining form ur(o) means urine or urinary tract. **Urology** is concerned with the urinary tract in both genders, as well as the male genital tract. A specialist in urology is a

urologist

_____.

   Urologic, urological, and **urinary** mean pertaining to the urine or the urinary system. A uro/logic examination is an examination of the urinary tract.

1-56 Immuno/logy is a rapidly expanding area of medicine, and immun(o) is the combining form for immune. This branch of science involves assessment of the patient's immune defense mechanism against disease, hypersensitivity, and many diseases now thought to be associated with the immune mechanism. This mechanism involves the natural defenses that protect the body from pathogenic organisms and malignancies, but it is also involved in allergies, excessive reactions to common and often harmless substances in the environment.

immunologist

   The specialist in immunology is an _____. Sometimes immunology is combined with the identification and treatment of allergies.

1-57 Almost all words that contain the combining form rheumat(o) pertain to rheumatism. **Rheumatology** is the branch of medicine that deals with rheumatic disorders. One may think of **rheumatism** as just one disease, but it is any of a variety of disorders marked by inflammation, degeneration, or other problems of the connective tissues of the body, especially the joints and related structures.

rheumatologist

A specialist in rheumatology is a _____.

> ➤ **BEYOND** THE BLUEPRINT Ancient Greeks thought humors (certain fluids within the body) became imbalanced. They believed that one's health was determined by the mixture of humors. The word *rheum* meant a watery discharge; rheumatism was thought to be caused by a flowing of humors in the body and was thus named.

1-58 Psych/iatry is a medical specialty that deals with the causes, treatment, and prevention of mental, emotional, and behavioral disorders. A physician who specializes in psychiatry is a **psychiatrist.**

psychologist

Clinical psycho/logy is concerned with the diagnosis, treatment, and prevention of a wide range of personality and behavioral disorders. One who is trained in this area is a **clinical** _____. Clinical psychology is a branch of psychology rather than a branch of medicine.

neurology

1-59 A **neuro/logist** is a physician who specializes in _____, the field of medicine that deals with the nervous system and its disorders.

The combining form neur(o) means nerve. A nerve cell is called a **neuron** (Fig. 1.11). In many words, neur(o) refers to the nervous system, which is composed of the brain, spinal cord, and nerves.

neurosurgeon

1-60 Neurosurgery is surgery involving the brain, spinal cord, and/or peripheral nerves. Build a word combining neur(o) with surgeon that means a surgeon who specializes in surgery of the nervous system: _____.

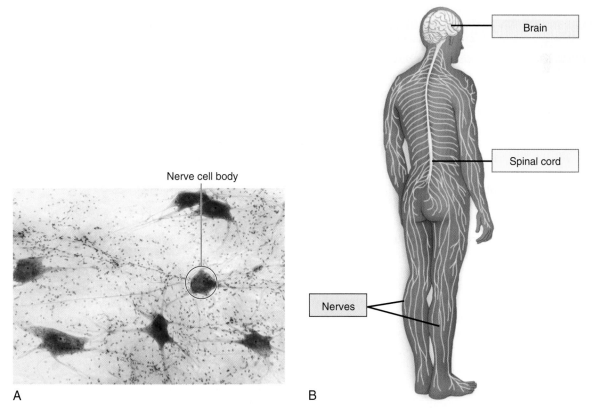

Figure 1.11 The nervous system. A, A stained preparation of nerve cells, neurons. **B,** The nervous system is made up of the brain, spinal cord, and nerves.

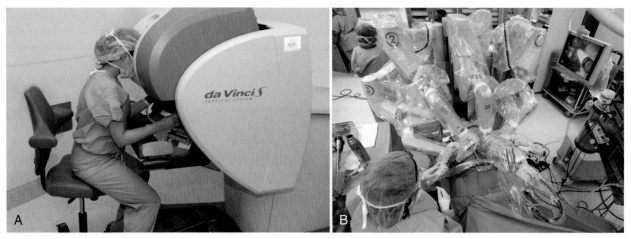

Figure 1.12 Robotic surgery. A, Surgeon seated at the surgical console. **B,** The surgical tower around the patient (view from the ceiling).

surgery

1-61 The term *surgery* is derived from a Greek word that means handwork. **Surgery** includes several branches of medicine that treat disease, injuries, and deformities by manual or operative procedures. The term *surgery* also refers to the work performed by a surgeon or the place where surgery is performed. Surgery that deals with operations of all kinds is called general _____. There are many surgical specialties. OR is the abbreviation for operating room, the place where surgeries are performed.

Small incisions through the skin and the use of scopes provide access to various body cavities, providing a faster, less painful recovery with fewer visible scars. In addition, more surgeries are being performed using the body's natural openings. Accessing abdominal organs through the mouth, nose, vagina, or rectum avoids the need to cut through sensitive tissues and generally provides faster recoveries.

> **BEYOND** THE BLUEPRINT The use of robotics has gained increasing popularity (Fig. 1.12). Robotic surgery offers advantages of minimally invasive surgery, decreased blood loss, faster recovery, decreased pain after surgery, and shorter hospital stays.

plastic

1-62 Plastic surgery is the repair or reconstruction of tissue or organs by means of surgery. The combining form plast(o) means repair. Reconstructive surgery is one aspect of plastic surgery. It includes procedures such as resetting broken facial bones, restoring parts of the body destroyed by cancer, and correcting birth defects.

Aesthetic plastic surgery has greatly increased in the last few years, particularly that involving the face and breasts. Another notable trend is the increasing number of men who are having cosmetic surgery, with hair replacement leading the list. The medical specialist who performs plastic surgery is called a _____ surgeon.

WORD ORIGIN
pes- *(L.)*
pes, foot

orthopedics

1-63 Ortho/pedics is a branch of surgery that deals with the preservation and restoration of the bones and associated structures. The specialist is called an **orthoped/ist** or an **orthopedic surgeon** (Fig. 1.13).

The combining form orth(o) means straight, and ped(o) refers to child or foot (pes-, pod[o], and -pod also refer to foot). The orthopedist originally straightened children's bones and corrected deformities. Today, an orthopedist specializes in disorders of the bones and associated structures in people of all ages. The specialty that is concerned with diseases and disorders of the bones and associated structures is _____.

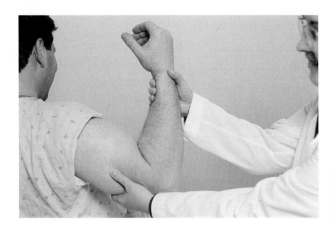

Figure 1.13 Orthopedist examining a patient. Orthopedics is a branch of medicine that specializes in the prevention and correction of disorders of the muscular and skeletal systems of the body.

BUILD IT! **EXERCISE 20**

Build medical terms for the following definitions by using the word parts you have learned.

1. rheumatology specialist _____/_____
2. specialist in immune disorders _____/_____
3. specialty for bones and associated structures _____/_____/_____
4. specialty practiced by psychiatrists _____/_____
5. surgical specialty for the nervous system _____/_____
6. urinary tract specialist _____/_____

---

epidemiologist

1-64 An **epidemic** attacks several people in a region at the same time. The field of medicine that studies the factors that determine the frequency and distribution of diseases is **epidemiology.** The specialist is an _____. A physician with this specialty may be assigned the responsibility of directing infection control programs within a hospital.

1-65 There are many other areas in which physicians specialize. **Preventive medicine** is concerned with preventing the occurrence of both mental and physical illness and disease. **Emergency physicians** specialize in **emergency medicine,** dealing with very ill or injured patients who require immediate medical treatment.

In the emergency room, patients are often prioritized according to their need for treatment. This method of sorting according to the patients' needs for care is called **triage.** A person who is hemorrhaging is given top priority. Likewise, a person with symptoms of a heart problem is a high priority because of the danger of cardiac arrest (stoppage of the heartbeat). Write the term that

triage

means the sorting and prioritizing of patients for treatment: _____.

Emergency department (ED) more accurately describes the place in a hospital where emergency physicians handle emergencies, and the terminology is evolving to reflect this fact.

1-66 Some physicians specialize in sports medicine, which is concerned with prevention, diagnosis, and treatment of sports injuries.

A specialist in **forensic medicine** deals with the legal aspects of health care. In forensic pathology, for example, the cause and time of an individual's death is determined by a pathologist.

WRITE IT! **EXERCISE 21**

Write a word in each blank to complete these sentences.

1. Sorting patients according to urgency of need for care is _____.
2. A disease that spreads rapidly through a population is called an _____.
3. The branch of medicine that specializes in the prevention of disease is _____ medicine.
4. The medical specialty that deals with acutely ill or injured persons who require immediate care on arrival at the hospital is _____ medicine.
5. A specialist in _____ medicine deals with the legal aspects of health care.

Write the specialty associated with the following conditions or situations:

1. heart attack _____

2. interpreting a radiograph _____

3. deficiency of the immune system _____

4. hormonal deficiency _____

5. nosebleed _____

6. miscarriage _____

7. irritable bowel disease _____

8. urinary infection _____

9. broken wrist _____

10. rheumatoid arthritis _____

CATEGORIES OF MEDICAL TERMS

1-67 All medical specialties follow a process to study an illness and then treat it. The process includes knowledge of anatomy, uses diagnostic tests, determines the probable cause, and treats the problem with surgical or other therapeutic means. **Therapy** is treatment of a disease or pathologic condition. As you study medical terminology, you will observe that terms are used in a variety of ways that correspond to this process. It will be helpful to keep the medical process in mind, as certain word parts indicate how a term is used.

KEY POINT **Here are the categories used in this book:**

• **Anatomy**, the science of the structure of the body and the relation of its parts: the names of structures and related words, such as colon (large intestine) and colonic (pertaining to the colon). Anatomy is presented by body systems in Chapters 4-13.

• **Diagnostic** tests and procedures: terms used to describe evidence of disease (for example, fever, headache) and the tests used to establish a **diagnosis,** the determination of the cause of a disease. Diagnostic tests include clinical studies (for example, measurement of blood pressure), laboratory tests (for example, determination of blood gases), and radiologic studies (for example, chest x-ray examination). You will learn many suffixes in Chapter 2 that form the basis of diagnostic terms.

• **Pathology** [path(o); disease]: the names of diseases or disorders (for example, influenza, leukemia). Several suffixes that form the basis of terms used to write pathologies are presented in Chapter 2.

• **Surgery:** operative procedures (for example, tonsillectomy, removal of the tonsils). You will learn many suffixes in Chapter 2 that form the basis of surgical terms.

• **Nonsurgical therapy:** treatment of a disease or abnormal condition without or in addition to surgery. Terms include prescribed drugs (such as, antibiotics) and physical treatments (such as, electric stimulation to enhance the healing process).

anatomy

The femur is commonly called the *thigh bone*. Femur is the name of a structure. The appropriate category for femur is _____.

BEYOND THE BLUEPRINT Anatomy and physiology, the study of processes and function, are often studied together. Dissection (*L. dissecare*, to cut apart), cutting a tissue apart, is used to study anatomy, whereas tests (for example, physical observation or chemical tests) determine the function of organs.

Categorize the terms in the left column by selecting A, B, C, D, or E.

_____ **1.** antibiotics

_____ **2.** colon

_____ **3.** blood gases

_____ **4.** leukemia

_____ **5.** removal of the tonsils

A. anatomy

B. diagnostic test or procedure

C. pathology

D. surgery

E. nonsurgical therapy

MEDICAL RECORDS

1-68 Medical specialties and other health professions use health records as written forms of communication to document information that is relevant to the care of the patient (Pt). Medical reports communicate the patient's health status to other health professionals and to insurance companies and federal and state agencies. Inpatients (IPs) are persons who have been admitted to a hospital or other health care facility for at least an overnight stay. Outpatients (OPs) are persons who are not admitted to a hospital and are being treated in an office, clinic, hospital, or other health care facility. Medical records must be maintained for OPs as well as IPs. The abbreviation IP means

inpatient _____.

🔑 **KEY** POINT **A health record must be maintained for every person who is assessed or treated in an approved health facility.** Diseases and procedures are translated into a system known as an ICD-10 code (International Classification of Diseases, 10th revision). Healthcare Common Procedure Coding System (HCPCS) and Current Procedural Terminology (CPT) are the standardized terminology and coding for medical services and procedures.

1-69 Medical coding is organizing information into categories that are assigned numbers for the purpose of sorting, storing, and retrieving data. Translation of a disease or disorder into an ICD code or a procedure into a CPT code requires knowing terms for anatomy and physiology, medical terminology (including disease processes, diagnostic terms, surgical procedures, and pharmacology), as well as coding rules and guidelines. Diagnosis-related groups (DRGs) are used by Medicare and others for reimbursement.

Organizing information into categories that are assigned numbers is called medical

coding _____.

1-70 The Health Insurance Portability and Accountability Act (HIPAA) is a federal privacy act that went into effect in 2003. It gives the patient certain rights, including the rights to request restrictions of protected health information and to receive confidential communications concerning one's own

privacy medical condition and treatment. HIPAA is a federal _____ act concerning a patient's medical records (Fig. 1.14).

1-71 The Affordable Care Act (ACA) was passed by Congress and then signed into law by the President in 2010, taking effect in 2014. It was designed to provide affordable health care options, increase the number of Americans covered by health insurance, and decrease the cost of health care. For additional information about ACA, go to *www.healthcare.gov/law/*.

1-72 There are many types of medical reports, including those for the history and physical (H&P) examination, operative (surgical) reports, consultation notes and letters, medication records, and laboratory and radiology reports. Medical reports often include demographic data (patient's legal name; date of birth [DOB]; file number, which may be the patient's social security number [SSN];

date physician's name, etc.) and a signature line. DOB means _____ of birth.

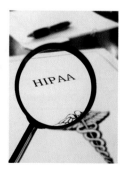

Figure 1.14 Health Insurance Portability and Accountability Act. This act not only gives access and privacy to patients regarding their medical records, but also includes continuity of insurance coverage when changing jobs.

Representative samples are included in this book in most chapters to give you experience understanding health care records. After you have learned several medical terms, you will be asked to read and explain various terms that are in medical reports and to apply terminology in practical situations. The following example, a history and physical (H&P) examination summary, documents the patient's medical history along with findings from the physical examination (PE). PE also means pulmonary embolism, blockage of an artery (a main blood vessel) in the lungs. Learn the common abbreviations that are shown on the report in Fig. 1.15.

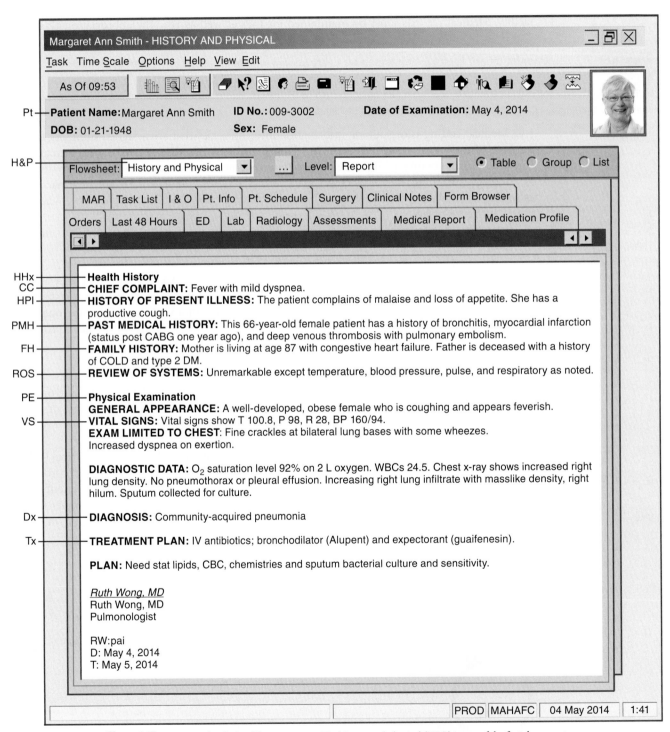

Figure 1.15 An example of a health care report. The history and physical (H&P) is one of the first documents prepared when a patient arrives for care.

WRITE IT! EXERCISE 24

Write a word in each blank space to answer these questions.

1. What is the term for persons who have been admitted to a hospital or other health care facility for at least an overnight stay? _____

2. What is the term for patients who are not hospitalized and are being treated in an office, clinic, or other health care facility? _____

3. What is the abbreviation for the federal privacy act that gives the patient certain rights concerning his or her own health information? _____

WRITE IT! EXERCISE 25

Write the meaning of these abbreviations.

1. CC _____

2. Dx _____

3. FH _____

4. H&P _____

5. HPI _____

6. HHx _____

7. OP _____

8. PE _____

9. PMH _____

10. ROS _____

11. Tx _____

12. VS _____

PHARMACOLOGY

1-73 Pharmaceutic means a drug or pertaining to drugs or pharmacy. **Pharmacology** is the science of drugs. This includes the origin, nature, chemistry, effects, and uses of drugs. A drug may modify one or more of the body's functions. Drugs are used in medicine to prevent, diagnose, or treat a disease or abnormal condition. Another term for drugs used in medicine is **pharmaceuticals.** Drugs used specifically to treat a condition are referred to as therapeutic agents, and drugs used to aid in identifying medical conditions are referred to as diagnostic agents. Another term for drugs is _____.

pharmaceuticals

1-74 Giving a drug to a patient is called drug administration. The route of administration is the method by which a drug is introduced to the body (Fig. 1.16). Although most drugs are administered orally (by mouth) or by injection, some can be administered via the skin, mucous membranes, lungs, and other methods. **Parenterals** are drugs not administered via the digestive tract; however, the term is most commonly used in reference to injectables. The method by which a drug is introduced to the body is the route of _____.

administration

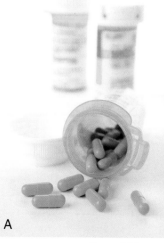
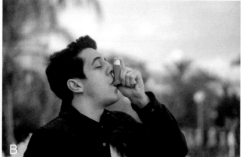
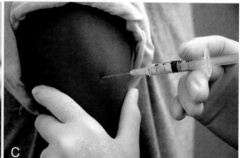

Figure 1.16 Examples of vehicles for drug administration. A, Capsules. **B,** An inhaler, a device for medication to be breathed in and absorbed in the lungs. **C,** Injection, administering liquid by means of a needle and syringe.

PHARMACOLOGY, cont'd

pharmacokinetics

1-75 Once administered, a drug may remain at the site of administration or it may enter the blood. The movement of the drug from the administration site into the blood is called absorption of the drug. The transportation of the drug to other body tissues is called the distribution of the drug. How the drug is used in the body after administration is referred to as **pharmacokinetics** and involves the drug's absorption, distribution, metabolism, and elimination. Kinetics involves movement or changes. The movement of the drug into the blood is called absorption, whereas how the drug is used after administration is called its _____.

local

1-76 How the drug affects the body is known as pharmacodynamics. Where and how a drug interacts with a site in the body is called the action of the drug. If the effect is confined to the site of administration, the drug has a **local effect.** If it acts on many sites away from the administration site, the effect is said to be **systemic.** The drug is eventually removed from the body in a process called elimination. When a drug is confined to the site of administration, it is called a _____ effect, whereas if a drug acts on many sites away from where it is administered, it is said to have a systemic effect.

potency

1-77 A measured amount of a drug is called a dose. Potency refers to the level of effect of a drug. The greater the effect with a single dose, the more potent a drug is. A placebo is an inactive mimic of another drug usually given as a control in a clinical drug study. Side effects are secondary consequences of taking a particular medication. Adverse drug reactions are harmful, unexpected responses to a drug. The more medicinally effective a single dose is refers to the _____ of the drug.

prescription

1-78 A prescription is an order for a drug with directions for use made by an authorized medical professional (a physician or nurse practitioner) for a specific patient. An over-the-counter (OTC) drug is available without a prescription and, like prescription drugs, is approved for safety and efficacy by the U.S. Food and Drug Administration (FDA). Herbal and dietary supplements are also available without a prescription but are not subject to the same regulations as drugs and are not classified as drugs. Written directions for a certain medication and how it is to be used is called a drug _____.

controlled

1-79 Drug abuse is the use of any drug in a way that deviates from the manner in which it was prescribed. Drug addiction is caused by excessive or continued use of habit-forming drugs. Any pharmaceutical with a potential for abuse or addiction is designated as a controlled substance, and is regulated by law with regard to possession and use. Pharmaceuticals with a potential for addiction or abuse are called _____ substances.

MATCH IT!

EXERCISE 26

Match the terms in the left column with their descriptions in the right column.

_____ **1.** local drug effect

_____ **2.** oral drug administration

_____ **3.** parenteral drug administration

_____ **4.** pharmaceuticals

_____ **5.** pharmacokinetics

_____ **6.** systemic drug effect

A. administering drugs by mouth

B. administering drugs in ways other than the digestive tract

C. drug action is confined to where it is administered

D. drug acts away from its administration site

E. drugs used in medicine

F. study of the movement and changing of drugs within the body

---

generic

1-80 The **generic name** (for example, acetaminophen) of a drug is the common name for the drug and is used by every company for consistent identification, whereas the **trade name** or **brand name** (for example, Tylenol) is the property of only one company and cannot be used by other companies. The first letter of the trade name is capitalized, whereas a generic name's first letter is not capitalized. For example: acetaminophen (Tylenol). A common drug name used by every company is the _____ name.

PHARMACOLOGY, cont'd

classes

1-81 Drugs are generally grouped into several *classes* based on their major effects or mechanisms of action, and some drugs may be categorized into multiple classes. Actions, reactions, and interactions with other drugs are often shared by drugs of the same class. Drugs are generally grouped into _____ based on their major effects.

1-82 A **pharmacist** is a trained medical expert in drug information. Pharmacists will provide information about a drug's actions, dosing, side effects, and potential interactions with other drugs, supplements, and food. A **pharmacy** is a licensed location that dispenses prescription drugs. A second meaning of pharmacy is the study of preparing and dispensing drugs.

It is more useful for the beginning health learner to focus on remembering the drug classes and their uses, rather than memorizing the name of every drug. The following drugs are listed by generic name with the trade name in parentheses. The listed trade name may be the only medication of its type available if no generic is on the market, but it still has to have a generic name. Sometimes there are multiple trade names for the same generic drug, but only one will be listed here. A few older drugs do not have a trade name. The following list indicates the classes of various drugs and gives some representative examples.

Anesthetics: Produce a loss of sensation

Local Anesthetics: *Local numbing effect at site of administration*
benzocaine (Orajel)   lidocaine (Xylocaine)   ropivacaine (Naropin)
bupivacaine (Marcaine)   prilocaine (Citanest)

General Anesthetics: *Loss of all body sensation, and some induce loss of consciousness*
desflurane (Suprane)   ketamine (Ketalar)   nitrous oxide (Nitronox)
etomidate (Amidate)   methohexital (Brevital)   propofol (Diprivan)

Opioid Antagonists: Block opioid receptors to treat opiate dependence or overdose
naloxone (Evzio)   naltrexone (Vivitrol)

WRITE IT! **EXERCISE 27**

Write a word in each blank space to complete these sentences.

1. The trade name of a drug is the property of one company, whereas the _____ name is used by every company for identification.

2. Grouping of drugs into classes is based on their major _____ or mechanisms of action.

3. In the example, "celecoxib (Celebrex)," the trade name is _____.

4. A person who formulates and dispenses prescription drugs is a _____.

CHAPTER ABBREVIATIONS*

Abbreviations are shortened forms of written words or phrases that are used in place of the whole. For example, MD means doctor of medicine. However, MD has other meanings, including medical department and maximum dose. Some abbreviations have been included in this chapter because of their common use, but there are many more in the following chapters.

Remember that certain abbreviations have been placed on a "Do Not Use" list when an error in reading could jeopardize patient safety (Table 1.7).

ACA	Affordable Care Act	GP	general practitioner	OP	outpatient
AMA	American Medical Association	HCPCS	Healthcare Common Procedure Coding System	ophth	ophthalmology
CC	chief complaint	H&P	history and physical	OR	operating room
CPT	Current Procedural Terminology	HHx	health history	OTC	over-the-counter
DOB	date of birth	HIPAA	Health Insurance Portability and Accountability Act	PACU	postanesthesia care unit
DRG	diagnosis-related group			PE	physical examination, pulmonary embolism
Dx	diagnosis	HPI	history of present illness	PMH	past medical history
ED	emergency department	ICD-9	International Classification of Diseases, 9th revision	Pt	patient
ENT	ear, nose, and throat	ICD-10	International Classification of Diseases, 10th revision	ROS	review of systems
FDA	Food and Drug Administration			SSN	social security number
		IP	inpatient	TJC	The Joint Commission
FH	family history	MD	doctor of medicine	Tx	treatment
		OB	obstetrics	VS	vital signs

*Many of these abbreviations share their meanings with other terms.

Table 1.7   The Joint Commission Official "Do Not Use" List*

Do Not Use	Potential Problem	Use Instead
U (unit)	Mistaken for "0" (zero), the number "4" (four) or "cc"	Write "unit"
IU (International Unit)	Mistaken for IV (intravenous) or the number 10 (ten)	Write "International Unit"
Q.D., QD, q.d., qd (daily)	Mistaken for each other	Write "daily"
Q.O.D., QOD, q.o.d, qod (every other day)	Period after the Q mistaken for "I" and the "O" mistaken for "I"	Write "every other day"
Trailing zero (X.0 mg)†	Decimal point is missed	Write "X mg"
Lack of leading zero (.X mg)	Decimal point is missed	Write "0.X mg"
MS	Can mean morphine sulfate or magnesium sulfate	Write "morphine sulfate"
MSO_4 and $MgSO_4$	Confused for each other	Write "magnesium sulfate"

*Applies to all orders and all medication-related documentation that is handwritten (including free-text computer entry) or on preprinted forms.

†Exception: a "trailing zero" may be used only where required to demonstrate the level of precision of the value being reported, such as for laboratory results, imaging studies that report size of lesions, or catheter or tube sizes. It may not be used in medication orders or other medication-related documentation.

© Joint Commission Resources. Oakbrook Terrace, IL: Joint Commission on Accreditation of Healthcare Organizations, 2016. Reprinted with permission.

PREPARING FOR A CHAPTER TEST

Measure your memory of what you learned in this chapter:
- Study the word parts for this chapter. Review all lists of word parts and their meanings using flash cards (on the Evolve website or make your own) before the test.
- Work the Self-Test. The review helps you know if you have learned the material. After completing all sections of the review, check your answers with the solutions found in Appendix IV.

Be Careful With These!

-ist (one who) vs. *-iatry* (medical profession or treatment)	*-logy* (study of) vs. *-logist* (one who studies; specialist) *ne(o)* (new) vs. *neur(o)* (nerve)	*or(o)* (mouth) vs. *ur(o)* (urinary tract or urine) vs. *ot(o)* (ear)	*intern* (one in postgraduate training) vs. *internist* (a physician)

Remember the Student Evolve Website at *http://evolve.elsevier.com/Leonard/building* Ⓔ

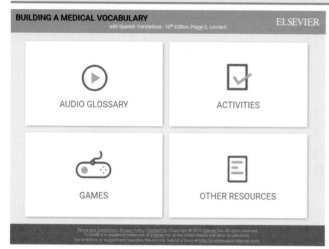

The games help you prepare for the test. However, the games on the website do not replace the Self-Test at the end of each chapter.

A Career as a Registered Nurse

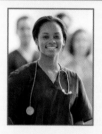

Chelsea Adkins is a registered nurse, working in pediatrics in a large metropolitan hospital where she has been employed for five years. She loves working with children and knowing that she makes a difference in their recovery as well as their attitudes toward other medical personnel. A registered nurse has graduated from a nursing program and met the requirements outlined by a licensing body in order to obtain a nursing license, and adheres to the laws and rules which govern nursing. RNs have a job growth rate well above the national average. In the U.S., registered nurses are employed in a wide variety of professional settings, often specializing in a field of practice. They may have supervisory responsibilities of licensed practical nurses, nursing students, and less-experienced RNs.

Nurses have many opportunities for meaningful and fulfilling careers as they provide direct assistance to people who are sick or may participate in education, assessment, diagnosis and treatment in a variety of settings. For more information, visit *www.nursingworld.org*.

 TOOL TIP!   *Career Highlights introduce you to possibilities in medical professions!*

 ## CHAPTER 1 SELF-TEST

Review the new word parts for this chapter. Work all of the following exercises to test your understanding of the material before checking your answers against Appendix IV.

BASIC UNDERSTANDING

Describing

I.   *Describe the role of each of the following word parts:*

1. combining form   _____

2. prefix   _____

3. suffix   _____

4. word root   _____

Identifying Word Parts

II. *Use slashes to divide the following terms into their component parts and identify the parts as WR (for word root), CF (for combining form), P (for prefix), or S (for suffix). Examples: neonatologist, obstetric = CF   CF   S   WR   S*
neo/nato/logist, obstetr/ic

1. cardiac _____

2. gastric _____

3. gerontology _____

4. neurology _____

5. oncology _____

6. ophthalmological _____

7. otic _____

8. pathology _____

9. psychiatry _____

10. urologic _____

Writing Plurals

III. *Write a singular or plural form for each term that is given.*

1. atrium _____

2. bulla _____

3. bursae _____

4. cervices _____

5. enchondromata _____

6. ganglion _____

7. indices _____

8. microvillus _____

9. septum _____

10. syndrome _____

Listing

IV. *List five categories used in this book for classifying medical terms.*

1. _____

2. _____

3. _____

4. _____

5. _____

Deconstructing Words

V. *Break the following terms into their word parts and define each word part. The first one is done as an example.*

Terms

1. anesthesiologist

2. cardiology

3. dermatologic

4. gastric

5. geriatrics

6. gynecology

7. neonatologist

8. neurology

9. obstetric

10. orthopedist

11. otic

12. oncology

13. ophthalmologic

14. pediatric

15. psychiatry

Meaning of Word Root/s

an-, without; esthesi/o, feeling; -logist, specialist _____

_____

_____

_____

_____

_____

_____

_____

_____

_____

_____

_____

_____

_____

_____

Finetuning Terms

VI. *In addition to spelling, describe at least one difference in the following:*

1. anatomic pathologist and clinical pathologist: _____

_____

2. a clinical psychologist and a psychiatrist: _____

_____

3. internist and a physician intern: _____

_____

4. primary health care provider and an emergency physician: _____

_____

5. therapy and triage: _____

_____

6. anesthetic and anesthesiologist: _____

_____

Using Vocabulary

VII. Circle the correct answer to the following questions.

1. A 65-year-old man has a history of heart problems. Which type of specialist should he see for care of his heart condition? (cardiologist, endocrinologist, laryngologist, orthopedist)

2. Cynthia is pregnant. Which type of specialist should she see to care for her during her pregnancy, labor, and delivery? (gerontologist, obstetrician, orthopedist, otologist)

3. Which term means a person who is not a physician but is trained in administering drugs that cause a loss of feeling? (anesthesiologist, anesthesist, anesthetics, anesthetist)

4. Which of the following physicians specializes in the diagnosis and treatment of newborns through the age of 28 days? (geriatrician, gynecologist, neonatologist, urologist)

5. Lorenzo suffers from persistent digestive problems. His primary care physician refers him to which of the following specialists? (gastroenterologist, immunologist, rheumatologist, toxicologist)

6. Sally injures her arm while ice skating. The emergency room physician orders an x-ray film. Which type of physician is a specialist in interpreting x-ray films? (gynecologist, ophthalmologist, plastic surgeon, radiologist)

7. Sally's x-ray film reveals a fractured radius, one of the bones of her forearm. Dr. Bonelly, a bone specialist, puts a cast on Sally's arm. Which type of specialist is Dr. Bonelly? (dermatologist, orthopedist, otologist, rhinologist)

8. What does the word *neuron* mean? (medical specialty that deals with the nervous system, nerve cell, neurosurgery, specialist in diseases of the nervous system)

9. Which physician specializes in diagnosis of disease using clinical laboratory results? (clinical pathologist, gastroenterologist, internist, surgical pathologist)

10. Which branch of medicine specializes in the legal aspects of health care? (diagnostic, forensic, geriatric, neurologic)

Writing Terms

VIII. Write a term for each of the following descriptions.

1. a specialist in internal medicine _____

2. determination of the cause of disease _____

3. method of prioritizing patients according to their need _____

4. pertaining to the heart _____

5. physician who specializes in caring for older persons _____

6. pertaining to newborns _____

7. study of endocrine glands and hormones _____

8. study of the characteristics, causes, and effects of disease _____

9. surgery of the nervous system _____

10. urinary tract specialty _____

GREATER COMPREHENSION

Spelling

IX. Circle all misspelled terms, and write their correct spellings:

cardiak   dermatologic   obstetrics   ofthalmic   sychiatry

Abbreviating

X.   Write a letter in each blank for abbreviations that correspond to these clues. (The first is done as an example.)

1. Affordable Care Act   _A_ _C_ _A_

2. Food and Drug Administration   — — —

3. history of a patient's present illness   — — —

4. over-the-counter   — — —

5. patient   — —

6. specialty concerning pregnancy and childbirth   — —

7. the date when one is born   — — —

8. therapy or treatment   — —

Pronouncing Terms

XI.   Write the correct term for the following phonetic spellings. (The first one is done as an example.)

1. an-us-thē-zē-**ol**-uh-jē   *anesthesiology*_____

2. fuh-**ren**-zik   _____

3. gas-trō-en-tur-**ol**-uh-jē   _____

4. or-thō-**pē**-diks   _____

5. pē-dē-**at**-rik   _____

6. ū-ruh-**loj**-i-kul   _____

Health Care Reporting

XII.   Circle the correct answer in Questions 1 through 5 after reading the following chart note.

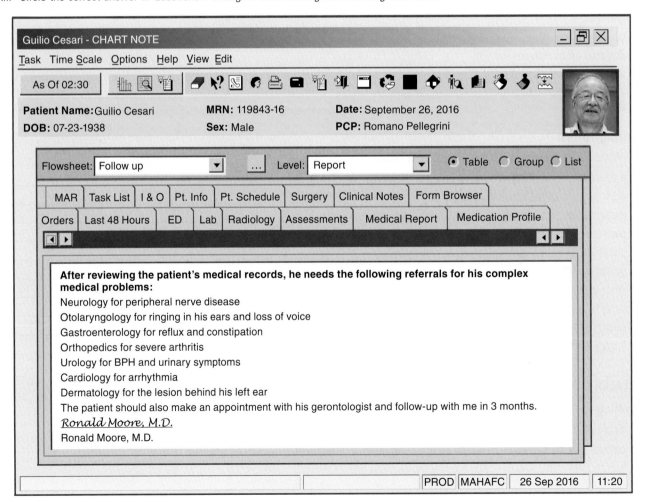

Circle the correct answer.

1. Dermatology is a medical specialty which involves treatment of disorders of the (glands, eyes, muscles, skin)
2. Otolaryngology is a medical specialty which does NOT involve treating of disorders of the (ears, lungs, nose, throat)
3. Which medical specialist deals with aging and issues encountered by older people? (cardiology, gerontologist, neurology, orthopedics)
4. Which of the following is NOT a meaning of a word part in the term "gastroenterology"? (intestines, kidneys, stomach, study of)
5. A common abbreviation for otolaryngology is (ED, ENT, OB, OR)

Using Pharmacologic Terms

XIII. Circle the correct answer to the following questions.

1. Which term is not a route of drug administration? (action, injection, orally, parenteral)
2. What is the correct term for the science that deals with the origin, nature, chemistry, effects, and uses of drugs? (pharmaceutical, pharmacology, pharmacy, pharmacokinetics)
3. Which term relates to a drug that acts on many sites away from the administration site? (action, biotransformation, local systemic)
4. An order for a drug made by an authorized medical professional is a (pharmacodynamics, pharmacokinetic, prescription, potency).
5. A measured amount of a drug is called a (distribution, dose, placebo, potency)

Categorizing Terms and Practicing Pronunciation

XIV. Match the following terms with their category (A, B, C, or D)

_____ **1.** anesthesiologist	_____ **11.** ophthalmology	**A.** adjective
_____ **2.** anesthetist	_____ **12.** orthopedist	**B.** medical specialist
_____ **3.** epidemiology	_____ **13.** otic	**C.** medical specialty
_____ **4.** gastroenterologist	_____ **14.** otolaryngology	**D.** another type of noun
_____ **5.** geriatrician	_____ **15.** pediatrician	
_____ **6.** gynecology	_____ **16.** psychiatry	
_____ **7.** holistic	_____ **17.** radiologist	
_____ **8.** neonatologist	_____ **18.** rheumatologist	
_____ **9.** obstetrician	_____ **19.** rhinology	
_____ **10.** oncology	_____ **20.** triage	

Be prepared to pronounce terms 1-20 in class after listening to Chapter 1 terms at *http://evolve.elsevier.com/Leonard/Building/.* In addition, practice categorizing all of the terms. You will discover that some terms fit more than one classification. "Anesthetic" is both a noun and an adjective, depending on its usage.

New Construction

XV. Mentally break these words into their component parts, then write their meanings. Even if you have not seen these terms before, you may be able to break them apart and determine their meanings. The first is done as an example.

1. orthopedic surgery   *medical treatment performed mainly by manipulative and operative methods*
2. endocrine therapy   _____
3. rhinopathy   _____
4. laryngologist   _____
5. pediatric cardiology   _____

(Use Appendix IV to check your answers to the exercises in the Self-Test. Pay particular attention to spelling. If most of your answers are correct, you are ready to move on to Chapter 2.)

 TOOL TIP!   ***Audio files for all boldface terms are found on the student Evolve website.***

Games, pronunciations, and more await you at *http://evolve.elsevier.com/Leonard/building.*

BMV LIST

Visit http://evolve.elsevier.com/Leonard/building/ *to listen to the boldface terms in Chapter 1. Look closely at the spelling of each term as it is pronounced.*

anatomic pathologist (an-uh-**tom**-ik puh-**thol**-uh-jist)
anatomic pathology (an-uh-**tom**-ik puh-**thol**-uh-jē)
anatomy (uh-**nat**-uh-mē)
anesthesiologist (an-us-thē-zē-**ol**-uh-jist)
anesthesiology (an-us-thē-zē-**ol**-uh-jē)
anesthetic (an-us-**thet**-ik)
anesthetics (an-us-**thet**-iks)
anesthetist (uh-**nes**-thuh-tist)
brand name (brand nām)
cardiac (**kahr**-dē-ak)
cardiologic (kahr-dē-ō-**loj**-ik)
cardiologist (kahr-dē-**ol**-uh-jist)
cardiology (kahr-dē-**ol**-uh-jē)
clinical pathologist (**klin**-i-kul puh-**thol**-uh-jist)
clinical pathology (**klin**-i-kul puh-**thol**-uh-jē)
clinical psychologist (**klin**-i-kul sī-**kol**-uh-jist)
clinical psychology (**klin**-i-kul sī-**kol**-uh-jē)
dermal (**dur**-mul)
dermatologic (dur-muh-tō-**loj**-ik)
dermatological (dur-muh-tō-**loj**-i-kul)
dermatologist (dur-muh-**tol**-uh-jist)
dermatology (dur-muh-**tol**-uh-jē)
diagnosis (dī-ug-**nō**-sis)
diagnostic (dī-ug-**nos**-tik)
emergency medicine (ē-**mur**-jun-sē **med**-i-sin)
emergency physician (ē-**mur**-jun-sē fi-**zish**-un)
endocrine (**en**-dō-krin, **en**-dō-krīn)
endocrinologist (en-dō-kri-**nol**-uh-jist)
endocrinology (en-dō-kri-**nol**-uh-jē)
epidemic (ep-i-**dem**-ik)
epidemiologist (ep-i-dē-mē-**ol**-uh-jist)
epidemiology (ep-i-dē-mē-**ol**-uh-jē)
family practice (**fam**-i-lē **prak**-tis)
forensic medicine (fuh-**ren**-zik **med**-i-sin)
gastric (**gas**-trik)
gastroenterologist (gas-trō-en-tur-**ol**-uh-jist)
gastroenterology (gas-trō-en-tur-**ol**-uh-jē)
generic name (juh-**ner**-ik nām)
geriatric (jer-ē-**at**-rik)
geriatrician (jer-ē-uh-**trish**-un)
geriatrics (jer-ē-**at**-riks)
gerontology (jer-on-**tol**-uh-jē)
gynecologist (gī-nuh-**kol**-uh-jist)
gynecology (gī-nuh-**kol**-uh-jē)
holistic health (hō-**lis**-tik helth)
immunologic (im-ū-nō-**log**-ik)
immunologist (im-ū-**nol**-uh-jist)
immunology (im-ū-**nol**-uh-jē)
internal medicine (in-**tur**-nul **med**-i-sin)
internist (in-**tur**-nist)
larynx (**lar**-inks)

local effect (**lō**-kul uh-**fekt**)
neonatologist (nē-ō-nā-**tol**-uh-jist)
neonatology (nē-ō-nā-**tol**-uh-jē)
neurologic (noor-ō-**loj**-ik)
neurological (noor-ō-**log**-i-kul)
neurologist (noo-**rol**-uh-jist)
neurology (noo-**rol**-uh-jē)
neuron (**noor**-on)
neurosurgeon (**noor**-ō-sur-jun)
neurosurgery (noor-ō-**sur**-jur-ē)
nonsurgical therapy (non-**sur**-ji-kul **ther**-uh-pē)
obstetric (ob-**stet**-rik)
obstetrical (ob-**stet**-ri-kul)
obstetrician (ob-stuh-**tri**-shun)
obstetrics (ob-**stet**-riks)
oncologist (ong-**kol**-uh-jist)
oncology (ong-**kol**-uh-jē)
ophthalmic (of-**thal**-mik)
ophthalmologic (of-thul-muh-**loj**-ik)
ophthalmological (of-thul-muh-**log**-i-kul)
ophthalmologist (of-thul-**mol**-uh-jist)
ophthalmology (of-thul-**mol**-uh-jē)
opioid antagonists (**ō**-pē-oid an-**tag**-uh-nists)
orthopedic (or-thō-**pē**-dik)
orthopedic surgeon (or-thō-**pē**-dik **sur**-jun)
orthopedics (or-thō-**pē**-diks)
orthopedist (or-thō-**pē**-dist)
otic (**ō**-tik)
otolaryngologist (ō-tō-lar-ing-**gol**-uh-jist)
otolaryngology (ō-tō-lar-ing-**gol**-uh-jē)
otologist (ō-**tol**-uh-jist)
otology (ō-**tol**-uh-jē)
parenteral (puh-**ren**-tur-ul)
pathologic (path-ō-**loj**-ik)
pathological (path-ō-**loj**-i-kul)
pathologist (puh-**thol**-uh-jist)
pathology (puh-**thol**-uh-jē)
pediatric (pē-dē-**at**-rik)
pediatrician (pē-dē-uh-**tri**-shun)
pediatrics (pē-dē-**at**-riks)
pharmaceutic (fahr-muh-**soo**-tik)
pharmaceutical (fahr-muh-**soo**-ti-kul)
pharmacist (**fahr**-muh-sist)
pharmacokinetics (fahr-muh-kō-ki-**net**-iks)
pharmacology (fahr-muh-**kol**-uh-jē)
pharmacy (**fahr**-muh-sē)
plastic surgery (**plas**-tik **sur**-jun)
preventive medicine (prē-**ven**-tiv **med**-i-sin)
primary health care provider (**prī**-mar-ē helth cār prō-**vī**-dur)
psychiatrist (sī-**kī**-uh-trist)
psychiatry (sī-**kī**-uh-trē)

radiologic (rā-dē-ō-**loj**-ik)
radiological (rā-dē-ō-**loj**-i-kul)
radiologist (rā-dē-**ol**-uh-jist)
radiology (rā-dē-**ol**-uh-jē)
rheumatism (roo-muh-tiz-um)
rheumatologist (roo-muh-**tol**-uh-jist)
rheumatology (roo-muh-**tol**-uh-jē)
rhinologist (rī-**nol**-uh-jist)
rhinology (rī-**nol**-uh-jē)
roentgenology (rent-gen-**ol**-uh-jē)

surgery (**sur**-jur-ē)
systemic (sis-**tem**-ik)
therapy (**ther**-uh-pē)
trade name (trād nām)
triage (trē-**ahzh, trē**-ahzh)
urinary (**ū**-ri-nar-ē)
urologic (ū-ruh-**loj**-ik)
urological (ū-ruh-**loj**-i-kul)
urologist (ū-**rol**-uh-jist)
urology (ū-**rol**-uh-jē)

ENHANCING SPANISH COMMUNICATION

Spanish translation of selected terms is presented at the end of each chapter. Appendix II has a comprehensive list of English-Spanish translations for easy reference.

Español ENHANCING SPANISH COMMUNICATION

The sounds of Spanish vowels do not vary and must be fully and distinctly pronounced. This does not apply to double vowels. Use these rules to pronounce vowels:

Spanish Vowel	Pronounce as
a	a in mama
u	u in rule or the sound of oo in spool (The u is generally silent in these syllables: que, gue, and gui.)
e	a in day
y	e in see, but sounds like j if it follows n
i	i in police
o	o in so

Some consonants have similar sounds in English and Spanish. A few significant differences are noted here:

Spanish	Pronunciation
c	k or s, except ch pronounced like church
d	sometimes as th
g	similar to g in go except pronounced as h before e or I
h	not pronounced
j	h
ll	blending of l and y, or simply y as in yet
ñ	blending of n and y as in canyon
q	k
r	trilled r
rr	strongly trilled r
z	s

Phonetic pronunciation is presented with the stressed syllable in uppercase letters, as in the example BO-cah. In this term, the first syllable is stressed. Boca is the Spanish word for mouth.

English	Spanish (Pronunciation)
aged	envejecido (en-vay-hay-SEE-do)
anatomy	anatomía (ah-nat-o-ME-ah)
anesthesiology	anestesología (an-es-te-se-o-lo-HE-ah)
anesthetic	anestésico (ah-nes-TAY-se-ko)
cancer	cáncer (KAHN-ser)
child	niña (NEE-nya), niño (NEE-nyo)
clinical	clinico (KLE-ne-ko)
diagnosis	el diagnostico (el de-ag-NOS-te-ko)
diagnostic	diagnóstico (de-ag-NOS-te-ko)
disease	enfermedad (en-fer-may-DAHD)
ear	oreja (o-RAY-hah)
emergency	emergencia (a-mar-han-SE-ah), urgencia (ur-han-SE-ah)
endocrine	endocrino (and-o-KRE-no)
epidemic	epidemia (ep-ah-day-ME-ah)
eye	ojo (O-ho)
female	mujer (mu-HAR)
foot (pl., feet)	pie (PE-ay), pies (PE-ays)
forensic	forense (fo-RAN-sa)
gastric	gástrico (GAS-tre-ko)
geriatrics	geriatriá (gay-re-ah-TRE-ah)
gynecology	ginecología (he-nay-ko-lo-HEE-ah)
heart	corazón (ko-rah-SON)
hormone	hormona (or-MOH-nah)
immunology	inmunologia (en-mu-no-lo-HE-ah)
internal medicine	medicina interna (may-de-SE-na in-TER-nah)
intestine	intestino (in-tes-TEE-no)
larynx	laringe (lah-REN-gay)
life	vida (VEE-dah)
mind	mente (MEN-te)
nerve	nervio (NERR-ve-o)
neurology	neurología (nay-oo-ro-lo-HEE-ah)
newborn	recién nacido (ray-see-AN nah-SEE-do)
nose	nariz (nah-REES)
nurse	enfermera(o) (en-fer-MAY-rah)
pathology	patología (pah-to-lo-HEE-ah)
pharmacist	farmacéutico (far-mah-SAY-oo-tee-koh)
pharmacy	farmacia (far-MAH-see-ah)
pregnancy	embarazo (em-bah-RAH-so)
prescription	receta (ray-SAY-tah)
psychiatry	psiquiatría (se-ke-ah-TREE-ah)
psychology	psicología (se-ko-lo-HEE-ah)
radiation	radiación (rah-de-ah-se-ON)
rheumatism	reumatismo (ru-may-TEZ-mo)
secrete	secretar (say-kra-TAR)
stomach	estómago (es-TOH-mah-go)
surgeon	cirujano(a) (se-roo-HAH-no) (na)
surgery	cirugía (se-roo-HEE-ah)
therapy	therapia (ther-ah-PEE-ah), tratamiento (trah-tah-me-EN-to)
throat	garganta (gar-GAHN-tah)
urinary system	sistema urinario (sis-TAY-mah oo-re-NAH-re-o)
urine	orina (o-REE-nah)
urology	urología (oo-ro-lo-HEE-ah)
x-ray	radiografía (rah-de-o-grah-FEE-ah)

CHAPTER 2

Diseases and Disorders: Diagnostic and Therapeutic Terms

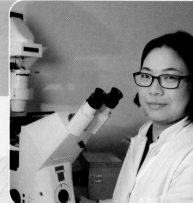

Surgeon using a video microscope for eye surgery.

CONTENTS

LEARNING OUTCOMES

Basic Understanding

1. List or recognize seven general causes of disease.
2. List or recognize four general types of microorganisms.
3. Recognize several terms associated with diseases and disorders or write their meanings.
4. Match word parts with their meanings.
5. Write the meanings of the word parts, and use them to build and analyze terms.
6. Identify the procedures used during a physical examination.
7. Recognize several types of diagnostic imaging procedures.
8. Write the meanings of surgical and nonsurgical therapeutic terms or match them with their meanings.

Greater Comprehension

9. Spell medical terms accurately.
10. Classify terms as anatomical, diagnostic imaging procedure, other diagnostic terms, surgical terms, or nonsurgical therapeutic term.
11. Write the meanings of the abbreviations.
12. Pronounce medical terms correctly.
13. Recognize the meanings of general pharmacological terms from this chapter as well as the drug classes and their uses.

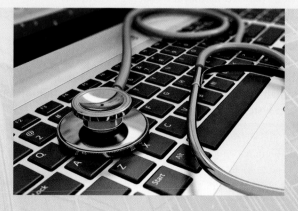

FUNCTION FIRST

Biology, the scientific study of life, has many branches (for example, genetics, the study of genes and heredity). Health is the condition of physical, mental, and social well-being and the absence of disease or other abnormal conditions. Illness occurs when any of these conditions change.

Pathology is the study of the characteristics, causes, and effects of disease. The adjective "pathologic" pertains to a condition that is caused by or involves a disease process. You'll soon begin to recognize several pathologies, as well as additional terms pertaining to diagnosis and treatment of diseases.

> **KEY** POINT **Most medical terms have one or more combining forms as their foundation.** The suffix that is added to a word part (mainly a combining form) generally determines its category. Some students find it helpful to know what types of words are formed by the use of various suffixes. It is logical that a suffix coincides with how its meaning is used in speech. For example, an instrument is a noun, so thermometer, an instrument for measuring temperature, is a noun.

CLASSIFICATION OF DISEASE

Diseases and Disorders

2-1 Illness is an abnormal process in which aspects of the social, physical, emotional, or intellectual condition or function of a person are diminished or impaired. A general term for impairments is "disease," and the specific illness is called a *disease* or a *disorder.*

> **KEY** POINT **Disease refers to either structurally or functionally abnormal processes, whereas a disorder tends to describe a disruption in function. Disease** is defined as a condition of abnormal structure or function of the body (for example, contagious disease), or the term can refer to a specific disorder or illness (for example, Lou Gehrig disease). A **disorder** is a disruption or interference with normal functions. See the websites of the National Institutes of Health (NIH) *www.nih.gov* and Centers for Disease Control and Prevention (CDC) *www.cdc.gov* for additional information.

function

A mental disorder is a disturbance of emotional equilibrium and represents a disturbance in

_____.

> **KEY** POINT **Acute and chronic have opposite meanings. Acute** means having a short and relatively severe course. The opposite of acute is **chronic**, which means persisting over a long period.

acute

A disease that lasts only a short time is a/n _____ disease.

2-2 There are several ways to classify diseases. A classification based on structure or function would be as follows:

- Organic diseases, which are associated with a demonstrable physical change in an organ or tissues (for example, a tumor)
- Functional disorders, which are marked by signs or symptoms but no physical changes (for example, most psychologic disorders)

physical

It is important to remember that organic diseases, unlike functional disorders, are associated with a demonstrable _____ change.

Classification of diseases according to cause includes the following:

- Infectious (caused by disease-causing organisms)
- Genetic (altered or mutated genes, the units of inheritance)
- Traumatic (caused by **trauma**, injury)
- Degenerative (deterioration of structure or function)
- Neoplastic (malignancies; abnormal tissue growths or tumors)
- Metabolic (endocrine imbalances or malnutrition)
- Inflammatory (abnormal or prolonged inflammation or **autoimmunity**, altered function of the immune system against one's own cell)

> **BEYOND** THE BLUEPRINT Marfan syndrome is a genetic disorder that affects the body's connective tissue, the tissue that holds all the body's cells, organs and tissue together. Every person's experience with Marfan syndrome is slightly different. A common Marfan feature is long arms, legs, and fingers as well as a curved spine. Some Marfan features — for example, aortic enlargement (expansion of the main blood vessel that carries blood away from the heart to the rest of the body) — can be life-threatening.

Match the types of diseases and disorders in the left column with their descriptions in the right column.

_____ **1.** functional disorder   **A.** caused by pathogenic organisms

_____ **2.** infectious disease   **B.** demonstrable physical change

_____ **3.** organic disease   **C.** signs or symptoms without physical change

Match the types of diseases or disorders with their descriptions in the right column.

_____ **1.** autoimmunity   **A.** altered function of immune system against one's own cells

_____ **2.** degenerative   **B.** pertaining to deterioration of structure or function

_____ **3.** metabolic   **C.** pertaining to endocrine imbalances or malnutrition

_____ **4.** neoplastic   **D.** pertaining to injury

_____ **5.** traumatic   **E.** pertaining to malignancies

(Use Appendix IV to check your answers.)

2-3 Other terms that are applied to various conditions:

- An **idiopathic disease** develops without an apparent or known cause (for example, high blood pressure for which there is no known cause) (idi[o] means individual).
- An **iatrogenic disorder** is an unfavorable response to medical treatment (for example, a transfusion reaction) (iatr[o] means physician or treatment).
- **Nosocomial infections** are hospital-acquired infections (for example, infection of a surgical wound). More specifically, this type of infection was not present or incubating before the patient's admission to the hospital and is acquired 72 hours or longer after admission (nos[o] means disease).
- **Congenital** conditions are those that exist at, or before, birth (for example, clubfoot: Fig. 2.1).
- An **anomaly** is a deviation from what is regarded as normal, especially as a result of congenital defects.

Study the meanings of the newly-introduced word parts.

WORD ORIGIN
nosocomial *(G.)*
nosokomeian, hospital

Word Parts

Combining Form	Meaning	Prefixes	Meaning
aut(o)	self	anti-	against
bi(o)	life or living	intra-	within
dipl(o)	double	micro-	small
gen(o)	beginning or origin	**Suffixes**	**Meaning**
iatr(o)	physician or treatment	-cidal	killing
idi(o)	individual	-emia	condition of the blood
nos(o), path(o)	disease	-gen	that which generates
		-genesis	producing or forming
		-genic	produced by or in

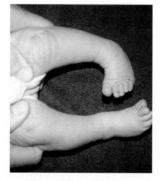

Figure 2.1 Clubfoot. This congenital anomaly of the foot sometimes results from constriction during development, and can affect one foot (as shown here) or both feet.

MATCH IT! EXERCISE 3

Match these terms with their descriptions.

_____ **1.** acute

_____ **2.** anomaly

_____ **3.** chronic

_____ **4.** congenital

_____ **5.** iatrogenic

_____ **6.** idiopathic

_____ **7.** nosocomial

A. a collapsed lung results from improper tube placement by a physician

B. a patient's wound becomes infected three days after surgery

C. a disease develops without an apparent cause

D. deviation from what is expected

E. having a short and severe course

F. persisting over a long period

G. present at birth

Infectious Diseases and Microorganisms

disease

Figure 2.2
Biohazard label.

small

2-4 You learned that pathology is the study of disease, including its characteristics and causes. **Patho/genic** (-genic, produced by or in) means capable of causing or producing a _____. Many organisms besides plants and animals are capable of carrying on life functions, including bacteria, viruses, fungi, protozoa, worms, parasites (living in or on another organism for nourishment) or arthropods (such as, ticks, spiders, and insects). Some of these can cause disease.

Laboratories, doctors' offices, and other organizations that work with radiation and/or possible disease-causing organisms that require special conditions for containment use **biohazard** labels (Fig. 2.2).

2-5 Micro/organisms (micro-, small) are tiny entities, which may or may not be pathogenic. The prefix micro- in microorganisms denotes that they are _____.

Micro/biology is the branch of science concerned with the study of microorganisms, which includes viruses, bacteria, fungi, and protozoa (Fig. 2.3).

If microorganisms are pathogenic, they are called **pathogens**. The degree to which they cause disease is referred to as **virulence** or **pathogenicity**.

2-6 Infectious diseases are caused by pathogenic organisms. **Contagious** means capable of being transmitted from one individual to another. When contagious diseases are passed from one person to another, there is transmission of the disease.

🔑 **KEY** POINT A **communicable disease** also called a *contagious disease*, is transmitted from one person or animal to another by one of these means:
- directly by contact with discharges or airborne droplets from an infected person
- indirectly via substances (for example, bloodborne transmission through contact with blood or body fluids that are contaminated with blood) or inanimate objects (such as, a contaminated spoon)
- via carriers called *vectors* (for example, mosquitoes, which transmit malaria)

communicable

A contagious disease is also called a _____ disease.

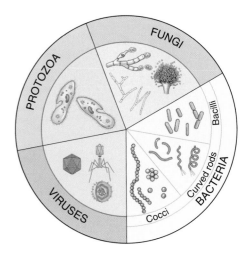

Figure 2.3 Major types of microorganisms. Major types of microorganisms include bacteria, viruses, fungi, and protozoa. Organisms that have characteristics of both viruses and bacteria, such as Rickettsia, are not included here (organisms are not drawn to scale).

Study the word parts that pertain to disease in the following list.

Word Parts: Infectious Disease

Combining Form	Meaning	Combining Form	Meaning
Infection		**Microorganisms**	
seps(o)	infection	bacter(i), bacteri(o)	bacteria
sept(i), sept(o)*	infection	fung(i), myc(o)	fungus
		parasit(o)	parasite
		staphyl(o)	grapelike cluster; uvula
		strept(o)	twisted
*Also means septum.		vir(o), virus(o)	virus

WRITE IT! EXERCISE 4

Write the combining form(s) for the following:

1. bacteria _____
2. fungi _____
3. grapelike cluster _____
4. infection _____
5. twisted _____
6. virus _____

blood

2-7 A number of infectious diseases will be studied in this book (Table 2.1). An **infection** is invasion of the body by pathogenic microorganisms. **Septic/emia** is an infection which has spread to the circulating blood from an infection in any part of the body. **Bacter/emia** is the presence of bacteria in the blood (which sometimes can be grown in the laboratory); **viremia** is the presence of viruses in the _____.

You are familiar with antibiotics that are generally used to treat bacterial infections. Most antibiotics are not effective treatment for viral infections, and physicians often try to avoid treating bacterial infections unless the patient has a fever.

> **BEYOND** THE BLUEPRINT Infections occur most often in high-risk patients, such as older persons and those with compromised immunity. Infection control within a health care facility is designed to reduce the risk of infection and follows monitoring of strict policies and procedures, which include hand hygiene, disinfection, and sterilization, as well as the use of isolation, gloves, and other contact precautions.

Viruses

viruses

2-8 A **virus** is a minute microorganism that replicates only within a cell of a living plant or animal, because viruses have no independent metabolic activity. Pathogenic viruses are responsible for human diseases, such as influenza, hepatitis, and fever blisters. The Zika virus is transmitted by a mosquito that primarily bites during the day (Fig. 2.4). Zika virus infection during pregnancy can cause microcephaly (smaller head of a newborn, often with a smaller brain). An infected man can also transmit the disease to a pregnant female. Microorganisms that can only replicate inside cells of another living organism are called _____.

Table 2.1 Transmission of Infectious Diseases and Selected Examples*

Direct Contact	Indirect Contact
Common cold (5)	Infected needles (acquired immunodeficiency syndrome [AIDS]; also direct contact, 8)
Genital warts (8)	Infected secretions or droplets (influenza, 5)
Infectious mononucleosis (3)	Infected food (salmonellosis, hepatitis A, 6)
Ringworm (13; also indirect contact)	Airborne (tuberculosis, 5)
	Insect bite (malaria, 2)
	Maternal-fetal infection (congenital syphilis, 8)

*The number within the parentheses indicates the chapter in which the condition is discussed.

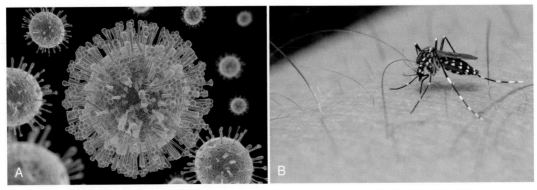

Figure 2.4 Zika virus and the female Aedes aegypti mosquito that transmits it. A, Artist's rendering of the virus, greatly enlarged. **B,** The mosquito that transmits the disease. The disease originated in Brazil, but is spreading to other countries, especially via persons who have traveled to areas of local transmission of Zika.

> 🔑 **KEY** POINT Typical laboratory microscopes provide low power and high power magnifications of 100x and 400x, meaning 100 times and 400 times the actual sizes of the objects viewed. Each microscopically-viewed area is called a *field of vision*. As an estimation of quantity, microscopy laboratory reports often cite the number of organisms per high-power field (HPF), not just in reporting bacteria but also in other areas such as the study of urine or in hematology. Sometimes the number of organisms or cells per low-power field (LPF) is reported.

Viruses are smaller than most bacteria, fungi, and protozoa. Because of their small size, viruses generally require the use of an electron microscope, which uses a beam of electrons rather than visible light. In contrast, a microbiologist uses a light microscope to view most bacteria, fungi, or protozoa.

The Ebola virus outbreak in West Africa captured worldwide attention in 2016 and killed more than 11,000 people. Medical personnel must isolate infected individuals and use proper protection. Human-to-human transmission occurs through exposure to body fluids such as saliva, urine, vomit, blood, semen, and feces. The virus can also be spread through needles or syringes used previously by an infected person.

Bacteria

2-9 Most **bacteria** (small unicellular organisms) are easy to study and grow in the laboratory (Fig. 2.5).

Microbiologists classify bacteria according to their shape. A special staining technique serves as a primary means of identifying and classifying bacteria into three major types: **cocci, bacilli,** or **spirilla** or **spirochetes** (Fig. 2.6). Gram stain is a special staining technique that serves as a primary means of identifying and classifying bacteria. The retention of the violet stain or the pink color of the counterstain classifies bacteria as Gram positive or Gram negative, respectively.

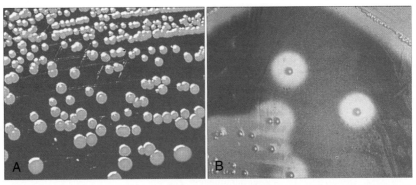

Figure 2.5 Bacterial colonies cultures in the laboratory in a Petri dish and culture media. Both **A** and **B** are grown on blood agar. Note that bacteria in **B** show zones of hemolysis (destruction of the blood) around the colonies.

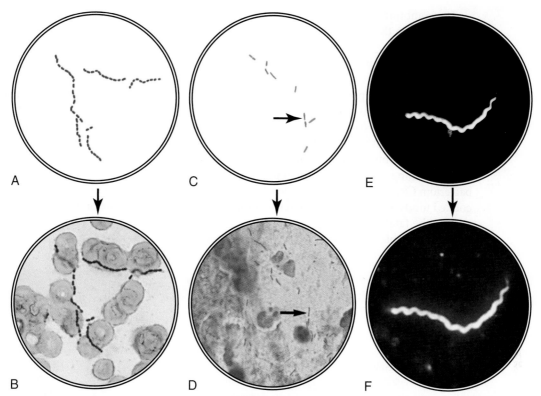

Figure 2.6 Bacteria in body fluids. A, Schematic drawing of Gram-positive cocci, which appear as tiny purple spheres. The cocci are in chains in this example. **B,** Gram-positive cocci in a Gram stain of a direct smear. Note the small size of the bacteria (which stain purple) compared with the much larger cells. **C,** Schematic of Gram-negative bacilli, which appear as tiny pinkish rods. **D,** Gram-negative bacilli *(arrow)* in the presence of numerous leukocytes in a Gram stain of a direct smear. **E,** Schematic of spirochetes, which appear as long, tightly coiled spirals. **F,** Spirochetes in material collected from a chancre, a skin lesion that occurs in syphilis, using special dark field illumination.

WRITE IT! EXERCISE 5	*Write a term in each blank.*
	1. Rod-shaped bacteria are called _____.
	2. Spherical-shaped bacteria are called _____.
	3. Coiled spiral bacteria are called _____.

streptococci

bacteria

2-10 Strep throat, caused by a type of bacteria, **streptococci,** is a common way of saying **strepto/coccal pharyng/itis.** Streptococcal means pertaining to _____. You may have heard of someone having a staph infection. Staph is an abbreviation for **staphylococci.** The number of methicillin-resistant *Staphylococcus aureus* (MRSA) infections has risen, and this potentially deadly infection is resistant to many of the most powerful antibiotics.

When bacteria are cultured in an artificial medium in a Petri dish, an antibiotic sensitivity test may also be performed to determine which antibiotics are effective against that particular pathogen (Fig. 2.7). This test is often ordered as a culture and sensitivity (C&S). Sensitivity pertains to the antibiotic which the _____ are sensitive.

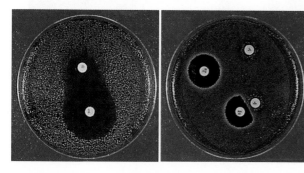

Figure 2.7 Bacterial culture and sensitivity testing. This is a common method of determining which antibiotics are effective against a particular bacteria. No growth around some of the antibiotic disks indicates effectiveness of that particular antibiotic.

bacteria

The combining form staphyl(o) is also used to mean uvula, a structure that hangs like a bunch of grapes from the soft palate in the back of the mouth. When staphyl(o) is joined to cocci, it refers to a type of _____. When it is not joined to cocci, you will have to decide which meaning is intended.

2-11 Bacterial food poisoning results from eating food that is contaminated by certain types of bacteria. One type is caused by various species of *Salmonella* and is characterized by fever and digestive signs and symptoms that include nausea, vomiting, and diarrhea beginning 8 to 48 hours after eating contaminated food. Similar symptoms caused by another type of bacteria, *Staphylococcus,* usually appear much sooner and usually last only a few hours. **Botulism,** an often fatal form of food poisoning, is caused by a toxin produced by the **anaerobic** (growing in the absence of oxygen) bacterium *Clostridium botulinum.* Most botulism occurs after eating improperly canned or improperly cooked foods. Of the types of bacterial food poisoning described, the one that is caused by a toxin

botulism

and can be fatal is called _____.

Refer to Table 2.2 for selected viral and bacterial diseases.

Table 2.2   Selected Viral and Bacterial Diseases

Viral		Bacterial	
fever blisters	measles	food poisoning by *Clostridia*	whooping cough
genital herpes	mumps	*Staphylococcus aureus* infection	tuberculosis
genital warts	pneumonia	tetanus	gonorrhea
hepatitis	poliomyelitis	diphtheria	syphilis
infectious mononucleosis	smallpox	pneumonia	typhoid fever
influenza	upper respiratory tract infections	meningitis	urinary tract infections

Fungi

2-12 Fungi are microorganisms that feed by absorbing organic molecules from their surroundings. They may be parasitic and may invade living organic substances. Yeasts and molds are included in this group.

➤ **BEYOND** THE BLUEPRINT Only a few of the known fungi are pathogenic to humans. *Candida albicans,* a microscopic fungus, is normally present in the mouth, intestinal tract, and vagina of healthy individuals. Infections may occur under certain circumstances, particularly when immunity is deficient (Fig. 2.8). Athlete's foot (Fig. 2.9) and ringworm (named because of the shape of the lesion on the skin) are other diseases caused by fungi.

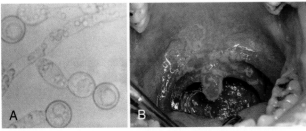

Figure 2.8 Oral infection caused by *Candida albicans,* a fungal organism. A, Appearance of the microscopic fungi, showing the way in which the fungi multiply by budding. **B,** Thrush, an oral infection of the mouth, caused by *C. albicans.*

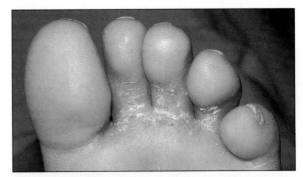

Figure 2.9 Athlete's foot. This fungal infection results in small blisters, cracking, and itching, especially between the toes.

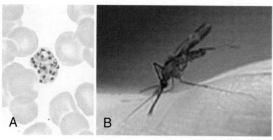

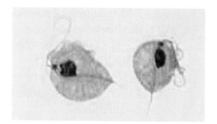

Figure 2.10 Malaria. A, Malarial parasites multiply inside immature red blood cells, which have a bluish color in stained smears. Note the cell with malarial parasites (in the center). **B,** A feeding female Anopheles mosquito.

Figure 2.11 Two *Trichomonas* **parasites.** Note the whiplike flagella that the organisms use for movement.

Protozoa

2-13 Protozoa are the simplest organisms of the animal kingdom. **Malaria,** an infectious illness, which infects the blood (Fig. 2.10, A) and can be spread by blood transfusion, is caused by one or more of several species of pathogenic protozoa, and is transmitted by the bite of an insect vector, the female *Anopheles* mosquito (Fig. 2.10, B). **Trichomoniasis,** another human protozoal infection, is a sexually transmitted disease. A stained preparation of these protozoa is shown in Fig. 2.11.

> **BEYOND** THE BLUEPRINT   Only a few species of protozoa are pathogenic to humans (example: malaria). In its acute form, malaria is characterized by anemia, enlarged spleen, chills, and fever.

WRITE IT!   EXERCISE 6

List four general types of microorganisms.

1. _____   3. _____

2. _____   4. _____

Bioterrorism

2-14 Bio/terrorism is the use of pathogenic biologic agents to cause terror in a population.

🔑 **KEY** POINT   **High-priority agents of bioterrorism pose a risk to national security.** Biologic agents are placed on this list largely for the following reasons:
- They can be easily disseminated (distributed over a general area) or transmitted from person to person.
- They cause high mortality and have a major public health impact.
- They can cause public panic and social disruption.
- They require special action for public health preparedness.

bioterrorism

The use of pathogenic biologic agents to cause terror in a population is known as _____. Several bioterrorism agents are listed by the CDC, including smallpox (Fig. 2.12). Many hospitals have implemented emergency preparedness plans to deal with threats or acts of bioterrorism.

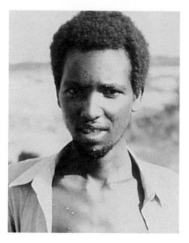

Figure 2.12 The last smallpox victim. The last known naturally occurring case of smallpox was in Somalia in 1977. Successful disease prevention techniques completely eradicated natural outbreaks of this disease that once killed millions worldwide. The World Health Organization (WHO) considers naturally occurring cases to be eradicated; thus the vaccine for smallpox is no longer required in the United States.

2-15 Weapons of mass destruction (WMD) have been a concern for many years but have come to the forefront in recent years. The Federal Emergency Management Agency (FEMA) and the CDC use the following categories to define weapons of mass destruction:

B Biologic

N Nuclear

I Incendiary (incendiaries, flammable substances used to ignite fires, or explosives)

C Chemical

E Explosive (A bomb constructed and deployed in a manner other than conventional military action is an improvised explosive device [IED]. These types of bombs may be partially composed of conventional military explosives attached to a detonating mechanism.)

Health care providers must be trained to recognize and deal with these emergencies. Biologic

living weapons of mass destruction use _____ organisms that are pathogenic to humans.

WRITE IT! EXERCISE 7

Write words in the blanks to complete these sentences.

1. WMD is the abbreviation for _____ of mass destruction.
2. CDC is the abbreviation for Centers for _____ Control and Prevention.
3. The use of pathogenic biologic agents to cause terror in a population is called _____.
4. A term that means scattered or distributed over a general area is _____.

INTRODUCTION TO DISEASES AND DISORDERS

Body Structures

2-16 It is sometimes easier to learn combining forms in groups, such as combining forms for body structures or those that describe colors. Adding various suffixes to combining forms determines how the resulting term is used in a sentence. Practice learning the combining forms in the same manner that you used previously.

Word Parts: Combining Forms for Selected Body Structures

Combining Form	Meaning	Combining Form	Meaning
aden(o)	gland	mamm(o), mast(o)	breast
angi(o)	vessel	muscul(o), my(o)	muscle
append(o), appendic(o)	appendix	nas(o), rhin(o)	nose
blephar(o)	eyelid	nephr(o), ren(o)	kidney
cephal(o)	head	or(o), stomat(o)	mouth
cerebr(o), encephal(o)	brain; cerebr(o) sometimes means cerebrum, the main portion of the brain	oste(o)	bone
		pod(o)	foot
		steth(o)	thorax (chest)
chir(o)	hand	tonsill(o)	tonsil
col(o), colon(o)	colon or large intestine	trache(o)	trachea (windpipe)
cutane(o), derm(a), dermat(o)	skin	vas(o)	vessel; ductus deferens (also called *vas deferens*, excretory duct of the testicle)
hist(o)	tissue		

MATCH IT! EXERCISE 8

Match meanings with their word parts in the right column.

_____ **1.** brain

_____ **2.** bone

_____ **3.** breast

_____ **4.** chest

_____ **5.** eyelid

_____ **6.** gland

_____ **7.** kidney

_____ **8.** vessel

A. aden(o)

B. angi(o)

C. blephar(o)

D. cerebr(o)

E. mamm(o)

F. nephr(o)

G. oste(o)

H. thorac(o)

WRITE IT! EXERCISE 9

Write a word part(s) for the following terms.

1. appendix _____

2. colon _____

3. foot _____

4. hand _____

5. head _____

6. mouth _____

7. muscle _____

8. nose _____

9. skin _____

10. tissue _____

11. tonsil _____

12. windpipe _____

---

vessels

2-17 An **angi/oma** is a benign tumor made up of blood _____ or lymph vessels (Fig. 2.13).

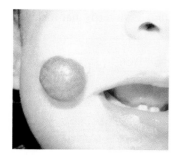

Figure 2.13 This type of angioma is filled with blood vessels. It is often called a _birthmark,_ because it is commonly found during infancy. It grows at first but may spontaneously disappear in early childhood. It can be surgically removed if bleeding or injury is a problem, or later for cosmetic reasons.

 Pathologies

diseases

2-18 Suffixes joined to combining forms are used to write the names of many diseases or disorders. Patho/logies are terms that represent the names of _____ or disorders. All the suffixes in the following list are used to write nouns.

Word Parts: Pathologies

Combining Form	Meaning	Suffix	Meaning
cancer(o), carcin(o)	cancer	-mania	excessive preoccupation
lith(o)	stone or calculus	-maniac	a person who shows excessive preoccupation
Suffix	**Meaning**	-oma	tumor
-cele	hernia (protrusion of all or part of an organ through the wall of the cavity that contains it)	-osis	condition (often an abnormal condition; sometimes an increase)
-emia	condition of the blood	-pathy	disease
-ia-, -iasis	condition	-phobia	abnormal fear
-itis	inflammation	-ptosis	prolapse (sagging)
-lith	stone or calculus		

Circle the correct answer to complete each sentence.

1. The suffix -iasis means (condition, dilatation, disease, excessive).
2. The suffix -itis means (deficiency, inflammation, sagging, soft).
3. The suffix -phobia means abnormal (bleeding, deficiency, fear, preoccupation).
4. The suffix -ptosis means (decreased, disease, fear, prolapse).
5. The suffix that means excessive preoccupation is (-mania, -maniac, -phobia, -ptosis).
6. The suffix that means tumor is (-oid, -oma, -osis, -rrhagia).
7. The suffix that means disease is (-pathy, -penia, -phobia, -ptosis).
8. The suffix that means hernia is (-cele, -megaly, -rrhea, -stasis).
9. The suffix that means a condition of blood is (-algia, -dynia, -emia, -emesis).
10. The suffix that means a stone or calculus is (-cele, -lith, -malacia, -megaly).

-oma

WORD ORIGIN
malignant *(L.)*
malignus, bad disposition
neoplasm *(G.)*
neos, new +
plasma, formation

cancer

hernia

herniation

2-19 You learned that onc(o) means tumor. The suffix that means tumor is _____. Tumor can sometimes mean a swelling, but it often means an uncontrolled growth of tissue. Tumors may be localized (remaining in one spot) or invasive (spreading to other organs or places), and benign or malignant (Fig. 2.14). A **benign tumor** does not spread or invade surrounding tissue. Compare this with a **malignant tumor,** which characteristically invades surrounding structures and spreads to distant sites. **Malignant** means tending to become worse, spread, and may cause death. Any new abnormal growth, either benign or malignant is a **neoplasm** (ne[o], new + -plasm, refers to repair). **Cancer** is a malignant neoplasm. Many tumors are benign.

    Carcin/oma is cancer or a cancer/ous tumor because carcin(o) means _____ and -oma means tumor.

2-20 In the list of suffixes that pertain to pathologies, a term that means protrusion of all or part of an organ through an abnormal opening is _____. This is also called **herniation**.

    An **encephalo/cele** is _____ of part of the brain through an opening in the skull, also called a **cerebral** hernia (Fig. 2.15).

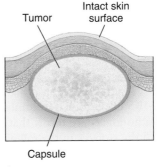
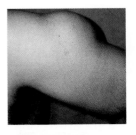

Tumor

Intact skin surface

Capsule

A

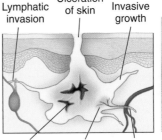

Lymphatic invasion

Ulceration of skin

Invasive growth

Death of tissue   Hemorrhage   Vessel invasion

B

Figure 2.14 Comparison of a benign and malignant tumor. A, Benign tumor. Drawing of its general characteristics and an example: a lipoma that consists of mature fat cells. **B,** Malignant tumor. Drawing of its general characteristics and an example: a malignant melanoma, which is a type of skin cancer.

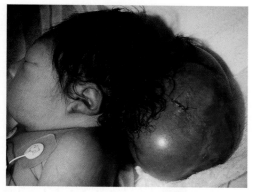

Figure 2.15 An encephalocele. Herniation of part of the brain and its covering through a defect in the skull.

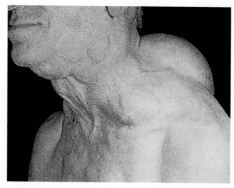

Figure 2.16 Enlarged lymph nodes. This particular type of adenopathy is enlargement of the cervical nodes, glands of the lymphatic system located in the neck.

gland

2-21 Literal interpretation of **adeno/pathy** is any disease of a _____; however, it means enlargement of a gland, especially a gland of the lymphatic system (Fig. 2.16).

FIND IT!   **EXERCISE 11**

Draw a slash between the combining forms and the suffixes in the following list of new terms. Then find the meanings of the word parts within the definition. (Draw the slash, and then perform the remainder of the activity as a mental exercise.) Think!

1. **adenitis** inflammation of a gland
2. **appendicitis** inflammation of the appendix
3. **cephalic** pertaining to the head
4. **mastitis** inflammation of the breast
5. **muscular** pertaining to or composed of muscles; having a well-developed musculature
6. **nasal** pertaining to the nose

7. **neuritis** inflammation of a nerve
8. **ophthalmitis** inflammation of the eye
9. **oral** pertaining to the mouth
10. **osteitis** inflammation of a bone
11. **otitis** inflammation of the ear
12. **tonsillitis** inflammation of the tonsils

skin

2-22 Dermat/itis is inflammation of the _____. One type of dermatitis is caused by an allergic reaction (Fig. 2.17).

fear

2-23 Phobia means any persistent and irrational fear of something. The suffix -phobia means abnormal _____.

sagging

2-24 As a suffix, -ptosis means prolapse or _____. As a term, **ptosis** has two meanings. It can mean the same as the suffix. It is also sometimes used to mean prolapse of one or both eyelids (Fig. 2.18).

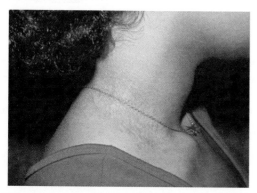

Figure 2.17 Allergic dermatitis caused by nickel in the necklace. Allergic dermatitis usually results from contact with jewelry, metal clasps, or coins. Other types of allergic dermatitis may be caused by contact with poison ivy, other metals, or chemicals, including latex, dyes, and perfumes.

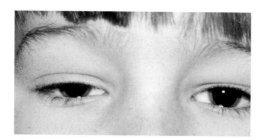

Figure 2.18 Blepharoptosis. Note the drooping of the right upper eyelid.

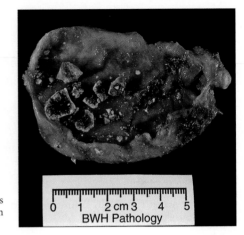

Figure 2.19 Gallstones in the gallbladder after removal. These stones may cause inflammation, jaundice, and pain and can lead to obstruction of the gallbladder.

-mania

2-25 A suffix that means excessive preoccupation is _____. **Mania** is a term that also means a psychologic disorder (see Chapter 10). In **klepto/mania** there is an excessive preoccupation that leads to an uncontrollable and recurrent urge to steal.

2-26 Several suffixes mean condition. **Hyster/ia** is a condition so named because ancient Greeks believed that hysterical women suffered from a disturbed condition of the uterus (hyster[o] means uterus). **Neur/osis** is a nervous _____ or disorder that is not caused by a demonstrable structural change. The suffix -iasis also means condition.

condition

disease

2-27 Both path(o) and the corresponding suffix -pathy mean _____.

2-28 **Ophthalmopathy** means any disease of the eye. Write a word that means any disease of the ear: _____.

otopathy

2-29 A calculus is a stone. **Calculi** are abnormal stones formed in body tissues and are usually associated with the urinary tract (kidney stones) or the gallbladder or its ducts (Fig. 2.19). Write a suffix that means a calculus: _____.

-lith

ANALYZE IT! EXERCISE 12

Break these words into their component parts. Then write the meaning of each term.
1. carcinoma   _____
2. dermatitis   _____
3. ophthalmopathy _____
4. otopathy   _____

Common Combining Forms and Suffixes

2-30 Read through the following list of word parts and their meanings. Thinking of familiar words that contain these word parts and using them on flash cards will help you remember their meanings.

Several suffixes mean *pertaining to*. Practice will help you remember which suffix to use. **Neur/al** means pertaining to a _____ or the nerves.

nerve

Word Parts: Common Suffixes and Combining Forms

Combining Form	Meaning	Suffix	Meaning
hem(o), hemat(o)	blood	-eum, -ium	membrane
lact(o)	milk	-ia, -ism	condition or theory
pyr(o)	fire	-iac	one who suffers
Suffix	**Meaning**	-opia	vision
-able, -ible	capable of, able to	-ose	sugar
-al, -ary, -eal, -ive, -tic	pertaining to	-ous	pertaining to or characterized by
-ase	enzyme	-y	state or condition
-crine	secrete		

MATCH IT! EXERCISE 13

Match suffixes in the left column with their meanings in the right column.

_____	**1.** -able	**A.**	capable of
_____	**2.** -ase	**B.**	condition or theory
_____	**3.** -eum	**C.**	enzyme
_____	**4.** -iac	**D.**	membrane
_____	**5.** -ism	**E.**	one who suffers
_____	**6.** -opia	**F.**	pertaining to
_____	**7.** -ose	**G.**	pertaining to or characterized by
_____	**8.** -ous	**H.**	state or condition
_____	**9.** -tic	**I.**	sugar
_____	**10.** -y	**J.**	vision

hematology

2-31 Hematology is the study of blood and blood-forming tissues. You need to remember to use hemat(o) to write the term that includes the study of blood. That term is _____.

one

2-32 Pyro/mania is a disorder characterized by excessive preoccupation with seeing or setting fires. Mania could be broken down further to mean mani-, meaning mental aberration or madness, +-ia, condition; however, we recognize -mania as excessive preoccupation. A **pyro/maniac** is _____ affected with a compulsion to set fires.

2-33 Enzymes are often named by changing -ose to -ase. **Enzymes** cause chemical changes in other substances (such as, sugars) and are usually named by adding -ase to the combining form of the substance on which they act.

🗝 **KEY** POINT **Two suffixes that may look similar but are very different are -ase and -ose.** Words ending in -ase usually refer to enzymes, and those that end in -ose are usually sugars.

lactase

The enzyme **lact/ase** acts on the sugar **lact/ose**. The combining form lact(o) means milk, and lactose is the main sugar found in milk. Lactose intolerance is a sensitivity disorder in which one cannot digest milk because of inadequate production of the enzyme _____.

pertaining

2-34 Divis/ive means _____ to something that causes division or dissension. Cyano/tic means pertaining to cyanosis.

capable

2-35 Preventable means capable of being prevented. Both -able and -ible are used to mean _____ of.

membrane

2-36 The suffixes -eum and -ium mean _____. Perhaps you have heard of the **peritoneum**, a membrane that lines the abdominal and pelvic cavities. (See also Fig. 3.25.)

FIND IT!

EXERCISE 14

Draw a slash between the combining forms and the suffixes in the following list of adjectives, all meaning "pertaining to" different structures or conditions. Then find the meanings of the word parts within the definitions. You may be wondering how you know which suffix to use, but this exercise will help you remember by visualizing the terms. (Draw the slash, and then perform the remainder of the activity as a mental exercise.) Think!

1. **blepharal** pertaining to the eyelids
2. **cancerous** pertaining to cancer
3. **cerebral** pertaining to the brain or the cerebrum
4. **mammary** pertaining to the breast
5. **tracheal** pertaining to the trachea (windpipe)

ANALYZE IT!

EXERCISE 15

Break these words into their component parts. Then write the meaning of each term.

1. lactase _____
2. lactose _____
3. pyromania _____
4. pyromaniac _____
5. neural _____

Using Combining Forms to Write Suffixes

specialist

2-37 A few combining forms and suffixes are so often combined that they remain fixed and easily recognized. For example, log(o) means knowledge or words. The suffix -logist, meaning one who studies or a specialist, results when log(o) is combined with -ist. You have already learned that the suffix -logist means one who studies or a _____.

2-38 Study the following list of word parts and their meanings. All the suffixes are used to form nouns with the exception of those ending in -ic and -tic. The suffixes -lytic, -phagic, and -trophic are used to form adjectives, words that modify or describe nouns. The suffix -ic can also be used to form words with several of the combining forms presented.

Word Parts: Selected Combining Forms and Related Suffixes

Combining Forms and Meanings	Suffixes and Meanings (if Different From the Combining Form)
cyt(o) means cell	-cyte
kinesi(o) means movement	-kinesia, -kinesis (movement, motion)
leps(o) means seizure	-lepsy
log(o) means knowledge or words	-logy (study or science of); -logist (one who studies)
lys(o) means destruction, dissolving	-lysin (that which destroys); -lysis (process of destroying); -lytic (capable of destroying; note the change in spelling)
megal(o) means large, enlarged	-megaly (enlargement)
metr(o) means measure; uterine tissue	-meter (instrument used to measure); -metry (process of measuring)
path(o) means disease	-pathy
phag(o) means eat, ingest	-phagia, -phagic, -phagy (eating, swallowing)
phas(o) means speech	-phasia
plas(o) means formation, development	-plasia (formation or development); -plasma (substance of cells)
plast(o) means repair	-plasty (surgical repair)
pleg(o) means paralysis	-plegia
schis(o), schiz(o), schist(o) mean split, cleft	-schisis
scler(o) means hard*	-sclerosis (hardening)
scop(o) means to examine, to view	-scope (instrument used for viewing); -scopy (process of visually examining)
troph(o) means nutrition	-trophic, -trophy

*Scler(o) sometimes means the sclera, the tough white outer coat of the eyeball.

MATCH IT!

EXERCISE 16

Match the following suffixes in the left column with their meanings in the right column.

_____ **1.** -cyte   **A.** capable of destroying
_____ **2.** -kinesia   **B.** cell
_____ **3.** -lepsy   **C.** instrument used for viewing
_____ **4.** -lysin   **D.** movement
_____ **5.** -lysis   **E.** process of destroying
_____ **6.** -lytic   **F.** process of examining visually
_____ **7.** -plasma   **G.** surgical repair
_____ **8.** -plasty   **H.** seizure
_____ **9.** -scope   **I.** substance of cells
_____ **10.** -scopy   **J.** that which destroys

MATCH IT!

EXERCISE 17

Match the following suffixes in the left column with their meanings in the right column.

_____ **1.** -megaly   **A.** disease
_____ **2.** -meter   **B.** eating or swallowing
_____ **3.** -metry   **C.** enlargement
_____ **4.** -pathy   **D.** hardening
_____ **5.** -phagia   **E.** instrument used to measure
_____ **6.** -phasia   **F.** nutrition
_____ **7.** -plegia   **G.** paralysis
_____ **8.** -schisis   **H.** process of measuring
_____ **9.** -sclerosis **I.** speech
_____ **10.** -trophy   **J.** split or cleft

microscopy

2-39 A **micro/scope** is an instrument for viewing objects that must be magnified so that they can be studied (Fig. 2.20). The process of viewing things with a microscope is _____.

hemolysin

2-40 Hemo/lysis is the destruction of red blood cells that results in the liberation of hemoglobin, a red pigment. A substance that causes hemolysis is a _____. This is also called a **hemolytic** substance or agent. **Hemolyze** is a verb that means to destroy red blood cells and cause them to release hemoglobin.

-megaly

2-41 The combining form megal(o) means large or enlarged. The suffix that means enlargement is _____.

carcinogenesis

2-42 A **carcino/gen** is a carcinogenic substance, one that produces cancer. The production or origin of cancer is called _____. Some commonly known carcinogens are listed in Chapter 14.

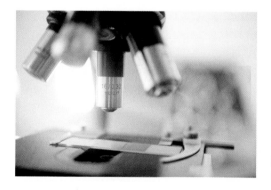

Figure 2.20 Microscopy. This microscope has a light source and different lenses for viewing very small objects, such as cells.

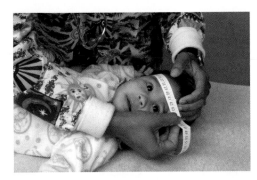

Figure 2.21 Cephalometry. This is an appropriate placement of the measuring tape to obtain the head circumference of a newborn (neonate).

cephalometer

2-43 Cephalo/metry (cephal[o] means head) is measurement of the dimensions of the head (Fig. 2.21). A device or instrument for measuring the head is a _____.

eating

2-44 Many words that contain the suffix -phagy have something to do with _____ or swallowing. A **phago/cyte** is a cell that can ingest and destroy particulate substances, such as bacteria. **Ingest** means to eat.

epilepsy

2-45 Epi/lepsy refers to a group of **neurologic disorders** characterized by seizures. Literal translation of this term does not give the full meaning. Write this term that refers to a group of neurologic disorders characterized by seizures: _____.

dystrophy

2-46 Dys/trophic muscle deteriorates because of defective nutrition or metabolism. Any disorder caused by defective nutrition or metabolism is called a _____.

movement

2-47 Kinesis is used both as a word and as the suffix -kinesis to mean _____.

2-48 It will be easier to remember the meaning of -megaly if you associate it with mega-. Write a word of your choice that begins with mega-: _____. It is likely that the word *large* is part of the word's meaning.

speech

2-49 The suffix -phasia means _____.

-plasia

2-50 Because plas(o) means formation or development, the corresponding suffix is _____.

-plegia

2-51 Pleg(o) means paralysis, and its corresponding suffix is _____.

-schisis

2-52 Schis(o), schiz(o), and schist(o) mean split or cleft, and the corresponding suffix is _____.

-sclerosis

2-53 Combine scler(o) and -osis to write a suffix that means hardening: _____. **Sclerosis** is also a term that means hardening.

WRITE IT! **EXERCISE 18**

Change the suffix in each underlined term to write a new word to complete these sentences. (#1 is done as an example.)

1. The instrument used in underlined{microscopy} is a *microscope.*
2. The term for a substance that causes underlined{hemolysis} is _____.
3. An adjective that means pertaining to underlined{hemolysis} is _____.
4. underlined{Ophthalmitis} is one type of a larger category that means any disease of the eye; this category is

_____.
5. A underlined{carcinogenic} substance is called a _____.
6. Measurement of the head using a underlined{cephalometer} is called _____.
7. A underlined{phagocytic} cell is called a _____.
8. A neurologic disorder in which underlined{epileptic} seizures occur is called _____

Colors

2-54 Study the following combining forms for colors with their meanings. Again, try to think of words that you know that will help you remember the combining forms. For example, it will be easy to remember that chlor(o) means green if you think of chlorophyll, the pigment that makes plants green.

Word Parts: Combining Forms for Color

Combining Form	Meaning	Combining Form	Meaning
alb(o), albin(o), leuk(o), occasionally leuc(o)	white	erythr(o)	red
		melan(o)	black
chlor(o)	green	xanth(o)	yellow
cyan(o)	blue		

WRITE IT! EXERCISE 19

Write the color associated with each of the following combining forms.

1. alb(o) _____
2. chlor(o) _____
3. cyan(o) _____
4. erythr(o) _____
5. leuk(o) _____
6. melan(o) _____
7. xanth(o) _____

white

2-55 An **albino** is an individual with congenital absence of pigment in the skin, hair, and eyes. The skin and hair appear _____ because of the lack of pigment. An albino has a hereditary condition known as **albinism**. Congenital conditions are those that exist at, or before, birth.

black

Albinism is characterized by partial or total lack of the pigment called melanin. **Melan/in** is a _____ or dark brown pigment that naturally occurs in the hair, skin, and eyes but is partially or totally lacking in albinos (Fig. 2.22).

2-56 **Cyan/osis** is a bluish discoloration of the skin and mucous membranes caused by a deficiency of oxygen in the blood (Fig. 2.23). The part of the term cyanosis that means blue is

cyan(o)

_____.

🔑 **KEY** POINT **Mucous membranes secrete mucus.** Because they secrete mucus, they are named *mucous membranes.* Membranes are sheets of tissue that cover or line various cavities or parts of the body that open to the outside, such as the lining of the mouth. (Note the different spelling of the body fluid mucus vs. the adjective mucous.) The mucous membrane is sometimes discolored in disease.

red

2-57 **Erythro/cytes** are _____ blood cells. (Erythrocytes are not actually red but are so named because they contain a red-pigmented protein.)

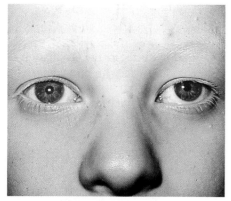

Figure 2.22 The white hair and pale skin of albinism. This condition is characterized by partial or total lack of melanin pigment in the body.

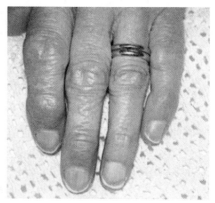

Figure 2.23 Cyanosis. The bluish discoloration is generally not as obvious as the extremely cyanotic skin of this patient.

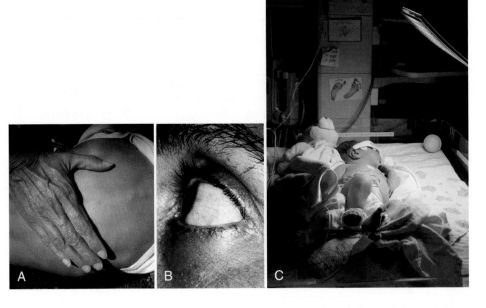

Figure 2.24 Jaundice. A, Note the contrast in the examiner's hand and the yellow discoloration of the skin of a patient with a chronic liver disorder. **B,** The sclera (the white outer part of the eyeball) has become yellow. **C,** A newborn with jaundice is placed under a special light.

yellow

2-58 Xantho/derma is a _____ coloration of the skin, as in jaundice. **Jaundice** is characterized by the yellow discoloration of the skin, mucous membranes, and **sclerae** (white outer part of the eyeballs) and is caused by an increased amount of bilirubin in the blood (Fig. 2.24A and B).

Jaundice of newborns is distinguished from other causes of jaundice, because it is temporary and usually harmless. It generally appears in the first week of life and disappears by 1-2 weeks. Bilirubin lights, also called bili lights or phototherapy, are a treatment for newborn jaundice (Fig. 2.24C).

BUILD IT!
EXERCISE 20

Use the following word parts to complete these sentences.
albin(o), cyan(o), erythr(o), xanth(o), -cyte, -derma, -ism, -osis
1. The literal translation of _____/_____ is yellow skin.
2. A bluish discoloration of the skin and mucous membranes is _____/_____.
3. A red blood cell, translated literally as red cell, is a(n) _____/_____.
4. An albino has a condition known as _____/_____.

DIAGNOSIS OF DISEASE

2-59 Diagnosis is the identification of a disease or condition by a scientific evaluation of physical signs, symptoms, history, tests, and procedures. Compare diagnosis with **prognosis,** which means the predicted outcome of a disease.

🔑 **KEY** POINT **Signs are objective; symptoms are subjective. Signs** are definitive evidence of an illness or disordered function. **Symptoms** are subjective evidence as perceived by the patient, such as pain.

sign
symptom

Indisputable evidence, such as a rash, is which—a sign or a symptom? _____
Is itching of the skin a sign or a symptom? _____
Itching and rash are both diagnostic terms.

2-60 Diagnostic terms are used to describe the signs and symptoms of disease (such as, rash and itching), as well as the tests used to establish a diagnosis.

KEY POINT **Diagnostic tests include basic examination procedures, clinical studies (such as, measuring blood pressure), laboratory tests (such as, determination of blood gases), and radio/logic studies, which relate to the use of radiant energy (such as, a chest x-ray study).** Laboratory (lab) tests, ranging from simple to sophisticated studies, identify and quantify substances to evaluate organ functions or establish a diagnosis. Within normal limits (WNL) is a phrase sometimes used by physicians to describe the results of a laboratory test.

diagnostic

Both laboratory and radiologic tests that are used to establish a diagnosis are _____ terms.

2-61 Suffixes that pertain to diagnosis are used to describe signs and symptoms, as well as tests and procedures that are used to diagnose disease. Some diseases are named for the diagnostic term. An abnormal condition of the respiratory system, bronchiectasis, is named for the dilation of the bronchial walls. Dilation, also called **dilatation,** is the condition of being stretched or dilated beyond the normal dimensions, or the process of being dilated. Write the term that is a synonym for dilation: _____.

dilatation

All the suffixes in the list below form nouns unless otherwise noted. Read and take time to study each word part and its meaning. (Note that two suffixes designate instruments.) It is also helpful to think of words that you may know that can help you to remember the meaning.

Word Parts: Prefixes and Suffixes in Diagnosis

Prefix	Meaning	Suffix	Meaning
endo-	inside	-rrhage, -rrhagia	excessive bleeding or hemorrhage
Suffix	**Meaning**	-rrhea	flow or discharge
Signs and Symptoms		-rrhexis	rupture
-algia, -dynia	pain	-spasm	twitching, cramp
-ectasia, -ectasis	dilatation or stretching of a structure or part	-stasis	stopping, controlling
-edema	swelling	**Procedures**	
-emesis	to vomit, vomiting	-gram	a record
-malacia	soft, softening	-graph	instrument used to record
-megaly	enlargement	-graphy	process of recording
-oid (forms adjectives and nouns)	resembling	-meter	instrument used to measure
		-scope	instrument used for viewing
-penia	deficiency	-scopy	visual examination

Match the suffixes in the left column with their meanings in the right column.

_____ **1.** -algia	**A.** controlling
_____ **2.** -ectasis	**B.** dilatation
_____ **3.** -edema	**C.** enlargement
_____ **4.** -emesis	**D.** excessive bleeding
_____ **5.** -malacia	**E.** pain
_____ **6.** -megaly	**F.** softening
_____ **7.** -rrhagia	**G.** swelling
_____ **8.** -stasis	**H.** vomiting

WRITE IT!
EXERCISE 22

Write the suffix that means the following:

1. deficiency _____
2. flow or discharge _____
3. resembling _____
4. rupture _____
5. twitching or cramp _____

---

bone

2-62 The combining form oste(o) means bone. If something is described as **oste/oid**, it resembles _____.

deficiency

2-63 The suffix -penia means _____. **Calci/penia** means a deficiency of calcium.

2-64 Several suffixes are also terms that can stand alone. **Malacia** means softening. Use a combining form before -malacia to write a word that means abnormal softening of the eye:

ophthalmomalacia

_____.

swelling

2-65 **Emesis** means the material expelled in vomiting, and **edema** is the presence of abnormally large amounts of fluid in the tissues, resulting in swelling. The suffix -edema means swelling.

Blephar(o) is a combining form that means eyelid. **Blephar/edema** is _____ of the eyelid.

An outstanding example of edema is seen in the late stages of **elephantiasis,** a parasitic disease generally seen in the tropics (Fig. 2.25). The excessive swelling is caused by obstruction of the lymphatic vessels by the parasites.

controlling

2-66 **Stasis,** the term, means the same as the suffix -stasis, which means stopping or _____. Stasis of hemorrhaging means controlling excessive bleeding (Fig. 2.26).

twitching

2-67 **Spasm** means cramp or twitching. **Blephuro/spasm** means _____ of the eyelid.

FIND IT!
EXERCISE 23

Draw a slash between the combining forms and the suffixes in the following list of terms. Then find the meanings of the word parts within the definition. (Draw the slash, and then perform the remainder of the activity as a mental exercise.) Think!

1. cardiomegaly enlarged heart
2. myalgia muscular pain
3. ophthalmalgia, ophthalmodynia painful eye
4. ophthalmorrhagia hemorrhage from the eye
5. otalgia, otodynia pain in the ear; earache
6. otorrhea discharge from the ear

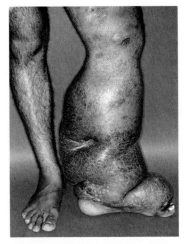

Figure 2.25 Lymphedema. Extensive swelling, caused by chronic obstruction of the lymphatic vessels, occurs in the late stages of elephantiasis.

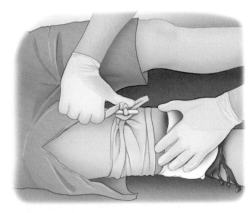

Figure 2.26 Controlling hemorrhage. Stasis of hemorrhaging is provided by compression (applying pressure) and a tourniquet (tight band). Tourniquets are used *only* when direct pressure applied or the wound or pressure points does not stop the bleeding.

Basic Examination Procedures

2-68 Basic examinations are performed to assess the patient's condition. Vital signs are measured and recorded for most patients.

> 🔑 **KEY** POINT **Vital signs actually include only the measurements of pulse rate, respiration rate, and body temperature.** However, they can vary and sometimes include other measurements. Although not strictly a vital sign, blood pressure is customarily included.

vital

The measurements of pulse rate, respiration rate, and body temperature are included when one checks the _____ signs of a patient.

2-69 The **pulse** (P) is the rhythmic expansion of an artery that occurs as the heart beats; it may be felt with a finger (Fig. 2.27). The pulse rate is the number of pulse beats per minute. A normal pulse rate in a resting state is 60 to 100 beats per minute. The rhythmic expansion of an artery that occurs as the heart beats is called the _____.

pulse

2-70 The **respiration rate** is the number of breaths per minute. Respiration (R), the rise and fall of the patient's chest, is observed while counting the number of breaths and noting the ease with which breathing is accomplished. The number of breaths per minute is the _____ rate.

respiration

2-71 The measurement of body temperature is also a vital sign. Therm(o), the combining form for heat, is used to write thermo/meter, which is an instrument for measuring temperature. Body temperature is the level of heat produced and sustained by the body processes. Variation and changes in body temperature may indicate disease. Normal adult body temperature as measured orally is 98.6° F or 37° C (F and C are abbreviations for Fahrenheit and Celsius). A thermo/meter is a(n) _____ for measuring temperature.

instrument

> 🔑 **KEY** POINT **Temperature (T) measurement can be accomplished by several means: most commonly oral, rectal, under the arm, or in the ear** (Fig. 2.28). Electronic measurement has decreased the time required for accurate measurement. One piece of equipment that contains a probe covered by a disposable sheath can be used to measure temperature under the tongue, in the rectum, or under the arm. For tympanic membrane (eardrum) temperature measurement, a specially designed probe similar to an otoscope is required.

mouth

2-72 An **oral thermometer** is placed in the _____. A **rectal thermometer** is inserted in the rectum. Rectal temperatures are generally slightly higher than oral temperatures. Measurements of temperature under the arm by **tympanic thermometers** vary somewhat from those obtained by oral or rectal means. Special under-the-arm **axillary** (axill[o] means armpit) **thermometers** for newborns are available.

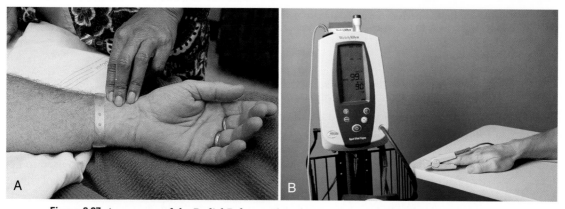

Figure 2.27 Assessment of the Radial Pulse. A, The pulse is an intermittent throbbing sensation felt when the fingers are pressed against an artery such as the radial artery. Radi(o) sometimes means radiant energy, but in this case it is used to mean radius, a bone of the forearm, for which the artery is named. **B,** Pulse can also be monitored electronically using a special clip-like device on the fingertip or earlobe. The oximeter shown indicates a blood oxygen level of 99 and a pulse rate of 90.

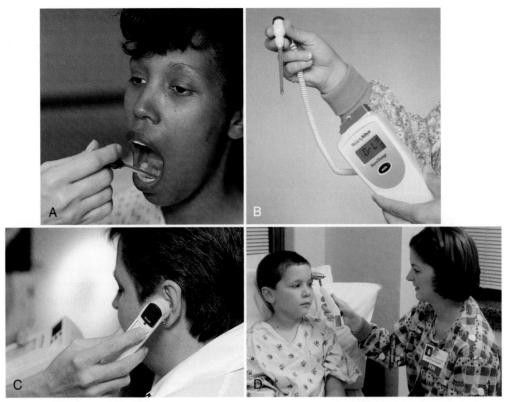

Figure 2.28 **Devices for electronic temperature measurement. A,** Original oral thermometer used sometimes at home, contains a liquid that expands or contracts according to changes in temperature. **B,** Thermometer for measuring temperature orally, rectally, or under the arm. **C,** Tympanic membrane thermometer that uses a probe placed in the ear. **D,** A temporal artery thermometer works well for use with babies or small children.

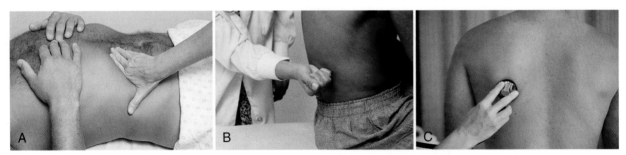

Figure 2.29 **Three aspects of the physical examination (PE).** These techniques help in assessing the internal organs. **A,** Palpation. **B,** Percussion. **C,** Auscultation with a stethoscope.

2-73 Blood pressure (BP) is the pressure exerted by the circulating volume of blood on the walls of the arteries and veins and on the chambers of the heart. Blood pressure is discussed in detail in Chapter 5.

One combining form for chest is steth(o). The **stetho/scope** is placed on the chest to listen to heart sounds, particularly closing of the heart valves. The stethoscope is also used to hear sounds of breathing and intestinal action and to take blood pressure. Write the name of the instrument placed on the chest to hear heart sounds: _____. A stethoscope is being used to listen to the patient's breathing in Fig. 2.29, C.

stethoscope

2-74 A physical examination (PE) is an investigation of the body to determine its state of health, using any of several techniques.

KEY POINT **A PE often includes the following:**
- **Inspection:** The examiner uses the eyes to observe the patient.
- **Palpation:** The examiner feels the texture, size, consistency, and location of certain body parts with the hands (see Fig. 2.29, A).
- **Percussion:** The examiner taps the body with the fingertips or fist to evaluate the size, borders, and consistency of internal organs and to determine the amount of fluid in a body cavity (see Fig. 2.29, B).
- **Auscultation:** The examiner listens for sounds within the body to evaluate the heart, blood vessels, lungs, intestines, or other organs or to detect the fetal heart sound in pregnant women. Auscultation is performed most commonly with a stethoscope (see Fig. 2.29, C).

palpation
percussion
auscultation

Using the hands to feel the location or size of the liver is an example of _____.
Tapping the chest with the fingertips is an example of _____.
Listening to the heart with a stethoscope is an example of _____.

walk

2-75 Ambulation means the act of walking. **Ambulant** describes a person who is able to _____. It is also accurate to say that a walking person is **ambulatory**. A person's ability to ambulate is one observation an examiner would make by inspection.

WRITE IT! EXERCISE 24

Write a word to complete each sentence.

1. The rhythmic expansion of an artery that occurs as the heart beats is called the _____.
2. Counting the number of breaths per minute measures the _____ rate.
3. The name of the procedure in which the physician listens with a stethoscope for sounds within the body is _____.
4. The name of the procedure in which the physician taps the patient's body with the fingertips to evaluate an internal organ is _____.
5. The name of the procedure in which the physician feels the texture, size, consistency, and location of body parts with the hands is _____.
6. The term for the act of walking is _____.

Other Diagnostic Procedures

Nonradiologic Terms

2-76 In addition to the basic examination, many tools are available to determine a person's health condition, which may include viewing internal structures with special instruments, data obtained from laboratory analysis of body fluids or tissue, and diagnostic radiology. Discussion will be grouped as either nonradiological (not involving use of radiology) or radiologic terms.

living

2-77 Bi/opsy is the examination of tissue from the _____ body. A biopsy is either removal of a small piece of living tissue or the tissue excised or aspirated. **Aspiration** is drawing in or out by suction, usually aided by the use of a syringe or a suction device. The term also means the drawing of a foreign substance, such as the gastric contents, into the respiratory tract while taking a breath.

KEY POINT **Know the difference between a biopsy and an autopsy.** In a **biopsy**, tissue is removed from a living body, sectioned, and viewed through a microscope to establish a precise diagnosis. In an **autopsy**, organs and tissues of a dead body are studied to determine the cause of death or pathologic conditions. An autopsy is the same as a **postmortem** examination.

histologist

2-78 Histo/logy is the study of the structure, composition, and function of tissues. A microscope is used to study the minute cells that make up tissue. Stated simply, histo/logy means the study of tissue. One who specializes in histology is a _____.

recording

record

electrocardiograph

2-79 Electro/cardio/graphy, the process of recording the electrical impulses of the heart, is one example of a diagnostic procedure. The suffix -graphy means the process of _____. An **electro/cardio/gram** is a record or tracing of the electrical impulses of the heart, because -gram means the _____ that is produced in this procedure. This is abbreviated as either ECG or EKG. The combining form electr(o) means electricity, and the suffix -graph means an instrument used for recording. Use electr(o) + cardi(o) + -graph to write the name of the instrument used in electrocardiography: _____ (Fig. 2.30).

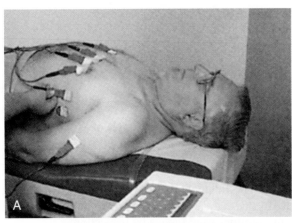

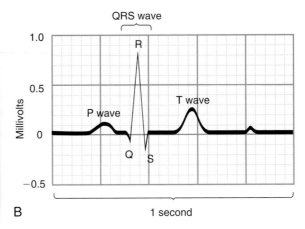

Figure 2.30 **Electrocardiography. A,** A patient undergoing electrocardiography, the study of graphic records produced by electrical activity of the heart muscle. The instrument, an electrocardiograph, is shown. The electrical impulses that are given off by the heart are picked up by electrodes (sensors) and conducted into the electrocardiograph through wires. **B,** An enlarged section of an ECG, a tracing that represents the heart's electrical impulses, which are picked up and conducted to the electrocardiograph by electrodes or leads connected to the body. The pattern of the graphic recording indicates the heart's rhythm and other actions. The normal ECG is composed of the labeled parts shown in the drawing. Each labeled segment represents a different part of the heartbeat. Electrocardiography is a valuable diagnostic tool.

➤ **BEYOND** THE BLUEPRINT In speaking, sometimes these terms are shortened to cardiogram, cardiograph, and cardiography. Don't confuse the terms: A cardiogram (a record) is produced by a cardiograph (a device that measures movements of the heart) in the process of cardiography.

otoscope

2-80 Oto/scopy means an examination of the outer ear, including the eardrum (Fig. 2.31). Write a word that means the lighted instrument used in otoscopy: _____.

➤ **BEYOND** THE BLUEPRINT Note that just one letter change in the suffix -scope (an instrument) produces -scopy, a suffix that means the process of viewing (for example, a *microscope* is used in *microscopy*).

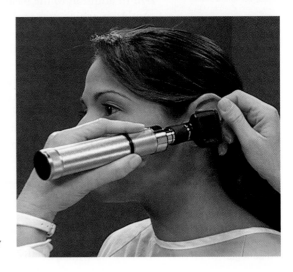

Figure 2.31 **Otoscopy.** An otoscope is being used to visually examine the ear, including the eardrum.

ophthalmoscopy

2-81 Using otoscopy as a model, write a term that means examination of the interior of the eye with an **ophthalmoscope**: _____ (Fig. 2.32).

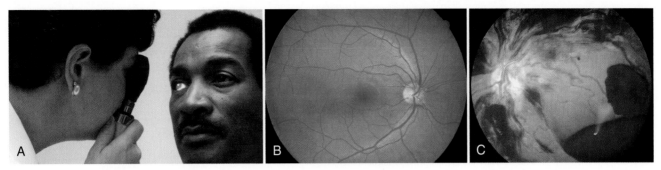

Figure 2.32 Ophthalmoscopy. A, Proper technique for ophthalmoscopic visualization of the interior of the eye. **B,** Normal ophthalmoscopic view. See Chapter 11 for additional information. **C,** Shaken baby syndrome. Ophthalmoscope view shows multiple hemorrhages typical of this type of child abuse.

2-82 An **endo/scope** is an illuminated optic instrument for the visualization of the interior of a body cavity or organ. Although the endoscope is generally introduced through a natural opening (for example, introduction of an endoscope into the mouth and through the esophagus to examine the interior of the stomach; Fig. 2.33), it may also be inserted through an incision (for example, insertion of an endoscope into the chest cavity through an incision in the chest wall).

Endoscopy is visual inspection of a cavity of the body by means of an endoscope. Write the term that means a diagnostic procedure that uses an endoscope: _____.

endoscopy

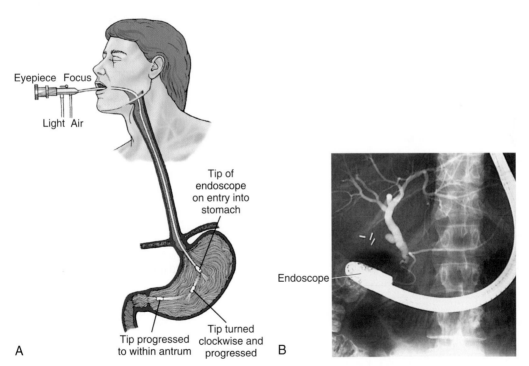

Figure 2.33 Example of a flexible endoscope. A, This endoscope is being used to examine the interior of the stomach through the esophagus. Depending on the structure to be examined, the physician chooses either a flexible or a rigid endoscope. Most of the interior stomach can be examined, including the antrum located in the lower part of the stomach. **B,** A radiographic view of the placement of the endoscope.

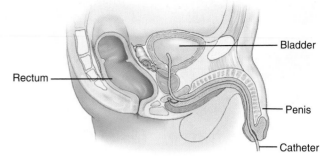

Bladder

Rectum

Penis

Catheter

Figure 2.34 Catheterization of the male bladder. This route of catheterization is insertion of the catheter through the external opening of the urethra and into the bladder, done to drain or remove fluid from the bladder, or to introduce fluids for various tests or treatments.

WORD ORIGIN
catheter (G.)
katheter, something lowered

catheter

2-83 A **catheter** is a hollow flexible tube that can be inserted into a cavity of the body to withdraw or to instill fluids, perform tests, or visualize a vessel or cavity (for example, to view inside blood vessels). The introduction of a catheter is **catheterization** (Fig. 2.34). To introduce a catheter within the body is to **catheterize**. Write the name of the device used in catheterization: _____.

▶ **BEYOND** THE BLUEPRINT   The earliest precursor to the present day Foley catheter (used to drain urine from the bladder and retained by means of a balloon at the tip, which is inflated with sterile water) is documented in 3000 BC by the Egyptians, probably using metal pipes to perform bladder catheterization. Benjamin Franklin invented a flexible catheter for his brother who had a urinary stone. The Foley catheter came into existence in the 1930s.

WORD ORIGIN
cannula (L.)
canna, "reed"

A Latin term **cannula** is also used to mean a hollow flexible tube that is inserted into vessels, ducts, or cavities, for delivery or removal of fluids. Common types are a venous cannula (for administration of fluids or medicine or obtaining blood samples) or a nasal cannula (for delivery of oxygen or gas mixture during anesthesia).

MATCH IT!   EXERCISE 25

Match these terms with their descriptions.

_____ **1.** blepharedema
_____ **2.** cannula
_____ **3.** catheterization
_____ **4.** catheterize
_____ **5.** electrocardiogram
_____ **6.** electrocardiograph
_____ **7.** electrocardiography
_____ **8.** ophthalmomalacia
_____ **9.** osteoid
_____ **10.** otoscope

A. a tracing of the electrical impulses of the heart
B. abnormal softening of the eye
C. hollow flexible tube inserted into vessels, ducts, or cavities
D. instrument used to record the electrical activity of the heart
E. introduction of a catheter into a body cavity
F. lighted instrument used to examine the ear
G. process of recording the electrical activity of the heart
H. resembling bone
I. swelling of the eye
J. to introduce a catheter into a body cavity

Diagnostic Radiology

2-84 Radiology is the branch of medicine concerned with x-rays and **radioactive** (giving off radiation as atomic nuclei disintegrate) substances and with the diagnosis and treatment of disease using any of the various sources of radiant energy. Diagnostic radiology is used to establish or confirm a diagnosis. Learn the following word parts and their meanings.

Word Parts: Radiology

Combining Form	Meaning	Prefix	Meaning
ech(o), son(o)	sound	ultra-	excessive
electr(o)	electricity		
fluor(o)	emitting or reflecting light		
radi(o)*	radiant energy		
tom(o)	to cut		

*Radi(o) sometimes means radius, a bone of the forearm.

WRITE IT!

EXERCISE 26

Match word parts with their meanings A-F. (One will be used more than once.)

_____ **1.** ech(o)   **A.** electricity

_____ **2.** electr(o)   **B.** emitting or reflecting light

_____ **3.** fluor(o)   **C.** excessive

_____ **4.** radi(o)   **D.** radiant energy

_____ **5.** son(o)   **E.** sound

_____ **6.** tom(o)   **F.** to cut

_____ **7.** ultra-

2-85 Radio/graphy was the predominant means of diagnostic imaging for many years, with x-rays providing film images of internal structures. Almost everyone is familiar with a chest x-ray examination (see Fig. 5.8).

This is a common type of diagnostic radiology. An x-ray image is a **radio/graph;** however, you have learned that -graph refers to an instrument used for recording. We see the same common usage in the word photograph, which refers to the picture obtained in photography. We commonly refer to a **radiographic** film as a _____ rather than a radiogram.

radiograph

WORD ORIGIN
opaque *(L.)*
opacus, dark, obscure.
lucent *(L.)*
lux, light

2-86 Substances that do not permit the passage of x-rays are described as **radiopaque**. When radi(o) is joined with the word opaque, one "o" is omitted to facilitate pronunciation. The combining form radi(o) is also joined with lucent to form the term **radiolucent**, which describes substances that readily permit the passage of x-rays.

Write the term that means not permitting the passage of x-rays or other radiant energy: _____.

radiopaque

🔑 **KEY** POINT **X-radiation passes through different substances in the body in varying degrees.** Where there is greater penetration, the image is black or darker; where the x-rays are absorbed by the subject, the image is white or light gray. Thus air appears black, fat appears dark gray, muscle tissue appears light gray, and bone appears very light or white. Heavy substances, such as lead or steel, appear white because they absorb the rays and prevent them from reaching the image receptor (see thumbtack in Fig. 2.35, A).

radiolucent

X-rays that pass through the patient expose the radiographic film or digital image receptor to create the image. X-radiation passes through different substances in the body to varying degrees, causing the image to appear dark, varying shades of gray, and white (see Fig. 2.35, C). You learned that substances that readily permit the passage of x-rays are described as _____.

2-87 Additional diagnostic imaging modalities include the following:
- Contrast imaging and fluoroscopy
- Computed tomography (CT), formerly known as **computed axial tomography** (CAT)
- Nuclear scans (placing radioactive materials into body organs for the purpose of imaging)
- Magnetic resonance imaging (MRI)
- Sono/graphy (also called ultra/sono/graphy, **echo/graphy**, or ultra/sound)

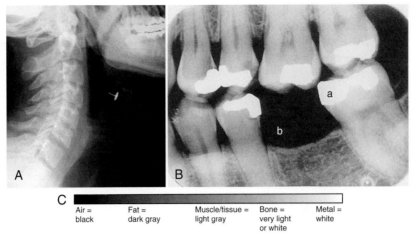

Figure 2.35 Penetration of x-radiation by various substances in an x-ray image. A, Radiograph of an aspirated thumbtack. The lodged tack appears white, because it absorbs most of the x-rays and prevents them from reaching the film or image receptor. Note also the different appearances of air, soft tissue, bone, and teeth. **B,** A dental radiograph. The white area *(a)* is an amalgam (filling) and the dark area *(b)* represents air. **C,** Schematic representation of how substances appear on an x-ray image, depending on the amount of x-radiation the substance absorbs.

contrast

2-88 Contrast imaging is the use of radiopaque materials to make internal organs visible on x-ray images. A contrast medium may be injected into a vessel, swallowed, or introduced into a body cavity, resulting in greater visibility of internal organs or cavities outlined by the contrast material. This type of imaging is _____ imaging. One example is a barium enema, which is the introduction of barium sulfate, a radiopaque contrast medium, into the rectum. A barium enema increases visibility of the inner contours of the lower intestinal tract (Fig. 2.36).

2-89 Fluoroscopy is the visual examination of an internal organ using a **fluoroscope** (Fig. 2.37). This technique offers continuous imaging of the motion of internal structures and immediate serial images, whereas radiology provides a record of the image at a particular point in time.

fluoroscope

Write the name of the instrument used in fluoroscopy: _____.
This device projects an x-ray image that can be seen on a monitor.

Digital imaging techniques can be used to achieve higher quality images in conventional and fluoroscopic images, and allows other professionals to see the images.

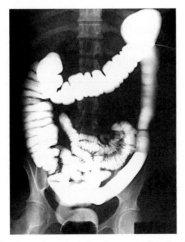

Figure 2.36 Contrast imaging. In this example of a barium enema, radiopaque barium sulfate is used to make the large intestine clearly visible.

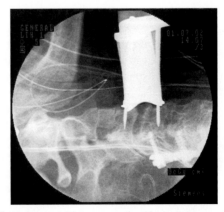

Figure 2.37 Fluoroscopy. The image produced by the fluoroscope is magnified and brightened electronically and projected on a monitor screen.

tomography

2-90 CT is the abbreviation for **computed** _____. This technique produces an image of a detailed cross-section of tissue similar to what one would see if the body or body part were actually cut into sections. The tom(o) in tomo/graphy means to cut. The procedure, however, is painless and non/invasive, meaning it does not require the skin to be broken or a cavity or organ of the body to be entered. A CT scanner and a **tomogram**, the record produced, are shown in Fig. 2.38.

Single-photo emission computed tomography (SPECT), a variation of computed tomography, involves an injection of radioactive tracer, rotation of the camera around the patient, and computer reconstruction of a 3D image.

🔑 **KEY** POINT **An integrated system often presents a more complete picture. Positron emission tomography** (PET) is a type of computerized radiographic technique using radioactive substances to examine the metabolic activity of various body structures, such as the brain (Fig. 2.39). A hybrid of both computed tomography and PET or emission scanning presents a more complete picture than attempting to correlate the two studies separately.

mouth

2-91 A PET scan is an example of nuclear medicine, which involves administering **radio/pharmaceuticals** to a patient orally, into the vein, or by having the patient breathe the material in vapor form. Computerized scanners called *gamma cameras* detect the radioactivity emitted by the patient and map its location to form an image of the organ or system (Fig. 2.40). You remember that oral administration is by _____. **Pharmaceuticals** are medicinal drugs, and radiopharmaceuticals are those that are radioactive.

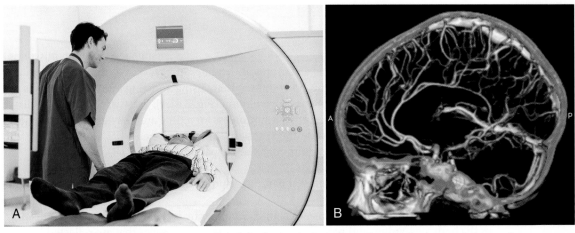

Figure 2.38 Computed tomography of the brain. A, Positioning of patient for computed tomography. **B,** Computed tomographic scan of blood vessels of the brain after injecting contrast dye.

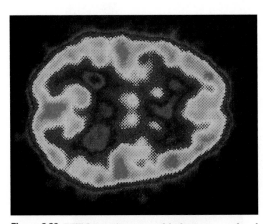

Figure 2.39 PET Scan. This image of the brain was produced after a seizure.

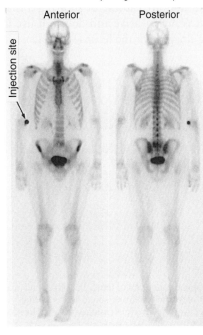

Figure 2.40 Nuclear medicine. Administering a radiopharmaceutical that accumulates in a specific organ or structure provides information about its function and, to some degree, its structure.

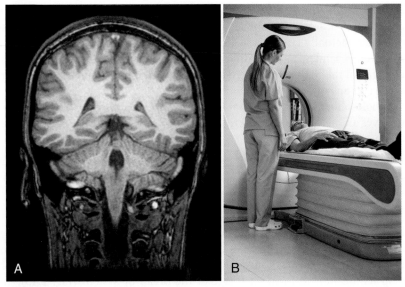

Figure 2.41 Magnetic resonance imaging (MRI). A, Midline sagittal view of the brain using MRI. **B,** Clinical setting for open magnetic resonance imaging.

magnetic

2-92 MRI is the abbreviation for _____ **resonance imaging**. It is a noninvasive technique for visualizing internal structures and creates images based on the magnetic properties of chemical elements within the body rather than using ionizing radiation such as x-rays. In addition, it produces superior soft-tissue resolution (Fig. 2.41A). Soft-tissue resolution distinguishes adjacent structures. Patients must remain motionless for a time and may experience anxiety because of being somewhat enclosed inside the scanner. The newer, open MRI scanners have eliminated much of the anxiety and can accommodate larger patients (Fig. 2.41B).

excessive

2-93 Sono/graphy is known by different names, including **ultrasonography** and diagnostic **ultrasound** (US). The prefix ultra- means _____. Most of these names use the combining form son(o), which means sound. Sonography is the process of imaging deep structures of the body by sending and receiving high-frequency sound waves that are reflected back as echoes from tissue interfaces. Conventional sonography provides two-dimensional images, but the more recent scanners are capable of showing a three-dimensional perspective. Sonography is very safe because it is not invasive and does not use ionizing radiation. It has many medical applications, including imaging of the fetus (Fig. 2.42).

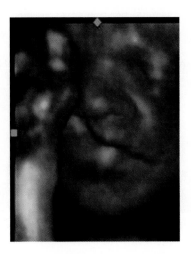

Figure 2.42 Three-dimensional sonogram of fetus. This ultrasound image shows a normal fetal face of late pregnancy. Utilizing sound waves at high frequency, ultrasound imaging provides two- and three-dimensional images of internal organs, including images of a developing fetus.

➤ **BEYOND** THE BLUEPRINT MR-guided focused ultrasound surgery incorporates nonionizing treatment with minimal discomfort and injury to surrounding tissue. It doesn't require hospitalization, and there is no cutting or scars; it is used primarily to treat breast and prostate cancers, as well as alleviation of bone cancer pain. Unfortunately, the procedure is not widely available at the time of this writing.

WRITE IT!

EXERCISE 27

Write a word in each blank to complete these sentences.

1. The use of radiopaque materials to make internal organs visible on x-ray examination is called _____ imaging.
2. CT means computed _____.
3. Nuclear medicine involves placing _____ materials into body organs for the purpose of imaging.
4. Creating images based on the magnetic properties of chemical elements within the body is MRI, which means magnetic _____ imaging.
5. Ultrasonography provides imaging of internal structures by measuring and recording _____ waves.

QUICK CASE STUDY

EXERCISE 28

Write an answer in each blank line.

Andrea Parker, a 66-year-old female, is a smoker and has a history of chronic bronchitis. She is coughing and short of breath. Vital Signs: T. 100.8; P 98; BP 160/94; R 28. ECG: Normal. Chest x-ray shows an unidentified opacity in the superior segment of the left lower lobe. CT scan of the chest with contrast: Multiple nodules throughout the left lung, as well as a well-defined nodular opacity (12 x 13 x 9 mm) in the superior segment of the left lower lobe. Dx: Upper respiratory tract infection; unidentified nodules in the left lung. Treatment Plan: Antibiotics for the respiratory tract infection; biopsy of the large pulmonary nodule, left lower lobe.

1. The abbreviations T, P, R, and BP mean _____, _____, _____, and _____, respectively.
2. Which radiologic abbreviation represents a test that uses contrast agents? _____
3. Is a chest x-ray invasive? _____

THERAPEUTIC INTERVENTIONS

treatment

2-94 The care and management of a patient to combat or prevent a disease is treatment or therapy. Strictly speaking, it includes both surgical and nonsurgical treatment (including counseling, prescribing medication, physical therapy, and radiation therapy).
   Therapeutic means pertaining to therapy or _____.

Nonsurgical Treatment

Learn these word parts.

Word Parts: Nonsurgical Treatment

Combining Form	Meaning	Combining Form	Meaning
algesi(o)	sensitivity to pain	therm(o)	heat
chem(o)	chemical	tox(o), toxic(o)	poison
cry(o)	cold		
esthesi(o)	feeling or sensation	**Prefix**	
narc(o)	stupor	an-	no, not, without
pharmac(o), pharmaceut(i)	drugs or medicine		
therapeut(o)	treatment	**Suffix**	
		-therapy	treatment

WRITE IT! **EXERCISE 29**

Write combining forms for the following meanings.

1. chemical _____
2. cold _____
3. drugs or medicine _____
4. feeling or sensation _____
5. heat _____
6. sensitivity to pain _____
7. stupor _____
8. treatment _____

---

tumors

2-95 **Radio/therapy**, radiation therapy, or **radiation oncology** mean the treatment of cancer using ionizing radiation (Fig. 2.43). The literal translation of onco/logy is the study of _____, but radiation oncology is treatment of tumors using ionizing radiation.

The source of radiation can be either external or internally implanted radioactive substances. Surgery is often a treatment, but radiation therapy is widely used before and after surgery. Radiotherapy can produce undesirable side effects because of incidental destruction of normal body tissues. Most of the side effects disappear with time and include nausea and vomiting, hair loss, ulceration or dryness of mucous membranes, and suppression of bone marrow activity.

KEY POINT **Radiation therapy is also called radiation oncology.** The **radiation oncologist** recommends one of several types of radiation that includes one of the following:
- High intensity radiation (radiation doses are directed at the tumor)
- Injection into the bloodstream
- Surgical implantation

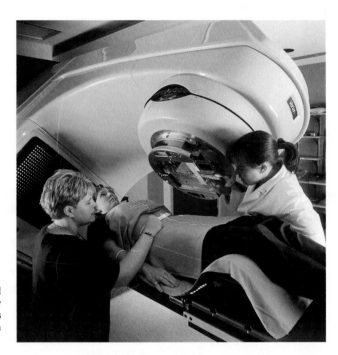

Figure 2.43 Radiation therapy. Also called *radiotherapy* or *radiation oncology*, radiation therapy treats neoplastic disease by using powerful x-rays or gamma rays to prevent the malignant cells from increasing in number.

cryotherapy

2-96 Heat and cold are used in various treatments. Treating with heat is called **thermotherapy**. Use cry(o) to write a term that means treating with cold temperatures: _____.

bacteria

2-97 An **anti/septic** is a substance that inhibits the growth of microorganisms without necessarily killing them. **Bacterio/static** means inhibiting the growth of bacteria. However, **bacteri/cidal** means killing _____. Both these terms can be written using either bacter(i) or bacteri(o), but note the more commonly used terms.

toxicologist

2-98 A **toxin** is a poison, produced by or occurring in a plant or microorganism. A **toxic dose** is the amount of a substance that may be expected to produce a toxic event. Pharmaceuticals taken in excessive amounts can cause toxic effects.

The scientific study of poisons is **toxicology**, and the specialist is a _____.

> **BEYOND** THE BLUEPRINT The use of tox(o) and toxic(o) originates with a Greek word that means archery or the archer's bow. Ancient Greeks smeared poison on arrowheads that were used in hunting. In a regular dictionary, you will find the word *toxophilite,* one fond of archery.

cells	**2-99** Cyt(o) is the combining form for cell, so **cyto/toxic** agents are those used to kill or poison _____, such as in cancer treatment. **Cytology** is the study of cells. Cells are discussed in Chapter 3.

WRITE IT! EXERCISE 30

Write a word in each blank to complete these sentences.
1. A word that means pertaining to treatment _____.
2. Treatment of cancer using ionizing radiation is called _____ oncology.
3. Treatment with heat is called _____.
4. Treatment with cold temperatures is _____.

Surgical Procedures

2-100 Surgery uses operative procedures to treat injuries and to diagnose and treat diseases. Invasive procedures are diagnostic or therapeutic techniques that require entry of a body cavity or interruption of normal body functions.

All the suffixes in the following list are used to name various surgical procedures and instruments, and all of them form nouns when combined with other word parts.

Word Parts: Suffixes in Surgical Procedures

Suffix	Meaning	Suffix	Meaning
-centesis	surgical puncture to aspirate or remove fluid	-scope	instrument used for viewing (also used in diagnostic procedures)
-ectomy	excision (surgical removal or cutting out)		
-lysis	process of loosening, freeing, or destroying	-scopy	visual examination with a lighted instrument (not always a surgical procedure)
-pexy	surgical fixation (fastening in a fixed position)		
-plasty	surgical repair	-stomy	formation of an opening
-rrhaphy	suture (uniting a wound by stitches)	-tome	an instrument used for cutting
		-tomy	incision (cutting into tissue)
		-tripsy	surgical crushing

suture	**2-101** Don't confuse -rrhaphy (meaning _____) with three other "look-alike" suffixes you have learned: -rrhagia (hemorrhage), -rrhea (flow or discharge) and -rrhexis (rupture).

MATCH IT! EXERCISE 31

Match the suffixes in the left column with their meanings in the right column.

_____	**1.** -centesis	**A.**	excision
_____	**2.** -ectomy	**B.**	formation of an opening
_____	**3.** -pexy	**C.**	incision
_____	**4.** -plasty	**D.**	instrument used for cutting
_____	**5.** -rrhaphy	**E.**	surgical crushing
_____	**6.** -scopy	**F.**	surgical fixation
_____	**7.** -stomy	**G.**	surgical puncture
_____	**8.** -tome	**H.**	surgical repair
_____	**9.** -tomy	**I.**	suture
_____	**10.** -tripsy	**J.**	visual examination

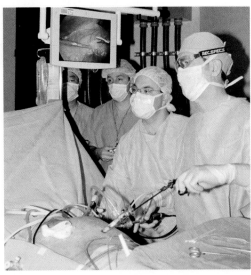

Figure 2.44 Minimally invasive endoscopic surgery. A telescope with a camera and long instruments are introduced into small incisions.

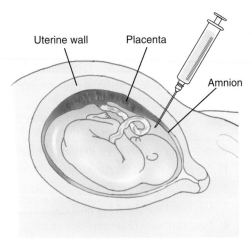

Uterine wall   Placenta   Amnion

Figure 2.45 Amniocentesis. Puncture of the amniotic sac is done to remove fluid for study of the fetal cells.

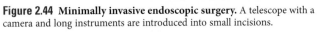

2-102 A minimally invasive surgery (MIS), endoscopic surgery, is done with only a small incision or no incision at all, such as through a cannula. A **trocar** is a solid rod with a tapered or sharp end that fits inside the hollow tube cannula and can be used to pierce the skin or the wall of a body cavity. When the trocar is in the correct position, the surgeon withdraws it, leaving the hollow cannula in place to receive endoscopic instruments. The sharp rod that fits inside the cannula is

trocar	a _____.
	Laparoscopy (lapar[o]) is endoscopic surgery of the abdomen (Fig. 2.44). The **laparoscope** is
instrument	an _____ used in laparoscopy.

2-103 The suffix -centesis means surgical puncture. **Amnio/centesis** is surgical _____
puncture

of the **amnion**, the thin membrane that surrounds the fetus during pregnancy (Fig. 2.45). A small amount of **amniotic** fluid is removed for analysis to aid in the diagnosis of fetal abnormalities.

2-104 You learned in the last chapter that neur(o) means _____.
nerve

  Neur/ectomy is partial or total excision of a nerve. (Note that partial or total is implied. Literal translation does not always indicate the full meaning.)

2-105 **Neuro/lysis** means destruction of nerve tissue or loosening of adhesions surrounding a nerve. Fibrous structures called **adhesions** form when two structures abnormally attach to each other.

  Change the suffix of neurolysis to form a word that specifically means surgical crushing of a
neurotripsy nerve: _____.

2-106 The suffix that means surgical fixation or fastening in a fixed position is _____.
-pexy

2-107 You learned earlier that ophthalm(o) means eye. Combine ophthalm(o) and -plasty to write
ophthalmoplasty a new term: _____. The term you just wrote means surgical repair of the eye.
incision   **Ophthalmo/tomy** is _____ of the eye (in this case, the eyeball).

2-108 Write the suffix that means an instrument used for cutting: _____.
-tome

🔑 **KEY** POINT Be sure you can distinguish between the words incision and excision. **Incision** is cutting into. **Excision** is cutting out or removal.

2-109 The suffix that means a visual examination with a lighted instrument is _____, and
-scopy the instrument used is a scope, which can also be a suffix.

2-110 Write a term that means surgical repair of the eyelid: _____.
blepharoplasty
hand   **Chiro/plasty** is plastic surgery on the _____.

suture

2-111 Angio/plasty means plastic surgery on vessels (in this case, blood vessels). **Angio/rrhaphy** means repair of a vessel by _____.

🔑 **KEY** POINT **Be careful not to misspell terms that contain rrh.** Note that angiorrhaphy is spelled with two r's.

ear

2-112 Oto/plasty is surgical repair of the_____.
   Rhinoplasty is surgical repair of the nose. This is either reconstructive or cosmetic plastic surgery of the nose (Fig. 2.46).

colonoscope

2-113 Both **colono/scopy** and **colo/scopy** mean an examination of the lining of the colon with a special instrument. The instrument is a _____, also called a **coloscope**.

suture

2-114 Colectomy is excision of the colon (or a portion of it). **Colo/pexy** is surgical fixation of the colon, and **colo/rrhaphy** is _____ of the colon.

-stomy

2-115 Perhaps you have heard of a **stoma**, which is a small opening, either natural or artificially created (Fig. 2.47). The suffix that means formation of an opening is _____ and is derived from the same root as stoma.

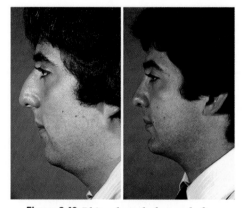

Figure 2.46 Rhinoplasty, before and after.

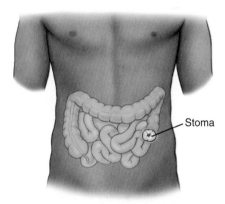

Stoma

Figure 2.47 Stoma. This is an example of surgical creation of a stoma, in this case an artificial anus, on the abdominal wall after removal of much of the large intestine.

-rrhaphy

2-116 Wounds are physical injuries to body tissue, whether caused by an accident or surgery. Where cutting or tearing has occurred, sutures or other materials (staples or wire) hold tissues together while wound healing takes place. To **suture** is to stitch together cut or torn edges of tissue with silk, catgut, wire, or synthetic material. Write the suffix that means suture: _____.
   Superficial wounds often heal on their own or by the use of an adhesive spray or skin closure tapes. Deep wounds or those located where movement opens the cut edges generally require stronger materials such as sutures or staples (Fig. 2.48).

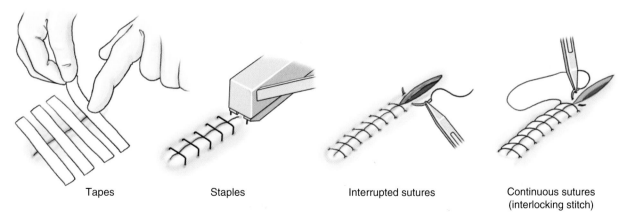

Tapes   Staples   Interrupted sutures   Continuous sutures (interlocking stitch)

Figure 2.48 Common skin closures.

> ► **BEYOND** THE BLUEPRINT Compare absorbable vs. nonabsorbable suture material. An *absorbable* suture is digested over time by body enzymes. Catgut, prepared from the intestines of mammals (originally cats), is one of the best examples of absorbable suture material. A *nonabsorbable* suture either is left in the body, where it becomes embedded in scar tissue, or is removed when healing is complete. Silk, cotton, wire, and certain synthetic materials are not absorbed by the body and are examples of nonabsorbable sutures.

approximate

2-117 Approximate means to bring close together by suture or other means. The act of bringing closer together is approximation. Tissue approximation can be accomplished with materials other than sutures, such as tape, clips, and staples. In some instances, special adhesives that bond almost instantly can be sprayed on a wound to _____ the skin, thus eliminating the need for stitches.

BUILD IT! EXERCISE 32

Use the following word parts to build terms. (Some word parts will be used more than once.)

amni(o), neur(o), ophthalm(o), ot(o), -centesis, -ectomy, -lysis, -plasty, -tripsy

1. excision of a nerve   _____/_____
2. surgical destruction of a nerve   _____/_____
3. surgical puncture of the amnion   _____/_____
4. surgical repair of the ear   _____/_____
5. surgical repair of the eye   _____/_____
6. surgical crushing of a nerve   _____/_____

osteotome

2-118 Osteo/tomy is cutting of a bone. Write a word that means the instrument used in osteotomy: _____.

incision

2-119 Tracheo/tomy is an _____ made into the **trachea** (windpipe) through the neck. This procedure may be performed as an emergency measure to gain access to the airway below a blockage. Use -stomy to build a word that means the opening into the trachea through which a tube may be inserted: _____.

tracheostomy

adenectomy

2-120 Combine aden(o) and -ectomy: _____. This new term means surgical removal of a gland.

2-121 Use append(o) to write a word that means surgical removal of the appendix: _____ _____.

appendectomy

incision

2-122 Encephalo/tomy and **cerebro/tomy** mean _____ of the brain. Not all word parts that have the same meaning are interchangeable. You will learn which version to use as you study them.

encephalotome

Write a word that means the instrument used in encephalotomy: _____.

mastectomy

2-123 Use mast(o) to write a term that means excision of a breast: _____. **Mammo/plasty** is surgical repair of the breast.

🔑 **KEY** POINT **Mammoplasty can enlarge or reduce the breasts.** Plastic surgery is performed to enlarge small breasts, to reduce or lift large or sagging breasts, or to reconstruct a breast after removal of a tumor. Enlarging the breasts is called augmentation mammoplasty (Fig. 2.49).

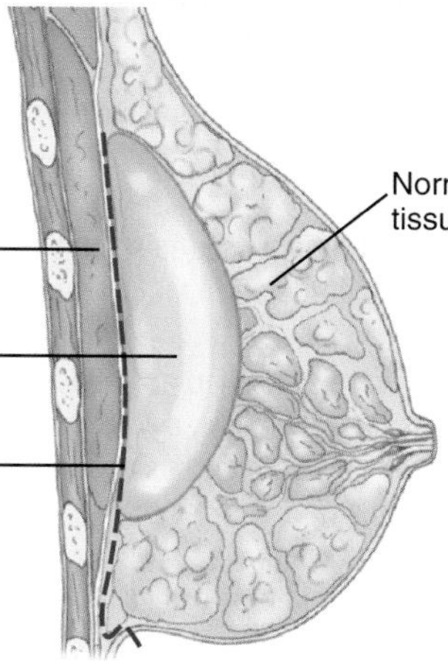

Pectoralis muscle

Normal breast tissue

Silicone implant

Incision

Figure 2.49 Augmentation mammoplasty. This type of augmentation is achieved by inserting envelopes filled with silicone gel *(shown here)* or saline beneath normal breast tissue or beneath the muscle of the chest. An incision below the breast causes the least obvious scarring.

WRITE IT! EXERCISE 33

Write the meaning of the underlined part in each of the following words.

1. neuro<u>lysis</u> _____
2. <u>ophthalmo</u>plasty _____
3. colo<u>rrhaphy</u> _____
4. <u>oto</u>plasty _____
5. <u>encephalo</u>tomy _____

6. mammo<u>plasty</u> _____
7. <u>angio</u>rrhaphy _____
8. <u>adenectomy</u> _____
9. cerebro<u>tomy</u> _____
10. <u>blepharo</u>plasty _____

BUILD IT! EXERCISE 34

Use the following word parts to build terms. (Some word parts will be used more than once.)

angi(o), append(o), blephar(o), chir(o), colon(o), encephal(o), mamm(o), oste(o), -ectomy, -plasty, -rrhaphy, -scopy, -tome, -tomy

1. examination using a colonoscope _____/_____
2. excision of the appendix _____/_____
3. incision of the brain _____/_____
4. instrument for cutting bone _____/_____
5. surgical repair of the breast _____/_____
6. surgical repair of the eyelid _____/_____
7. surgical repair of the hand _____/_____
8. suture of a vessel _____/_____

PHARMACOLOGY

medicine (drugs)

2-124 Pharmaco/therapy is the treatment of diseases with _____. A medication is a drug or medicine. Over-the-counter (OTC) medications can be obtained without a prescription, but a prescription drug (Rx) can be dispensed to the public only with an order by a properly authorized person. Some abbreviations that are commonly used by physicians when writing prescriptions follow.

Common Abbreviations Used in Writing Prescriptions

Abbreviation	Meaning	Abbreviation	Meaning
a.c.	before meals *(ante cibum)*	p.r.n.	as the occasion arises, as needed *(pro re nata)*
ad lib.	freely as needed, at pleasure *(ad libitum)*		
aq.	water *(aqua)*	q.	every *(quaque)*
b.i.d.	twice a day *(bis in die)*	q.i.d.	four times a day *(quater in die)*
NPO	nothing by mouth *(nil per os)*	stat.	immediately *(statim)*
p.o.	orally *(per os)*	t.i.d.	three times a day *(ter in die)*

PHARMACOLOGY, cont'd

chemical

2-125 Chemo/therapy is a general term for treatment of disease by chemical agents. The combining form chem(o) means _____.

neoplasms

2-126 Anti/neo/plastics are medications that are used to treat malignant _____. Many malignant tumors are curable if detected and treated in the early stage.

without

2-127 You have heard of the word *esthetic*, also spelled aesthetic, which pertains to the sense of beauty or to sensation (feeling). The prefix an- means not or without; esthesi(o) refers to feeling (nervous sensation). **An/esthetic** means characterized by or producing anesthesia, and the same term is applied to a drug that brings about this numbing effect. Literal translation of an/esthesia is _____ feeling, but **anesthesia** means loss of sensation or loss of the ability to feel pain.

The term anesthesia is formed by combining an- + esthesi(o) + -ia. (An "i" is dropped to avoid double "i" and to facilitate pronunciation.)

general

2-128 Anesthesia can occur with or without loss of consciousness. Anesthesia may be local, regional, or general. Local anesthesia is confined to one area of the body. Brief surgical or dental procedures can be performed when anesthesia is administered to a localized area; therefore, it is called *local anesthesia*. When an anesthetic blocks a group of nerve fibers, regional anesthesia occurs. In this case, loss of feeling occurs in a certain region of the body. For this reason, it is called *regional anesthesia*.

General anesthesia produces a state of unconsciousness with absence of sensation over the entire body. The drugs producing this state are called _____ _____ anesthetics. Compare local vs. general anesthesia (Fig. 2.50).

➤ **BEYOND** THE BLUEPRINT In mild sedation, also called twilight sleep, the patient maintains normal heart function during impaired consciousness while minor surgery or procedures are performed.

nerves

2-129 Certain drugs called *neuromuscular blocking agents* may be used to stop muscle contraction during surgery. **Neuro/muscul/ar** means pertaining to the _____ and muscles. Later you will study how the nerves and muscles interact to bring about movement.

pain

2-130 An **an/alges/ic** is a drug that relieves pain. Notice that one "i" is omitted to facilitate pronunciation.

The combining form algesi(o) means sensitivity to _____. An analgesic (such as, aspirin) is a type of pharmaceutical.

stupor

2-131 A **narcotic** is a substance that produces insensibility or _____. The term also means a narcotic drug. Narcotic analgesics alter perception of pain, induce a feeling of euphoria, and may induce sleep. Repeated use of narcotics may result in physical and psychological dependence. In large amounts (for example, in an overdose [OD]), narcotics can depress respiration.

The following list of pharmaceuticals affects multiple systems throughout the body. You are expected to remember only the drug classes and their uses.

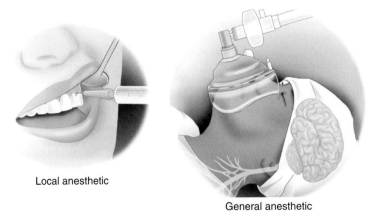

Local anesthetic

General anesthetic

Figure 2.50 Local vs. general anesthetic. Local anesthetics eliminate sensation in a defined area of the body. General anesthetics are inhaled or are given by intravenous injection, and they act on the brain, causing absence of sensation and consciousness.

PHARMACOLOGY, cont'd

Drug Class: Effects and uses

Analgesics: Relieve pain

Narcotic Analgesics: *Potential for addiction or abuse*

fentanyl (Duragesic)
meperidine (Demerol)

methadone (Dolophine)
morphine (MS Contin)

oxycodone (Percocet, OxyContin)
tramadol (Ultram)

Nonnarcotic Analgesics: *No potential for addiction or abuse*

acetaminophen (Tylenol)

Nonsteroidal antiinflammatory drugs (NSAIDs): Mild to moderate pain relief

aspirin (Bayer)

celecoxib (Celebrex)

ibuprofen (Motrin)

Radiopharmaceuticals: *Assess various internal functions (diagnostic) or treat certain cancers or tissue hyperfunction (therapeutic)*

iodine-131 sodium iodide (Hicon)
strontium-89 chloride (Metastron)

technetium-99m MDP (Technescan MDP)
technetium-99m tetrofosmin (Myoview)

thallium-201 thallous chloride

Minerals: *Essential inorganic substances for proper growth and function*

calcium
iodine
iron

magnesium
phosphorus
potassium

sodium
zinc

Vitamins: *Essential organic substances for proper growth and function*

A: Beta-carotene, retinol
B: Thiamine (B_1), riboflavin (B_2), niacin (B_3), pantothenic acid (B_5), pyridoxine (B_6), biotin (B_7), folic acid (B_9), cyanocobalamin (B_{12})
C: Ascorbic acid
D: Ergocalciferol (D_2), cholecalciferol (D_3)
E: Alpha-tocopherol
K: Phylloquinone (K_1), menaquinone (K_2), menadione (K_3)

WRITE IT!

EXERCISE 35

Write a word in each blank to complete these sentences.

1. A drug that relieves pain is a/an _____.
2. Partial or complete loss of sensation is _____.
3. Drugs that are used to stop muscle contraction are _____ blocking agents.
4. A(n) _____ is a substance that produces insensibility or stupor.
5. Radioactive drugs that are used in diagnosis and treatment as well as research are _____.
6. The abbreviation p.o. means _____.
7. The abbreviation aq. means _____.
8. The abbreviation stat. means _____.
9. The abbreviation t.i.d. means _____ times a day.
10. The abbreviation q. means _____.

CHAPTER ABBREVIATIONS*

a.c.	before meals (*ante cibum*)	F	Fahrenheit
ACS	American Cancer Society	FEMA	Federal Emergency Management Agency
ad lib.	freely as needed, at pleasure (*ad libitum*)	HPF	high-power field
aq.	water (*aqua*)	IED	improvised explosive device
b.i.d.	twice a day (*bis in die*)	lab	laboratory
BP	blood pressure	LPF	low-power field
C	Celsius	MIS	minimally invasive surgery
CDC	Centers for Disease Control and Prevention	MRI	magnetic resonance imaging
CT, CAT	computed tomography, computed axial tomography	MRSA	methicillin-resistant *Staphylococcus aureus*
ECG, EKG	electrocardiogram	NIH	National Institutes of Health
		NPO	nothing by mouth (*nil per os*)

OD	overdose; right eye *(oculus dexter)*	staph	staphylococci
P	pulse	stat.	immediately *(statim)*
PET	positron emission tomography	strep	streptococci
p.o.	orally *(per os)*	T	temperature
p.r.n.	as the occasion arises, as needed *(pro re nata)*	t.i.d.	three times a day *(ter in die)*
q.	every *(quaque)*	TNM	a system used in cancer staging
q.i.d.	four times a day *(quater in die)*	US	ultrasound
R	respiration	WHO	World Health Organization
Rx	prescription	WMD	weapons of mass destruction
SPECT	single-photon emission computed tomography	WNL	within normal limits

*Many of these abbreviations share their meanings with other terms.

! Be Careful With These!

-*ase* (enzyme) vs. -*ose* (sugar)

diagnosis (identification of disease) vs. *prognosis* (predicted outcome)

-*gram* (a record) vs. -*graph* (an instrument) vs. -*graphy* (a process)

-*ia* (condition) vs. -*iac* (one who suffers)

iatrogenic (unfavorable response to medical treatment) vs. *idiopathic* (disease without an apparent or known cause)

incision (cutting into) vs. *excision* (cutting out, removal)

-*lysin* (that which destroys) vs. -*lytic* (capable of destroying)

-*phagia* (eating, swallowing) vs. -*phasia* (speech)

-*plasia* (formation, development) vs. -*plasty* (surgical repair)

-*rrhage* (excessive bleeding) vs. -*rrhea* (discharge) vs. -*rrhexis* (rupture)

sign (objective) vs. *symptom* (subjective)

-*tome* (cutting instrument) vs. -*tomy* (cutting into)

-*tomy* (cutting into) vs. -*stomy* (formation of an opening)

A Career as a Radiologic Technologist

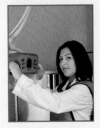

Radiologic technologists (RTs) play a vital role in diagnosis. They perform diagnostic imaging examinations, creating the images that radiologists evaluate. RTs work with many types of imaging, including plain x-ray examinations, magnetic resonance imaging (MRI), computed tomography (CT), mammography, sonography, and fluoroscopy. RTs can also be trained to administer radiation therapy treatments. Meet Jeanne Jones, an RT who works at a community hospital. She is positioning a patient for an x-ray examination of the abdomen. Jeanne loves her work, because she knows that radiologists, as well as patients, count on her to provide the best diagnostic tools possible. To learn more, visit the website *www.asrt.org*.

CHAPTER 2 SELF-TEST

Review the word parts for this chapter. Work all of the following exercises to test your understanding of the material before checking your answers against those in Appendix IV.

BASIC UNDERSTANDING

Matching

I.   Match suffixes in the left column with their meanings in the right column.

_____ **1.** -cele

_____ **2.** -emia

_____ **3.** -iasis

_____ **4.** -lith

_____ **5.** -mania

_____ **6.** -oma

_____ **7.** -phobia

_____ **8.** -ptosis

A. abnormal fear

B. calculus

C. condition

D. condition of the blood

E. excessive preoccupation

F. hernia

G. prolapse

H. tumor

II.   *Match combining forms for colors and their meanings.*

_____ **1.** alb(o)   **A.** black
_____ **2.** chlor(o)   **B.** blue
_____ **3.** cyan(o)   **C.** green
_____ **4.** erythr(o)   **D.** red
_____ **5.** melan(o)   **E.** white
_____ **6.** xanth(o)   **F.** yellow

III.   *Match the following surgical suffixes with their meanings.*

_____ **1.** -centesis   **A.** excision
_____ **2.** -ectomy   **B.** formation of an opening
_____ **3.** -pexy   **C.** surgical crushing
_____ **4.** -plasty   **D.** surgical fixation
_____ **5.** -rrhaphy   **E.** surgical puncture
_____ **6.** -scopy   **F.** surgical repair
_____ **7.** -stomy   **G.** suture
_____ **8.** -tripsy   **H.** visual examination

Matching

IV.   *Match the following diagnostic suffixes with their meanings.*

_____ **1.** -algia   **A.** dilatation
_____ **2.** -ectasia   **B.** enlargement
_____ **3.** -edema   **C.** excessive bleeding
_____ **4.** -emesis   **D.** flow or discharge
_____ **5.** -malacia   **E.** pain
_____ **6.** -megaly   **F.** resembling
_____ **7.** -oid   **G.** rupture
_____ **8.** -rrhagia   **H.** softening
_____ **9.** -rrhea   **I.** swelling
_____ **10.** -rrhexis   **J.** vomiting

Using Vocabulary

V.   *Circle one answer for each of the following questions.*

1. Susie tells the doctor that she has a sore throat. Which term describes the sore throat? (diagnosis, prognosis, sign, symptom)
2. Mr. Jones has plastic surgery on his hand. What is the name of this procedure? (carpectomy, chiroplasty, ophthalmoplasty, otoplasty)
3. Which word means stopping or controlling? (phobia, ptosis, spasm, stasis)
4. A 70-year-old man is told he has an enlarged heart. Which term describes his condition? (cardiomegaly, carditis, coronary artery disease, megalomania)
5. Which term means a record of the electrical impulses of the heart? (echography, electrocardiogram, electrocardiograph, electrocardiography)
6. Which term specifically means an opening into the trachea through which a tube may be inserted? (tracheoplasty, tracheostomy, tracheotome, tracheotomy)
7. Which term means removal of a gland? (adenectomy, adenotomy, appendotomy, appendectomy)
8. Which term means abnormal softening of the eye? (ophthalmalgia, ophthalmomalacia, ophthalmoscopy, ophthalmotomy)
9. Which term means an earache? (otodynia, otology, otoscope, otoscopy)
10. Which diagnostic procedure produces an image of a detailed cross-section of tissue similar to what one would see if the organ were actually cut into sections? (computed tomography, contrast imaging, electrocardiography, nuclear medicine imaging)
11. Julie experiences redness of the skin around her recently acquired earrings. What is Julie's condition called? (dermatitis, malacia, mastitis, ptosis)

12. When James and Cynthia's baby is born, it has a yellow discoloration of the skin and mucous membranes. Which condition is most likely? (albinism, cyanosis, jaundice, myalgia)

13. Manuel, a college student, sees the physician and is told that his appendix is inflamed. What is the name of his condition? (appendectomy, appendicitis, appendorrhexis, appendotomy)

14. Karen sustains a severe head injury in which there is herniation of the brain through an opening in the skull. What is the name of this pathology? (cerebritis, cerebrotomy, encephalocele, encephaloplasty)

15. Ken suffers an abnormal fear of heights. What type of pathology does he have? (dilatation, mania, phobia, ptosis)

16. Which word is missing? As an outpatient, Mrs. Harrison had an incisional _____ of tissue from the mass in her left breast. (autopsy, biopsy, postmortem, ptosis)

17. A 3-year-old is treated for otitis media. Which type of disorder does she have? (adenopathy, ophthalmopathy, osteopathy, otopathy)

18. Susan's job includes staining tissues and studying cells from various organs. In which type of laboratory does Susan work? (histology, microbiology, ophthalmology, otology)

19. Which of the following means a cell that can ingest and destroy particulate substances? (carcinogen, erythrocyte, leukocytosis, phagocyte)

20. Which of the following is a verb that means to destroy red blood cells and cause them to release hemoglobin? (hemolysin, hemolysis, hemolytic, hemolyze)

21. Which of the following is a general term for a disease associated with a demonstrable physical change? (autoimmune disease, communicable disease, functional disorder, organic disease)

22. Which of the following terms applies to a hospital-acquired infection? (iatrogenic, idiopathic, nosocomial, therapeutic)

Listing

VI. Name four general types of microorganisms, and describe at least one outstanding feature.

1. _____

2. _____

3. _____

4. _____

Deconstructing Words

VII. Break the following terms into their component parts and state the meaning of each word part. The first one is done as an example.

1. amniocentesis   *amnio/centesis: amnion; surgical puncture* _____

2. blepharoplasty   _____

3. coloscopy   _____

4. echography   _____

5. electrocardiograph   _____

6. fluoroscope   _____

7. osteoid   _____

8. tomogram   _____

Writing Terms

VIII. Write a term for each clue that is given.

1. excessive bleeding   _____

2. excision of the colon   _____

3. incision of the eye   _____

4. instrument used in encephalotomy   _____

5. plastic surgery of the ear   _____

6. a red (blood) cell   _____

7. a disruption of normal function   _____

8. a substance that produces cancer   _____

9. any disease of the eye   _____

10. excessive preoccupation with fires   _____

11. surgical crushing of a nerve _____

12. surgical fixation of the colon   _____

13. suture of a vessel   _____

14. swelling of the eyelid   _____

15. visual examination of the ear   _____

16. inflammation of a bone   _____

17. muscular pain   _____

18. pertaining to the nose   _____

19. stones   _____

20. viewing things with a microscope   _____

Writing the Meanings

IX.   *Write the meanings of these types of therapeutic terms:*

1. antineoplastics   _____

2. chemotherapy   _____

3. pharmacotherapy   _____

4. thermotherapy   _____

Labeling

X.   *Label these three aspects of the physical examination.*

1. _____   **2.** _____   **3.** _____

Identifying Illustrations

XI.   *Identify the following illustrations using one of these terms: albinism, blepharoptosis, dermatitis, encephalocele*

1. _____   **2.** _____

3. _____   **4.** _____

Making Connections

XII.   *All of the following terms end in the suffix -plasty and mean surgical repair of different parts of the body. Circle each combining form, and write its meaning.*

Term	Meaning of Combining Form	Term	Meaning of Combining Form
1. angioplasty	_____	**4.** mammoplasty	_____
2. blepharoplasty	_____	**5.** ophthalmoplasty	_____
3. chiroplasty	_____	**6.** otoplasty	_____

Finetuning Terms

XIII. In addition to spelling, describe at least one difference in the following:

1. mania and phobia: _____

_____

2. lactase and lactose: _____

_____

3. biopsy and autopsy: _____

_____

4. ophthalmoscope and ophthalmoscopy: _____

_____

5. incision and excision: _____

_____

6. electrocardiogram and electrocardiograph: _____

_____

7. encephalotome and encephalotomy: _____

_____

GREATER COMPREHENSION

Health Care Reporting

XIV. Read the following Office Note. Then circle the correct answer to the questions that follow the report.

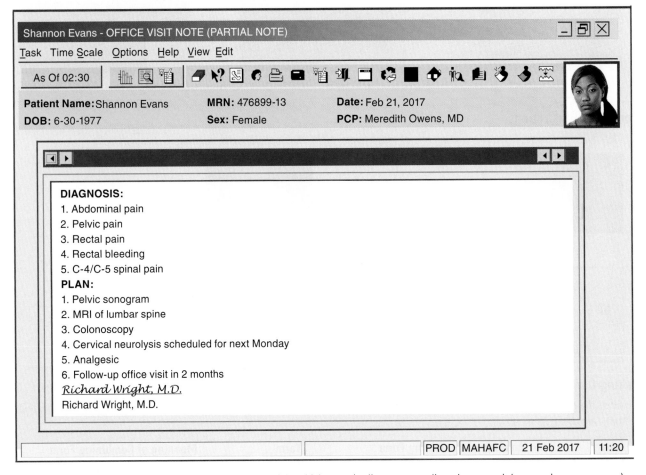

1. The patient is having a medical imaging exam of her pelvis which uses (radio waves, radioactive materials, sound waves, x-rays).
2. The patient was prescribed medication to treat (cancer, inflammation, fever, pain).
3. The "M" in the abbreviation "MRI" stands for (magnetic, medical, motion, muscular).
4. The patient will be scheduled for a treatment designed to destroy (intestine, nerve, pelvis, spine) tissue.
5. An alternate term for sonography is (fluoroscopy, radiography, tomography, ultrasound).

Health Care Reporting

XV. Read the following Office Note. Then circle the correct answer to the questions that follow the note.

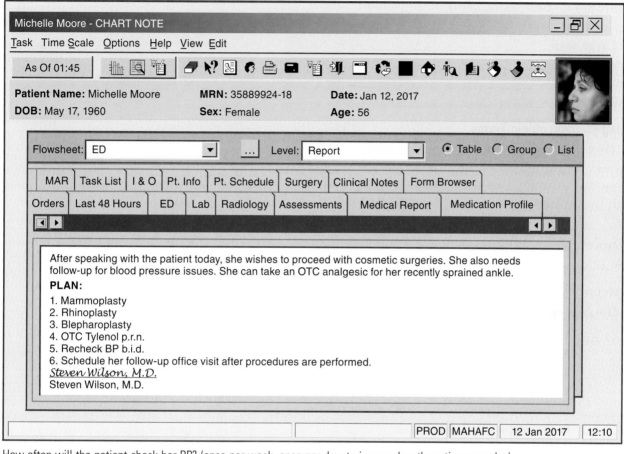

1. How often will the patient check her BP? (once per week, once per day, twice per day, three times per day)
2. The "C" in the abbreviation "OTC" stands for (cancer, Celsius, computed, counter)
3. Which body structure is not included for surgical repair? (abdomen, breast, eyelid, nose)
4. How often can the patient take Tylenol? (as needed, every hour, four times per day, immediately)
5. The "P" in the abbreviation "BP" stands for (positron, power, pressure, pulse)

Spelling

XVI. Circle all misspelled terms, and write their correct spellings.

angioma   blepharal   cefalic   cerebrotomy   colorrhaphy   nurotripsy   ofthalmoplasty   serebral   simptom   trauma

Abbreviating

XVII. Write a letter in each blank that corresponds to each clue.

1. blood pressure   ____ ____
2. Federal Emergency Management Agency   ____ ____ ____ ____
3. high-power field   ____ ____ ____
4. minimally invasive surgery   ____ ____ ____
5. nothing by mouth   ____ ____ ____
6. prescription   ____ ____
7. single-photo emission CT   ____ ____ ____ ____ ____
8. weapons of mass destruction   ____ ____ ____
9. ultrasound   ____ ____
10. World Health Organization   ____ ____ ____

Pronouncing Terms

XVIII. Write the correct term for the following phonetic spellings. (The first one is done as an example.)

1. ap-en-**dek**-tuh-mē   *appendectomy* _____

2. en-sef-uh-**lot**-uh-mē   _____

3. kal-si-**pē**-nē-uh)   _____

4. noo-**rol**-i-sis   _____

5. suh-**nog**-ruh-fē   _____

6. **vir**-ū-lens   _____

Using Pharmacologic Terms

XIX. Write one word in each blank to complete the sentence.

1. A PET scan is an example of nuclear medicine that involves administering _____, either orally, into the veins, or in vapor form.

2. Medications that are used to treat malignant neoplasms are _____.

3. Treatment of disease by chemical agents is _____.

4. Drugs that are used to relieve pain are _____.

5. A _____ is a substance that produces insensibility or stupor.

Categorizing Terms and Practicing Pronunciation

XX. Categorize the terms in the left column by selecting A, B, C, D, or E.

_____ **1.** analgesics

_____ **2.** angiorrhaphy

_____ **3.** cephalic

_____ **4.** coloscopy

_____ **5.** electrocardiography

_____ **6.** fluoroscopy

_____ **7.** mammary

_____ **8.** ophthalmoscopy

_____ **9.** osteotomy

_____ **10.** thermotherapy

A. anatomical

B. diagnostic imaging term

C. diagnostic term that is not related to imaging

D. surgical term

E. nonsurgical therapeutic term

(Be prepared to pronounce terms 1-10 in class after listening to the Chapter 2 terms at *http://evolve.elsevier.com/Leonard/building/*. In addition, practice categorizing all end-of-chapter terms.)

NEW CONSTRUCTION

XXI. Break these words into their component parts and write their meanings. Even if you have not seen these terms before, you may be able to break them apart and determine their meanings. The first is done as an example.

1. appendicitis   *appendic/itis: inflammation of the appendix* _____

2. blepharitis _____

3. chirospasm _____

4. encephalitis _____

5. leukocyte _____

6. myocele _____

7. neurogenic _____

8. rhinoplasty _____

9. tracheoscopy _____

10. xanthous _____

(Use Appendix IV to check your answers to the exercises.)

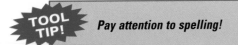
Pay attention to spelling!

BMV LIST

Visit *http://evolve.elsevier.com/Leonard/building/* to listen to the boldface terms in Chapter 2. Look closely at the spelling of each term as it is pronounced.

acute (uh-**kūt**)
adenectomy (ad-uh-**nek**-tuh-mē)
adenitis (ad-uh-**nī**-tis)
adenopathy (ad-uh-**nop**-uh-thē)
adhesions (ad-**hē**-zhunz)
albinism (**al**-bi-niz-um)
albino (al-**bī**-no)
ambulant (**am**-bū-lunt)
ambulation (am-bū-**lā**-shun)
ambulatory (**am**-bū-luh-tor-ē)
amniocentesis (am-nē-ō-sen-**tē**-sis)
amnion (**am**-nē-on)
amniotic (am-nē-**ot**-ik)
anaerobic (an-uh-**rō**-bik)
analgesic (an-ul-**jē**-zik)
analgesics (an-ul-**jē**-ziks)
anesthesia (an-es-**thē**-zhuh)
anesthetic (an-us-**thet**-ik)
angioma (an-jē-**ō**-muh)
angioplasty (**an**-jē-ō-plas-tē)
angiorrhaphy (an-jē-**or**-uh-fē)
anomaly (uh-**nom**-uh-lē)
antineoplastic (an-tē-nē-ō-**plas**-tik)
antiseptic (an-ti-**sep**-tik)
appendectomy (ap-en-**dek**-tuh-mē)
appendicitis (uh-pen-di-**sī**-tis)
approximate (uh-**prok**-si-māt)
aspiration (as-pi-**rā**-shun)
auscultation (aws-kul-**tā**-shun)
autoimmunity (aw-tō-i-**mūn**-i-tē)
autopsy (**aw**-top-sē)
axillary thermometer (**ak**-si-lar-ē thur-**mom**-uh-tur)
bacilli (buh-**sil**-ī)
bacteremia (bak-tur-**ē**-mē-uh)
bacteria (bac-**tēr**-ē-uh)
bactericidal (bak-tēr-i-**sī**-dul)
bacteriostatic (bak-tēr-ē-ō-**stat**-ik)
benign tumor (buh-**nīn tōō**-mur)
biohazard (**bī**-ō-haz-urd)
biology (bī-**ol**-uh-jē)
biopsy (**bī**-op-sē)
bioterrorism (bī-ō-**ter**-ur-izm)
blepharal (**blef**-uh-rul)
blepharedema (blef-uh-ri-**dē**-muh)
blepharoplasty (**blef**-uh-rō-plas-tē)
blepharospasm (**blef**-uh-rō-spaz-um)
botulism (**boch**-uh-liz-um)
calcipenia (kal-si-**pē**-nē-uh)
calculi (**kal**-kū-lī)
cancer (**kan**-sur)
cancerous (**kan**-sur-us)
cannula (**kan**-ū-luh)

carcinogen (kahr-**sin**-uh-jen)
carcinogenesis (kahr-si-nō-**jen**-uh-sis)
carcinoma (kahr-si-**nō**-muh)
cardiomegaly (kahr-dē-ō-**meg**-uh-lē)
catheter (**kath**-uh-tur)
catheterization (kath-uh-tur-i-**zā**-shun)
catheterize (**kath**-uh-ter-īz)
cephalic (suh-**fal**-ik)
cephalometer (sef-uh-**lom**-uh-tur)
cephalometry (sef-uh-**lom**-uh-trē)
cerebral (suh-**rē**-brul, **ser**-uh-brul)
cerebrotomy (ser-uh-**brot**-uh-mē)
chemotherapy (kē-mō-**ther**-uh-pē)
chiroplasty (**kī**-rō-plas-tē)
chronic (**kron**-ik)
cocci (**kok**-sī)
colectomy (kō-**lek**-tuh-mē)
colonoscope (kō-**lon**-ō-skōp)
colonoscopy (kō-lun-**os**-kuh-pē)
colopexy (**kō**-lō-pek-sē)
colorrhaphy (kō-**lor**-uh-fē)
coloscope (**kol**-ō-skōp)
coloscopy (kō-**los**-kō-pē)
communicable disease (kuh-**mū**-ni-kuh-bul di-**zēz**)
computed axial tomography (kom-**pū**-tid **ak**-sē-ul tō-**mog**-ruh-fē)
computed tomography (kom-**pū**-tid tō-**mog**-ruh-fē)
congenital (kun-**jen**-i-tul)
contagious (kun-**tā**-jus)
cryotherapy (krī-ō-**ther**-uh-pē)
cyanosis (sī-uh-**nō**-sis)
cytology (sī-**tol**-uh-jē)
cytotoxic (sī-tō-**tok**-sik)
dermatitis (dur-muh-**tī**-tis)
diagnosis (dī-ug-**nō**-sis)
dilatation (dil-uh-**tā**-shun)
disease (di-**zēz**)
disorder (dis-**or**-dur)
dystrophic (dis-**trō**-fik)
dystrophy (**dis**-truh-fē)
echography (uh-**kog**-ruh-fē)
edema (uh-**dē**-muh)
electrocardiogram (ē-lek-trō-**kahr**-dē-ō-gram)
electrocardiograph (ē-lek-trō-**kahr**-dē-ō-graf)
electrocardiography (ē-lek-trō-kahr-dē-**og**-ruh-fē)
elephantiasis (el-uh-fun-**tī**-uh-sis)
emesis (**em**-uh-sis)
encephalocele (en-**sef**-uh-lō-sēl)
encephalotome (en-**sef**-uh-luh-tōm)
encephalotomy (en-sef-uh-**lot**-uh-mē)
endoscope (**en**-dō-skōp)
endoscopy (en-**dos**-kuh-pē)

enzyme (**en**-zīm)
epilepsy (**ep**-i-lep-sē)
erythrocyte (uh-**rith**-rō-sīt)
excision (ek-**sizh**-un)
fluoroscope (**floor**-ō-skōp)
fluoroscopy (floo-**ros**-kuh-pē)
fungi (**fun**-jī)
hematology (hē-muh-**tol**-uh-jē)
hemolysin (hē-**mol**-uh-sin)
hemolysis (hē-**mol**-uh-sis)
hemolytic (hē-mō-**lit**-ik)
hemolyze (**hē**-mō-līz)
hernia (**hur**-nē-uh)
herniation (hur-nē-**ā**-shun)
histologist (his-**tol**-uh-jist)
histology (his-**tol**-uh-jē)
hysteria (his-**ter**-ē-uh)
iatrogenic disorder (ī-at-rō-**jen**-ik dis-**or**-dur)
idiopathic disease (id-ē-ō-**path**-ik di-**zēz**)
incision (in-**sizh**-un)
infection (in-**fek**-shun)
ingest (in-**jest**)
inspection (in-**spek**-shun)
jaundice (**jawn**-dis)
kleptomania (klep-tō-**mā**-nē-uh)
lactase (**lak**-tās)
lactose (**lak**-tōs)
laparoscope (**lap**-uh-rō-skōp)
laparoscopy (lap-uh-**ros**-kuh-pē)
magnetic resonance imaging (mag-**net**-ik **rez**-ō-nuns
    im-uh-jing)
malacia (muh-**lā**-shuh)
malaria (muh-**lar**-ē-uh)
malignant (muh-**lig**-nunt)
malignant tumor (muh-**lig**-nunt **too**-mur)
mammary (**mam**-uh-rē)
mammoplasty (**mam**-ō-plas-tē)
mania (**mā**-nē-uh)
mastectomy (mas-**tek**-tuh-mē)
mastitis (mas-**tī**-tis)
melanin (**mel**-uh-nin)
microbiology (mī-krō-bī-**ol**-uh-jē)
microorganisms (mī-krō-**or**-gan-iz-umz)
microscope (**mī**-krō-skōp)
microscopy (mī-**kros**-kuh-pē)
minerals (**min**-ur-ulz)
muscular (**mus**-kū-lur)
myalgia (mī-**al**-juh)
narcotic (nahr-**kot**-ik)
nasal (**nā**-zul)
neoplasm (**nē**-ō-plaz-um)
neural (**noor**-ul)
neurectomy (noo-**rek**-tuh-mē)
neuritis (noo-**rī**-tis)
neurologic disorders (noor-uh-**loj**-ik dis-**or**-durz)
neurolysis (noo-**rol**-i-sis)
neuromuscular (noor-ō-**mus**-kū-lur)

neurosis (noo-**rō**-sis)
neurotripsy (noor-ō-**trip**-sē)
nosocomial infections (nos-ō-**kō**-mē-ul in-**fek**-shunz)
ophthalmalgia (of-thul-**mal**-juh)
ophthalmitis (of-thul-**mī**-tis)
ophthalmodynia (of-thal-mō-**din**-ē-uh)
ophthalmomalacia (of-thal-mō-muh-**lā**-shuh)
ophthalmopathy (of-thul-**mop**-uh-thē)
ophthalmoplasty (of-**thal**-mō-plas-tē)
ophthalmorrhagia (of-thal-mō-**rā**-juh)
ophthalmoscope (of-**thal**-mō-skōp)
ophthalmoscopy (of-thul-**mos**-kuh-pē)
ophthalmotomy (of-thul-**mot**-uh-mē)
oral (**or**-ul)
oral thermometer (**or**-ul thur-**mom**-uh-tur)
osteitis (os-tē-**ī**-tis)
osteoid (**os**-tē-oid)
osteotome (**os**-tē-ō-tōm)
osteotomy (os-tē-**ot**-uh-mē)
otalgia (ō-**tal**-juh)
otitis (ō-**tī**-tis)
otodynia (ō-tō-**din**-ē-uh)
otopathy (ō-**top**-uh-thē)
otoplasty (**ō**-tō-plas-tē)
otorrhea (ō-tō-**rē**-uh)
otoscope (**ō**-tō-skōp)
otoscopy (ō-**tos**-kuh-pē)
palpation (pal-**pā**-shun)
pathogen (**path**-ō-jun)
pathogenic (path-ō-**jen**-ik)
pathogenicity (path-ō-juh-**nis**-i-tē)
percussion (pur-**kuh**-shun)
peritoneum (per-i-tō-**nē**-um)
phagocyte (**fā**-gō-sīt)
pharmaceutical (fahr-muh-**soo**-ti-kul)
pharmacotherapy (fahr-muh-kō-**ther**-uh-pē)
phobia (**fō**-bē-uh)
positron emission tomography (**poz**-i-tron ē-**mish**-un
    tō-**mog**-ruh-fē)
postmortem (pōst-**mor**-tum)
prognosis (prog-**nō**-sis)
protozoa (prō-tō-**zō**-uh)
ptosis (**tō**-sis)
pulse (puls)
pyromania (pī-rō-**mā**-nē-uh)
pyromaniac (pī-rō-**mā**-nē-ak)
radiation oncologist (rā-dē-**ā**-shun ong-**kol**-uh-jist)
radiation oncology (rā-dē-**ā**-shun ong-**kol**-uh-jē)
radioactive (rā-dē-ō-**ak**-tiv)
radiograph (**rā**-dē-ō-graf)
radiographic (rā-dē-ō-**graf**-ik)
radiolucent (rā-dē-ō-**loo**-sunt)
radiopaque (rā-dē-ō-**pāk**)
radiopharmaceuticals (rā-dē-ō-fahr-muh-**soo**-ti-kulz)
radiotherapy (rā-dē-ō-**ther**-uh-pē)
rectal thermometer (**rek**-tul thur-**mom**-uh-tur)
respiration rate (res-pi-**rā**-shun rāt)

rhinoplasty (**rī**-nō-plas-tē)
sclera (**sklēr**-uh)
sclerosis (skluh-**rō**-sis)
septicemia (sep-ti-**sē**-mē-uh)
signs (sīnz)
sonography (suh-**nog**-ruh-fē)
spasm (**spaz**-um)
spirilla (spī-**ril**-uh)
spirochetes (**spī**-rō-kēts)
staphylococci (staf-uh-lō-**kok**-sī)
stasis (**stā**-sis)
stethoscope (**steth**-ō-skōp)
stoma (**stō**-muh)
streptococcal pharyngitis (strep-tō-**kok**-ul far-in-**jī**-tis)
streptococci (strep-tō-**kok**-sī)
suture (**soo**-chur)
symptoms (**simp**-tumz)
therapeutic (ther-uh-**pū**-tik)
thermotherapy (thur-mō-**ther**-uh-pē)
tomogram (**tō**-mō-gram)
tonsillitis (ton-si-**lī**-tis)

toxic dose (**tok**-sik dōs)
toxicologist (tok-si-**kol**-uh-jist)
toxicology (tok-si-**kol**-uh-jē)
toxin (**tok**-sin)
trachea (**trā**-kē-uh)
tracheal (**trā**-kē-ul)
tracheostomy (trā-kē-**os**-tuh-mē)
tracheotomy (trā-kē-**ot**-uh-mē)
trauma (**traw**-muh)
trichomoniasis (trik-ō-mō-**nī**-uh-sis)
trocar (**trō**-kahr)
tympanic thermometer (tim-**pan**-ik thur-**mom**-uh-tur)
ultrasonography (ul-truh-suh-**nog**-ruh-fē)
ultrasound (**ul**-truh-sound)
viremia (vī-**rē**-mē-uh)
virulence (**vir**-ū-luns)
virus (**vī**-rus)
vitamins (**vī**-tuh-minz)
xanthoderma (zan-thō-**der**-muh)

Español   ENHANCING SPANISH COMMUNICATION

English	Spanish (Pronunciation)
acute	agudo (ah-GOO-do)
anesthesia	anestesia (ah-nes-TAY-se-ah)
appendix	apéndice (ah-PEN-de-say)
bacilli	bacilos (bah-SE-los)
benign	benign (bay-NEEG-no)
biopsy	biopsia (be-OP-see-ah)
blood	sangre (SAHN-gray)
bone	hueso (oo-AY-so)
brain	cerebro (say-RAY-bro)
breast	seno (SAY-no)
calculus	cálculo (KAHL-coo-lo)
cells	célula (SAY-LU-AH)
chronic	crónico (KRO-ne-ko)
cold	frio (FRE-o)
congenital	congénito (kon-HE-ne-to)
contagious	contagioso (kon-tay-HEYO-so)
destruction	destrucción (des-strook-se-ON)
dilatation	dilatación (de-lah-tah-se-ON)
edema	hidropesía (e-dro-pay-SEE-ah)
electricity	electricidad (ay-lec-tre-se-DAHD)
endoscopy	endoscopía (an-do-sko-PEE-ah)
enlargement	aumento (ah-oo-MEN-to)
enzyme	enzima (en-SEE-mah)
eyelid	párpado (PAR-pah-do)
fear	miedo (me-AY-do)
fever	fiebre (fe-AY-bray)
fire	fuego (foo-AY-go)
fungus	hongo (ONG-go)
genetic	genetic (he-NE-te-kah)
gland	glándula (GLAN-doo-lah)

English	Spanish (Pronunciation)
hand	mano (MAH-no)
head	cabeza (kah-BAY-sah)
heat	calor (kah-LOR)
hemorrhage	hemorragia (ay-mor-RAH-he-ah)
hernia	hernia (AYR-ne-ah), quebradura (kay-brah-DOO-rah)
infection	infección (en-fek-SYON)
infectious	infeccioso (en-fek-SYO-so)
inflammation	inflamación (in-flah-mah-se-ON)
influenza	gripe (GREE-pay)
instrument	instrumento (ins-troo-MEN-to)
kidney	riñon (ree-NYOHN)
malignant	maligno (mah-LEEG-no)
membrane	membrana (mem-BRAH-nah)
microscope	microscopio (me-kros-KO-pe-o)
movement	movimiento (mo-ve-me-EN-to)
muscle	músculo (MOOS-koo-lo)
narcotic	narcótico (nar-KO-te-ko)
nutrition	nutrición (noo-tre-se-ON)
pain	dolor (do-LOR)
paralysis	parálisis (pah-RAH-le-sis)
parasite	parásito (pah-RAH-se-to)
physical examination	examen físico (ek-SAH-men FEE-se-co)
procedure	procedimiento (pro-se-de-MYEN-to)
prolapse	prolapso (pro-LAHP-so)
pulse	pulso (POOL-so)
puncture	perferación (per-fo-ra-SYON)
repair (to)	reparar (ray-puh-rahr)
rupture	ruptura (roop-TOO-rah)

English	Spanish (Pronunciation)	English	Spanish (Pronunciation)
seizure	ataque (ah-TAH-kay)	trauma	daño (DAH-nyo), herida (ay-REE-dah)
signs	signos (SAYG-nos)		
sound	sonido (so-NE-do)	treatment	tratamiento (trah-tah-MYEN-to)
spasm	espasmo (es-PAHS-mo)	twisted	torcido (tor-SE-do)
speech	habla (AH-blah), lenguaje (len-goo-AH-hay)	ultrasonic	ultrasonic (ul-trah-SO-ne-ko)
		ultrasound	ultrasonido (ul-trah-so-NEE-do)
stone	cálculo (KAHL-koo-lo)	vessel	vaso (VAH-so)
sugar	azúcar (ah-SOO-kar)	vomiting	vómito (VO-me-to)
suture	sutura (soo-TOO-rah)	wound	lesión (lay-se-ON)
swelling	hinchar (in-CHAR)		
symptom	síntoma (SEEN-to-mah)	**Colors**	**Los Colores**
temperature	temperatura (tem-pay-rah-TOO-rah)	black	negro (NAY-gro)
tests	pruebas (proo-AY-bahs)	blue	azul (ah-SOOL)
tissue	tejido (TAY-he-do)	green	verde (VERR-day)
tonsil	tonsila (ton-SEE-lah), amígdala (ah-MEEG-dah-lah)	red	rojo (RO-ho)
		white	blanco (BLAHN-ko)
trachea	tráquea (TRAH-kay-ah)	yellow	amarillo (ah-mah-REEL-lyo)

Organization of the Body

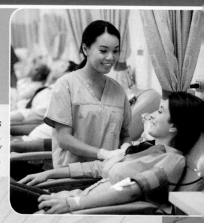

A blood bank is responsible for collecting, processing, and storing blood. Donation of whole blood is the most common type of blood donation, but other types include red cells, platelets, and plasma. Blood components are obtained by apheresis, also called pheresis, a process whereby blood is temporarily withdrawn, one or more components are selectively removed, and the rest is reinfused into the donor.

CONTENTS

LEARNING OUTCOMES

Basic Understanding

In this chapter you will learn to do the following:

1. Recognize the relationship of cells, tissues, and organs.
2. Name four main types of tissue.
3. Match or write the meanings of prefixes, and use them to build and analyze terms.
4. Write or match combining forms for position and direction with their meanings.
5. Label the directional terms and planes of the body.
6. Write or match combining forms for body regions and body cavities.
7. Identify the clinical and anatomic divisions of the abdomen.
8. Write or match terms that relate to the body as a whole with their meanings.
9. Recognize general facts about body fluids and analyze associated terms.
10. Recognize types of body fluids and some kinds of metabolic imbalances.
11. Write the meanings of word parts pertaining to body fluids and immunity, and use them to build and analyze terms.
12. Name the functions of the formed elements of the blood, and recognize the meaning of several signs and symptoms of anemia.
13. Write or match the name of blood pathologies with their descriptions.
14. Write terms that describe coagulation or match the terms with their descriptions.
15. List several body defense mechanisms, define active versus passive immunity, and natural versus artificial immunity.

Greater Comprehension

16. Write the meanings of the abbreviations.
17. Spell medical terms accurately.
18. Pronounce medical terms correctly.
19. Categorize terms as anatomy, diagnostic test or procedure, pathology, surgery or nonsurgical therapy.
20. Recognize the meanings of general pharmacological terms from this chapter as well as the drug classes and their uses.

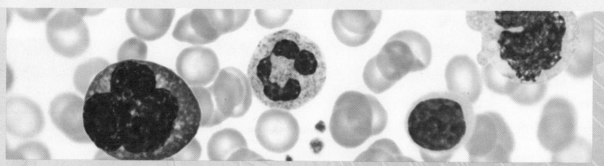

FUNCTION FIRST

Order and organization are outstanding features of the human body. All its parts, from tiny atoms to visible structures, work together as a functioning whole. Before learning to navigate around the body (inside, outside, regions, specific organs), it is extremely helpful to have a good foundation in prefixes and their meanings. For this reason, several pages are dedicated to prefixes early in the chapter. Some will be familiar through commonly-used words (allowing you to speed through them), while others will be new.

Body fluids normally constitute more than half of an adult's weight. Although these fluids are vital in transporting oxygen and nutrients throughout the body, they are also involved in eliminating wastes and transporting other essentials, including immune substances, enzymes, and hormones. Immunity is the body's ability to resist foreign organisms and toxins. The immune system protects the body initially by creating local barriers (for example, the skin) to foreign substances, but an important part of our immunity depends on substances in body fluids, especially cells and antibodies in the blood.

STRUCTURAL ORGANIZATION

3-1 The human body consists of trillions of cells.

🔑 **KEY** POINT **The cell is the fundamental unit of all living matter.** The typical cell in humans consists of a nucleus and cytoplasm, surrounded by a cell membrane. Chromosomes, the determinants of inherited characteristics, are in the nucleus (Fig. 3.1).

WRITE IT! EXERCISE 1	*Name the three major parts of a cell.*
	1. _____ **2.** _____ **3.** _____
	(Use Appendix IV to check your answers.)

DNA

There are numerous types of body cells (blood cells, bone cells, liver cells, and many others), but they all share certain characteristics, such as metabolism, building up of substances, and breaking down of substances for the body's use. Chromosomes, threadlike structures within the nucleus of a cell, contain deoxyribonucleic acid (DNA), which functions in the transmission of genetic information. Write the abbreviation for the material in cells that contains genetic information: _____.

3-2 Human body cells, except for the egg and sperm, contain 23 pairs of chromosomes. An egg and a sperm each have 23 unpaired chromosomes until the sperm cell penetrates the egg to form the embryo, which then has 46 chromosomes, 23 pairs (Fig. 3.2). That single cell replicates into two cells, then four, eight, and so on, until maturity. During development, cells become specialized. Cells that have the ability to divide without limit and give rise to specialized cells are called **stem cells.** They are abundant in a fetus and in cord blood of a newborn. Stem cells are used in bone marrow transplants and can be used in research for organ or tissue regeneration. These undifferentiated cells that can give rise to other types of cells are called _____ cells.

stem

3-3 In humans, each somatic cell has 23 pairs of chromosomes. The combining forms somat(o) and som(a) mean body. **Somatic cells** are all the cells of the body except the sex cells, sperm and ova (singular: ovum). Somat/ic means pertaining to the _____.

body

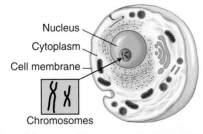

Figure 3.1 Basic cell structure, diagrammatic representation. Chromosomes are threadlike structures in the nucleus of a cell that function in the transmission of genetic information. Each chromosome consists of a double strand of deoxyribonucleic acid (DNA).

Nucleus
Cytoplasm
Cell membrane
Chromosomes

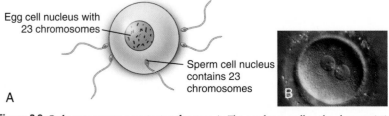

Egg cell nucleus with 23 chromosomes

Sperm cell nucleus contains 23 chromosomes

A

B

Figure 3.2 Only one sperm penetrates the egg. A, The gender as well as the characteristics of the individual are determined by the joining of the male and female nuclei. **B,** Human embryo.

WORD ORIGIN
congenital *(L.)*
congenitus, born together

Down

An abnormality in the chromosomes themselves, or too many chromosomes, usually results in defects. **Down syndrome,** the most common chromosomal abnormality of a generalized syndrome, is a congenital condition characterized by varying degrees of mental retardation and multiple defects (see Fig. 8.48). The incidence can be associated with advanced age of the mother. Congenital means existing at, and usually before, birth. One example of a congenital defect, usually caused by an extra chromosome 21, is _____ syndrome.

🔑 **KEY** POINT **Each chromosome has a double strand of DNA.** Genes, the biologic units of inheritance, are arranged in a linear pattern along the length of each strand of DNA. A **genetic disorder** (also called an *inherited disorder*) is a disease or condition that is determined by one's genes or a change in the number or structure of the chromosomes. Some genetic disorders are listed in Table 3.1.

Table 3.1 Selected Genetic Disorders		
albinism (2)*	gout (9)	muscular dystrophy (9)
cystic fibrosis (5)	hemophilia (3)	rheumatoid arthritis (9)
diabetes mellitus (6, 12)	Huntington disease (10)	sickle cell anemia (3)
Down syndrome (3, 8)		

*The number in parentheses indicates the chapter in which the disorder is explained.

3-4 The body's organizational structure has several levels. These are illustrated in Fig. 3.3. From simplest to complex, the levels are as follows:
- Atoms or ions (for example, carbon, oxygen, hydrogen, nitrogen, chloride)
- Molecules (for example, proteins, sugars, water)
- Organelles (specialized structures within cells—for example, the nucleus)
- Cells (fundamental units of life)
- Tissues (similar cells acting together to perform a function)
- Organs (tissue types working together to perform one or more functions, such as the lungs)
- Body systems (several organs working together to accomplish a set of functions)
- Total organism (a human capable of carrying on life functions)

atom or ion

The simplest level is the _____ level.

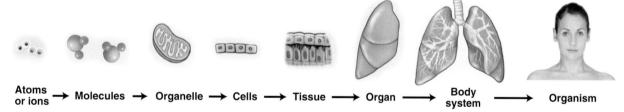

Atoms or ions → Molecules → Organelle → Cells → Tissue → Organ → Body system → Organism

Figure 3.3 Organizational scheme of the body. The formation of the human organism progresses from different levels of complexity. All its parts, from tiny atoms to visible structures, work together to make a functioning whole.

WRITE IT! EXERCISE 2
Four levels of human organization are cells, organelles, organs, and tissues. List these levels in order from simple to more complex levels: _____
_____

3-5 A **tissue** is a group of cells that have similar structure and function as a unit.

🔑 **KEY** POINT **Learn the four types of tissues:**
- Fig. 3.4, A: **epithelial tissue** forms the covering of body surfaces, both inside and on the body surface, e.g., the outer layer of the skin.
- Fig. 3.4, B: **connective tissue** supports and binds other body tissues and parts; examples are bone and fat.
- Fig. 3.4, C: **nervous tissue** coordinates and controls many body activities; it is found in the brain, spinal cord, and nerves.
- Fig. 3.4, D: **muscle tissue** produces movement; an example is skeletal muscle that makes bending of the arm possible.

tissue

A group of cells with similar structure that function as a unit is called a _____.

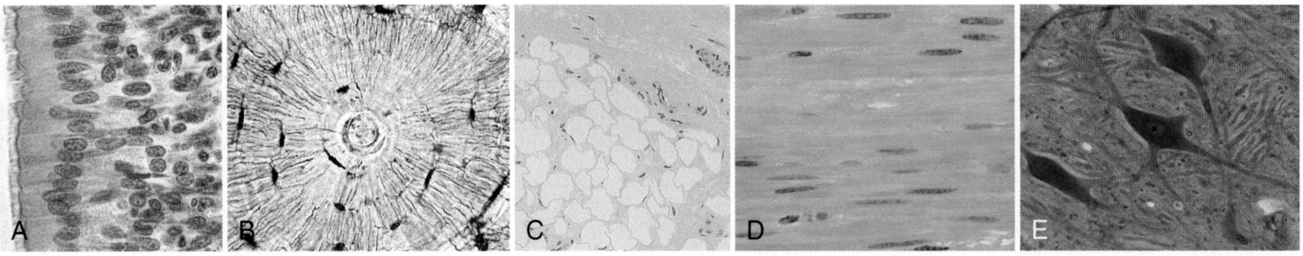

Figure 3.4 Stained Histology Slides Representing the Major Types of Tissue. A, Epithelial cells of the type shown are made of several layers of cells, such as those found on the outer layers of skin. **B and C,** Two types of connective tissue are shown: bone (B) and adipose (fat) tissue (C). Note the center of the compact bone has a canal that carries blood vessels throughout the bone. Adipose tissue is composed of large fat cells. **D,** Muscle tissue showing more than a dozen long, slender central nuclei within narrow cells that lie parallel to each other. **E,** Note the large nerve cells with pale nuclei and numerous cytoplasmic extensions.

3-6 Organs are made up of two or more tissue types that work together to perform one or more functions and form a more complex structure. You are familiar with many organs, such as the liver, the lungs, and the reproductive organs.

A body system consists of several organs that work together to accomplish a set of functions. See Table 3.2 for a listing of the major body systems and their functions. Body systems will be covered in Chapters 4 through 13 of this book. Some systems will be combined in the same chapter; for example, the cardiovascular and lymphatic systems are presented in Chapter 4. You have already learned that cardi(o) means the _____.

heart

Table 3.2   Functions of Major Body Systems

Body System	Major Functions
Cardiovascular system	Delivers oxygen, nutrients, and vital substances throughout the body; transports cellular waste products to the lungs and kidneys for excretion
Lymphatic system	Helps maintain the internal fluid environment; produces some types of blood cells; regulates immunity
Respiratory system	Brings oxygen into the body and removes carbon dioxide and some water waste
Digestive system	Provides the body with water, nutrients, and minerals; removes solid wastes
Urinary system	Filters blood to remove wastes of cellular metabolism; maintains the electrolyte and fluid balance
Reproductive system	Produces offspring
Muscular system	Makes movement possible
Skeletal system	Provides protection, form, and shape for the body; stores minerals and forms some blood cells
Nervous system	Coordinates the reception of stimuli; transmits messages to stimulate movement
Integumentary system	Provides external covering for protection; regulates the body temperature and water content
Endocrine system	Secretes hormones and helps regulate body activities

WRITE IT!   EXERCISE 3

Write a word in each of the blanks to complete these sentences.

1. Every individual begins life as a single _____.

2. Similar cells acting together to perform a function are called _____.

3. Tissue types working together to perform a function are called a/an _____.

4. The type of tissue that supports and binds other body tissues is called _____ tissue.

5. The tissue type that forms the covering of body surfaces is _____ tissue.

6. The type of tissue that produces movement is _____ tissue.

7. The tissue type that coordinates and controls many body activities is _____ tissue.

8. All cells of the body except the sex cells are called _____ cells.

9. Undifferentiated cells that give rise to specialized cells are called _____ cells.

10. The term that means existing at or before birth is _____.

USING PREFIXES TO WRITE TERMS

3-7 You'll need to learn several prefixes to understand body positions and directional terms. Most prefixes can be added to the remainder of the word without change. You will, however encounter some exceptions. Prefixes will be grouped as those pertaining to numbers or quantity, to position or direction, and to negation; you will also learn some miscellaneous prefixes. Study the following prefixes that pertain to numbers or quantity. Many of the prefixes in the list are used in everyday language, so think of words you may know that can help you remember their meanings.

Word Parts: Prefixes for Numbers or Quantity

Prefix	Meaning	Example (Meaning)
Specific Numbers		
mono-, uni-	one	**mononeuropathy** (disease affecting a single nerve); **uniglandular** (affecting only one gland)
bi-, di-	two	**binuclear** (having two nuclei); **dioxide** (an oxygen compound that contains two oxygen atoms)
tri-	three	**triceps** (used in naming a muscle that has three heads)
quad-, quadri-, tetra-	four	**quadruplets** (four offspring born of a single pregnancy); **tetralogy** (a combination of four elements or factors, for example, tetralogy of Fallot, a cardiac condition)
centi-	one hundred or one hundredth (1/100)	**centimeter** (unit of length equal to 1/100 of a meter; cm)
deci-	one tenth (1/10)	A **deciliter** (dL) is one-tenth of a liter
milli-	one thousandth (1/1000)	**milliliter** (unit of volume equal to 1/1000 of a liter; mL). A liter (L) is 1000 mL, which is slightly more than a quart.
Quantities		
ana-	excessive, upward or again	**analeptic** (invigorating or a drug that acts as a central nervous system stimulant, such as coffee)
diplo-	double	**diplopia** (double vision or having two images of a single object; note that one "o" is dropped to avoid double o)
hemi-, semi-	half, partly	**hemicolectomy** (excision of approximately half of the colon); **semicoma** (a stupor from which the patient may be aroused)
hyper-	excessive, more than normal	**hyperactive** (excessively active)
hypo-	beneath or below normal	**hypothyroidism** (below normal thyroid activity)
multi-, poly-	many	**multicellular** (composed of many cells, for example, humans); **polydactyly** (a developmental abnormality characterized by the presence of more than the usual number of fingers or toes, Fig. 3.5, A)
nulli-	none	**nullipara** (a woman who has never born a viable child; para, woman who has borne viable offspring)
pan-	all	**pandemic** (widespread epidemic of a disease, occurring widely throughout a region)
primi-	first	**primigravida** (a woman pregnant for the first time; gravida means a pregnant woman)
super-, ultra-	excessive	**supersensitivity** (excessive sensitivity, as that following damage of a nerve supply to a body part); **ultraviolet** (beyond the violet end of the light spectrum)

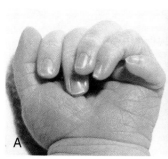 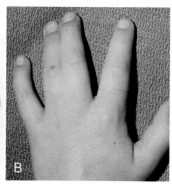

Figure 3.5 Comparison of the fingers in polydactyly and syndactyly. **A,** Polydactyly. Note the presence of six fingers. **B,** Syndactyly. Note the webbing of the third and fourth phalanges.

MATCH IT!

EXERCISE 4

Match the prefixes in the left column with their meaning(s) in the right column. (A choice on the right may be used more than once.)

_____ **1.** bi-   **A.** one
_____ **2.** di-   **B.** two
_____ **3.** centi-   **C.** three
_____ **4.** milli-   **D.** four
_____ **5.** mono-   **E.** one hundredth or 1/100
_____ **6.** quad-   **F.** 1/1000
_____ **7.** tri-
_____ **8.** uni-

one

3-8 A **mono/cyte** is a special type of white blood cell that has _____ nucleus.

3-9 A **bi/focal** lens in glasses or contact lenses has one part of the lens for near vision and the other part for distant vision.

two

3-10 Carbon di/oxide (CO_2) contains _____ atoms of oxygen.

> **BEYOND** THE BLUEPRINT Different prefixes change the meaning of a word. For example, some prefixes identify the type of cycle, and they are named according to the number of wheels (unicycle, bicycle, and tricycle). That's a memory jogger!

four

3-11 Carbon tetra/chloride (CCl_4) has _____ chloride atoms.

3-12 When trying to remember the meaning of **centi/grade,** it is helpful to remember that centigrade is a temperature scale in which 0° is the freezing point and 100° is the boiling point of water at sea level (Fig. 3.6). Centigrade is the same as **Celsius,** named after the Swedish scientist, Anders Celsius. Write the prefix used to write the term *centigrade,* which means 100:

centi-

_____

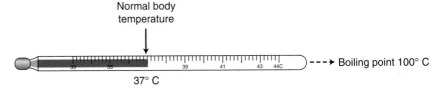

Figure 3.6 Degrees centigrade. Centigrade, or degrees Celsius, is so named because 0° is the freezing point and 100° is the boiling point of water at sea level using this temperature scale. The normal adult body temperature, as measured orally, is 37° centigrade.

Normal body temperature

37° C

Boiling point 100° C

milligram

3-13 If a millimeter is one thousandth of a meter, write a term that means one thousandth of a gram: _____ .

3-14 Ultrasonic is descriptive of sound frequencies so high that they cannot be perceived by the human ear. In ultra/sonography, images of deep structures of the body are obtained by measuring and recording the reflection of high-frequency sound waves.

Ultra/violet describes light beyond the visible spectrum at its violet end. These rays have powerful properties, including sunburn and tanning of the skin, as well as uses in medicine in the diagnosis and treatment of disease.

In both ultrasonic and ultraviolet, you need to remember that ultra- means

excessive

_____ .

10% glucose   20% glucose   15% glucose   15% glucose

Semipermeable
membrane
(permeable to
H_2O and glucose)

Insoluble fat
molecule

Glucose

Water

Diffusion ──────────────► Equilibrium
          Time

Glucose

Water

Figure 3.7 Semipermeable membrane. Some particles in a fluid move from an area of higher concentration to an area of lower concentration, but other particles cannot move across the membrane because of size, charge, or solubility.

semipermeable

3-15 Semi- sometimes means partial, as in semi/dry, or moderately dry. Add a prefix to permeable to write a term that means partially but not wholly permeable: _____.

A semipermeable membrane is one that allows the passage of some substances but prevents the passage of others based on differences in the size, charge, or solubility (Fig. 3.7).

nulli-

3-16 Null is a word that means having no value, nothing, or equal to zero. Write the prefix that means none: _____.

three

3-17 Bi/ceps refers to a muscle having two heads. The biceps brachii is the long muscle of the upper arm, arising in two heads from the shoulder blade. The triceps brachii is a large muscle of the upper arm that has _____ heads that converge in a long tendon. These two muscles are commonly called the *biceps* and *triceps*. Compare them in Fig. 3.8. Biceps and triceps reflex testing check normal deep tendon reflexes (Fig. 3.8, B and C).

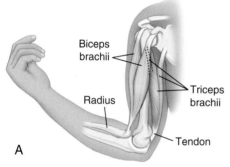
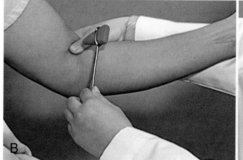
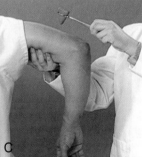

Biceps
brachii

Radius

Triceps
brachii

Tendon

A   B   C

Figure 3.8 The biceps and triceps muscles of the upper arm. A, Drawing of the biceps and triceps brachii of the upper arm. The third head of the triceps brachii is shown as a *dotted line,* because it is visible only from the back. **B,** Biceps reflex testing. Contraction of a biceps muscle produced when the tendon is tapped with a percussor, a percussion instrument, tests deep tendon response. Tendons attach muscles to bones. **C,** Triceps reflex testing. A deep tendon reflex elicited by tapping the triceps tendon near the elbow. Deep tendon responses vary from none, to sluggish, to normal, to slightly hyperactive, to hyperactive.

FIND IT! EXERCISE 5

Draw a slash between the word parts in the following terms. Then, find the meanings of the word parts within the definition. Draw the slash, and then perform the remainder of the activity as a mental exercise. Think!

1. **bipedal** having two feet or pertaining to both feet
2. **monovision** vision resulting from correction of one eye for near vision and the other eye for far vision, especially with contact lens
3. **triplegia** paralysis of three limbs (example, both legs and one arm)
4. **supervitaminosis** a condition resulting from excessive ingestion (swallowing or taking by mouth) of vitamins

3-18 Several important prefixes pertain to position or direction. Study the following list. Again, think of familiar words to help you remember their meanings, and practice with flash cards.

Word Parts: Prefixes for Position or Direction

Prefix	Meaning	Example (Meaning)
ab-	away from	**abduct** (to move away from the axis of the body, Fig. 3.9, A); to carry away by force
ad-	toward	**adduct** (to move toward the middle axis of the body, see Fig. 3.9, B) Memory aid: Tape adheres to a surface.
ante-, pre-, pro-	before in time or in place	**antemortem** (before death); **prenatal** (before birth, or occurring before or existing at birth); **provitamin** (precursor of a vitamin)
circum-, peri-	around or circular	**circumduction** (circular movement of a limb, see Fig. 3.9, C); **pericolitis** (inflammation of the connective tissue around the colon)
dia-	through	**diarrhea** (frequent passage of loose, watery stools)
ecto-, ex-, exo-, extra-	out, without, away from	**ectopic** (situated in an unusual place; sometimes occurring at the wrong time)
en-, end-, endo-	inside	**endoscopy** (visualization of the interior of organs and cavities; see Fig. 2.33)
epi-	above, on	**epidermis** (the outermost layer of the skin, see Fig. 13.1)
hypo-, infra-, sub-	beneath, under	**hypoalgesia** (reduced sensitivity to pain) **infrasonic** (below the range of sound waves normally perceived by the human ear)
inter-	between	**interrenal** (situated between the kidneys)
intra-	within	**intramuscular** (situated in the muscle)
ipsi-	same	**ipsilateral** (pertaining to or affecting the same side of the body)
meso-, mid-, medio-	middle	**mesoderm** (the middle layer of the early layers in development of an embryo); **midsection** (a cut through the middle of an organ or part)
para-	near, beside, or abnormal	**paramedic** (a person who acts as an assistant to a physician or acts in place of a physician until the physician is available); **paranormal** (beyond normal or natural; example, extrasensory perception)
per-	through or by	**perspire** (to excrete through the pores of the skin)
post-	after, behind	**postnatal** (occurring after birth); **postnasal** (occurring behind the nose)
retro-	behind, backward	**retrocolic** (behind the large intestine)
super-, supra-	above, beyond	**superficial** (situated on or near the surface); **suprarenal** (above the kidney)
sym-, syn-	joined, together	**symmetry** (correspondence of parts on opposite sides of a dividing line; **syndrome** (a set of symptoms that occur together and collectively characterize a particular disease or condition); **syndactyly** (fusion or joining of the fingers or toes; see Fig. 3.5, B)
trans-	across	**transdermal** (entering through or passing across the skin)

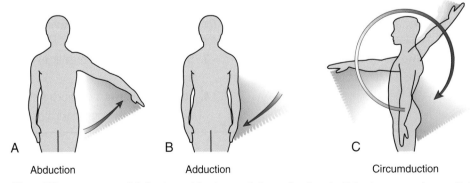

A Abduction   B Adduction   C Circumduction

Figure 3.9 **Comparison of abduction, adduction, and circumduction. A,** Abduction moves a bone or limb away from the midline of the body. **B,** Adduction moves a bone or limb toward the midline of the body. **C,** Circumduction is circular movement of a limb.

MATCH IT!
EXERCISE 6

Match the prefixes with their meanings.

_____ **1.** ab-   **A.** away from

_____ **2.** dia-   **B.** between

_____ **3.** epi-   **C.** near, beside, or abnormal

_____ **4.** infra-   **D.** same

_____ **5.** inter-   **E.** through

_____ **6.** intra-   **F.** under

_____ **7.** ipsi-   **G.** upon

_____ **8.** para-   **H.** within

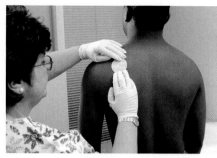

Figure 3.10 Transdermal drug delivery. Application of a nitroglycerin patch.

before

3-19 The prefixes ante-, pre-, and pro- mean before in time. **Pre/cancerous** is a term that is used to describe an abnormal growth that is likely to become cancerous. Preadmission certification is a system whereby physicians are required to obtain advance approval for nonemergency admission for many patients. With pre/admission, the approval is obtained _____ the person is admitted to the hospital.

adduct

3-20 Ab/duct means to carry away by force or draw away from a given position. Write the term that is opposite of abduct: _____. In **chemical addiction,** a person has a compulsive need for a certain drug or, in other words, is drawn toward a habit-forming drug.

across

3-21 A **trans/dermal** drug is one that can be absorbed through unbroken skin. An example is the patch to prevent motion sickness. The literal translation of trans/dermal is _____ the skin (Fig. 3.10).

circular

3-22 A **circumcision** generally means a surgical procedure in which the foreskin of the penis is excised. Remember that circum- means circular or around. In a circum/cision, a _____ incision is performed to remove the foreskin of the penis.

outside

3-23 An **ectopic pregnancy** is an abnormal pregnancy in which the embryo implants _____ the uterus. Ecto/top/ic comes from ecto- (outside) + top(o), place, + -ic, pertaining to. (One "o" is omitted to facilitate pronunciation.) Types of ectopic pregnancy are implantations within the abdomen, an ovary, or a fallopian tube.

> **BEYOND** THE BLUEPRINT Ectopic pregnancy was first described more than 1000 years ago. Before surgery was performed for ectopic pregnancy, the mortality rate was extremely high due to rupture of a fallopian tube (uterine tube), which is the most common site of abnormal implantation. With earlier detection, many women with ectopic pregnancy are successfully treated before it becomes life-threatening.

between

3-24 Extra-, intra-, and inter- are added to the same root to change the meanings of terms to outside, within, and _____, respectively.

KEY POINT **Know the difference in these terms: intracellular vs. intercellular vs. extracellular. Intracellular** means within the cell, and **extracellular** means situated outside a cell or the cells of the body. **Intercellular** means located between cells. For example, the space between cells is called the *intercellular space.*

post-

3-25 The prefix that means after in time is _____.
   Post/anesthetic describes the time after anesthetic is administered, and **post/infectious** describes the time after an infection.

together

3-26 Both sym- and syn- mean joined or _____. A **syn/drome** is a set of symptoms that occur together and collectively characterize a particular disease or condition.

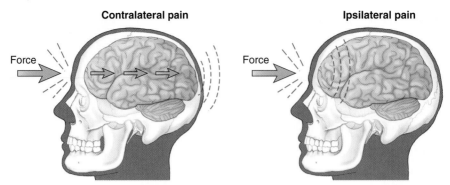

Figure 3.11 **Contralateral and ipsilateral are opposites.** If an injury to the forehead causes pain in the back of the skull, that is contralateral pain; however, if the same injury caused pain in the front of the skull, that is ipsilateral pain.

same

3-27 Only a few terms contain ipsi-. Ipsi/lateral means pertaining to or affecting the _____ side of the body. The opposite of this term, **contra/lateral** means affecting the opposite side. Compare the two terms (Fig. 3.11). The prefix contra- means against, but here it is used to mean opposite or opposed to a particular side of the body.

above

3-28 Superficial means on or near the surface, because super means _____ or beyond. See how superficial sensation is tested (Fig. 3.12).

under

3-29 You have learned that intra- means within. The prefixes hypo-, infra-, and sub- mean beneath or _____. **Hypo/dermic** means beneath the skin. A hypodermic needle is used to inject a drug or medication under the skin or into blood vessels or is used for withdrawing a fluid, such as blood. Study four important types of injections in Fig. 3.13:
- **sub/cutaneous**
- **intra/muscular**
- **intra/dermal** (The dermis is the layer of skin that contains the blood vessels.)
- **intra/venous,** IV

under

The literal translation of subcutaneous is _____ the skin.
In a subcutaneous injection, the needle is placed into the subcutaneous tissue beneath the skin.

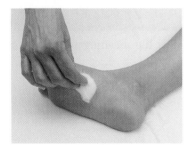

Figure 3.12 **Testing for superficial tactile sensation.** Superficial sensation is the perception of feelings in the superficial layers of the skin, responding in this case to slight touch of a cotton ball.

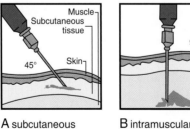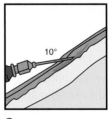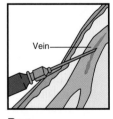

A subcutaneous   B intramuscular   C intradermal   D intravenous

Figure 3.13 **Using prefixes in naming types of injections.** Note how the prefixes sub- and intra- are added to terms and used to describe the correct position of a needle: **A,** A subcutaneous injection places a small amount (0.5 mL to 2 mL) of medication below the skin layer into the subcutaneous tissue. The needle is inserted at a 45° angle. **B,** An intramuscular injection deposits medication into a muscular layer. As much as 3 mL to 5 mL may be administered in one injection, and depending on the size of the patient, a needle 1 to 3 inches in length is used. **C,** An intradermal injection places very small amounts into the outer layers of the skin with a short, fine-gauge needle. This type of injection is often used to test allergic reactions. **D,** An intravenous injection is used to administer medications directly into the bloodstream for immediate effect. A few milliliters of medication, or much larger amounts given over a long period, may be administered after venipuncture of the selected vein has been performed.

WRITE IT! EXERCISE 7

Write answers in the blank lines to complete the sentences. (Although an answer may require more than one word, it is represented by a single line.)

1. The prefix ab- means _____, but ad- means _____.
2. Postnasal pertains to the region _____ the nose.
3. Two prefixes that have opposite meanings are endo- and ecto-. An abbreviated meaning of ecto- is outside, and endo- means _____.
4. Intercellular means _____ cells.
5. Suprarenal glands are located _____ each kidney.
6. Both peri- and circum- mean _____.
7. The opposite of prenatal is _____.
8. If intracellular means within the cell, _____ is outside the cell.
9. Ipsilateral means affecting the _____ side of the body.
10. The literal meaning of transdermal is _____ the skin.

symptoms

3-30 When a prefix of negation is placed before a term, it forms a new word with the opposite meaning. For example, **symptomatic** means having symptoms, and **asymptomatic** means without (not having) _____.

Word Parts: Prefixes: Negation

Prefix	Meaning
a-, an-	no, not, without
in-	not or inside (in)

3-31 Hydrous means containing water. **Anhydrous** means absence of water.

🔑 **KEY POINT Learn these rules for using a- or an- to write words that mean the opposite.**
- Use a- before a consonant.
- Use an- before a vowel or the letter h.
(If unsure, use a medical dictionary.)

atraumatic

3-32 You know that trauma means a wound or injury, whether physical or emotional. **Traumatic** means pertaining to or occurring as the result of trauma (injury).
   Write a word that means not inflicting or causing damage or injury: _____.

in-

3-33 Another prefix that means not, as in the term inconsistent, is _____.
   Sometimes in- means inside, as in the terms include and **inhale,** which means to breathe in.

WRITE IT! EXERCISE 8

Use either a- or an- to write words that have the opposite meanings of these terms.

1. The opposite of esthesia is _____.
2. The opposite of hydrous is _____.
3. The opposite of plastic is _____.
4. The opposite of traumatic is _____.
5. The opposite of symptomatic is _____.

WRITE IT! EXERCISE 9

Use in- to write words that have the opposite meaning.

1. The opposite of compatible is _____.
2. The opposite of digestion is _____.
3. The opposite of attentive is _____.
4. The opposite of capable is _____.
5. The opposite of operable is _____.

3-34 There are additional prefixes that you need to know. Their meanings should be easy to remember, because many of them are used in everyday language. Note that some prefixes have more than one meaning and may pertain to two classifications, such as position and time. An example is post-, which means *after* to describe time or *behind* to describe position. Study the list of miscellaneous prefixes, using word association to help you remember their meanings.

Word Parts: Miscellaneous Prefixes

Prefix	Meaning	Prefix	Meaning
Related to Size		**Related to Description**	
macro-, mega-, megalo-	large or great	anti-, contra-	against
micro-	small	brady-	slow
		dys-	bad, difficult
		eu-	good, normal
		mal-	bad
		pro-	favoring, supporting
		tachy-	fast

MATCH IT! **EXERCISE 10**

Match the prefixes in the left column with their meaning(s) in the right column. The choices on the right may be used more than once.

_____ **1.** anti-   **A.** against
_____ **2.** brady-   **B.** bad
_____ **3.** contra-   **C.** fast
_____ **4.** dys-   **D.** good or normal
_____ **5.** eu-   **E.** large
_____ **6.** mal-   **F.** slow
_____ **7.** micro-   **G.** small
_____ **8.** macro-
_____ **9.** megalo-
_____ **10.** tachy-

microscopic

3-35 When referring to size, **macro/scopic** structures are large enough to be seen by the naked eye. If the structures are so small that they can be seen only with a microscope, they are called _____ structures.

small

3-36 Micr/ot/ia is an unusually small size of the external ear (one "o" is omitted to facilitate pronunciation). The literal translation of microtia is _____ ear (Fig. 3.14).

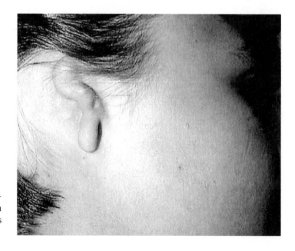

Figure 3.14 Microtia. This example shows the unusual shape that resulted from underdevelopment of the external ear. Perhaps you can see an inked pattern behind the ear, which indicates the size of the ear after otoplasty, reconstructive surgery of the ear, is performed.

destruction

3-37 Analysis means the separation of substances into their component parts or elements. It is also an informal term for **psychoanalysis.** The literal translation of ana/lysis is: ana- (again) + -lysis, _____ or destroying something.

> **BEYOND** THE BLUEPRINT Psychoanalysis is a theory of human phenomena and behavior developed by Freud. It focuses on the influence that unconscious forces, such as repressed impulses, internal conflicts, and childhood trauma have on the mental state, to furnish hints for psychotherapeutic procedures.

against

3-38 Both anti- and contra- mean _____, as in the terms **anti/perspirant** and **contra/ceptive.** An antiperspirant inhibits or prevents perspiration (sweating). A contraceptive prevents conception or diminishes the likelihood of conception.

The prefix that means the opposite of against is pro-, which means favoring or supporting (in other words, for). "Weighing the pros and cons" is commonly understood.

fast

slow

3-39 The prefixes brady- and tachy- have opposite meanings, slow and _____, respectively. You learned that -phasia means speech. **Brady/phasia** means an abnormally _____ manner of speech, often associated with mental illness. The opposite of bradyphasia is **tachy/phasia,** rapid speech, as may be present in the manic phase of bipolar disorder. Compare bradycardia, abnormal slowness of the heart, with an increased heart rate, tachycardia (Fig. 3.15). These terms correspond to a decreased pulse, and increased pulse, respectively.

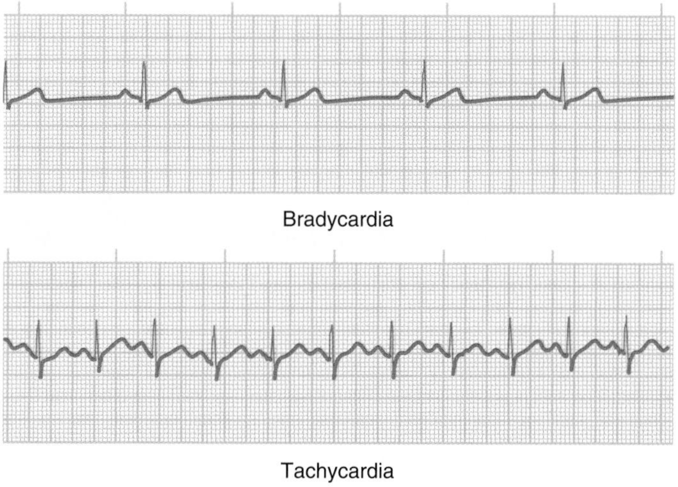

Bradycardia

Tachycardia

Figure 3.15 Bradycardia and tachycardia are opposites. A graphic record of the heartbeats (an electrocardiogram) shows many abnormalities including abnormal slowness (bradycardia). Each record represents slightly more than 6 seconds of heart activity.

bad

3-40 Both dys- and mal- mean _____, but dys- can also mean difficult, as in the term **dys/lexia,** which means difficulty in reading, often reversing letters or having difficulty distinguishing letter sequences. **Malaise** is a vague feeling of bodily discomfort and fatigue.

3-41 Fatigue is a state of exhaustion or a loss of strength or endurance. A second definition of fatigue is loss of the ability to respond to stimuli that normally evoke muscular contraction or other activity. **Lethargy,** more severe than fatigue, is a state of dullness, sluggishness, or prolonged sleepiness or drowsiness. A person suffering _____ is said to be

lethargy

lethargic.

normal

3-42 The prefix eu- means good or _____. **Eu/phoria** is a feeling or state of well-being, and **dys/phoria** is characterized by depression and anguish.

BUILD IT!

EXERCISE 11

Use the following prefixes to complete these sentences.

brady-, contra-, dys-, eu-, macro-, mal-, micro-, post-, pre-, tachy-

1. An abnormally fast manner of speech is _____phasia.
2. A vague feeling of bodily discomfort and fatigue is _____aise.
3. An abnormal growth that is likely to become cancerous is described as _____cancerous.
4. Objects that are large enough to be seen by the naked eye are described as _____scopic structures.
5. A feeling of well-being is _____phoria.
6. The description of the time after anesthetic is administered is _____anesthetic.
7. An unusually small size of the external ear is _____otia.
8. Difficulty in reading is _____lexia.
9. The term for a device or technique that prevents conception is _____ceptive.
10. Abnormally slow speech is _____phasia.

FIND IT!

EXERCISE 12

Draw a slash between the word parts in the following terms. Then, find the meanings of the word parts within the definition. Draw the slash, and then perform the remainder of the activity as a mental exercise.

1. **malnutrition** any disorder of nutrition
2. **macrocyte** an abnormally large cell (usually a large erythrocyte)
3. **megadose** a dose that greatly exceeds the amount prescribed or recommended
4. **megalocyte** an extremely large erythrocyte
5. **microcyte** an abnormally small erythrocyte

ANATOMIC POSITION AND DIRECTIONAL TERMS

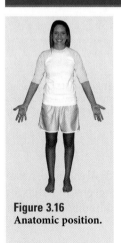

**Figure 3.16
Anatomic position.**

lower

3-43 Anatomy is the study, description, and classification of structures and organs of the body.

> 🔑 **KEY** POINT **Anatomists use directional terms and planes to describe the position and direction of the body.** Locations and positions are always described relative to the body in the **anatomic position**—that is, the position that a person has while standing erect with the face directed to the front, with the arms at the sides and the palms turned forward, as shown in Fig. 3.16.

3-44 Anatomic planes, imaginary flat surfaces, are used to aid in visualizing spatial relationships of internal body parts (Fig. 3.17). Locations and positions are described relative to the body in the anatomic position. Study Fig. 3.17 as you read the following sentences:

The **frontal plane** divides the body into front and back portions. This plane is also called the *coronal plane.*

A **sagittal plane** divides the body into right and left sides. If the right and left sides are equal, the plane is a **midsagittal plane.**

The **transverse plane** divides the body into upper and _____ portions.

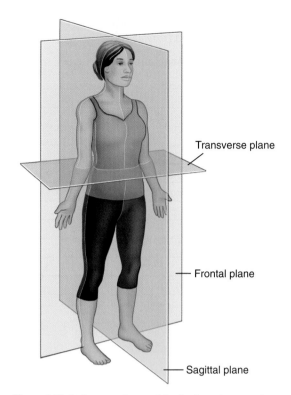

Figure 3.17 Reference planes of the body. Color is used to distinguish the frontal (coronal), transverse, and midsagittal planes. The midsagittal plane is a special sagittal plane that is located in the center to create two equal portions.

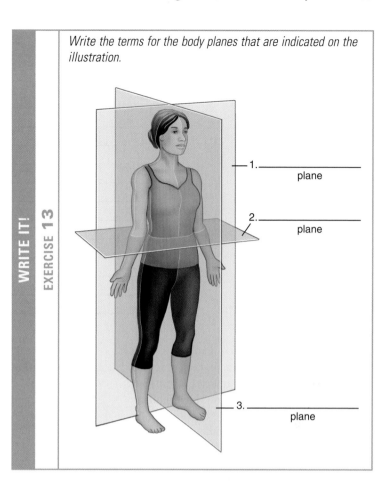

WRITE IT!

EXERCISE 13

Write the terms for the body planes that are indicated on the illustration.

1. _____ plane

2. _____ plane

3. _____ plane

Study the following combining forms used in directional terms. Associate the combining forms with words you already know. For example, it may be easier to remember that tel(e) means far or distant if you think of a telephone, which allows you to talk with someone distant from you.

Word Parts: Combining Forms for Directional Terms

Combining Form	Term	Meaning
anter(o)	**anterior**	nearer to or toward the front
poster(o)	**posterior**	nearer to or toward the back
ventr(o)	**ventral**	belly side
dors(o)	**dorsal**	directed toward or situated on the back side
medi(o)	**medial, median**	middle or nearer the middle
later(o)	**lateral**	farther from the midline of the body or from a structure
super(o)	**superior**	uppermost or above
infer(o)	**inferior**	lowermost or below
proxim(o)	**proximal**	nearer the origin or point of attachment
dist(o), tel(e)	**distal**	far or distant from the origin or point of attachment
caud(o)	**caudad** or **caudal**	in an inferior position; tail or toward the tail
cephal(o)	**cephalad**	toward the head

Complete the table by writing the meaning of each word part that is listed. Also write the corresponding anatomic term for 1 through 12. (Numbers 2 and 8 have two anatomic terms each.) Number 1 is done as an example.

Combining Form	Meaning	Anatomic Term
1. anter(o)	*front*	*anterior*
2. caud(o)		
3. cephal(o)		
4. dist(o)		
5. dors(o)		
6. infer(o)		
7. later(o)		
8. medi(o)		
9. poster(o)		
10. proxim(o)		
11. super(o)		
12. ventr(o)		

3-45 Six important aspects are shown in Fig. 3.18 and are used to describe locations:

- anterior (front)
- posterior (behind)
- lateral (side)
- medial (middle)
- superior (uppermost)
- inferior (lowermost)

side

The lateral aspect is the view of the _____ of the structure or of an organ or part.

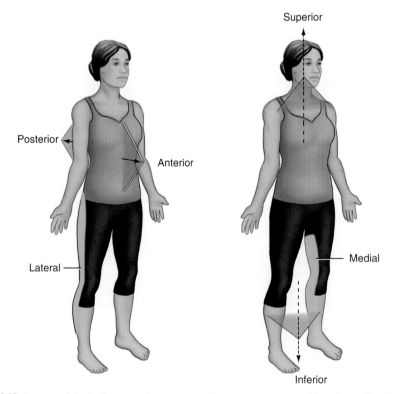

Figure 3.18 Aspects of the body. Locate the six aspects: **A,** anterior, posterior, and lateral, as well as **B,** superior, inferior, and medial.

Write the terms for the aspects that are indicated on the illustration.

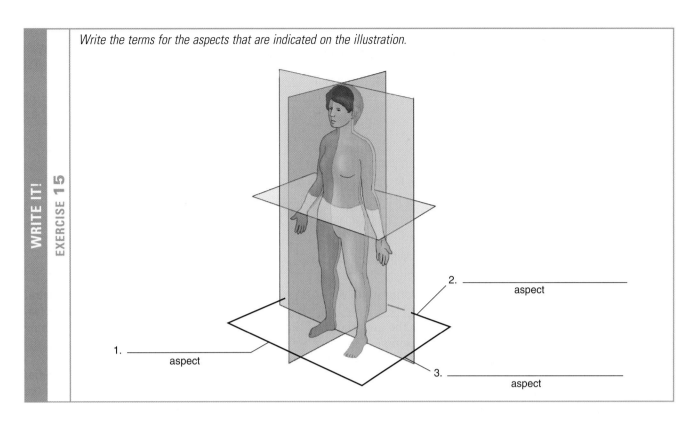

1. _____
   aspect

2. _____
   aspect

3. _____
   aspect

ventral

3-46 In humans, the **anterior** or front side is the same as the belly side or _____ surface. In dogs, however, the ventral surface is not the front side.

3-47 The opposite of anterior is posterior. Posterior means directed toward or situated at the back. Another term for this is **dorsal.**

front
back
front

3-48 In radiology, directional terms are used to specify the direction of the x-ray beam from its source to its exit surface before striking the image receptor. **Lateral** means side, and "left lateral" and "right lateral" are used to describe patient positioning. In an anteroposterior projection, the x-ray beam strikes the anterior aspect of the body first. In other words, the beam passes from _____ to back. **Postero/anterior,** abbreviated PA, means from the posterior to the anterior surface, or, in other words, from _____ to front.
    Antero/posterior (AP) pertains to both the _____ and the back sides, or from the front to the back of the body.
    Positions for some common radiographic projections of the chest are shown in Fig. 3.19.

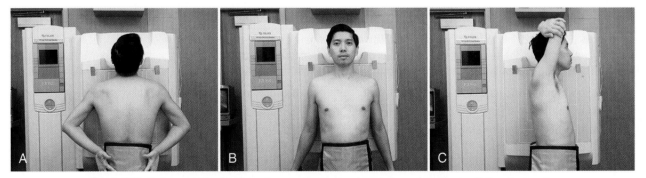

Figure 3.19 Patient positioning for a chest x-ray examination. A, In a posteroanterior (PA) projection, the anterior aspect of the chest is closest to the image receptor. **B,** In an anteroposterior (AP) projection, the posterior aspect of the chest is closest to the image receptor. **C,** In a left lateral chest projection, the left side of the patient is placed against the image receptor.

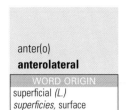

anter(o)
anterolateral
WORD ORIGIN
superficial *(L.)*
superficies, surface

3-49 Unilateral means involving only one side. **Bilateral** pertains to both sides of the body. Write the combining form for anterior: _____. Write a new word using lateral that means situated in front and to one side: _____.

   Superficial means situated on or near the surface, and sometimes means not grave or dangerous.

WRITE IT!   **EXERCISE 16**

Case Study. *Write a term from the report to complete each sentence.*

Emily's physician ordered chest x-rays. In the first image, she was positioned with her chest nearest the image receptor. In the second image, she was standing with her left side against the image receptor. Choose from the following directional terms to describe the projections: anteroposterior, posteroanterior, left lateral, right lateral

1. Which term is correct for the first position? _____

2. Which term is correct for the second position? _____

---

belly (front)

side

3-50 Both **dorsal** and **posterior** mean directed toward or situated on the back side. **Dorso/ventral** pertains to the back and _____ surfaces. (Note the order in which the two word parts are presented. The importance of the order becomes obvious when one is describing the path of a bullet, for example. Dorsoventral sometimes means passing from the back to the belly surface.) **Dorso/cephalad** means situated toward the back of the head.

   Medial and **median** mean pertaining to the middle or midline of a body or structure. **Medio/lateral** means from the middle to one _____. This term also denotes the direction of a line, as in the path of a bullet or an x-ray beam.

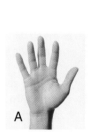
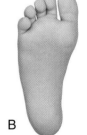

Figure 3.20 Palmar vs. plantar. A, Palmar pertains to the inside surface of the hands. **B,** Plantar pertains to the sole of the foot.

palm
WORD ORIGIN
palm *(L.)*
palma, palm.
plantar *(L.)*
planta, sole.

3-51 In the anatomic position, the palms are forward. The palm is the hollow of the hand. **Palm/ar** pertains to the _____.

   Plantar pertains to the sole, or bottom of the foot. Compare palmar and plantar (Fig. 3.20).

FIND IT!   **EXERCISE 17**

Draw a slash between the word parts in the following list of new terms. Then find the meanings of the combining forms within the definitions. (Draw the slash, and then perform the remainder of the activity as a mental exercise.) Think!

1. anteromedial located in front and to the middle

2. anterosuperior situated in front of and higher

3. cephalic pertaining to the head

4. dorsolateral, posterolateral located behind and to one side

5. inferomedian situated in the middle of the underside

6. posteroexternal located on the outer side of a posterior part

7. posteromedial situated in the middle of the back

8. posterosuperior situated behind and above

9. posterointernal located within and toward the posterior surface

10. ventromedian both ventral and medial

WORD ORIGIN
prone *(L.)*
pronus, inclined forward.
supine *(L.)*
supinus, lying on the back, face upward.

up

side

3-52 Most locations and directions pertaining to the whole organism are described relative to the body in the anatomic position. Physicians rely on additional positions for examination or surgery. **Prone** and **supine** are terms used to describe the position of persons who are lying face downward or lying on the back, respectively (Fig. 3.21, A and B).

Pronation and **supination** are generally used to indicate positioning of the hands and feet, but their complete meanings include the act of lying prone or face downward and assumption of a supine position. Pronation of the arm is the rotation of the forearm so that the palm faces downward.

Supination is the rotation of a joint that allows the hand or foot to turn upward. Supination of the wrist allows the palm to turn _____. Compare pronation and supination of the wrist in Fig. 3.21, C.

Recumbent means lying down. The lateral recumbent position (see Fig. 3.21, D) is assumed by the patient lying on the side, because lateral means pertaining to the _____.

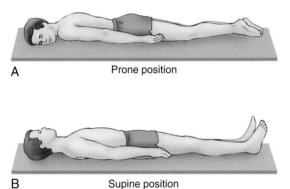

A   Prone position

B   Supine position

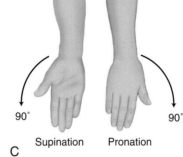

90°   90°

C   Supination   Pronation

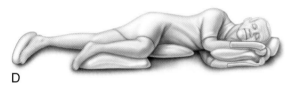

D

Lateral (recumbent) position

Figure 3.21 Comparison of pronation and supination. A, Prone, lying face down. **B,** Supine, lying on the back. **C,** Supination and pronation, turning of the hand upward (supination) or downward (pronation), respectively. **D,** The lateral recumbent position (sometimes called the *Sims position*) is sometimes used in surgery. The patient is lying on the left side with the right knee and thigh flexed (bent) and the upper limb parallel along the back.

WRITE IT!   **EXERCISE 18**

Label the body positions with one of these two terms: prone or supine.

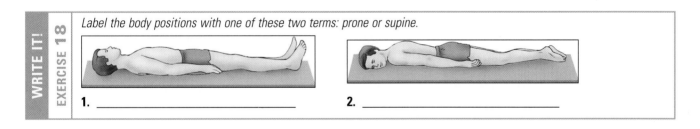

1. _____   2. _____

BODY REGIONS AND BODY CAVITIES

trunk

3-53 The body is made up of two major regions:
- head, neck, and trunk (chest, abdomen, and pelvis)
- extremities (arms and legs)

The chest, abdomen, and pelvis make up the body's _____. The trunk has two major cavities that contain internal organs.

Learn the following combining forms that are used to describe the body.

Word Parts: Selected Combining Forms for the Body

Combining Form	Meaning	Combining Form	Meaning
abdomin(o)	abdomen	omphal(o), umbilic(o)	umbilicus (navel)
acr(o)	extremities (arms and legs)	pelv(i)	pelvis
axill(o)	armpit	periton(o)	peritoneum
cephal(o)	head	pod(o)	foot
crani(o)	cranium (skull)	som(a), somat(o)	body
dactyl(o)	finger or toe	spin(o)	spine
encephal(o)	brain	thorac(o), steth(o)	thorax (chest)
herni(o)	hernia	viscer(o)	viscera (large abdominal organs)

MATCH IT!
EXERCISE 19

Match the parts of the body with their combining forms.

_____	**1.** armpit	**A.**	acr(o)
_____	**2.** arms and legs	**B.**	axill(o)
_____	**3.** chest	**C.**	cephal(o)
_____	**4.** finger or toe	**D.**	crani(o)
_____	**5.** foot	**E.**	dactyl(o)
_____	**6.** head	**F.**	omphal(o)
_____	**7.** skull	**G.**	pod(o)
_____	**8.** umbilicus	**H.**	thorac(o)

chest

3-54 The **thorax** is the chest. **Thoracotomy** refers to any incision of the chest wall. The thorac/ic region is the area of the chest. **Thoracic** means pertaining to the _____.

abdominothoracic

3-55 The **abdomen** is that part of the body lying between the thorax and the pelvis. Write a word that means pertaining to the abdomen and thorax by combining abdomin(o) + thorac(o) + -ic: _____.

3-56 Because of its large area and numerous internal organs, the abdomen is frequently subdivided using imaginary lines to indicate points of reference. There are two methods of using imaginary lines to divide the abdomen into regions. Dividing the abdomen into four quadrants is a convenient way to designate areas in the abdominal cavity (Fig. 3.22). Refer to the diagram to answer the following:

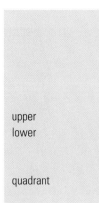
upper
lower

quadrant

Quadrant is a term that means any one of four corresponding parts. RUQ and LUQ refer to the right and left _____ quadrants, respectively. RLQ and LLQ refer to the right and left _____ quadrants.

Abdominal quadrants are used to describe the location of pain or of body structures. The system of naming four abdominal areas that are determined by drawing two imaginary lines through the umbilicus is the four-_____ system. Principal organs contained in the four abdominal quadrants are shown in Table 3.3.

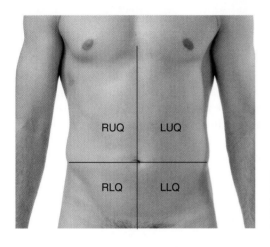

Figure 3.22 One of two systems of using imaginary lines to divide the abdomen into regions. Quadrants of the abdomen: four divisions of the abdomen determined by drawing a vertical line and a horizontal line through the umbilicus. *RUQ, LUQ, RLQ,* and *LLQ* are abbreviations for right upper quadrant, left upper quadrant, right lower quadrant, and left lower quadrant, respectively.

Table 3.3 Abdominal Quadrants and Their Contents	
Right upper quadrant (RUQ): *Contains the right lobe of the liver, gallbladder, right kidney, and parts of the large and small intestines*	Left upper quadrant (LUQ): *Contains the left lobe of the liver, stomach, pancreas, left kidney, spleen, and parts of the large and small intestines*
Right lower quadrant (RLQ): *Contains the right ureter, right ovary and uterine tube, appendix, and parts of the large and small intestines*	Left lower quadrant (LLQ): *Contains the left ureter, left ovary and uterine tube, and parts of the large and small intestines*

WRITE IT!   EXERCISE 20

Label the abdominal quadrants that are indicated on the diagram with these abbreviations; LLQ, LUQ, RLQ, RUQ.

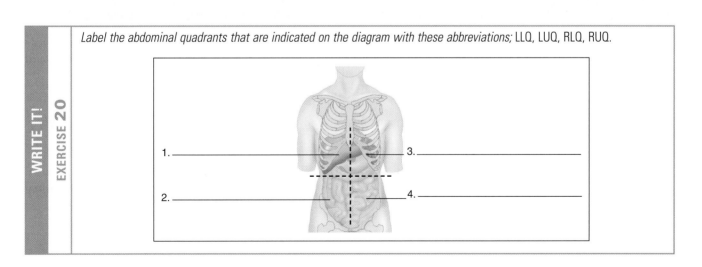

1. _____   3. _____

2. _____   4. _____

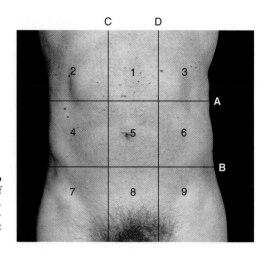

Figure 3.23 Second of two systems using imaginary lines to divide the abdomen into regions. The nine anatomic regions of the abdomen, determined by four imaginary lines *A*, *B*, *C*, and *D*. The regions are *1*, epigastric; *2*, right hypochondriac; *3*, left hypochondriac; *4*, right lumbar; *5*, umbilical; *6*, left lumbar; *7*, right inguinal (or iliac); *8*, hypogastric; *9*, left inguinal (or iliac).

3-57 Anatomists describe the abdomen as having nine regions, shown in Fig. 3.23. The nine-region system is also used in clinical and surgical settings. Some of the terms may be unfamiliar, but try to remember the divisions. It may be helpful to label the nine regions in Fig. 3.23. When the terms are studied in more detail in later chapters, they will acquire more meaning. Look at Fig. 3.23 while working this frame.

hypochondriac

The upper lateral regions beneath the ribs are the right and left _____ **regions.**

epigastric

Between the hypochondriac regions lies the _____ **region**. The stomach is in this region.

umbilical

The _____ region lies just below the epigastric region. The **umbilical region** is that of the navel, or umbilicus.

lumbar

The right and left _____ **regions** lie on each side of the umbilical region.

hypogastric

The lower middle region is called the _____ **region.**

iliac

inguinal

Finally, the two lower lateral regions are the right and left _____ or _____ **regions.**

3-58 The first abdominal region you named in the preceding frame was the hypochondriac region.

abdomen

In discussing abdominal regions, **abdomin/al** means pertaining to the _____.

> **BEYOND** THE BLUEPRINT You have probably also heard the term **hypochondriac** applied to a person who has a false belief of suffering from some disease. Ancient Greeks believed that organs in the hypochondriac region of the abdomen were the cause of melancholy and imaginary diseases, hence the term *hypochondriac*.

3-59 The body has two major cavities, spaces that contain internal organs. The two principal cavities are the dorsal cavity and the ventral cavity. We learned previously that dorsal means situated toward

back (posterior)
front (belly)

the _____ surface of the body.

Ventral means situated toward the _____ surface.

3-60 The dorsal and ventral cavities are subdivided as shown in Fig. 3.24. The **dorsal cavity** is

cranial, spinal

divided into the _____ cavity and the _____ cavity.

Cranial means pertaining to the skull. The **cranial cavity** contains the brain, and the spinal cavity contains the spinal cord and the beginnings of the spinal nerves. The cranial and spinal

dorsal

cavities are divisions of the body's _____ cavity.

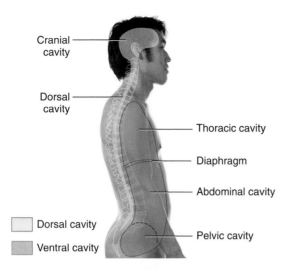

Cranial cavity

Dorsal cavity

Thoracic cavity

Diaphragm

Abdominal cavity

Dorsal cavity

Ventral cavity

Pelvic cavity

Figure 3.24 The body has two principal body cavities, the dorsal and ventral cavities, each further subdivided. The dorsal cavity is divided into the cranial cavity and the spinal cavity. The ventral cavity is divided into the thoracic cavity and the abdominopelvic cavity, which is subdivided into the abdominal cavity and the pelvic cavity.

thorax (chest)

3-61 The **ventral cavity** is the anterior body cavity. It is subdivided into the thoracic, abdominal, and pelvic cavities. You have learned that thoracic means pertaining to the _____.

(The combining form steth[o] is used in the term *stethoscope*, but thorac[o] is used in referring to the thoracic or chest cavity.) The thoracic cavity is surrounded by the ribs. The abdominal and pelvic cavities are not separated by a muscular partition, and together they are often called the **abdomino/pelvic cavity.** The muscular **diaphragm** separates the thoracic cavity from the abdominopelvic cavity.

pelvic

3-62 The **pelvis** is the lower portion of the trunk of the body. You learned that pelv(i) is the combining form for pelvis. The cavity formed by the pelvis is the _____ cavity.

The major body cavities and their principal organs are summarized in Table 3.4.

Table 3.4   Major Body Cavities and Principal Organs
Dorsal Body Cavity (Two Cavities Separated by the Diaphragm) Cranial cavity (contains the brain) Spinal cavity (contains the spine)
Ventral Body Cavity Thoracic cavity (contains the heart and blood vessels, trachea, and esophagus) Abdominopelvic cavity (no physical partition between the abdominal and pelvic cavities) Abdominal cavity (contains the liver, stomach, small intestine, colon, spleen, gallbladder, kidneys) Pelvic cavity (contains the bladder, reproductive organs, part of the large intestine, rectum)

WRITE IT!   **EXERCISE 21**

Label the abdominopelvic, cranial, and thoracic cavities.

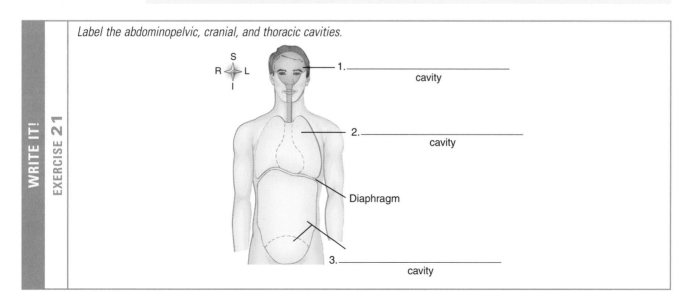

1. _____ cavity

2. _____ cavity

Diaphragm

3. _____ cavity

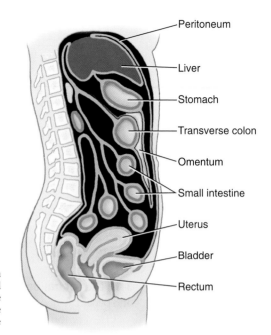
Peritoneum
Liver
Stomach
Transverse colon
Omentum
Small intestine
Uterus
Bladder
Rectum

Figure 3.25 The peritoneum (tan) in a median sagittal section of a female. This extensive membrane lines the entire abdominal wall and is reflected over the viscera. The free surface of the peritoneum is smooth and lubricated by a fluid that permits the viscera to glide easily against the abdominal wall and against one another.

3-63 The abdominopelvic cavity is lined with a membrane called the **peritoneum.** This membrane also covers the internal organs (Fig. 3.25). Write the name of the membrane that lines the abdominopelvic cavity and covers the internal organs: _____.

peritoneum

There are two types of peritoneum:
- The **parietal peritoneum** lines the abdominal and pelvic walls.
- The **visceral peritoneum** contains large folds that weave in between the organs, binding them to one another and to the walls of the cavity.

parietal

The peritoneum that lines the abdominopelvic cavity is _____ peritoneum.
Organs within the ventral body cavity, especially the abdominal organs, are called **viscera.**

visceral

Peritoneum that invests the viscera is called _____ peritoneum.

3-64 Build a word that means pertaining to the peritoneum using the suffix -eal: _____.

peritoneal

Serous membranes, such as the peritoneum, secrete a lubricating fluid that allows the organs to slide against one another or against the cavity wall. The peritoneal cavity is the space between the parietal peritoneum and the visceral peritoneum.

➤ **BEYOND** THE BLUEPRINT The peritoneum extends into the center of the abdominopelvic cavity as the omentum, which supports the stomach and hangs down as a fatty apron to cover and protect the small intestine. The peritoneum is a closed membranous sac in males, but is perforated by the uterine tubes in females.

3-65 Thoraco/dynia is a type of chest pain. (It differs from **angina pectoris,** a heart disease in which the chest pain results from interference with the supply of oxygen to the heart muscle.) A term for pain in the chest is _____. It is likely that a person experiencing chest pains would have an electrocardiogram to determine if there are cardiac abnormalities. A **tele/cardio/gram** is a heart tracing that registers distant from the patient by means of electrical sending of the signal.

thoracodynia

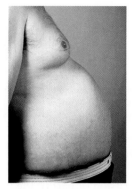

Figure 3.26 **Ascites.** This abnormal accumulation of a fluid in the peritoneal cavity is treated with dietary therapy and drugs. Abdominal paracentesis may be performed to relieve the pressure of the accumulated fluid.

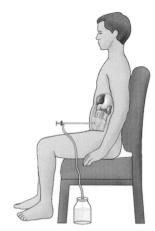

Figure 3.27 **Paracentesis.** This procedure in which fluid is withdrawn from a body cavity is performed to remove excess fluid from the abdomen.

abdomen

paracentesis

abdominoplasty

incisional

femoral

inguinal

3-66 Ascites is abnormal accumulation of serous fluid in the peritoneal cavity, sometimes resulting in considerable **distension** (enlargement, stretching) of the abdomen (Fig. 3.26).

Abdomino/centesis is surgical puncture of the _____.

Abdominal paracentesis is another name for abdominocentesis. This procedure is performed to remove fluids or to inject a therapeutic agent. It is most often done to remove excess fluid, ascites, from the peritoneal cavity (Fig. 3.27). The removal of the excess fluid in the peritoneal cavity is called abdominal _____.

3-67 Write a word using -plasty that means surgical repair of the abdomen: _____.

(This type of plastic surgery, when done for aesthetic reasons to tighten the abdominal muscles, is commonly called a *tummy tuck*.)

3-68 A hernia can occur through any weakness or defect in the peritoneum that lines the abdominal or pelvic cavities. In addition to the umbilicus, frequent sites of such weaknesses are old surgical scars and the inguinal (groin) and **femoral** (thigh) canals (Fig. 3.28). A hernia that occurs through an inadequately healed surgical site is an _____ hernia.

The type of hernia that occurs if a loop of intestine descends through the femoral canal into the groin is a _____ hernia.

A direct or indirect hernia that occurs in the groin is an _____ hernia.

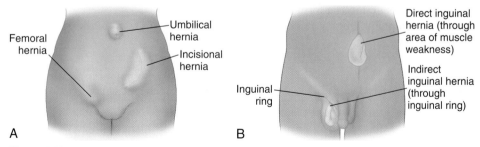

Figure 3.28 **Common types of abdominal hernias. A,** Umbilical hernias result from a weakness in the abdominal wall around the umbilicus. An incisional hernia is herniation through inadequately healed surgery. In a femoral hernia, a loop of intestine descends through the femoral canal into the groin. **B,** Inguinal hernias are of two types. A *direct hernia* occurs through an area of weakness in the abdominal wall. In an *indirect hernia,* a loop of intestine descends through the inguinal canal, an opening in the abdominal wall for passage of the spermatic cord in males and a ligament of the uterus in females.

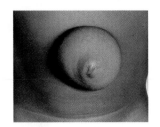

Figure 3.29 Omphalocele. An umbilical hernia is a skin-covered protrusion of intestine through a weakness in the abdominal wall around the umbilicus. The hernia often closes spontaneously within 2 years, but large hernias may require surgical closure.

umbilicus

3-69 Omphalus is another name for the **umbilicus** or navel.
　　An **omphalo/cele** is a congenital hernia of the _____.
　　Babies are sometimes born with an omphalocele, protrusion of part of the intestine through a defect in the abdominal wall at the umbilicus (Fig. 3.29). Write the formal name for an umbilical

omphalocele

hernia: _____.

> **BEYOND** THE BLUEPRINT Inguinal hernias are more common in men; femoral hernias are more common in women, especially older women. Hernias that easily return to the abdominal cavity are called reducible (reduced manually or reduce spontaneously when the person lies down). If the hernia cannot be placed back in the body cavity, it is called an irreducible or incarcerated hernia.

hernia

3-70 Hernio/plasty, surgical repair of a _____, is sometimes used specifically to denote repair using a mesh patch or plug to reinforce the area of the defect.

3-71 The body's **extremities** are the four limbs. Each arm, elbow, forearm, wrist, hand, and associated fingers make up one of the body's upper extremities. Each thigh, knee, leg, ankle, foot, and associated toes make up one of the lower extremities. Fingers and toes are digits. When referring to the bones of the digits, *phalanges* is the proper term. When referring to a digit in its entirety (multiple phalanges plus surrounding soft tissues), *digit, finger,* or *toe* should be used. Many medical terms use combining forms for the body extremities—hands, feet, and phalanges (bones of the fingers

extremities

and toes). In **acro/paralysis,** movement of the _____ is impaired.
　　Acro/cyanosis is an intermittent cyanosis of the extremities, caused by exposure to cold or emotional stimuli. Acrocyanosis is also called **Raynaud phenomenon** or sign (Fig. 3.30). (The literal translation of acrocyanosis is a blue condition of the extremities.)

3-72 The combining form dactyl(o) usually refers to a finger but sometimes to a toe. Fingers and toes are also called **digits.** Whenever you see dactyl(o) or digit, immediately think of a finger or toe. A **dactylo/gram** is a mark or record of a fingerprint. The part of the word that refers to the

dactylography

finger is dactyl(o). The process of taking fingerprints is _____.
　　Dactylo/spasm is a cramping or twitching of a digit. Write the word that means cramping of a

dactylospasm

finger or toe: _____.

chirospasm

3-73 Use chir(o) and -spasm to write a new word: _____.
　　Writer's cramp is a form of **chirospasm.**

hands

　　Chiro/pod/y literally refers to the _____ and feet and was once a term for podiatry.

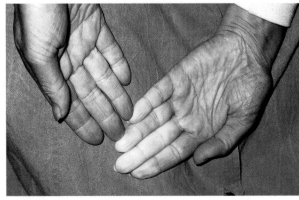

Figure 3.30 Raynaud phenomenon occurs in Raynaud disease. This intermittent lack of circulation of the fingers, toes, and sometimes ears and nose, with severe paleness, often accompanied by pain, is usually brought on by cold or emotional stimuli.

feet

podiatry

A **pod/iatrist** specializes in the care of _____.

The specialized field dealing with the foot, ankle, and lower leg, including their anatomy, pathology, and medical and surgical treatment, is _____.

A **podo/gram** is a print or record of the foot; however, the term *footprint* is more commonly used.

> **BEYOND** THE BLUEPRINT The professional care of feet was in existence even in ancient Egypt. The term "podiatry" came into use first in the early twentieth century United States, where it now denotes a Doctor of Podiatric Medicine (DPM), who diagnoses and treats conditions affecting the foot, ankle, and related structures of the leg. Within the field of podiatry, practitioners can specialize in many areas. The older title of "chiropodist" is gradually falling from use.

FIND IT!   EXERCISE 22

Draw a slash between the word parts in the following list of new terms. Think! Then find the meanings of the word parts within the definitions. (Draw the slash, and then perform the remainder of the activity as a mental exercise.)

1. **dactylitis** inflammation of a finger or toe
2. **chiroplasty** plastic surgery (surgical repair) of the hand
3. **omphalic** pertaining to the umbilicus; umbilical
4. **omphalitis** inflammation of the umbilicus
5. **omphaloma** umbilical tumor
6. **omphalorrhagia** hemorrhage from the umbilicus
7. **omphalorrhexis** rupture of the umbilicus
8. **pelvic** pertaining to the pelvis
9. **transthoracic** performed through the chest wall cavity, or through the thoracic cavity
10. **suprathoracic** superior to the thorax

TERMS RELATED TO THE BODY AS A WHOLE

WORD ORIGIN
pyrexia *(G.)*
pyretos, fever

without

fever

3-74 A disease or a disorder in one structure can affect the functioning of the body as a whole. In Chapter 2, you learned how an infectious disease such as influenza can spread from one person to someone else. Infections occur when the body is invaded by pathogenic microorganisms. Infection is just one of several causes of an abnormal elevation of the body temperature, which is called fever or **pyrexia**.

Febrile pertains to fever. **A/febrile** means _____ fever.

An **anti/pyretic** is an agent that is effective against _____.

Anti/febrile and antipyretic both mean effective against fever. Aspirin is a well-known antipyretic.

hyperpyrexia

3-75 A **pyro/gen** is a substance or agent that produces fever, such as some bacterial toxins. **Hyperpyrexia** denotes a highly elevated body temperature because hyper- means excessive or more than normal. This can be produced by physical agents, such as hot baths or hot air, or by reaction to infection. A body temperature that is much greater than normal is called _____.

An abnormally high temperature is considered to be **hyperpyrexial.**

against

3-76 **Anti/infective** means capable of killing infectious micro/organisms or of preventing them from spreading. An agent that is capable of this action is also called an *antiinfective*. The literal translation of antiinfective is acting _____ infection.

Anti/microb/ial agents act against **microbes,** another name for microorganisms. Antimicrobial means the same as antiinfective.

living

There are many types of antiinfectives. The term anti/bio/tic pertains to the ability to destroy living organisms. Also, **antibiotics** act against _____ microscopic organisms. They are derived from microorganisms, or they are produced semisynthetically and are used to treat infections, largely bacterial infections. Read more about other types of antiinfectives in the Pharmacology section later in this chapter.

against

3-77 The suffix -osis means condition but sometimes implies a disease or abnormal increase. It usually indicates an abnormal noninflammatory condition. **Inflammation** is tissue reaction to injury and is recognized by pain, heat, redness, and swelling. **Antiinflammatory** means acting _____ inflammation.

In other words, it means counteracting or reducing inflammation.

without

3-78 Earlier in this chapter, you studied how tissue is a collection of similar cells acting together to perform a particular function. The suffix -plasia means formation. Several terms that contain -plasia are used to describe abnormal tissue formation. **Dys/plasia** is the abnormal development of tissues or organs. **A/plasia** is the lack of development of an organ or tissue. Translated literally, aplasia means _____ development. **An/otia,** congenital absence of one or both ears, is an example of aplasia.

Hypo/plasia is less severe than aplasia; it is underdevelopment of an organ or tissue and usually results from fewer than the normal number of cells. For example, hypoplastic bone marrow is hypo/cellular, having fewer cells than normal (Fig. 3.31).

hyperplasia

3-79 Write a new term by combining hyper- and -plasia: _____. Literal translation of the word parts yields "increased development," but you will need to remember that **hyper/plasia** means an abnormal increase in the number of normal cells in tissue. Hyperplasia contrasts with another term, **hyper/trophy** (hyper-, increased; -trophy, nutrition), which means an increase in the size of an organ caused by an increase in the size of the cells rather than the number of cells. Fig. 3.32 will help you understand the difference between hyperplasia and hypertrophy. It may be helpful to note that, despite the technical difference between hyperplasia and hypertrophy, these terms are sometimes used interchangeably to indicate increased size of a body part.

Cells of the heart are particularly prone to hypertrophy. In other words, the heart increases in size by enlarging individual cells. An enlargement of the adult heart may be caused by an increased workload. This differs from hyperplasia, in which the number of cells increases. (The new cells may be either benign or malignant, so hyperplasia does not necessarily mean that the new cells are cancerous.)

malignancy

3-80 However, a change in the structure and orientation of cells, characterized by a loss of differentiation and reversal to a more primitive form, is characteristic of malignancy. This change in cell structure is called **ana/plasia.** The prefix ana- means upward, excessive, or again. The important thing to remember about anaplasia is that it is especially characteristic of _____.

Normal somatic cells divide to produce two identical daughter cells in a predictable manner. Cell growth or function is changed in aplasia, anaplasia, dysplasia, hypoplasia, or hyperplasia, but an important difference is that anaplastic cells are characteristic of carcinoma. Study Table 3.5 to understand the difference in these terms.

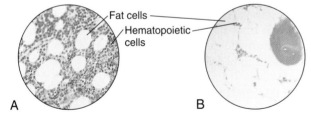

Figure 3.31 Biopsy smears help compare normal versus hypoplastic bone marrow tissue. A, Stained normal bone marrow tissue shows many hematopoietic cells (precursors of blood cells). **B,** Stained hypoplastic bone marrow tissue has few cells, and many of those may be abnormal in appearance.

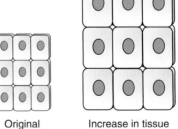 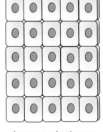

Original tissue   Increase in tissue size by hypertrophy   Increase in tissue size by hyperplasia

Figure 3.32 A representation of tissue enlargement by hypertrophy and hyperplasia.

Table 3.5 Comparison of Abnormal Tissue Formation

Term	Cell Division	Significance	Metastasis
aplasia	Essentially absent	Organ or tissue does not develop	No
hypoplasia	Reduced	Underdevelopment of organ or tissue	No
hyperplasia	Increased	More tissue development; enlargement of organ	No
dysplasia	Continuous or inappropriate	Cellular deviation from the normal, which may progress to anaplasia in certain organs (for example, the uterus)	No
anaplasia	Rapid and abnormal cells	Characteristic of malignancy	Possible

3-81 Wounds are physical injury to body tissue, whether caused by accident (burns, cuts, or bruises, for example) or surgery.

KEY POINT Several factors slow the process of healing:
- infection
- presence of foreign material
- decaying tissue
- movement (lack of immobilization) of the wound
- poor blood circulation
- decreased number of white blood cells
- deficiency of antibodies
- malnutrition in the individual

3-82 Deep wounds or those in an area of movement, such as near a joint, may require sutures or another means of holding the tissue together while healing occurs. Movement retards healing and can lead to **dehiscence,** a splitting open or rupture of a wound after it has closed. It also means the separation of a surgical incision, typically an abdominal incision. Write this term that means a splitting open: _____.

dehiscence

evisceration

Evisceration is the protrusion of internal organs through an open wound. If an internal organ protrudes through a dehiscence, this is called _____. Compare dehiscence and evisceration (Fig. 3.33).

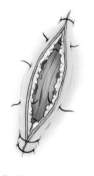
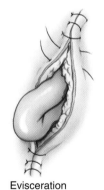

Dehiscence   Evisceration

Figure 3.33 Dehiscence and evisceration. Both are complications of wound healing and involve a splitting open of the wound, but evisceration is the total separation of all wound layers and protrusion of internal organs (for example, part of the intestine) through the open wound.

BUILD IT!

EXERCISE 23

Use these word parts to write terms to complete these sentences. (Some will be used more than once.)

pyr(o), a-, ana-, dys-, hyper-, hypo-, -gen, -plasia

1. An agent that causes fever is a/an _____/_____.
2. Abnormal development of tissue or organs is called _____/_____.
3. Lack of development of an organ or tissue is _____/_____.
4. Underdevelopment of an organ or tissue is _____/_____.
5. Abnormal increase in the number of normal cells in tissue is _____/_____.
6. A change in the structure and orientation of cells that is characteristic of malignancy is _____/_____.

body

somat(o)

3-83 Both som(a) and somat(o) refer to the body in general. **Somato/genic** means originating in the _____.

The part of somatogenic that means body is _____.

The death of a person, **somatic death,** is usually defined as absence of electrical activity of the brain for a specified period under rigidly defined circumstances.

> **BEYOND** THE BLUEPRINT For legal and medical purposes, the following definition of death has been proposed—the irreversible cessation of all of the following:
> • Total cerebral function
> • Spontaneous function of the respiratory system
> • Spontaneous function of the circulatory system

head

3-84 You have already learned that cephal(o) refers to the head and that cephal/ad means toward the _____.

The combining form encephal(o) means the brain and is so called because the brain is located inside the head. **Electro/encephalo/graphy** is the process of recording electrical activity of the brain and can be used to determine somatic death.

brain

inflammation

3-85 An **electro/encephalo/gram** is a record produced by the electrical impulses of the _____. (You see why the abbreviation EEG is commonly used!)

The instrument used to record electrical impulses of the brain is an **electroencephalograph.**
Encephal/itis is _____ of the brain.

There are many types of encephalitis, but a large percentage of cases are caused by viruses. The symptoms include mild to severe convulsions, coma, and even death in some cases.

disease

Encephalo/pathy is any _____ of the brain.

body

3-86 Som/esthetic pertains to the general feeling of one's _____.

The "a" is dropped from som(a) to facilitate pronunciation. A particular part of the brain, the somesthetic area, is responsible for receiving and pinpointing where and what sensations occur in the body. A lesion in this part of the brain could affect one's ability to read, write, or speak and also one's ability to recognize objects by touch. A lesion is a wound or other pathologic change in body tissue.

mind

3-87 Somato/psych/ic pertains to both body and _____.

Somatopsychic disorders are physical disorders that influence mental activity. A brain lesion (physical disorder) often produces significant intellectual difficulties and memory loss (mental activities).

Physiology is the study of the function of the body. **Psycho/physio/logic,** also called **psycho/somatic,** disorders are the opposite of somatopsychic. Extreme or prolonged emotional states that influence the physical body's functioning are psychophysiologic disorders. Emotional factors may precipitate conditions, such as high blood pressure. You learned that physi(o) means nature. In psychophysiologic disorders, the natural functioning of the body is influenced by emotional factors.

mind

3-88 Psychosomatic is also the commonly used term that refers to the interaction of the mind, or psyche, and the body. You have learned that psych(o) means _____.

Psych/ic has two meanings: Psychic means pertaining to the mind, or the term refers to a person with the ability to read the minds of others.

extremities

3-89 Acro/megaly is a disorder in which there is enlargement of the _____.

In acromegaly there is enlargement of many parts of the skeleton, particularly the distal portions, such as the nose, ears, jaws, fingers, and toes (see Fig. 12.16). It is caused by increased secretion of growth hormone by the pituitary gland.

skin

extremities

dermatoplasty

3-90 Literal translation of **dermat/osis** is a _____ condition.
Its true meaning is any disease of the skin in which inflammation is not present. Inflammation of the skin is called **dermatitis. Acro/dermat/itis** is inflammation of the skin of the _____, especially the hands and feet.
Write another word that, translated literally, means surgical repair of the skin: _____. In this surgery, skin grafts are used to cover destroyed or lost skin.

WRITE IT! EXERCISE 24

Write a word in each blank to complete the sentences.
1. The death of a person is called _____ death.
2. Electroencephalography is the process of recording electrical activity of the _____.
3. A term that means pertaining to the body and the mind is psychosomatic or _____.
4. A splitting open of a wound is called _____.
5. The protrusion of internal organs through an open wound is _____.

CELLULAR NEEDS AND BODY FLUIDS

within

water

3-91 Body fluids are classified as one of the following:
• plasma (liquid part of the circulating blood)
• intracellular fluid
• intercellular fluid
Intra/cellular fluid is located _____ cells. In contrast, **inter/cellular fluid** is located between (or among) cells.

3-92 Water is the most important component of body fluids. Body fluids are not distributed evenly throughout the body, and they move back and forth between compartments that are separated by cell membranes. The most important component of body fluids is _____.
Chemical and microscopic studies are performed on various body fluids to determine the body's internal status. Laboratory tests are commonly used to detect, identify, and quantify substances; evaluate organ functions; help establish or confirm a diagnosis; and aid in the management of disease.

3-93 A healthy adult's body weight is approximately 50% to 60% fluid. However, water accounts for much of a newborn's body weight, thus explaining why fluid imbalance in infants can quickly lead to dehydration (Fig. 3.34).

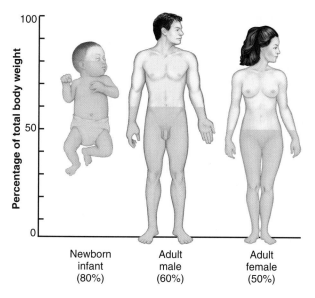

Figure 3.34 **Water content varies with age, gender, and body mass.**

Newborn infant (80%)   Adult male (60%)   Adult female (50%)

Percentage of total body weight

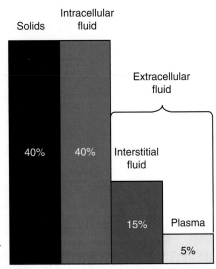

Figure 3.35 The body's fluid compartments. Fluid makes up 60% of the adult's body weight, and most of that is intracellular fluid. Two types of extracellular fluid are interstitial fluid and plasma.

intracellular

Compare the balance of solids vs. fluids in a healthy adult (Fig. 3.35). You see that most of the fluid is _____ fluid, meaning that it is located within the cells. **Cellul/ar** means pertaining to (or consisting of) cells, because cellul(o) means little cell or compartment. You know that *intracellular* and *extracellular* are terms that describe location either within or outside the cell.

extracellular

3-94 Fluid that is not contained within the cells, the _____ **fluid,** is either plasma or interstitial fluid. Only about one fourth of the extracellular fluid is **plasma,** the liquid part of the blood.

> **KEY** POINT The **interstitial fluid** is intercellular and fills the spaces between most of the cells of the body and is transported away from the tissues by the lymphatic system. If anything interferes with that transportation, the fluid accumulates in the interstitial spaces, resulting in a condition called *edema*, which you studied in Chapter 2.

WORD ORIGIN
interstitial *(L.)*
interstitium, space or gap
in a tissue or structure

BUILD IT!
EXERCISE 25

Use these prefixes to build terms to complete these sentences.
extra-, inter-, intra-
1. More than half of all body fluid is contained within cells and is called _____cellular fluid.
2. Fluid outside cells is called _____cellular fluid.
3. The fluid that fills the spaces between most of the body cells is _____stitial fluid.

Fluid Balance

fluid

3-95 The regulation of the amount of water in the body is called *fluid balance.*
Fluid balance depends on proper functioning of several body systems, particularly the urinary system. **Dehydration** (excessive loss of water from body tissue) or generalized edema (swelling caused by excessive accumulation of fluid in the body tissues) can occur if the body cannot maintain fluid balance. This regulation of the amount of water in the body is called _____ balance.

> **KEY** POINT **Fluid balance is maintained through intake and output of water.** Water is obtained by drinking fluids and eating foods. Water leaves the body via urine, feces, sweat, tears, and other fluid discharges. This balance depends on the proper intake of water and the elimination (output) of body wastes, including excess water (Fig. 3.36). Note that most of the fluid gained by the body is through drinking water, and most of the fluid is excreted in the urine.

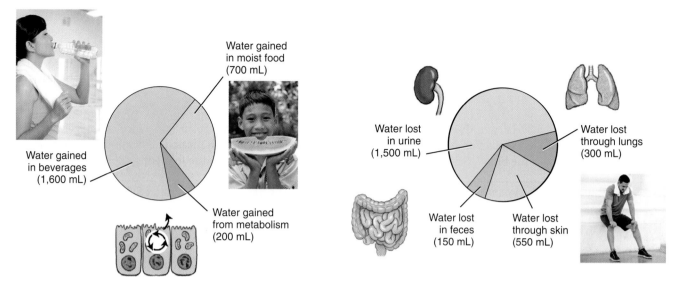

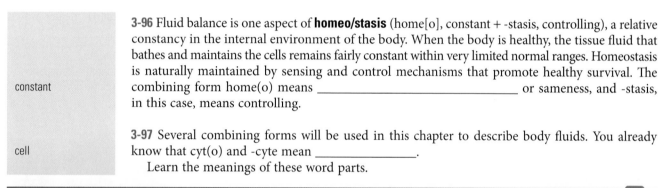

Figure 3.36 Avenues of fluid intake and output. The kidneys are the main regulators of fluid loss. Generally, fluid intake equals fluid output so that the total amount of fluid in the body remains constant. Water is the most important constituent of the body and is essential to every body process. Depriving the body of needed water eventually leads to dehydration.

constant

3-96 Fluid balance is one aspect of **homeo/stasis** (home[o], constant + -stasis, controlling), a relative constancy in the internal environment of the body. When the body is healthy, the tissue fluid that bathes and maintains the cells remains fairly constant within very limited normal ranges. Homeostasis is naturally maintained by sensing and control mechanisms that promote healthy survival. The combining form home(o) means _____ or sameness, and -stasis, in this case, means controlling.

cell

3-97 Several combining forms will be used in this chapter to describe body fluids. You already know that cyt(o) and -cyte mean _____.
Learn the meanings of these word parts.

Word Parts: Body Fluids

Combining Form	Meaning	Combining Form	Meaning
Selected Compartments		**Selected Electrolytes**	
angi(o), vascul(o)	vessel	calc(i)	calcium
cellul(o)	little cell or compartment	kal(i)	potassium
		natr(o)	sodium
Miscellaneous			
home(o)	sameness; constant		
hydr(o)	water		

MATCH IT! **EXERCISE 26**

Match each word part in the left column with its meaning in the right column. (Choices A through G may be used more than once.)

_____ **1.** angi(o)

_____ **2.** calc(i)

_____ **3.** cellul(o)

_____ **4.** home(o)

_____ **5.** hydr(o)

_____ **6.** kal(i)

_____ **7.** natr(o)

_____ **8.** vascul(o)

A. calcium

B. little cell or compartment

C. potassium

D. sameness or constant

E. sodium

F. vessel

G. water

3-98 The nervous system and endocrine system work together to bring about homeostasis by affecting various functions, including the heartbeat, respiration, blood pressure, body temperature, and the concentration of electrolytes in the body fluids. **Electrolytes** are molecules that conduct an electric charge. Some examples of electrolytes in body fluids are calcium, potassium, and sodium. To remember that electrolytes conduct an electric charge, it may be helpful to recall that electr(o) means _____.

electricity

3-99 Certain diseases, conditions, and medications may lead to an imbalance of the electrolytes. Deficiencies or excesses are detected by laboratory tests, which measure the amount of electrolytes in the blood. Selected electrolyte imbalances are presented in the following exercise.

FIND IT!
EXERCISE 27

Draw a slash between the word parts in the following list of new terms. Then find the meanings of the word parts within the definitions. Think! (Draw the slash, and then perform the remainder of the activity as a mental exercise.)

1. **hypercalcemia** greater than normal concentration of calcium in the blood
2. **hyperkalemia** greater than normal concentration of potassium in the blood
3. **hypernatremia** greater than normal concentration of sodium in the blood
4. **hypocalcemia** less than normal concentration of calcium in the blood
5. **hypokalemia** less than normal concentration of potassium in the blood
6. **hyponatremia** less than normal concentration of sodium in the blood

---

water, head

3-100 In chemistry, hydr(o) refers to hydrogen, but more commonly hydr(o) means water. Hydro/cephaly appears to mean _____ in the _____.

🔑 **KEY** POINT **In medical terms, some interpretation is needed in dividing words into their components.** **Hydrocephaly** is more commonly called **hydrocephalus.** Hydrocephalus means a condition characterized by abnormal accumulation of cerebrospinal fluid (see Chapter 10) within the skull, causing enlargement of the head, mental retardation, and convulsions (Fig. 3.37).

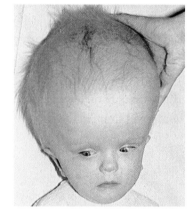

Figure 3.37 Four-month-old child with hydrocephalus. Hydrocephalus is usually caused by obstruction of the flow of cerebrospinal fluid. If hydrocephalus occurs in an infant, the soft bones of the skull push apart as the head increases progressively in size.

Treatment of hydrocephalus generally consists of surgical intervention to correct the cause or to shunt the excess fluid away from the skull. **Shunt,** as a verb, means to redirect the flow of a body fluid from one cavity or vessel to another. The device that is implanted in the body to redirect the fluid is also called a shunt (noun). Write this new term for what is often used in treating hydrocephalus: _____. Remember, the word can be used as a verb or a noun.

shunt

WRITE IT!
EXERCISE 28

In your own words, describe the following terms:

1. dehydration _____
2. edema _____
3. electrolytes _____
4. fluid balance _____
5. shunt _____

Major Types of Body Fluids

fluids

3-101 Although one may first think of blood when speaking of body fluids, there are many others, including **lymph,** saliva, urine, mucus, spinal fluid, tears, gastric juices, perspiration, and pus. The proper functioning of all body systems is dependent on body fluids. Blood, lymph, saliva, and urine are all examples of body _____.

KEY POINT **Several body fluids are associated with specific body systems.** For example, cerebrospinal fluid bathes the brain and spinal cord and is associated with the nervous system. Urine is formed and excreted by the urinary system.

intravascular

3-102 As blood circulates, it remains inside blood vessels in humans, so it is an **intra/vascular** fluid. Write this term that means within a vessel by combining intra-, vascul(o), and -ar: _____.

3-103 Blood and lymph are the fluids that we generally associate with the **cardio/vascul/ar** (cardi[o], heart; vascul[o], vessel; -ar, pertaining to) and lymphatic systems. These fluids circulate throughout the body, providing nutrients for cells and transporting wastes for removal.

KEY POINT **Lymph is the fluid that circulates through the lymphatic vessels.** As blood circulates, needed substances move across the vessel walls into the fluid that surrounds the body cells and fluid accumulates in the tissue spaces. This excess fluid is normally transported away from the tissues by the **lymphatic system.** The fluid is called *lymph.*

blood
lymph

The fluid _____ is carried by the cardiovascular system, and the fluid _____ is carried by the lymphatic system. Compare blood circulation with lymph circulation (Fig. 3.38).

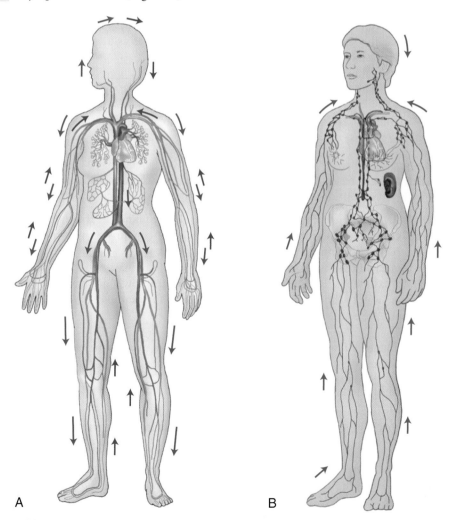

Figure 3.38 Blood circulation vs. lymph circulation. A, Blood is carried away from the heart by arteries *(red)* to all cells in the body. The veins *(blue)* carry blood back to the heart. **B,** Lymph is a thin watery fluid that is transported by lymphatic vessels *(green)* back toward the heart. Lymph nodes, knotty structures along the way, filter the lymph, which eventually is returned to the bloodstream.

Study the word parts and their meanings in the following list.

Word Parts: Selected Body Fluids

Combining Form	Meaning	Combining Form	Meaning
hem(a), hem(o), hemat(o), -emia	blood	muc(o)	mucus
		py(o)	pus
hidr(o)	sweat, perspiration	sial(o)	saliva; salivary glands
hydr(o)	water	ur(o)	urine; urinary tract

MATCH IT! **EXERCISE 29**

Match each combining form in the left column with the correct body fluid in the right column. (Choices A through G may be used more than once.)

_____ **1.** hem(o)   **A.** blood
_____ **2.** hemat(o)   **B.** mucus
_____ **3.** hidr(o)   **C.** perspiration
_____ **4.** hydr(o)   **D.** pus
_____ **5.** muc(o)   **E.** saliva
_____ **6.** py(o)   **F.** urine
_____ **7.** sial(o)   **G.** water
_____ **8.** ur(o)

hidr(o)

3-104 More than a million tiny structures called *sweat glands* are found in the skin. Sweat, or **perspiration,** contains water, salts, and other waste products. These substances are excreted through pores in the skin when one perspires, and this serves as a means of ridding the body of wastes and regulating the body temperature.

The combining form for sweat is _____. Do not confuse this combining form with hydr(o), which has the same pronunciation.

3-105 Substances that are secreted or excreted are called *secretions* or *excretions,* respectively. It is easy to confuse the terms excrete and secrete.

🔑 **KEY POINT Excretion is the body's way of eliminating waste substances.** (Remember that ex- means out.) Perspiration is excreted through pores in the skin (to the outside). **Secretion** is the process of discharging a chemical substance needed by the body into a cavity. For example, saliva is secreted into the mouth to keep the mouth moist, along with other functions.

sial(o)

Saliva is the clear fluid secreted by the salivary glands in the mouth. It serves to moisten the oral cavity, aids in chewing and swallowing, and contains an enzyme that initiates digestion of starch. The combining form that means saliva is _____. This combining form also means the salivary glands.

An **exudate** is fluid, cells, or substances that are slowly discharged from cells or blood vessels. **Serum** (watery fluid from more solid elements: for example, the fluid in a blister), perspiration, and pus are exudates.

mucus

3-106 Mucus is the slippery secretion of glands within mucous membranes. **Muc/ous** means composed of or secreting _____. Mucous membranes line cavities or canals of the body that open to the outside, such as the digestive tract. Note the difference in spelling and meaning of the terms *mucus* (noun) and *mucous* (adjective).

py(o)

3-107 Pus is the liquid product of infection. The combining form that means pus is _____.

🔑 **KEY POINT Bacterial infection is the most common cause of pus production.** Pus is a thick fluid that is made up of the remains of liquefied infected tissue, usually by bacteria. Pus is composed of protein substances, fluid, bacteria, and white blood cells (or their remains). It is generally yellow; if it is red, this suggests blood from the rupture of small vessels.

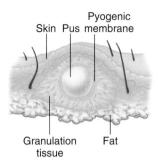

Skin Pus
Pyogenic
membrane

Granulation
tissue
Fat

Figure 3.39 **An abscess.** The pus is contained within a thin pyogenic membrane that is surrounded by harder granulation tissue, the tissue's response to the infection.

3-108 A localized collection of pus in a cavity surrounded by inflamed tissue is called an **abscess** (Fig. 3.39). The inflamed tissue may disintegrate and become necrotic, which increases the difficulty of delivering medication to the site of infection and slows the healing process. The combining form necr(o) means death. In **necrosis,** there is localized tissue death in response to either injury or disease, and the tissue is described as **necrotic.** Abscesses may need to be excised or surgically drained for healing to occur.

abscess

A localized collection of pus in a cavity is an _____.

3-109 Discharges from infected tissue are described as **purulent** or **suppurative.** Both terms mean pertaining to, consisting of, or producing pus. **Sanguinous** means containing blood.

Write the term that begins with a "p" that is used to describe infected tissue:

purulent

_____.

Write the term that begins with an "s" that is used to describe infected tissue:

suppurative

blood

_____.

Sanguinous means containing _____.

3-110 A **hemat/oma** is a localized collection of blood, usually clotted, in an organ, space, or tissue, resulting from a break in the wall of a blood vessel. The term *hematoma* (hemat[o], blood + -oma, tumor) is derived from the old meaning of tumor, a swelling, because there is a raised area wherever a hematoma exists. Hematomas can occur almost anywhere in the body. They are especially dangerous when they occur inside the skull, but most hematomas are not serious (Fig. 3.40). Bruises are familiar forms of hematomas.

You will use the suffix -oma to write words for tumors of many kinds, but you'll also need to remember that a localized collection of blood in an organ, tissue, or space is called a

hematoma

_____.

blood

3-111 Translated literally, hyper/emia means excessive _____.

You need to know that **hyperemia** is an excess of blood in part of the body caused by increased blood flow, as one often sees in inflammation. In hyperemia, the overlying skin usually becomes reddened and warm.

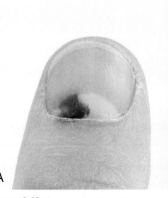

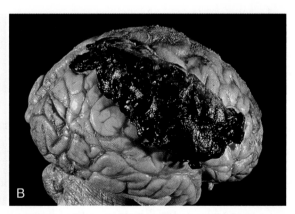

A

B

Figure 3.40 **Two examples of hematomas.** A hematoma forms when blood escapes a vessel and collects as a clot. **A,** A hematoma under the nail is not considered serious. **B,** A cerebral hematoma is serious, as noted by this postmortem photograph of the brain.

MATCH IT!   EXERCISE 30

Match the terms in the left column with the descriptions in the right column.

_____ **1.** excretion   **A.** containing blood

_____ **2.** hematoma   **B.** excess of blood in some part that is caused by increased blood flow

_____ **3.** hyperemia   **C.** localized collection of blood in an organ, space, or tissue

_____ **4.** pus   **D.** pertaining to or consisting of pus

_____ **5.** sanguinous   **E.** process of discharging a substance into a cavity

_____ **6.** secretion   **F.** process of eliminating waste substances

_____ **7.** suppurative   **G.** the liquid product of infection

COMPOSITION OF BLOOD

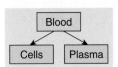

3-112 Blood, the most studied of all body fluids, is composed of a liquid portion, plasma, and several formed elements (cells or cell fragments).

🔑 **KEY POINT Hematology is the study of blood and blood-forming tissues.** The combining form hemat(o) means blood, but in the word *hematology*, the definition includes the blood-forming tissues, in other words, the bone marrow and lymphoid tissue (spleen, thymus, tonsils, and lymph nodes). **Hemato/logic** means pertaining to hematology or the study of the blood.

Learn these word parts.

Word Parts: Aspects of the Blood and Related Functions

Combining Form	Meaning	Suffix	Meaning
Blood Cells		-ant	that which causes
cyt(o), -cyte	cell	-ate	to cause an action or the result of an action
hemoglobin(o)	hemoglobin		
kary(o), nucle(o)	nucleus	-cidal	killing
Blood Clotting		-poiesis	production
coagul(o)	coagulation	-poietin	that which causes production
fibrin(o)	fibrin		
thromb(o)	thrombus; clot		
Miscellaneous			
necr(o)	death		
phil(o)	attraction		

MATCH IT!   EXERCISE 31

Match the word parts in the left column with the descriptions in the right column.

_____ **1.** -ant   **A.** attraction

_____ **2.** -ate   **B.** cell

_____ **3.** coagul(o)   **C.** coagulation

_____ **4.** -cyte   **D.** death

_____ **5.** necr(o)   **E.** production

_____ **6.** phil(o)   **F.** that which causes

_____ **7.** -poiesis   **G.** that which causes production

_____ **8.** -poietin   **H.** to cause an action or result of the action

3-113 Hemato/poiesis is the production of blood, specifically the formation and development of its cells. Hematopoiesis occurs in the bone marrow (specifically, the red bone marrow), the soft, spongelike material in the cavity of bones. When you hear the term *bone marrow failure*, it is failure of the **hemato/poietic** function of the bone marrow. In other words, in bone marrow failure, the red bone marrow does not produce _____ cells.

blood

These three terms look similar. Divide them into their component parts, and explain the differences in their meanings.
1. hematologic _____
2. hematopoiesis _____
3. hematopoietic _____

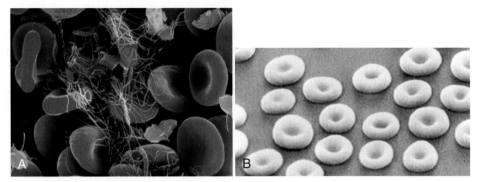

Figure 3.41 Blood coagulation. A, This scanning electron micrograph has been colored to emphasize the different structures. Red blood cells *(red)* are entangled with the fibrin *(yellow)*. Note the thin center and the thick edges that give red blood cells a concave appearance. The platelets *(blue)*, which initiate clotting, are also visible. **B,** Appearance of red blood cells in electron microscopy.

coagulation

3-114 Blood clots when it is removed from the body. **Coagulation** is the formation of a clot (Fig. 3.41A). Blood coagulation, blood clotting, is a series of chemical reactions in which special fibers (fibrin) entrap blood cells, resulting in a blood clot. Write this word that means blood clotting:
_____.

3-115 Look again at Fig. 3.41A, and notice the red donut-shaped cells, which are red blood cells. A red blood cell (RBC), often shortened to red cell, is an **erythro/cyte** (erythr[o] means red). The blood platelets (which are involved in coagulation) are stained blue. An important blood cell that is missing in Fig. 3.41A is a **leukocyte,** also called a *white blood cell,* often shortened to white cell or WBC. Note the biconcave appearance of red blood cells seen with an electron microscope (Fig. 3.41B).

Draw a slash between the word parts in the following list of new terms. Then find the meanings of the word parts within the definitions. Think! (Draw the slash, and then perform the remainder of the activity as a mental exercise).
1. anticoagulant a substance that prevents or delays coagulation (noun)
2. coagulant an agent that causes coagulation (noun)
3. coagulate to cause to clot; to undergo coagulation (verb)
4. coagulopathy any disorder of blood coagulation (noun)

KEY POINT Red cells and white cells are sometimes called *corpuscles.* A **corpuscle** is defined as any small mass or cell.

fibrin

fibrinolysin

3-116 Coagulation of the blood is a series of chemical reactions that result in a blood clot. **Fibrin** is formed when blood clots. Composed of stringy protein fibers, fibrin entraps blood cells in blood clotting. Fibrino/gen is a precursor of _____. **Fibrinogen** is a protein that is changed into fibrin in the process of coagulation.
   Fibrino/lysis is the destruction of fibrin. Write a word that means a substance that can dissolve fibrin: _____.

KEY POINT **Learn the difference between internal vs. external blood clots.** The combining form thromb(o) means **thrombus,** a blood clot that is attached to a vessel wall and that tends to obstruct a blood vessel or a cavity of the heart. Be aware that some specialists differentiate between a blood clot (occurring in a test tube) and a thrombus (occurring internally).

thrombus

A fibrinolysin can dissolve a blood clot, which is another name for a _____.
Heparin and warfarin (Coumadin) are in vivo anticoagulants that are used to prevent blood clots.

> **BEYOND** THE BLUEPRINT Warfarin in large doses causes massive hemorrhage and death and was initially marketed as a pesticide against rats and mice. A few years after its introduction, warfarin was found to be effective and relatively safe in preventing thrombosis and embolism, but the level of anticoagulant must be strictly maintained.

The blood of persons taking anticoagulants is tested regularly using laboratory tests, such as prothrombin time (PT) and partial thromboplastin time (PTT). **Prothrombin** and **thromboplastin** are factors involved in different parts of the coagulation process, and the tests provide information about various stages of the coagulation process. The importance of accurate and reliable PT measurements has resulted in a standardized reporting system for PTs called the *International Normalized Ratio (INR)*.

BUILD IT!
EXERCISE 34

Use the following word parts to build terms to complete these sentences. (Some word parts will be used more than once.)
coagul(o), fibrin(o), hem(o), -ation, -gen, -lysin, -lysis, -stasis
1. Destruction of fibrin is _____.
2. A series of chemical reactions that result in a blood clot is _____.
3. Special fibers that entrap blood cells in blood clotting are called _____.
4. The term for a substance that can dissolve a blood clot is _____.
5. A term for a protein that is changed into fibrin when coagulation takes place is _____.

anticoagulant

3-117 A circulating anticoagulant normally prevents blood from clotting within the body. However, when blood is removed from the body, a series of chemical reactions occur to cause coagulation (not exposure to air) unless one uses an anticoagulant.
Transfusions and many hematologic studies require blood that has not clotted; therefore, the blood is treated with an _____ as soon as it is removed from the body.

in vitro

WORD ORIGIN
in vitro (L.)
in, within; *vitreus,*
   glassware
in vivo (L.)
in, within; *vivo,* alive

3-118 In vitro means occurring in a laboratory test tube (or glass) or occurring in an artificial environment. Because the anticoagulant is placed in the blood in an artificial environment (outside the body), this is in vitro use of an anticoagulant. A Latin term meaning in an artificial environment or outside the body is _____.
Some patients tend to form clots within blood vessels, a serious condition that can result in death. For these patients, a physician prescribes in vivo anticoagulant therapy to suppress blood clot formation. **In vivo** is a Latin term that means occurring in a living organism.

3-119 Laboratory tests often require treating blood with an anticoagulant to prevent clotting. The blood in the tube in Fig. 3.42 has been treated with an anticoagulant. The formed elements are
• erythrocytes—red blood cells
• leukocytes—white blood cells
• blood platelets—also called thrombocytes
The layer that is made up of leukocytes and platelets is sometimes called the *buffy coat.*

hemat(o)

3-120 The **hemato/crit** measures the percentage of red blood cells in a volume of blood. The part of hematocrit that means blood is _____. (Hematocrit is often abbreviated Hct.)
The hematocrit is not a difficult concept. It simply tells us what percentage of the blood is made up of red blood cells. Normal values are based on packed red cell volume, which is determined by centrifuging the blood. Exact normal values vary among children, men, and women, but they usually range between 37% and 54%. (The hematocrit can also be calculated based on the size and number of red cells in a minute sample of blood.)

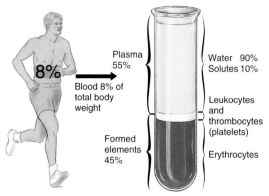

Figure 3.42 **Blood components.** The blood in this test tube has been treated with anticoagulant to prevent clotting and has been centrifuged to separate its components. Red blood cells, the heaviest of the three components, make up the bottom layer. The middle layer of white blood cells (WBCs) and platelets is often called the *buffy coat*. The liquid part of treated blood (plasma) constitutes the upper layer. Any of these blood components can be given in a transfusion.

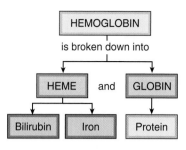

Figure 3.43 **Hemoglobin is a protein that is broken down into two parts, heme and globin.** The heme portion is broken down into bilirubin and iron (combines with oxygen and renders the blood red). The globin portion is broken down into protein molecules.

white
red

3-121 The blood of healthy persons has normal numbers of erythrocytes and leukocytes. This number is determined by blood counts. A leukocyte count is a determination of the number of _____ blood cells. An erythrocyte count is the evaluation of the number of _____ blood cells.

3-122 Erythrocytes, leukocytes, and **thrombocytes** (more commonly called **blood platelets**) are the formed elements of the blood.

thrombocyte

A thrombo/cyte is not a cell that has clotted. It is a cell fragment that initiates the formation of a clot. You need to remember that another name for a blood platelet is a _____.

3-123 Erythrocytes, leukocytes, and blood platelets have different functions. Erythrocytes transport oxygen to body tissue cells and pick up carbon dioxide to be excreted by the lungs. Erythrocytes are able to accomplish this because they contain the protein **hemoglobin**, which enables them to carry oxygen. The "heme" portion of hemoglobin combines with oxygen and produces the bright red color of blood (Fig. 3.43).

The primary function of leukocytes is to protect the body against pathogenic organisms, and blood platelets play an important role in blood coagulation. Review these functions:

oxygen
harmful (pathogenic)
coagulation

Erythrocytes transport _____ to body cells and pick up carbon dioxide for excretion. Leukocytes protect the body against _____ organisms. Blood platelets initiate the formation of a blood clot in blood _____.

Our blood types are determined by inherited genetic material on the erythrocytes. The most important blood types are the ABO and Rh blood groups. The ABO blood groups contain A, B, AB, and O antigens, proteins that are described later in this chapter (Table 3.6). Type O is known as the universal donor, because it does not contain A or B antigens and is not likely to cause a transfusion reaction. The Rh blood group is complex and has many different antigens.

Table 3.6 ABO Blood Groups	
Blood Type	**Antigen on the Erythrocytes**
A	A
B	B
AB	A and B
O	Neither A nor B

WRITE IT! EXERCISE 35

Write the medical term, as well as the common name of the formed elements of the blood.

Medical Term	Common Name
1. ________	________
2. ________	________
3. ________	________

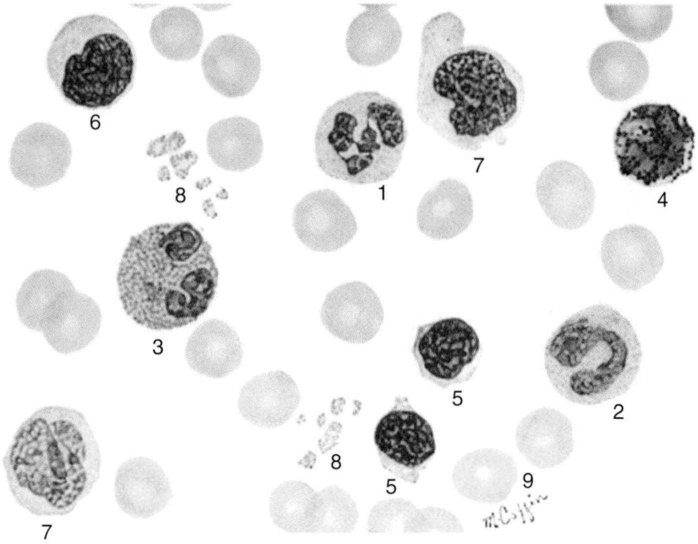

Figure 3.44 Human blood, stained (drawing). All of these elements are normally present. Representatives are a segmented neutrophil *(1)*, a neutrophilic band lacking the segments *(2)*, an eosinophil *(3)*, a basophil *(4)*, small lymphocytes *(5)*, a large lymphocyte *(6)*, and monocytes *(7)*. Platelets *(8)* and many erythrocytes *(9)* are also present. A normal range exists for the frequency of each type of leukocyte in a sample, and increases or decreases are sometimes helpful in the diagnosis.

3-124 A stained blood smear allows microscopic examination of the erythrocytes, leukocytes, and blood platelets. A normal red cell in circulating blood has matured and lost its nucleus; however, a WBC still has a nucleus. There are five major types of leukocytes (shown in Fig. 3.44):

- **neutrophil,** sometimes abbreviated neut
- **eosinophil,** abbreviated eos
- **basophil,** abbreviated baso
- **lymphocyte,** abbreviated lymph
- **monocyte,** abbreviated mono

A differential white cell count is a microscopic examination and enumeration of the distribution of leukocytes in a stained blood smear. This laboratory test provides information related to infections and various diseases and is included in a complete blood cell count (CBC).

WRITE IT! EXERCISE 36

List the five major types of WBCs.

1. ________
2. ________
3. ________
4. ________
5. ________

FIND IT! EXERCISE 37

Draw a slash between the word parts in the following list of new terms. Then find the meanings of the word parts within the definitions. Think! (Draw the slash, and then perform the remainder of the activity as a mental exercise.)

1. **erythrocytic** pertaining to erythrocytes (adjective)
2. **erythropoiesis** production of erythrocytes (noun)
3. **erythropoietin** a hormone that is produced in the kidneys and acts on stem cells in the bone marrow to stimulate erythropoiesis (noun)
4. **karyomegaly** abnormal enlargement of a cell nucleus
5. **nucleoid** resembling a nucleus

BLOOD DISORDERS

clot

3-125 Terminology associated with selected hematologic disorders is presented in this section. Hematologic disorders range from a mild anemia to a life-threatening blood clot. Thromb(o) means a thrombus or a blood clot. **Thrombo/genesis** is the formation of a blood _____ or a thromb/us (plural: **thrombi**).

embolus

3-126 A piece of a thrombus, a bit of tissue or tumor, or a bubble of gas or air that circulates in the bloodstream until it becomes lodged in a vessel is an **embolus. Embolism** is the presence of an _____.

FIND IT! EXERCISE 38

Draw a slash between the word parts in the following list of new terms. Then find the meanings of the word parts within the definitions. Think! (Draw the slash, and then perform the remainder of the activity as a mental exercise.)

1. **thrombocytopenia** decrease in the number of blood platelets (noun)
2. **thrombocytosis** an increase in the number of thrombocytes in the circulating blood (noun)
3. **thrombolysis** destruction of a blood clot (noun)
4. **thrombolytic** dissolving of a blood clot (adjective); an agent that dissolves a blood clot (noun)
5. **thrombosis** formation, development, or presence of a blood clot (noun)

excised (removed)

3-127 A blood clot sometimes dissolves spontaneously, or a thrombolytic agent may be used. If therapeutic measures are not successful, a **thromb/ectomy** may be performed. In a thrombectomy, the blood clot is _____.

decreased

3-128 In **thrombopenia,** same as thrombocytopenia, the number of platelets are _____. Because blood platelets are an important part of blood coagulation, severe thrombopenia results in a bleeding disorder.

blood

destruction (hemolysis)

3-129 Literal translation of hemo/lysis is destruction of _____.
     Hemolysis is destruction of the red blood cell membrane, resulting in the release of hemoglobin, the oxygen-carrying red pigment of blood. Because you have learned three combining forms that mean blood, you may be wondering how one knows which form to use. Common usage determines the proper form. Even though hemato/lysis is a good word, hemolysis is much better known.
     A **hemo/lysin** is a substance that causes _____ of red blood cells. When blood is placed in water or another substance that hemolyzes it, the destruction refers to the dissolving of the erythrocytes, which burst and release their red pigment.

> **BEYOND** THE BLUEPRINT Hemolysins are produced by some bacteria and are present in the venom of some poisonous snakes. Rattlesnake venom contains hemotoxins, which hemolyze the blood.

bacteria
streptococci

3-130 The blood is normally free of microorganisms. **Bacter/emia** is the presence of _____ in the blood. **Staphylo/cocc/emia** is staphylococci, a type of bacteria, in the blood. **Streptococc/emia,** a type of bacter/emia, is the presence of _____ in the blood. A blood culture is helpful in detecting and identifying many types of bacteria that cause bacteremia. A sensitivity test provides information about which antibiotic is likely to be most effective for treatment.

KEY POINT **Systemic means pertaining to the whole body rather than to a specific area of the body. Septic/emia** (sept[i], infection + -emia, blood) is a systemic infection in which pathogens have spread from some part of the body and not only are present in the circulating blood but also are multiplying and causing blood infection. This is also called *sepsis,* and the patient is described as *septic.*

The presence of microbial toxins in the blood is **tox/emia,** a serious condition. A unique type of toxemia is seen in toxic shock syndrome (TSS). The severity of the disease is caused by toxins of a pathogenic strain of *Staphylococcus* and can become life-threatening unless it is recognized and treated. It is most common in menstruating females using high-absorbency tampons but has been seen in other persons. Although toxemia is generally reserved to describe the presence of toxins in the blood, it is sometimes used to mean severe and progressive (for example, toxemia of pregnancy).

3-131 Anemia is a deficiency in the number of red blood cells, a deficiency in hemoglobin, or sometimes a reduction in both red cells and hemoglobin. The literal translation of the parts of an/emia is *without blood.* Because no one can live without blood, the name anemia is an exaggeration of the condition.

KEY POINT Anemia is not a disease but a sign of various diseases. The severity of signs and symptoms depends on the severity of the anemia. Severe anemia may be accompanied by signs and symptoms that stem from diminished oxygen-carrying capacity of the blood.

fast

Table 3.7 lists classic signs and symptoms of severe anemia. Several new terms are included in the table. **Tachycardia** means an increased pulse rate; it will be studied in the next chapter. Analyzing its word parts, tachy- means _____, cardi(o) means heart, and -ia means condition. One "i" is omitted to facilitate pronunciation.

difficult

Dys/pnea means _____ breathing, because the suffix -pnea means breathing. You will learn more about dyspnea in Chapter 5. Note that **pallor,** named after the Latin term, refers to an unnatural paleness or absence of color. **Syncope** is fainting, and **tinnitus** is ringing in the ears.

> **WORD ORIGIN**
> syncope *(G.)*
> *synkoptein,* to cut short
> tinnitus *(L.)*
> *tinnire,* to tinkle

Table 3.7 **Classic Signs and Symptoms of Severe Anemia**	
• Pallor (color of nail beds, palms, and mucous membranes of the mouth and conjunctivae are more reliable than skin color for assessing paleness) • Tachycardia (increased pulse rate) • Heart murmur • Angina (chest pain) • Decreased number of erythrocytes, hemoglobin, or both • Congestive heart failure	• Dyspnea (difficult breathing) • Shortness of breath • Fatigue on exertion • Headache • Dizziness • Syncope (fainting) • Tinnitus (ringing in the ears) • Gastrointestinal symptoms (anorexia, nausea, sore tongue and mouth) • Constipation or diarrhea

3-132 Iron deficiency anemia results when there is a greater demand for iron than the body can supply. It can be caused by blood loss or insufficient intake or absorption of iron from the intestinal tract. Iron deficiency anemia is often treated successfully with iron tablets and a balanced diet.

> **BEYOND THE BLUEPRINT** Ancient Greeks drank water in which iron swords had been allowed to rust, thinking that they derived strength from the sword. The French steeped iron filings in wine and then drank it! Like the French wine with added iron, some modern products contain iron and vitamins with substantial alcohol. It is said that long ago, people stuck nails in apples and let the nails rust. They removed the nails and fed the apples to their children.

iron

A greater demand for iron than the body can supply results in _____ deficiency anemia.

deficiency

3-133 Erythro/cyto/penia is a _____ of erythrocytes. Erythrocytopenia can be shortened to **erythropenia.** Either word means a deficiency in the number of red blood cells.

erythrocytes

3-134 Erythro/cyt/osis means an increase in the number of _____. There is an increase in the number of erythrocytes in **polycythemia.** There are two forms of this condition, primary polycythemia (also called **polycythemia vera**) and secondary polycythemia. In both, there is a marked increase in the number of erythrocytes.

WRITE IT!   EXERCISE 39

Write a word in each blank to complete these sentences.
1. Another name for a blood platelet is _____.
2. A clot in a vessel or the heart is _____.
3. Thrombogenesis is the formation of a blood _____.
4. Destruction of a thrombus is _____.
5. Destruction of red blood cells, resulting in the release of hemoglobin, is called _____.
6. An increase in the number of thrombocytes is called _____.
7. A term for a deficiency in the number of red blood cells, a deficiency in hemoglobin, or sometimes a reduction in both red cells and hemoglobin is _____.
8. The meaning of syncope is _____.

---

blood

3-135 Literal translation of leuk/emia is white _____, and it is so called because of the large number of WBCs in the blood of patients with this disease. **Leukemia** is a progressive, malignant disease of the hematopoietic (blood-forming) organs, characterized by a sharp increase in the number of leukocytes, as well as the presence of immature forms of leukocytes in the blood and bone marrow. A malignancy in which there is a sharp increase in the number of leukocytes

leukemia

is _____.

> **BEYOND** THE BLUEPRINT Myelocytes, precursor cells of neutrophils, eosinophils, and basophils are normally found only in the bone marrow. Myelogenous pertains to the cells produced in the bone marrow or the tissue from which these cells originate. Immature leukocytes appear in the blood in leukemia or occasionally in severe infection. There are four types of leukemia: acute myelogenous (myelocytic), acute lymphocytic, chronic myelogenous (myelocytic), and chronic lymphocytic.

white

3-136 Leukocytosis means an increase in the number of _____ blood cells. There is a major difference between leukemia and most conditions that cause leukocytosis. In leukemia, the production of leukocytes is uncontrolled, and many of the leukocytes produced are immature and nonfunctional.

Leukocytosis may be transitory and often accompanies a bacterial, but not usually a viral, infection. Because the main function of leukocytes is protection against harmful invading micro-organisms (such as bacteria), this should help you remember which type of cell is likely to increase

leukocytes

during a bacterial infection: _____.

3-137 Infectious mononucleosis is an acute viral infection that affects mainly young people. Unlike most viral infections, infectious mononucleosis is characterized by leukocytosis with atypical lymphocytes, fever, sore throat, swollen lymph glands, abnormal liver function, and enlarged spleen. The name may not help in remembering the disease, infectious _____

mononucleosis

(referring to one type of cell with a single nucleus, the lymphocyte).

Treatment is primarily symptomatic with analgesics to control pain and enforced bed rest to prevent complications of the liver or spleen. The disease is caused by the Epstein-Barr virus (EBV), which resides in the salivary glands, and continues to be shed indefinitely.

leukocytopenia

3-138 Write a word using leuk(o), cyt(o), and -penia: _____. This is often shortened to **leukopenia.** Either word means a decrease or deficiency in the number of leukocytes.

3-139 Leukocytosis is common when infection is present, because leukocytes are part of the body's natural defense mechanisms. Don't confuse infection (the invasion of the body by a pathogenic organism) with inflammation (a protective response of body tissues to irritation or injury). Inflammation occurs in other conditions besides infection and may be acute or chronic, lasting for months or even years.

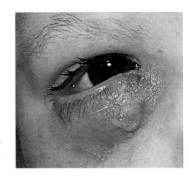

Figure 3.45 Sty. This infection of a gland of the eyelid shows two of the cardinal signs of inflammation: redness and swelling. It is not difficult to imagine that the sty has the other two signs of inflammation, pain and warmth, in the area around the sty.

🔑 **KEY** POINT **The cardinal signs of acute inflammation are redness, heat, swelling, and pain, sometimes accompanied by loss of function** (Fig. 3.45). Pain is actually a symptom rather than a sign but is included as one of the four cardinal signs.

3-140 Bleeding disorders can result from a number of deficiencies, including a deficiency of vitamin K.

🔑 **KEY** POINT **Classic hemo/philia is a hereditary bleeding disorder in which there is deficiency of one coagulation factor called *anti/hemophilic factor (AHF) VIII.*** Other types of hemophilia may result from the deficiencies of other coagulation or clotting factors. In hemophilia there is spontaneous bleeding or prolonged bleeding after a minor injury. Perhaps the naming of hemophilia came about because of excessive and prolonged bleeding that occurs in the disorder, leading to an inaccurate conclusion that affected individuals had an affinity or attraction to blood. The word parts (hem[o], blood + -philia, attraction) are not especially helpful in remembering the term, hemophilia.

anemia

Prolonged bleeding leads to a deficiency of both red blood cells and hemoglobin. This condition is called _____.

3-141 In summary, principal conditions that are associated with abnormalities in the number of blood cells and platelets are listed in Table 3.8.

Table 3.8   Principal Conditions Affecting the Number of Blood Cells and Platelets

Conditions Involving Erythrocytes	Conditions Involving Leukocytes	Conditions Involving Blood Platelets
anemia	leukocytosis	disseminated intravascular coagulation
bone marrow failure	leukopenia	thrombocytopenia
hemolysis	leukemia (acute or chronic)	thrombocytosis
polycythemia		

coagulation

Disseminated means scattered or distributed over a considerable area; disseminated intra/vascul/ar coagulation (DIC) is a grave coagulopathy in which there is generalized intravascular clotting. A coagulo/pathy is any disorder of _____.

WRITE IT! EXERCISE 40

Describe the difference in these terms.
1. leukocytosis and leukemia _____
_____

2. infection and inflammation _____
_____

Anemias and Abnormal Hemoglobins

hemoglobinopathy

3-142 Hemoglobin (Hb, Hgb), the iron-containing pigment of erythrocytes, carries oxygen from the lungs to tissues throughout the body. Use hemoglobin(o) to write a word that literally means any disease of the hemoglobins: _____.

The hemoglobinopathies are a group of diseases caused by or associated with the presence of abnormal hemoglobin in the blood. Some anemias are hereditary and are caused by abnormal hemoglobins.

3-143 Because hemoglobins are proteins, they move at various speeds across paper or starch gel, based on their electric charge, their size, and their mobility. **Hemoglobin electrophoresis** is used to identify abnormal hemoglobin.

Hemoglobins are generally identified by letters or sometimes by their place of occurrence and discovery. Normal adult hemoglobin is designated hemoglobin A. There are many abnormal types. One type of abnormal hemoglobin, S, is found in sickle cell anemia. Abnormal hemoglobins, such as Hb S, generally result in distortion and fragility of the erythrocytes, causing them to hemolyze more readily. Hemo/lyze means that the erythrocytes _____.

dissolve

3-144 Hemo/lytic anemia is a disorder characterized by premature destruction of the erythrocytes. This type of anemia may be an inherited disorder; may be associated with some infectious diseases; or may occur as a response to drugs, various toxic agents, or certain incompatibilities in blood or tissue types. The disorder in which erythrocytes are destroyed prematurely is called _____ anemia.

hemolytic

Hemolytic disease of the newborn (HDN) is also called **erythro/blast/osis fetalis.** The blood of infants who are born with this type of hemolytic anemia contains **erythro/blasts** (immature erythrocytes), and it is for this reason the condition was named erythroblastosis fetalis.

🔑 **KEY** POINT **The cause of erythroblastosis fetalis may be an Rh factor incompatibility of the mother and the fetus** (for example, an Rh negative mother carrying an Rh positive fetus.) The disease results from an incompatibility of the blood groups of the mother and fetus, such as the rhesus (Rh) factor, ABO blood groups, or other blood incompatibilities. Diagnosis is confirmed during pregnancy by amniocentesis and analysis of the amniotic fluid. See Chapter 8, the section, "Pregnancy and Childbirth," for more information.

Treatment may consist of an **intrauterine** (within the uterus) **transfusion** or immediate exchange transfusions after birth. In Rh factor incompatibility, sensitization to the Rh factor can be prevented by injection of the mother with a preparation, such as RhoGAM. Hemolytic reactions involving the ABO blood groups are generally less severe than those involving the Rh factor.

aplastic

3-145 Write a word that means the opposite of plastic by using either a- or an-: _____. You previously learned that plast(o) means repair. **Aplastic** means having no tendency to develop new tissue. In aplastic anemia, the bone marrow is diseased and produces few cells.

WORD ORIGIN
dyscrasia (G.)
dys, bad; *krasis,* mingling

Irregularities in the blood often indicate abnormal conditions of various body systems; however, certain diseases or disorders are associated mainly with the blood or bone marrow and are called **dyscrasias.** Some examples of the latter are leukemia and aplastic anemia.

WRITE IT!
EXERCISE 41

Write a word for the following descriptions.
1. a group of diseases associated with abnormal hemoglobin _____
2. anemia in which erythrocytes are destroyed prematurely _____
3. anemia in which bone marrow produces few cells _____

Learn these word parts.

Word Parts: Descriptive Aspects of Erythrocytes

Combining Form	Meaning	Combining Form	Meaning
chrom(o)	color	morph(o)	shape
is(o)	equal	norm(o)	normal

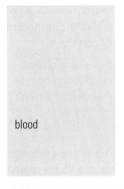

normocyte

3-146 Microscopic variations in the erythrocytes are often observed in anemias and can be seen on a stained smear. Normal erythrocytes are **normo/cyt/ic** (normal + cell + pertaining to), meaning normal size, and **normo/chrom/ic** (normal + color + pertaining to), meaning containing a normal amount of hemoglobin. A cell that is normocytic is called a _____. Now you're ready to test your understanding of the following nouns associated with abnormal appearances of erythrocytes in a stained smear. Anemia is often present when these types of cells are seen.

FIND IT!

EXERCISE 42

Draw a slash between the word parts in the following list of new terms. Then find the meanings of the word parts within the definitions. Think! (Draw the slash, and then perform the remainder of the activity as a mental exercise.)

1. **macrocyte** larger than normal erythrocyte
2. **megalocyte** a very large cell, usually an erythrocyte
3. **macrocytosis** the presence of larger than normal erythrocytes
4. **microcyte** undersized erythrocyte
5. **microcytosis** a condition characterized by the presence of many undersized cells

blood

3-147 The erythrocytes of persons with sickle cell anemia appear elongated and sickled. **Sickle cell anemia** is a hereditary anemia that mainly afflicts blacks who inherit an abnormal type of hemoglobin. In vivo hemolysis occurs, resulting in hemolytic anemia. Compare normal cells with sickle cells in Fig. 3.46.

3-148 Hemoglobin is the red pigment found inside erythrocytes that gives blood its red color. Globins or globulins are types of proteins; therefore hemoglobin is a type of protein found in _____. Hemoglobin is often abbreviated Hb or Hgb.

You learned earlier that a cell with the normal amount of hemoglobin, like those in Fig. 3.46, are normochromic. Test your skills by discovering the abnormalities of the erythrocyte's hemoglobin content in the following exercise.

FIND IT!

EXERCISE 43

Draw a slash between the word parts in the following list of new terms. Then find the meanings of the word parts within the definitions. Think! (Draw the slash, and then perform the remainder of the activity as a mental exercise.)

1. **hypochromia** a condition in which the erythrocytes have less than the normal amount of color (noun)
2. **hypochromic** pertaining to less than normal color, usually an erythrocyte, and characterizes anemia with decreased synthesis of hemoglobin (adjective)
3. **hyperchromic** having a greater density of color or pigment; descriptive of erythrocytes with more color than normal (adjective)

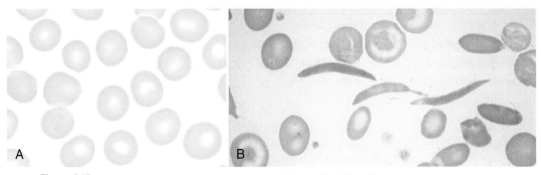

A   B

Figure 3.46 Comparison of normal erythrocytes with those of sickle cell anemia. A, Normocytic normochromic erythrocytes. **B,** Erythrocytes in sickle cell disease. Three erythrocytes are elongated and sickle-shaped. Note the fewer erythrocytes and their variation in size and color, which is also typical in sickle cell anemia.

COAGULATION, TRANSFUSION, AND BONE MARROW TRANSPLANTS

platelets

3-149 Blood coagulation saves lives when it occurs in response to injury. It can result in death, however, if it occurs in the circulating blood. An internal blood clot, a thrombus, usually starts with tissue damage and is particularly life-threatening if the clot occurs in the heart or if it breaks off and is taken by the bloodstream to the brain or heart. Thrombocyt/osis, an increase in the number of blood _____, can also cause thrombosis. Blood coagulation brings about hemo/stasis. Stasis means stoppage of flow. **Hemo/stasis** can mean arrest of bleeding or interruption of blood flow through a vessel or to any part of the body.

It can be natural by clotting, or artificial, by compression or suturing of a wound. Perhaps you have heard of a hemostat, a clamp that is used to stop hemorrhage (Fig. 3.47).

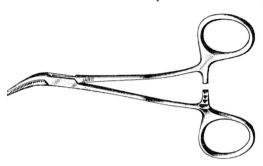

Figure 3.47 Hemostat. A surgical clamp, a hemostat, is used to control blood flow. This is a type of artificial hemostasis.

🔑 **KEY** POINT **Bleeding disorders can be as serious a problem of blood coagulation as thrombosis.** The most common cause of bleeding disorders is thrombocyto/penia, an insufficiency of blood platelets, resulting from either decreased production or survival or increased destruction. In addition, malfunction or absence of any of the coagulation factors causes at least some degree of bleeding tendency. Hemostasis may be delayed in these cases, which could result in the loss of large amounts of blood. A transfusion may be necessary to replace the lost blood.

across

3-150 The prefix trans- means through or across. The introduction of whole blood or blood components into the bloodstream of a person is called a **blood transfusion.** In the earliest transfusions, blood was passed directly _____ from one person to another.

🔑 **KEY** POINT **Blood from a donor to be used in a transfusion is first screened to be sure that it does not carry a bloodborne disease, such as hepatitis.** Then, blood typing determines if the blood is Rh positive or Rh negative. (The Rh factor, a factor that is found also in the rhesus monkey, is reported as Rh positive or Rh negative). Grouping determines if the blood group is group O, A, B, or AB. Cross-matching of blood is done by mixing the cells of the patient with the donor's serum (liquid part of blood that has been separated from its cellular component.) If no agglutination or hemolysis occurs, the donor's blood is considered safe for the patient.

In the laboratory, one's blood type is determined by mixing blood with commercially prepared sera and observing for **agglutination,** aggregates or small clumps of erythrocytes, which may be visible macro/scopically (Fig. 3.48) or perhaps only micro/scopically.

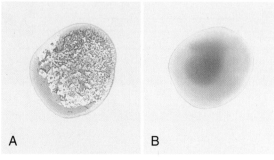

Blood Type	Agglutination with Anti-A antiserum	Agglutination with Anti-B antiserum
A	Yes	No
B	No	Yes
AB	Yes	Yes
O	No	No

A   B   C

Agglutination   No agglutination

Figure 3.48 Observing macroscopic agglutination in the laboratory and agglutination patterns for ABO blood types. A, Agglutination. This test on a glass slide using blood and commercially-prepared serum results in visible small clumps, agglutination. **B,** No macroscopic agglutination. No visible clumping but microscopic examination is required to verify that agglutination has not occurred. **C,** Agglutination patterns for ABO blood types.

> **BEYOND** THE BLUEPRINT ABO and Rh factors on the surface of red blood cells are genetically determined and are considered antigens, because some of the factors may be antigenic to a person who does not have that particular factor. For more information, visit *http://www.ncbi.nlm.nih.gov/books/NBK2264*.

3-151 A transfusion reaction is an adverse reaction to the blood a person receives in a transfusion. Among the most common reactions are those that result from blood group incompatibilities. In other words, something in the donor's blood is not compatible with the blood of the recipient. Symptoms of transfusion reactions vary in degree from mild to severe. Some are manifested immediately, whereas others may not occur for several days. Blood group incompatibilities often result in agglutination or hemolysis of the erythrocytes. Hemo/lysis is _____

destruction

of the erythrocytes.

🔑 **KEY** POINT **Certain diseases can be transmitted to the recipient through blood transfusion.** Various screening tests are performed to avoid using infected blood. Screening generally includes testing for several types of **hepatitis**—hepatitis A, B, C, and D; human **immunodeficiency** virus (the agent that causes acquired immunodeficiency syndrome [AIDS]); cytomegalovirus (CMV); and syphilis (rapid plasma reagin [RPR] test is commonly used). Certain areas of the United States also test for the West Nile virus, which causes West Nile encephalitis.

3-152 Autologous and homologous are terms that are often associated with blood transfusions or skin grafts. In an **autologous transfusion,** blood is removed from a donor and stored for a variable period before it is returned to the donor's circulation. In an _____ **graft,** tissue is transferred from one site to another on the same body.

autologous

WORD ORIGIN
autologous *(G.)*
autos, self
homologous *(G.)*
homos, same

In contrast, a **homologous graft** is a tissue removed from a donor for transplantation to a recipient of the same species. This is also called an **allograft.** A transplant from one's identical twin is an **iso/graft,** but a transplantation from all other individuals of one's species is an allo/graft. Best results occur with an isograft or when the donor is closely related to the recipient. Transplantation of certain organs, such as kidneys, has a high degree of success.

3-153 Bone marrow transplants are used in treating patients with leukemia or aplastic anemia. **Allo/gene/ic,** also called **allo/genic,** bone marrow transplants (from a donor with a close leukocyte antigen type) have a lower success rate than many organ transplants, such as transplant of the kidneys. For this reason, autologous transplants are preferred, using marrow previously obtained from the patient and stored, then reinfused when needed.

WRITE IT! **EXERCISE 44**

Write words in the blanks to complete these sentences.
1. A term for aggregation of cells into clumps or masses is _____.
2. A/An _____ reaction is an adverse reaction to the blood a person receives.
3. The term for the transfusion of a person's own blood after it has been collected in advance and stored is a/an _____ transfusion.
4. A/An _____ graft is tissue removed from a donor for transplantation to a recipient of the same species.
5. In vivo anticoagulants are given to persons to prevent blood _____.
6. Arrest of bleeding is called _____.

IMMUNITY

disease

3-154 Our bodies have many defenses, including immunity, which usually protect us from pathogenic organisms and other foreign substances. **Immunity** is the protection against infectious disease conferred by immunization, previous infection, or other factors. The immune reaction that can occur in a blood transfusion is part of the same system that provides protection against disease-causing organisms. We are continually exposed to pathogens and other harmful substances. Patho/gens are microorganisms that are capable of causing _____.

Study the word parts for immunity.

Word Parts: Immunity

Combining Form	Meaning	Suffix/Prefix	Meaning
aut(o)	self	-phylaxis	protection
immun(o)	immune	ana-	upward, excessive, or again

KEY POINT **Any substance that is capable, under appropriate conditions, of inducing a specific immune response is an antigen.** Antigens may be bacteria, tissue cells, toxins, or foreign proteins. The body's natural ability to counteract microorganisms or toxins is called **resistance. Susceptibility** is a lack of resistance. For example, when we are exposed to the influenza virus, we do not become ill if our body has sufficient resistance.

susceptibility

The term for lacking resistance (or being susceptible) is _____.

3-155 The body's defense against pathogens is not contained within a single set of organs, but depends on several body systems acting simultaneously. Undamaged skin, acids of the stomach or other organs, cilia (hairlike projections in the nasal passages), mucus, phagocytes, **complement** (complex serum proteins), and **interferon** (a special protein that reacts to viruses) help protect against pathogens.

phagocytic

Phagocytosis is the ingestion and destruction of microorganisms and cellular debris by certain cells, mainly leukocytes and large **phago/cytic** tissue cells called **macro/phages.** Which adjective in the last sentence means "capable of phagocytosis?" _____

Immunity against specific pathogens is brought about by complex systems involved in antibodies and special lymphocytes called *T lymphocytes* (or *T-cells*).

autoimmune

3-156 Anti/bodies are formed against antigens. When faced with a threat, our bodies usually make antibodies to counteract the invader. People do not generally form antibodies against their own body cells; however, this happens in **autoimmune diseases,** a group of diseases characterized by production of antibodies against one's own cells. The condition in which one forms antibodies against one's own cells is an _____ disease.

against

3-157 Antibodies are immunoglobulins and are classified as IgA, IgD, IgE, IgG, or IgM. The combining form immun(o) means immune. An antibody interacts with the antigen that induced its synthesis. **Immuno/globulins,** or antibodies, are found in the blood plasma and act _____ harmful invading microorganisms.

antibodies

Specific antibodies provide us with immunity against disease-causing organisms. We generally acquire antibodies either by having a disease or by receiving a vaccination. A vaccination causes our bodies to produce _____.

3-158 Immunization is the process by which resistance to an infectious disease is induced or augmented.

KEY POINT **Remember the difference between active and passive immunity.** Active immunity occurs when the individual's own body produces an immune response to a harmful antigen. Passive immunity results when the immune agents develop in another person or animal and then are transferred to an individual who was not previously immune. This second type of immunity is borrowed immunity (for example, receiving a transfusion of antibodies from a donor) that provides immediate protection but is effective for only a short time.

Natural | Artificial

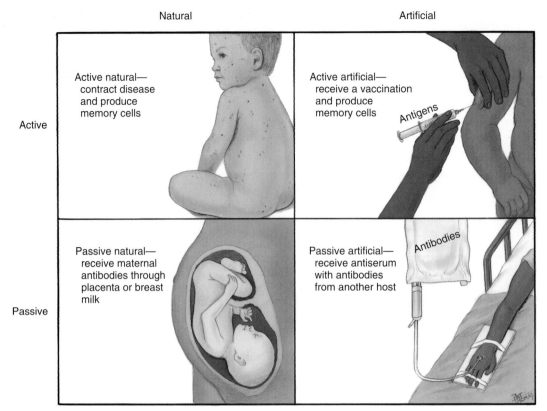

Active

Active natural—
contract disease
and produce
memory cells

Active artificial—
receive a vaccination
and produce
memory cells

Antigens

Passive

Passive natural—
receive maternal
antibodies through
placenta or breast
milk

Passive artificial—
receive antiserum
with antibodies
from another host

Antibodies

Figure 3.49 Four types of specific immunity. Active natural and passive natural immunities, as the names imply, occur through the normal activities of either an individual contracting a disease or a fetus being exposed to maternal antibodies. Both active artificial and passive artificial immunities require deliberate actions of receiving vaccinations or antibodies.

active
passive

Immunity that an individual develops in response to a harmful antigen is _____ immunity. Borrowed immunity that is effective for only a short time is _____ immunity.

3-159 In both active and passive immunity, the recognition of specific antigens is called *specific immunity.* The terms *natural* and *artificial* refer to how the immunity is obtained (Fig. 3.49).

A **vaccination** is any injection or ingestion of inactivated or killed microbes or their products that is administered to induce immunity. Vaccinations are available to immunize against many diseases, such as typhoid, diphtheria, polio, measles, and mumps. Depending on its type, vaccine is administered orally or by injection. Vaccination is a form of **prophylaxis,** prevention of or protection against disease. Which type of immunity (active or passive) results from having a disease or receiving a vaccination to prevent disease? _____

active

KEY POINT The toxins of toxoids are antigens, which cause our bodies to produce antibodies. A **toxoid** is a toxin that has been treated to eliminate its harmful properties without destroying its ability to stimulate antibody production.

antibodies

3-160 Polio vaccine contains polio antigen, which causes the formation of polio _____. After receiving the polio vaccine, one is immunized against poliomyelitis for a specific length of time.

Occasionally, the interaction of our defense mechanisms with an antigen results in an excessive reaction called **hyper/sensitivity.** Write this word that means a heightened reaction to an antigen: _____.

hypersensitivity

Anaphylaxis or **anaphylactic reactions** are exaggerated, life-threatening hypersensitivity reactions to a previously encountered antigen. The suffix -phylaxis means protection, and ana- means upward, excessive, or again. With a wide range in the severity of symptoms, the reactions may include generalized itching, difficult breathing, airway obstruction, and shock. Insect stings and penicillin are two common causes of anaphylactic shock, a severe and sometimes fatal systemic hypersensitivity reaction.

3-161 Allergies are conditions in which the body reacts with an exaggerated immune response to common, harmless substances, most of which are found in the environment.

🔑 **KEY** POINT An **allergen** is a substance that can produce an allergic reaction but is not otherwise harmful. Some common allergens are certain foods, pollen, animal dander, feathers, and house dust.

allergens

Essentially harmless substances that cause allergies are called _____. Allergy testing is used to identify the specific allergens. The most common is skin testing, which exposes the patient to small quantities of the suspected allergens.

In an allergic reaction, injured cells release a substance called **histamine,** which causes dilation of the capillaries (the smallest blood vessels), an increase in gastric secretion, and contraction of smooth muscle of several internal organs. Histamine is responsible for the symptoms of hay fever: teary eyes, sneezing, and swollen membranes of the upper respiratory tract. An **anti/histamine,** a

against

preparation that acts _____ histamine, usually relieves the symptoms.

3-162 Immuno/compromised pertains to an immune response that has been weakened by a disease or an **immuno/suppressive** agent. Radiation and certain drugs are **immuno/suppressants,** meaning

immune

that they suppress the _____ response.

In a broad sense, **immunotherapy** is treatment of disease by enhancing or suppressing an immune response. Cancer immunotherapy uses man-made antibodies designed to attach to cancer cells and mark them for destruction by our immune systems. The drugs allow the immune system to recognize the tumor; but unfortunately, the therapy is not always effective.

➤ **BEYOND** THE BLUEPRINT David Vetter, "The Boy in the Bubble," was born with a rare immunodeficiency disease. He spent his 12 years of life inside a sterile isolator with a layer of plastic shielding him from microorganisms. He died 2 weeks after being removed from the "bubble." Read David's story that was presented on the American Experience at *www.pbs.org*.

3-163 To **transplant** is to transfer tissue. The tissue that is transplanted is called a *transplant*. The pronunciation of the term depends on its usage as a verb or a noun. When tissue is transplanted from one person to another, rejection is often a problem. **Rejection** is an immune reaction to the donor's tissue cells with ultimate destruction of the transplanted tissue. Medications are used to suppress immune reactions, but the drugs have side effects. Rejection is still the most common problem encountered in transplantation of tissue from one person to another.

3-164 Immunodeficiency diseases are a group of diseases caused by a defect in the immune system and are generally characterized by susceptibility to infections and chronic diseases. Acquired immune deficiency syndrome or **acquired immunodeficiency syndrome** (AIDS) is a disease of the human immune system caused by the **human immunodeficiency virus** (HIV). Latter stages of AIDS leave individuals susceptible to opportunistic infections and tumors. Although treatments can slow the course of AIDS, there is currently no known cure or vaccine. AIDS means acquired

immunodeficiency

_____ syndrome.

🔑 **KEY** POINT AIDS occurs throughout the world, but more than three-fourths of the deaths in 2007 due to AIDS occurred in sub-Saharan Africa. HIV is transmitted through direct contact of a mucous membrane or body fluid of an infected person, such as vaginal fluid, semen, blood, and breast milk. Transmission can involve vaginal, anal, or oral sex, blood transfusion, contaminated hypodermic needles, or exchange between mother and fetus during pregnancy, childbirth, or breastfeeding.

cells

3-165 Although a toxoid is a helpful form of toxin, be aware that many words containing tox(o) refer to substances that have an adverse effect. For example, a **cyto/toxin** has harmful effects on _____. **Cyto/tox/icity** is the degree to which an agent possesses a specific destructive action on cells. This term is used in referring to the lysis of cells by immune phenomena, and it is also used to describe the activity of antineoplastic drugs that selectively kill cells. Anti/neo/plastic means inhibiting or preventing development of neoplasms, malignant tumors.

Tox/icity is the degree to which something is poisonous or a condition that results from exposure to a toxin or to toxic amounts of a substance that does not cause adverse effects in smaller amounts.

Write words in the blanks to complete these sentences.

1. A foreign substance that induces production of antibodies is called a/an _____.

2. Lacking resistance is being _____ to a disease.

3. Another name for "antibody" is _____.

4. A special protein of the body that specifically reacts to viruses is _____.

5. _____ immunity occurs when an individual's body produces an immune response to a harmful antigen.

6. AIDS is an abbreviation for acquired _____ syndrome.

PHARMACOLOGY

The pharmaceuticals in the following list affect multiple systems throughout the body.

In vivo Anticoagulants: *Prevent clotting of blood*

enoxaparin (Lovenox) heparin (Panheprin) warfarin (Coumadin)

Antihistamines: *Block histamine-1 receptors to relieve allergy symptoms*

cetirizine (Zyrtec) diphenhydramine (Benadryl) loratadine (Claritin)
chlorpheniramine (Chlor-Trimeton) fexofenadine (Allegra) promethazine (Phenergan)

Antiinflammatory Drugs: *Reduce inflammation*
Corticosteroids: *Glucocorticoid-acting steroids suppress inflammation and immunity, while mineralocorticoid-acting steroids regulate the balance of salt and water in the body*

dexamethasone (Decadron) hydrocortisone (Cortef) prednisone (Rayos)
fludrocortisone (Florinef) methylprednisolone (Medrol) triamcinolone (Kenalog)

Nonsteroidal Antiinflammatory Drugs (NSAIDs): *Mild to moderate pain relief; reduction of inflammation without steroids*

aspirin (Bayer) indomethacin (Indocin) naproxen (Aleve)
celecoxib (Celebrex) ketoprofen (Orudis) oxaprozin (Daypro)
diclofenac (Arthrotec) ketorolac (Toradol) sulindac (Clinoril)
ibuprofen (Motrin) nabumetone (Relafen)

Antineoplastic/Cytotoxic/Chemotherapeutic Agents: *Destroy or inhibit growth of cancerous cells*
Subclasses include alkylating agents, anthracyclines, antimetabolites, terpenoids, plant alkaloids, topoisomerase inhibitors, and monoclonal antibodies

cisplatin (Platinol) melphalan (Alkeran) tamoxifen (Soltamox)
cyclophosphamide (Cytoxan) methotrexate (Trexall) vincristine (Oncovin)
doxorubicin (Doxil) paclitaxel (Taxol)
fluorouracil (Efudex) rituximab (Rituxan)

Antipyretics: *Reduce fever*

acetaminophen (Tylenol) aspirin (Bayer) ibuprofen (Motrin)

Immunosuppressants: *Inhibit immune system*

azathioprine (Imuran) everolimus (Zortress) mycophenolate (CellCept)
cyclosporine (Neoral) glatiramer (Copaxone) tacrolimus (Prograf)

PHARMACOLOGY, cont'd

Antiinfectives/Antimicrobials: Kill or stop growth of microbes to fight infection
Antibiotics: Kill or inhibit growth of bacteria, fungi, or protozoa

Antibacterials: *Treat bacterial infections*
Antibacterials are grouped into many subclasses such as aminoglycosides, cephalosporins, fluoroquinolones, macrolides, penicillins, sulfonamides, and tetracyclines based on chemical structure, method of action, and the type of bacteria they are effective against

amoxicillin (Amoxil)	ciprofloxacin (Cipro)	nitrofurantoin (Macrobid)
ampicillin (Principen)	clarithromycin (Biaxin)	penicillin V (Veetids)
azithromycin (Zithromax)	erythromycin (Ery-Tab)	sulfamethoxazole/trimethoprim (Septra)
cefaclor (Ceclor)	fidaxomicin (Dificid)	tetracycline (Sumycin)
cefpodoxime (Vantin)	gentamicin (Garamycin)	tobramycin (Nebcin)
ceftazidime (Fortaz)	levofloxacin (Levaquin)	vancomycin (Vancocin)
cephalexin (Keflex)	minocycline (Minocin)	

Antifungals: *Treat fungal infections*

amphotericin B (Abelcet)	ketoconazole (Nizoral)	terbinafine (Lamisil)
fluconazole (Diflucan)	nystatin (Mycostatin)	

Antiprotozoals: *Treat protozoal infections*
Antimalarials are antiprotozoals that specifically treat malaria

atovaquone (Mepron)	mefloquine (Lariam)	pyrimethamine (Daraprim)
hydroxychloroquine (Plaquenil)	metronidazole (Flagyl)	

Antitubercular Agents: *Antibacterials that specifically treat tuberculosis*

ethambutol (Myambutol)	pyrazinamide (Rifater, in combination)
isoniazid (Laniazid)	rifampin (Rifadin)

Anthelmintics: *Destroy or expel parasitic worms*

ivermectin (Stromectol)	mebendazole (Vermox)

Antivirals: *Treat viral infections*

acyclovir (Zovirax)	famciclovir (Famvir)	ganciclovir (Cytovene)
amantadine (Symmetrel)	foscarnet (Foscavir)	oseltamivir (Tamiflu)

Vaccine/Immunization: *Modified version of a disease-causing agent that induces resistance to that disease*

cholera vaccine (Shanchol)	human papillomavirus quadrivalent vaccine (Gardasil)	meningitis vaccine (Menveo)
diphtheria, tetanus toxoids, acellular pertussis vaccine (DTaP)	inactivated poliovirus (IPV)	pneumococcal conjugate vaccine (Prevnar)
hepatitis B vaccine (Recombivax HB)	influenza vaccine (Fluzone)	rotavirus vaccine (Rotarix)
	measles, mumps, rubella vaccine (MMR)	typhoid fever vaccine (Vivotif)
		varicella vaccine (Varivax)

MATCH IT!
EXERCISE 46

___ **1.** antibiotics

___ **2.** antiinflammatories

___ **3.** antihelmintics

___ **4.** antihistamines

___ **5.** immunosuppressants

___ **6.** antineoplastics

A. block histamines and relieve allergy symptoms

B. destroy or inhibit growth of cancer cells

C. destroy parasitic worms

D. inhibit the immune system

E. kill or inhibit growth of bacteria, fungi, or protozoa

F. reduce inflammation

COMMON ABBREVIATIONS IN MEDICAL RECORDS

3-166 You will encounter dozens of abbreviations in medical records such as DOB, meaning date of birth. Many are concerned with medication administration, units of measure, or information obtained from the history (Hx) or examinations. Study the Chapter Abbreviations list on page 145 to complete the next frames and exercises and use the abbreviations you've already learned. Practice using flash cards of the abbreviations and their meanings, or use the electronic flash cards available on the Evolve website.

3-167 You have already learned several abbreviations, but one that is commonly seen is HEENT, a convenient way of referring to the head, eye, ear, nose, and throat. WD/WN is an easy way to describe a child who appears appropriately developed and well nourished (WD/WN) for his or her age.

The patient's state of mind and ability to correctly perceive the environment may be reported as A&O (alert and oriented). If one's parents are still living with only minor health concerns, the examiner may note the parents as L&W (living and well). So, recognize these new abbreviations, including HEENT, an abbreviation for the head, eye, ear, nose, and _____.

throat

Also, the patient may be described as A&O, alert and _____.

oriented

3-168 WD/WN means well developed, well _____.

nourished

3-169 L&W means living and _____.

well

> **BEYOND** THE BLUEPRINT Some references list more than 20,000 medical abbreviations and acronyms. However, use great care in both reading and writing abbreviations, and use them sparingly because of the danger of misinterpreting (for example, the dosage of medicine to be given a patient).

3-170 Abbreviations used in measuring length are cm (1/1000 of a meter) and m, which mean centimeter and _____, respectively.

meter

3-171 Abbreviations used in measuring weight are g, mg, and mcg, which mean _____, milligram (1/1000 of a gram), and microgram (1/1,000,000 of a gram), respectively.

gram

3-172 Common liquid measures include liter, deciliter, and milliliter, using the abbreviations L, dL, and _____, respectively.

milliliter

WRITE IT! EXERCISE 47

Write the meanings of the abbreviations for questions 1-20.

1. cm _____
2. dL _____
3. g _____
4. kg _____
5. L _____
6. mcg _____
7. mg _____
8. mL _____
9. A&O _____
10. BP _____
11. CC _____
12. DOB _____
13. Dx _____
14. Hx _____
15. P _____
16. PE _____
17. R _____
18. ROM _____
19. RUQ _____
20. T _____

WRITE IT! EXERCISE 48

Write the abbreviation for each of the following:

1. twice per day _____
2. hour _____
3. intravenous _____
4. minutes _____
5. orally _____
6. alert and oriented _____
7. head, eyes, ears, nose, throat _____
8. living and well _____
9. well-developed, well nourished _____

CHAPTER ABBREVIATIONS*

A&O	alert and oriented	**min**	minutes
AHF	antihemophilic factor	**mono**	monocyte
AIDS	acquired immunodeficiency syndrome	**neut**	neutrophil
AP	anteroposterior (also others)	**PA**	posteroanterior (also others)
baso	basophil	**PT**	prothrombin time (also physical therapy)
CBC, cbc	complete blood count	**PTT**	partial thromboplastin time
CMV	cytomegalovirus	**RBC**	red blood cell, red blood cell count
DIC	disseminated intravascular coagulation	**Rh**	rhesus (a blood group)
DNA	deoxyribonucleic acid	**RLQ**	right lower quadrant
EBV	Epstein-Barr virus	**ROM**	range of motion
EEG	electroencephalogram	**RPR**	rapid plasma reagin
eos	eosinophil	**RUQ**	right upper quadrant
h	hour *(hora)*	**WBC**	white blood cell, white blood cell count
Hb, Hgb	hemoglobin	**WD, WN**	well developed, well nourished
HCT, Hct	hematocrit		

Units of Measure

HDN	hemolytic disease of the newborn	**cm**	centimeter
HEENT	head, eye, ear, nose, throat	**dL**	deciliter
HIV	human immunodeficiency virus	**g**	gram
Hx	history	**kg**	kilogram
INR	International Normalized Ratio	**L**	liter
IV	intravenous	**mcg**	microgram
L&W	living and well	**mg**	milligram
LLQ	left lower quadrant	**mL**	milliliter
LUQ	left upper quadrant		
lymph	lymphocyte		

*Many of these abbreviations share their meanings with other terms.

! Be Careful With These!

hidr(o) vs. *hydr(o)*	*immunity* vs. *immunocompromised*	*en-, end-, endo-* (inside) vs. *ecto-, exo-, extra-* (outside)
in- (not) vs. *in-* (inside)	*intracellular* vs. *extracellular*	
infra- (under) vs. *intra-* (within)	*leukopenia* vs. *leukocytosis*	*hyper-* (more than normal) vs. *hypo-* (less than normal)
autologous vs. *homologous*	*microcyte* vs. *macrocyte* or *megalocyte*	
coagulant vs. *anticoagulant*	*mucus* vs. *mucous*	*macro-* (large) vs. *micro-* (small)
erythropenia vs. *erythrocytosis*	*resistance* vs. *susceptibility*	*nulli-* (none) vs. *pan-* (all)
excretion vs. *secretion*	**Opposites**	*proxim(o)* vs. *dist(o)*
hyperkalemia vs. *hypokalemia*	*ab-* (away from) vs. *ad-* (toward)	*prone* vs. *supine*
hypocalcemia vs. *hypercalcemia*	*febrile* vs. *afebrile*	*super-, supra-* (above) vs. *hypo-, infra-, sub-* (below)
hypochromic vs. *hyperchromic*	*ante-, pre-* (before) vs. *post-* (after)	
hyponatremia vs. *hypernatremia*	*anter(o)* vs. *poster(o)*	*ventr(o)* vs. *dors(o)*

A Career as a Medical Technologist

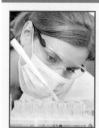

Bethany Euclid loves her job as a medical technologist. She works in a usually quiet environment, but also has unpredictable tests to run on a "stat" or emergent basis. She completed a bachelor's degree to prepare for the certification exam, and is employed in a hospital lab. She mainly runs tests on body fluids (blood, sputum, urine, etc.), and uses equipment to run many of the analyses. Her favorite part is when the results help the physician establish a diagnosis and quickly begin treating a very sick patient. Bethany knows she is an integral part of the diagnostic medical process. For more information, visit *ascp.org* or *www.americanmedtech.org*.

CHAPTER 3 SELF-TEST

Review the new word parts for this chapter. Work all of the following exercises to test your understanding of the material before checking your answers against those in Appendix IV.

BASIC UNDERSTANDING

Matching

I. Match the prefixes on the left with their meanings on the right.

_____ **1.** di-	**A.** all
_____ **2.** diplo-	**B.** below normal
_____ **3.** hyper-	**C.** double
_____ **4.** hypo-	**D.** four
_____ **5.** nulli-	**E.** many
_____ **6.** pan-	**F.** more than normal
_____ **7.** poly-	**G.** none
_____ **8.** quad-	**H.** one
_____ **9.** tri-	**I.** three
_____ **10.** uni-	**J.** two

II. Match the prefixes on the left with their meanings on the right. All choices will not be used, and some will be used more than once.

_____ **1.** ab-	**A.** away from
_____ **2.** di-	**B.** excessive
_____ **3.** hemi-	**C.** half, partly
_____ **4.** milli-	**D.** many
_____ **5.** mono-	**E.** one
_____ **6.** multi-	**F.** one hundred or one hundredth
_____ **7.** poly-	**G.** one thousandth
_____ **8.** semi-	**H.** toward
_____ **9.** super-	**I.** two
_____ **10.** supra-	**J.** three
_____ **11.** tetra-	**K.** four

III. Match descriptions in the left column with A, B, or C.

_____ **1.** body defense	**A.** leukocyte
_____ **2.** blood platelet	**B.** erythrocyte
_____ **3.** contains hemoglobin	**C.** thrombocyte
_____ **4.** initiates coagulation	
_____ **5.** transports oxygen	

IV. Match each type of immunity with its description in the right column.

_____ **1.** active natural	**A.** contracting a disease
_____ **2.** active artificial	**B.** exposure of the fetus to maternal antibodies
_____ **3.** passive artificial	**C.** receiving a vaccination
_____ **4.** passive natural	**D.** receiving an injection of antibodies

V. *Match the signs and symptoms of anemia in the left column with their meanings in the right column.*

_____ **1.** angina   **A.** chest pain

_____ **2.** dyspnea   **B.** difficult breathing

_____ **3.** pallor   **C.** fainting

_____ **4.** syncope   **D.** increased pulse rate

_____ **5.** tachycardia   **E.** paleness

_____ **6.** tinnitus   **F.** ringing in the ears

Labeling

VI. *Use the following terms to label planes #1 through #3 (frontal, sagittal, transverse) and aspects #4 through #6 (inferior, lateral, superior) in the illustration.*

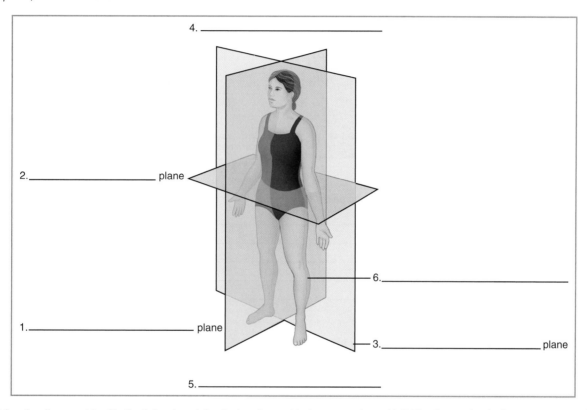

4. _____

2. _____ plane

1. _____ plane

6. _____

3. _____ plane

5. _____

VII. *Using the diagram, identify the following abdominal regions with the correct letter (A-I). The first region is done as an example.*

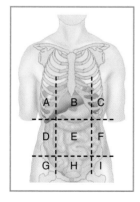

1. epigastric   _B_

2. hypogastric   _____

3. left hypochondriac   _____

4. left iliac   _____

5. left lumbar   _____

6. right hypochondriac   _____

7. right iliac   _____

8. right lumbar   _____

9. umbilical   _____

VIII. Build terms using these word parts to identify these illustrations. (Prefixes may be used more than once.)
hyper-, -plasia, -trophy

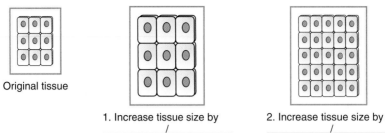

Original tissue

1. Increase tissue size by _____/_____

2. Increase tissue size by _____/_____

IX.   Use word parts to write terms to label 1 to 3.

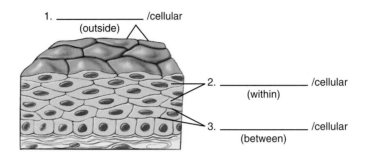

1. _____ /cellular
(outside)

2. _____ /cellular
(within)

3. _____ /cellular
(between)

Listing

X.   Name five body defenses that react to pathogens, in general.

1. _____

2. _____

3. _____

4. _____

5. _____

Deconstructing Words

XI.   Divide these terms into their component parts, and define the terms.

1. cellular _____

2. coagulant _____

3. postnasal _____

4. tachyphasia _____

5. transdermal _____

XII.   Circle the prefixes in each grouping. Then write the common meaning of the prefixes.

1. antemortem, prenatal   _____

2. macrocyte, macroscopic, megadose   _____

3. monocyte, mononeuropathy, uniglandular   _____

4. quadruplets, tetralogy   _____

XIII. The following terms end in -plasia and describe abnormal tissue formation. Write the meaning of each term.

Term	**Meaning**
1. aplasia	_____
2. anaplasia	_____
3. dysplasia	_____
4. hyperplasia	_____
5. hypoplasia	_____

Using Vocabulary

XIV. Circle the correct answer in each of the following questions.

1. Mrs. Hill is told that the type of disorder which she has affects a single nerve. Which term describes Mrs. Hill's disorder? (monocyte, mononeuropathy, nullipara, uniglandular)

2. Which term is used in naming a muscle that has three heads? (bipedal, dipedal, triceps, triplegia)

3. What is the name of the substance from which fibrin originates? (fibrinogen, fibrinolysis, thrombogen, thrombolysis)

4. An epidemiologist was concerned that an influenza virus would spread and infect a large proportion of the human population. What is the term for this type of epidemic? (endemic, isolated epidemic, pandemic, sporadic epidemic)

5. An infant is born with six fingers on one hand. What is the term for this developmental abnormality? (diplopia, hypothyroidism, polydactyly, symmetry)

6. The physical therapist has Joan move each arm in a circular movement. What is the term for this movement? (abduction, adduction, circumduction, extension)

7. A microbiologist is studying a pathogenic microorganism. What is the term for the degree of disease-causing capability of the organism? (resistance, sensitivity, susceptibility, virulence)

8. Dr. Hoffmann prescribes a special patch for Natalie to wear to avoid seasickness on her 3-day cruise. What type of drug delivery is provided in the patch? (intramuscular, intravenous, subcutaneous, transdermal)

9. In studying embryology, Clark learns the names of the embryonic layers in development. What is the name of the middle layer? (blastoderm, ectoderm, endoderm, mesoderm)

10. The physician examines Mr. White's spine and determines that the spine is straight and both sides of his back appear normal. What is the term for correspondence of parts on opposite sides of a dividing line? (endoscopy, midsection, symmetry, syndrome)

11. Which of the following means a collection of similar cells acting together to perform a function? (body system, organ, organism, tissue)

12. Mrs. Coffee's bone marrow study indicates that her bone marrow cells are not developing into new blood cells, resulting in a deficiency of all the formed elements in the blood, especially the erythrocytes. Which term best describes Mrs. Coffee's type of anemia? (analytic, anisocytosis, aplastic, hemolytic)

13. The autopsy report states, "The bullet is missing, but damage to the abdomen indicates an anteroposterior trajectory." What is the trajectory of the bullet? (back to front, back to side, front to back, front to side)

14. Dr. Ray explains in a radiology report that a fracture has occurred in the distal portion of the thigh bone. What is meant by "distal"? (farther from the origin, in the middle of the bone, nearer the origin, on the side of the bone)

15. Alison's resistance prevented her from getting influenza when she was exposed to the H1N1 virus. Which of the following may have been part of her specific resistance to the H1N1 virus? (antibodies, intact skin, interferon, phagocytosis)

16. Eddie falls and skins his knee, which later shows swelling and redness. The pediatrician says the redness and swelling is part of the body's normal defensive response to injury. Which is the cause of the swelling and redness? (erythropenia, infection, inflammation, xanthoderma)

17. The instructions are to "place the child in a prone position." Which is true of the child's position? (lying face downward, lying on the back, lying on the left side, lying on the right side)

18. Shelley has a noninflammatory skin condition. What is the skin condition called? (dermatitis, dermatosis, pyosis, pyrexia)

19. Which of the following is the most abundant body fluid? (extracellular, interstitial, intracellular, plasma)

20. Which of these terms means a muscular partition that separates the thoracic and abdominopelvic cavities? (diaphragm, paracentesis, peritoneum, pyrogen)

Identifying Illustrations

XV. Identify the illustrations using one of these terms: abduction, adduction, hydrocephalus, paracentesis, polydactyly, syndactylism.

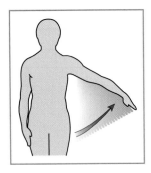 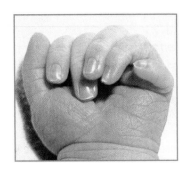 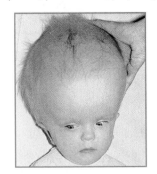

1. _____ **2.** _____ **3.** _____

Opting for Opposites

XVI. Use a- or an- to write terms that have the opposite meanings of these words.

1. esthesia vs. _____
2. hydrous vs. _____
3. plastic vs. _____
4. symptomatic vs. _____
5. traumatic vs. _____

Writing Terms

XVII. Write a term for each of the following meanings.

1. a homologous graft _____
2. a record of electrical impulses of the brain _____
3. a small erythrocyte _____
4. abnormal development of tissue _____
5. affecting only one side _____
6. below normal sodium in the blood _____
7. body's ability to resist infectious disease _____
8. cramping of the hand _____
9. dissolving of a thrombus _____
10. formation of a thrombus _____
11. inflammation of the skin _____
12. localized collection of pus in a cavity _____
13. lying flat on the back _____
14. most abundant blood cell _____
15. pertaining to above the chest _____
16. pertaining to the abdomen and pelvis _____
17. pertaining to the peritoneum _____
18. pertaining to the sole _____
19. production of blood _____
20. within cells _____

Making Connections

XVIII. The following terms describe types of tissue grafts. Write the meaning of each term.

1. autologous _____

_____

2. homologous _____

_____

Finetuning Terms

XIX. In addition to spelling, describe at least one difference in the following:

1. afebrile and antifebrile _____

_____

2. agglutination vs. coagulation _____

_____

3. erythropoiesis vs. erythropoietin _____

_____

4. excretion vs. secretion _____

_____

5. inflammation vs. infection _____

_____

6. parietal vs. visceral peritoneum _____

_____

7. plasma vs. interstitial fluid _____

_____

8. prone vs. supine _____

_____

9. somatic cells vs. stem cells _____

_____

Describing Differences

XX. Describe the difference in the use of prefixes in these terms.

1. postnatal and postnasal _____

_____

2. supervitaminosis and suprarenal _____

_____

3. macrocyte and megalocyte _____

_____

Opting for Opposites

XXI. Write a term that you learned that means the opposite of these words.

1. adduct _____   **8.** hyperplasia _____

2. bradyphasia _____   **9.** hypokalemia _____

3. coagulant _____   **10.** inferior _____

4. compatible _____   **11.** intracellular _____

5. contralateral _____   **12.** megalocyte _____

6. febrile _____   **13.** prenatal _____

7. hyperchromic _____   **14.** proximal _____

GREATER COMPREHENSION

Health Care Reporting

XXII. Read the following consultation report. Then write the term or abbreviation from the report that is described in questions 1-8. Although you may be unfamiliar with some of the terms, you should be able to determine their meanings by considering their word parts.

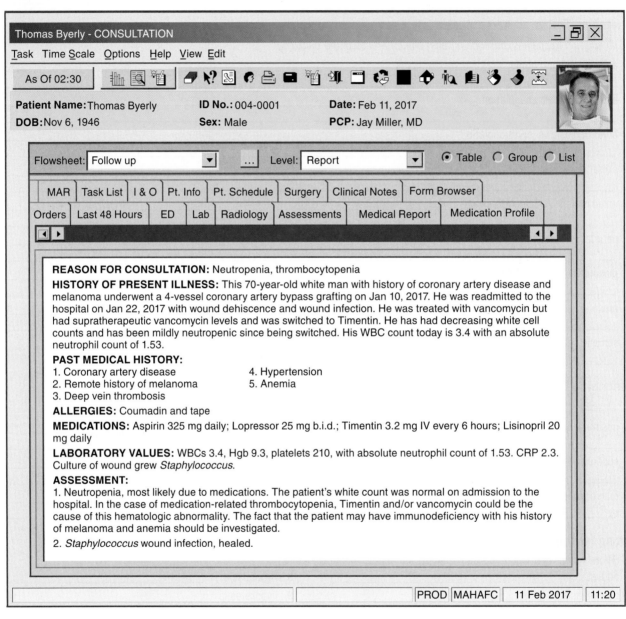

Write the term.

1. a bursting open, splitting or gaping of a wound _____

2. above the normal dosage needed for treatment _____

3. decrease in the number of blood platelets _____

4. deficiency in erythrocytes, hemoglobin, or both _____

5. internal blood clot _____

6. lack of body's natural ability to ward off infectious disease(s) _____

7. pertaining to hematology _____

8. twice a day _____

XXIII. Read the following physical examination report, and define the terms or abbreviations that follow the report. Although you may be unfamiliar with some terms, you should be able to determine their meanings by considering their word parts.

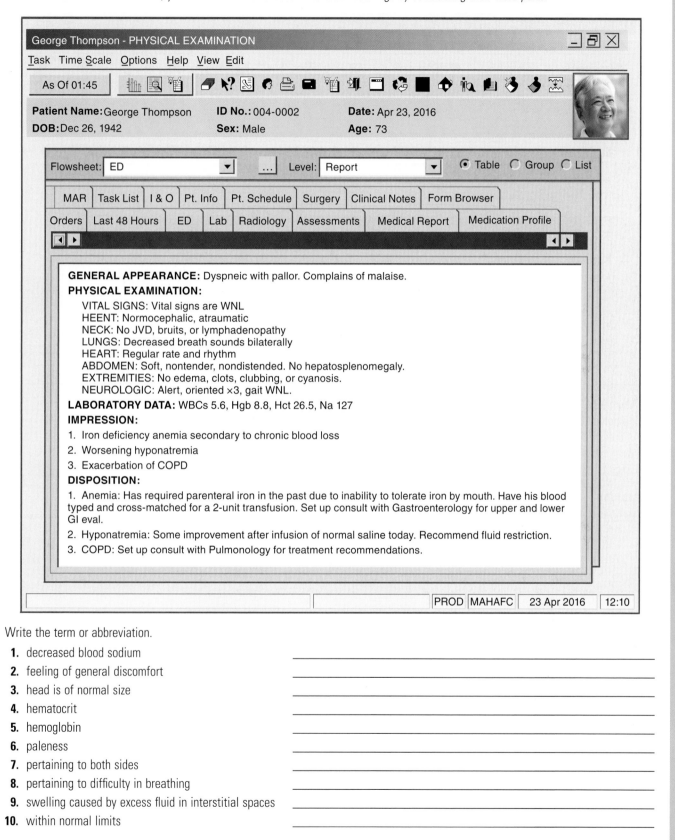

George Thompson - PHYSICAL EXAMINATION

Task Time Scale Options Help View Edit

As Of 01:45

Patient Name: George Thompson   **ID No.:** 004-0002   **Date:** Apr 23, 2016
DOB: Dec 26, 1942   **Sex:** Male   **Age:** 73

Flowsheet: ED ... Level: Report ● Table ○ Group ○ List

MAR | Task List | I & O | Pt. Info | Pt. Schedule | Surgery | Clinical Notes | Form Browser

Orders | Last 48 Hours | ED | Lab | Radiology | Assessments | Medical Report | Medication Profile

GENERAL APPEARANCE: Dyspneic with pallor. Complains of malaise.
PHYSICAL EXAMINATION:
    VITAL SIGNS: Vital signs are WNL
    HEENT: Normocephalic, atraumatic
    NECK: No JVD, bruits, or lymphadenopathy
    LUNGS: Decreased breath sounds bilaterally
    HEART: Regular rate and rhythm
    ABDOMEN: Soft, nontender, nondistended. No hepatosplenomegaly.
    EXTREMITIES: No edema, clots, clubbing, or cyanosis.
    NEUROLOGIC: Alert, oriented ×3, gait WNL.
LABORATORY DATA: WBCs 5.6, Hgb 8.8, Hct 26.5, Na 127
IMPRESSION:
1. Iron deficiency anemia secondary to chronic blood loss
2. Worsening hyponatremia
3. Exacerbation of COPD
DISPOSITION:
1. Anemia: Has required parenteral iron in the past due to inability to tolerate iron by mouth. Have his blood typed and cross-matched for a 2-unit transfusion. Set up consult with Gastroenterology for upper and lower GI eval.
2. Hyponatremia: Some improvement after infusion of normal saline today. Recommend fluid restriction.
3. COPD: Set up consult with Pulmonology for treatment recommendations.

PROD | MAHAFC | 23 Apr 2016 | 12:10

Write the term or abbreviation.

1. decreased blood sodium   _____

2. feeling of general discomfort   _____

3. head is of normal size   _____

4. hematocrit   _____

5. hemoglobin   _____

6. paleness   _____

7. pertaining to both sides   _____

8. pertaining to difficulty in breathing   _____

9. swelling caused by excess fluid in interstitial spaces   _____

10. within normal limits   _____

XXIV. Read the following postoperative note and circle the correct answer in the statements or questions that follow.

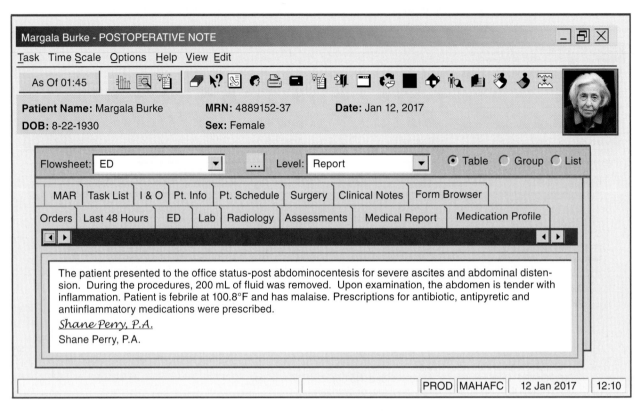

Margala Burke - POSTOPERATIVE NOTE

Task Time Scale Options Help View Edit

As Of 01:45

Patient Name: Margala Burke   **MRN:** 4889152-37   **Date:** Jan 12, 2017
DOB: 8-22-1930   **Sex:** Female

Flowsheet: ED   ...   Level: Report   ⦿ Table ○ Group ○ List

MAR | Task List | I & O | Pt. Info | Pt. Schedule | Surgery | Clinical Notes | Form Browser
Orders | Last 48 Hours | ED | Lab | Radiology | Assessments | Medical Report | Medication Profile

> The patient presented to the office status-post abdominocentesis for severe ascites and abdominal disten-sion. During the procedures, 200 mL of fluid was removed. Upon examination, the abdomen is tender with inflammation. Patient is febrile at 100.8°F and has malaise. Prescriptions for antibiotic, antipyretic and antiinflammatory medications were prescribed.
>
> *Shane Perry, P.A.*
> Shane Perry, P.A.

PROD | MAHAFC | 12 Jan 2017 | 12:10

1. Which term describes the patient's fever? (ascites, distension, febrile, malaise)
2. The patient had undergone an abdominal procedure that involved surgical (incision, puncture, removal, repair).
3. An antipyretic is prescribed for which of the following? (ascites, fever, infection, pain)
4. Which medication was prescribed to act against living microscopic organisms? (antibiotics, antiinflammatory, antipyretic)
5. Which term indicates that the abdomen is enlarged? (abdominocentesis, distension, inflammation, status-post)

Matching

XXV. Match the signs and symptoms of severe anemia in the left column with the correct meaning in the right column: (Not all choices will be used.)

_____ **1.** dyspnea   **A.** difficult breathing
_____ **2.** pallor   **B.** fainting
_____ **3.** syncope   **C.** loss of appetite
_____ **4.** tinnitus   **D.** nausea
                             E. paleness
                             F. ringing in the ears

Spelling

XXVI. Circle all misspelled terms, and write their correct spellings.

abdomin   acrosyanosis   adiction   antiperspirant   hydrosephalus   ipselateral   palmar   phagocytosis   toxisity   suprarenal

Abbreviating

XXVII. Write three-letter abbreviations that correspond to the following clues.

1. carrier of genetic information   ___ ___ ___   6. iron-containing pigment in an erythrocyte   ___ ___ ___
2. complete blood count   ___ ___ ___   7. leukocyte   ___ ___ ___
3. electroencephalogram   ___ ___ ___   8. quadrant below the right upper quadrant   ___ ___ ___
4. extent of circular movement of a joint   ___ ___ ___   9. screening test for syphilis   ___ ___ ___
5. hematocrit   ___ ___ ___   10. virus that causes AIDS   ___ ___ ___

Pronouncing Terms

XXVIII. Write the correct term for the following phonetic spellings.

1. an-uh-fuh-**lak**-sis _____
2. an-**ō**-shuh _____
3. **eks**-ū-dāt _____
4. **kī**-rō-plas-tē _____
5. hi-pur-pī-**rek**-sē-uh _____
6. im-ū-nō-**kom**-pruh-mīzd _____
7. in-tur-**stish**-ul _____
8. puh-**rī**-uh-tul _____
9. staf-uh-lō-kok-**sē**-mē-uh _____
10. **om**-fuh-lō-sēl _____

Using Pharmacologic Terms

XXIX. Circle the correct answer to the following questions.

1. Which of the following are modified versions of a disease-causing agent that induce resistance in that disease? (antiinfectives/ antimicrobials, immunosuppressants, cytotoxic agents, vaccine/immunization)
2. Which is used specifically to inhibit the immune system? (antihistamines, antiinflammatory drugs, immunosuppressants, antineoplastics)
3. Which of the following are used specifically to reduce fever? (antibiotics, antipyretics, antituberculars, antihelmintics)
4. Which of the following are used to destroy or expel parasitic worms? (antihelmintics, antimalarials, antibiotics, chemotherapeutics)
5. Which of the following are grouped into many subclasses such as cephalosporins and tetracyclines? (antibacterials, antiprotozoals, antituberculars, antivirals)

Categorizing Terms and Practicing Pronunciation

XXX. Categorize the terms in the left column by selecting A, B, C, D, or E

_____ **1.** abscess	**A.** anatomical term
_____ **2.** antiinfectives	**B.** diagnostic test or procedure
_____ **3.** corpuscle	**C.** a disease or disorder
_____ **4.** diaphragm	**D.** surgical term
_____ **5.** dyscrasia	**E.** nonsurgical therapeutic term
_____ **6.** electrocardiography	
_____ **7.** hematocrit	
_____ **8.** midsagittal plane	
_____ **9.** omphalocele	
_____ **10.** thrombectomy	
_____ **11.** tinnitus	
_____ **12.** transplant (of tissue, for example)	
_____ **13.** ultraviolet therapy	
_____ **14.** vaccination	

(Be prepared to pronounce terms 1-14 in class after listening to the Chapter 3 terms at *http://evolve.elsevier.com/Leonard/building/*. In addition, practice categorizing all terms in the BMV List.)

New Construction

XXXI. Break these words into their components parts, and write their meanings. Even if you have not seen these terms before, you may be able to break them apart and determine their meanings.

1. cephalocentesis _____
2. dactyledema _____
3. dorsodynia _____
4. erythroid _____
5. extraperitoneal _____
6. hemoglobinometer _____
7. leukopoiesis _____
8. otitis media _____
9. periappendicitis _____
10. thromboid _____

Use Appendix IV to check your answers to the exercises.

TOOL TIP! *Pay attention to spelling!*

BMV LIST

Visit **http://evolve.elsevier.com/Leonard/building/** *to listen to the boldface terms in Chapter 3. Look closely at the spelling of each term as it is pronounced.*

abdomen (**ab**-duh-mun)
abdominal (ab-**dom**-i-nul)
abdominal paracentesis (ab-**dom**-i-nul par-uh-sun-**tē**-sis)
abdominocentesis (ab-dom-i-nō-sen-**tē**-sis)
abdominopelvic cavity (ab-dom-i-nō-**pel**-vik **kav**-i-tē)
abdominoplasty (ab-**dom**-i-nō-plas-tē)
abdominothoracic (ab-dom-i-nō-thuh-**ras**-ik)
abduct (ab-**dukt**)
abscess (**ab**-ses)
acquired immunodeficiency syndrome (uh-**kwīrd** im-ū-nō-duh-**fish**-un-sē **sin**-drōm)
acrocyanosis (ak-rō-sī-uh-**nō**-sis)
acrodermatitis (ak-rō-dur-muh-**tī**-tis)
acromegaly (ak-rō-**meg**-uh-lē)
acroparalysis (ak-rō-puh-**ral**-i-sis)
adduct (uh-**dukt**)
afebrile (ā-**feb**-ril)
agglutination (uh-glōō-ti-**nā**-shun)
allergen (**al**-ur-jen)
allergies (**al**-ur-jēz)
allogeneic (al-ō-juh-**nē**-ik)
allogenic (al-ō-**jen**-ik)
allograft (**al**-ō-graft)
analeptic (an-uh-**lep**-tik)
anaphylactic reactions (an-uh-fuh-**lak**-tik rē-**ak**-shunz)
anaphylaxis (an-uh-fuh-**lak**-sis)
anaplasia (an-uh-**plā**-zhuh)
anatomic plane (an-uh-**tom**-ik plān)
anatomic position (an-uh-**tom**-ik puh-**zish**-un)
anatomy (uh-**nat**-uh-mē)

anemia (uh-**nē**-mē-uh)
angina pectoris (an-**jī**-nuh **pek**-tuh-ris)
anhydrous (an-**hī**-drus)
anotia (an-**ō**-shuh)
antemortem (an-tē-**mor**-tum)
anterior (an-**tēr**-ē-ur)
anterolateral (an-tur-ō-**lat**-ur-ul)
anteromedial (an-tur-ō-**mē**-dē-ul)
anteroposterior (an-tur-ō-pos-**tēr**-ē-ur)
anterosuperior (an-tur-ō-soo-**pēr**-ē-ur)
antibiotics (an-tē-bī-**ot**-iks)
antibodies (**an**-ti-bod-ēz)
anticoagulant (an-tē-kō-**ag**-ū-lunt)
antifebrile (an-tē-**feb**-ril)
antigen (**an**-ti-jun)
antihistamine (an-tē-**his**-tuh-mēn)
antihistamines (an-tē-**his**-tuh-mēnz)
antiinfective (an-tē-in-**fek**-tiv)
antiinflammatory (an-tē-in-**flam**-uh-tor-ē)
antiinflammatory drugs (an-tē-in-**flam**-uh-tor-ē drugz)
antimicrobial (an-tē-mī-**krō**-bē-ul)
antineoplastic agents (an-tē-nē-ō-**plas**-tik **ā**-junts)
antiperspirant (an-tē-**pur**-spur-unt)
antipyretics (an-tē-pī-**ret**-iks)
aplasia (uh-**plā**-zhuh)
aplastic (ā-**plas**-tik)
ascites (uh-**sī**-tēz)
asymptomatic (ā-simp-tō-**mat**-ik)
atraumatic (ā-traw-**mat**-ik)
autoimmune diseases (aw-tō-i-**mūn** di-**zēz**-uz)

autologous graft (aw-**tol**-uh-gus graft)
autologous transfusion (aw-**tol**-uh-gus trans-**fū**-zhun)
bacteremia (bak-tur-**ē**-mē-uh)
basophil (**bā**-sō-fil)
biceps (**bī**-seps)
bifocal (bī-**fō**-kul)
bilateral (bī-**lat**-ur-ul)
binuclear (bī-**noo**-klē-ur)
bipedal (bī-**ped**-ul)
blood platelets (blud **plāt**-luts)
blood transfusion (blud trans-**fū**-zhun)
bradyphasia (brad-i-**fā**-zhuh)
cardiovascular (kahr-dē-ō-**vas**-kū-lur)
caudad (**kaw**-dad)
caudal (**kaw**-dul)
cellular (**sel**-ū-lur)
Celsius (**sel**-sē-us)
centigrade (**sen**-ti-grād)
centimeter (**sen**-ti-mē-tur)
cephalad (**sef**-uh-lad)
cephalic (suh-**fal**-ik)
chemical addiction (**kem**-i-kul uh-**dik**-shun)
chemotherapeutic agents (kē-mō-ther-uh-**pū**-tik **ā**-junts)
chiroplasty (**kī**-rō-plas-tē)
chiropody (kī-**rop**-uh-dē)
chirospasm (**kī**-rō-spaz-um)
circumcision (sur-kum-**sizh**-un)
circumduction (sur-kum-**duk**-shun)
coagulant (kō-**ag**-ū-lunt)
coagulate (kō-**ag**-ū-lāt)
coagulation (kō-ag-ū-**lā**-shun)
coagulopathy (kō-ag-ū-**lop**-uh-thē)
complement (**kom**-pluh-munt)
connective tissue (kuh-**nek**-tiv tish-**oo**)
contraceptive (kon-truh-**sep**-tiv)
contralateral (kon-truh-**lat**-ur-ul)
corpuscle (**kor**-pus-ul)
cranial (**krā**-nē-ul)
cranial cavity (**krā**-nē-ul **kav**-i-tē)
cytotoxic agents (sī-tō-**tok**-sik **ā**-junts)
cytotoxicity (sī-tō-tok-**sis**-i-tē)
cytotoxin (**sī**-tō-tok-sin)
dactylitis (dak-tuh-**lī**-tis)
dactylogram (dak-**til**-ō-gram)
dactylography (dak-tuh-**log**-ruh-fē)
dactylospasm (**dak**-tuh-lō-spaz-um)
deciliter (**des**-i-lē-tur)
dehiscence (dē-**his**-uns)
dehydration (dē-hī-**drā**-shun)
dermatitis (dur-muh-**tī**-tis)
dermatoplasty (**dur**-muh-tō-plas-tē)
dermatosis (dur-muh-**tō**-sis)
diaphragm (**dī**-uh-fram)
diarrhea (dī-uh-**rē**-uh)
digits (**dij**-its)
dioxide (dī-**ok**-sīd)
diplopia (di-**plō**-pē-uh)

disseminated (di-**sem**-i-nāt-ud)
distal (**dis**-tul)
distension (dis-**ten**-shun)
dorsal (**dor**-sul)
dorsal cavity (**dor**-sul **kav**-i-tē)
dorsocephalad (dor-sō-**sef**-uh-lad)
dorsolateral (dor-sō-**lat**-ur-ul)
dorsoventral (dor-sō-**ven**-trul)
Down syndrome (doun **sin**-drōm)
dyscrasias (dis-**krā**-zhuz)
dyslexia (dis-**lek**-sē-uh)
dysphoria (dis-**for**-ē-uh)
dysplasia (dis-**plā**-zhuh)
dyspnea (disp-**nē**-uh)
ectopic (ek-**top**-ik)
ectopic pregnancy (ek-**top**-ik **preg**-nun-sē)
electroencephalogram (ē-lek-trō-en-**sef**-uh-lō-gram)
electroencephalograph (ē-lek-trō-en-**sef**-uh-lō-graf)
electroencephalography (ē-lek-trō-un-sef-uh-**log**-ruh-fē)
electrolytes (ē-**lek**-trō-līts)
embolism (**em**-buh-liz-um)
embolus (**em**-bō-lus)
encephalitis (en-sef-uh-**lī**-tis)
encephalopathy (en-sef-uh-**lop**-uh-thē)
endoscopy (en-**dos**-kuh-pē)
eosinophil (ē-ō-**sin**-ō-fil)
epidermis (ep-i-**dur**-mis)
epigastric region (ep-i-**gas**-trik **rē**-jun)
epithelial tissue (ep-i-**thē**-lē-ul tish-**oo**)
erythroblastosis fetalis (uh-rith-rō-blas-**tō**-sis fi-**ta**-lus)
erythroblasts (uh-**rith**-rō-blasts)
erythrocyte (uh-**rith**-rō-sīt)
erythrocytic (uh-rith-rō-**sit**-ik)
erythrocytopenia (uh-rith-rō-sī-tō-**pē**-nē-uh)
erythrocytosis (uh-rith-rō-sī-**tō**-sis)
erythropenia (uh-rith-rō-**pē**-nē-uh)
erythropoiesis (uh-rith-rō-poi-**ē**-sis)
erythropoietin (uh-rith-rō-**poi**-uh-tin)
euphoria (ū-**for**-ē-uh)
evisceration (ē-vis-ur-**ā**-shun)
excretion (eks-**krē**-shun)
extracellular (eks-truh-**sel**-ū-lur)
extracellular fluid (ex-truh-**sel**-ū-lur **floo**-id)
extremities (ek-**strem**-i-tēz)
exudate (**eks**-ū-dāt)
fatigue (fuh-**tēg**)
febrile (**feb**-ril)
femoral (**fem**-uh-rul)
fibrin (**fī**-brin)
fibrinogen (fī-**brin**-ō-jun)
fibrinolysin (fī-bri-**nol**-uh-sin)
fibrinolysis (fī-bri-**nol**-uh-sis)
frontal plane (**frun**-tul plān)
genetic disorder (juh-**net**-ik dis-**or**-dur)
hematocrit (hē-**mat**-uh-krit)
hematologic (hē-muh-tō-**loj**-ik)
hematology (hē-muh-**tol**-uh-jē)

hematoma (hē-muh-**tō**-muh)

hematopoiesis (hē-muh-tō-poi-**ē**-sis)

hematopoietic (hē-muh-tō-, hem-uh-tō-poi-**et**-ik)

hemicolectomy (hem-ē-kō-**lek**-tuh-mē)

hemoglobin (**hē**-mō-glō-bin)

hemoglobin electrophoresis (**hē**-mō-glō-bin ē-lek-trō-fuh-**rē**-sis)

hemoglobinopathy (hē-mō-glō-bin-**op**-uh-thē)

hemolysin (hē-**mol**-uh-sin)

hemolysis (hē-**mol**-uh-sis)

hemophilia (hē-mō-**fil**-ē-uh)

hemostasis (hē-mō-**stā**-sis, hē-**mos**-tuh-sis)

hepatitis (hep-uh-**tī**-tis)

hernioplasty (**hur**-nē-ō-plas-tē)

histamine (**his**-tuh-mēn)

homeostasis (hō-mē-ō-**stā**-sis)

homologous graft (hō-**mol**-uh-gus graft)

human immunodeficiency virus (**hū**-mun im-ū-nō-duh-**fish**-un-sē **vī**-rus)

hydrocephalus (hī-drō-**sef**-uh-lus)

hydrocephaly (hī-drō-**sef**-uh-lē)

hydrous (**hī**-drus)

hyperactive (hī-pur-**ak**-tiv)

hypercalcemia (hī-pur-kal-**sē**-mē-uh)

hyperchromic (hī-pur-**krō**-mik)

hyperemia (hī-pur-ē-**mē**-uh)

hyperkalemia (hī-pur-kuh-**lē**-mē-uh)

hypernatremia (hī-pur-nuh-**trē**-mē-uh)

hyperplasia (hī-pur-**plā**-zhuh)

hyperpyrexia (hi-pur-pī-**rek**-sē-uh)

hyperpyrexial (hi-pur-pī-**rek**-sē-ul)

hypersensitivity (hī-pur-sen-si-**tiv**-i-tē)

hypertrophy (hī-**pur**-truh-fē)

hypoalgesia (hī-pō-al-**jē**-zē-uh)

hypocalcemia (hī-pō-kal-**sē**-mē-uh)

hypochondriac (hī-pō-**kon**-drē-ak)

hypochondriac regions (hī-pō-**kon**-drē-ak **rē**-junz)

hypochromia (hī-pō-**krō**-mē-uh)

hypochromic (hī-pō-**krō**-mik)

hypodermic (hī-pō-**dur**-mik)

hypogastric region (hī-pō-**gas**-trik **rē**-jun)

hypokalemia (hī-pō-kuh-**lē**-mē-uh)

hyponatremia (hī-pō-nuh-**trē**-mē-uh)

hypoplasia (hī-pō-**plā**-zhuh)

hypothyroidism (hī-pō-**thī**-roid-iz-um)

iliac regions (**il**-ē-ak **rē**-junz)

immunity (i-**mū**-ni-tē)

immunization (im-ū-ni-**zā**-shun)

immunocompromised (im-ū-nō-**kom**-pruh-mīzd)

immunodeficiency (im-ū-nō-duh-**fish**-un-sē)

immunoglobulins (im-ū-nō-**glob**-ū-linz)

immunosuppressant (im-ū-nō-suh-**pres**-unt)

immunosuppressants (im-ū-nō-suh-**pres**-unts)

immunosuppressive (im-ū-nō-suh-**pres**-iv)

immunotherapy (im-mū-nō-**ther**-uh-pē)

in vitro (in **vē**-trō)

in vivo (in **vē**-vo)

infectious mononucleosis (in-**fek**-shus mōn-ō-nōō-klē-**ō**-sis)

inferior (in-**fēr**-ē-ur)

inferomedian (in-fur-ō-**mē**-dē-un)

inflammation (in-fluh-**mā**-shun)

infrasonic (in-fruh-**son**-ik)

inguinal regions (**ing**-gwi-nul **rē**-junz)

inhale (in-**hāl**)

intercellular (in-tur-**sel**-ū-lur)

intercellular fluid (in-tur-**sel**-ū-lur **flōō**-id)

interferon (in-tur-**fēr**-on)

interrenal (in-tur-**rē**-nul)

interstitial fluid (in-tur-**stish**-ul **flōō**-id)

intracellular (in-truh-**sel**-ū-lur)

intracellular fluid (in-truh-**sel**-ū-lur **flōō**-id)

intradermal (in-truh-**dur**-mul)

intramuscular (in-truh-**mus**-kū-lur)

intravenous (in-truh-**vē**-nus)

intrauterine transfusion (in-truh-**ū**-tur-in trans-**fū**-zhun)

intravascular (in-truh-**vas**-kyū-lur)

ipsilateral (ip-si-**lat**-ur-ul)

isograft (**ī**-sō-graft)

karyomegaly (kar-ē-ō-**meg**-uh-lē)

lateral (**lat**-ur-ul)

lethargic (le-**thar**-jik)

lethargy (**leth**-ur-jē)

leukemia (lōō-**kē**-mē-uh)

leukocyte (**lōō**-kō-sīt)

leukocytopenia (lōō-kō-sī-tō-**pē**-nē-uh)

leukocytosis (lōō-kō-sī-**tō**-sis)

leukopenia (lōō-kō-**pē**-nē-uh)

lumbar regions (**lum**-bur, **lum**-bahr **rē**-junz)

lymph (limf)

lymphatic system (lim-**fat**-ik **sis**-tum)

lymphocyte (**lim**-fō-sīt)

macrocyte (**mak**-rō-sīt)

macrocytosis (mak-rō-sī-**tō**-sis)

macrophage (**mak**-rō-fāj)

macroscopic (mak-rō-**skop**-ik)

malaise (ma-**lāz**)

malnutrition (mal-nōō-**trish**-un)

medial (**mē**-dē-ul)

median (**mē**-dē-un)

mediolateral (mē-dē-ō-**lat**-ur-ul)

megadose (**meg**-uh-dōs)

megalocyte (**meg**-uh-lō-sīt)

mesoderm (**mez**-ō-durm)

microbes (**mī**-krōbz)

microcyte (**mī**-krō-sīt)

microcytosis (mī-krō-sī-**tō**-sis)

microscopic (mī-krō-**skop**-ik)

microtia (mī-**krō**-shuh)

midsagittal plane (mid-**saj**-i-tul plān)

midsection (mid-**sek**-shun)

milligram (**mil**-i-gram)

milliliter (**mil**-i-lē-tur)

monocyte (**mon**-ō-sīt)

mononeuropathy (mon-ō-noo-**rop**-thē)

monovision (**mon**-ō-vish-un)
mucous (**mū**-kus)
mucus (**mū**-kus)
multicellular (mul-tē-**sel**-ū-lur)
muscle tissue (**mus**-ul **tish**-o͞o)
necrosis (nuh-**krō**-sis)
necrotic (nuh-**krot**-ik)
nervous tissue (**nur**-vus **tish**-o͞o)
neutrophil (**no͞o**-trō-fil)
normochromic (nor-mō-**krō**-mik)
normocytes (**nor**-mō-sīts)
normocytic (nor-mō-**sit**-ik)
nucleoid (**no͞o**-klē-oid)
nullipara (nuh-**lip**-uh-ruh)
omphalic (om-**fal**-ik)
omphalitis (om-fuh-**lī**-tis)
omphalocele (**om**-fuh-lō-sēl)
omphaloma (om-fuh-**lō**-muh)
omphalorrhagia (om-fuh-lō-**rā**-juh)
omphalorrhexis (om-fuh-lō-**rek**-sis)
omphalus (**om**-fuh-lus)
pallor (**pal**-ur)
palmar (**pahl**-mur)
pandemic (pan-**dem**-ik)
paramedic (par-uh-**med**-ik)
paranormal (par-uh-**nor**-mul)
parietal peritoneum (puh-**rī**-uh-tul per-i-tō-**nē**-um)
pelvic (**pel**-vik)
pelvis (**pel**-vis)
pericolitis (per-ē-kō-**lī**-tis)
peritoneal (per-i-tō-**nē**-ul)
peritoneum (per-i-tō-**nē**-um)
perspiration (pur-spi-**rā**-shun)
perspire (pur-**spīr**)
phagocytic (fā-gō-**sit**-ik)
phagocytosis (fā-gō-sī-**tō**-sis)
plantar (**plan**-tur)
plasma (**plaz**-muh)
podiatrist (pō-**dī**-uh-trist)
podiatry (pō-**dī**-uh-trē)
podogram (**pod**-ō-gram)
polycythemia (pol-ē-sī-**thē**-mē-uh)
polycythemia vera (pol-ē-sī-**thē**-mē-uh **vē**-ruh)
polydactyly (pol-ē-**dak**-tuh-lē)
postanesthetic (pōst-an-us-**thet**-ik)
posterior (pos-**tēr**-ē-ur)
posteroanterior (pos-tur-ō-an-**tēr**-ē-ur)
posteroexternal (pos-tur-ō-ek-**stur**-nul)
posterointernal (pos-tur-ō-in-**tur**-nul)
posterolateral (pos-tur-ō-**lat**-ur-ul)
posteromedial (pos-tur-ō-**mē**-dē-ul)
posterosuperior (pos-tur-ō-so͞o-**pēr**-ē-ur)
postinfectious (pōst-in-**fek**-shus)
postnasal (pōst-**nā**-zul)
postnatal (pōst-**nā**-tul)
precancerous (prē-**kan**-sur-us)
prenatal (prē-**nā**-tul)

primigravida (prī-mi-**grav**-i-duh)
pronation (prō-**nā**-shun)
prone (prōn)
prophylaxis (prō-fuh-**lak**-sis)
prothrombin (prō-**throm**-bin)
provitamin (prō-**vī**-tuh-min)
proximal (**prok**-si-mul)
psychic (**sī**-kik)
psychoanalysis (sī-kō-uh-**nal**-i-sis)
psychophysiologic (sī-kō-fiz-ē-ō-**loj**-ik)
psychosomatic (sī-kō-sō-**mat**-ik)
purulent (**pū**-ro͞o-lunt)
pus (pus)
pyrexia (pī-**rek**-sē-uh)
pyrogen (**pī**-rō-jun)
quadrant (**kwod**-runt)
quadruplets (kwod-**ro͞o**-pluts)
Raynaud phenomenon (rā-**nō** fuh-**nom**-uh-non)
recumbent (rē-**kum**-bunt)
rejection (rē-**jek**-shun)
resistance (rē-**zis**-tuns)
retrocolic (ret-rō-**kol**-ik)
sagittal plane (**saj**-i-tul plān)
saliva (suh-**lī**-vuh)
sanguinous (**sang**-gwi-nus)
secretion (sē-**krē**-shun)
semicoma (sem-ē-**kō**-muh)
semipermeable (sem-ē-**pur**-mē-uh-bul)
septicemia (sep-ti-**sē**-mē-uh)
serum (**sēr**-um)
shunt (shunt)
sickle cell anemia (**sik**-ul sel uh-**nē**-mē-uh)
somatic cells (sō-**mat**-ik selz)
somatic death (sō-**mat**-ik deth)
somatogenic (sō-muh-tō-**jen**-ik)
somatopsychic (sō-muh-tō-**sī**-kik)
somesthetic (sō-mes-**thet**-ik)
staphylococcemia (staf-uh-lō-kok-**sē**-mē-uh)
stem cells (stem selz)
streptococcemia (strep-tō-kok-**sē**-mē-uh)
subcutaneous (sub-kū-**tā**-nē-us)
superficial (so͞o-pur-**tish**-ul)
superior (so͞o-**pēr**-ē-ur)
supersensitivity (so͞o-pur-sen-si-**tiv**-i-tē)
supervitaminosis (so͞o-pur-vī-tuh-min-**ō**-sis)
supination (so͞o-pi-**nā**-shun)
supine (**so͞o**-pīn, so͞o-**pīn**)
suppurative (**sup**-ū-rā-tiv)
suprarenal (so͞o-pruh-**rē**-nul)
suprathoracic (so͞o-pruh-thuh-**ras**-ik)
susceptibility (suh-sep-ti-**bil**-i-tē)
symmetry (**sim**-uh-trē)
symptomatic (simp-tō-**mat**-ik)
syncope (**sing**-kuh-pē)
syndactyly (sin-**dak**-tuh-lē)
syndrome (**sin**-drōm)
systemic (sis-**tem**-ik)

tachycardia (tak-i-**kahr**-dē-uh)

tachyphasia (tak-ē-**fā**-zhuh)

telecardiogram (tel-uh-**kahr**-dē-ō-gram)

tetralogy (te-**tral**-uh-jē)

thoracic (thuh-**ras**-ik)

thoracodynia (thor-uh-kō-**din**-ē-uh)

thoracotomy (thor-uh-**kot**-uh-mē)

thorax (**thor**-aks)

thrombectomy (throm-**bek**-tuh-mē)

thrombi (**throm**-bī)

thrombocyte (**throm**-bō-sīt)

thrombocytopenia (throm-bō-sī-tō-**pē**-nē-uh)

thrombocytosis (throm-bō-sī-**tō**-sis)

thrombogenesis (throm-bō-**jen**-uh-sis)

thrombolysis (throm-**bol**-i-sis)

thrombolytic (throm-bō-**lit**-ik)

thrombopenia (throm-bō-**pē**-nē-uh)

thromboplastin (throm-bō-**plas**-tin)

thrombosis (throm-**bō**-sis)

thrombus (**throm**-bus)

tinnitus (**tin**-i-tus, ti-**nī**-tus)

tissue (**tish**-o͞o)

toxemia (tok-**sē**-mē-uh)

toxicity (tok-**sis**-i-tē)

toxoid (**tok**-soid)

transdermal (trans-**dur**-mul)

transplant ([verb] trans-**plant**; [noun] **trans**-plant)

transthoracic (trans-thuh-**ras**-ik)

transverse plane (trans-**vurs** plān)

traumatic (traw-**mat**-ik)

triceps (**trī**-seps)

triplegia (trī-**plē**-juh)

ultrasonic (ul-truh-**son**-ik)

ultraviolet (ul-truh-**vī**-uh-lut)

umbilical region (um-**bil**-i-kul **rē**-jun)

umbilicus (um-**bil**-i-kus)

uniglandular (ū-ni-**glan**-dū-lur)

unilateral (ū-ni-**lat**-ur-ul)

vaccination (vak-si-**nā**-shun)

vaccine (vak-**sēn**)

ventral (**ven**-trul)

ventral cavity (**ven**-trul **kav**-i-tē)

ventromedian (ven-trō-**mē**-dē-un)

viscera (**vis**-ur-uh)

visceral peritoneum (**vis**-ur-ul per-i-tō-**nē**-um)

Español ENHANCING SPANISH COMMUNICATION

English	Spanish (pronunciation)	English	Spanish (pronunciation)
abdomen	abdomen (ab-DOH-men), vientre (ve-EN-tray)	clot	coágulo (ko-AH-goo-lo)
abscess	absceso (ab-SAY-so), apostema (ah-pos-TAY-ma)	coagulant	coagulante (ko-ah-goo-LAHN-tay)
		coagulation	coagulación (ko-ag-oo-lahse-ON), coágulo (ko-AH-goo-lo)
allergy	alergia (ah-LEHR-he-ah)	constipation	estreñimiento (es-tray-nye-me-EN-to)
anatomy	anatomía (ah-nah-to-MEE-ah)		
anemia	anemia (ah-NAY-me-ah)	dehydration	deshidración (des-e-dra-se-ON)
antibiotic	antibiótico (an-te-be-O-te-ko)	destruction	destrucción (des-trook-se-ON)
anticoagulant	anticoagulante (an-te-ko-ah-goo-LAHN-tay)	diarrhea	diarrea (de-ar-RAY-ah)
		disseminate	diseminar (de-say-me-NAR)
antigen	antígeno (an-TEE-hay-no)	dizziness	vértigo (VERR-te-go)
antihistamine	antihistamina (an-te-es-tay-MEnah)	dyspnea	disnea (dis-NAY-ah)
		embolus	émbolo (EM-bo-lo)
arm	brazo (BRAH-so)	erythrocyte	erithrocito (a-rith-ro-SEE-to)
aspirate	aspirar (as-pe-RAR)	excretion	excreción (ex-kray-se-ON)
belly	barriga (bar-REE-gah)	face	cara (KAH-rah)
blood	sangre (SAHN-gray)	fainting	languidez (lan-gee-DES), desmayo (des-MAH-yo)
blood sample	muestra de sangre (moo-AYStrah day SAHN-gray)		
		fatigue	fatiga (fah-TEE-gah)
blood transfusion	transfusión de sangre (trans-foo-se-ON day SAHN-gray)	fever	fiebre (fe-AY-bray)
		fiber	fibra (FEE-brah)
blood vessel	vaso sanguine (VAH-so san-GEE-nay)	fibrin	fibrina (fe-BREE-nah)
		finger	dedo (DAY-do)
body	cuerpo (koo-ERR-po)	fingerprint	impresión digital (im-pray-se-ON de-he-TAHL)
breathing	respiración (res-pe-rah-se-ON)		
chest	pecho (PAY-cho)	fluid	fluido (floo-EE-do)

English	Spanish (pronunciation)	English	Spanish (pronunciation)
headache	dolor de cabeza (do-LOR day kah-BAY-sa)	resistance	resistencia (ray-sis-TEN-se-ah)
		rib	costilla (kos-TEEL-lyah)
hemophilia	hemophilia (ay-mo-FEE-le-ah)	ringing	zumbido (zoom-BEE-do)
hip	cadera (kah-DAY-rah)	saliva	saliva (sah-LEE-vah)
hydrocephalus	hidrocéfalo (e-dro-SAY-fah-lo)	sanguinous	sanguineo, nea (san-GEE-nay-o, san-GEE-nay-ah)
hypodermic	hipodérmico (e-po-DER-me-co)		
immunity	inmunidad (in-moo-ne-DAHD)	secretion	secreción (say-kray-se-ON)
injury	daño (DAH-nyo)	serum	suero (soo-AY-ro)
kidney	riñon (ree-NYOHN)	skull	cráneo (KRAH-nay-o)
leg	pierna (pe-ERR-nah)	sole	planta (PLAHN-tah)
leukemia	leucemia (lay-oo-SAY-me-ah)	susceptibility	susceptibilidad (soos-sep-te-be-le-DAHD)
liver	hígado (EE-ga-do)		
lymph	linfa (LEEN-fa)	sweat	sudor (soo-DOR)
lymphatic	linfático (lin-FAH-te-ko)	swelling	prominencia (pro-me-NEN-se-ah)
microscope	microscopio (me-kros-KO-pe-o)		
mucous	mucoso (moo-KO-so)	syncope	síncope (SEEN-ko-pay)
mucus	moco (MO-ko)	tears	lágrimas (LAH-gre-mahs)
navel	ombligo (om-BLEE-go)	thigh	muslo (MOOS-lo)
oxygen	oxígeno (ok-SEE-hay-no)	toe	dedo del pie (DAY-do del PE-ay)
pallor	palidez (pah-le-DAS)	toxin	toxina (tox-SEE-nah)
palm	palma (PAHL-mah)	transfusion	transfusión (trans-foo-se-ON)
perspiration	sudor (soo-DOR)	urinary	bladder vejiga (vah-HEE-gah)
perspire	sudar (soo-DAR)	uterus	útero (OO-tay-ro)
phagocyte	fagocito (fah-go-SEE-to)	vaccination	vacunación (vah-koo-nah-se-ON)
protection	proteccion (pro-tek-se-ON)	water	agua (AH-goo-ah)
purulent	purulento (poo-roo-LEN-to)	wound	lesión (lay-se-ON)
redness	rojo (RO-ho)	wrist	muñeca (moo-NYAY-kah)

Congratulations! You have completed the foundation upon which you will build many medical words.

Circulatory System
Cardiovascular and Lymphatic Systems

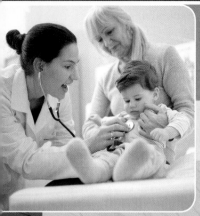

Cardiology is the study of the anatomy, normal functions, and disorders of the heart. This patient has been referred to a cardiologist by his pediatrician.

CONTENTS

Basic Understanding

In this chapter you will learn to do the following:

1. State the meaning of the circulatory system and its function.
2. State the functions of the cardiovascular and lymphatic systems, and analyze associated terminology.
3. Write the meanings of the word parts associated with the cardiovascular and lymphatic systems, and use them to build and analyze terms.
4. Write the names of the structures of the cardiovascular and lymphatic systems, and define the terms associated with these structures.
5. Sequence the flow of blood from when it enters the heart until it returns to the heart.

6. Write the names of the diagnostic tests and procedures for assessment of the cardiovascular and lymphatic systems when given their descriptions, or match procedures with their descriptions.
7. Write the names of cardiovascular and lymphatic pathologies when given their descriptions, or match pathologies with their meanings.
8. Match surgical and nonsurgical therapeutic interventions with their descriptions, or write the names of the interventions when given their descriptions.
9. Build terms using word parts to label illustrations.

Greater Comprehension

10. Use word parts from this chapter to determine the meaning of terms in a health care report.
11. Spell the terms accurately.
12. Pronounce the terms correctly.
13. Write the meanings of the abbreviations.

14. Categorize terms as anatomy, diagnostic test or procedure, pathology, surgery, or nonsurgical therapy.
15. Recognize the meanings of general pharmacological terms from this chapter as well as the drug classes and their uses.

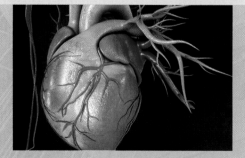

FUNCTION FIRST

The **circulatory system** consists of the **cardio/vascul/ar** system (heart and blood vessels) and the lymphatic system (structures involved in the conveyance of the fluid, **lymph**). The circulatory system cooperates with other body systems to maintain homeostasis.

Body cells must have a constant supply of food, oxygen, and other substances to function properly. Blood circulates through the heart and blood vessels, carrying oxygen, nutrients, vitamins, antibodies, and other substances. It carries away waste and carbon dioxide.

The cardiovascular system supplies body cells with needed substances, transports waste products for disposal,

maintains the acid–base balance of the body, prevents hemorrhage through blood clotting, protects against disease, and helps regulate temperature.

As blood circulates, interstitial fluid accumulates in the tissue spaces. This excess fluid is normally transported away from the tissues by another vascular network that helps maintain the internal fluid environment—the lymphatic system. The lymphatic system helps maintain the internal fluid environment of the body by returning proteins and tissue fluids to the blood, aids in the absorption of fats into the bloodstream, and helps to defend the body against microorganisms and disease.

WRITE IT! EXERCISE 1

Write words in the blanks to complete the sentences.

1. The circulatory system consists of the lymphatic and the _____ systems.

2. Body cells must have a constant supply of the gas _____.

3. Waste products carried away from tissue include carbon _____.

4. The lymphatic system transports excess _____ from the tissues.

CARDIOVASCULAR SYSTEM
ANATOMY AND PHYSIOLOGY

4-1 The heart and blood vessels make up the **cardio/vascul/ar** (cardi[o], heart + vascul[o], vessel + -ar, pertaining to) **system.** Hear heart beats, as well as breath sounds, at *www.easyauscultation.com.*

🔑 **KEY** POINT **The vast network of blood vessels delivers oxygen, nutrients, and vital substances to the interstitial fluids surrounding all the body's cells.** Blood vessels include arteries, arterioles, capillaries, venules, and veins. Arteries, veins, and capillaries are the main types of blood vessels. Arteries have thicker walls to withstand the high pressure of the heart's pumping action, veins have thinner walls, and microscopic capillaries are one cell thick (Fig. 4.1).

Learn the word parts that describe the anatomy and physiology of the cardiovascular system.

Word Parts: Cardiovascular Anatomy and Physiology

Combining Form	Meaning	Combining Form	Meaning
Main Components of the Cardiovascular System		**Other Word Parts**	
angi(o), vas(o), vascul(o)	vessel	atri(o)	atrium
aort(o)	aorta	coron(o)	crown
arter(o), arteri(o)	artery	mediastin(o)	mediastinum
arteriol(o)	arteriole	ox(i)	oxygen
cardi(o)	heart	pulmon(o)	lung
phleb(o), ven(i), ven(o)	vein	sept(o)*	septum; partition
venul(o)	venule	sin(o)	sinus
		steth(o), thorac(o)	chest
Tissues of the Heart		valv(o), valvul(o)	valve
endocardi(o)	endocardium	ventricul(o)	ventricle
myocardi(o)	myocardium	**Suffix**	
pericardi(o)	pericardium	-ole	small
*Sept(o) sometimes means infection.			

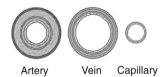

Artery   Vein   Capillary

Figure 4.1 Major types of blood vessels. Note the difference in thickness of walls of arteries, veins, and capillaries (which are only one cell thick). The elastic walls of arteries withstand high pressure of the heartbeat and allow them to expand as the heart beats.

vessel

Vascul/ar means pertaining to a _____, specifically a blood vessel. A simplified drawing of the cardiovascular system includes the heart and main blood vessels that circulate blood throughout the body (Fig. 4.2).

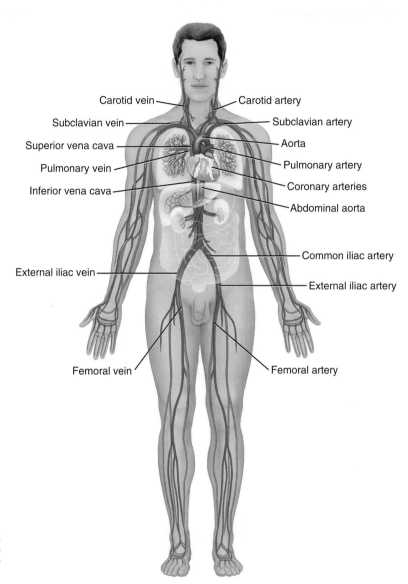

Carotid vein
Carotid artery
Subclavian vein
Subclavian artery
Superior vena cava
Aorta
Pulmonary vein
Pulmonary artery
Inferior vena cava
Coronary arteries
Abdominal aorta
Common iliac artery
External iliac vein
External iliac artery
Femoral vein
Femoral artery

Figure 4.2 The cardiovascular system: the heart and blood vessels. Two major components of the vascular network are shown, the arteries *(red)* and the veins *(blue)*. Only the larger or more common blood vessels are labeled.

MATCH IT! **EXERCISE 2**

Match the combining forms in the left column with the structures in the right column.

_____ **1.** arter(o)   **A.** arteriole
_____ **2.** arteriol(o)   **B.** artery
_____ **3.** phleb(o)   **C.** lung
_____ **4.** pulmon(o)   **D.** vein
_____ **5.** venul(o)   **E.** venule

WORD ORIGIN
capillaries *(L.)*
hairlike

4-2 The arteries are shown in red and the veins are shown in blue in Fig. 4.2. This oversimplifies blood circulation, but it will help you remember that, in general, **arteries** carry oxygen-rich blood to body tissues and **veins** carry oxygen-poor blood back to the heart.

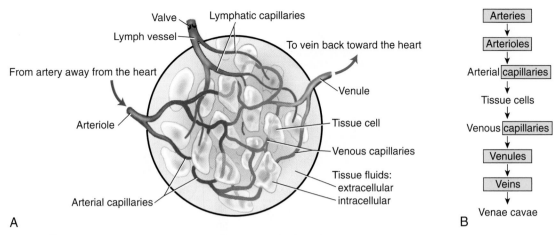

Figure 4.3 A capillary bed showing the relationship of blood vessels. A, Relationship of blood flow through blood vessels. Blood that is rich in oxygen is carried by the arteries, which branch many times to become arterioles. Arterioles branch to become capillaries, the site of oxygen and carbon dioxide exchange. Oxygen-poor blood is returned to the heart through the venules, which flow into the veins. The veins carry the blood to the two largest veins, the superior and inferior venae cavae, which empty into the heart. Venae cavae is plural for vena cava. **B,** Schematic showing relationship of blood flow through vessels. Main types of vessels are highlighted.

little

Arteri/ole means little artery when translated literally because -ole means _____.
Capillaries are microscopic blood vessels that receive blood from the arterioles. Capillaries are so small that erythrocytes must pass through them in single file. Blood and tissue fluids exchange various substances across the capillary walls. The capillaries join arterioles and venules (Fig. 4.3). **Venules** join the capillaries and veins.

WORD ORIGIN
venule *(L.)*
venula, small vein

WRITE IT! EXERCISE 3

Write the meaning of the following combining forms.

1. angi(o) _____

2. atri(o) _____

3. coron(o) _____

4. mediastin(o) _____

5. sept(o) _____

6. steth(o) _____

7. valvul(o) _____

8. ventricul(o) _____

4-3 Blood circulation is the circuit of blood through the body, from the heart through the arteries, arterioles, capillaries, venules, and veins and back to the heart. Circulation means movement in a regular or circular fashion. If you study blood circulation more closely, you learn that it consists of many events that occur simultaneously. Label and study Fig. 4.4 as you read about the two types of circulation.

🔑 **KEY** POINT **Two important types of circulation occur each time the heart beats:**
- **Systemic circulation:** The general circulation that carries oxygenated blood from the heart to the tissues of the body and returns the blood with much of its oxygen exchanged for carbon dioxide back to the heart
- **Pulmonary circulation:** The circuit that the blood makes from the heart to the lungs for the purpose of ridding the body of carbon dioxide and picking up oxygen

systemic

The general circulation that transports oxygen to all tissues of the body is _____ circulation.

4-4 All tissues of the body, including heart tissue and lung tissue, receive oxygen via the systemic circulation. However, you will need to remember that pulmonary circulation provides the means for the blood to take on oxygen from air that we take into our lungs.

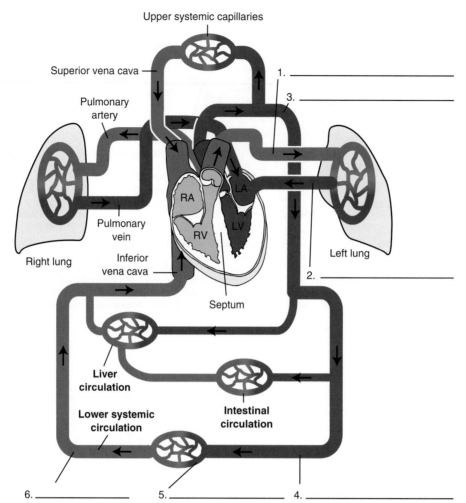

Upper systemic capillaries

Superior vena cava

1. _____

3. _____

Pulmonary artery

RA

LA

LV

RV

Pulmonary vein

Inferior vena cava

Right lung

Left lung

2. _____

Septum

Liver circulation

Lower systemic circulation

Intestinal circulation

6. _____   5. _____   4. _____

Figure 4.4 **Schematic drawing of blood circulation and the relationship of blood vessels.** *Arrows* indicate the direction of blood flow through the heart to the lungs and the major vessels of the cardiovascular system. *RA, RV, LA,* and *LV* are abbreviations for the four chambers of the heart. Blood circulation consists of two types of circulation: pulmonary circulation and systemic circulation. Label the diagram as indicated. **Pulmonary circulation:** Pulmonary arteries carry oxygen-deficient blood *(blue)* to the lungs, where it is oxygenated. Label the left pulmonary artery *(1)*. Oxygenated blood is returned to the heart via pulmonary veins. Label the left pulmonary vein *(2)*. **Systemic circulation:** Oxygen-rich blood *(red)* is pumped from the heart into the aorta *(3)* and is routed to arteries that branch to become arterioles, which branch to become capillaries. Label the artery *(4)* and capillary *(5)*. In the capillaries, blood is provided to the tissues of the body and the blood, with much of its oxygen exchanged for carbon dioxide, passes into the venules, and then the veins. Label the vein indicated by number 6. Blood then returns to the heart via veins called the *superior* and *inferior venae cavae.*

🔑 **KEY** POINT **The naming of pulmonary arteries and veins is different from that of other arteries and veins in the body.** You have learned that, in general, arteries transport blood rich in oxygen, and veins transport blood that has had much of its oxygen removed. Pulmonary arteries transport deoxygenated blood to the lungs. After the blood absorbs oxygen in the lungs, the pulmonary veins transport the blood back to the heart before it is pumped throughout the body.

arteries	Oxygen-deficient blood leaves the heart via the pulmonary _____.
	After oxygenation, which takes place in the lungs, the blood is returned to the heart via the
veins	pulmonary _____.

4-5 The heart has four chambers: right **atrium** (RA), right **ventricle** (RV), left atrium (LA), and left ventricle (LV).

Beginning with artery, list the six components of the cardiovascular system (2 through 5) to indicate the flow of blood in systemic circulation as it circulates back toward the heart. Numbers 1 and 6 are done as examples.

1. _artery_

2. _____

3. _____

4. _____

5. _____

6. _superior and inferior venae cavae_

4-6 As you read Frames 4-6 through 4-7, use Fig. 4.4 to help you visualize the pattern of blood flow. Blood that is rich in oxygen is pumped throughout the body, providing oxygen to all body cells. Then oxygen-poor blood, **deoxygenated blood,** returns to the heart.

🔑 **KEY** POINT A simple explanation of the circuit of blood flow is this: Oxygen-poor blood enters the right side of the heart→lungs (to pick up oxygen)→left side of the heart→pumped throughout the body→back to the heart to complete the circuit. Deoxygenated blood enters the heart on the right side of the body through its two largest veins. These veins are the inferior and superior vena cava. Collectively, the two veins are called the *venae cavae.*

atrium

Blood from the trunk and legs enters the heart via the **inferior vena cava.** Blood from the head and arms enters the heart by way of the large vein, the **superior vena cava.** The venae cavae bring the blood to the right _____.

WORD ORIGIN
vena cava *(L.)*
vena, veins; *cava,* cavity

lungs

4-7 The right atrium contracts to force blood through the **tricuspid valve** into the right ventricle. Contraction of the right ventricle forces blood through the pulmonary artery, which branches and carries blood to the _____.

🔑 **KEY** POINT As blood flows through the lungs, it becomes **oxygenated** (having additional oxygen) and returns to the left side of the heart by way of the pulmonary veins, which bring the blood to the left atrium. This is an extraordinary situation in which a vein (pulmonary vein) is carrying blood that is rich in oxygen.

The left atrium contracts and forces blood into the left ventricle via the **mitral valve,** also called the **bicuspid valve.** This richly oxygenated blood is then pumped into the **aorta** from the left ventricle. The aorta is the largest artery of the body, and it branches into smaller arteries to carry blood throughout the body. In summary, the right side of the heart receives oxygen-poor blood, the lungs oxygenate the blood, and the left side of the heart sends oxygen-rich blood to the aorta (Fig. 4.5).

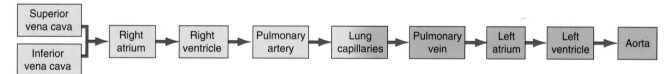

Figure 4.5 Pathway of blood through the heart. Valves open and close to prevent backflow.

WORD ORIGIN
valvula *(L.)*
valva, valve

4-8 In normal heart function, valves close and prevent backflow of blood when the heart contracts. (Be aware that certain small valves in the body are called **valvula.**)

🔑 **KEY** POINT Valves between the atria and ventricles are **atrioventricular valves**. The tricuspid valve is the name of the valve between the right atrium and the right ventricle, and the bicuspid, or mitral, valve is the valve between the left atrium and left ventricle (see Fig. 4.7, B). Cuspid refers to the little flaps of tissue that make up the valve. The left atrioventricular valve is generally called the *mitral valve* in medicine and is so named because the two valve flaps are shaped somewhat like the mitered corner joints of a picture frame.

two

Remembering that bi- means two, the bi/cuspid valve has _____ flaps. The tricuspid valve has three flaps of tissue.

pulmonary

veins

4-9 The pulmonary valve regulates the flow of blood from the right ventricle to the pulmonary trunk, which divides into _____ arteries that lead to the lungs. Pulmonary means pertaining to the lungs, and vessels that carry blood from the heart to the lungs are **pulmonary arteries**. Note that vessels that carry blood from the lungs back to the heart are **pulmonary** _____.

After flowing from the left atrium to the left ventricle, blood leaves the heart by way of the **aortic valve,** which regulates the flow of blood into the aorta. The pulmonary and aortic valves are also called **semilunar valves** (because of the half-moon appearance of the cusps).

MATCH IT! EXERCISE 5

Match the term with its meaning. Each term is used only once.

_____ **1.** large vein by which blood enters the heart

_____ **2.** structure that closes and prevents backflow of blood

_____ **3.** type of valves located between the atria and the ventricles

_____ **4.** valve leading to the aorta from the left ventricle

_____ **5.** valves with a half-moon appearance of the cusps

A. aortic
B. atrioventricular
C. semilunar
D. valve
E. vena cava

chest

4-10 The muscular heart is the center of the cardiovascular system. It beats normally about 70 times per minute, or more than 100,000 times per day. In the adult, it weighs 230 to 340 grams (about ½ pound) and is the size of a clenched fist. The heart lies in the thoracic cavity. You learned earlier that the thoracic cavity is the _____ cavity.

KEY POINT The heart lies just left of the midline of the body, between the lungs, in a space called the **mediastinum.** The **media/stinum** is an area in the chest cavity between the lungs. The mediastinum contains the heart and its large vessels, the trachea, the esophagus, and nearby structures, such as the lymph nodes.

coronary

4-11 Special arteries supply blood to the heart itself. **Coronary** means encircling in the manner of a crown. Blood vessels that supply oxygen to the heart encircle it in a crownlike fashion (Fig. 4.6). Arteries that supply blood to the heart are _____ **arteries.**

around

4-12 The heart is enclosed in **pericardium,** a membranous sac (Fig. 4.6, A). Literal translation of peri/cardium is a membrane _____ the heart. Terms ending in -cardium (cardi(o) + -ium) can be confusing because one i is dropped to facilitate pronunciation, and their literal translation is heart membrane.

KEY POINT The tissue layers of the heart, starting from the outside, are the **epicardium**, the **myocardium**, and the **endocardium.** The myocardium, the thick, contractile, middle layer is made up of muscle fibers that contract, which results in a wringing type of movement that squeezes blood from the heart. Translated literally, the endo/cardium is the membrane inside the heart. Locate these structures in the Fig. 4.6, B inset.

endocardium

The myocardium is the middle layer of the heart, and the innermost layer is the _____.

4-13 The pericardium, a tough fibrous tissue that constitutes the outermost sac, fits loosely around the heart and protects it. The pericardium is composed of an inner, visceral layer (**visceral pericardium,** also called *epicardium*) and an outer, tougher layer (**parietal pericardium**). Epi/cardium is so named because it lies on the surface of the heart. The space between the two layers is the **pericardial cavity.** Locate the two types of pericardium in the Fig. 4.6 inset.

4-14 The four-chambered heart is separated into right and left chambers by a partition called the **septum.**

KEY POINT The combining form sept(o) has two meanings, either septum or infection. However, the term septum always means a dividing wall or partition. Septum may be used in describing structures other than the heart, but the word always means a dividing wall or partition.

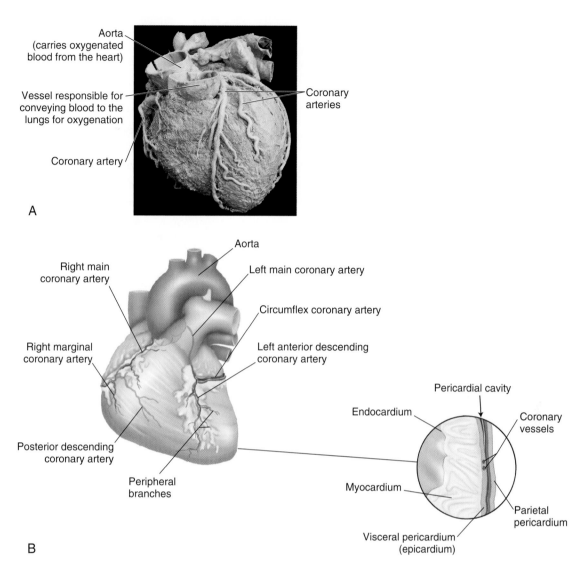

Figure 4.6 **Gross heart anatomy, coronary arteries, and heart tissues. A,** Anterior photograph of the external heart. **B,** The two main coronary arteries are the left coronary artery (LCA) and right coronary artery (RCA). The three tissue layers of the heart, beginning with the innermost layer, are endocardium, myocardium, and epicardium (also called the *visceral pericardium*).

In addition to being divided longitudinally into right and left chambers by a septum, each side of the heart is further divided into an atrium (plural: atria) and a ventricle. This can be seen in the simple drawing of blood circulation in Fig. 4.4, but you will also be able to see these features in later drawings.

The two upper chambers of the heart are the right and left atria. The two lower chambers of the heart are the right and left _____.

ventricles

4-15 The heart has both a left ventricle and a right ventricle. **Ventricular** means pertaining to a ventricle. Combine atri(o) and ventricular to write a term that is abbreviated AV or A-V and means pertaining to an atrium and a ventricle of the heart: _____.

atrioventricular

➤ **BEYOND** THE BLUEPRINT The term ventricle is also applied to a chamber of the brain. Therefore ventricul(o) refers to a ventricle of either the heart or the brain. By analyzing other parts of the term or the sentence, one can often determine which organ is affected, the brain or the heart.

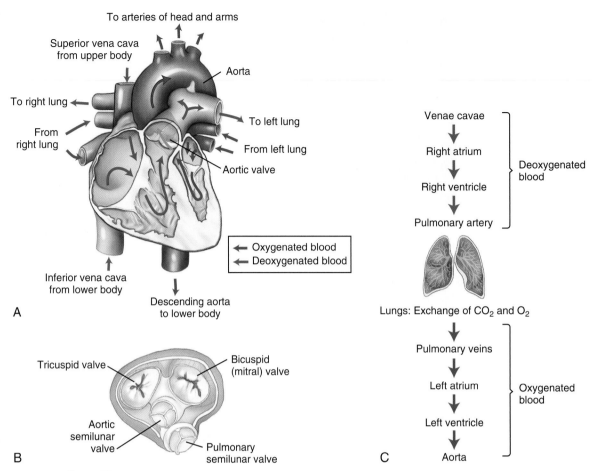

Figure 4.7 Circulation of blood through the heart. A, Anterior cross-section showing the heart chambers. *Arrows* indicate the direction of blood flow through the heart. **B,** Heart valves (viewed from above), the structures that prevent backflow of blood by opening and closing with each heartbeat. **C,** Schematic representation of deoxygenated or oxygenated status of the blood as it flows through the heart.

4-16 Circulation of blood through the heart is a coordination of nerve impulses and muscular contraction (Fig. 4.7). It is important to remember that both atria contract simultaneously, followed by simultaneous contraction of both ventricles. The cardiac conduction system is composed of highly specialized tissue that is capable of producing and conveying electric impulses.

Look at Fig. 4.8, and find the **sino/atrial (SA) node,** located at the junction of the right atrium and the superior vena cava. Electric impulses arise spontaneously in the SA node and stimulate contraction. The SA node is the natural pacemaker of the heart. The SA node is also called the *sinus node.*

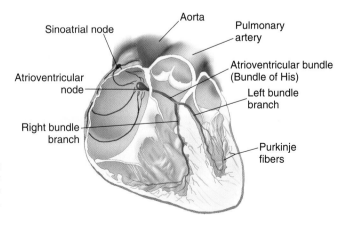

Figure 4.8 Conduction system of the heart (shown in cross-section). The electrical impulse originates in the heart, and contraction of the heart's chambers is coordinated by specialized heart tissues.

> **BEYOND** THE BLUEPRINT The combining form sin(o) means sinus. A sinus is a cavity or channel. Perhaps you are more familiar with the sinuses near the nose (air cavities that sometimes drain or become inflamed in sinus/itis). The term *sinusitis* does not use the combining form.

sinoatrial

Use sin(o) atrial to write the name of the natural pacemaker of the heart, the _____ node.

4-17 The electric impulse generated by the SA node travels through both atria to the **atrio/ventricul/ar** (AV) **node,** which in turn conducts the impulse to the atrioventricular bundle (AV bundle, also called the *bundle of His*) and then to the **Purkinje fibers** and walls of the ventricles. This highly specialized system results in simultaneous contraction of the atria, followed by contraction of the ventricles.

atrioventricular

AV node means the _____ node. This special type of cardiac tissue is located near the septal wall between the left and right atria. The atria contract while the electric impulse is briefly delayed in the AV node.

4-18 Blood vessels play an important role in providing a continuous supply of oxygen and nutrients to cells. A capillary, where the exchange of oxygen for carbon dioxide takes place, consists of a single layer of endothelial cells, yet blood vessels (especially the arteries) are subjected to great pressure with each heartbeat.

KEY POINT **Arteries, veins, and capillaries are lined with endothelium, a layer of epithelial cells, which secretes substances that prevent blood clotting and regulate the tone of the vessels.** Arteries and veins have three additional layers: an inner layer, a muscular layer, and a white fibrous outer layer. Arteries are thicker than veins, and their outer layer is elastic, allowing them to expand as the heartbeat forces blood into them.

arteries

Arteries carry blood away from the heart. For this reason, blood pressure is much higher in _____ than in veins. Veins also contain valves at various intervals to control the direction of the blood flow back to the heart.

FIND IT!

EXERCISE 6

Draw a slash between the word parts in the following list of new terms. Then find the meanings of the word parts within the definitions. (Draw the slash, and then perform the remainder of the activity as a mental exercise. Think!)

1. **arterial** pertaining to one or more arteries
2. **venous** pertaining to, composed of, or affecting veins
3. **arteriovenous** pertaining to both arteries and veins
4. **atrial** pertaining to an atrium
5. **cardiopulmonary** pertaining to the heart and lungs
6. **septal** pertaining to a septum
7. **pericardial** pertaining to the pericardium

8. **endocardial** pertaining to the endocardium
9. **myocardial** pertaining to the myocardium
10. **pulmonary** pertaining to the lungs
11. **phlebotomist** a person with special training in the practice of drawing blood
12. **phlebotomy, venipuncture** opening of a vein to draw blood for laboratory analysis

---

BUILD IT!

EXERCISE 7

Use the following word parts to build terms. (Some word parts will be used more than once.)

endo-, peri-, arteri(o), atri(o), cardi(o), my(o), sept(o), ven(o), ventricul(o), -al, -ar, -ium, -ous

1. cardiac muscle tissue _____/_____/_____
2. inner lining of the heart _____/_____/_____
3. outer membranous sac of the heart _____/_____/_____
4. pertaining to both arteries and veins _____/_____
5. pertaining to the inner lining of the heart _____/_____/_____
6. pertaining to the lower heart chambers _____/_____
7. pertaining to the septum _____/_____
8. pertaining to the upper heart chambers _____/_____

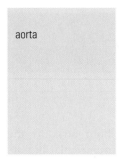

aorta

4-19 The aorta is the main trunk of the systemic arterial system. Arteries branch out either directly or indirectly from the _____, and each artery is responsible for conveying oxygen and nutrients to specific organs and tissues. To identify and discuss location, anatomists divide the aorta into three major portions:

- ascending aorta
- aortic arch
- descending aorta (which is further divided into the thoracic aorta and the abdominal aorta)

    Use the color coding of the labels in Fig. 4.9 to compare the flow of blood to your right arm versus the flow of blood to your right leg.

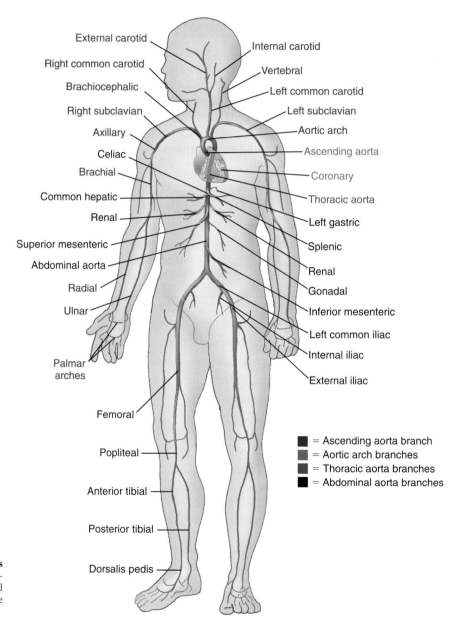

Figure 4.9 Anterior view of the aorta and its principal arterial branches. Labels for the ascending aorta, aortic arch, thoracic aorta, and abdominal aorta are shown. Names of respective arteries are shown in _red, green, purple,_ and _black._

FIND IT! EXERCISE 8

Draw a slash between the word parts in the following list of new terms. Then find the meanings of the word parts within the definitions. (Draw the slash, and then perform the remainder of the activity as a mental exercise. Think!)

1. aortic pertaining to the aorta

2. intraaortic within the aorta

3. valval, valvar pertaining to a valve

4. valvate, valvular pertaining to or having valves

WRITE IT! **EXERCISE 9**

Write a word in each blank to complete these sentences that describe circulation.

Oxygen-poor blood is delivered to the right side of the heart via the two largest veins, the superior and inferior (1) _____ _____. The blood from these two largest veins is emptied into the chamber of the heart called the right (2) _____. When the heart contracts, blood is forced through the tricuspid valve to the lower chamber, called the (3) _____ _____. Another contraction of the heart forces the blood into the pulmonary artery, which branches and carries blood to the (4) _____, where it picks up oxygen. The pulmonary veins take blood back to the heart chamber called the (5) _____ _____. The flow of blood from the left atrium to the left ventricle is controlled by the (6) _____ valve. Blood is then pumped into the largest artery in the body, the (7) _____. This vessel branches many times to become arteries, which again branch many times to become the smallest arteries, called (8) _____, which in turn branch to become the smallest vessels, where oxygen is delivered to body tissues. These vessels, called (9) _____, are composed of only a single layer of cells and are continuous with venules, which in turn are continuous with larger vessels called (10) _____. These vessels are directly or indirectly connected with the venae cavae.

DIAGNOSTIC TESTS AND PROCEDURES

4-20 The heart rate **(pulse rate)** and blood pressure (BP) give a preliminary indication of how well the heart is functioning. **Blood pressure** is the pressure exerted by the circulating volume of blood on the walls of the arteries and veins and on the chambers of the heart. A direct measurement can be obtained only by measuring pressure within a vessel of the heart itself, as in heart catheterization, which is described later in this chapter.

Indirect measurement is made with a stethoscope and a sphygmomanometer (a blood pressure cuff and pressure gauge). With the upper arm at the level of the heart, the cuff is placed around the upper arm and inflated to a pressure that occludes (closes off) the brachial artery, the principal artery of the upper arm. The pressure in the compressed artery is estimated by the column of mercury when the cuff is inflated (Fig. 4.10).

WORD ORIGIN
sphygmomanometer *(G.)*
sphygmos, pulse; *manos,*
thin; *metron,* measure

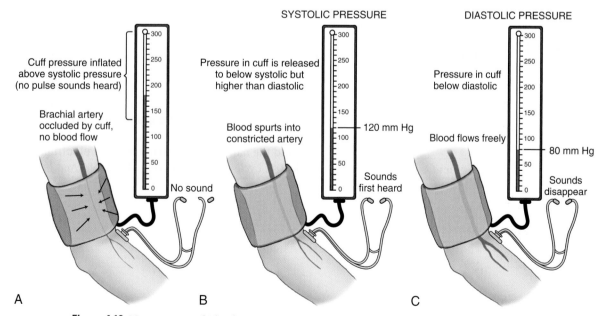

Figure 4.10 Measurement of Blood Pressure. A to C, Drawings of the mercury manometer apparatus, an older method of measuring blood pressure, facilitate the understanding of blood pressure readings. In **A,** No sounds are heard because the pressure in the cuff is higher than the systolic pressure. **B,** The first sound heard (a systolic pressure of 120 mm Hg) is noted. **C,** The last sound heard (80 mm Hg) represents the diastolic pressure. This example represents a normal blood pressure reading of 120/80 mm Hg (the height of mercury in a graduated column on the blood pressure apparatus).

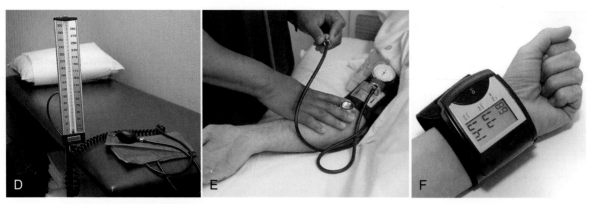

Figure 4.10 **Measurement of Blood Pressure (cont.)** **D to F,** Three types of instruments for indirect measurement of blood pressure: mercury, aneroid, and automatic digital. **D,** This type of apparatus has been used in health care for more than a century. **E,** Anaeroid types have an easy-to-read dial and wall-mounted models are recommended, because mechanical jarring may result in less accurate readings. **F,** An automatic digital instrument that a person can use at home. It also records the pulse (smaller reading of "68" in this illustration).

> **KEY POINT** Indirect blood pressure readings consist of two numbers expressed as a fraction; the first number represents the maximum pressure on the artery, and the second number represents the amount of pressure that still exists when the heart is relaxed (in other words, not contracting). Observe the drawings in Fig. 4.10 to understand indirect blood pressure readings. The standard unit of measurement is millimeters of mercury (mm Hg). For example, a healthy young person has a blood pressure of approximately 120/80 mm Hg. The higher reading indicates the **systolic pressure,** and the lower reading indicates the **diastolic pressure.** Likewise, blood pressure is at its highest point (when the ventricles contract) during **systole;** relaxation of the ventricles is **diastole.** Three types of instruments are shown in Fig. 4.10, D–F.

WORD ORIGIN
diastole *(G.)*
diastole, expansion

Arteries are popularly used to measure blood pressure, and the reading is a reflection of cardiac output and arterial resistance. Four factors that increase blood pressure are the following:
- increased cardiac output
- increased blood volume
- increased blood viscosity
- loss of elasticity of the arterial walls

In other words, blood pressure readings reflect the quantity of blood flow through the heart and resistance in the walls of the _____.

arteries

4-21 Hyper/tension, abbreviated HTN, is increased blood pressure. Decreased blood pressure is

_____.

hypotension

4-22 The electric impulses arising in the SA node and carried by the cardiac conduction system produce electric currents that can be measured in **electro/cardio/graphy,** the process of recording the electrical currents of the heart. The record produced in electrocardiography is an

_____, and the name of the instrument is an **electrocardiograph.** Each segment of the ECG shows the electric cycle of the heart (Fig. 4.11). Normal heart rhythm is called *sinus rhythm.*

electrocardiogram

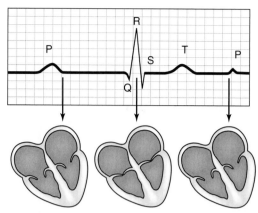

Figure 4.11 Electrocardiogram showing the location of the major waves. The P wave begins the cycle and represents the contraction of the atria when forcing the blood into the ventricles. The QRS complex represents the contraction of the ventricles when forcing the blood into both the pulmonary and systemic circulation. Relaxation of the heart occurs at the T wave. The cycle begins again with the new P wave.

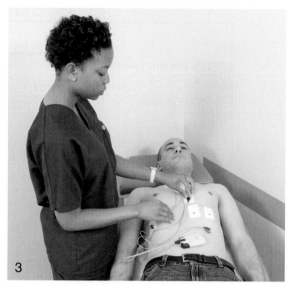

Figure 4.12 Placement of the leads on the chest in Holter monitoring.

🔑 **KEY** POINT **Electrocardiograms may be recorded in places other than a hospital or a doctor's office. Tele/cardio/ graphy** is the recording of a telecardiogram by transmission of impulses to a site that is distant from the patient; it is now regularly done via a telephone to a referral center or a physician's office. A **Holter monitor** is a portable electrocardiograph that a person can wear while conducting normal daily activities (Fig. 4.12). This device records heart activity over time and during various activities to aid in the diagnosis of cardiac problems that occur intermittently.

An increased pulse rate (greater than 100 beats per minute) is **tachy/cardia.** Using brady-, write a word that means a decreased pulse rate (less than 60 beats per minute): _____.

bradycardia

4-23 Laboratory tests for cardiovascular disorders include testing for fats and cardiac enzymes in the blood. **Lipids** are fatty substances in the body and include **cholesterol** and **triglycerides.** High levels of these two lipids are associated with greater risk of **arteriosclerosis,** hardening of the arteries. Two lipids associated with a greater risk of cardiovascular disease are triglycerides and

cholesterol

_____.

Lipo/proteins are special proteins that transport lipids in the blood. The elevation of **low-density lipoproteins** (LDLs) is associated with an increased risk of cardiovascular disease. High levels of **high-density lipoproteins** (HDLs) are associated with decreased cardiac risk profiles. A lipid profile report shows the amounts of LDLs and HDLs (Fig. 4.13). **Hypercholesterolemia** and **hyperlipidemia** mean greater than normal amounts of cholesterol and lipids in the blood, respectively. Either of these may lead to atherosclerosis, which you will study in the section "Blood Vessel Pathologies."

4-24 Certain enzymes are released into the bloodstream by damaged heart muscle. Levels of these enzymes can be measured in blood tests called the *lactate dehydrogenase (LDH) test* and *creatine kinase (CK) test,* also called *creatine phosphokinase (CPK).* Levels of these enzymes usually rise within a few hours after a heart attack. LDH and CPK are blood tests to assess _____ damage.

heart

PARTICLE CONCENTRATION AND SIZE

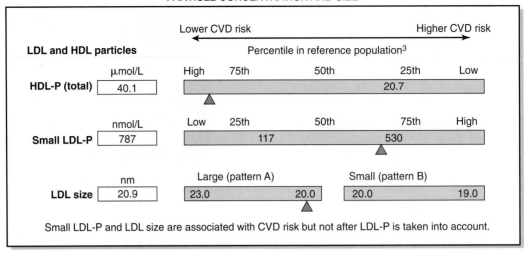

LDL and HDL particles		Lower CVD risk ← Percentile in reference population[3] → Higher CVD risk				
HDL-P (total)	μmol/L 40.1	High	75th	50th	25th ▲ 20.7	Low
Small LDL-P	nmol/L 787	Low	25th 117	50th	75th 530 ▲	High
LDL size	nm 20.9	Large (pattern A) 23.0 20.0 ▲			Small (pattern B) 20.0 19.0	

Small LDL-P and LDL size are associated with CVD risk but not after LDL-P is taken into account.

Figure 4.13 Small portion of a lipid profile report.

WRITE IT!
EXERCISE 10

Write a word in each blank to complete these sentences.

1. Increased blood pressure is _____.
2. Decreased pulse is _____.
3. Relaxation of the ventricles is called _____.
4. Blood pressure that is measured when the ventricles contract is the _____ pressure.
5. A portable electrocardiograph that a person can wear is a _____ monitor.
6. Cholesterol and triglycerides are fatty substances called _____.
7. LDL and HDL are special proteins called _____.

Additional diagnostic procedures are used to help assess heart diseases, and many of them are noninvasive. For example, examination of a chest x-ray gives information about the size and position of the heart. Additional noninvasive procedures include the following:

cardiac computed tomography Produces cross-sectional images of the heart.

cardiac MRI Magnetic resonance imaging of the heart.

echo/cardio/graphy A noninvasive procedure using ultrasonic waves, ultrasonography, in diagnosing heart disease (Fig. 4.14, A). The graphic record of the heart obtained during echocardiography is an **echocardiogram. Doppler echocardiography** is a technique in which Doppler ultrasonography is used to evaluate the direction and pattern of blood flow within the heart (Fig. 4.14, B). A **transesophageal echocardiogram** (TEE) is an endoscopic ultrasound test that provides ultrasonic imaging of the heart from a retrocardiac vantage point (inside the esophagus).

positron emission tomography A computerized radiographic technique that uses radioactive substances to examine the myocardial metabolic activity.

stress tests Tests that measure the heart's response during controlled physiologic stress, usually exercise. In the treadmill exercise test (or **treadmill stress test**), an ECG and other measurements are taken

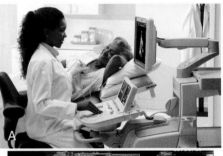
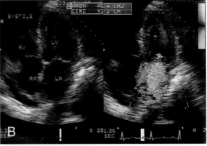

Figure 4.14 Echocardiography. A, An echocardiographer demonstrates the procedure. **B,** Color Doppler image of the heart. The chambers of the heart are labeled in the black and white image on the left.

while the patient walks on an inclined treadmill at varying speeds and inclines. The **thallium stress test** and other nuclear medicine procedures also measure cardiovascular function, particularly in coronary artery disease.

Invasive procedures include the following:

arterio/graphy Radiography of arteries after injection of radiopaque material into the bloodstream. Literally, this word means recording of the arteries. The film produced in arteriography is an arteriogram (Fig. 4.15). Through common usage, **arteriograph** is used interchangeably with **arteriogram,** just as photo/graph is used to mean the record (picture) produced in photography. **Coronary arteriography** is a radiographic procedure used to study coronary arteries. **Aorto/graphy** is radiography of the aorta after introduction of a contrast medium. The film produced by aortography is an **aortogram.** Different areas of the aorta are generally studied, rather than visualization of all of its divisions. Thoracic, abdominal, and renal aortography are examples of areas of the aorta that are studied.

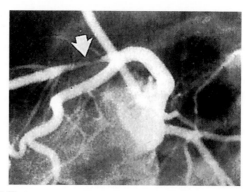

Figure 4.15 Arteriogram. Radiographic image after injection of a radiopaque contrast medium reveals blockage of an artery *(arrow).*

cardiac catheterization A diagnostic procedure in which a catheter is introduced through an incision into a large blood vessel of the arm, leg, or neck and threaded through the circulatory system to the heart. Pressures and patterns of blood flow can be determined in catheterization (Fig. 4.16). The catheter enables the use of contrast media that enhance x-ray images of the heart and its vessels.

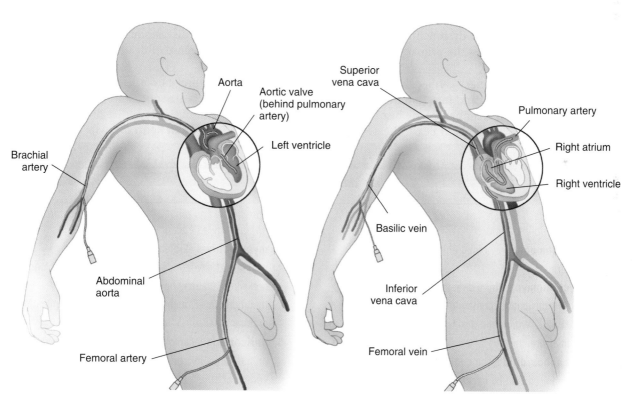

Figure 4.16 Heart catheterization. A, Left-sided. **B,** Right-sided. Progress of the catheter is monitored by fluoroscopy as it is threaded through blood vessels to reach the heart. Fluoroscopy gives the physician immediate images of the location of the catheter throughout the procedure. The right side of the heart may be the only side examined because left-sided heart catheterization is riskier than that of the right.

coronary angiography Radiography of the heart and its vessels by injection of radiopaque contrast medium directly into coronary arteries using the same procedure as that used for cardiac catheterization. The record produced is a **coronary angiogram.** This is also called **angiocardiography. Digital subtraction angiography** (DSA) provides computer-enhanced radiographic images of blood vessels filled with contrast material.

electrophysiology studies Use electrode catheters inserted into the right side of the heart to identify disturbances in different cardiac structures.

BUILD IT!

EXERCISE 11

Use the following word parts to build terms. (Some word parts will be used more than once.)

aort(o), arteri(o), cardi(o), ech(o), -gram, -graphy

1. ultrasonography of the heart   _____/_____/_____
2. radiography of the aorta   _____/_____
3. image produced in radiography of the arteries   _____/_____

PATHOLOGIES

Heart Pathologies

cardiovascular

4-25 Cardiovascular disease is any abnormal condition characterized by dysfunction of the heart and blood vessels. Diagnosis and treatment of cardiovascular disorders have improved, but cardiovascular disease still ranks slightly higher than cancer as the major cause of death in the United States.

Heart disease can be classified in many ways. One method is based on whether the cause of the heart dysfunction developed away from the heart (as in diseases of the arteries) or the heart itself was the primary site of the dysfunction. The leading cause of death in the United States is _____ disease.

Primary cardiac diseases include those caused by structural cardiac defects, as well as inflammation and infection that originate within the heart. Defects are sometimes present in one of the four chambers of the heart, in one of the heart valves, or in the septum that divides the two sides of the heart. If heart disease is present at birth, it is a **congenital heart disease.**

> **BEYOND** THE BLUEPRINT Spontaneous coronary artery dissection (SCAD) is a rare type of heart attack in which blood pools between the layers of the arterial wall, blocks blood flow from the heart, leading to a tear inside an artery.

FIND IT!

EXERCISE 12

Draw a slash between the word parts in the following list of new terms. Then find the meanings of the word parts within the definitions. (Draw the slash, and then perform the remainder of the activity as a mental exercise. Think!)

1. **atriomegaly** abnormal enlargement of an atrium.
2. **cardiomyopathy** a general diagnostic term that designates primary myocardial disease. In other words, the disease originated in the myocardium.
3. **endocarditis** inflammation of the inner lining of the heart, caused by infectious microorganisms.
4. **myocarditis** a cardiomyopathy that results in insufficient oxygen, damaged valves, or high blood pressure. This may be caused by an infection, rheumatic fever, a chemical agent, or a complication of another disease.
5. **pericarditis** inflammation of the pericardium owing to an infectious microorganism, a cancerous growth, or a variety of other causes.

Learn these word parts that are used to describe heart abnormalities.

Additional Word Parts: Heart Pathologies

Word Part	Meaning	Word Part	Meaning
rhythm(o), rrhythm(o)	rhythm	scler(o), -sclerosis	hard, hardening
de-	down, from, or reversing	-stenosis	narrowing, stricture

atria

4-26 A **ventricular septal defect** is an abnormal opening in the septum dividing the right and the left ventricles (Fig. 4.17). This defect is a type of congenital heart disease. An **atrial septal defect** is also a congenital heart disease. An atrial septal defect is an abnormal opening in the part of the septum that separates the right and the left _____.

4-27 There are other congenital heart diseases, but atrial septal defects and ventricular septal defects account for 30% to 40% of heart diseases that are present at birth. Almost all congenital heart defects (those present at birth) interrupt the normal flow of blood through the heart and vessels. **Heart murmurs**—abnormal heart sounds—are often heard. Cyanosis may also be present.

blue (or bluish)

Cyan/osis is a _____ discoloration of the skin and mucous membranes that results from insufficient oxygen to the tissues.

It may be difficult to remember specifics of the following defects, but it is important to remember that these three are also congenital heart diseases and that surgery may be indicated:
- **patent ductus arteriosus** (PDA), an abnormal opening between the pulmonary artery and the aorta
- **coarctation of the aorta** narrowing of a part of the aorta
- **tetralogy of Fallot**, four congenital heart defects, named for the French physician

without

4-28 Normally the intervals between pulses are of equal length. Remembering that a- means no or without, **a/rrhythmia** is _____ rhythm. The combining forms rrhythm(o) and rhythm(o) mean rhythm. Arrhythmia is the same as arhythmia and is the more common spelling.

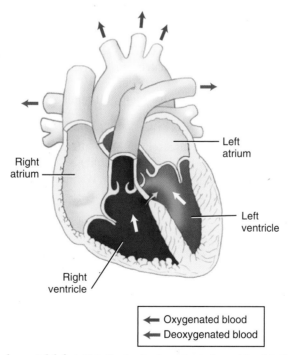

Right atrium

Left atrium

Left ventricle

Right ventricle

← Oxygenated blood
← Deoxygenated blood

Figure 4.17 Ventricular septal defect. Note the abnormal opening in the septal wall *(yellow arrow)* that divides the left and right ventricles. The direction of abnormal blood flow (left to right or right to left) depends on the severity of the septal defect. Dilution of oxygenated blood results in cyanosis or a bluish discoloration of the skin.

A variation in the normal rhythm of the heartbeat is an arrhythmia. Although this term is more commonly used, **dys/rhythm/ia** would be more technically correct. Dysrhythmia is a disturbance of rhythm. Common usage generally determines whether one uses one "r" or two in medical terms that pertain to rhythm. Write the new term that means an abnormal, disordered, or disturbed rhythm: _____.

dysrhythmia

Heart flutters are rapid contractions of either the atria or the ventricles and can be seen on the electrocardiogram. Heart **palpitations,** however, are subjective sensations of a pounding or racing heart. It can be associated with heart disease, but some persons experience palpitations and yet have no evidence of heart disease. In these cases, the palpitations are believed to be emotional responses to stress.

4-29 Ventricular fibrillation is a severe cardiac arrhythmia in which ventricular contractions are too rapid and uncoordinated for effective blood circulation. A cardiac arrhythmia marked by rapid, uncoordinated contractions is called _____.

fibrillation

Sometimes a defibrillator is used to alleviate fibrillation. (The prefix de- is used to mean down, from, or reversing. It is in the latter sense that it is used here.) A **defibrillator** is an electronic apparatus that has defibrillator paddles that are used to make contact with the patient and deliver a preset voltage of electricity to shock the heart (Fig. 4.18). **Defibrillation** stops _____. Ventricular fibrillation is often a cause of cardiac arrest. Another name for cardiac arrest is **a/systole,** which means absence of heartbeat or contraction.

fibrillation

4-30 You learned earlier that the heart has a special structure, the SA node, where electric impulses arise and stimulate contraction. Impairment in the conduction of the impulse from the SA node to other parts of the heart is known as a **heart block.** When the electric impulse is not conducted throughout the heart, normal heart contraction does not occur. This condition is known as a heart _____. The condition may be asymptomatic and require no intervention, but implantation of an artificial pacemaker (described later in the Surgical and Therapeutic Intervention section) may be necessary in complete heart block.

block

4-31 Atrial fibrillation (AFib)**,** a cardiac arrhythmia characterized by disorganized electric activity in the atria, results in reduced stroke volume (the amount of blood ejected by a ventricle during contraction) but is not as life-threatening as ventricular fibrillation. Other arrhythmias that can be detected by electrocardiography include bradycardia, tachycardia, premature ventricular contractions (PVCs), and atrioventricular block (AVB).

In **paroxysmal atrial tachycardia** (PAT), the patient may detect palpitations and a racing heartbeat (150 to 250 beats per minute) that occur and stop suddenly. Paroxysmal means occurring in sudden, repeated episodes.

Atrioventricular block is a disorder of impulse transmission between the atria and the _____.

ventricles

4-32 In many types of heart disease, the heart attempts to compensate for its deficit by working harder. Cardio/megaly may result. **Cardiomegaly** is _____ of the heart.

Micro/cardia, the opposite of cardiomegaly, is abnormal _____ of the heart.

enlargement
smallness

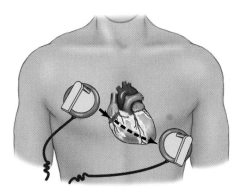

Figure 4.18 Flow of current when defibrillator paddles are applied. The paddles, usually applied over special defibrillator pads on the patient's chest, deliver an electric shock at a preset voltage to the myocardium. *Arrows* indicate the flow of the electric current as it passes through the heart.

ischemia

WORD ORIGIN

angina pectoris *(L.)*
angor, strangling; *pectus,*
breast or chest

oxygen

WORD ORIGIN

infarct *(L.)*
infarcire, to stuff

infarction

4-33 Insufficient blood flow to an area is termed **ischemia.** If the myocardial demand for oxygen exceeds the capability of diseased coronary arteries, myocardial _____ results. The patient may experience chest pain, often called **angina pectoris,** or simply angina. The pain usually radiates along the neck, jaw, and shoulder and down the left arm. The pain of angina is often relieved by rest and the use of a coronary vasodilator, **nitroglyerin** tablets, placed under the tongue.

4-34 An/ox/ia means an abnormal condition characterized by absence of _____. A localized area of damaged tissue resulting from anoxia is called an **infarct. Myocardial infarction** (MI) is necrosis of a portion of cardiac muscle caused by an obstruction or a blood clot in a coronary artery. Cells die when deprived of oxygen. The death of cells in an area of the myocardium because of oxygen deprivation is myocardial infarction (Fig. 4.19). A myocardial infarction is a heart attack. It is important to call an emergency medical service (EMS) at the first sign of chest pain or a suspected heart pain to avoid damage to the heart by myocardial infarction.

Whether death occurs after MI largely depends on the resulting damage to the myocardium. Those who survive often have complications of heart function. When areas of the myocardium die because of lack of oxygen, this is called myocardial _____.

Rest is an important part of recovery after a heart attack. The patient is usually left with some heart damage, often resulting in failure of the heart to function normally. This deficiency of the heart is called **cardiac insufficiency.** If the damage is too severe, surgical intervention may be necessary. An acute coronary syndrome (ACS) is a classification that can range from unstable angina to myocardial infarction.

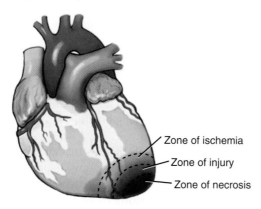

Zone of ischemia
Zone of injury
Zone of necrosis

Figure 4.19 Myocardial infarction. Also called a *heart attack,* myocardial infarction is necrosis of a portion of cardiac muscle. It is usually caused by an obstruction in a coronary artery.

BUILD IT!   EXERCISE 13

Use the following word parts to build terms. (Some word parts will be used more than once.)

an-, dys-, micro-, atri(o), cardi(o), cyan(o), ox(i), rhythm(o), -ia, -megaly, -osis

1. Enlargement of an atrium of the heart   _____/_____
2. Bluish discoloration of the skin and mucous membranes   _____/_____
3. A variation in the normal rhythm of the heartbeat   _____/_____/_____
4. Abnormal smallness of the heart   _____/_____/_____
5. Abnormal condition of absence of oxygen   _____/_____/_____

WRITE IT!   EXERCISE 14

Case Study. *Define the terms as indicated.*

Marshall is seen in the emergency department with pain in the chest and left arm. He has shortness of breath, tachycardia, hypotension, dysrhythmia, elevation of the S-T segment on the electrocardiogram, and a normal chest x-ray, except for moderate cardiomegaly. Miguel is placed on heparin and admitted for further testing in the AM.

1. tachycardia   _____
2. hypotension   _____
3. dysrhythmia   _____
4. electrocardiogram _____
5. cardiomegaly   _____

4-35 MI and other disorders in which there is insufficient oxygen to the heart may lead to **congestive heart failure** (CHF), also called *congestive heart disease*. CHF is an abnormal condition that reflects impaired cardiac function. The patient experiences weakness, breathlessness, and edema. Edema is an abnormal accumulation of fluid in the interstitial spaces of tissue. This condition is called _____ heart failure.

congestive

4-36 Heart valves can also be defective, resulting in the valves not opening fully, as in **valvul/ar stenosis. Stenosis** means narrowing. When a valve is stenosed, it becomes constricted or narrower. Valvular stenosis is _____ of the opening created by the valve. Stenosis of any of the heart's valves can decrease blood circulation.

narrowing

Valves may also become infected and inflamed. **Valvul/itis** is inflammation of a valve, especially a heart valve. Build a new word that specifically means inflammation of the valves of the heart by using a combining form that means heart + valvulitis: _____.

cardiovalvulitis

Weakening of one or both mitral cusps when the heart contracts is called **mitral valve prolapse** (MVP). When a valve prolapses, such as in MVP, the valve sags rather than opening fully and also permits leakage because of the faulty valve flaps. Symptoms vary from absent to severe, and the condition may be associated with sounds heard through a stethoscope, including a clicking sound or heart murmur.

4-37 Rheumatic fever, usually occurring in childhood, may develop as a delayed reaction to an inadequately treated infection of the upper respiratory tract by certain pathogenic streptococci (group A beta-hemolytic). The disease may affect the brain, heart, joints, or skin. **Rheumatic heart disease** is damage to heart muscle and heart valves caused by episodes of rheumatic fever. Permanent damage to the heart or the valves may occur. This type of damage is called _____ heart disease.

rheumatic

WORD ORIGIN
effusion *(L.)*
effusion, pour out

4-38 **Hemo/pericardium** is an effusion of blood into the pericardial space. **Effusion** means the escape of fluid into a part, such as a cavity. Blood in the pericardial space is called _____. An accumulation of fluid in the pericardial space can lead to compression of the heart, which is called **cardiac tamponade.**

hemopericardium

4-39 **Shock** is a life-threatening condition in which there is inadequate blood flow to the body's tissues. It is usually associated with inadequate cardiac output, hypotension, and tissue damage. Causes of shock include hemorrhage or dehydration resulting in hypo/vol/emia. The term **hypovolemia** means an abnormally _____ circulating blood volume.

low

WRITE IT!   **EXERCISE 15**

Write the names of the cardiac pathologies represented by the following definitions. The first letter of each term is given as a clue.

1. enlarged heart *c* _____

2. rapid and uncoordinated ventricular contractions *f* _____

3. absence of heart contractions *a* _____

4. a localized area of damaged tissue resulting from insufficient oxygen *i* _____

5. insufficient blood flow to an area *i* _____

6. inflammation of the valves of the heart *c* _____

7. inflammation of the pericardium *p* _____

8. a word that means narrowing *s* _____

9. inflammation of the lining of the heart *e* _____

10. a life-threatening condition in which blood flow is inadequate *s* _____

Blood Vessel Pathologies

4-40 Arteries, arterioles, capillaries, venules, and veins make up the network of blood vessels that carry blood. The dilation and constriction of blood vessels influence blood pressure and the distribution of blood to various parts of the body. The **vaso/motor** center located in the brain regulates vasoconstriction and vasodilation, thus influencing the diameter of the blood vessels.

vasodilation

Vaso/dilation is stretching or dilation of a vessel. In the word vasodilation, dilation means expansion or stretching. An increase in the diameter of a blood vessel is _____.

The opposite of vasodilation is **vaso/constriction.** When blood vessels constrict, they become narrow. A decrease in the diameter of blood vessels is vasoconstriction.

Learn the meaning of these word parts used to describe disorders of the blood vessels.

Additional Word Parts: Blood Vessel Pathologies

Combining Form	Meaning
aneurysm(o)	aneurysm
ather(o)	yellowish, fatty plaque
embol(o)	embolus

Read about selected pathologies of blood vessels.

aneurysm A localized dilation or ballooning out of the wall of a blood vessel. Aneurysms can occur in many blood vessels, but most aneurysms are arterial (because pressure is higher in the arteries, particularly the aorta). An aneurysm may rupture, causing hemorrhage, or thrombi may form in the dilated vessel and give rise to emboli that may obstruct smaller vessels. Aneurysms tend to occur at specific sites (Fig. 4.20).

angi/oma A benign tumor of either blood **(hem/angi/oma)** or lymph **(lymph/angi/oma)** vessels. Angiomas are not malignant and sometimes disappear spontaneously. Whether a hemangioma or a lymphangioma, the tumor consists of a mass of blood vessels (see Fig. 2.13). (Note that the vowel is dropped from hem[a] and lymph[o] when they are joined with combining forms that begin with a vowel.) A lymphangioma is a tumor composed of a mass of lymphatic vessels.

angio/stenosis Narrowing of the diameter of a vessel. Narrowing of the aorta is **aortic stenosis,** in which blood cannot flow efficiently from the left ventricle into the aorta, and the condition may lead to congestive heart failure. Stenosis, as well as **stricture,** means an abnormal condition characterized by narrowing or constriction of an opening or passageway. (Two terms often have the

same meaning because words are derived from both the Latin and the Greek languages.)

aortic regurgitation Blood flows back into the left ventricle during diastole because the aortic valve does not close completely. The heart will work harder in an attempt to deliver needed oxygen and nutrients to all the body's cells. Also called **aortic insufficiency** (AI).

arterio/scler/osis A thickening and loss of elasticity of the walls of the arteries. Literal interpretation of arterio/scler/osis is hardening of the arteries. Scler/osis means abnormal hardening of tissue.

arterio/sclero/tic heart disease (ASHD) Hardening and thickening of the walls of the coronary arteries. This reduces the oxygen supply to the myocardium and may lead to a heart attack.

athero/sclerosis A form of arteriosclerosis, characterized by the formation of fatty deposits on the walls of arteries (Fig. 4.21). The yellowish plaques in atherosclerosis are cholesterol, other lipids, and cellular debris that accumulate in the inner walls of arteries. As atherosclerosis progresses, the vessel walls become fibrotic and calcified and the **lumen** (cavity) narrows, which results in reduced blood flow. Plaque is one of the major causes of coronary heart disease, angina pectoris, myocardial infarction, and other cardiac disorders.

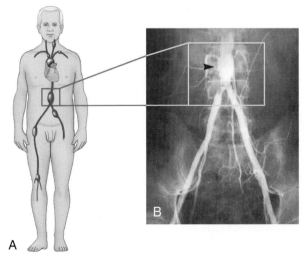

Figure 4.20 Common sites of aneurysms. A, Common anatomic sites of arterial aneurysms. **B,** Arteriogram of an abdominal aortic aneurysm. Note the abnormal dilation (bulging out) of the site indicated by the *arrow.*

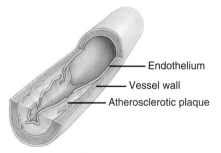

Figure 4.21 Partial blockage of an artery by plaque in atherosclerosis. The endothelium is a layer of epithelial cells that lines blood and lymph vessels as well as the heart and many closed cavities of the body. As lipids, calcium, fibrin, and other cellular substances are deposited within the lining of the arteries, an inflammatory response results from the efforts to heal the endothelium.

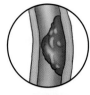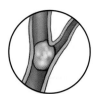

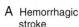

A Hemorrhagic   B Thrombotic   C Embolic (embolitic)
   stroke   stroke   stroke

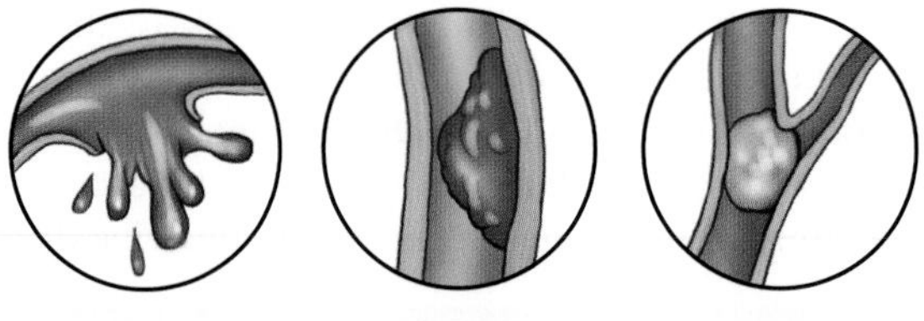

Figure 4.22 Types of stroke. A, Hemorrhagic stroke. Blood vessel bursts and allows blood to seep into brain tissue until clotting stops the seepage. **B,** Thrombotic stroke. Plaque can cause a clot that blocks blood flow to brain tissue. **C,** Embolic stroke. A blood clot or other embolus reaches an artery in the brain, lodges there, and blocks the flow of blood.

cerebro/vascular accident (CVA) An abnormal condition characterized by occlusion of a vessel of the brain by an embolus, thrombus, or cerebrovascular hemorrhage or spasm that results in ischemia of the brain tissues, also called a *stroke* (Fig. 4.22).

coronary artery disease (CAD) An abnormal condition of the coronary arteries that causes a reduced flow of oxygen and nutrients to the myocardium; may precede a heart attack.

coronary occlusion Obstruction or blockage of a coronary artery. The occlusion may result from a thrombus, but

it is more likely to be caused by a narrowing of the lumen of the blood vessel by plaque.

coronary thrombosis Formation of a blood clot in a coronary artery.

peripheral vascular disease Blockage or narrowing of arteries, especially those conditions affecting the lower extremities and resulting in interference of adequate blood flow to the extremities. Atherosclerosis is one cause of this condition.

FIND IT!   EXERCISE 16

Draw a slash between the word parts in the following new terms. Then find the meanings of the word parts within the definition. (Draw the slash, and then perform the remainder of the activity as a mental exercise. Think!)

1. **aortitis** inflammation of the aorta
2. **aortosclerosis** hardening of the aorta
3. **aneurysmal** pertaining to an aneurysm
4. **angiocarditis** inflammation of the heart and large blood vessels
5. **arteritis** inflammation of an artery
6. **arteriopathy** any disease of the arteries

BUILD IT!   EXERCISE 17

Use the following word parts to build terms. (Some word parts will be used more than once.)

aneurysm(o), angi(o), arteri(o), cardi(o), lymph(o), -al, -itis, -oma, -sclerosis, -stenosis

1. narrowing of the diameter of a vessel _____/_____
2. pertaining to a localized dilation of the wall of a blood vessel _____/_____
3. a tumor composed of lymph vessels _____/_____/_____
4. thickening and loss of elasticity of the arteries _____/_____
5. inflammation of the heart and large blood vessels _____/_____/_____

WRITE IT!   EXERCISE 18

Write a word in each blank to complete these sentences.

1. A term for a localized dilation or ballooning out of the wall of a blood vessel is _____.
2. CAD is an abbreviation that means _____ artery disease.
3. A closing off of a coronary artery is called coronary _____.
4. Formation of a blood clot in a coronary artery is coronary _____.
5. Formation of fatty deposits on the walls of arteries is a form of arteriosclerosis, called _____.
6. Hardening of the aorta is _____.
7. Narrowing of the diameter of the aorta is called aortic _____.

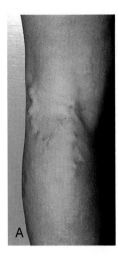

A

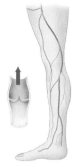

NORMAL VEINS
Functional valves aid
in flow of venous blood
back to heart

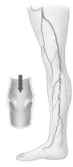

VARICOSE VEINS
Failure of valves and
pooling of blood in
superficial veins

B

Figure 4.23 **Varicose veins. A,** The appearance of superficial varicose veins. **B,** Comparison of normal veins and varicose veins. Sluggish blood flow, weakened walls, and incompetent valves contribute to varicose veins in the legs, a common location for these enlarged and twisted veins near the surface of the skin.

varicose

4-41 Varicose veins are swollen and knotted and occur most often in the legs. They result from sluggish blood flow in combination with weakened walls and incompetent valves in the veins. Unlike arteries, which have substantially more muscle and elastic tissue, veins have flaplike valves that prevent blood from flowing backward. Defective valves allow the blood to collect in the veins, which become swollen and knotted (Fig. 4.23). This condition is called _____ veins.

phlebitis

4-42 Using phleb(o), build a word that means inflammation of a vein: _____ .
   Thrombo/phleb/itis is inflammation of a vein associated with a blood clot. Deep vein thrombophlebitis involves a thrombus in one of the deep veins of the body, most commonly the iliac or femoral veins. **Venous thrombosis,** formation of a thrombus within a vein, may be a complication of phleb/itis. It may also result from an injury to the leg or prolonged bed confinement.
   Hemorrhoids are a type of varicose veins in the lower rectum or anus (see Fig. 6.22, B).

4-43 Phlebo/stasis may be a spontaneous slowing down of blood flow in a vein or the result of a deliberate act in which one compresses the vein to control the flow of blood temporarily. In many words, -stasis will be used for either of these two meanings.

vein

   You will need to remember that phlebostasis means either a spontaneous venous stasis or stopping the flow of blood in a _____ by application of a tourniquet on an extremity. A **tourniquet** is a device applied around an extremity to control the circulation and prevent the flow of blood to or from the distal area.

**MATCH IT!
EXERCISE 19**

Match the terms in the left column with the descriptions in the right column.

_____ **1.** phlebitis
_____ **2.** phlebostasis
_____ **3.** thrombophlebitis
_____ **4.** venous thrombosis

A. formation of a blood clot within a vein
B. inflammation of a vein
C. slowing down of blood flow in a vein
D. inflammation of a vein associated with a blood clot

SURGICAL AND THERAPEUTIC INTERVENTIONS

4-44 Cardio/pulmonary resuscitation (CPR) is a basic emergency procedure for life support, consisting of manual external cardiac massage and artificial respiration. The artificial respiration can be mouth-to-mouth breathing or a mechanical form of ventilation.
   CPR is used in cases of cardiac arrest to establish effective circulation and ventilation to prevent irreversible cerebral and cardiac damage resulting from anoxia. CPR is an abbreviation for

cardiopulmonary

_____ resuscitation.

pacemaker

4-45 You learned earlier that the SA node is called the pacemaker of the heart. A second meaning of pacemaker is an artificial **cardiac pacemaker,** a small battery-powered device that is generally used to increase the heart rate by electrically stimulating the heart muscle. Depending on the patient's need, a cardiac pacemaker may be permanent or temporary and may fire only on demand or at a constant rate (Fig. 4.24). Severe bradycardia may indicate the need for an artificial cardiac

_____.

Arrhythmias that do not respond to medications are sometimes treated using catheter ablation, in which an area of the heart causing the arrhythmia is destroyed using radiofrequency.

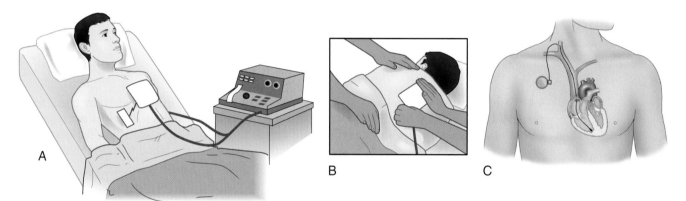

A   B   C

Figure 4.24 Artificial cardiac pacemaker. An *external* pacemaker is used temporarily in a hospital setting to deliver electric current through the skin. Electrodes are placed on the patient's anterior (**A**) and posterior (**B**) chest walls and attached to an external pacing unit. **C,** An *internal* artificial cardiac pacemaker provides an electric current that travels from the battery through a conducting wire to the myocardium and stimulates the heart to beat.

cardioverter

4-46 Cardio/version uses electric shock to restore the normal rhythm of the heart with a device that delivers a direct-current shock. An automatic implantable **cardioverter** is a device that detects sustained ventricular tachycardia or fibrillation and terminates it by a shock that restores the normal rhythm (Fig. 4.25). **Defibrillation** stops fibrillation. This implanted device is called an automatic implantable _____.

cardioplegic

4-47 Surgical repair may be indicated in aortic stenosis, narrowing of the aortic valve. The replacement may be an open heart surgery, in which the chest is opened, or more recently, a catheter-based surgery. In a transcatheter aortic valve replacement, a catheter is guided into the heart through the femoral artery and a stent valve is inserted through the catheter.

If surgery is to be performed on the heart, **cardio/plegia** may be necessary to stop myocardial contractions. Solutions used to stop the heart's action so that surgery may be performed on the heart are called _____ **solutions.**

🔑 **KEY** POINT Surgeries involving the heart and major vessels generally require **cardiopulmonary bypass**, a procedure in which the heart is bypassed by providing an **extra/corporeal** (outside the body) device to pump blood. The blood is diverted from the heart and lungs to a pump oxygenator, then returned directly to the aorta and pumped to the rest of the body (Fig. 4.26). Developments in cardiac surgery are heart transplantation and use of an artificial heart.

bypass

4-48 The term **bypass** is also used to mean bypass surgery. A **coronary artery bypass** is an open heart surgery in which a prosthesis or a section of a blood vessel is grafted onto one of the coronary arteries, bypassing a blocked or narrowed coronary artery in coronary artery disease. If a vessel from elsewhere in the patient's body is used to provide an alternate route for the blood to circumvent the obstructed coronary artery, the surgery is called a **coronary artery bypass graft** (CABG), pronounced "cabbage" (Fig. 4.27).

The vessels that are generally used are a segment of the saphenous vein from the patient's leg or the mammary artery. A bypass is also called a **shunt.** One that circumvents a vessel that supplies blood to the heart is called a coronary artery _____.

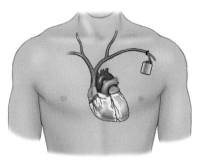

Figure 4.25 Implantable cardioverter-defibrillator. This surgically implanted electric device automatically terminates arrhythmias by delivering low-energy shocks to the heart, restoring proper rhythm when the heart begins beating too fast or erratically. It is generally attached to the chest wall and has a wire lead embedded in the heart.

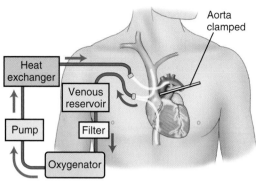

Figure 4.26 Components of a cardiopulmonary bypass system used during heart surgery.

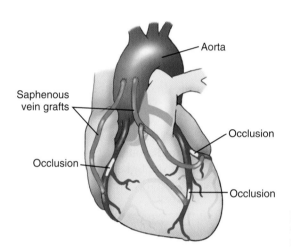

Figure 4.27 **Coronary artery bypass graft using saphenous vein grafts.** Sections of the patient's own saphenous veins located in the legs are grafted onto the coronary arteries to bypass the blocked coronary arteries.

🔑 **KEY** POINT **Depending on the patient, there may be less-invasive surgeries for coronary artery disease that do not require cardiopulmonary bypass.** Options for traditional CABG include minimally invasive direct coronary artery bypass (MIDCAB), off-pump coronary artery bypass (OPCAB), and port-access and video-assisted CABGs.

percutaneous

4-49 Modification of risk factors (cessation of smoking, physical activity, and diet control) is often a necessary part of management of cardiovascular disease. A variety of procedures, some not requiring extensive surgery, are available for treating vascular insufficiencies. Per/cutane/ous means performed through the skin. Percutaneous procedures to improve blood flow in a particular vessel involve the use of a catheter, monitored by fluoroscopy, that is introduced through a blood vessel. The management of coronary artery occlusions by any of the catheter-based techniques is called **percutaneous coronary intervention** (PCI). These procedures include the compression or removal of plaque that may be preventing adequate blood flow. PCI is _____ coronary intervention and applies to a coronary artery.

🔑 **KEY** POINT **PCI is invasive management of coronary arteries, but doesn't involve the trauma of regular surgery.** PCI involves the use of catheters inserted into occluded or stenosed arteries. Plaque is compressed, destroyed, or cut away and removed. Procedures include laser-assisted angioplasty, percutaneous transluminal coronary angioplasty, implantation of coronary stents to keep the vessel open, and atherectomy.

repair

As a term written alone, angio/plasty means surgical _____ of a blood vessel that has become damaged by disease or injury.

artery

4-50 **Laser-assisted angioplasty** applies to arteries in general and is the opening of an occluded artery with laser energy delivered to the site through a fiberoptic probe. One type of PCI, **excimer laser coronary angioplasty,** is used to remove blockage in a coronary _____.

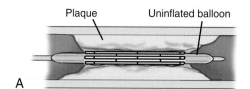

Plaque   Uninflated balloon

A

Figure 4.28 Balloon angioplasty and placement of a coronary artery stent. A small, balloon-tipped catheter is threaded into a coronary artery and inflated to compress the plaque. A stent, an expandable meshlike structure, is placed over the angioplasty site to keep the coronary artery open. **A,** The stent and uninflated balloon catheter are positioned in the artery. **B,** The stent expands as the balloon is inflated. **C,** The balloon is then deflated and removed, leaving the implanted stent.

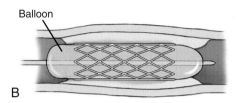

Balloon

B

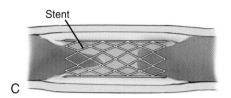

Stent

C

4-51 In **percutaneous transluminal coronary angioplasty** (PTCA), a catheter equipped with an inflatable balloon tip is inserted into a partially occluded coronary artery. After the catheter is passed through and just past the appropriate area, the balloon at the tip of the catheter is inflated, and the atherosclerotic plaque is compressed **(balloon angioplasty).** PTCA means percutaneous transluminal coronary _____.

angioplasty

An **intracoronary stent** is sometimes inserted during PTCA to treat abrupt or threatened closure of a coronary artery. **Stents,** sometimes containing drugs to discourage blood clots, are expandable meshlike structures that are placed over the angioplasty site to keep the vessel open by compressing the arterial walls (Fig. 4.28). Intra/coronary pertains to the interior of a coronary

artery

_____.

➤ **BEYOND** THE BLUEPRINT Angio/genesis occurs in a healthy body for healing wounds and restoring blood flow to tissues after injury. Therapeutic angiogenesis is treatment of ischemic organs or tissues; for example, puncturing an ischemic heart to stimulate the creation of new blood vessels; however, controversy exists regarding the value of this procedure.

4-52 Atherectomy uses a specially designed catheter for cutting away plaque from the lining of an artery. Some atherectomies use a rotational blade to shave off the plaque, which is simultaneously extracted by suction (Fig. 4.29). Cutting away plaque from the interior of an artery with a rotational blade is a type of _____.

atherectomy

4-53 If less invasive procedures are either unsuccessful or not recommended (for example, total occlusion of a blood vessel), it may be possible to surgically remove plaque that has accumulated in an artery. In the case of coronary arteries, you read earlier that CABG or one of its options is often performed.

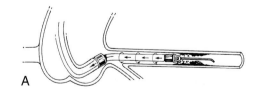

A

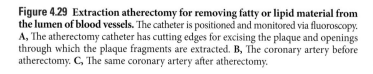
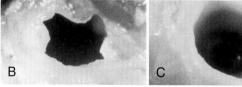

B   C

Figure 4.29 Extraction atherectomy for removing fatty or lipid material from the lumen of blood vessels. The catheter is positioned and monitored via fluoroscopy. **A,** The atherectomy catheter has cutting edges for excising the plaque and openings through which the plaque fragments are extracted. **B,** The coronary artery before atherectomy. **C,** The same coronary artery after atherectomy.

artery

endarterectomy

thrombolysis

vein

End/arter/ectomy is surgical excision of arteriosclerotic plaque from the inner wall of an obstructed _____. Endarterectomy does not designate a particular artery. There are several sites in the body where plaque commonly forms. One of these is the carotid artery, and this occlusion causes restricted blood flow to the brain. Removal of arteriosclerotic plaque from an obstructed carotid artery, usually done to prevent stroke, is called **carotid** _____.

4-54 The formation of a blood clot is often prevented by administration of an oral anticoagulant. Once a thrombus (blood clot) in an artery is formed, it is sometimes treated with a thrombo/lytic agent to dissolve the clot. This procedure may be recommended for a blood clot in a coronary artery in a patient with acute myocardial infarction. In this procedure, called **intra/vascular thrombo/lysis,** the thrombolytic agent is delivered through a catheter and infused into the clot, which often dissolves over a period of time. The use of a catheter to deliver a thrombolytic agent to dissolve a blood clot is called intravascular _____.

4-55 Discomfort from varicose veins varies widely. Superficial varicose veins may primarily present a cosmetic problem. In such situations **sclero/therapy,** direct injection of a sclerosing agent, can be performed in an office setting and causes minimal discomfort. It successfully eliminates unsightly superficial varicose veins (see Fig. 4.23) but does not prevent development of further varicosities.

Conservative treatment of varicose veins includes elevation of the limb, compression stockings, and exercise. Surgical intervention for varicose veins involves tying off the entire vein and removing its incompetent tributaries. In selected patients the use of laser therapy delivered through a catheter may be an option in the treatment of varicosities.

Phleb/ectomy is surgical removal of a _____. This procedure may involve removing only a segment of the vein. Phlebectomy may be necessary for treatment of varicose veins. Continue learning about surgical terms pertaining to the cardiovascular system by working the next exercise. _Want more information? Go to http://www.heart.org._

FIND IT!
EXERCISE 20

Draw a slash between the word parts in the following new terms. Then find the meanings of the word parts within the definition. (Draw the slash, and then perform the remainder of the activity as a mental exercise. Think!)

1. **phleboplasty** plastic surgery of a vein
2. **pericardiocentesis** surgical puncture of the pericardium. This is done to draw off fluid that has accumulated in the pericardial space.
3. **atrioseptoplasty** surgical repair of the septum in the area between the right and left atria. This is performed when necessary for surgical closure of the abnormal opening between the atria.
4. **angiostomy** formation of a new opening into a blood vessel
5. **angiotomy** incision of a blood or lymphatic vessel
6. **angiectomy** excision of a vessel
7. **embolectomy** excision of an embolus

MATCH IT!
EXERCISE 21

Read the surgical schedule, and match the diagnoses in the left column with the surgical interventions in the right column. (All selections are used.)

Surgical Schedule:

_____ **1.** arrhythmia

_____ **2.** atrial septal defect

_____ **3.** blocked coronary artery

_____ **4.** plaque in a peripheral artery

_____ **5.** severe bradycardia

_____ **6.** varicose veins

A. atherectomy

B. atrioseptoplasty

C. cardiac pacemaker

D. internal cardioverter

E. phlebectomy

F. PTCA

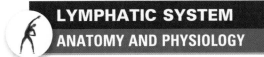

LYMPHATIC SYSTEM
ANATOMY AND PHYSIOLOGY

4-56 The lymphatic system has several important functions:
- Helps protect and maintain the internal fluid environment of the body by producing, filtering, and conveying lymph
- Absorbs and transports fats to the blood system
- Serves as an important part of the immune system: Lymph nodes filter lymph and trap substances, helping prevent the spread of infection or cancer cells. In addition, lymph nodes contain macro/phages that can phagocytize foreign substances. Lymphocytes undergo maturation in lymphatic tissue to become B lymphocytes (B cells) or T lymphocytes (T cells). B cells and T cells are involved in antibody- and cell-mediated immunity, respectively.

🔑 **KEY** POINT **The lymphatic system is also called the lymphatics.** This system is composed of lymphatic vessels, a fluid called **lymph, lymph nodes,** and three organs: the spleen, thymus, and tonsils.

lymph

The fluid transported by the lymphatic vessels is _____.
Learn the meaning of the following word parts.

Word Parts: Lymphatic System

Combining Form	Meaning	Combining Form	Meaning
aden(o)	gland	lymphat(o)	lymphatics
adenoid(o)	adenoids	splen(o)	spleen
lymph(o)	lymph, lymphatics	thym(o)	thymus
lymphaden(o)	lymph node	tonsill(o)	tonsil
lymphangi(o)	lymph vessel		

WRITE IT!   EXERCISE 22

Write the combining form for these structures of the lymphatic system.

1. gland _____
2. lymph node _____
3. lymph vessel _____
4. spleen _____
5. thymus _____
6. tonsil _____

lymphogenous

4-57 Lympho/genous means either producing lymph or produced from lymph or the lymphatics. Write the word that means originating in the lymphatics: _____.

4-58 Study the major parts of the lymphatic system (Fig. 4.30). Only the major lymph vessels and nodes are shown. The smallest vessels of this system are lymph capillaries, which are found in almost all regions of the body. Look at the detailed drawing of the proximity of the lymphatic capillaries to the cardiovascular capillaries, venules, and arterioles. The lymphatic capillaries pick up _____ fluid that has collected from the normal course of blood circulation.

interstitial

4-59 Note the bean-shaped lymph nodes along the course of the lymph vessels shown in Fig. 4.30. The **cisterna chyli** and the ducts are structures that are formed by the merging of many lymph vessels and their trunks.
    As its name indicates, the thorac/ic duct is located in the _____.

chest

4-60 Three types of lymph nodes are shown in the drawing. The combining form that you will use to write terms about lymph nodes is _____.
    The **cervic/al lymph nodes** are located in the area of the _____.
    In other chapters, you will study the combining forms cervic(o), axill(o), and inguin(o), which mean neck, armpit, and groin, respectively, as used here. For now, remember the locations of the cervical, **axillary,** and **inguinal** lymph **nodes.**

lymphaden(o)

neck

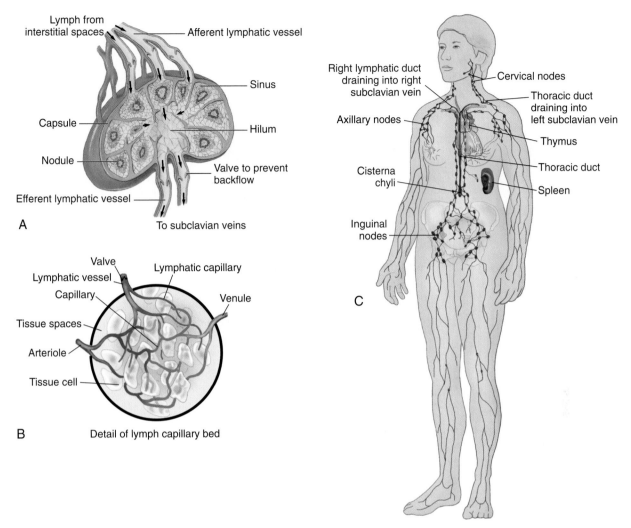

Figure 4.30 Lymphatic system. A, Lymph nodes filter lymph and fight infection. They range in size from pinhead to the size of a bean. Lymph flows into the node through afferent lymphatic vessels, where many harmful substances in the fluid are trapped, then the filtered lymph exits by efferent lymphatic vessels. **B,** Detailed drawing showing the close relationship of the lymphatic and cardiovascular systems. **C,** Major lymph nodes and vessels of the lymphatic system.

4-61 Fluid enters the lymph vessels and is transported back to the cardiovascular system because of valves that carry the fluid away from the tissue. The system depends on muscular contraction, because there is no pump, and transport of fluid is slow. Lymph ducts eventually empty the lymph into the subclavian veins, thus returning the fluid to the systemic circulation (Fig. 4.31).

Lymph is the fluid transported by the lymphatic vessels. Sometimes lymph(o) is used to mean lymphatics, but it is also a combining form for lymph. The combining form that you will use to write terms about lymph vessels is _____.

lymphangi(o)

4-62 Cells from malignant tumors may escape and be transported by the lymphatic circulation or the bloodstream to implant in lymph nodes and other organs far from the primary tumor. Cancer cells that wander into a lymph vessel may be trapped by the lymph nodes and begin growing there, or the cells may be carried to sites far from their origin. Lymph nodes are often examined to determine if cancer has spread to the lymphatics.

4-63 The **spleen,** the **tonsils,** and the **thymus** contain lymphatic tissue and are specialized lymphatic organs. The spleen is a large organ situated in the upper left part of the abdominal cavity. Splen/ic refers to the _____. Although one can live without the spleen, it performs important tasks, such as defense, production of lymphocytes and plasma cells, blood storage, and destruction and recycling of red blood cells and platelets. Write a new word that means pertaining to the spleen by combining splen(o) + -ic: _____. **Spleno/lymphatic** pertains to the spleen and the lymph nodes.

spleen

splenic

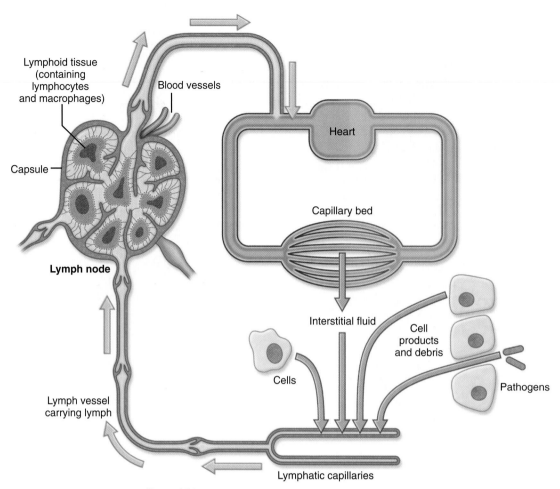

Figure 4.31 Circulation of lymph in the lymphatic system.

4-64 The thymus is also called the *thymus gland*, because it is a glandlike body. It is located in the anterior mediastinal cavity and is important in the maturation of T cells, lymphocytes that are involved in cell-mediated immunity. The thymus usually obtains its greatest absolute size at puberty and then becomes smaller. Use thym(o) + -ic to write a new word that means pertaining to the thymus: _____.

thymic

4-65 When we see the word tonsil, we think of the pair of small, almond-shaped masses located at the back of the throat. These are the **palatine tonsils** (the palate is the roof of the mouth, the bony partition between the oral and nasal cavities) and are usually what one is referring to when the term tonsil is used. But one should be aware that the tonsils are small masses of lymphatic tissue of several types, including the palatine and **lingual** (lingu[o], tongue + -al, pertaining to) **tonsils,** as well as the **adenoids** (also called pharyngeal tonsils). **Tonsill/ar** means pertaining to a _____. The combining form adenoid(o) means adenoids.

tonsil

WRITE IT! **EXERCISE 23**

Write a word in each blank to complete this paragraph.

As blood circulates, interstitial fluid accumulates in the tissue spaces. This excess fluid is normally transported away from the tissues by a vascular network called the (1) _____ system. The system is composed of vessels, nodes, the spleen, thymus, tonsils, and a fluid called (2) _____. The fluid flows in one direction only, away from the tissue, and is eventually emptied into the subclavian (3) _____, thus returning the fluid to the (4) _____ circulation. The spleen, the tonsils, and the thymus are specialized lymphatic organs. A term that means pertaining to the spleen is (5) _____. Pertaining to the thymus is (6) _____. Pertaining to the palatine tonsils is (7) _____.

DIAGNOSTIC TESTS AND PROCEDURES

lymphogram

4-66 The lymphatic channels and lymph nodes can be x-rayed after injection of radiopaque material into a lymphatic vessel. This procedure is called **lympho/graphy**. Write a word that means the picture produced in lymphography: _____.

nodes

4-67 The lymphatic vessels are the focus of study in **lymph/angio/graphy,** radiology of the lymphatic vessels after the injection of a contrast medium. In lymphadeno/graphy, the lymph _____ are the focus of study.

Imaging of lymphoid organs can also be accomplished using computed tomography, magnetic resonance imaging, and nuclear magnetic imaging.

4-68 Biopsies of the lymph nodes are important tools for diagnosis of the spread of cancer and are routine during many surgeries in which cancerous organs are removed.

> **BEYOND** THE BLUEPRINT The first lymph node to receive lymphatic drainage from a malignant tumor is termed the *sentinel node*. This node is identified using radioactive dye, which causes the node to "light up" like a sentinel, indicating that the node is the most appropriate one for examination, thus the term *sentinel node biopsy*. If the sentinel nodes do not contain malignant cells, this usually eliminates the necessity of removing more distal nodes.

lymph

Biopsy of _____ nodes near cancerous organs is an important tool to determine whether cancer has spread.

Blood tests provide additional information about the lymphatic system, especially tests related to immunity and specialized studies of the lymphocytes.

WRITE IT! **EXERCISE 24**

Write a word in each blank to complete these sentences.

1. Radiography of the lymphatic vessels and nodes after injection of radiopaque material is

_____.

2. Radiology of the lymphatic vessels after injection of a contrast medium is _____.

3. Removal of tissue from the lymph nodes to determine whether cancer has spread from a nearby organ is called _____ of the lymph nodes.

PATHOLOGIES

Selected disorders of the lymphatic system are presented.

Adenoids

adenoid/itis Inflammation of the adenoids. When the adenoids are enlarged as a result of frequent infection, they can obstruct the passageway, and removal may be indicated.

Lymphatic Vessels and Lymph Nodes

lymph/aden/itis Inflammation of a lymph gland. This inflammatory condition can result from a bacterial or viral infection or other inflammatory condition, and the location of the affected node is indicative of the site of the infection. For example, inflammation of a cervical lymph node indicates infection of a tooth; the mouth, throat, ear, or somewhere else in the head (Fig. 4.32). Antibiotics are generally indicated when bacterial infection is present. Swelling of several lymph glands is characteristic of infectious mononucleosis, an acute viral infection that was discussed in the previous chapter.

lymph/adeno/pathy Any disorder characterized by a localized or generalized enlargement of the lymph nodes or lymph vessels. However, a lymphangioma, composed of a mass of dilated lymph vessels, is benign.

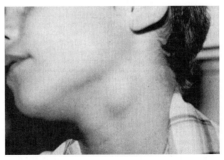

Figure 4.32 Lymphadenitis. The cervical lymph node is enlarged, firm, and freely movable. The node may resolve without treatment or may eventually rupture and drain.

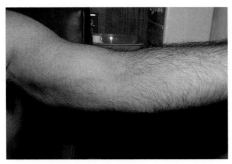

Figure 4.33 Streptococcal lymphangitis. This type of inflammatory condition of the lymph nodes is caused by streptococcal bacteria. Examination of the area distal to the affected node usually reveals the source of the infection.

lymph/ang/itis Inflammation of a lymphatic vessel, often the result of an acute streptococcal infection of one of the extremities (Fig. 4.33). (Note the spelling of lymphangitis, which uses the combining forms for lymph, vessel, and inflammation. Some of the vowels are omitted in the spelling of lymphangitis to facilitate pronunciation.)

lymph/edema Swelling of the subcutaneous tissue of an extremity as a result of obstruction of the lymphatics. The meaning of lymphedema is implied. Primary lymphedema is hypoplasia and maldevelopment of the lymphatic system resulting in swelling and sometimes grotesque distortion of the extremities. Acquired lymphedema results from trauma to the lymphatic ducts, such as surgical removal of lymph channels in mastectomy, obstruction of lymph drainage by malignant tumors, or the infestation of lymph vessels with parasites (Fig. 4.34).

lymph/oma A type of neoplasm (tumor) of lymphoid tissue that originates in the system itself and is usually malignant. Two main types of lymphomas are Hodgkin disease and non-Hodgkin lymphoma. Not all malignancies of the lymphatic system originate in the system itself. Cancer cells may be brought to the lymphatics via lymph and may result in lymphatic carcinoma.

lympho/stasis Stoppage of lymph flow.

thrombo/lymphang/itis Inflammation of a lymph vessel caused by a blood clot.

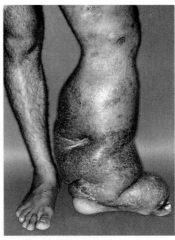

Figure 4.34 Lymphedema. Extensive swelling, caused by chronic obstruction of the lymphatic vessels, occurs in the late stages of elephantiasis.

Spleen

spleno/megaly Enlargement of the spleen.

spleno/pathy Any disease of the spleen.

spleno/ptosis A downward displacement (sagging) of the spleen.

spleno/rrhagia Hemorrhage from the spleen. Because of its anatomic location, the spleen is often injured in abdominal trauma. Rupture of the spleen can occur from blunt trauma, such as a blow from a car accident.

Thymus

thym/oma A tumor, usually benign, of the thymus.

thymo/pathy Any disease of the thymus.

Tonsils

tonsill/itis Inflammation of the palatine tonsils.

MATCH IT! **EXERCISE 25**

Match pathologies in the left column with the correct terms in the right column.

_____ **1.** enlarged spleen

_____ **2.** inflammation of a lymph vessel

_____ **3.** inflammation of a lymph node

_____ **4.** inflammation of the palatine tonsils

_____ **5.** tumor originating in the lymphatics

A. lymphadenitis
B. lymphangitis
C. lymphoma
D. splenomegaly
E. tonsillitis

SURGICAL AND THERAPEUTIC INTERVENTIONS

excision

4-69 Penicillin and hot soaks are usually prescribed for lymphangitis. Infected lymph nodes often respond to antibiotic therapy or resolve on their own. **Lymphaden/ectomy** is _____ of a lymph node. This term is often accompanied by an adjective referring to the location of the node that is removed, such as cervical (referring to the neck) lymphadenectomy.

radiation

4-70 Treatment of lymphoma is determined by the type of lymphoma but can include intensive radiotherapy, chemotherapy, and biological therapies, including interferon. Radio/therapy is treatment of tumors using _____ to kill malignant cells and deter their proliferation.

4-71 Splenoptosis, prolapse of the spleen, can be corrected by surgical fixation of the spleen. This surgery is called **spleno/pexy.**

splenectomy

A ruptured spleen often requires surgical intervention. **Spleno/rrhaphy** is suture of the spleen. Surgical removal of the spleen is _____.

tonsillectomy

4-72 Thymectomy means removal of the thymus.

Excision of the tonsils is a _____. A tonsillectomy is performed to treat a chronic infection of the tonsils. An **adenoidectomy** is performed because the adenoids are enlarged, chronically infected, or causing obstruction. They are sometimes removed at the same time as a tonsillectomy as a prophylactic measure. A procedure in which tonsillectomy and adenoidectomy are performed at the same time is called a **tonsilloadenoidectomy.**

MATCH IT!
EXERCISE 26

Match interventions in the left column with the correct terms in the right column. (Not all selections will be used.)

_____ **1.** excision of the adenoids

_____ **2.** excision of a lymph node

_____ **3.** excision of the tonsils

_____ **4.** removal of the thymus

_____ **5.** suture of the spleen

_____ **6.** surgical fixation of the spleen

A. adenoidectomy

B. adenoidopathy

C. lymphadenectomy

D. lymphangiectomy

E. splenopexy

F. splenorrhaphy

G. thymectomy

H. tonsillectomy

BUILD IT!
EXERCISE 27

Use the following word parts to build terms. (Some word parts will be used more than once.)

lymph(o), splen(o), thym(o), tonsill(o), lymphaden(o), -ectomy, -edema, -ic, -pathy, -rrhagia

1. pertaining to the thymus _____/_____

2. swelling from obstruction of the lymphatics _____/_____

3. hemorrhage from the spleen _____/_____

4. surgical removal of the tonsils _____/_____

5. any disorder characterized by enlargement of the lymph nodes _____/_____

PHARMACOLOGY

Many of the agents in this chapter may be found together in combination drugs to treat multiple facets of a disease at once.

Drug Class: Effects and Uses

Antianginal Drugs: Relax blood vessels of the heart to treat and prevent angina

isosorbide dinitrate (Isordil)
isosorbide mononitrate (Imdur)
nitroglycerin (Nitrostat)
ranolazine (Ranexa)

Antiarrhythmics: Regulate cardiac rhythm to treat arrhythmias
- Categorized into five subclasses based on primary mechanism of action, but some drugs have multiple actions: Class I (a, b, c) affects sodium channels; Class II: Beta-blockers; Class III affects potassium channels; Class IV affects calcium channel blockers; Class V (miscellaneous)

adenosine (Adenocard)
amiodarone (Pacerone)
digoxin (Lanoxin)
disopyramide (Norpace)
dronedarone (Multaq)
flecainide (Tambocor)
ibutilide (Corvert)
lidocaine (Xylocaine)
procainamide (Pronestyl)
propafenone (Rythmol)

Anticoagulants: Prevent clotting of blood

enoxaparin (Lovenox)
heparin (Panheprin)
warfarin (Coumadin)

Antihyperlipidemics: Reduce cholesterol in the blood to treat hyperlipidemia or dyslipidemia
- Subclasses include fibrates, HMG-CoA reductase inhibitors ("statins"), bile-acid sequestrants, niacin, and selective cholesterol absorption inhibitors

atorvastatin (Lipitor)
cholestyramine (Questran)
ezetimibe (Zetia)
fenofibric acid (Trilipix)
gemfibrozil (Lopid)
niacin (Niaspan)
pitavastatin (Livalo)
simvastatin (Zocor)

Antihypertensives: Reduce high blood pressure

Angiotensin-Converting Enzyme Inhibitors (ACE Inhibitors): Block formation of angiotensin II (a vasoconstricting hormone) to treat hypertension, heart failure, or kidney disease

captopril (Capoten)
ramipril (Altace)
lisinopril (Zestril)
quinapril (Accupril)
enalapril (Vasotec)
trandolapril (Mavik)

Angiotensin-II Receptor Blockers (ARBs): Block the action of angiotensin II (a vasoconstricting hormone) to treat hypertension, heart failure, or kidney disease

azilsartan (Edarbi)
candesartan (Atacand)
irbesartan (Avapro)
losartan (Cozaar)
valsartan (Diovan)

Beta-Blockers: Block neurotransmitters from binding beta-I receptors to decrease heart rate and force of contractility in the heart
- Cardiovascular uses: hypertension, heart failure, angina, cardiac arrhythmia, and heart attack
- Other uses: glaucoma, migraine prophylaxis, anxiety, and essential tremor

atenolol (Tenormin)
carvedilol (Coreg)
esmolol (Brevibloc)
metoprolol (Lopressor)
nadolol (Corgard)
propranolol (Inderal)

Calcium Channel Blockers (CCBs): Inhibit movement of calcium ions across cell membranes to relax the heart muscles and blood vessels to treat angina, hypertension, and arrhythmias

amlodipine (Norvasc)
clevidipine (Cleviprex)
diltiazem (Cardizem)
felodipine (Plendil)
nifedipine (Procardia)
nisoldipine (Sular)
verapamil (Calan)

Diuretics: Increase excretion of water and sodium as urine to treat edema and hypertension

hydrochlorothiazide (Oretic)
metolazone (Zaroxolyn)
furosemide (Lasix)
bumetanide (Bumex)
spironolactone (Aldactone)
triamterene (Dyrenium)
torsemide (Demadex)

Renin Inhibitors: Suppress renin-angiotensin system to treat hypertension and prevent cardiovascular events
aliskiren (Tekturna)

PHARMACOLOGY, cont'd

Antiplatelet Drugs/Antiaggregants: Inhibit function or reduce number of platelets to prevent thrombosis

abciximab (ReoPro)   clopidogrel (Plavix)   prasugrel (Effient)
aspirin (Bayer)   dipyridamole (Persantine)   tirofiban (Aggrastat)

Blood Flow Agents: Improve peripheral blood supply to treat claudication (leg cramps), symptoms of cerebral vascular insufficiency, nighttime leg cramping, or arteriosclerosis

cilostazol (Pletal)   isoxsuprine (Vasodilan)   pentoxifylline (Trental)

Cardiac Stimulants: Support circulation to treat cardiogenic shock, hypotension, or congestive heart failure

Inotropes: Increase heart's force of contraction to improve cardiac output

dobutamine (Dobutrex)   inamrinone (Inocor)
epinephrine (Adrenaclick)   metaraminol (Aramine)

Vasoconstrictors, Vasopressors: Constrict blood vessels to raise blood pressure

dobutamine (Dobutrex)   epinephrine (Adrenaclick)   vasopressin (Vasostrict)

Hemostatics: Stop bleeding

aminocaproic acid (Amicar) phytonadione (Vitamin K_1)

Thrombolytics: Dissolve blood clots, commonly referred to as "clot busters"

alteplase (Activase)   reteplase (Retavase)   tenectaplase (TNKase)

> **BEYOND** THE BLUEPRINT Research and treatments for heart disease are historically designed for men, yet gender-specific research on heart disease continues to show differences between the two genders. Because of this gap, physicians lack information about how best to diagnose and treat female heart disease. Go Red for Women and other initiatives are helping better educate about women's risks and recognition of this leading cause of women's death. Clinical trials need to include an equal number of females in this equal-opportunity killer.

CIRCLE IT! EXERCISE 28

Circle the correct answer to complete these sentences.

1. Drugs that relax blood vessels of the heart to treat or prevent angina are (antianginals, antiaggregants, antihypertensives, vasoconstrictors).
2. Drugs known as "clot busters" are (anticoagulants, antihyperlipidemics, antihypertensives, thrombolytics).
3. The drug class used to stop bleeding is (anticoagulants, beta blockers, hemostatics, vasoconstrictors).
4. The drug class used to prevent clotting of blood is (antianginal drugs, anticoagulants, antihyperlipidemics, beta blockers).
5. The drug class used to reduce high blood pressure is (antihypertensives, antiaggregants, hemostatics, vasopressors).

CHAPTER ABBREVIATIONS*

ACS	acute coronary syndrome
AFib	atrial fibrillation
AI	aortic insufficiency (and several others)
ASHD	arteriosclerotic heart disease
AV, A-V	atrioventricular
AVB	atrioventricular block
BP	blood pressure
CABG	coronary artery bypass graft
CAD	coronary artery disease
CHF	congestive heart failure
CK (CPK)	creatine kinase (formerly called creatine phosphokinase)
CPR	cardiopulmonary resuscitation
CVA	cerebrovascular accident (also costovertebral angle)
DSA	digital subtraction angiography
EMS	emergency medical service
HDL	high-density lipoprotein
HTN	hypertension
LA	left atrium
LDH	lactate dehydrogenase (enzyme elevated after MI)

LDL	low-density lipoprotein
LV	left ventricle
MI	myocardial infarction
MIDCAB	minimally invasive direct coronary artery bypass
mm Hg	millimeters of mercury
MVP	mitral valve prolapse
OPCAB	off-pump coronary artery bypass
PAT	paroxysmal atrial tachycardia
PCI	percutaneous coronary intervention
PDA	patent ductus arteriosus (also posterior descending [coronary] artery)
PTCA	percutaneous transluminal coronary angioplasty
PVC	premature ventricular contraction
RA	right atrium (also rheumatoid arthritis)
RV	right ventricle
SA	sinoatrial
TEE	transesophageal echocardiogram

*Many of these abbreviations share their meanings with other terms.

 Be Careful With These!

bradycardia vs. *tachycardia*   *hypertension* vs. *hypotension*   *lymphangi(o)* vs. *lymphaden(o)*

diastole vs. *systole*   *vasodilation* vs. *vasoconstriction*

A Career as an Echocardiographer

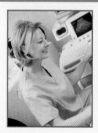

Meet Marsha Brown, an echocardiographer who works at a cardiologist's office. Marsha is a radiologic technologist who has specialized in echocardiography (echo). Echo is a type of ultrasonography that can show "moving" pictures of the heart during contractions. An ECG is done at the same time as the echo examination, and the results are coordinated to compare the physical motion and electric activity of the heart. Marsha also uses echo to test the effects of stress on the heart. For more information on this important career in diagnostic imaging, visit *www.asecho.org* or view this video on the Internet: *http://www.asrt.org/main/careers/careers-in-radiologic-technology/career-videos.*

CHAPTER 4 SELF-TEST

Review the new word parts for this chapter. Work all of the following exercises to test your understanding of the material before checking your answers against those in Appendix IV.

BASIC UNDERSTANDING

Labeling

I. Using this illustration of a capillary bed, write combining forms for the structures that are indicated. (Line 1 is done as an example.) Write two combining forms for line 2 (artery) and three combining forms for line 4 (vein), as indicated on the drawing.

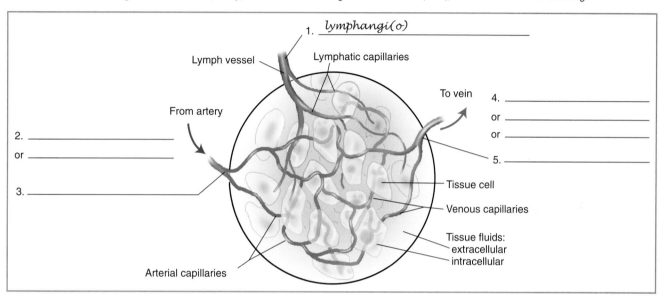

II. Write combining forms for the structures that are indicated on the diagram: lymph node, lymph vessel, spleen, thymus, tonsil.

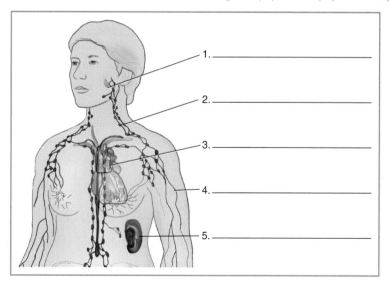

Matching

III. Use all selections to match terms in the left column with their descriptions in the right column.

_____	**1.** arterioles	**A.** lower chambers of the heart
_____	**2.** aorta	**B.** the largest artery
_____	**3.** atria	**C.** two large veins that communicate with the right atrium
_____	**4.** capillaries	**D.** upper chambers of the heart
_____	**5.** pulmonary arteries	**E.** vessels that carry blood from the heart to the lungs
_____	**6.** pulmonary veins	**F.** vessels that carry blood from the lungs to the heart
_____	**7.** veins	**G.** vessels that convey blood from the venules toward the heart
_____	**8.** venae cavae	**H.** vessels that join arteries and capillaries
_____	**9.** venules	**I.** vessels that join arterioles and venules
_____	**10.** ventricles	**J.** vessels that join capillaries and veins

IV. Match terms in the left column with their descriptions in the right column.

_____	**1.** cardiac septum	**A.** area in the chest cavity that contains the heart
_____	**2.** endocardium	**B.** cardiac muscle tissue
_____	**3.** mediastinum	**C.** inner lining of the heart
_____	**4.** myocardium	**D.** sac which encloses the heart
_____	**5.** pericardium	**E.** wall between the left and right sides of the heart

Listing

V. Name three functions of the lymphatic system.

1. _____

2. _____

3. _____

Deconstructing Words

VI. Divide these terms into their component parts, and state the meaning of each term.

1. adenoidectomy _____

2. angiography _____

3. anoxia _____

4. atriomegaly _____

5. cardiovascular _____

6. echocardiography _____

7. endarterectomy _____

8. hemopericardium _____

9. phlebectomy _____

10. thrombophlebitis _____

Opting for Opposites

VII. Write a term that you learned that means the opposite of these words.

1. bradycardia _____

2. cardiomegaly _____

3. hypotension _____

4. vasodilation _____

Identifying Illustrations

VIII. Label these illustrations using one of the following: aneurysm, echocardiography, elephantiasis, lymphangitis, lymphadenitis, phlebotomy

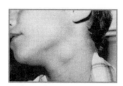

1. _____

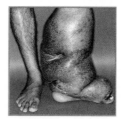

2. _____

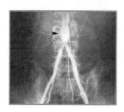

3. _____

4. _____

Writing Terms

IX. Write one word for each of the following clues.

1. a tumor of the thymus   _____

2. abnormal hardening of the aorta   _____

3. absence of a heartbeat   _____

4. agent that causes dilation of blood vessels _____

5. increased blood pressure   _____

6. increased pulse   _____

7. inflammation of a lymphatic vessel   _____

8. narrowing of the diameter of a vessel   _____

9. removal of the tonsils   _____

10. suture of the spleen   _____

Using Vocabulary

X. Circle the correct answer for each of the following questions.

1. Charlie, a 60-year-old man, has just been diagnosed as having a coronary occlusion. He is most at risk for which of the following? (atrioventricular block, congenital heart disease, myocardial infarction, rheumatic fever)

2. Charlie is told that he has a form of arteriosclerosis in which yellowish plaque has accumulated on the walls of the arteries. What is the name of this form of arteriosclerosis? (aortostenosis, atherosclerosis, cardiomyopathy, coarctation)

3. Charlie's physician advises surgery. Which surgery is generally prescribed for coronary occlusion? (automatic implantable cardiopulmonary bypass, cardioverter, coronary artery bypass, pericardiocentesis)

4. Kristen, a 25-year-old woman, is told she has inflammation of the lining of the heart. What is the medical term for this heart pathology? (coronary heart disease, endocarditis, myocarditis, pericarditis)

5. Jayne suffered ventricular fibrillation during coronary angiography. What procedure did the physician use to stop fibrillation? (atherectomy, endarterectomy, cardiopulmonary resuscitation, defibrillation)

6. Jim developed a blood clot in a coronary artery. What is Jim's condition called? (myocardial infarction, coronary artery bypass, coronary thrombosis, fibrillation)

7. Baby Seth is born with cyanosis and a heart murmur. Which congenital heart disease does the neonatologist think is more likely? (atrial septal defect, atrioventricular block, megalocardia, pericarditis)

8. Ten-year-old Zack had a sore throat for several days before he developed painful joints and a fever. Which disease does the physician suspect that can cause damage to the heart valves? (aortic valve sclerosis, aortic valve stenosis, mitral valve prolapse, rheumatic fever)

9. Ed experiences pain in his legs that is caused by blockage of arteries in the lower extremities. What is the name of his condition? (angiocarditis, lymphangioma, peripheral artery disease, varicose veins)

10. Carol has an angiogram that shows a ballooning out of the wall of a cerebrovascular artery. Which condition does Carol have? (aneurysm, angioma, arteriosclerosis, coronary thrombosis)

Making Connections

XI.   Describe the relationship of these terms.

1. embolus and cerebrovascular accident _____

_____

2. angioplasty and intracoronary stent _____

_____

Finetuning Terms

XII. In addition to spelling, describe at least one difference in the following:

1. systemic circulation and pulmonary circulation _____

_____

2. angiogram and angiography _____

_____

GREATER COMPREHENSION

Using Pharmacologic Terms

XIII. Matching

Use all selections to match terms in the left column with terms in the right column.

_____	1. antiaggregants	**A.** dissolve blood clots
_____	2. anticoagulants	**B.** prevent clotting of blood
_____	3. antihyperlipidemics	**C.** prevent thrombosis by reducing number of platelets
_____	4. antihypertensives	**D.** reduce cholesterol in the blood
_____	5. hemostatics	**E.** reduce high blood pressure
_____	6. thrombolytics	**F.** stop hemorrhage

Challenge: New Construction

XIV. Break these words into their component parts, and write their meanings. Even if you have not seen these terms before, you may be able to break them apart and determine their meanings.

1. aneurysmectomy   _____
2. epicardial   _____
3. lymphangiectasia _____
4. pericardiostomy _____
5. vasculitis   _____

Health Care Reports

XV. Read the following partial Emergency Treatment Record; then write the terms from the report that are described in numbers 1 through 6.

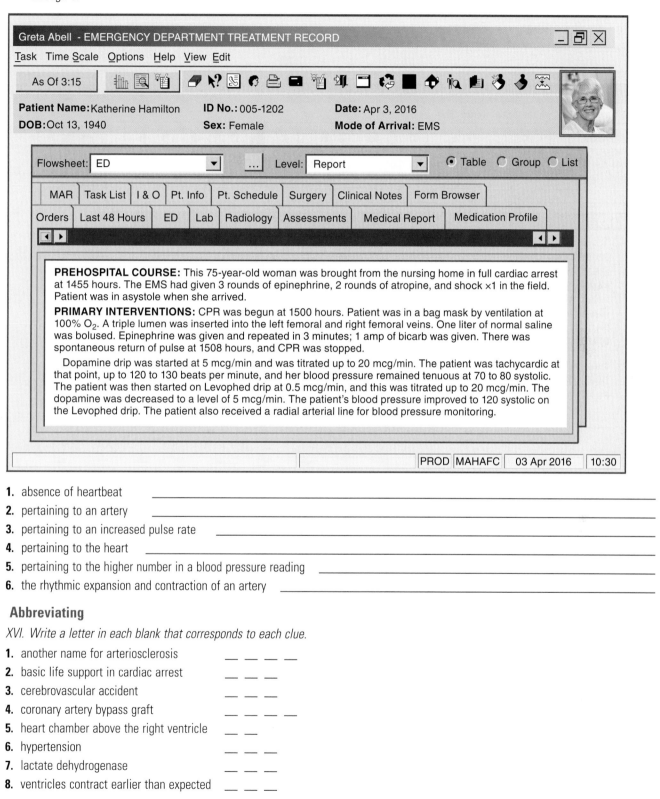

Greta Abell - EMERGENCY DEPARTMENT TREATMENT RECORD

Task   Time Scale   Options   Help   View   Edit

As Of 3:15

Patient Name: Katherine Hamilton   **ID No.:** 005-1202   **Date:** Apr 3, 2016
DOB: Oct 13, 1940   **Sex:** Female   **Mode of Arrival:** EMS

Flowsheet: ED   Level: Report   ⦿ Table ○ Group ○ List

MAR   Task List   I & O   Pt. Info   Pt. Schedule   Surgery   Clinical Notes   Form Browser

Orders   Last 48 Hours   ED   Lab   Radiology   Assessments   Medical Report   Medication Profile

PREHOSPITAL COURSE: This 75-year-old woman was brought from the nursing home in full cardiac arrest at 1455 hours. The EMS had given 3 rounds of epinephrine, 2 rounds of atropine, and shock ×1 in the field. Patient was in asystole when she arrived.

PRIMARY INTERVENTIONS: CPR was begun at 1500 hours. Patient was in a bag mask by ventilation at 100% O_2. A triple lumen was inserted into the left femoral and right femoral veins. One liter of normal saline was bolused. Epinephrine was given and repeated in 3 minutes; 1 amp of bicarb was given. There was spontaneous return of pulse at 1508 hours, and CPR was stopped.

Dopamine drip was started at 5 mcg/min and was titrated up to 20 mcg/min. The patient was tachycardic at that point, up to 120 to 130 beats per minute, and her blood pressure remained tenuous at 70 to 80 systolic. The patient was then started on Levophed drip at 0.5 mcg/min, and this was titrated up to 20 mcg/min. The dopamine was decreased to a level of 5 mcg/min. The patient's blood pressure improved to 120 systolic on the Levophed drip. The patient also received a radial arterial line for blood pressure monitoring.

PROD   MAHAFC   03 Apr 2016   10:30

1. absence of heartbeat _____

2. pertaining to an artery _____

3. pertaining to an increased pulse rate _____

4. pertaining to the heart _____

5. pertaining to the higher number in a blood pressure reading _____

6. the rhythmic expansion and contraction of an artery _____

Abbreviating

XVI. Write a letter in each blank that corresponds to each clue.

1. another name for arteriosclerosis   _ _ _ _

2. basic life support in cardiac arrest   _ _ _

3. cerebrovascular accident   _ _ _

4. coronary artery bypass graft   _ _ _ _

5. heart chamber above the right ventricle   _ _

6. hypertension   _ _ _

7. lactate dehydrogenase   _ _ _

8. ventricles contract earlier than expected   _ _ _

Spelling

XVII. Circle all misspelled terms and write their correct spelling:

adenoidectomy   athrosclerosis   diastole   iskemia   mediastinum

Health Care Reporting

XVIII. Read the Office Visit Note and circle the correct answer in numbers 1-5.

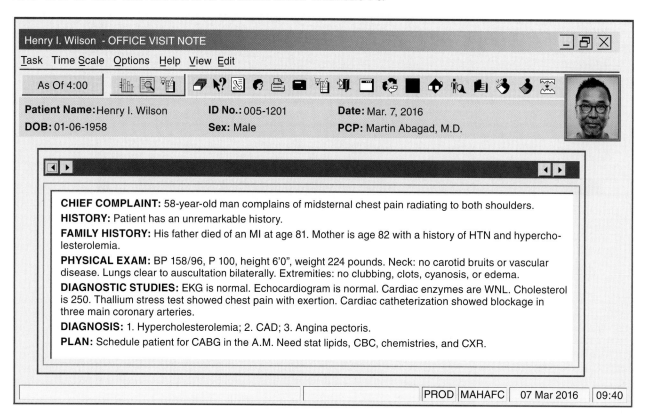

Henry I. Wilson - OFFICE VISIT NOTE

Task   Time Scale   Options   Help   View   Edit

As Of 4:00

Patient Name: Henry I. Wilson   **ID No.:** 005-1201   **Date:** Mar. 7, 2016
DOB: 01-06-1958   **Sex:** Male   **PCP:** Martin Abagad, M.D.

CHIEF COMPLAINT: 58-year-old man complains of midsternal chest pain radiating to both shoulders.
HISTORY: Patient has an unremarkable history.
FAMILY HISTORY: His father died of an MI at age 81. Mother is age 82 with a history of HTN and hypercholesterolemia.
PHYSICAL EXAM: BP 158/96, P 100, height 6'0", weight 224 pounds. Neck: no carotid bruits or vascular disease. Lungs clear to auscultation bilaterally. Extremities: no clubbing, clots, cyanosis, or edema.
DIAGNOSTIC STUDIES: EKG is normal. Echocardiogram is normal. Cardiac enzymes are WNL. Cholesterol is 250. Thallium stress test showed chest pain with exertion. Cardiac catheterization showed blockage in three main coronary arteries.
DIAGNOSIS: 1. Hypercholesterolemia; 2. CAD; 3. Angina pectoris.
PLAN: Schedule patient for CABG in the A.M. Need stat lipids, CBC, chemistries, and CXR.

PROD   MAHAFC   07 Mar 2016   09:40

1. Which term or phrase indicates the patient is suffering from chest pain? (angina pectoris, coronary, cyanosis midsternal)

2. Which abbreviation indicates blockage of the arteries which supply blood to the heart? (CABG, CAD, CBC, CXR)

3. Which of the following is indicated as the father's cause of death? (blood clot, heart attack, hypercholesterolemia, hypertension)

4. Which abbreviation indicates abnormally high blood pressure? (CAD, EKG, HTN, WNL)

5. Which term means an excessive level of cholesterol in the blood? (angina, cyanosis, hypercholesterolemia, hypertension, vascular)

Pronouncing Terms

XIX. Write the correct term for the follo wing phonetic spellings.

1. an-tē-hī-pur-lip-i-**dē**-mik   _____

2. kahr-dē-ō-mī-**op**-uh-thē   _____

3. lim-**fog**-ruh-fē   _____

4. per-i-**kahr**-dē-um   _____

5. throm-bō-**lit**-iks   _____

6. vā-zō-dī-**lā**-shun   _____

Health Care Reporting

XX. Read the Office Visit Note and circle the correct answer in numbers 1-5.

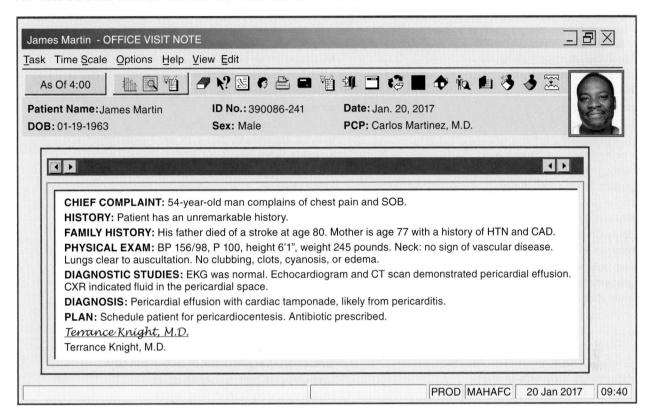

James Martin - OFFICE VISIT NOTE

Task Time Scale Options Help View Edit

As Of 4:00

Patient Name: James Martin   **ID No.:** 390086-241   **Date:** Jan. 20, 2017
DOB: 01-19-1963   **Sex:** Male   **PCP:** Carlos Martinez, M.D.

CHIEF COMPLAINT: 54-year-old man complains of chest pain and SOB.
HISTORY: Patient has an unremarkable history.
FAMILY HISTORY: His father died of a stroke at age 80. Mother is age 77 with a history of HTN and CAD.
PHYSICAL EXAM: BP 156/98, P 100, height 6'1", weight 245 pounds. Neck: no sign of vascular disease. Lungs clear to auscultation. No clubbing, clots, cyanosis, or edema.
DIAGNOSTIC STUDIES: EKG was normal. Echocardiogram and CT scan demonstrated pericardial effusion. CXR indicated fluid in the pericardial space.
DIAGNOSIS: Pericardial effusion with cardiac tamponade, likely from pericarditis.
PLAN: Schedule patient for pericardiocentesis. Antibiotic prescribed.
Terrance Knight, M.D.
Terrance Knight, M.D.

PROD MAHAFC 20 Jan 2017 09:40

1. Which layer of the patient's heart tissue was affected by disease? (inner layer, middle layer, outer layer)
2. Which term describes the compression of the patient's heart? (cardiac tamponade, cyanosis, pericardial effusion, pericarditis)
3. Which abbreviation refers to the patient's abnormally high blood pressure? (BP, EKG, HTN, SOB)
4. Which procedure involving the pericardium is the patient scheduled for? (surgical incision, surgical puncture, surgical removal, surgical repair)
5. The probable cause of the patient's mother's CAD is (atherosclerosis, cardioversion, coronary thrombosis, thrombophlebitis)

Categorizing Terms and Practicing Pronunciation

XXI. Classify the terms in the left column (1-10) by selecting A, B, C, D, or E.

_____ **1.** angiography   **A.** anatomical term

_____ **2.** angiostenosis   **B.** diagnostic test or procedure

_____ **3.** atrioseptoplasty   **C.** disease or disorder

_____ **4.** aortosclerosis   **D.** surgical term

_____ **5.** lymphoma   **E.** nonsurgical therapeutic term

_____ **6.** lymphangitis

_____ **7.** lymphography

_____ **8.** phlebectomy

_____ **9.** vasodilators

_____ **10.** venule

(Be prepared to pronounce terms 1-10 in class after listening to the Chapter 4 terms at *http://evolve.elsevier.com/Leonard/building/*. In addition, practice categorizing all boldfaced terms in this chapter.)
(Use Appendix IV to check your answers to the exercises.)

BMV LIST

Visit *http://evolve.elsevier.com/Leonard/building/* to listen to the boldface terms in Chapter 4. Look closely at the spelling of each term as it is pronounced.

adenoidectomy (ad-uh-noid-**ek**-tuh-mē)
adenoiditis (ad-uh-noid-**ī**-tis)
adenoids (**ad**-uh-noidz)
aneurysm (**an**-ū-riz-um)
aneurysmal (an-ū-**riz**-mul)
angiectomy (an-jē-**ek**-tuh-mē)
angina pectoris (an-**jī**-nuh **pek**-tuh-ris)
angiocardiography (an-jē-ō-kahr-dē-**og**-ruh-fē)
angiocarditis (an-jē-ō-kahr-**dī**-tus)
angioma (an-jē-**ō**-muh)
angiostenosis (an-jē-ō-stuh-**nō**-sis)
angiostomy (an-jē-**os**-tuh-mē)
angiotomy (an-jē-**ot**-uh-mē)
anoxia (uh-**nok**-sē-uh)
antiaggregants (an-tē-**ag**-ruh-gunts)
antianginal drugs (an-tē-an-**jī**-nul drugz)
antiarrhythmics (an-tē-uh-**rith**-miks)
anticoagulants (an-tē-kō-**ag**-ū-lunts)
antihyperlipidemics (an-tē-hī-pur-lip-i-**dē**-miks)
antihypertensive drugs (an-tē-hī-pur-**ten**-siv drugz)
antiplatelet drugs (an-tē-**plāt**-lut drugz)
aorta (ā-**or**-tuh)
aortic (ā-**or**-tik)
aortic insufficiency (ā-**or**-tik **in**-suh-**fish**-un-sē)
aortic regurgitation (ā-**or**-tik rē-gur-ji-**tā**-shun)
aortic stenosis (ā-**or**-tik stuh-**nō**-sis)
aortic valve (ā-**or**-tik valv)
aortitis (ā-or-**tī**-tis)
aortogram (ā-**or**-tō-gram)
aortography (ā-or-**tog**-ruh-fē)
aortosclerosis (ā-or-tō-skluh-**rō**-sis)
arrhythmia (uh-**rith**-mē-uh)
arterial (ahr-**tēr**-ē-ul)
arteries (**ahr**-tuh-rēz)
arteriogram (ahr-**tēr**-ē-ō-gram)
arteriograph (ahr-**tēr**-ē-ō-graf)
arteriography (ahr-tēr-ē-**og**-ruh-fē)
arteriole (ahr-**tēr**-ē-ōl)
arteriopathy (ahr-tēr-ē-**op**-uh-thē)
arteriosclerosis (ahr-tēr-ē-ō-skluh-**rō**-sis)
arteriosclerotic heart disease (ahr-tēr-ē-ō-skluh-**rot**-ik hahrt di-**zēz**)
arteriovenous (ahr-tēr-ē-ō-**vē**-nus)
arteritis (ahr-tuh-**rī**-tis)
asystole (ā-**sis**-tō-lē)
atherectomy (ath-er-**ek**-tuh-mē)
atherosclerosis (ath-ur-ō-skluh-**rō**-sis)
atrial (**ā**-trē-ul)
atrial fibrillation (**ā**-trē-ul fib-ri-**lā**-shun)
atrial septal defect (**ā**-trē-ul **sep**-tul **dē**-fekt)
atriomegaly (ā-trē-ō-**meg**-uh-lē)
atrioseptoplasty (ā-trē-ō-**sep**-tō-plas-tē)
atrioventricular (ā-trē-ō-ven-**trik**-ū-lur)

atrioventricular block (ā-trē-ō-ven-**trik**-ū-lur blok)
atrioventricular node (ā-trē-ō-ven-**trik**-ū-lur nōd)
atrioventricular valves (ā-trē-ō-ven-**trik**-ū-lur valvz)
atrium (**ā**-trē-um)
axillary nodes (**ak**-si-lar-ē nōdz)
balloon angioplasty (buh-**loon** **an**-jē-ō-plas-tē)
bicuspid valve (bī-**kus**-pid valv)
blood flow agents (blud flō **ā**-junts)
blood pressure (blud **presh**-ur)
bradycardia (brad-ē-**kahr**-dē-uh)
bypass (**bī**-pas)
capillaries (**kap**-i-lar-ēz)
cardiac catheterization (**kahr**-dē-ak kath-uh-tur-i-**zā**-shun)
cardiac computed tomography (**kahr**-dē-ak kom-**pū**-tid rā-dē-**og**-ruh-fē)
cardiac insufficiency (**kahr**-dē-ak in-suh-**fish**-un-sē)
cardiac MRI (**kahr**-dē-ak MRI)
cardiac pacemaker (**kahr**-dē-ak **pās**-mā-kur)
cardiac stimulants (**kahr**-dē-ak **stim**-ū-lunts)
cardiac tamponade (**kahr**-dē-ak tam-pon-**ād**)
cardiomegaly (kahr-dē-ō-**meg**-uh-lē)
cardiomyopathy (kahr-dē-ō-mī-**op**-uh-thē)
cardioplegia (kahr-dē-ō-**plē**-juh)
cardioplegic solutions (kahr-dē-ō-**plē**-jik suh-**loo**-shunz)
cardiopulmonary (kahr-dē-ō-**pool**-muh-nar-ē)
cardiopulmonary bypass (kahr-dē-ō-**pool**-muh-nar-ē **bī**-pas)
cardiopulmonary resuscitation (kahr-dē-ō-**pool**-muh-nar-ē rē-sus-i-**tā**-shun)
cardiovalvulitis (kahr-dē-ō-val-vū-**lī**-tis)
cardiovascular (kahr-dē-ō-**vas**-kū-lur)
cardiovascular system (kahr-dē-ō-**vas**-kū-lur **sis**-tum)
cardioversion (**kahr**-dē-ō-vur-zhun)
cardioverter (kahr-dē-ō-**vur**-tur)
carotid endarterectomy (kuh-**rot**-id end-ahr-tur-**ek**-tuh-mē)
cerebrovascular accident (ser-uh-brō-**vas**-kū-lur **ak**-si-dunt)
cervical lymph nodes (**sur**-vi-kul limf nōdz)
cholesterol (kuh-**les**-tur-ol)
circulatory system (**sur**-kū-luh-tor-ē **sis**-tum)
cisterna chyli (sis-**tur**-nuh **kī**-lī)
coarctation of the aorta (kō-ahrk-**tā**-shun uv thē ā-**or**-tuh)
congenital heart disease (kun-**jen**-i-tul hahrt di-**zēz**)
congestive heart failure (kun-**jes**-tiv hahrt **fāl**-yur)
coronary (**kor**-uh-nar-ē)
coronary angiogram (**kor**-uh-nar-ē **an**-jē-ō-gram)
coronary angiography (**kor**-uh-nar-ē an-jē-**og**-ruh-fē)
coronary arteries (**kor**-uh-nar-ē **ahr**-tuh-rēz)
coronary arteriography (**kor**-uh-nar-ē ahr-tēr-ē-**og**-ruh-fē)
coronary artery bypass (**kor**-uh-nar-ē **ahr**-tuh-rē **bī**-pas)
coronary artery bypass graft (**kor**-uh-nar-ē **ahr**-tuh-rē **bī**-pas graft)
coronary artery disease (**kor**-uh-nar-ē **ahr**-tuh-rē di-**zēz**)
coronary occlusion (**kor**-uh-nar-ē uh-**kloo**-zhun)
coronary thrombosis (**kor**-uh-nar-ē throm-**bō**-sis)

defibrillation (dē-fib-ri-**lā**-shun)

defibrillator (dē-**fib**-ri-lā-tur)

deoxygenated blood (dē-**ok**-si-juh-nā-tud blud)

diastole (dī-**as**-tō-lē)

diastolic pressure (dī-uh-**stol**-ik **presh**-ur)

digital subtraction angiography (**dij**-i-tul sub-**trak**-shun an-jē-**og**-ruh-fē)

Doppler echocardiography (**dop**-lur ek-ō-kahr-dē-**og**-ruh-fē)

dysrhythmia (dis-**rith**-mē-uh)

echocardiogram (ek-ō-**kahr**-dē-ō-gram)

echocardiography (ek-ō-kahr-dē-**og**-ruh-fē)

effusion (uh-**fū**-zhun)

electrocardiogram (ē-lek-trō-**kahr**-dē-ō-gram)

electrocardiograph (ē-lek-trō-**kahr**-dē-ō-graf)

electrocardiography (ē-lek-trō-kahr-dē-**og**-ruh-fē)

electrophysiology studies (ē-lek-trō-fiz-ē-**ol**-uh-jē **stud**-ēz)

embolectomy (em-buh-**lek**-tuh-mē)

endarterectomy (end-ahr-tur-**ek**-tuh-mē)

endocardial (en-dō-**kahr**-dē-ul)

endocarditis (en-dō-kahr-**dī**-tis)

endocardium (en-dō-**kahr**-dē-um)

epicardium (ep-i-**kahr**-dē-um)

excimer laser coronary angioplasty (**ek**-si-mur **lā**-zur **kor**-uh-nar-ē **an**-jē-ō-plas-tē)

extracorporeal (eks-truh-kor-**por**-ē-ul)

fibrillation (fib-ri-**lā**-shun)

heart block (hahrt blok)

heart flutters (hahrt **flut**-urz)

heart murmur (hahrt **mur**-mur)

hemangioma (hē-man-jē-**ō**-muh)

hemopericardium (hē-mō-per-i-**kahr**-dē-um)

hemostatics (hē-mō-**stat**-iks)

high-density lipoproteins (hī-**den**-si-tē lip-ō, lī-pō-**prō**-tēnz)

Holter monitor (**hōl**-tur **mon**-i-tur)

hypercholesterolemia (hī-pur-kō-les-tur-ol-**ē**-mē-uh)

hyperlipidemia (hī-pur-li-pi-**dē**-mē-uh)

hypertension (hī-pur-**ten**-shun)

hypotension (hī-pō-**ten**-shun)

hypovolemia (hī-pō-vō-**lē**-mē-uh)

infarct (**in**-fahrkt)

inferior vena cava (in-**fēr**-ē-ur **vē**-nuh **kā**-vuh)

inguinal nodes (**ing**-gwi-nul nōdz)

intraaortic (in-truh-ā-**or**-tik)

intracoronary stent (in-truh-**kor**-uh-nar-ē stent)

intravascular thrombolysis (in-truh-**vas**-kyū-lur throm-**bol**-i-sis)

ischemia (is-**kē**-mē-uh)

laser-assisted angioplasty (**lā**-zur uh-**sis**-tud **an**-jē-ō-plas-tē)

lingual tonsils (**ling**-gwul **ton**-silz)

lipids (**lip**-idz)

lipoproteins (lip-ō, lī-pō-**prō**-tēnz)

low-density lipoproteins (lō-**den**-si-tē lip-ō, lī-pō-**prō**-tēnz)

lumen (**loo**-mun)

lymph (limf)

lymph nodes (limf nōdz)

lymphadenectomy (lim-fad-uh-**nek**-tuh-mē)

lymphadenitis (lim-fad-uh-**nī**-tis)

lymphadenopathy (lim-fad-uh-**nop**-uh-thē)

lymphangiography (lim-fan-jē-**og**-ruh-fē)

lymphangioma (lim-fan-jē-**ō**-muh)

lymphangitis (lim-fan-**jī**-tis)

lymphatic system (lim-**fat**-ik **sis**-tum)

lymphatics (lim-**fat**-iks)

lymphedema (lim-fuh-**dē**-muh)

lymphogenous (lim-**foj**-uh-nus)

lymphogram (**lim**-fō-gram)

lymphography (lim-**fog**-ruh-fē)

lymphoma (lim-**fō**-muh)

lymphostasis (lim-**fos**-tuh-sis)

mediastinum (mē-dē-uh-**stī**-num)

microcardia (mī-krō-**kahr**-dē-uh)

mitral valve (**mī**-trul valv)

mitral valve prolapse (**mī**-trul valv **prō**-laps)

myocardial (mī-ō-**kahr**-dē-ul)

myocardial infarction (mī-ō-**kahr**-dē-ul in-**fahrk**-shun)

myocarditis (mī-ō-kahr-**dī**-tis)

myocardium (mī-ō-**kahr**-dē-um)

nitroglycerin (nī-trō-**glis**-ur-in)

oxygenated (**ok**-si-juh-nāt-ud)

palatine tonsils (**pal**-uh-tīn **ton**-silz)

palpitations (pal-pi-**tā**-shunz)

parietal pericardium (puh-**rī**-uh-tul per-i-**kahr**-dē-um)

paroxysmal atrial tachycardia (par-ok-**siz**-mul **ā**-trē-ul tak-i-**kahr**-dē-uh)

patent ductus arteriosus (**pā**-tunt **duk**-tus ahr-tēr-ē-**ō**-sus)

percutaneous coronary intervention (pur-kū-**tā**-nē-us **kor**-uh-nar-ē in-tur-**ven**-shun)

percutaneous transluminal coronary angioplasty (pur-kū-**tā**-nē-us trans-**loo**-mi-nul **kor**-uh-nar-ē **an**-jē-ō-plas-tē)

pericardial (per-ē-**kahr**-dē-ul)

pericardial cavity (per-ē-**kahr**-dē-ul **kav**-i-tē)

pericardiocentesis (per-ē-kahr-dē-ō-sen-**tē**-sis)

pericarditis (per-i-kahr-**dī**-tis)

pericardium (per-i-**kahr**-dē-um)

peripheral vascular disease (puh-**rif**-ur-ul **vas**-kū-lur di-**zēz**)

phlebectomy (fluh-**bek**-tuh-mē)

phlebitis (fluh-**bī**-tis)

phleboplasty (**fleb**-ō-plas-tē)

phlebostasis (fluh-**bos**-tuh-sis)

phlebotomist (fluh-**bot**-uh-mist)

phlebotomy (fluh-**bot**-uh-mē)

positron emission tomography (**poz**-i-tron ē-**mish**-un tō-**mog**-ruh-fē)

pulmonary (**pool**-mō-nar-ē)

pulmonary arteries (**pool**-mō-nar-ē **ahr**-tuh-rēz)

pulmonary circulation (**pool**-mō-nar-ē sur-kū-**lā**-shun)

pulmonary veins (**pool**-mō-nar-ē vānz)

pulse rate (puls rāt)

Purkinje fibers (pur-**kin**-jē **fī**-burz)

rheumatic heart disease (roo-**mat**-ik hahrt di-**zēz**)

sclerotherapy (sklēr-ō-**ther**-uh-pē)

semilunar valves (sem-ē-**loo**-nur valvz)

septal (**sep**-tul)

septum (**sep**-tum)

shock (shok)

shunt (shunt)

sinoatrial node (sī-nō-**ā**-trē-ul nōd)

spleen (splēn)
splenectomy (splē-**nek**-tuh-mē)
splenic (**splen**-ik)
splenolymphatic (splē-nō-lim-**fat**-ik)
splenomegaly (splē-nō-**meg**-uh-lē)
splenopathy (splē-**nop**-uh-thē)
splenopexy (**splē**-nō-pek-sē)
splenoptosis (splē-nop-**tō**-sis, splē-nō-**tō**-sis)
splenorrhagia (splē-nō-**rā**-juh)
splenorrhaphy (splē-**nor**-uh-fē)
stenosis (stuh-**nō**-sis)
stents (stents)
stress tests (stres tests)
stricture (**strik**-chur)
superior vena cava (soo̅-**pēr**-ē-ur **vē**-nuh **kā**-vuh)
systemic circulation (sis-**tem**-ik sur-kū-**lā**-shun)
systole (**sis**-tō-lē)
systolic pressure (sis-**tol**-ik **presh**-ur)
tachycardia (tak-i-**kahr**-dē-uh)
telecardiography (tel-uh-kahr-dē-**og**-ruh-fē)
tetralogy of Fallot (te-**tral**-uh-jē ov fuh-**lō**)
thallium stress test (**thal**-ē-um stres test)
thrombolymphangitis (thromb-bō-lim-fan-**jī**-tis)
thrombolytics (throm-bō-**lit**-iks)
thrombophlebitis (throm-bō-fluh-**bī**-tis)
thymectomy (thī-**mek**-tuh-mē)
thymic (**thī**-mik)
thymoma (thī-**mō**-muh)
thymopathy (thī-**mop**-uh-thē)
thymus (**thī**-mus)
tonsillar (**ton**-si-lur)

tonsillectomy (ton-si-**lek**-tuh-mē)
tonsillitis (ton-si-**lī**-tis)
tonsilloadenoidectomy (ton-si-lō-ad-uh-noid-**ek**-tuh-mē)
tonsils (**ton**-silz)
tourniquet (**toor**-ni-kut)
transesophageal echocardiogram (trans-uh-sof-uh-**jē**-ul ek-ō-**kahr**-dē-ō-gram)
treadmill stress test (**tred**-mil stres test)
tricuspid valve (trī-**kus**-pid valv)
triglycerides (trī-**glis**-ur-īdz)
valval (**val**-vul)
valvar (**val**-vur)
valvate (**val**-vāt)
valvula (**val**-vū-luh)
valvular (**val**-vū-lur)
valvular stenosis (**val**-vū-lur stuh-**nō**-sis)
valvulitis (val-vū-**lī**-tis)
varicose veins (**var**-i-kōs vānz)
vascular (**vas**-kū-lur)
vasoconstriction (vā-zō-kun-**strik**-shun)
vasodilation (vā-zō-dī-**lā**-shun)
veins (vānz)
venipuncture (**ven**-i-punk-chur)
venous (**vē**-nus)
venous thrombosis (**vē**-nus throm-**bō**-sis)
ventricle (**ven**-tri-kul)
ventricular (ven-**trik**-ū-lur)
ventricular fibrillation (ven-**trik**-ū-lur fib-ri-**lā**-shun)
ventricular septal defect (ven-**trik**-ū-lur **sep**-tul **dē**-fekt)
venules (**ven**-ūlz)
visceral pericardium (**vis**-ur-ul per-i-**kahr**-dē-um)

Español ENHANCING SPANISH COMMUNICATION

English	Spanish (pronunciation)	English	Spanish (pronunciation)
angina	angina (ahn-HEE-nah)	murmur	murmullo (moor-MOOL-lyo)
aneurysm	aneurisma (ah-neh-REES-mah)	narrow	estrecho (es-TRAY-cho)
artery	arteria (ar-TAY-re-ah)	obstruction	obstrucción (obs-trook-se-ON)
blood pressure	presión sanguínea (pray-se-ON san-GEE-nay-ah)	pulse	pulso (POOL-so)
capillary	capilar (kah-pe-LAR)	rheumatic fever	fiebre reumática (fe-AY-bray ray-oo-MAT-e-kah)
catheter	catéter (kah-TAY-ter)	rhythm	ritmo (REET-mo)
chest pain	dolor en el pecho (do-LOR en el PAY-cho)	spleen	bazo (BAH-so)
		thrombus	coágulo (ko-AG-goo-loh)
cholesterol	colesterol (ko-les-tay-ROL)	tonsil	tonsila (ton-SEE-lah), amígdala (ah-MEEG-dah-lah)
electrocardiogram	electrocardiograma (a-lek-tro-kahr-de-o-GRAH-ma)	varicose veins	venas varicosas (VAH-nahs vah-re-KO-sas)
high blood pressure	hipertensión, presión alta (e-per-ten-se-ON, pray-se-ON AHL-tah)	vein	vena (VAY-nah)
		weakness	debilidad (day-be-le-DAHD)

Respiratory System

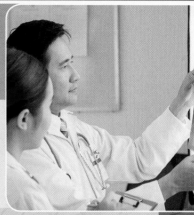

A pulmonologist, a specialist in pulmonary medicine, depends on observation and diagnostic tests to evaluate a patient's respiratory functions. He or she is assisted by a pulmonary function technologist, who provides pulmonary function testing, assists with several procedures, and monitors patients after treatment.

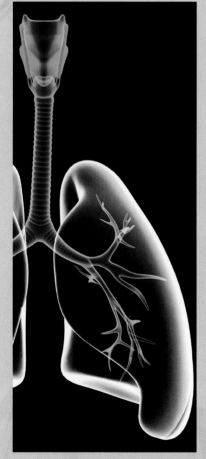

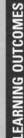

CONTENTS

LEARNING OUTCOMES

Basic Understanding

In this chapter you will learn to do the following:

1. State the function of the respiratory system, and analyze associated terminology.
2. Write the names of the structures of the respiratory system when given their descriptions, define the terms associated with these structures, and label the structures.
3. Write the meaning of the word parts associated with the respiratory system, and use the word parts to build and analyze terms.
4. Distinguish between structures of the upper respiratory tract and those of the lower respiratory tract.
5. Write or recognize the sequence of the flow of air from the atmosphere through the respiratory structures.
6. Match structures of the respiratory system with the instruments and procedures that are used to study them, or write the names of the procedures when given their descriptions.
7. Match terms for respiratory system pathologies with their meanings, or write the names of the pathologies when given their descriptions.
8. Match terms for surgical and other therapeutic interventions for respiratory system pathologies with descriptions of the interventions, or write the names of the interventions when given their descriptions.
9. Build terms from word parts to label illustrations.

Greater Comprehension

10. Use word parts from this chapter to define terms in a health care report.
11. Spell the terms accurately.
12. Pronounce the terms correctly.
13. Write the meanings of the abbreviations.
14. Categorize terms as anatomy, diagnostic test or procedure, pathology, surgery, or nonsurgical therapy.
15. Recognize the meanings of general pharmacological terms from this chapter as well as the drug classes and their uses.

FUNCTION FIRST

The primary function of the respiratory system is to provide oxygen for the body and remove the gaseous waste carbon dioxide. Secondary functions are maintaining the acid–base balance, producing speech, facilitating smell, and maintaining the body's heat and water balances.

KEY POINT **External respiration moves oxygen from the air into the blood; internal respiration moves oxygen from the blood to the tissues.** External respiration is the process involved in breathing, the ventilation of the lungs, and the exchange of oxygen (O_2) and carbon dioxide (CO_2) between the air in the lungs and the blood. Internally, this exchange of O_2 and CO_2 is called cellular respiration.

ANATOMY AND PHYSIOLOGY

oxygen

5-1 The **respiratory system** cooperates with the circulatory system to provide _____ for body cells and to expel waste carbon dioxide through breathing. The exchange of these gases is involved in both internal and external respiration. This chapter focuses on external respiration.

5-2 Breathing is alternate inspiration and expiration of air into and out of the lungs. **Inspiration** (in, into + spir[o], to breathe + -ation, process) is the process of breathing in. The drawing of air into the lungs is _____. It is also called **in/halation.**

Expelling air from the lungs, the act of breathing out or letting out one's breath, is **expiration.** This is the same as **exhalation.**

WRITE IT!
EXERCISE 1

Write words that are associated with the functions of the respiratory system; the first letter is provided. (Question number 1 is done as an example.)

The respiratory system cooperates with the (1) _(c)irculatory_____ system to provide

(2) _o_____ for body cells. Expelling waste

(3) _c_____dioxide is also part of respiration. Breathing in is inhalation or

(4) _i_____ ; breathing out is exhalation or (5) _e_____ .

lungs

5-3 A **pulmono/logist** is a physician specializing in evaluating and treating lung disorders. In studying the respiratory system, you will often see breathing referred to as pulmonary ventilation, or simply, **ventilation. Pulmon/ary** pertains to the _____.

The respiratory tract is the complex of organs and structures that perform pulmonary ventilation and the exchange of oxygen and carbon dioxide between the air and the blood as it circulates through the lungs. See the names and locations of the structures in Fig. 5.1. The conducting passages are known as the upper respiratory tract and the lower respiratory tract. Label the numbered structures as you read the information that accompanies the drawing.

WORD ORIGIN
ventilation *(L.)*
ventilare, to fan

5-4 Within the body, the lungs are separated from each other by other organs in the chest, especially the heart. You are able to recognize the trachea (windpipe), the two branches (bronchi) and the spongy lungs in the illustration (Fig. 5.2, A). The nose, nasal cavity, paranasal sinuses, pharynx, and larynx comprise the upper respiratory tract. The trachea, bronchi, bronchioles, alveoli, and lungs belong to the _____ respiratory tract. Gas exchange of carbon dioxide for oxygen occurs in the alveoli (Fig. 5.2, B). Also note that the top of the lung is referred to as the apex, and the bottom of the lung is broader and is called the base.

lower

WRITE IT!
EXERCISE 2

List the five structures that make up the upper respiratory tract (in any order).

1. _____   4. _____

2. _____   5. _____

3. _____

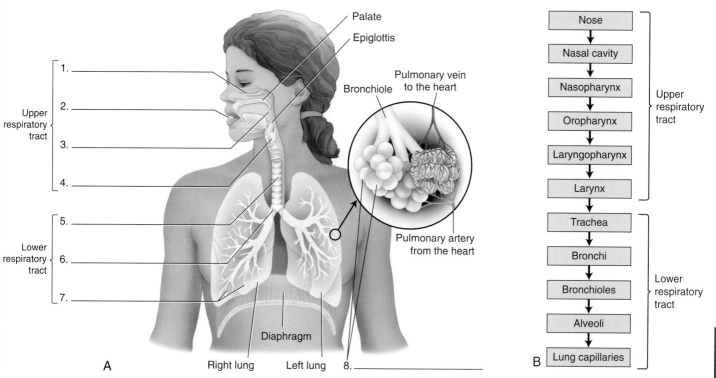

Figure 5.1 The organs of respiration. A, Air first enters the body through the nose and passes through the nasal cavity *(1)*, or it enters through the mouth and passes through the oral cavity *(2)*. The air reaches the pharynx *(3)* and passes to the larynx *(4)* and the trachea *(5)*. The trachea divides into a left and a right bronchus *(6)*. Each bronchus divides into smaller tubes called *bronchioles (7)*. At the end of each bronchiole are clusters of air sacs called *alveoli (8)*, where oxygen is exchanged for waste carbon dioxide. The insert shows a bronchiole tree. Normal quiet breathing is accomplished almost entirely by movement of the diaphragm. The epiglottis (not part of the respiratory system) covers the larynx during swallowing to prevent food from entering the larynx and trachea. **B,** Pathway of air from the nose to the capillaries of the lungs.

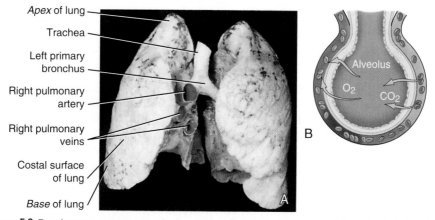

Figure 5.2 Respiratory anatomy. A, The lungs, bronchi, and trachea, removed from the body for clarity. Descriptions often include the *apex* (top) as well as the *base* of the lung. The pulmonary artery and vein (part of the cardiovascular system) are involved in oxygenation of the blood by the lungs. **B,** A diagram of the exchange of gases between an alveolus and a lung capillary.

WRITE IT! EXERCISE 3

List five structures that make up the lower respiratory tract.

1. _____   4. _____
2. _____   5. _____
3. _____

Study the following word parts and be sure you know their meanings.

Word Parts: Respiratory Anatomy and Physiology

Combining Form	Meaning
Upper Respiratory Tract	
epiglott(o)	epiglottis
laryng(o)	larynx
nas(o), rhin(o)	nose
palat(o)	palate
pharyng(o)	pharynx
sin(o), sinus(o)	sinus
Lower Respiratory Tract	
alveol(o)	alveoli
apic(o)	apex
bronch(o), bronchi(o)	bronchi
bronchiol(o)	bronchioles
lacrim(o)	tears (as in crying)
lob(o)	lobe
mediastin(o)	mediastinum
phren(o)	diaphragm or mind

Combining Form	Meaning
pleur(o)	pleura
pneum(o)	lungs or air
pneumon(o), pulm(o), pulmon(o)	lungs
thorac(o)	chest
trache(o)	trachea
Word Parts Used to Describe Function	
acid(o)	acid
alkal(o)	alkaline; basic
ox(i)	oxygen
phas(o)	speech
phon(o)	voice
spir(o)	to breathe
Suffix	
-ation	process
-capnia	carbon dioxide
-pnea	breathing
-ptysis	spitting

WRITE IT! EXERCISE 4

Write the combining form for these terms.

1. diaphragm or mind _____   4. pharynx _____
2. larynx _____   5. speech _____
3. lungs or air _____   6. to breathe _____

Upper Respiratory Passageways

nose (or mouth)

5-5 Looking at Fig. 5.1, follow the passage of air through the respiratory system by writing the names of respiratory structures in the blanks: Air first enters the body through the _____, where it is warmed, moistened, and filtered. Regardless of whether air is taken in by the nose or the mouth, it passes to the pharynx, a muscular tube about 13 cm (5 inches) long in an adult. The pharynx also functions as part of the digestive system in the swallowing of food. Air then passes over the vocal cords in the larynx before reaching the **trachea,** also known as the windpipe. The trachea divides into two primary bronchi, which divide further into many _____. Oxygen and carbon dioxide are exchanged within the alveoli.

bronchioles

WRITE IT! EXERCISE 5

Arrows in Figure 5.1B represent the pathway of air from the nose to the lung capillaries. Write the names of the structures represented by the blanks.

Nose → Nasal cavity → Nasopharynx → **1.** _____ → Laryngopharynx →

2. _____ → Trachea → **3.** _____ → Bronchioles →

4. _____ → Lung capillaries

nose

5-6 The respiratory tract is lined with mucous membranes. Organs of the upper respiratory tract filter, moisten, and warm the air as it is inhaled. The combining forms nas(o) and rhin(o) mean _____. Common names for the **larynx** and pharynx are voice box and throat, respectively.

Both cartilage and bone give structure to the nose. The external part of the nose contains two openings, the nostrils, also called the **nares,** singular **naris.** The hollow interior of the nose is separated into right and left cavities by the **nasal septum,** which is composed of cartilage. Literal interpretation of **para/nas/al sinuses** means the air cavities _____ the nose. The paranasal sinuses are pairs of air cavities around the nose (Fig. 5.3).

near

🔑 **KEY** POINT **The nose has nerve endings that detect many odors. Olfactory** pertains to the sense of smell. **Olfaction,** the sense of smell, is a function of the nose. Olfactory is derived from *olfacere (L.),* to smell.

palate

5-7 The anterior portion of the **palate,** or roof of the mouth, separates the nasal cavity and the oral cavity. The palate consists of bone and the membrane that covers it. Because the anterior portion contains bone, it is called the *hard palate.* The soft palate is the fleshy posterior portion of the palate. The pendant, fleshy tissue that hangs from the soft palate is the palatine **uvula.** The combining form palat(o) means palate. **Palatine** refers to the _____.

nasal

5-8 The naso/lacrimal duct opens into the nasal cavity. The **nasolacrimal duct** is a tubular passage that carries fluid (tears) from the eye to the _____ cavity. Now you can understand why the nose fills with fluid when a person cries. **Lacrimal** pertains to tears.

FIND IT! **EXERCISE 6**

Draw a slash between the word parts in the following list of new terms. Then find the meanings of the word parts within the definitions. Think! (Draw the slash, and then perform the remainder of the activity as a mental exercise.)

1. **endonasal** within the nose
2. **nasal** pertaining to the nose
3. **nasolacrimal** pertaining to the nose and tearing apparatus
4. **oral** pertaining to the mouth
5. **retronasal** behind the nose
6. **supranasal** above the nose

5-9 The **pharynx** serves as a passageway for both the respiratory and digestive tracts. In referring to parts of the pharynx, three divisions are recognized (see Fig. 5.1B):

- **nasopharynx,** located behind the nasal cavity; it is the uppermost of the three regions of the pharynx
- **oropharynx** that part of the pharynx that lies posterior to the mouth
- **laryngopharynx** the lowermost part of the pharynx; it lies near the larynx

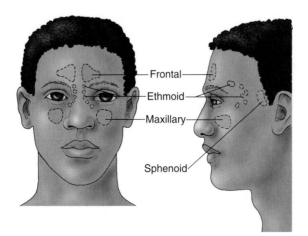

—Frontal—
—Ethmoid—
—Maxillary—

Sphenoid

Figure 5.3 Paranasal sinuses. These air-filled, paired cavities in various bones around the nose are lined with mucous membranes. Their openings into the nasal cavity are easily obstructed.

pharynx

Pharyng/eal means pertaining to the pharynx. **Oro/pharyngeal** means pertaining to the mouth and _____. This term also pertains to the oropharynx. The oropharynx contains the palatine tonsils, which are visible when the mouth is open wide. At the level of the larynx, the pharynx divides into the larynx and the esophagus. Air passes through the larynx, and food passes through the esophagus.

5-10 The nasopharynx is the upper part of the pharynx and is continuous with the nasal passages. The **auditory tube,** formerly called the **eustachian tube,** is a narrow channel connecting the middle ear and the nasopharynx. The opening to the auditory tube is in the nasopharynx. The adenoids are also located in the nasopharynx.

nasopharynx

Naso/pharyng/eal pertains to the _____.

larynx, pharynx

5-11 Laryngeal means pertaining to the larynx. **Laryngo/pharyng/eal** pertains to the _____ and the _____.

The **glottis** is the vocal apparatus of the larynx. It consists of the vocal cords and the opening between them. The **vocal cords,** also called *vocal folds,* are a pair of strong bands of elastic tissue with a mouthlike opening through which air passes, creating sound.

🔑 **KEY** POINT **Muscles open and close the glottis during inspiration and expiration, and they regulate the vocal cords during the production of sound.** Muscles also close off a lidlike structure that covers the glottis during swallowing. The lidlike structure, the **epiglottis,** is composed of cartilage and covers the larynx during the swallowing of food.

epiglottis

5-12 Foreign bodies may be aspirated into the nose, throat, or lungs on inspiration. If a person inspires while attempting to swallow, food may be accidentally aspirated into the larynx. Spontaneous coughing is the body's effort to clear the obstructed airway. Respiration stops if complete obstruction of the airway occurs.

In usual situations, food does not enter the larynx but passes on to the esophagus. Food does not enter the larynx, because a lidlike structure, the _____, is closed. **Epiglottides** is the plural of epiglottis; hence we have the term *epiglottiditis.*

ANALYZE IT!
EXERCISE 7

Divide the following words into their component parts, and write the meaning of each term.
1. inspiration _____
2. paranasal _____
3. pharyngeal _____
4. pulmonary _____
5. retronasal _____

WRITE IT!
EXERCISE 8

Write the names of respiratory structures to complete these sentences.
1. The structure that is commonly called the throat is the _____.
2. The hollow interior of the nose is separated into two cavities by the nasal _____.
3. The glottis is the vocal apparatus of the _____.
4. The upper respiratory tract consists of the nose, nasal cavity, paranasal _____, pharynx, and larynx.
5. The lidlike structure called the _____ covers the larynx during the swallowing of food.

Lower Respiratory Passageways

5-13 Infections of the upper respiratory tract are common and often spread to the lower respiratory tract. The lower respiratory tract, a continuation of the upper respiratory tract, begins with the trachea.

In addition to the trachea, the lower respiratory tract includes two primary bronchi and several secondary bronchi, bronchioles, alveolar ducts, and alveoli. The two lungs are composed of millions of alveoli and their related ducts, bronchioles, and bronchi. The trachea branches into the right and left primary _____.

bronchi

Bronchi are lined with cilia, hairlike projections that propel mucus up and away from the lower airway. Bronchi branch to become **bronchioles,** structures that lead to alveolar ducts. At the ends of the ducts are the **alveoli,** small pockets where carbon dioxide and oxygen are exchanged between the inspired air and capillary blood.

5-14 Most of the lower respiratory passageways are located in the chest cavity.

🔑 **KEY** POINT **The mediastinum is the middle portion of the thoracic cavity between the two lungs.** In the mediastinum, the trachea (windpipe) divides into the right and left primary bronchi; bronch(o) and bronchi(o) mean bronchi. *Bronchial tubes* is another term for bronchi (singular is bronchus).

bronchus

Bronchioles are small airways that extend from the bronchi into the lungs. Translated literally, bronchi/ole means little _____.

FIND IT!
EXERCISE 9

Draw a slash between the word parts in the following list of new terms. Then find the meanings of the word parts within the definitions. Think! (Draw the slash, and then perform the remainder of the activity as a mental exercise.)

1. **alveolar** pertaining to the alveoli
2. **bronchial** pertaining to the bronchi
3. **bronchoalveolar** pertaining to a bronchus and alveoli
4. **endotracheal** within the trachea
5. **interalveolar** pertaining to the area between alveoli
6. **tracheal** pertaining to the trachea

5-15 Both lungs are composed of millions of alveoli and their related ducts, bronchioles, and bronchi.

🔑 **KEY** POINT **The two lungs have similar characteristics but have a different number of lobes.** Each lung is conical and has an apex (pointed top) and a base (lower portion). Note in Fig. 5.1 that the left lung has two lobes and the right lung has three lobes.

apex

Apical refers to the _____. The depression where blood vessels enter and leave the lung is called the **hilum.**

WORD ORIGIN
visceral *(L.)*
viscus, internal organ
parietal *(L.)*
paries, wall

lungs

5-16 Each lung is surrounded by a membrane called the **pleura** (plural is pleurae). One layer of the membrane, the **visceral pleura,** covers the lung's surface. The other layer, the **parietal pleura,** lines the walls of the thoracic cavity. **Visceral** means pertaining to the viscera, the large internal organs enclosed within a body cavity, especially the abdominal cavity. Parietal pertains to the outer wall of a cavity or organ.

The visceral pleura surrounds the _____, and the parietal pleura lines the walls of the thoracic cavity. The **pleural cavity** is a space between the pleurae, which contains a thin film of pleural fluid that acts as a lubricant as the lungs expand and contract during respiration.

FIND IT!
EXERCISE 10

Draw a slash between the word parts in the following list of new terms. Then find the meanings of the word parts within the definitions. Think! (Draw the slash, and then perform the remainder of the activity as a mental exercise.)

1. **extrapleural** outside the pleural cavity
2. **extrapulmonary** outside of or unrelated to the lungs
3. **pleural** pertaining to the pleura
4. **pulmonic** pertaining to the lungs or the respiratory system
5. **subpulmonary** below the lung

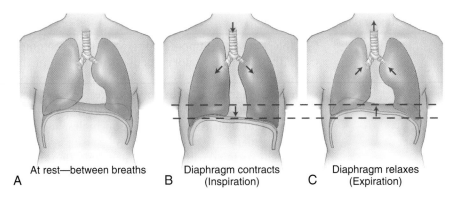

Figure 5.4 Changes in the lungs and diaphragm during respiration. A, Diaphragm relaxed, just before inspiration. **B,** Inspiration. The diaphragm contracts, moving downward and increasing the size of the thoracic cavity. Inspiration is also aided by contraction of the intercostal muscles, which are between the ribs. Air moves into the lungs until pressure inside the lungs equals atmospheric pressure. **C,** Expiration. Respiratory muscles relax, and the chest cavity decreases in size as air moves from the lungs out into the atmosphere.

A   At rest—between breaths   B   Diaphragm contracts (Inspiration)   C   Diaphragm relaxes (Expiration)

5-17 Normal lungs are highly elastic and fill the chest cavity during inspiration. The **diaphragm,** the muscular partition that separates the thoracic and abdominal cavities, contracts and increases the size of the thoracic cavity during inspiration. It aids respiration by moving up and down as we exhale and inhale (Fig. 5.4).

diaphragm

The formal anatomic name for the diaphragm is **diaphragma. Diaphragma/tic** means pertaining to the _____. The diaphragm is pierced by several openings through which pass the aorta, the inferior vena cava, and the esophagus.

➤ **BEYOND** THE BLUEPRINT The combining form phren(o) means both diaphragm and mind. Ancient Greeks believed that the midriff was the seat of emotions; the Greek word *phren* was applied to this area as a structure, as well as the center of emotions. For this reason diaphragm and mind have the same combining form, phren(o).

Phren/ic has two meanings, either pertaining to the diaphragm or pertaining to the mind. **Sub/phrenic** means located beneath the diaphragm. When studying respiration, phren(o) probably refers to the muscular partition that separates the chest and abdominal cavities, the

diaphragm

_____.

WRITE IT! **EXERCISE 11**

Write a word in each blank to complete these sentences.

1. Tiny structures of the respiratory system where carbon dioxide and oxygen are exchanged between the inspired air and capillary blood are _____.

2. Each lung is surrounded by a membrane called the _____.

3. The pointed top of the lung is called the _____.

4. The divisions into which lungs are anatomically divided are called _____.

5. The muscular partition that separates the thoracic and abdominal cavities is the _____.

DIAGNOSTIC TESTS AND PROCEDURES

5-18 The **respiratory rate** (number of breaths per minute) varies by age, but is easily measured as the examiner watches a quietly sitting patient, and should be approximately 12 to 30 breaths per minute in adults. Oxygen content of the blood is measured using a **pulse oximeter,** a photo/electric device for determining the oxygen saturation of the blood in a pulsating capillary bed (Fig. 5.5). The finger probe is most commonly used for monitoring the patient's oxygenation status in a physician's office, a hospital, during pulmonary rehabilitation programs, or during stress testing; however, an ear oximeter is sometimes used. The name of the procedure that determines the oxygen saturation of the blood in a capillary bed is **pulse** _____.

oximetry

5-19 The use of percussion, described in Chapter 2, is helpful in assessing the lungs (see Fig. 2.29, B). Chest auscultation (see Fig. 2.28, C), listening to breath sounds, provides information about the flow of air through the tracheo/bronchial tree. Abnormal sounds that are heard during inspiration include rhonchi, wheezes, crackles (also called **rales**), and friction rub (Fig. 5.6).

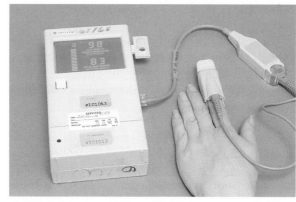

Figure 5.5 Oximetry, noninvasive monitoring of oxygen saturation. The oximeter shows an oxygen saturation of 98%. The finger probe is most frequently used for stationary measurements.

auscultation

WORD ORIGIN
rhonchus *(G.)*
rhonchos, snore
stridor *(L.)*
stridor, harsh sound

stridor

Abnormal sounds can be heard when a stethoscope is used to evaluate the sound of air moving in and out of the lungs. This procedure is called _____.

5-20 A **rhonchus** is an abnormal sound consisting of a continuous rumbling sound that clears on coughing. A **wheeze** is a musical noise that sounds like a squeak. **Crackles** are discontinuous bubbling noises during inspiration that are not cleared by coughing. A **friction rub** is a dry, grating sound. If the friction rub is heard over the pleural area, it may be a sign of lung disease, although it may be normal if heard over another area, such as the liver.

Practice enables development of the ability to distinguish these abnormal sounds. Another sound, **stridor,** is an abnormal high-pitched musical sound caused by an obstruction in the trachea or larynx, most often heard during inspiration. Write the term that is an abnormal high-pitched sound associated with an obstruction in the trachea or larynx: _____.

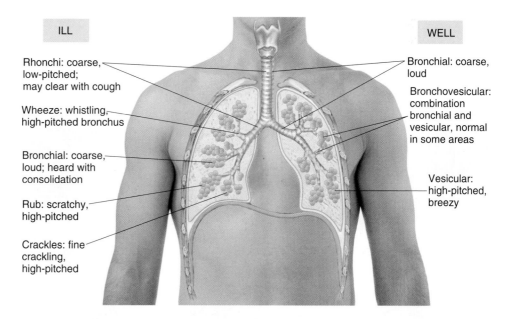

Figure 5.6 Breath sounds in the ill and well patient. Common terms used to describe sounds heard in the ill patient are rhonchi, wheeze, friction rub, and crackles, as well as coarse, loud bronchial sounds heard with consolidation. Consolidation means the process of becoming solid, as when the lungs become firm and inelastic in pneumonia.

nasal

5-21 A nasal speculum, a **naso/scope,** is one of various types of specula that is used for inspecting the _____ cavity.

The color of the mucous membranes and the presence of swelling, bleeding, or discharge are noted. One finding is septal deviation, a structural defect of the nasal septum in which it is shifted toward one side of the nose or the other.

pharynx

A **pharyngoscope** is an instrument for examining the lining of the structure that is commonly called the throat, the _____.

arterial

5-22 Arterial blood gas (ABG) analysis is a blood test that measures the amount of oxygen, carbon dioxide, and pH in a blood sample collected from an artery. ABG is the abbreviation for _____ blood gas.

Other laboratory tests include cultures for bacteria or fungi in sputum or material collected from throat swabs. **Phlegm** is abnormally thick mucus secreted by the membranes of the respiratory passages. **Sputum** is phlegm or other material that is coughed up from the lungs.

5-23 The lung volume in normal quiet breathing is approximately 500 mL; however, forced maximum inspiration raises this level considerably. **Spiro/metry** is a measurement of the amount of air taken into and expelled from the lungs (Fig. 5.7). The combining form spir(o) as used here means breath or breathing. The instrument used is a _____.

spirometer

The largest volume of air that can be exhaled after maximal inspiration is the vital capacity (VC). A reduction in vital capacity often indicates a loss of functioning lung tissue.

Spirometry measures ventilation (the ability of the lungs to move air) and is one type of pulmonary function test (PFT) that helps determine the capacity of the lungs to exchange oxygen and carbon dioxide effectively.

5-24 Radiography of the chest, commonly called a *chest x-ray,* is a valuable tool in studying the lungs as well as nearby structures. Examine the chest x-ray in Fig. 5.8, and study the relationship of the lungs with other structures in the chest cavity.

KEY POINT In looking at the respiratory structures in a chest x-ray, it is understandable why the trachea and bronchial branches are referred to as the tracheobronchial tree. The air in the lungs appears black. Note also the white appearance of bone (collarbone, breastbone, and ribs). The breasts and other soft tissues appear gray.

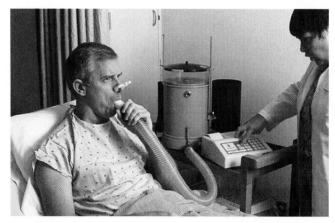

Figure 5.7 Spirometry. Evaluation of the air capacity of the lungs uses a spirometer, such as the one shown. The spirometer is used to assess pulmonary function by measuring and recording the volume of inhaled and exhaled air.

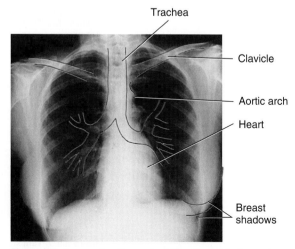

Figure 5.8 A normal radiograph of the chest with the tracheobronchial tube outlined. Do not be concerned about the meanings of all the terms in the chest x-ray film. The clavicle is the collarbone.

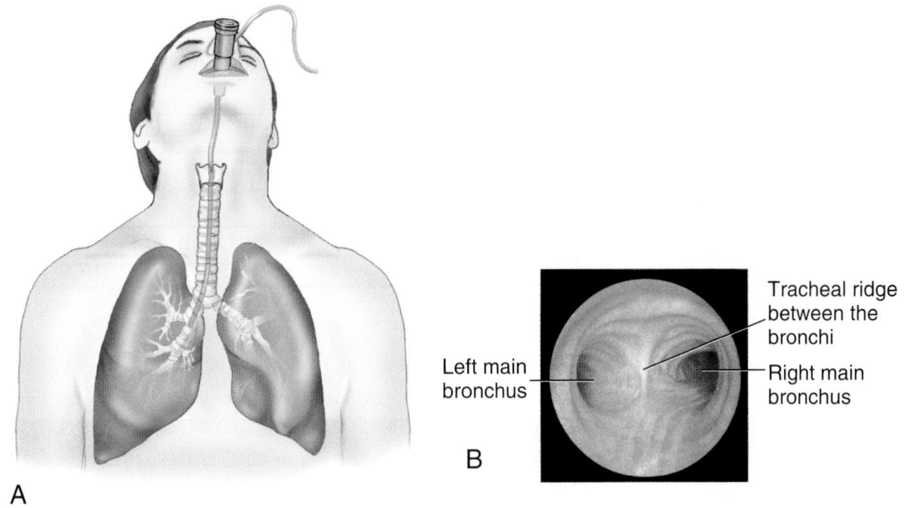

Figure 5.9 Bronchoscopy. **A,** Visual examination of the tracheobronchial tree using a bronchoscope. Other uses for this procedure include suctioning, obtaining a biopsy specimen or fluid, or removing foreign bodies. **B,** Endoscopic view of the lower end of the trachea and the beginning of the bronchi.

bronchogram

5-25 Broncho/scopy or **broncho/scopic examination** is direct viewing of the bronchi using a **bronchoscope** (Fig. 5.9). **Broncho/graphy** involves the use of x-rays after instillation of contrast media. The film obtained by broncho/graphy is a _____. This procedure is seldom used, having been replaced by computed tomography.

vessels

5-26 Pulmonary angio/graphy is radiography of the _____ of the lungs after injection of a contrast medium. Pulmonary angiography is primarily performed on patients with suspected thromboembolic disease. A thrombus is an internal blood clot. If part of it breaks off, the clot fragment can travel in the bloodstream to another site. Any foreign object that circulates in the bloodstream and becomes lodged in a vessel is called an *embolus*. **Thrombo/embol/ic** pertains to obstruction of a blood vessel with material from a blood clot that is carried by the bloodstream from its site of origin.

Other diagnostic radiologic studies of respiratory organs include computed tomography, magnetic resonance imaging, and lung scans. A lung scan uses radioactive material to test blood flow or air distribution in the lungs. Information about the flow of blood in the lungs is helpful in diagnosing pulmonary embo/lism, the presence of an embolus in the lungs.

FIND IT! **EXERCISE 12**

Draw a slash between the word parts in the following list of new terms. Then find the meanings of the word parts within the definitions. Think! (Draw the slash, and then perform the remainder of the activity as a mental exercise.)

1. **laryngography** radiographic examination of the larynx that usually also includes the pharynx
2. **laryngoscope** an endoscope used to examine the larynx
3. **laryngoscopy** examination of the larynx with a laryngoscope
4. **mediastinoscope** an endoscope used to examine the mediastinum
5. **mediastinoscopy** examination of the mediastinum by means of a mediastinoscope inserted through a chest incision
6. **tracheoscopy** viewing the interior of the trachea with the use of a tracheoscope

---

MATCH IT! **EXERCISE 13**

Match these structures with the instrument or procedure that is used to study them.

_____ **1.** blood vessels of the lung   **A.** laryngoscope
_____ **2.** nose   **B.** nasoscope
_____ **3.** throat   **C.** pharyngoscope
_____ **4.** voice box   **D.** pulmonary angiography
_____ **5.** windpipe   **E.** tracheoscope

Use the following word parts to build terms.

bronch(o), laryng(o), ox(i), pharyng(o), spir(o), -graphy, -meter, -metry, -scope, -scopy

1. a device that determines oxygen saturation _____/_____
2. measurement of the amount of air taken into and expelled from the lung _____/_____
3. process of visualizing the bronchi with x-rays _____/_____
4. examination of the larynx with an endoscope _____/_____
5. instrument for examining the pharynx _____/_____

PATHOLOGIES

Disordered Breathing

apnea

5-27 Disorders of the respiratory system are a major cause of illness and death. Acute or chronic respiratory problems can progress rapidly and become life-threatening emergencies. Chronic lung disease often causes heart disease because of the lungs' functional role in circulation. Pulmonary hypertension is a condition of abnormally high blood pressure in the pulmonary circulation, caused by resistance of blood flow in the vessels of the lung. This brings about an increased workload for the heart and eventually leads to heart failure.

You learned earlier that -pnea is a suffix that means breathing. Choose either a- or an- to write a word that means absence of spontaneous breathing: _____.

5-28 Sleep apnea is a sleep disorder characterized by transient periods of cessation of breathing. The two primary types are central sleep apnea (from failure of stimulation by the nervous system) and obstructive sleep apnea (from collapse or obstruction of the airway).

Cheyne-Stokes respiration (CSR) is an abnormal pattern of respiration that is characterized by alternating periods of apnea and deep, rapid breathing, occurring more frequently during sleep.

breathing

5-29 Many pathologies can cause shortness of breath (SOB). Remembering that dys- means bad or difficult, **dys/pnea** is labored or difficult _____.

Dys/pne/ic is an adjective that means pertaining to or caused by dyspnea.

WORD ORIGIN
asphyxia *(G.)*
a-, no; *phyxis*, pulse
extrinsic *(L.)*
extrinsecus, on the outside
intrinsic *(L.)*
intrinsecus, on the inside

5-30 **Asphyxia** or **asphyxiation** is a condition caused by insufficient intake of oxygen. Extrinsic causes, those originating outside the body, include drowning, crushing injuries of the chest, and inhalation of carbon monoxide. Intrinsic causes include hemorrhage into the lungs or pleural cavity, foreign bodies in the throat, and diseases of the air passages.

KEY POINT Anoxia is more severe than hypoxia. An/ox/ia means an absence or deficiency of oxygen in body tissues below the level needed for proper functioning. **Hypoxia** is a reduction of oxygen in body tissues to levels below those required for normal metabolic functioning. Note the spelling of hyp/ox/ia (the "o" of hypo- has been dropped). Anoxia is more severe than hypoxia, but both mean oxygen deficiency.

asphyxia or asphyxiation

Cyanosis, dyspnea, and tachycardia accompanied by mental disturbances are seen in asphyxia. In extreme cases, convulsions, unconsciousness, and death may occur. **Tachy/cardia** means an increased heart rate.

Write the term that means a condition caused by insufficient intake of oxygen (be careful with the spelling): _____.

> **BEYOND** THE BLUEPRINT Scuba diving buddies must be aware of the possibility of hypoxia in themselves as well as their diving partner. Mild hypoxia or asphyxia in divers has many causes, including poorly-functioning equipment, ascending to the surface too quickly, or an improper air mixture. Hypoxia leads to confusion and impaired judgment, and diving buddies must be alert to its signs.

5-31 Hyper/pnea is an exaggerated deep, rapid, or labored respiration. It occurs normally with exercise and abnormally in several conditions, including pain, fever, hysteria, or inadequate oxygen. The latter can occur in cardiac or respiratory disease. A literal translation of hyper/pnea is excessive

breathing

_____.

Hyper/pnea may lead to **hyper/ventilation**—excessive aeration of the lungs—that commonly reduces carbon dioxide levels in the body. Carbon dioxide contributes to the acidity of body fluids, and if too much carbon dioxide is lost, alkalosis results. **Alkal/osis** is a pathologic condition resulting from the accumulation of basic substances or from the loss of acid by the body. Transient alkalosis can be caused by hyperventilation. Transient means not lasting or of brief duration.

WORD ORIGIN
transient *(L.)*
trans, to go by

5-32 The abbreviation pH means potential hydrogen and is the symbol for hydrogen ion concentration, a calculated scale that represents the relative acidity or alkalinity of a solution; a value of 7.0 is neutral, below 7.0 is acidic, and above 7.0 is alkaline. The normal pH of body fluids (plasma and intracellular and interstitial fluids) is 7.35 to 7.45. Is normal plasma slightly acid or alkaline?

alkaline

_____

🔑➡ **KEY POINT The state of equilibrium of the blood pH is called the acid–base balance.** Cellular metabolism produces substances (such as, excess carbon dioxide) that would upset the pH balance were it not for buffer systems of the blood, along with respiratory and urinary functions that help keep the pH constant. The expelling of carbon dioxide during exhalation is part of the regulatory mechanism that maintains the constancy of the pH—that is, the acid-base balance.

5-33 The combining form alkal(o) means alkaline or basic. Alkal/osis is an alkaline condition. **Alkal/emia** is increased alkalinity of the blood. Alkal/emia is an aspect of alkalosis, the general term for accumulation of basic substances in the body fluids. The opposite of alkalosis is **acid/osis.** The combining form acid(o) means acid. A pathologic condition that results from

acidosis

accumulation of acid or depletion of alkaline substances is called _____.

5-34 The suffix -capnia refers to carbon dioxide. **Hyper/capnia** means greater than normal amounts of carbon dioxide in the blood. **Hypo/ventilation,** a reduced amount of air entering the pulmonary alveoli, results in hypercapnia. Carbon dioxide contributes to the acidity of blood. Does hypercapnia

lowering

result in lowering or increasing blood pH? _____

Within minutes, the lungs begin to compensate for any acid–base imbalance by increasing the excretion of carbon dioxide through faster or deeper breathing.

5-35 Hypo/capnia is the opposite of hypercapnia and means an abnormally low level of carbon dioxide in the blood. **A/capnia** is a synonym for hypocapnia, although in its strictest sense a/capnia

absence

hypocapnia

means _____ of carbon dioxide.

Would hyperventilation lead to hypercapnia or hypocapnia? _____

5-36 Acid/emia is an arterial blood pH below 7.35, whereas alkal/emia is recognized as a blood pH above 7.45. Either of these conditions can be considered an acid–base imbalance. Look at some conditions listed in Table 5.1 that can lead to an acid–base imbalance.

acidemia

Asphyxia leads to which condition, alkalemia or acidemia? _____

Table 5.1   Potential Causes of Acid–Base Imbalances

Acidemia	Alkalemia
Ingestion of highly acidic drugs	Ingestion of alkaline drugs
Severe diarrhea	Intense hyperventilation
Severe diabetes	Vomiting of gastric acid
Asphyxia	Metabolic problems
Vomiting	
Disease, particularly respiratory or kidney failure	

BUILD IT!   EXERCISE 15

Use the following word parts to build terms. (Some word parts will be used more than once.)

a-, an-, dys-, hypo-, alkal(o), ox(i), -capnia, -ia, -osis, -pnea

1. absence or deficiency of oxygen _____/_____/_____
2. abnormally low level of carbon dioxide _____/_____
3. labored or difficult breathing _____/_____
4. cessation of breathing _____/_____
5. condition of accumulation of basic substances in the body _____/_____

WRITE IT!   EXERCISE 16

Write a word in each blank to complete these sentences.

1. Asphyxia is a condition caused by insufficient intake of _____.
2. Exaggerated deep or rapid breathing is _____.
3. Increased aeration of the lungs is _____.
4. A greater than normal amount of carbon dioxide is _____.
5. A term for an arterial blood pH below 7.35 is _____.

5-37 Acute respiratory failure is a sudden inability of the lungs to maintain normal respiratory function. It may be caused by an obstruction in the airways or failure of the lungs. Respiratory failure leads to hyp/ox/ia. Acute (or adult) respiratory distress syndrome (ARDS) is severe pulmonary congestion characterized by respiratory insufficiency and hypoxemia and can result in acute respiratory failure.

blood

Hyp/ox/emia is decreased oxygen in the _____.

Once again, notice the spelling. You learned earlier that asphyxia is caused by insufficient intake of oxygen. This leads to hypoxemia, hypercapnia, loss of consciousness, and death, if not corrected.

5-38 In **ortho/pnea,** breathing is difficult except in an upright position. Analyze ortho/pnea (orth[o], straight + -pnea, breathing). In orthopnea, the person experiences chronic airflow limitation (CAL) and is unable to breathe when lying flat. Write the term that means a condition in which breathing

orthopnea

is difficult except in an upright position: _____.

Two comfortable positions that help orthopneic patients breathe more comfortably are shown in Fig. 5.10.

5-39 Abnormalities in the diaphragm will affect breathing, because the diaphragm normally moves downward as the lungs expand during inspiration. **Phreno/dynia** is pain in the diaphragm. Paralysis of the diaphragm is **phreno/plegia. Phreno/ptosis** is a prolapsed or downward displacement of the diaphragm. Use phren(o) to write a word that means inflammation of the diaphragm:

phrenitis

_____.

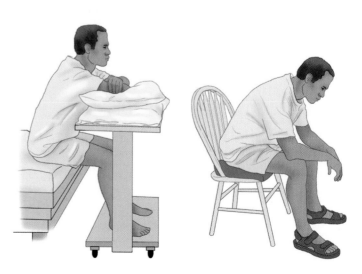

Figure 5.10 Two positions for the orthopneic patient. These positions ease the work of breathing for persons with chronic airflow limitation (CAL). This "tripod position" is often assumed by the patient with respiratory insufficiency.

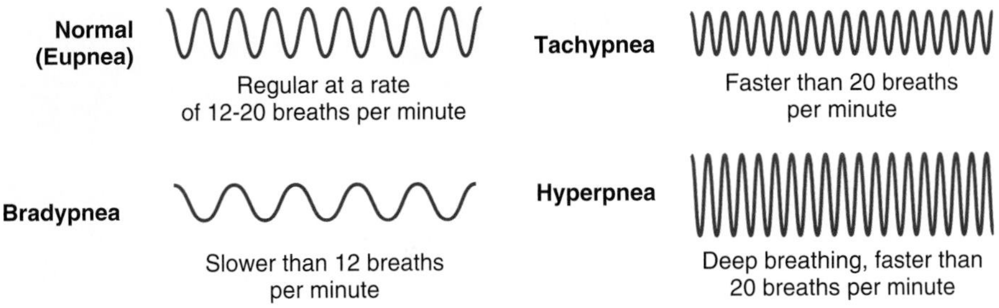

Normal (Eupnea)

Regular at a rate of 12-20 breaths per minute

Bradypnea

Slower than 12 breaths per minute

Tachypnea

Faster than 20 breaths per minute

Hyperpnea

Deep breathing, faster than 20 breaths per minute

Figure 5.11 Selected patterns of respiration. An example of normal respiration is compared with those seen in bradypnea, tachypnea, and hyperpnea.

5-40 Adults normally have a respiration rate of about 12 to 20 breaths per minute. **Eu/pnea** means normal breathing. If a person were breathing at a rate of 25 breaths per minute at rest, this would be **tachypnea.** The word tachy/pnea means breathing _____.

fast

bradypnea

The opposite of this is slow breathing, or _____. A graphic representation of various patterns of breathing is shown in Fig. 5.11.

In another condition, **hypo/pnea,** the breathing is shallow, in addition to being slow. This can occur if it is painful to breathe or if there is damage to the brain stem. Hypopnea may be appropriate in a well-conditioned athlete.

ANALYZE IT!

EXERCISE 17

Break the following terms into their component parts. Then write the meaning of each term.
1. bradypnea _____
2. eupnea _____
3. hypoxemia _____
4. orthopnea _____
5. phrenoplegia _____
6. tachypnea _____

Upper Respiratory Abnormalities

5-41 An upper airway obstruction is any significant interruption in the airflow through the nose, mouth, pharynx, or larynx. Laryngoscopy may be helpful in locating and removing the cause of the obstruction. If the cause is not removed, respiratory arrest occurs. Respiratory arrest is cessation of _____.

respiration (or breathing)

5-42 It may be possible to see a **nasal polyp** with the help of a nasoscope (Fig. 5.12). A polyp is a growth or mass protruding from a mucous membrane. Polyps are usually (but not always) benign. They can grow on almost any mucous membrane. If such a growth occurs in the nasal cavity or in the sinuses, it is called a nasal _____.

polyp

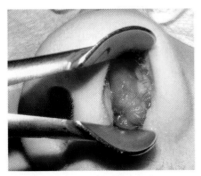

Figure 5.12 Nasal polyps. Note the rounded pieces of mucosa projecting into the nasal cavity.

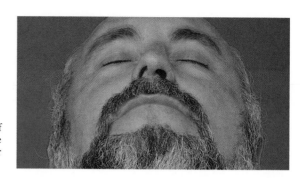

Figure 5.13 Deviated septum. This shifted partition of the nasal cavity may obstruct the nasal passages. Severe septal deviation may be corrected by rhinoplasty or septoplasty.

inflammation

5-43 During infections and allergies, swelling may block the passages and cause fluid to accumulate in the sinuses. A sinus headache can result from the pressure within the sinuses. **Sinus/itis** is _____ of one or more paranasal sinuses. A structural defect (such as a deviated septum [Fig. 5.13]) of the nose can also result in sinusitis.

rhinitis

WORD ORIGIN
coryza *(G.)*
koryza, catarrh

nose

5-44 Build a word using rhin(o) that means inflammation of the mucous membranes of the nose: _____. Acute rhinitis is also called **coryza,** meaning a profuse discharge of the mucous membranes of the nose.

Rhino/rrhea is discharge from the _____. This is commonly called a runny nose.

hemorrhage

WORD ORIGIN
epistaxis *(G.)*
staxis, dripping

pharynx

5-45 Nosebleeds have many causes, including irritation of the nasal membranes, fragility of these membranes, violent sneezing, trauma, high blood pressure, vitamin K deficiency, or (particularly in children) picking the nose. **Rhinorrhagia** means profuse bleeding from the nose. Literal translation of rhino/rrhagia is _____ from the nose. Another medical term for nosebleed is **epistaxis.**

5-46 **Pharyng/itis** is inflammation or infection of the _____, usually causing symptoms of a sore throat. Canker sores are ulcerations, especially inside the mouth.

Tonsill/itis is one reason for a sore throat. The tonsils are located in the oropharynx. Enlarged tonsils can fill the space behind the nares and may completely block the passage of air from the nose into the throat.

Other causes of a sore throat include streptococcal infections, **herpes simplex virus** (HSV), or infectious mononucleosis. It is important to receive an antibiotic for strep infections, because untreated strep infections sometimes lead to rheumatic fever (see Chapter 4). Herpes simplex, caused by the herpes simplex virus, usually produces small, transient, irritating, and sometimes fluid-filled blisters on the skin and mucous membranes. Infections tend to occur particularly around the nose and mouth.

speech

dysphasia

5-47 The combining form phas(o) means speech. Literal translation of dys/phas/ia is difficult _____. **Dysphasia** is impairment of speech, characterized by a lack of coordination and an inability to arrange words in their proper order, a problem resulting from a brain lesion. Difficulty in speech caused by a brain lesion is called _____.

absence

5-48 **A/phasia** is the _____ of speech. Aphasia is an inability to communicate through speech or writing, as a result of dysfunction of the brain. A person who has aphasia is said to be aphasic.

Read about additional pathologies and associated terms of the upper respiratory tract.

aphonia A condition characterized by the inability to produce normal speech sounds, resulting from overuse of the vocal cords, organic disease, or emotional problems, such as anxiety.

dysphonia Hoarseness or abnormality in the speaking voice that may precede aphonia.

laryngalgia Laryngeal pain; same as laryngodynia, but this term is not generally used.

laryngitis Inflammation of the larynx that would likely result in temporary loss of voice. It may be caused not only by infectious microorganisms but also by overuse of the voice, allergies, or irritants.

nasopharyngitis Inflammation of the nasopharynx.

palatitis Inflammation of the hard palate, the bony portion of the roof of the mouth.

pharyngalgia Sore throat (pharyngeal pain); same as **pharyngodynia.**

pharyngomycosis A fungal infection of the pharynx.

pharyngopathy Any disease of the pharynx.

rhinolithiasis The presence of a calculus or stone in the nasal cavity. A nasal calculus, a **rhinolith,** can interfere with breathing through the nose.

BUILD IT!

EXERCISE 18

Use the following word parts to build terms. (Some word parts will be used more than once.)

a-, dys-, pharyng(o), phas(o), rhin(o), sinus(o), -dynia, -ia, -itis, -rrhea

1. discharge from the nose   _____/_____

2. impairment of speech   _____/_____/_____

3. inflammation of one or more paranasal sinuses   _____/_____

4. throat pain   _____/_____

5. inability to communicate   _____/_____/_____

---

polyp

5-49 You learned earlier that a polyp is a tumor-like growth, usually benign, that projects from a mucous membrane. A growth of this type on the vocal cords is called a laryngeal _____ (Fig. 5.14).

Although painless, laryngeal polyps cause hoarseness. They are generally caused by smoking, allergies, or abuse of the voice, and eliminating the cause often relieves the hoarseness. Surgery can be performed using direct laryngoscopy if rest does not correct the problem.

discharge

5-50 The common cold is a contagious viral infection of the upper respiratory tract. Some of its major characteristics are rhinitis, rhinorrhea, tearing and eye discomfort, and sometimes low-grade fever. **Rhin/itis** is inflammation of the nasal membranes. **Rhino/rrhea** is _____ from the nasal membranes.

The barking cough of **croup** is often accompanied by difficulty in breathing and stridor. Croup is an acute viral infection of the upper and lower respiratory tract that occurs primarily in infants and young children. Upper respiratory tract infections (URIs) include the common cold, pharyngitis, laryngitis, rhinitis, sinusitis, and tonsillitis.

diphtheria

5-51 Diphtheria and **pertussis** are two acute contagious respiratory diseases. They are both caused by specific pathogenic bacteria and are both preventable by vaccination. Immunization for diphtheria and pertussis is usually begun in conjunction with tetanus immunization early in infancy. It is easy to misspell the term *diphtheria*. Write the term here: _____. The exotoxin of the tetanus bacillus affects the nervous system, resulting in paralysis. For this reason, the common name of tetanus is lockjaw.

Pertussis is commonly called *whooping cough,* named for the coughing that ends in a loud whooping inspiration. It occurs primarily in infants and young children but can occur in anyone who has not been immunized.

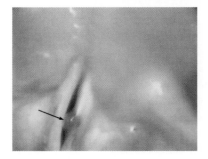

Figure 5.14 A laryngeal polyp. This hemorrhagic polyp *(arrow)* on the vocal cord occurs most commonly in adults who smoke, have many allergies, live in dry climates, or abuse the voice.

severe

5-52 A **corona/virus,** named for its appearance under an electron microscope, has been identified as the organism responsible for severe acute respiratory syndrome (SARS). It is spread by close contact with an infected person. Illness generally begins with a fever and body aches, and some people experience mild respiratory symptoms. After 3 to 7 days, a lower respiratory phase begins and patients may develop a dry cough and have trouble breathing.

Severity of the disease ranges from causing mild illness to death. The Centers for Disease Control and Prevention reports a fatality rate of approximately 3%. SARS is the abbreviation for _____ acute respiratory syndrome.

5-53 Influenza is a highly contagious respiratory infection that is caused by various strains of influenza virus. Three main types (type A, type B, and type C) have been identified, but new strains emerge at regular intervals (for example, Asian flu virus, bird flu, and H1N1 influenza). The 2009 H1N1 spreads from person to person, and while many infected persons have recovered without needing medical treatment, hospitalizations and deaths from infection with this virus have occurred. H1N1 influenza was originally thought to be the same as the virus found in swine and was called "swine flu." Influenza is characterized by a fever, sore throat, coughing, muscle aches, and weakness. Yearly vaccination is recommended for health care personnel, the elderly, and debilitated persons.

influenza

This highly contagious disease that is characterized by fever, respiratory symptoms, muscle aches, and weakness is _____.

FIND IT! **EXERCISE 19**

Draw a slash between the word parts in the following list of new terms. Then find the meanings of the word parts within the definitions. Think! (Draw the slash, and then perform the remainder of the activity as a mental exercise.)

1. **epiglottitis** inflammation of the epiglottis, the structure that overhangs the larynx like a lid and prevents food from entering the larynx and trachea while swallowing
2. **laryngopathy** any disease of the larynx
3. **laryngoplegia** paralysis of the laryngeal muscles
4. **larygospasm** spasmodic closure of the larynx

Lower Respiratory Abnormalities

5-54 The lower respiratory tract is a common site of infections, obstructive conditions, and malignancies. As explained in Chapter 14, lung cancer accounts for more deaths in the United States than any other cancer in both men and women, although cancer of the lung and bronchi are not the most common types.

➤ BEYOND THE BLUEPRINT The majority of pulmonary malignancies are attributable to cigarette smoking. Lung cancer develops most often in scarred or chronically diseased lungs. Compare the appearance of healthy lung tissue to that of a cigarette smoker (Fig. 5.15).

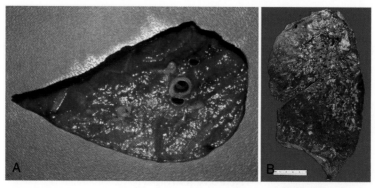

Figure 5.15 **Healthy lung tissue (sectioned) vs. the lungs of a smoker. A,** Healthy lung tissue is pink and highly elastic. **B,** A lung damaged by cigarette smoking is scarred, dark, and has lost much of its elasticity.

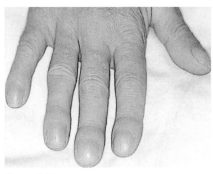

Figure 5.16 **Clubbing.** Abnormal enlargement of the distal phalanges is seen in advanced chronic pulmonary disease but may be associated with other disorders, such as cyanotic heart disease, chronic kidney disease, and cystic fibrosis.

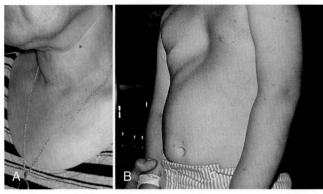

Figure 5.17 **Comparison of two structural problems of the chest, pigeon chest and funnel chest. A,** Pigeon chest, a congenital structural defect characterized by prominent sternal protrusion. **B,** Funnel chest, indentation of the lower sternum.

Fatigue is common in chronic respiratory conditions. Clubbing is a sign that is often associated with advanced chronic pulmonary disease. An abnormal enlargement of the distal fingers and toes, clubbing is most easily seen in the distal fingers (Fig. 5.16).

Several unnatural surface features of the chest can be seen during a physical examination. Both pigeon chest and funnel chest are skeletal abnormalities of the chest. The breastbone has a prominent anterior projection in pigeon chest, and it is depressed in funnel chest (Fig. 5.17). Breathing is generally not affected in either of these structural defects. A prominent anterior projection of the breastbone is characteristic of which skeletal abnormality, pigeon chest or funnel chest?

pigeon

_____ chest

5-55 Flail chest occurs when multiple rib fractures cause instability of the chest wall. The lung underlying the injury contracts and bulges with each inspiration and expiration. This condition must be surgically corrected to prevent hypoxia.

Barrel chest—a large, rounded thorax—may be normal in some individuals but may also be a sign of pulmonary emphysema. The common name for a large, rounded thorax is

barrel

_____ chest.

Match the following unnatural chest features with their outstanding characteristics.

_____ **1.** barrel chest   **A.** contracting and bulging of the lung during inspiration and expiration

_____ **2.** flail chest   **B.** depression of the breastbone

_____ **3.** funnel chest   **C.** prominent anterior projection of the breastbone

_____ **4.** pigeon chest   **D.** rounded chest

Learn the meanings of the word parts in the following list.

Word Parts: Respiratory Pathologies

Combining Form	Meaning	Prefix	Meaning
anthrac(o)	coal	meta-	change; next, as in a series
atel(o)	imperfect or incomplete	**Suffix**	
coni(o)	dust	-ation	process
embol(o)	embolus	-pnea	breathing
fibr(o)	fiber or fibrous	-ptosis	prolapse
thromb(o)	thrombus	-ptysis	spitting
		-stenosis	narrowing

Match the word parts in the left column with the descriptions in the right column.

_____ **1.** anthrac(o)   **A.** breathing
_____ **2.** atel(o)   **B.** change or next
_____ **3.** -ation   **C.** coal
_____ **4.** coni(o)   **D.** dust
_____ **5.** meta-   **E.** imperfect
_____ **6.** -pnea   **F.** narrowing
_____ **7.** -ptysis   **G.** process
_____ **8.** -stenosis   **H.** spitting

aplasia

5-56 The suffix -plasia means formation or development. **A/plasia** means absence of formation or development. Incomplete formation or development of the lung is the same as _____ of the lung.

5-57 Adult respiratory distress syndrome, also called acute respiratory distress syndrome (ARDS), is respiratory failure as a result of disease or injury, characterized by severe pulmonary congestion. Respiratory distress syndrome (RDS) of the newborn is an acute lung disease of the newborn that occurs most often in premature babies. In most cases, the infant dies only a few days after birth or recovers with no after effects. Sudden infant death syndrome (SIDS) is the unexpected and sudden death of an apparently normal and healthy infant that occurs during sleep and may be linked with

infant

respiration. SIDS means sudden _____ death syndrome.

dilation

5-58 Literal translation of **bronchi/ectasis** is _____ of the bronchi; however, bronchiectasis is an abnormal condition of the bronchial tree that is characterized by irreversible dilation and destruction of the bronchial walls. Signs and symptoms include chronic sinusitis, a constant cough producing a great deal of sputum, hemoptysis (hem[o], blood + -ptysis, spitting), and persistent crackles.

5-59 **Broncho/spasm** means bronchial spasm. Bronchospasm brings about **broncho/constriction,** resulting in an acute narrowing and obstruction of the respiratory airway. There is usually a cough with generalized wheezing, a chief characteristic of asthma and bronchitis.

    Asthma is characterized by recurring episodes of paroxysmal wheezing and dyspnea, constriction of the bronchi, coughing, and viscous bronchial secretions. It is also called *bronchial asthma.* **Paroxysmal** refers to a sudden recurrence or intensity of symptoms.

lungs

5-60 The highly elastic lungs are the main components of the respiratory system. **Pneumon/ia,** or **pneumonitis,** means inflammation of the _____.

    Acute pneumonia involving both lungs is double pneumonia. Several microorganisms including bacteria, viruses, and fungi have been identified as causes of pneumonia, but the disease is often caused by pneumo/cocci, a type of pathogenic coccal bacteria. This type of pneumonia is called **pneumo/coccal pneumonia.** A vaccine is available for pneumococcal pneumonia and is recommended for persons older than 65 years of age and/or those with immunodeficiencies.

    Broncho/pneumon/ia involves both the bronchi and the lungs and is usually a result of the spread of infection from the upper to the lower respiratory tract. Lobar pneumonia involves one or more of the five major lobes of the lungs.

chest

5-61 **Hydrothorax** is a noninflammatory accumulation of fluid in one or both pleural cavities. Literal interpretation of hydro/thorax is watery _____.

    An accumulation of blood and fluid in the pleural cavity is called **hemo/thorax.** Trauma, such as a knife wound, is the most common cause of hemothorax, but it can occur as a result of inflammation or tumors. Write this new term that means blood and fluid in the pleural cavity:

hemothorax

_____.

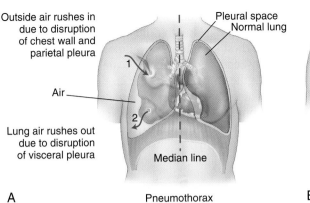

Outside air rushes in due to disruption of chest wall and parietal pleura

Air

Lung air rushes out due to disruption of visceral pleura

Pleural space
Normal lung

Median line

A   Pneumothorax

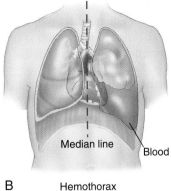

Median line

Blood

B   Hemothorax

Figure 5.18 **Two abnormal conditions of the chest cavity. A,** Pneumothorax. The *arrows* indicate the two situations that result in pneumothorax. *Arrow 1* represents an open chest wound that permits the entrance of air into the pleural space. *Arrow 2* represents a tear within the lung that allows air to enter the pleural space. **B,** Hemothorax. The massive hemothorax shown has caused much of the left lung to collapse.

5-62 Pneumo/thorax is air or gas in the pleural cavity; it leads to collapse of the lung. This may be the result of an open chest wound that permits the entrance of air, rupture of a vesicle on the surface of the lung, or a severe bout of coughing; it may even occur spontaneously without apparent cause. (Both pneumothorax and hemothorax are illustrated in Fig. 5.18.)

blood
    Pneumo/hemo/thorax is an accumulation of air and _____ in the pleural cavity.

pleura
5-63 Pleur/itis is inflammation of the _____.
    Pleurisy is another name for pleuritis. Pleurisy may be caused by an infection, injury, tumor, or a complication of certain lung diseases. A sharp pain on inspiration is characteristic of pleurisy.

pleuritis
Pleurisy is another name for _____.

5-64 Pleuro/pneumon/ia is a combination of pleurisy and pneumonia. You will need to remember

lungs
that pleuropneumonia is inflammation of both the pleura and the _____.

pleural
5-65 Pleural effusion is a collection of nonpurulent fluid in the _____ cavity (Fig. 5.19). Non/purulent means not containing pus. If pleural effusion contains pus, it is called **pyo/thorax** or **empyema.** This condition is an extension of infection from nearby structures.
    Untreated empyema can lead to **pulmonary fibrosis** (fibrosis of the lungs). The combining form fibr(o) means fiber or fibrous (tough, threadlike). Aplasia results in the absence of an organ or tissue and it applies also to failure of normal cell generation and development in the bone marrow.

fibrous
Pulmonary fibrosis is a _____ condition of the connective tissue of the lungs, resulting from the formation of scar tissue.

5-66 Pleuro/dynia is pain of the pleura. This can be caused by inflammation of the pleura or by **pleural adhesions,** in which the pleural membranes stick together or to the wall of the chest and produce pain on movement or breathing. Adhesion means a sticking together of two surfaces that are normally separated. Pleural adhesion may be associated with pleur/itis, which is inflammation

pleura
of the _____.

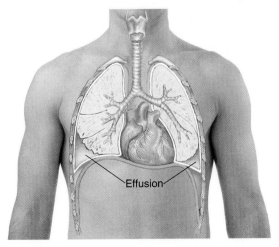

Effusion

Figure 5.19 **Pleural effusion.** Abnormal accumulation of fluid in the pleural space is characterized by fever, chest pain, dyspnea, and nonproductive cough.

lung

5-67 Pulmonary edema is an accumulation of extravascular fluid in _____ tissue. Pulmonary edema also involves the alveoli and progresses to fluid entering the bronchioles and bronchi. Dyspnea on exertion is one of the earliest symptoms of pulmonary edema. As the condition becomes more advanced, the patient may become orthopneic. Acute pulmonary edema is an emergency situation. Congestive heart failure is the most common cause of pulmonary edema.

In **congestive heart failure,** the work demanded of the heart is greater than its ability to perform. Decreased output of blood by the left ventricle produces congestion and engorgement of the pulmonary vessels with escape of fluid into pulmonary tissues. Congestive heart failure can result in the lung disorder, _____ edema.

pulmonary

pulmonary

5-68 A **pulmon/ary embolus** is an obstruction of the _____ artery or one of its branches by a blood clot (Fig. 5.20). Obstruction of a large pulmonary vessel can cause sudden death.

Match these pathologies with their descriptions.

_____ **1.** accumulation of extravascular fluid in lung tissue

_____ **2.** air or gas in the pleural cavity

_____ **3.** blood and fluid in the pleural cavity

_____ **4.** inflammation of the lungs

_____ **5.** localized pus-containing cavity surrounded by inflamed lung tissue

_____ **6.** noninflammatory accumulation of fluid in one or both pleural cavities

_____ **7.** nonpurulent fluid in the pleural cavity

_____ **8.** obstruction of a pulmonary artery or one of its branches

A. hemothorax

B. hydrothorax

C. pleural effusion

D. pneumonia

E. pneumothorax

F. pulmonary abscess

G. pulmonary edema

H. pulmonary embolus

5-69 The lungs of a newborn are pink. The adult lung darkens as a result of dust, soot, or other environmental pollutants. **Pneumo/coni/osis** is any disease of the lung caused by chronic inhalation of dust, usually mineral dust of either occupational or environmental origin.

dust

The combining form coni(o) means dust. Pneumoconiosis is a condition (disease) of the lungs caused by inhalation of _____.

5-70 Anthracosis, asbestosis, and silicosis are three kinds of pneumoconiosis. The combining form anthrac(o) means coal. **Anthrac/osis** is a chronic lung disease characterized by the deposit of _____ dust in the lungs. It occurs in coal miners and is aggravated by cigarette smoking.

coal

Asbest/osis is a chronic lung disease that results from prolonged exposure to _____. It may occur in asbestos miners and workers or those exposed to asbestos building materials (Fig. 5.21). **Mesothelioma,** a rare malignant tumor, is associated with exposure to asbestos and is almost always fatal. The mesothelium is a layer of epithelial cells that covers the pleura and the peritoneum.

asbestos

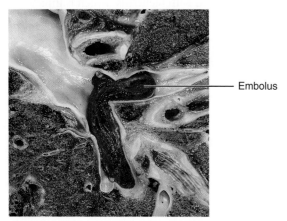

Figure 5.20 — Embolus

Figure 5.20 **Pulmonary embolus.** This particular internal blood clot broke loose and traveled from a lower extremity and is now located in a pulmonary artery branch.

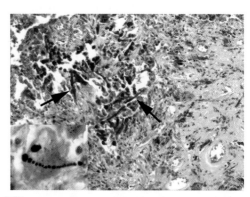

Figure 5.21 **Asbestos fibers in stained lung tissue sample.** Arrows point to asbestos fibers.

pneumoconiosis

Silic/osis is a lung disorder caused by long-term inhalation of silica dust, which is found in sands, quartzes, and many other stones. This lung disorder is a type of _____.

5-71 Chronic obstructive pulmonary disease (COPD), also called *chronic obstructive lung disease (COLD),* is a nonspecific designation that includes a group of progressive and irreversible respiratory problems in which dyspnea and a chronic cough are prominent features. The mechanism of air trapping is explained in Fig. 5.22. Airflow obstruction ultimately occurs. Emphysema, chronic bronchitis, asthmatic bronchitis, bronchiectasis, and cystic fibrosis are often included in this group. COPD is aggravated by cigarette smoking and air pollution.

WORD ORIGIN
emphysema *(G.)* *en,* inside; *physema,* a blowing

emphysema

Emphysema, characterized by overinflation and destructive changes in alveolar walls, is probably the most severe COPD (Fig. 5.23). Permanent hyperinflation of the lungs occurs as alveoli are destroyed, and alveolar air is trapped, thus interfering with exchange of carbon dioxide and oxygen.

Overinflation and destruction of the alveolar walls are major characteristics of _____.

lungs

5-72 Tuberculosis (TB) is an infectious disease that often is chronic and commonly affects the lungs, although it may occur in other parts of the body. Pulmonary tuberculosis affects the _____.

Resistance to tuberculosis depends a great deal on a person's general health. The disease is named after **tubercles,** which are small, round nodules produced in the lungs by the infective bacteria.

5-73 Liquefaction of the tubercles not only results in tubercular cavities in the lungs but can also cause the production of a large quantity of highly infectious sputum that is raised when the infected person coughs.

out

To **ex/pectorate** is to cough up and spit _____ material from the lungs and air passages. (The material coughed up from the lungs is sputum.) Blood-stained sputum is often produced in tuberculosis. **Hemo/ptysis** is the spitting of blood or blood-stained sputum.

5-74 Cystic fibrosis is an inherited disorder of the exocrine glands that involves the lungs, pancreas, and sweat glands. Heavy secretion of thick mucus clogs the bronchi and leads to a chronic cough and persistent upper respiratory infections. Excessive salt loss (three to six times the normal concentrations) in the perspiration of persons who have cystic fibrosis forms the basis of the sweat test, a laboratory test to determine the amount of sodium and chloride excretion from the sweat

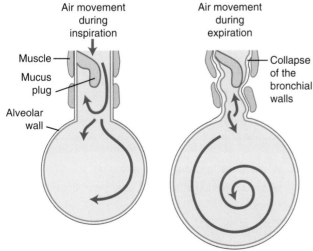

Figure 5.22 **Mechanisms of air trapping in chronic obstructive pulmonary disease.** Air trapping is the result of an inefficient expiratory effort. As the rate of respiration increases, breathing becomes shallower and the amount of trapped air increases.

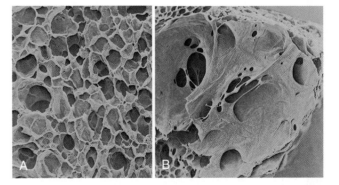

Figure 5.23 **A,** Normal lung tissue. **B,** Emphysema. Notice the overinflation of air sacs with destruction of alveolar walls.

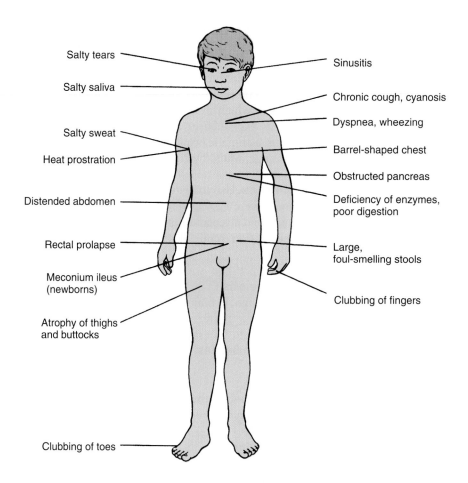

Salty tears

Salty saliva

Salty sweat

Heat prostration

Distended abdomen

Rectal prolapse

Meconium ileus
(newborns)

Atrophy of thighs
and buttocks

Clubbing of toes

Sinusitis

Chronic cough, cyanosis

Dyspnea, wheezing

Barrel-shaped chest

Obstructed pancreas

Deficiency of enzymes,
poor digestion

Large,
foul-smelling stools

Clubbing of fingers

Figure 5.24 Manifestations of cystic fibrosis.

fibrosis

glands. The disease is usually diagnosed in infancy or early childhood (Fig. 5.24). The sweat test is performed to diagnose cystic _____.

5-75 Atel/ectasis (atel[o], imperfect + -ectasis, stretching) is an abnormal condition characterized by the collapse of all or part of a lung. Failure of the lungs to expand fully at birth is called *primary atelectasis*. Other causes of atelectasis include obstructions of the airways, compression of the lung as a result of fluid or air, and pressure from a tumor.

atelectasis

Write the name of this abnormal condition in which there is incomplete expansion of a lung at birth or airlessness of a lung that once functioned: _____.

WRITE IT! **EXERCISE 23**

Write terms for the following meanings.
1. a lung disease characterized by the deposit of coal dust in the lungs _____
2. any disease of the lung characterized by chronic inhalation of dust _____
3. collapse of all or part of a lung _____
4. spitting of blood or blood-stained sputum _____

CIRCLE IT! **EXERCISE 24**

Circle the correct answer.
1. Overinflation and destructive changes in alveolar walls are characteristics of which of the following? (congenital atelectasis, emphysema, mesothelioma, pleuropneumonia)
2. Which of the following represents a group of progressive and irreversible respiratory problems in which dyspnea is a prominent feature? (COPD, cystic fibrosis, embolism, pulmonary edema)
3. Which of the following is not a type of pneumoconiosis? (anthracosis, asbestosis, emphysema, silicosis)
4. Which of the following is an inherited disorder of the exocrine glands that involves the lungs, pancreas, and sweat glands? (congestive heart failure, cystic fibrosis, pneumohemothorax, pulmonary edema)

Additional lower respiratory pathologies and associated terms include the following:

bronchiolectasis Dilation of the bronchioles
bronchiolitis Inflammation of the bronchioles
bronchitis Inflammation of the bronchi
bronchogenic Originating in a bronchus
broncholithiasis A condition in which stones are present in the lining of the bronchi
bronchopathy Any disease of the bronchi
bronchopulmonary Pertaining to the bronchi and lungs
laryngotracheal Pertaining to the larynx and the trachea
laryngotracheitis Inflammation of the larynx and trachea

laryngotracheobronchitis Inflammation of the larynx, trachea, and bronchi
pulmonary abscess A localized cavity containing pus and surrounded by inflamed lung tissue
trachealgia Pain of the trachea
tracheitis Inflammation of the trachea, a type of lower respiratory tract infection, which also includes bronchitis, bronchiolitis, and pneumonia.
tracheomalacia Softening of the trachea
tracheostenosis Narrowing of the lumen of the trachea

WRITE IT! **EXERCISE 25**

Case Study. *Define the terms listed after the case study.*

Valesca Morales, age 2, is seen by Dr. Wong, in the ED. She presents with fever, tachycardia, hyperpnea, severe coughing, and dyspnea. Radiograph indicates bronchopneumonia. Antibiotics and oxygen therapy are initiated, and the patient is admitted, transferred immediately to an isolation unit, and referred to Dr. Walter Smith, pulmonologist.

1. tachycardia _____

2. hyperpnea _____

3. dyspnea _____

4. bronchopneumonia _____

5. pulmonologist _____

BUILD IT! **EXERCISE 26**

Use the following word parts to build terms. (Some word parts will be used more than once.)

bronch(o), bronchiol(o), laryng(o), pulmon(o), trache(o), -algia, -ary, -ectasis, -itis

1. dilation of the bronchioles _____/_____

2. inflammation of the larynx and trachea _____/_____/_____

3. inflammation of the bronchioles _____/_____

4. pain of the trachea _____/_____

5. pertaining to the bronchi and lungs _____/_____/_____

SURGICAL AND THERAPEUTIC INTERVENTIONS

5-76 Asphyxiation, the inability to breathe, requires immediate corrective measures to prevent damage or death. Removal of a foreign body in the airway may be needed before oxygen and artificial respiration are administered. One method of dislodging food or other obstruction from the windpipe is the **Heimlich maneuver** (Fig. 5.25).

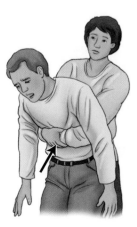

Figure 5.25 Heimlich maneuver. The rescuer grasps the choking person from behind, placing the thumb side of the fist against the victim's abdomen, in the midline, slightly above the navel and well below the breastbone. Abruptly pulling the fist firmly upward will often force the obstruction up the windpipe.

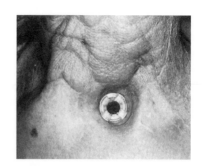

Figure 5.26 Healed tracheostomy after laryngectomy.

🔑 **KEY** POINT **Artificial respiration may be manual, as in the lifesaving procedure cardiopulmonary resuscitation (CPR), or provided by a mechanical ventilator, a device used to provide assisted respiration and usually temporary life support.** CPR consists of artificial respiration and external cardiac massage.

opening

A **tracheo/stomy,** surgical creation of an _____ in the trachea, may be necessary in upper airway obstruction. A tracheostomy requires a **tracheo/tomy,** an incision into the trachea through the neck below the larynx.

5-77 Sometimes a person has a stoma at the base of the neck. Surgical creation of this type of opening into the trachea is called a tracheostomy. A general term for a mouthlike opening is a

stoma _____.

🔑 **KEY** POINT **A tracheostomy is not always an emergency procedure and can be temporary or permanent.** A tracheostomy is performed after a **laryngectomy** or when prolonged mechanical ventilation is needed. A tube is inserted through an incision in the neck into the trachea. There are many types of tracheostomy tubes; some permit speech (Fig. 5.26).

5-78 In COPD or other problems in hypoxic patients, oxygen therapy may be prescribed by the physician. Oxygen is sometimes administered after general surgery. In patients who can breathe but are hypoxic, oxygen is delivered through tubing via:
- a simple face mask
- **nasal cannulae,** small tubes inserted into the nares
- a **Venturi mask**
- **trans/tracheal oxygen** (TTO) delivery

A Venturi mask and a transtracheal oxygen system deliver a more consistent and accurate oxygen concentration. Compare the four types of airway management shown in Fig. 5.27.

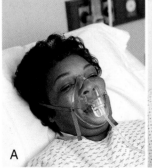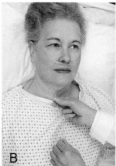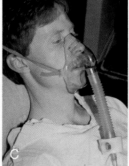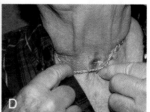

A B C D

Figure 5.27 Four means of administering oxygen. A, A simple oxygen mask delivers high concentrations of oxygen and is used for short-term oxygen therapy or in an emergency. **B,** The nasal cannula, a device that delivers oxygen by way of two small tubes that are inserted into the nostrils. **C,** The Venturi mask, a face mask designed to allow inspired air to mix with oxygen. **D,** Transtracheal oxygen is a long-term method of delivering oxygen directly into the lungs.

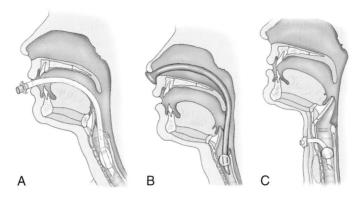

Figure 5.28 Comparison of endotracheal intubation and a tracheostomy tube. A, Orotracheal intubation for short-term airway management. **B,** Nasotracheal intubation for short-term airway management. **C,** Tracheostomy tube for longer maintenance of the airway.

5-79 Oxygen is administered in hypoxic patients to increase the amount of oxygen in circulating blood. It is also administered during anesthesia because oxygen functions as a carrier gas for the delivery of anesthetic agents to the tissues of the body. An overdose of oxygen can have toxic effects, which include respiratory depression and damage to the lungs. Using hyp/ox/emia as a model, write a word that means increased oxygen content of the blood: _____.

hyperoxemia

5-80 Receiving oxygen by intubation (insertion of a tube into a body canal or cavity) is one of the following types:

- Transtracheal oxygen delivered through a **tracheostomy tube** is used for prolonged airway management.
- **Endotracheal intubation** (an airway catheter inserted through the mouth or nose).

Oro/tracheal intubation and **naso/tracheal intubation** are insertion of a tube through the mouth or nose into the trachea. Compare these two types of intubation with transtracheal oxygen via a tracheostomy tube (Fig. 5.28).

Nasotracheal intubation is insertion of a nasotracheal tube through the _____

nose

into the trachea.

KEY POINT **Mechanical ventilation is the use of an artificial device to assist in breathing.** It is a means of supporting patients until either they recover sufficiently to breathe independently or the decision is made to withdraw respiratory support (Fig. 5.29).

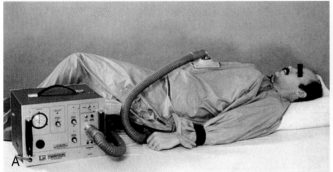
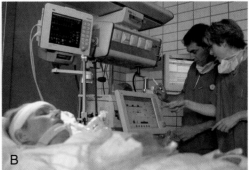

Figure 5.29 Mechanical ventilation. This treatment cares for patients until they recover the ability to breathe independently or can serve as a bridge to long-term mechanical ventilation. **A,** Noninvasive negative pressure ventilation pulls the chest outward, producing ventilation similar to normal breathing. An early type was the "iron lung" developed during the polio epidemic in the United States in the 1950s. **B,** Positive pressure ventilation. This type of ventilation requires an artificial airway and is the primary method used with acutely ill patients. It pushes air into the lungs under positive pressure.

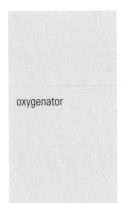
oxygenator

5-81 Oxygenation means the act or process of adding oxygen. Extra/corpor/eal means outside the body. **Extracorporeal membrane oxygenator** (ECMO) is a device used in a hospital to provide respiratory support by circulating the blood through an artificial lung, then returning the blood to the patient's circulatory system. It is used in newborns and occasionally in adults with acute respiratory distress syndrome.

ECMO is the abbreviation for extracorporeal membrane _____.

5-82 Surgery is often the most effective treatment for lung cancer, but most lung cancers are far advanced when detected. **Pneumonectomy (pneumectomy)** is the excision of lung tissue, either a complete lung (total pneumonectomy) or part of it (partial pneumonectomy). Removal of a lobe of the lung is called **pulmonary lobectomy**. Wedge resection is the removal of a small, localized area of diseased tissue; however, the cancer must be near the lung's surface.

Read about additional surgical interventions:

adenoid/ectomy Excision of the adenoids.

palatoplasty Surgical repair (reconstruction) of the palate. Along with additional plastic surgery, palatoplasty is used to correct cleft palate, a congenital defect characterized by a fissure (split) in the midline of the palate.

pneumo/centesis Puncturing of the lung to drain fluid that has accumulated in the organ itself.

thoracentesis Surgical puncture of the chest wall and pleural space with a needle to aspirate fluid or to obtain a specimen for biopsy. It has both therapeutic and diagnostic uses and can be used in the treatment of pleural effusion (Fig. 5.30); shortened form of **thoracocentesis.**

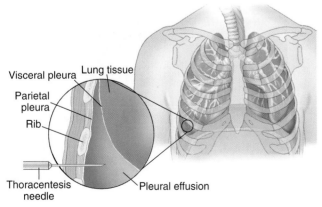
B

Figure 5.30 **Thoracentesis. A,** Common position for thoracentesis. **B,** Insertion of the needle in thoracentesis. The insertion site depends on the location of the fluid.

thoraco/stomy An opening into the chest wall for insertion of a chest tube. A chest tube is inserted into the pleural space to remove air and/or fluid and is commonly used after chest surgery (Fig. 5.31).

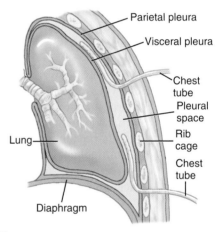

Figure 5.31 **Placement of chest tube.** A chest tube is a catheter that is inserted through the thorax into the pleural space and is attached to a water-seal chest drainage device. The chest tube is used to remove fluid or air after chest surgery and lung collapse.

rhinoplasty Plastic surgery of the nose, for trauma of the head and face, but usually done for cosmetic reasons.

tracheoplasty Plastic surgery to repair the trachea.

septoplasty Surgical reconstruction of the nasal septum.

septorhinoplasty Plastic surgery of the nasal septum and the external nose.

thoraco/plasty Surgical procedure that involves removing ribs and allowing the chest wall to collapse a lung. The procedure is sometimes done to gain access during thoracic surgery.

uvul/ectomy Excision of the uvula, the pendant tissue in the back of the pharynx, either by conventional or laser surgery.

BUILD IT!
EXERCISE 27

Use the following word parts to build terms. (Some word parts will be used more than once.)

laryng(o), pneumon(o), sept(o), thorac(o), trache(o), -centesis, -ectomy, -plasty

1. surgical removal of the voice box   _____/_____
2. surgical puncture of the chest wall and pleural space to aspirate fluid   _____/_____
3. plastic surgery to repair the trachea   _____/_____
4. surgical reconstruction of the nasal septum   _____/_____
5. partial or complete surgical removal of a lung   _____/_____

5-83 Surgery is not always necessary for sleep apnea. For mild sleep apnea, weight loss or a change in sleeping position may reduce or correct the problem. A common nonsurgical method to prevent airway collapse is the use of continuous positive airway pressure (CPAP) ventilation. A small electric compressor delivers positive pressure through a face mask during sleep (Fig. 5.32).

neoplasms

An anti/neoplas/tic is a treatment that acts against _____.

Either radiation or chemo/therapy or both may be used to destroy tumor cells or may be used in certain types of localized malignancies.

🔑 **KEY POINT Many malignant lesions may be curable if detected in the early stage.** Treatment selection depends on the site, stage of the cancer, and unique characteristics of the individual. Some anti/cancer treatments include surgery, irradiation, and chemotherapy with antineoplastic agents. Irradiation uses radiant energy, such as x-rays and radioactive substances, to treat cancer.

5-84 A method of encouraging voluntary deep breathing after surgery or with patients who have chronic air obstruction involves use of an incentive spirometer, a small apparatus that provides visual feedback about the inspired volume of air (Fig. 5.33). While in the hospital, a registered pulmonary function therapist (RPFT) is involved in respiratory treatments and evaluating progress.

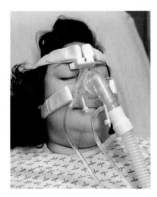

Figure 5.32 Noninvasive use of continuous positive airway pressure (CPAP) to alleviate mild sleep apnea. This machine may be used in the home setting to maintain adequate blood oxygen levels while sleeping.

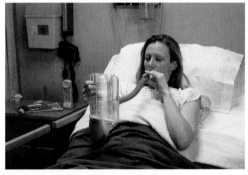

Figure 5.33 Incentive spirometry. A therapeutic means of encouraging deep breathing using a specially designed spirometer that provides visual feedback.

WRITE IT!
EXERCISE 28

Write words in the blanks to complete these sentences. The first letters of the answers are given as clues.

1. The inability to breathe is _a_____ .
2. Artificial respiration and external cardiac massage are administered in cardiopulmonary
   _r_____ .
3. In a hospital setting, artificial respiration is supplied by a mechanical _v_____ .
4. Surgical creation of an opening into the trachea is called a _t_____ .
5. COPD means chronic _o_____ pulmonary disease.
6. TTO is the abbreviation for _t_____ oxygen, which is a means of delivering oxygen to the lungs.
7. Insertion of a tube through the mouth into the trachea is called _o_____ intubation.
8. Pneumocentesis is surgical puncture of a _l_____ to drain fluid contents.
9. A _t_____ is an opening into the chest wall for insertion of a chest tube.
10. Removal of a lobe of the lung is pulmonary _l_____ .

PHARMACOLOGY

Respiratory infections are generally treated with antibiotics, along with other medications that individual patients need.

An **inhaler** is a device for administering medications that are breathed in, such as vapors or fine powders. Hand-held **nebulizers** are powered devices that convert a liquid into a fine spray before delivering it into the respiratory passages, either with or without oxygen to carry it into the lungs.

Drug Class: Effects and Uses

Antiasthmastics: *Prevent or treat the symptoms of asthma.*

Therapy types: bronchodilators, leukotriene receptor antagonists, corticosteroids, and mast cell stabilizers

Antihistamines: *Block histamine-1 to reduce allergic response; reduce the effects of histamine*
Used to treat or prevent allergic rhinitis or asthma; some inhalation formulations available
azelastine (Astelin)
olopatadine (Patanase)

> **WORD ORIGIN**
> antitussive *(L.)*
> anti-, against; tussis, cough

Antitussives: Suppress coughing
benzonatate (Tessalon)
codeine (in combination, e.g., Robitussin AC)
dextromethorphan (Delsym, combination products)

Bronchodilators: Open the airways to improve respiration to treat asthma, chronic obstructive pulmonary disease (COPD), or symptoms of bronchitis. Many combination products now available

Anticholinergics: Dilate the bronchi and bronchioles
ipratropium (Atrovent)   *tiotropium (Spiriva)*

Beta-2 Agonists: Relax smooth muscle in airways
albuterol (Proventil)   *metaproterenol (Alupent)*   *terbutaline (Brethaire)*
arformoterol (Brovana)   *salmeterol (Serevent)*

Inhaled Corticosteroids: Reduce inflammation of the airways. Used for allergic rhinitis when available as a nasal spray
beclomethasone (QVAR)   *fluticasone (Flovent)*   *triamcinolone (Nasacort)*
ciclesonide (Alvesco)   *mometasone (Asmanex)*

Methylxanthines: Relax airway muscles to open airways, increase diaphragm contractions to draw more air into the lungs, and mildly reduce inflammation
aminophylline (Phyllocontin)   *theophylline (Theo-24)*

> **WORD ORIGIN**
> decongestant *(L.)*
> de-, away or remove; congerere, to pile up

Decongestants: Reduce swelling of mucous membranes to treat nasal and sinus congestion
phenylephrine (in combination products)
pseudoephedrine (Sudafed, combination products)

Expectorants: Improve expulsion of mucus from lungs
ammonium chloride (in combination products)
guaifenesin (Mucinex)

Leukotriene Receptor Antagonists (LTRAs): *Block leukotrienes in the long-acting inflammatory response to allergens*
Montelukast (Singulair)   *Zileuton (Zyflo)*

Mast Cell Stabilizers: Prevent mast cell's release of histamine
Used to prevent allergic rhinitis or asthma
cromolyn (Intal)   *nedocromil (Tilade)*

Mucolytics: Break up mucus in the lungs
acetylcysteine (Mucomyst)

PHARMACOLOGY, cont'd

Smoking Cessation Drugs: Aid in quitting smoking or the use of other tobacco products
Therapy types: nicotine replacement therapy or reduction of cravings and/or withdrawal symptoms with a drug that acts on the brain
bupropion (Zyban)
nicotine polacrilex (Nicorette)
varenicline (Chantix)

WRITE IT!   EXERCISE 29

Write one term in each blank.

1. A general term for drugs which break up mucus in the lungs is _____.
2. A term for drugs used to prevent asthma are _____.
3. Drugs used to block histamines are called _____.
4. Drugs used to suppress coughing are called _____.
5. Medications that open the airways to improve respiration are _____.

CHAPTER ABBREVIATIONS*

ABG	arterial blood gas	O_2	oxygen
ARDS	acute (or adult) respiratory distress syndrome	PFT	pulmonary function test
CAL	chronic airflow limitation	pH	potential hydrogen; hydrogen ion concentration
CO_2	carbon dioxide	RDS	respiratory distress syndrome
COLD	chronic obstructive lung disease	RPFT	registered pulmonary function therapist
COPD	chronic obstructive pulmonary disease	SARS	severe acute respiratory syndrome
CPAP	continuous positive airway pressure (for sleep apnea)	SIDS	sudden infant death syndrome
		SOB	shortness of breath
CPR	cardiopulmonary resuscitation	TB	tuberculosis
CSR	Cheyne-Stokes respiration	TTO	transtracheal oxygen
ECMO	extracorporeal membrane oxygenator	URI	upper respiratory infection
HSV	herpes simplex virus	VC	vital capacity
LTRA	leukotriene receptor antagonist		

*Many of these abbreviations share their meanings with other terms. CO_2 and O_2 are chemical symbols.

! Be Careful With These!

anoxia vs. *hypoxia* vs. *hypoxemia*	*hyperpnea* vs. *hyperventilation*	*larynx* vs. *pharynx*	*pneumocentesis* vs.
aphasia vs. *aphonia*	*inhalation* vs. *exhalation*	*nasotracheal intubation* vs.	*thoracentesis*
dysphasia vs. *dysphonia*	*inspiration* vs. *expiration*	*orotracheal intubation*	*pneumothorax* vs. *hemothorax*
endotracheal intubation vs.	*internal respiration* vs. *external*	*pneum(o)* vs. *pneumat(o),*	*rhonchi* vs. *rales* vs. *wheeze*
ECMO	*respiration*	*pulm(o), pulmon(o)*	vs. *friction rub*

A Career as a Respiratory Therapist

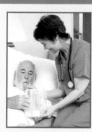

Dawn Robertson is a respiratory therapist in a hospital, working with physicians to establish and evaluate breathing therapies. She combines information about technology with patient physiology to develop individualized respiratory therapy programs. Dawn's work is rewarding, because she can see the success of her efforts as patients improve. She had the option of working in the intensive care unit or in the emergency department, but Dawn prefers helping patients who have asthma, are recovering from infections, or who have COPD. Certified respiratory therapists may specialize in pulmonary testing, newborns, etc. For more information, visit the website of the American Association for Respiratory Care: *www.aarc.org/career/be_an_rt.*

CHAPTER 5 SELF-TEST

Review the new word parts for this chapter. Work all of the following exercises to test your understanding of the material before checking your answers against those in Appendix IV.

BASIC UNDERSTANDING

Matching

I. Match structures in the left column (1-7) with their characteristics or functions in the right column (A-G).

_____ **1.** alveolus   **A.** a branch of the trachea

_____ **2.** bronchus   **B.** a muscular partition that facilitates breathing

_____ **3.** diaphragm   **C.** commonly called the windpipe

_____ **4.** larynx   **D.** connected with the paranasal sinuses

_____ **5.** nose   **E.** contains the palatine tonsils

_____ **6.** pharynx   **F.** contains the vocal cords

_____ **7.** trachea   **G.** where oxygen and carbon dioxide exchange occurs

II. Match diseases or disorders in the left column (1-7) with their characteristics in the right column (A-G).

_____ **1.** anthracosis   **A.** accumulation of coal dust in the lungs

_____ **2.** asthma   **B.** can result from disorders such as chronic bronchitis and chronic asthma

_____ **3.** atelectasis   **C.** chronic respiratory infection and disorders of the pancreas and sweat glands

_____ **4.** COPD   **D.** congenital, incomplete expansion of a lung or a portion of a lung

_____ **5.** cystic fibrosis   **E.** destruction of the alveolar walls that leads to hindered gas exchange

_____ **6.** emphysema   **F.** paroxysmal cough, ending in a whooping inspiration

_____ **7.** pertussis   **G.** paroxysmal dyspnea accompanied by wheezing

Labeling

III. Label structures in the diagram with the corresponding combining form. The first one is done as an example. Note that number 2 and number 6 have two answers.

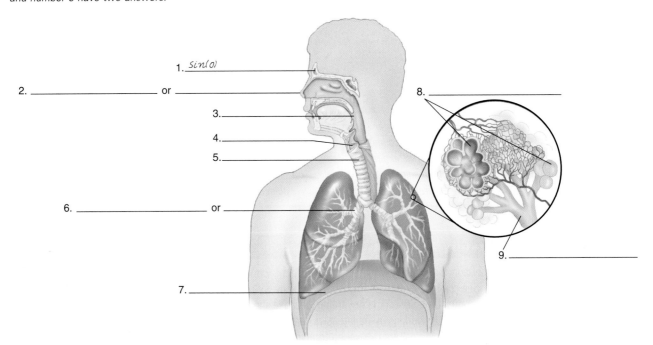

1. _sin(o)_

2. _____ or _____

3. _____

4. _____

5. _____

6. _____ or _____

7. _____

8. _____

9. _____

Sequencing

IV. *Number the following structures to show the sequence of passage of air from the nose to the lungs. The first one is done as an example.*

nasal cavity *1*_____   bronchi _____   larynx _____   pharynx_____

trachea _____   alveoli _____   bronchioles_____

Listing

V. *List five functions of the respiratory system.*

1. _____
2. _____
3. _____
4. _____
5. _____

Matching

VI. *Select A (upper respiratory tract) or B (lower respiratory tract) to identify the locations of these structures.*

_____ **1.** alveolus   _____ **5.** nose   **A.** upper respiratory tract

_____ **2.** bronchiole   _____ **6.** pharynx   **B.** lower respiratory tract

_____ **3.** bronchus   _____ **7.** trachea

_____ **4.** larynx

Identifying Illustrations

VII. *Label these illustrations using one of the following: bronchoscopy, hemothorax, palatoplasty, pneumothorax, thoracentesis, thoracoplasty.*

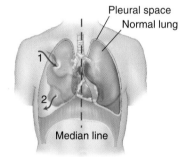

Pleural space
Normal lung
Median line

1. _____

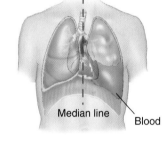

Median line   Blood

2. _____

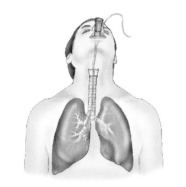

3. _____

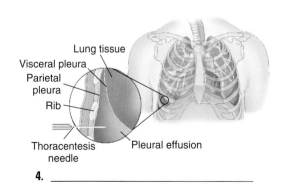

Lung tissue
Visceral pleura
Parietal pleura
Rib
Thoracentesis needle
Pleural effusion

4. _____

VIII. Label these patterns of respiration.

WWWWWWW
Regular at a rate
of 12-20 breaths per minute

1. _____

WWWWW
Slower than 12 breaths
per minute

2. _____

WWWWWWWWWWW
Faster than 20 breaths
per minute

3. _____

WWWWWWWWWWW

Deep breathing, faster than
20 breaths per minute

4. _____

Using Vocabulary

IX. Circle one answer for each of the following multiple choice questions.

1. Mrs. Nguyen's doctor tells her that she has pneumonia. What is another name for her diagnosis? (congestive heart disease, pneumonitis, pulmonary edema, pulmonary insufficiency)

2. Harry, diagnosed with tuberculosis, coughed up and spit out sputum. What is this sign called? (expectoration, expiration, exhalation, extrapleural)

3. John Rodriguez is told that he suffers periodic absence of breathing. What is the name of his condition? (apnea, dyspnea, hyperpnea, hypopnea)

4. Which of the following activities is the respiratory system's greatest contribution to the acid–base balance? (exchange of CO_2 for O_2, maintaining body temperature, regulating water loss, taking in water)

5. Medical students are viewing a chest surgery. What is the term for the serous membrane that lines the walls of the thoracic cavity? (parietal pleura, rhinorrhea, silicosis, visceral pleura)

6. Which term refers to the sudden recurrence or intensity of Sara's asthmatic symptoms? (atelectasis, extracorporeal, hypoventilation, paroxysmal)

7. Mrs. Kamala has difficulty breathing except when sitting in an upright position. What is the term for her condition? (anoxia, hypocapnia, inspiration, orthopnea)

8. What is the term for reduced acidity of the body fluids, such as may occur in hyperventilation? (acid-base balance, acid-base compensation, acidosis, alkalosis)

9. The pulmonologist orders a test to measure the amount of air taken into and expelled from the lungs. What is the name of the test? (laryngoscopy, mediastinoscopy, spirometry, thoracometry)

10. What is effusion of fluid into the air spaces and tissue spaces of the lungs called? (pleuropneumonia, pneumonitis, pulmonary edema, pulmonary insufficiency)

Writing Terms

X.   Write a term for each of the following.

1. an internal blood clot   _____

2. difficult or weak voice   _____

3. direct visualization of the bronchi   _____

4. within the nose   _____

5. inflammation of the throat   _____

6. presence of nasal calculi   _____

7. pertaining to the air sacs of the lung   _____

8. radiographic examination of the larynx   _____

9. profuse nosebleed   _____

10. within the nose   _____

Making Connections

XI.   Describe the relationship of these terms.

1. mild sleep apnea and Cheyne-Stokes respiration _____

_____

2. laryngopharynx and oropharynx _____

_____

Finetuning Terms

XII.   In addition to spelling, describe at least one difference in the following:

1. internal respiration vs. external respiration _____

_____

2. expiration and inspiration _____

_____

3. pneumocentesis and thoracentesis _____

_____

4. glottis and epiglottis _____

_____

5. pneumothorax and hemothorax _____

_____

Opting for Opposites

XIII. Write a term that you learned that means the opposite of these words.

1. bradypnea   _____

2. bronchodilation   _____

3. hypercapnia   _____

4. inhalation   _____

GREATER COMPREHENSION

Health Care Reports

XIV. During her hospitalization, Valesca asked for a copy of her pulmonary report. She has underlined some of the terms and asked you, her attending nurse, to explain them. Write underlined terms or abbreviations from the report that match questions 1-10.

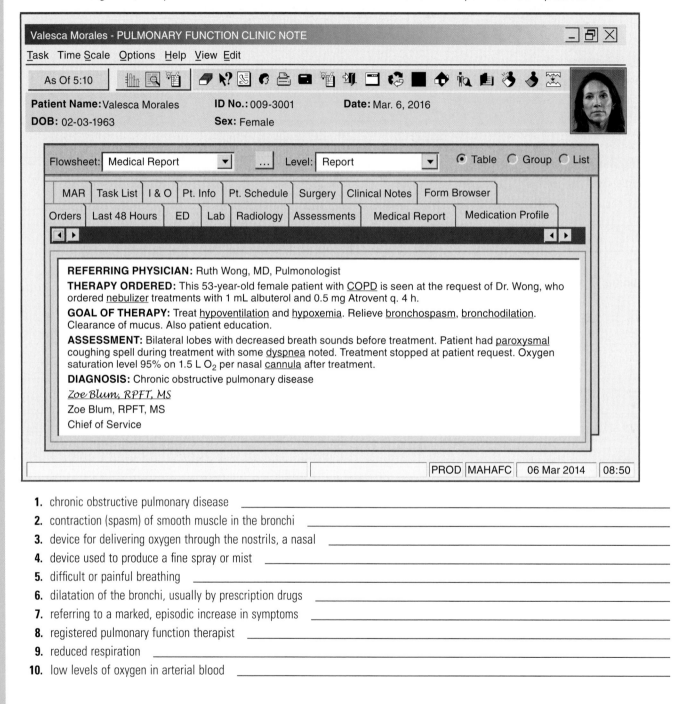

Valesca Morales - PULMONARY FUNCTION CLINIC NOTE

Task Time Scale Options Help View Edit

As Of 5:10

Patient Name: Valesca Morales   **ID No.:** 009-3001   **Date:** Mar. 6, 2016
DOB: 02-03-1963   **Sex:** Female

Flowsheet: Medical Report   Level: Report   ● Table ○ Group ○ List

MAR | Task List | I & O | Pt. Info | Pt. Schedule | Surgery | Clinical Notes | Form Browser

Orders | Last 48 Hours | ED | Lab | Radiology | Assessments | Medical Report | Medication Profile

REFERRING PHYSICIAN: Ruth Wong, MD, Pulmonologist

THERAPY ORDERED: This 53-year-old female patient with COPD is seen at the request of Dr. Wong, who ordered nebulizer treatments with 1 mL albuterol and 0.5 mg Atrovent q. 4 h.

GOAL OF THERAPY: Treat hypoventilation and hypoxemia. Relieve bronchospasm, bronchodilation. Clearance of mucus. Also patient education.

ASSESSMENT: Bilateral lobes with decreased breath sounds before treatment. Patient had paroxysmal coughing spell during treatment with some dyspnea noted. Treatment stopped at patient request. Oxygen saturation level 95% on 1.5 L O_2 per nasal cannula after treatment.

DIAGNOSIS: Chronic obstructive pulmonary disease

Zoe Blum, RPFT, MS
Zoe Blum, RPFT, MS
Chief of Service

PROD | MAHAFC | 06 Mar 2014 | 08:50

1. chronic obstructive pulmonary disease   _____

2. contraction (spasm) of smooth muscle in the bronchi   _____

3. device for delivering oxygen through the nostrils, a nasal   _____

4. device used to produce a fine spray or mist   _____

5. difficult or painful breathing   _____

6. dilatation of the bronchi, usually by prescription drugs   _____

7. referring to a marked, episodic increase in symptoms   _____

8. registered pulmonary function therapist   _____

9. reduced respiration   _____

10. low levels of oxygen in arterial blood   _____

XV. *Read the following History and Physical, and then write the abbreviations or terms that are indicated.*

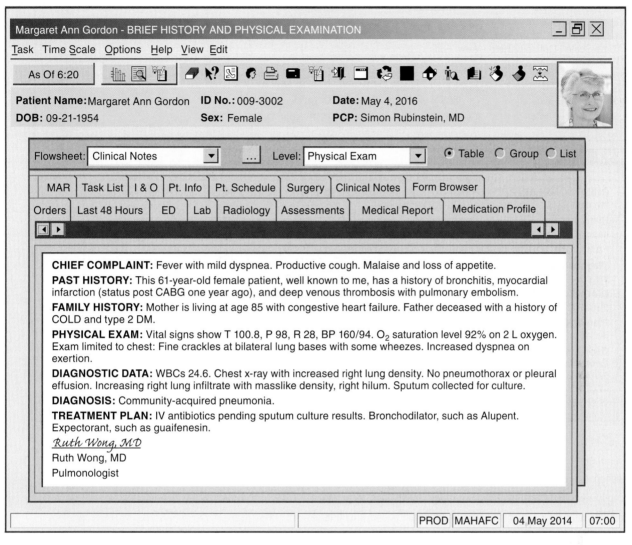

Margaret Ann Gordon - BRIEF HISTORY AND PHYSICAL EXAMINATION

Task Time Scale Options Help View Edit

As Of 6:20

Patient Name: Margaret Ann Gordon   **ID No.:** 009-3002   **Date:** May 4, 2016
DOB: 09-21-1954   **Sex:** Female   **PCP:** Simon Rubinstein, MD

Flowsheet: Clinical Notes   ...   Level: Physical Exam   ● Table ○ Group ○ List

MAR | Task List | I & O | Pt. Info | Pt. Schedule | Surgery | Clinical Notes | Form Browser

Orders | Last 48 Hours | ED | Lab | Radiology | Assessments | Medical Report | Medication Profile

CHIEF COMPLAINT: Fever with mild dyspnea. Productive cough. Malaise and loss of appetite.

PAST HISTORY: This 61-year-old female patient, well known to me, has a history of bronchitis, myocardial infarction (status post CABG one year ago), and deep venous thrombosis with pulmonary embolism.

FAMILY HISTORY: Mother is living at age 85 with congestive heart failure. Father deceased with a history of COLD and type 2 DM.

PHYSICAL EXAM: Vital signs show T 100.8, P 98, R 28, BP 160/94. O_2 saturation level 92% on 2 L oxygen. Exam limited to chest: Fine crackles at bilateral lung bases with some wheezes. Increased dyspnea on exertion.

DIAGNOSTIC DATA: WBCs 24.6. Chest x-ray with increased right lung density. No pneumothorax or pleural effusion. Increasing right lung infiltrate with masslike density, right hilum. Sputum collected for culture.

DIAGNOSIS: Community-acquired pneumonia.

TREATMENT PLAN: IV antibiotics pending sputum culture results. Bronchodilator, such as Alupent. Expectorant, such as guaifenesin.

Ruth Wong, MD
Ruth Wong, MD
Pulmonologist

PROD | MAHAFC | 04 May 2014 | 07:00

Write terms or abbreviations from the report that correspond to each of these descriptions.

1. a vague feeling of discomfort and fatigue _____

2. abnormal accumulation of fluid in the pleural space _____

3. abnormal musical respiratory sounds _____

4. abnormal respiratory sounds that consist of discontinuous bubbling noise _____

5. the presence of air or gas in the pleural space _____

6. inflammation of the bronchi _____

7. chronic obstructive lung disease _____

8. the lodging in a blood vessel of a substance brought by the circulating blood _____

9. therapeutic agent that relaxes the bronchioles _____

10. therapeutic agent that assists in the coughing up of sputum _____

XVI. Read the following note from an Office Visit; then circle the correct answer in the statements that follow the report.

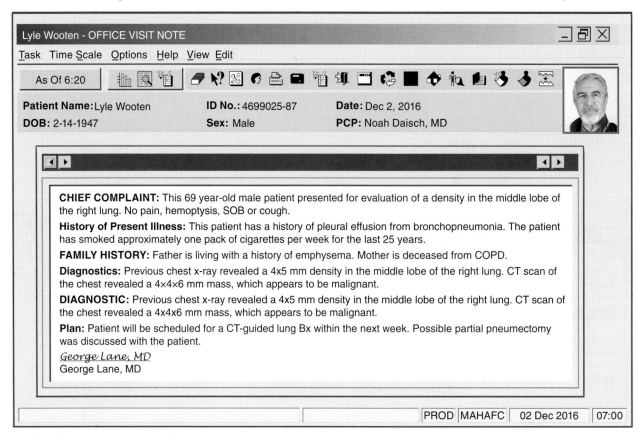

1. The "S" in the abbreviation "SOB" stands for: (shortness, stridor, subphrenic, surgical)
2. The term in the report that refers to blood in the sputum is
(bronchopneumonia, emphysema, hemoptysis, malignant)
3. Effusion refers to an abnormal amount of (air, blood, fluid, infection)
4. A pneumectomy indicates a complete or partial portion of a lung is
(surgically incised, surgically punctured, surgically removed, surgically repaired).
5. A pulmonary disease characterized by destruction of many of the alveolar walls is indicated by (hemoptysis, effusion, bronchopneumonia, emphysema)

Pronouncing Terms

XVII. Write the correct term for the following phonetic spellings.

1. fuh-**rin**-jē-ul _____
2. lar-ing-**gop**-uh-thē _____
3. mē-zō-thē-lē-**ō**-muh _____
4. puh-**rī**-uh-tul _____
5. spī-**rom**-uh-tur _____
6. trā-kē-**os**-tuh-mē _____

Spelling

XVIII. Circle all misspelled terms and write their correct spellings:

acapnia   auscultation   bronchiectasis   laryngografy   pnumonitis

Abbreviating

XIX. Write a letter in each blank that corresponds to the clue.

1. continuous positive airway pressure   — — — —

2. delivering of oxygen via the trachea   — — —

3. infection of the upper respiratory tract   — — —

4. manual artificial respiration   — — —

5. oxygenator which circulates blood through artificial lung   — — — —

6. therapist involved in respiratory treatments & progress   — — — —

Using Pharmacologic Terms

XX. Match descriptions in the right column with terms in the left column.

___ **1.** antihistamines   **A.** break up mucus in the lungs

___ **2.** antitussives   **B.** improve expulsion of mucus from the lungs

___ **3.** bronchodilators   **C.** open the airways to improve respiration

___ **4.** decongestants   **D.** reduce swelling of mucous membranes to treat congestion

___ **5.** expectorants   **E.** suppress coughing

___ **6.** mucolytics   **F.** used to treat or prevent allergic rhinitis or asthma

Categorizing Terms and Practicing Pronunciation

XXI. Categorize the terms by selecting category A, B, C, D, or E.

_____ **1.** anthracosis   **A.** anatomy

_____ **2.** bronchography   **B.** diagnostic test or procedure

_____ **3.** coryza   **C.** pathology

_____ **4.** epiglottis   **D.** surgery

_____ **5.** incentive spirometry   **E.** nonsurgical therapy

_____ **6.** naris

_____ **7.** oximeter

_____ **8.** palatoplasty

_____ **9.** percussion

_____ **10.** rhonchus

Be prepared to pronounce terms 1-10 in class after listening to the Chapter 5 terms at *http://evolve.elsevier.com/Leonard/building*. In addition, practice categorizing all boldface terms in this chapter.

Challenge

XXII. Break these words into their component parts, and write their meanings. Even if you have not seen these terms before, you may be able to break them apart and determine their meanings.

1. bronchospirometry _____

2. laryngostomy _____

3. pharyngoplegia _____

4. pneumomycosis _____

5. sinoscopy _____

(Use Appendix IV to check your answers to the exercises.)

BMV LIST

Visit *http://evolve.elsevier.com/Leonard/building* to listen to the boldface terms in Chapter 5. Look closely at the spelling of each term as it is pronounced.

acapnia (ā-**kap**-nē-uh)
acidemia (as-i-**dē**-mē-uh)
acidosis (as-i-**dō**-sis)
adenoidectomy (ad-uh-noid-**ek**-tuh-mē)
alkalemia (al-kuh-**lē**-mē-uh)
alkalosis (al-kuh-**lō**-sis)
alveolar (al-**vē**-uh-lur)
alveoli (al-**vē**-ō-lī)
anoxia (uh-**nok**-se-uh)
anthracosis (an-thruh-**kō**-sis)
antiasthmatics (an-tē-az-**mat**-iks)
antihistamines (an-tē-**his**-tuh-mēnz)
antitussive (an-tē-**tus**-iv)
aphasia (uh-**fā**-zhuh)
aphonia (ā-**fō**-nē-uh)
apical (**ap**-i-kul)
aplasia (uh-**plā**-zhuh)
apnea (**ap**-nē-uh)
asbestosis (as-bes-**tō**-sis)
asphyxia (as-**fik**-sē-uh)
asphyxiation (as-fik-sē-**ā**-shun)
asthma (**az**-muh)
atelectasis (at-uh-**lek**-tuh-sis)
auditory tube (**aw**-di-tor-ē tŏōb)
bradypnea (brad-ē-**nē**-uh, brad-**ip**-nē-uh)
bronchi (**brong**-kī)
bronchial (**brong**-kē-ul)
bronchiectasis (brong-kē-**ek**-tuh-sis)
bronchiolectasis (brong-kē-ō-**lek**-tuh-sis)
bronchioles (**brong**-kē-ōlz)
bronchiolitis (brong-kē-ō-**lī**-tis)
bronchitis (brong-**kī**-tis)
bronchoalveolar (brong-kō-al-**vē**-uh-lur)
bronchoconstriction (brong-kō-kun-**strik**-shun)
bronchodilators (brong-kō-**dī**-lā-turz, -dī-**lā**-turz)
bronchogenic (brong-kō-**jen**-ik)
bronchogram (**brong**-kō-gram)
bronchography (brong-**kog**-ruh-fē)
broncholithiasis (brong-kō-li-**thī**-uh-sis)
bronchopathy (brong-**kop**-uh-thē)
bronchopneumonia (brong-kō-noo-**mō**-nyuh)
bronchopulmonary (brong-kō-**pool**-muh-nar-ē)
bronchoscope (**brong**-kō-skōp)
bronchoscopic examination (brong-kō-**skop**-ik
  eg-zam-i-**nā**-shun)
bronchoscopy (brong-**kos**-kuh-pē)
bronchospasm (**brong**-kō-spaz-um)
cardiopulmonary resuscitation (kahr-dē-ō-**pool**-muh-nar-ē
  rē-sus-i-**tā**-shun)
Cheyne-Stokes respiration (chān stōks res-pi-**rā**-shun)
congestive heart failure (kun-**jes**-tiv hahrt **fāl**-yur)

coronavirus (kuh-**rō**-nuh-vī-rus)
coryza (kō-**rī**-zuh)
crackles (**krak**-ulz)
croup (krŏōp)
cystic fibrosis (**sis**-tik fī-**brō**-sis)
decongestants (dē-kun-**jes**-tunts)
diaphragm (**dī**-uh-fram)
diaphragma (**dī**-uh-frag-muh)
diaphragmatic (dī-uh-frag-**mat**-ik)
diphtheria (dif-**thēr**-ē-uh)
dysphasia (dis-**fā**-zhuh)
dysphonia (dis-**fō**-nē-uh)
dyspnea (disp-**nē**-uh)
dyspneic (disp-**nē**-ik)
emphysema (em-fuh-**sē**-muh)
empyema (em-pī-**ē**-muh)
endonasal (en-dō-**nā**-zul)
endotracheal (en-dō-**trā**-kē-ul)
endotracheal intubation (en-dō-**trā**-kē-ul in-tŏō-**bā**-shun)
epiglottides (ep-i-**glot**-i-dēs)
epiglottis (ep-i-**glot**-is)
epiglottitis (ep-i-glo-**tī**-tis)
epistaxis (ep-i-**stak**-sis)
eupnea (yŏōp-**nē**-uh)
eustachian tube (ū-**stā**-kē-un tŏōb)
exhalation (eks-huh-**lā**-shun)
expectorants (ek-**spek**-tuh-runts)
expectorate (ek-**spek**-tuh-rāt)
expiration (ek-spi-**rā**-shun)
extracorporeal membrane oxygenator (eks-truh-kor-**por**-ē-ul
  mem-brān **ok**-si-juh-nā-tur)
extrapleural (eks-truh-**ploor**-ul)
extrapulmonary (eks-truh-**pool**-mō-nar-ē)
friction rub (**frik**-shun rub)
glottis (**glot**-is)
Heimlich maneuver (**hīm**-lik muh-**nŏō**-vur)
hemoptysis (hē-**mop**-ti-sis)
hemothorax (hē-mō-**thor**-aks)
herpes simplex virus (**hur**-pēz **sim**-pleks **vī**-rus)
hilum (**hī**-lum)
hydrothorax (hī-drō-**thor**-aks)
hypercapnia (hī-pur-**kap**-nē-uh)
hyperoxemia (hī-pur-ok-**sē**-mē-uh)
hyperpnea (hī-pur-**nē**-uh, hī-purp-**nē**-uh)
hyperventilation (hī-pur-ven-ti-**lā**-shun)
hypocapnia (hī-pō-**kap**-nē-uh)
hypopnea (hī-**pop**-nē-uh)
hypoventilation (hī-pō-ven-ti-**lā**-shun)
hypoxemia (hī-pok-**sē**-mē-uh)
hypoxia (hī-**pok**-sē-uh)
influenza (in-flŏō-**en**-zuh)

inhalation (in-huh-**lā**-shun)
inhaler (in-**hāl**-ur)
inspiration (in-spi-**rā**-shun)
interalveolar (in-tur-al-**vē**-uh-lur)
lacrimal (**lak**-ri-mul)
laryngalgia (lar-in-**gal**-juh)
laryngeal (luh-**rin**-jē-ul)
laryngectomy (lar-in-**jek**-tuh-mē)
laryngitis (lar-in-**jī**-tis)
laryngography (lar-ing-**gog**-ruh-fē)
laryngopathy (lar-ing-**gop**-uh-thē)
laryngopharyngeal (luh-ring-gō-fuh-**rin**-jē-ul)
laryngopharynx (luh-ring-gō-**far**-inks)
laryngoplegia (luh-ring-gō-**plē**-juh)
laryngoscope (luh-**ring**-gō-skōp)
laryngoscopy (lar-ing-**gos**-kuh-pē)
laryngospasm (luh-**ring**-gō-spaz-um)
laryngotracheal (luh-ring-gō-**trā**-kē-ul)
laryngotracheitis (luh-ring-gō-trā-kē-**ī**-tis)
laryngotracheobronchitis (luh-ring-gō-trā-kē-ō-brong-**kī**-tis)
larynx (**lar**-inks)
leukotriene receptor antagonists (lōō-kō-**trī**-ēn rē-**sep**-tur an-**tag**-uh-nists)
mast cell stabilizers (mast sel **stā**-buh-lī-zurz)
mediastinoscope (mē-dē-uh-**stī**-nō-skōp)
mediastinoscopy (mē-dē-as-ti-**nos**-kuh-pē)
mediastinum (mē-dē-uh-**stī**-num)
mesothelioma (mē-zō-thē-lē-**ō**-muh)
mucolytic (mū-kō-**lit**-ik)
nares (**nā**-rēz)
naris (**nā**-ris)
nasal (**nā**-zul)
nasal cannulae (**nā**-zul **kan**-ū-lē)
nasal polyp (**nā**-zul **pol**-ip)
nasal septum (**nā**-zul **sep**-tum)
nasolacrimal (nā-zō-**lak**-ri-mul)
nasolacrimal duct (nā-zō-**lak**-ri-mul dukt)
nasopharyngeal (nā-zō-fuh-**rin**-je-ul)
nasopharyngitis (nā-zō-far-in-**jī**-tis)
nasopharynx (nā-zō-**far**-inks)
nasoscope (**nā**-zō-skōp)
nasotracheal intubation (nā-zō-**trā**-kē-ul in-tōō-**bā**-shun)
nebulizers (**neb**-ū-lī-zurz)
olfaction (ol-**fak**-shun)
olfactory (ol-**fak**-tuh-rē)
oral (**or**-ul)
oropharyngeal (or-ō-fuh-**rin**-jē-ul)
oropharynx (or-ō-**far**-inks)
orotracheal intubation (or-ō-**trā**-kē-ul in-tōō-**bā**-shun)
orthopnea (or-thop-**nē**-uh)
oxygenation (ok-si-juh-**nā**-shun)
palate (**pal**-ut)
palatine (**pal**-uh-tīn)
palatitis (pal-uh-**tī**-tis)
palatoplasty (**pal**-uh-tō-plas-tē)
paranasal sinuses (par-uh-**nā**-zul **sī**-nus-uz)
parietal pleura (puh-**rī**-uh-tul **ploor**-uh)

paroxysmal (par-ok-**siz**-mul)
pertussis (pur-**tus**-is)
pharyngalgia (far-in-**gal**-juh)
pharyngeal (fuh-**rin**-jē-ul)
pharyngitis (far-in-**jī**-tis)
pharyngodynia (fuh-ring-gō-**din**-ē-uh)
pharyngomycosis (fuh-ring-gō-mī-**kō**-sis)
pharyngopathy (far-ing-**gop**-uh-thē)
pharyngoscope (fuh-**ring**-gō-skōp)
pharynx (**far**-inks)
phlegm (flem)
phrenic (**fren**-ik)
phrenitis (fruh-**nī**-tis)
phrenodynia (fren-ō-**din**-ē-uh)
phrenoplegia (fren-ō-**plē**-juh)
phrenoptosis (fren-op-**tō**-sis, fren-ō-**tō**-sis)
pleura (**ploor**-uh)
pleural (**ploor**-ul)
pleural adhesions (**ploor**-ul ad-**hē**-zhunz)
pleural cavity (**ploor**-ul **kav**-i-tē)
pleural effusion (**ploor**-ul uh-**fū**-zhun)
pleurisy (**ploor**-i-sē)
pleuritis (ploo-**rī**-tis)
pleurodynia (ploor-ō-**din**-ē-uh)
pleuropneumonia (ploor-ō-noo-**mō**-nē-uh)
pneumectomy (nōō-**mek**-tuh-mē)
pneumocentesis (nōō-mō-sen-**tē**-sis)
pneumococcal pneumonia (nōō-mō-**kok**-ul nōō-**mōn**-yuh)
pneumoconiosis (nōō-mō-kō-nē-**ō**-sis)
pneumohemothorax (nōō-mō-hē-mō-**thor**-aks)
pneumonectomy (nōō-mō-**nek**-tuh-mē)
pneumonia (nōō-**mōn**-yuh)
pneumonitis (nōō-mo-**nī**-tis)
pneumothorax (nōō-mō-**thor**-aks)
pulmonary (**pool**-mō-nar-ē)
pulmonary abscess (**pool**-mō-nar-ē **ab**-ses)
pulmonary angiography (**pool**-mō-nar-ē an-jē-**og**-ruh-fē)
pulmonary edema (**pool**-mō-nar-ē uh-**dē**-muh)
pulmonary embolus (**pool**-mō-nar-ē **em**-bō-lus)
pulmonary fibrosis (**pool**-mō-nar-ē fī-**brō**-sis)
pulmonary lobectomy (**pool**-mō-nar-ē lō-**bek**-tuh-mē)
pulmonic (pul-**mon**-ik)
pulmonologist (pool-muh-**nol**-uh-jist)
pulse oximeter (puls ok-**sim**-uh-tur)
pulse oximetry (puls ok-**sim**-uh-trē)
pyothorax (pī-ō-**thor**-aks)
rales (rahlz)
respiratory rate (**res**-pur-uh-tor-ē rāt)
respiratory system (**res**-pur-uh-tor-ē **sis**-tum)
retronasal (ret-rō-**nā**-zul)
rhinitis (rī-**nī**-tis)
rhinolith (**rī**-nō-lith)
rhinolithiasis (rī-nō-li-**thī**-uh-sis)
rhinoplasty (**rī**-nō-plas-tē)
rhinorrhagia (rī-nō-**rā**-juh)
rhinorrhea (rī-nō-**rē**-uh)
rhonchus (**rong**-kus)

septoplasty (**sep**-tō-plas-tē)
septorhinoplasty (sep-tō-**rī**-nō-plas-tē)
silicosis (sil-i-**kō**-sis)
sinusitis (sī-nus-**ī**-tis)
smoking cessation drugs (**smōk**-ing suh-**sā**-shun drugz)
spirometer (spī-**rom**-uh-tur)
spirometry (spī-**rom**-uh-trē)
sputum (**spū**-tum)
stridor (**strī**-dur)
subphrenic (sub-**fren**-ik)
subpulmonary (sub-**pool**-mō-nar-ē)
supranasal (soo-pruh-**nā**-zul)
tachycardia (tak-i-**kahr**-dē-uh)
tachypnea (tak-ip-**nē**-uh, tak-ē-**nē**-uh)
thoracentesis (thor-uh-sen-**tē**-sis)
thoracocentesis (thor-uh-kō-sen-**tē**-sis)
thoracoplasty (**thor**-uh-kō-plas-tē)
thoracostomy (thor-uh-**kos**-tuh-mē)
thromboembolic (throm-bō-em-**bol**-ik)
tonsillitis (ton-si-**lī**-tis)
trachea (**trā**-kē-uh)

tracheal (**trā**-kē-ul)
trachealgia (trā-kē-**al**-juh)
tracheitis (trā-kē-**ī**-tus)
tracheomalacia (trā-kē-ō-muh-**lā**-shuh)
tracheoplasty (**trā**-kē-ō-plas-tē)
tracheoscopy (trā-kē-**os**-kuh-pē)
tracheostenosis (trā-kē-ō-stuh-**nō**-sis)
tracheostomy (trā-kē-**os**-tuh-mē)
tracheostomy tube (trā-kē-**os**-tuh-mē toob)
tracheotomy (trā-kē-**ot**-uh-mē)
transtracheal oxygen (trans-**trā**-kē-ul **ok**-si-jun)
tubercles (**too**-bur-kulz)
tuberculosis (too-bur-kū-**lō**-sis)
uvula (**ū**-vū-luh)
uvulectomy (ū-vū-**lek**-tuh-mē)
ventilation (ven-ti-**lā**-shun)
Venturi mask (ven-**too**-rē mask)
visceral (**vis**-ur-ul)
visceral pleura (**vis**-ur-ul **ploor**-uh)
vocal cords (**vō**-kul kordz)
wheeze (hwēz)

Español | ENHANCING SPANISH COMMUNICATION

English	Spanish (Pronunciation)
acidity	acidez (ah-se-DES)
asphyxia	asfixia (as-FEEK-se-ah)
asthma	asma (AHS-mah)
breathe	alentar (ah-len-TAR), respirar (res-pe-RAR)
breathing	respiración (res-pe-rah-se-ON)
cough	tos (tos)
diaphragm	diafragma (de-ah-FRAHG-mah)
erect, straight	derecho (day-RAY-cho)
imperfect	imperfecto (im-per-FEK-to)
influenza	gripe (GREE-pay)
lobe	lóbulo (LO-boo-lo)
lung	pulmón (pool-MON)
nose	nariz (nah-REES)
nostril	orificio de la nariz (or-e-FEE-se-o day lah nah-REES)
obstruction	obstrucción (obs-trook-se-ON)
pertussis	tos ferina (TOS fay-REE-nah)
pneumonia	neumonía (nay-oo-mo-NEE-ah), pulmonía (pool-mo-NEE-ah)
pulmonary	pulmonar (pool-mo-NAR)
pulmonary thrombosis	thrombosis pulmonar (throm-BO-ses pool-mo-NAR)
respiration	respiración (res-pe-rah-se-ON)
sputum	esputo (es-POO-to)
throat	garganta (gar-GAHN-tah)
tonsil	tonsila (ton-SEE-lah), amígdala (ah-MEEG-dah-lah)
trachea	tráquea (TRAH-kay-ah)
voice	voz (vos)
whisper	voz baja (voz BAH-hah)

Digestive System

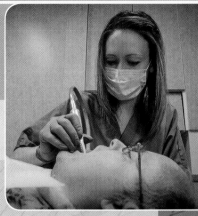

Dental hygienists work under the supervision of dentists and provide dental prophylaxis (protection against dental disease) by cleaning the teeth and inspection of the mouth and gums, radiography, administration of medications, and dental education.

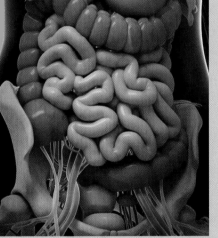

CONTENTS

Basic Understanding

In this chapter, you will learn to do the following:

1. State the four major functions of the digestive system, and analyze associated terms.
2. List the three classes of nutrients and their functions.
3. Write the names of the major structures of the digestive system, define the terms associated with these structures, and label the structures.
4. Write the meanings of the word parts associated with the upper and lower digestive tract, and use them to build and analyze terms.
5. State the function of the accessory organs of digestion, and analyze associated terms.
6. Write the names of the diagnostic tests and procedures for assessment of the digestive system when given their descriptions, and match them with the digestive structures.
7. Match terms for digestive system pathologies with their meanings, or write the names of the pathologies when given their descriptions.
8. Match the pathologies of accessory organs of digestion with their meanings, or write the names of the pathologies when given their descriptions.
9. Match terms for surgical and other therapeutic interventions for digestive tract and accessory organ pathologies with descriptions of the interventions, or write the names of the interventions when given their descriptions.
10. Build terms from word parts to label illustrations.

Greater Comprehension

11. Use word parts from this chapter to determine the meanings or answer questions about the terms in a health care report.
12. Spell the terms accurately.
13. Pronounce the terms correctly.
14. Write the meanings of the abbreviations.
15. Categorize terms as anatomy, diagnostic test or procedure, pathology, surgery, or nonsurgical therapy.
16. Recognize the meanings of general pharmacological terms from this chapter as well as the drug classes and their uses.

FUNCTION FIRST

Four major functions of the digestive system are ingestion of food, digestion of food, absorption of nutrients, and elimination of wastes. Accessory organs of digestion have additional functions, including the production or storage of secretions that aid in the chemical breakdown of food, filtration of the blood and breakdown of toxic compounds, storage of iron and certain vitamins, synthesis of plasma proteins, and regulation of blood glucose levels.

ANATOMY AND PHYSIOLOGY

6-1 The digestive system is known by many names, including the digestive tract, the **alimentary tract**, and the gastrointestinal or GI system. **Gastro/intestin/al** refers to the stomach and the

intestines

_____.

🔑 **KEY** POINT **The digestive tract is a long, muscular tube, lined with mucous membrane, that extends from the mouth to the anus.** The upper GI (UGI) tract consists of the mouth (oral cavity), **pharynx** (called the _throat_ in nonmedical language), esophagus, and stomach. The lower GI tract is made up of the small and large intestines. The accessory organs (salivary glands, liver, gallbladder, and pancreas) secrete fluids that aid in digestion and absorption of nutrients.

WRITE IT! EXERCISE 1

Write four major functions of the digestive system.

1. _____   3. _____

2. _____   4. _____

WRITE IT! EXERCISE 2

List four accessory organs of the digestive system.

1. _____   3. _____

2. _____   4. _____

Digestion and Nutrition

WORD ORIGIN
nutrition _(L.)_
nutriens, food that
nourishes

6-2 Nutrition is the sum of the processes involved in the taking in, digestion, absorption, and use of food substances by the body. The digestive system provides the body with water, nutrients, and minerals and eliminates undigested food particles.

🔑 **KEY** POINT **Nutrition can be divided into four stages.** The stages from beginning to end can be divided into four separate functions: ingestion, digestion, absorption, and elimination.

Stage 1: **ingestion:** Swallowing, orally taking substances into the body
Stage 2: **digestion:** Conversion of food into substances that can be absorbed; actually begins in the mouth!
Stage 3: **absorption:** Digested food molecules pass through the lining of the small intestine into the blood or lymph
Stage 4: **elimination:** Excretion of undigested food particles (wastes) through the anus

6-3 After swallowing, food particles are moved along the digestive tract and mixed with enzymes and digestive fluids. Movements are brought about by the contractions of smooth muscles of the digestive system.

The presence of food in the digestive tube stimulates a coordinated, rhythmic muscular contraction called **peristalsis.** You learned earlier that peri- means _____. The suffix -stalsis means contraction.

around

🔑 **KEY** POINT **Digestion consists of mechanical and chemical processes.** Mechanical digestion begins in the mouth with chewing and continues with churning actions in the stomach. Carbohydrates, proteins, and fats are transformed into smaller molecules through chemical digestion. The accessory organs contribute digestive fluids to aid this process.

absorption

6-4 Numerous folds in the small intestine increase the speed of transfer of nutrient molecules in the third stage of digestion, _____. Assimilation is the process of incorporating nutritive material into living tissue and occurs either after or simultaneously with absorption.

6-5 Wastes are excreted (eliminated) through the anus in the form of **feces.** The anus is the opening of the large intestine to the outside. This last function of the digestive system is called

elimination

_____.

> **BEYOND** THE BLUEPRINT The elimination of undigested food particles is only one type of elimination of body wastes. Other body wastes include carbon dioxide excreted by the lungs and excess water and other substances excreted in the urine and through perspiration.

dietary

6-6 Alimentation is the process of providing nourishment, or nutrition, for the body. Good nutrition is essential for **metabolism,** the sum of all the physical and chemical processes that take place in living organisms and result in growth, generation of energy, elimination of wastes, and other body functions as they relate to the distribution of nutrients in the blood after digestion.

A balanced diet is one that is adequate in energy-providing substances (carbohydrates and fats), tissue-building compounds (proteins), inorganic chemicals (water and mineral salts), vitamins, and certain other substances, such as bulk for promoting movement of the contents of the digestive tract. The dietary reference intakes (DRIs) are the levels of daily intake of essential nutrients that are considered adequate to meet nutritional needs. DRI means _____ reference intake.

Homeostasis, equilibrium of the internal environment of the body, is maintained even though the amounts of various food substances and water that we take in vary.

Learn the meanings of the following word parts that are used in discussing digestion and nutrition.

Word Parts: Digestion and Nutrition

Combining Form	Meaning	Suffix	Meaning
Substances		**Functions**	
amyl(o)	starch	-dipsia	thirst
bil(i), chol(e)	bile or gall	-orexia	appetite
glyc(o)	sugar	-pepsia	digestion
lact(o)	milk	-stalsis	contraction
lip(o)	fats		
prote(o)	protein		

WRITE IT! EXERCISE 3

Write the meanings of these word parts.

1. amyl(o) _____ **6.** prote(o) _____
2. chol(e) _____ **7.** -dipsia _____
3. glyc(o) _____ **8.** -orexia _____
4. lact(o) _____ **9.** -pepsia _____
5. lip(o) _____ **10.** -stalsis _____

sugar

6-7 The three classes of nutrients and their functions are the following:
- carbohydrates (includes starches and sugars), the basic source of cell energy
- proteins (nitrogenous compounds), provide amino acids and building material for development, growth, and maintenance
- fats (lipids), energy reserve

The combining form glyc(o) means sugar. **Glyco/lysis** is the breaking down of _____.

KEY POINT **Glucose, a simple sugar, is the major source of energy for the body's cells.** It is found in certain foods, especially fruits, and it is also formed when more complex sugars and starches are broken down by the digestive system. The concentration of glucose in the blood in healthy individuals is maintained at a fairly constant level.

destruction

6-8 Starches, a second type of carbohydrate, break down easily and are eventually reduced to glucose before being absorbed into the blood. The combining form amyl(o) means starch. The digestive process whereby starch is converted into sugars is called **amylolysis.** The literal translation of amylo/lysis is _____ of starch.

protein

6-9 Proteo/lysis is breaking down (destruction, digestion) of _____. Proteolysis is necessary for digestion because proteins must be chemically broken down before they can be absorbed.

fats

6-10 Fats, also called *lipids,* serve as an energy reserve. When stored in fat cells, they form lipoid tissue that helps to cushion and insulate vital organs. Although **lipids** also include steroids, waxes, and fatty acids, lip(o) usually refers to fats. **Lip/oid** means resembling _____.

   Bile is a digestive chemical that breaks fats into smaller particles, preparing them for further action by lipases and absorption.

6-11 Calories are units that are used to denote the energy value of food or the heat expenditure of an organism. Proteins, carbohydrates, and fats contain calories. Having about twice as many calories per gram as carbohydrates and proteins, fats are well suited for storage of unused calories.

-pepsia

   The normal desire for food is called the *appetite.* The suffix that means digestion is _____. Normal digestion is **eu/pepsia.**

KEY POINT **Digestive enzymes act on food substances, causing them to break down into simpler compounds.** Enzymes are usually named by adding -ase to the combining form of the substance on which they act. For example, **lip/ase** breaks down lipids.

lactase

6-12 The enzyme that breaks down lactose, the main sugar in the milk of mammals, is _____.

   Lactose intolerance is a disorder caused by inadequate production of, or defect in, the enzyme lactase.

   Amylase is an enzyme that breaks down starch. **Proteinase** or **protease** is an enzyme that breaks down protein.

-dipsia

6-13 Thirst is the desire for fluid, especially for water. Not only does water serve to transport food in the digestive tract but it is also the principal medium in which chemical reactions occur. The suffix that means thirst is _____.

MATCH IT! EXERCISE 4

Match the terms in the left column with their descriptions in the right column.

_____ **1.** absorption
_____ **2.** alimentation
_____ **3.** calories
_____ **4.** carbohydrate
_____ **5.** digestion
_____ **6.** elimination
_____ **7.** gastrointestinal
_____ **8.** ingestion
_____ **9.** lipids
_____ **10.** proteolysis

A. breaking down of protein
B. conversion of food into substances that can be absorbed
C. fats
D. how the body takes in nutrients
E. pertaining to the stomach and intestines
F. removal of undigested food particles
G. the basic source of energy for human cells; includes glucose and starches
H. the process in which digested food molecules pass through the small intestine lining into the blood or lymph capillaries
I. the process of providing nourishment or nutrition for the body
J. units that denote the energy value of food

Major Structures of the Digestive System

resembling

lower

6-14 The digestive tract is lined with a mucous membrane, which secretes mucus for lubrication. **Mucosa** is the same as a mucous membrane. The adjective used to describe a membrane that secretes mucus is **mucous**. **Muc/oid** means _____ mucus.

The structures that you are about to label make up the muscular tube portion of the digestive tract, which consists of the upper GI tract and the _____ GI tract.

The salivary glands, liver, gallbladder, and pancreas (the accessory organs) are already labeled. Note their locations in relation to the other structures.

6-15 Label the structures in Fig. 6.1, A, as you read the following information:
- Digestion begins in the mouth *(1)*. The teeth grind and chew the food before it is swallowed. The mass of chewed food is called a **bolus**.
- The pharynx *(2)* passes the bolus to the **esophagus** *(3)*, which leads to the stomach *(4)*, where food is churned and broken down chemically and mechanically.
- The liquid mass, called **chyme**, is passed to the small intestine, where digestion continues and absorption of nutrients occurs. The three parts of the small intestine are shown: duodenum *(5)*, jejunum *(6)*, and ileum *(7)*.
- Undigested food passes to the large intestine *(8)*, where much of the water is absorbed. It is stored in the rectum until it is eliminated through the anus *(9)*.
Study the schematic of the pathway of food through the digestive tract (Fig. 6.1, B).

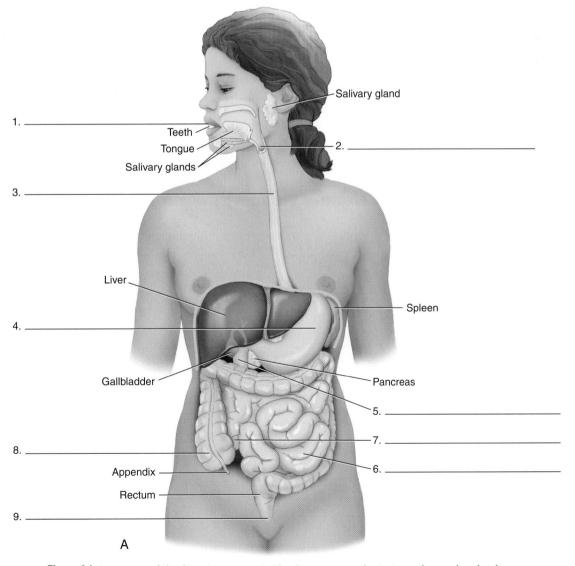

Salivary gland

1. _____

Teeth
Tongue
Salivary glands

2. _____

3. _____

Liver

Spleen

4. _____

Gallbladder

Pancreas

5. _____

7. _____

8. _____

6. _____

Appendix

Rectum

9. _____

A

Figure 6.1 Structures of the digestive system. A, The alimentary tract, beginning at the mouth and ending at the anus, is basically a long, muscular tube. Several accessory organs (salivary glands, liver, gallbladder, and pancreas) are also shown. *Continued*

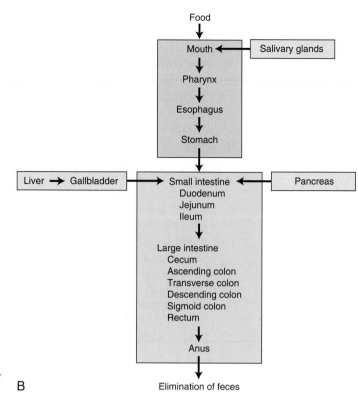

Figure 6.1, cont'd B, Summary of the pathway of food through the upper and lower digestive tract.

B

Learn the meanings of the following word parts.

Word Parts: Major Structures of the Digestive System

Structure	Combining Form	Structure	Combining Form
Upper GI Tract		**Lower GI Tract**	
mouth	or(o), stomat(o)	intestine, in general	intestin(o)
esophagus	esophag(o)	small intestine	enter(o)†
pharynx	pharyng(o)	duodenum	duoden(o)
stomach	gastr(o)	jejunum	jejun(o)
		ileum	ile(o)
Accessory Organs of Digestion		large intestine	col(o), colon(o)‡
gallbladder	cholecyst(o)	rectum	rect(o)
common bile duct	choledoch(o)	anus	an(o)
liver	hepat(o)		
pancreas	pancreat(o)		
salivary glands	sialaden(o)*		

*Sometimes sial(o).
†Enter(o) sometimes means the intestines in general.
‡Col(o) and colon(o) sometimes refer specifically to the colon, the larger portion of the large intestine.

WRITE IT!   EXERCISE 5

Write the meaning of these combining forms.

1. an(o) _____

2. cholecyst(o) _____

3. choledoch(o) _____

4. col(o) _____

5. duoden(o) _____

6. enter(o) _____

7. esophag(o) _____

8. gastr(o) _____

9. hepat(o) _____

10. ile(o) _____

11. jejun(o) _____

12. or(o) _____

13. pancreat(o) _____

14. rect(o) _____

15. sialaden(o) _____

16. stomat(o) _____

Draw a slash between the word parts in the following list. Then find the meanings of the word parts within the definitions. Think! (Draw the slash, and then perform the remainder of the activity as a mental exercise.)

1. **esophageal** pertaining to the esophagus
2. **gastric** pertaining to the stomach
3. **oropharyngeal** pertaining to the mouth and pharynx or pertaining to the oropharynx
4. **pharyngeal** pertaining to the pharynx

intestine

6-16 Both **intestin/al** and **enter/ic** mean pertaining to the _____. Most medical words concerning the intestines are formed using enter(o), but a few terms use enter(o) to specifically mean the small intestine (for example, **enter/itis**).

intestine

6-17 **Enter/al** means within, by way of, or pertaining to the small intestine. Although enter(o) is used to write terms about the small intestine, you need to remember that enter(o) means either the small intestine or the _____ in general. Enteral tube feeding introduces food directly into the gastrointestinal tract.

colonic

6-18 The combining form col(o) means the large intestine. This combining form can also mean the **colon,** the structure that comprises most of the large intestine and where much of the water is absorbed as the wastes are moved along to the rectum. An adjective that means pertaining to the colon uses colon(o). Join colon(o) and -ic to write this term: _____.
  Colic means pertaining to the large intestine, but it also means spasm in any hollow or tubular soft organ accompanied by pain. You may be most familiar with infantile colic, which is colic occurring during the first few months of life.

6-19 The **rectum** is the lower part of the large intestine. The **anus** is the outlet of the rectum, and it lies in the fold between the buttocks. The anal canal is about 4 cm long. Solid wastes are eliminated via the anus. **Rectal** and **anal** mean pertaining to the rectum and anus, respectively.

Use the following word parts to build terms. (Some word parts will be used more than once.)

colon(o), enter(o), gastr(o), muc(o), or(o), pharyng(o), -eal, -ic, -itis, -oid

1. inflammation of the small intestines _____/_____
2. pertaining to the stomach _____/_____
3. pertaining to the mouth and throat _____/_____/_____
4. pertaining to the large intestines _____/_____
5. resembling mucus _____/_____

Upper Digestive Tract

stomach

6-20 The **oral cavity** is the beginning of the digestive tract and, along with the esophagus and _____, comprises the upper digestive tract.
  Learn the following word parts that pertain to structures of the upper digestive tract.

Word Parts: Additional Structures of the Upper Digestive Tract

Combining Form	Meaning	Combining Form	Meaning
Structures of the Mouth		palat(o)	palate
bucc(o)	cheek	sial(o)	saliva, salivary glands
cheil(o)	lip	sialaden(o)	salivary gland
dent(i), dent(o), odont(o)	teeth	uvul(o)	uvula
gingiv(o)	gums	**Other Structures**	
gloss(o), lingu(o)	tongue	pylor(o)	pylorus
mandibul(o)	mandible	vag(o)	vagus nerve
maxill(o)	maxilla		

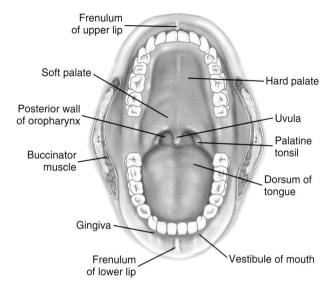

Frenulum
of upper lip

Soft palate

Hard palate

Posterior wall
of oropharynx

Uvula

Palatine
tonsil

Buccinator
muscle

Dorsum of
tongue

Gingiva

Vestibule of mouth

Frenulum
of lower lip

Figure 6.2 Mouth structures. The mouth is bounded anteriorly by the lips and contains the tongue and teeth. The roof of the mouth is the hard palate. Other aspects of the mouth include the gums, the uvula (the fleshy appendage in the back of the throat), the oropharynx, and the buccinator muscle (the main muscle of the cheek that is involved in chewing).

WRITE IT!   EXERCISE 8

Write the meaning of the following combining forms.

1. bucc(o)   _____
2. cheil(o)   _____
3. gastr(o)   _____
4. gingiv(o)   _____
5. odont(o)   _____
6. sialaden(o)   _____
7. stomat(o)   _____
8. vag(o)   _____

---

palate

6-21 The **mandible** is the lower jaw bone, and the **maxilla** is the upper jaw bone. The mouth contains many structures that hold the food in place and facilitate chewing (Fig. 6.2). The roof of the mouth is formed by the bony arch of the hard palate and the fibrous soft palate. **Palat/ine** pertains to the

_____.

The combining form bucc(o) means cheek, and the **bucc/al cavity** pertains to the area between the teeth and the cheeks.

under

6-22 The tongue muscle, covered with mucous membrane, is the principal organ of taste (see Chapter 11) and assists in chewing and swallowing food. Both gloss(o) and lingu(o) mean the tongue; therefore, **gloss/al** and **lingu/al** mean pertaining to the tongue. Most words involving the tongue use the combining form gloss(o). However, both **hypo/glossal** and **sub/lingual** mean _____ the tongue. Some medications are designed to be placed under the tongue, where they dissolve.

teeth

6-23 The mucous membrane that provides support for the teeth is the gum. Another name for the gum is **gingiva**. A **dent/ure** refers to a set of teeth, either natural or artificial, but is ordinarily used to designate artificial ones.
   Dent/al pertains to the _____.

mandibular

6-24 There are 32 permanent teeth in a full set. The mouth has an upper and a lower dental arch, the curving shape formed by the arrangement of a normal set of teeth in the jaw.
   A complete set has 16 teeth in each dental arch. Study the dental arch in Fig. 6.3. Note that the illustration shows the teeth of the lower jaw, or _____ arch. The eight teeth on each side of the dental arch make up a quadrant. Label the teeth in a quadrant as you read the information that follows.
   There are two **incisors** *(1),* one **cuspid** *(2)* or canine, two **bicuspids** *(3)* or premolars, and three **molars** *(4)* in each quadrant. Anterior teeth generally fall out and are replaced sooner than posterior ones. The last molar, which is posterior to all other teeth, is known as the *wisdom tooth.*

➤ **BEYOND** THE BLUEPRINT The primary or deciduous teeth, often called "baby teeth," begin to fall out and to be replaced with permanent teeth when a child is about 6 years of age. The wisdom teeth are the last to erupt, usually between 17 and 25 years of age.

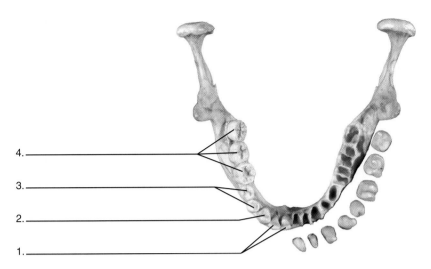

4.
3.
2.
1.

Figure 6.3 Designations of permanent teeth. Teeth of the lower jaw (mandibular arch). Half of the teeth are removed to demonstrate the sockets.

6-25 All teeth consist of two basic parts: the crown (portion of the tooth that normally projects above the gums) and the root or roots (embedded in the bony socket).

The crown is covered by enamel, the hardest substance in the body. The soft tissue inside the tooth is the dental pulp, also called the **endodontium.**

The tissue investing and supporting the teeth is **periodontium.** You learned that peri- means around, so peri/odont/ium is the tissue _____ the teeth. **Peri/odont/al** means around a tooth, or pertaining to the periodontium.

around

6-26 Dentistry is the art and science of diagnosing, preventing, and treating diseases and disorders of the _____ and surrounding structures of the oral cavity. There are several specialties within dentistry; each requires additional training after graduation from a school of dentistry.

teeth

Specialties in dentistry include the following:
- **endodontics:** Diagnosis and treatment of diseases of the dental pulp, tooth root, and surrounding tissues and the associated practice of root canal therapy; specialist is an **endodontist.**
- **orthodontics:** Diagnosis and treatment of irregularities of the teeth, including straightening. An **orthodontist** often uses braces to straighten the teeth (one "o" is dropped when orth[o] is combined with odont[o]).
- **periodontics:** Study and treatment of the periodontium by a **periodontist.**
- **gerodontics:** Dental diagnosis, prevention, and treatment of older persons; the specialist is a **gerondontist.**
- **pedodontics:** Study and treatment of children's dental needs; the specialist is a **pedodontist.**

FIND IT!
EXERCISE 9

Draw a slash between the word parts in the following list. Then find the meanings of the word parts within the definitions. (Draw the slash, and then perform the remainder of the activity as a mental exercise.)

1. **dentilingual** pertaining to the teeth and the tongue
2. **gingival** pertaining to the gums
3. **glossopharyngeal** pertaining to the tongue and pharynx
4. **interdental** pertaining to between the teeth
5. **maxillary** pertaining to the maxilla (upper jaw)

BUILD IT!
EXERCISE 10

Use the following word parts to build terms. (Some word parts will be used more than once.)

inter-, peri-, dent(o), lingu(o), mandibul(o), odont(o), palat(o), -al, -ar, -ine, -ist

1. pertaining to the tongue   _____/_____
2. pertaining to the lower jaw   _____/_____
3. practitioner who specializes in the gums and other tissues that support the teeth
                                                _____/_____/_____
4. pertaining to the roof of the mouth   _____/_____
5. pertaining to between the teeth   _____/_____/_____

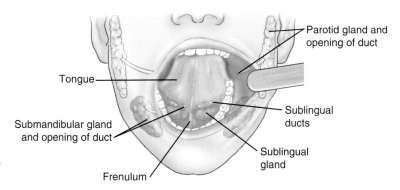

Figure 6.4 Salivary glands. Three pairs of salivary glands (parotid, sublingual, and submandibular glands) consist of numerous lobes connected by vessels and ducts.

starch

6-27 Salivary glands, which are accessory organs of digestion, secrete saliva into the oral cavity. The mouth tastes what we consume and performs other functions of digestion by mixing the food with saliva, chewing, and voluntarily swallowing it. In addition, saliva contains amylase, which begins digestion of _____ in the mouth.
     The salivary glands are three paired glands (Fig. 6.4).

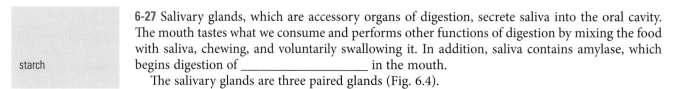

KEY POINT **The names of the salivary glands indicate their location.** The **par/otid glands,** the largest salivary glands, are near the ears. The suffix -id means either having the shape of or a structure. The **sub/lingual glands** are located under the tongue. The **sub/mandibular glands** are located in the tissue of the lower jaw, rather than beneath it as the name implies.

6-28 Food that is swallowed passes from the mouth to the pharynx and the esophagus. Both the pharynx and the esophagus are muscular structures that move food along on its way to the stomach.

KEY POINT **The esophagus is a muscular canal extending from the pharynx to the stomach.** The esophagus, about 24 cm (about 9½ inches) long, secretes mucus to facilitate the movement of food into the stomach. Upper and lower esophag/eal sphincters control the movement of food into and out of the esophagus. The **sphincter** *(/G.] that which binds tight)* consists of circular muscle that constricts a passage or closes a natural opening in the body.

behind

Post/esophag/eal means situated _____ the esophagus.

6-29 Examine Fig. 6.5, A, to learn more about the structure of the stomach. Regions of the stomach are the **cardiac region,** the **fundus,** the body, and the **pyloric region,** or **pylorus.**

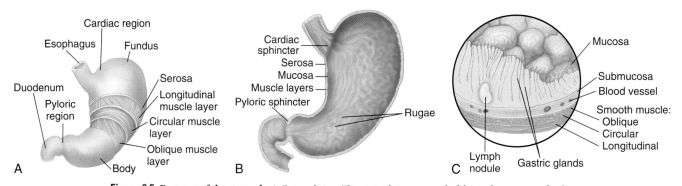

Figure 6.5 Features of the stomach. A, External view: The stomach is composed of the cardiac region, a fundus or round part, a body or middle portion, and a pyloric portion, which is the small distal end. The stomach has a serous coat (serosa) and three muscular layers. **B,** Internal view: The cardiac sphincter guards the opening of the esophagus into the stomach and prevents backflow of material into the esophagus. The stomach ends with the pyloric sphincter, which regulates outflow. The lining of the stomach, the mucosa, is arranged in temporary folds called *rugae* (visible in the empty stomach), which allow expansion as the stomach fills. **C,** Structure of the stomach wall: Longitudinal, circular, and oblique smooth muscle lie just beneath the serosa. All stomach layers are richly supplied with blood vessels and nerves. Gastric glands secrete gastric juice through gastric pits, tiny holes in the mucosa.

The stomach ends with the pyloric sphincter, which regulates the outflow of stomach contents into the **duodenum,** the first part of the small intestine. Look at Fig. 6.5, B. The mucosa that lines the stomach is arranged in temporary folds called **rugae.** Ruga (singular of rugae) means ridge, wrinkle, or fold. The rugae, most apparent when the stomach is empty, allow the stomach to expand as it fills. Three muscle layers are present in the stomach, rather than two, which are found in other structures of the digestive tract (see Fig. 6.5, C).

serosa

The outer layer of the stomach is the _____. This type of visceral peritoneum holds the stomach in position by folding back on and over the structure.

endogastric

6-30 Place a prefix before gastric to write a word that means pertaining to the inside (interior) of the stomach: _____.

The stomach is a temporary reservoir for food and is the first major site of digestion. After digestion, the stomach gradually feeds liquefied food (chyme) into the small intestine.

WRITE IT!
EXERCISE 11

Write a term for each meaning.
1. lower jaw _____
2. upper jaw _____
3. roof of the mouth _____
4. gums _____
5. beneath the tongue _____
6. dental pulp _____

Lower Digestive Tract

6-31 The intestines make up the lower digestive tract. The intestines are sometimes called the *bowels.* Extending from the pyloric opening to the anus, the intestinal tract is about 7.5 to 8.5 meters (about 24½ to 28 feet) long.

🔑 **KEY** POINT **The intestines include the small intestine and the large intestine.** The adult small intestine, comprising more than three fourths of the length of the intestines, is 6 to 7 meters (about 20 to 23 feet) long. The large intestine is so named because it is larger in diameter than the small intestine, but it is less than one fourth as long.

small

Which is longer, the small intestine or the large intestine? _____ intestine. The small intestine finishes the process of digestion, absorbs the nutrients, and passes the residue on to the large intestine. In other words, the small intestine is responsible for two successive processes, digestion and absorption, before passing the residue to the large intestine.

6-32 The small intestine consists of three parts: the duodenum, the jejunum, and the ileum. The structure of the small intestine is shown in Fig. 6.6. Read the information that accompanies the drawing, and label the three parts of the small intestine.

The duodenum is about 25 cm, less than a foot long. The part of the small intestine below the duodenum is the **jejunum.** It is about 2.4 meters (about 8 feet) long and joins the ileum, which is the twisted end of the small intestine.

ileum

The **ileum** is the distal portion of the small intestine. Both **ile/ac** and **ile/al** mean pertaining to the _____. **Duodenal** and **jejunal** mean pertaining to the duodenum and jejunum, respectively.

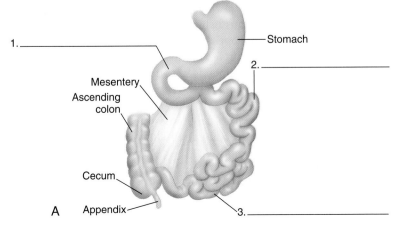

Stomach

1. _____
2. _____

Mesentery
Ascending colon
Cecum
Appendix
3. _____

A

Figure 6.6 Characteristics of the small intestine. A, Label the three parts of the small intestine (1 to 3) as you read. The first portion, the duodenum *(1),* begins at the pyloric sphincter and is the shorter section. The second portion is the jejunum *(2),* which is continuous with the third portion, the ileum *(3).* The ileum is the longest of the three parts of the small intestine. Note that the small intestine decreases in diameter from its beginning at the duodenum to its ending, at the ileum.

Continued

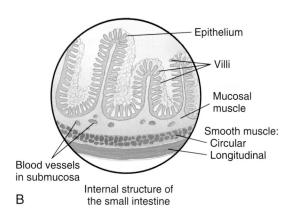

Epithelium

Villi

Mucosal muscle

Smooth muscle:
Circular
Longitudinal

Blood vessels in submucosa

B

Internal structure of the small intestine

Figure 6.6, cont'd B, The internal structure of the small intestine is similar throughout its length. The wall has an inner lining of mucosa, two layers of muscle, and an outer layer of serosa. The mesentery, the fan-shaped fold of peritoneum, suspends the jejunum and the ileum from the dorsal wall of the abdomen.

villi

WORD ORIGIN
villus *(L.)*
villi (pl.); tuft of hair

large

6-33 Study the layers of the wall of the small intestine to write answers in these blanks. The innermost membrane is called the *mucosa.* Both the mucosa and submucosa have many folds and fingerlike projections called _____. Both of these features increase the surface area of the mucosa. In addition, the **villi** function to absorb nutrients.

There are two layers of muscle and an outer membrane called the **serosa.**

6-34 The large intestine is only about 1.5 meters (about 5 feet) long. The combining forms col(o) and colon(o) mean the colon or the _____ intestine. The colon is only that portion of the large intestine extending from the cecum to the rectum, but colon is sometimes used to mean the large intestine in general.

The large intestine is anatomically divided into the cecum, colon, rectum, and anal canal. Learn the combining forms for the following structures.

Word Parts: Large Intestine

Combining Form	Meaning	Combining Form	Meaning
Structures		proct(o)	anus, rectum
append(o), appendic(o)	appendix	sigmoid(o)	sigmoid colon
cec(o)	cecum	**Pathology**	
col(o), colon(o)	large intestine or colon	diverticul(o)	diverticula

WRITE IT! **EXERCISE 12**

Write a combining form for these structures.

1. anus or rectum _____
2. cecum _____
3. diverticulum _____
4. sigmoid colon _____

cecum

6-35 Study the location of the parts of the large intestine in Fig. 6.7.

The **cecum** forms the first portion of the large intestine and is located just distal to the ileum. The combining form cec(o) means cecum. The **ileo/cecal valve** is located between the ileum and the _____. **Retro/cecal** means behind the cecum.

The **vermiform appendix** is a wormlike structure that opens into the cecum. An appendix simply means an appendage, but its most common usage is in referring to the vermiform appendix just described. **Appendicular** means either pertaining to an appendage or pertaining to the vermiform _____.

appendix

sigmoid

6-36 The colon makes up most of the 1.5 meters (5 feet) of large intestine. Different parts of the colon are designated as the ascending, transverse, descending, and **sigmoid colon.** The last part of the colon is the _____ colon.

Retro/col/ic means behind the colon. **Pericolic** means pertaining to the tissue around the colon. In this term, "the tissue around the structure" is implied.

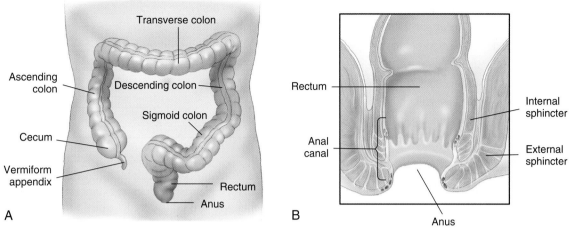

Figure 6.7 Features of the large intestine: the cecum, appendix, colon, and rectum. A, The colon is anatomically divided into four parts. The first part rises upward and is called the *ascending colon*. The transverse colon is the part that crosses the abdomen. The colon then descends on the left side of the abdomen and thus is called the *descending colon*. The last part is S-shaped and is called the *sigmoid colon*. **B,** The internal structure of a portion of the rectum and the anus are shown on the right.

rectum

6-37 The lower part of the large intestine is the rectum, which terminates in a narrow anal canal. This canal in turn opens to the exterior at the anus. **Feces** are body waste that is discharged from the bowels by way of the anus where feces are discharged. Feces are also called *stool* or *fecal material*. **Defecation** is the elimination of feces from the rectum.

    Colo/rectal means pertaining to or affecting the colon and the _____.

rect(o)

6-38 The combining form proct(o) refers to the anus or rectum. You have now learned two combining forms for rectum: proct(o) and _____. A **procto/logist** specializes in treating disorders of the colon, rectum, and anus.

anus

    Most medical terms that refer to the anus use proct(o), but you need to remember that an(o) also means anus. An/al refers to the _____, as in the phrases *anal opening* and *anal canal*.

intestines

6-39 The combining form enter(o) means intestines, sometimes referring to the small intestine only, but the term **gastro/entero/logy** is the study of the stomach and _____ and associated diseases.

6-40 Structural features of both the small intestine and large intestine are well suited for their roles in the digestive system.

🔑 **KEY POINT The large intestine has several important functions:**
- While moving wastes along its length, the large intestine absorbs water, sodium, and chloride. The large intestine is capable of absorbing 90% of the water and sodium it receives.
- The large intestine secretes mucus, which binds fecal particles into a formed mass and lubricates the mucosa.
- Bacteria in the large intestine are responsible for the production of several vitamins.
- Feces are formed and expelled from the body.

MATCH IT! EXERCISE 13

Match the structures in the left columns with either (A) small intestine, or (B) large intestine.

___ **1.** anal canal   ___ **5.** ileum   **A.** small intestine
___ **2.** cecum   ___ **6.** jejunum   **B.** large intestine
___ **3.** colon   ___ **7.** rectum
___ **4.** duodenum

Use the following word parts to build terms. (Some word parts will be used more than once.)

peri-, retro-, cec(o), col(o), duoden(o), ile(o), proct(o), -al, -ic, -logist

1. pertaining to the first part of the small intestine   _____/_____

2. specialist in treating disorders of the colon, rectum, and anus   _____/_____

3. pertaining to behind the first portion of the large intestine   _____/_____/_____

4. pertaining to the third part of the small intestine   _____/_____

5. pertaining to the tissue around the colon   _____/_____/_____

Accessory Organs of Digestion

accessory

6-41 The liver, gallbladder, pancreas, and salivary glands produce substances that are needed for proper digestion and absorption of nutrients and are considered to be _____ organs of the digestive system.

🔑 **KEY** POINT **Accessory organs of digestion are digestive glands.** These organs lie outside the digestive tract, yet they produce or store secretions that are conveyed to the digestive tract by ducts. The secretions aid in the breakdown of food.

The liver, gallbladder, and pancreas are located near the other digestive structures within the abdominal cavity. See these structures in Fig. 6.8. The liver is the largest gland of the body and is essential for the maintenance of life.

6-42 Production of bile is a major function of the liver. The bile is then transported to the gallbladder for storage.

🔑 **KEY** POINT **The liver has several important functions.** In addition to production of bile, liver functions include the following:
- Breakdown of toxic compounds
- Involvement in the regulation of blood glucose
- Lipid metabolism
- Synthesis of plasma proteins
- Storage of iron and certain vitamins
- Filtering of the blood
- Excretion of bile pigments from the breakdown of hemoglobin
- Excretion of hormones and cholesterol

bile

A major function of the liver is the production of _____, which is transported to the gallbladder for storage. Bile aids in the digestion of fats.

bile

6-43 The combining forms chol(e) and bil(i) refer to bile or gall. **Biliary** means pertaining to _____, but chol(e) is used more often to write terms. The organs and ducts that participate in the secretion, storage, and delivery of bile make up the biliary tract. Bile leaves the liver by the hepatic duct and is taken to the gallbladder for storage until it is needed. The combining form cholecyst(o) often forms part of a term that refers to the gallbladder.

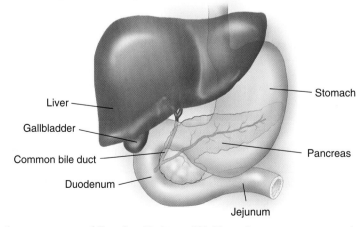

Liver
Gallbladder
Common bile duct
Duodenum
Jejunum
Stomach
Pancreas

Figure 6.8 Accessory organs of digestion. The liver, gallbladder, and pancreas are accessory digestive organs. The liver and pancreas have additional functions as well. More than 500 functions of the liver have been identified. The formation and excretion of bile for digestion of fats is one of its most commonly known activities. Bile is stored in the gallbladder and released when fats are ingested. The pancreas secretes many substances, including digestive enzymes and insulin.

6-44 The pancreas has both digestive and hormonal functions. This elongated gland stretches transversely across the posterior abdominal wall (See Fig. 6.8).

🔑 **KEY** POINT **Pancreatic juice plays an important role in the digestion of all classes of food.** Pancreatic juice contains lipase, amylase, and several other enzymes that are essential to normal digestion. The pancreas also produces hormones (including insulin) that play a primary role in the regulation of carbohydrate metabolism.

blood

6-45 Clusters of cells in the pancreas, the islets of Langerhans, produce glucagon and insulin. **Glucagon** increases blood glucose levels, and **insulin** lowers blood glucose levels. The two hormones, glucagon and insulin, work together to regulate blood glucose. Secretion of glucagon is stimulated by hypoglycemia. **Hypo/glycemia** is a decreased level of glucose in the _____. Small amounts of insulin are secreted continuously in the fasting state, but secretion rises in response to an increase in blood glucose levels.

Hyper/glyc/emia (see Fig. 12.10) is a greater than normal amount of sugar in the blood. This condition is most often associated with **diabetes mellitus** (DM), primarily a result of insufficient production or improper use of insulin.

Want more information? Go to *www.diabetes.org*.

FIND IT! **EXERCISE 15**

Draw a slash between the word parts in the following list. Then find the meanings of the word parts within the definitions. (Draw the slash, and then perform the remainder of the activity as a mental exercise.)

1. **cholecystic** pertaining to the gallbladder
2. **cholecystogastric** pertaining to the gallbladder and the stomach
3. **choledochal** pertaining to the common bile duct
4. **extrahepatic** situated or occurring outside the liver
5. **hepatic** pertaining to the liver
6. **hepatotoxic** destructive to the liver; sometimes called **hepatolytic**
7. **pancreatic** pertaining to the pancreas
8. **suprahepatic** situated above the liver

BUILD IT! **EXERCISE 16**

Use the following word parts to build terms. (Some word parts will be used more than once.)

extra-, hyper-, hypo-, cholecyst(o), gastr(o), glyc(o), hepat(o), -emia, -ic, -lytic

1. pertaining to the gallbladder and the stomach _____/_____/_____
2. destructive to the liver _____/_____
3. decreased level of blood sugar _____/_____/_____
4. increased level of blood sugar _____/_____/_____
5. situated outside the liver _____/_____

DIAGNOSTIC TESTS AND PROCEDURES

auscultation

6-46 Physical assessment of the GI system often begins with an examination of the patient's mouth, pharynx, and abdomen. A systematic assessment of the internal abdominal organs can be made using auscultation, percussion, and palpation (see Fig. 2.29). Which of these procedures is usually performed using a stethoscope? _____

6-47 Assessment of the intestinal tract has been greatly facilitated by radiology and endoscopy (direct visualization of internal organs using an endoscope), revealing abnormalities, such as masses, tumors, and obstructions. An abdominal x-ray is usually one of the first radiographic studies performed.

Computed tomography, sonography, and endoscopic procedures are often used to detect gallstones. Each of the instruments used in endoscopy is specially designed for the examination of particular organs. The instruments used in endoscopy are called _____.

endoscopes

Other instruments can be inserted through the endoscope to remove small pieces of tissue, to collect samples of tissue for study, to inject agents, or to perform laser surgery.

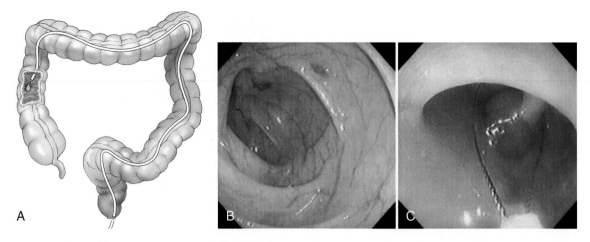

Figure 6.9 Colonoscopy. A, Endoscopic examination of the colon using a flexible colonoscope. **B,** View of a normal colon through the colonoscope. **C,** Colonic polyps often can be removed with the use of a snare (wire noose) that fits through the colonoscope.

Read about various endoscopic examinations of the digestive tract.

colonoscopy Visual examination of the mucosal lining of the colon; same as **coloscopy,** but colonoscopy is more common. Instrument used is a **colonoscope;** tissue biopsy specimens or polyps can often be removed (Fig. 6.9).

duodenoscopy Endoscopic examination of the duodenum using a **duodenoscope.**

esophagogastroscopy Endoscopic examination of the esophagus and the stomach using a **gastroscope.**

esophagogastroduodenoscopy (EGD) Endoscopic examination of the esophagus, stomach, and duodenum (Fig. 6.10). If the esophagus is the focus of the examination, the procedure is called **esophagoscopy;** if the stomach is the focus, the procedure is a **gastroscopy.**

proctosigmoidoscopy Endoscopic examination of the rectum and sigmoid colon using a **sigmoidoscope;** also called **sigmoidoscopy.**

pyloroscopy Endoscopic examination of the pyloric region of the stomach.

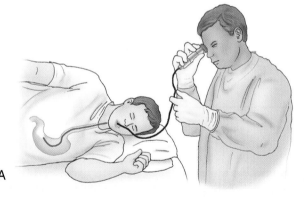
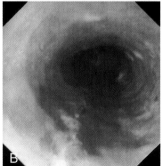

Figure 6.10 Esophagogastroduodenoscopy. A, This endoscopic procedure permits visualization of the upper GI tract. **B,** Endoscopic view of the gastroesophageal junction shows a mucosal tear at about six o'clock. The patient was admitted to the hospital with hematemesis after an alcoholic binge.

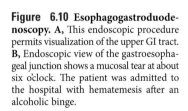

liver

fluoroscope

6-48 Sonography is less invasive than endoscopy and can be used to image soft tissues, such as the liver, the spleen, and the pancreas.

Nuclear imaging can be used to evaluate the size of organs and vessels as well as to detect the presence of tumors or abscesses. One of the more common tests of this type is a liver scan, which involves intravenous injection of a radioactive compound that is readily absorbed by certain cells of the liver. The radiation emitted by the compound provides information about the size, shape, and consistency of the _____.

Fluoroscopy permits both structural and functional visualization of internal body structures and is used to provide visualization of the digestive tract. With the use of contrast media, the motion of a body part can be viewed, and the image can be permanently recorded. The equipment used in fluoro/scopy is a specialized type of x-ray machine called a _____.

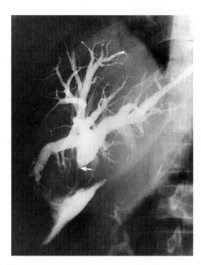

Figure 6.11 Percutaneous transhepatic cholangiography. This radiographic procedure allowed radiographic examination of the bile duct via a needle passed through the skin and showed stenosis *(arrow)* of the common bile duct.

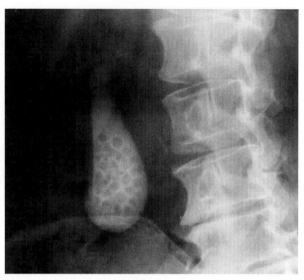

Figure 6.12 Oral cholecystogram. Numerous gallstones are evident on this cholecystogram. In oral cholecystography, radiography of the gallbladder is obtained 12 to 15 hours after ingestion of contrast medium. Because nausea, vomiting, and diarrhea are fairly common with this means of diagnosing biliary disease, it has been largely replaced by ultrasound.

cholangiography

6-49 Cholangio/graphy is radiography of the major bile ducts and is useful in demonstrating gallstones and tumors. Percutaneous transhepatic cholangiography produces images of the bile duct by injecting a contrast medium directly into a hepatic duct via the skin (Fig. 6.11). One type of cholangiography is performed during surgery to detect residual calculi in the biliary tract, after the gallbladder has been removed. This radiographic procedure is called operative _____, and the contrast material is injected into the common bile duct.

operative

6-50 Operative cholangiography is performed by injecting a contrast medium into the common bile duct through a catheter called a *T-tube*. This allows residual stones in the bile ducts to be seen. This type of angiography is called _____ cholangiography. It is not unusual for the incision to be closed with the T-tube left temporarily in the common bile duct and extending through the skin. The T-tube allows for drainage and postoperative study.

Additional radiographic procedures include the following:

cholecystography Radiographic examination of the gallbladder accomplished by rendering the gallbladder and ducts opaque with a contrast medium. In an oral **cholecystogram,** the patient is given a contrast agent in tablet form. Examine the appearance of several gallstones in Fig. 6.12. Oral cholecystograms were the principal method for determining the presence of gallstones until the advent of ultrasound.

esophagram X-ray image of the esophagus taken after swallowing a liquid barium suspension; called also an **esophagogram** or a barium swallow.

pancreatography Visualization of the pancreas by various means, including CT and sonography.

sialography Radiographic examination of the salivary glands after injection of a radiopaque contrast medium.

upper and lower gastrointestinal series Examination of the upper GI tract (esophagus, stomach, and duodenum) and lower GI tract using barium as the contrast medium. A barium meal is ingested in a UGI series, also called *barium swallow*. A barium enema is administered in a **lower gastrointestinal series.**

liver

6-51 Several blood tests provide information about functions of the liver, and these are aptly named liver function tests (LFTs). Examples include serum bilirubin, alkaline phosphatase, aspartate aminotransferase (AST or SGOT), and alanine aminotransferase (ALT or SGPT). Increases in these laboratory values often indicate liver disease. LFT is an abbreviation for _____ function test.

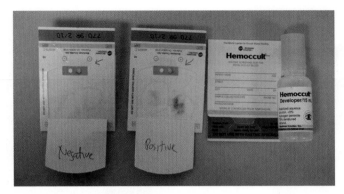

Figure 6.13 Occult blood test.

WORD ORIGIN
hematochezia *(G.)*
haima, blood; *chezo,* feces

hematochezia

WORD ORIGIN
occult *(L.)*
occultus, to hide

bad

6-52 Additional blood tests are helpful in the diagnosis of disorders of the liver as well as other organs of the digestive system. Urine tests and stool examinations are also used.

The presence of blood in the stool is **hematochezia.** Using hemat(o), which you know means blood, write the term that means blood in the stool: _____.

Occult blood is blood that is not obvious on examination but can be detected by chemical tests, guaiac tests (for example, the Hemoccult test). An occult blood test of the stool (Fig. 6.13) in healthy individuals is usually negative. The presence of occult blood in the stool may indicate gastrointestinal bleeding, a finding associated with ulcers, ulcerative colitis, or cancer.

6-53 Stool samples are tested for fats as an indication of pancreatic disease or mal/absorption, impaired absorption. Fat is normally absorbed in the small intestine, giving a negative test result for fecal fats. The presence of fat in stool samples is an abnormal finding. Literal translation of malabsorption is poor or _____ absorption.

Stool samples are also tested for ova and parasites to aid in the diagnosis of parasitic infection.

BUILD IT! EXERCISE 17

Use the following word parts to build terms. (Some word parts will be used more than once.)

cholecyst(o), col(o), esophag(o), fluor(o), gastr(o), sial(o), -gram, -graphy, -scopy

1. direct visualization of the large intestine _____/_____
2. radiographic examination of the salivary glands _____/_____
3. visual examination of the esophagus and stomach _____/_____/_____
4. radiographic record of the gallbladder _____/_____
5. visual examination using a fluoroscope _____/_____

MATCH IT! EXERCISE 18

Match the diagnostic test, procedure, or instrument in the left column with the digestive structure in the right column that is the focus of study. (Use all terms once.)

____ **1.** cholangiography
____ **2.** cholecystography
____ **3.** duodenoscopy
____ **4.** esophagram
____ **5.** gastroscope
____ **6.** pancreatography
____ **7.** pyloroscopy
____ **8.** sialography

A. bile ducts
B. duodenum
C. esophagus
D. gallbladder
E. lower region of the stomach
F. pancreas
G. salivary ducts
H. stomach

PATHOLOGIES

appetite

without

6-54 Nausea and vomiting (N&V) often occur together; however nausea is the urge to vomit, whether or not vomiting occurs. Many disturbances of the digestive system can give a feeling of malaise sometimes accompanied by **anorexia,** lack or loss of _____. Basic functions, such as eating, can be severely impaired by problems of the digestive system, but not all eating or nutritional disorders are caused by malfunction of the digestive system. For example, **anorexia nervosa** is a sometimes life-threatening illness that is self-induced starvation (Chapter 10). Literal translation of an/orexia is _____ appetite.

This clinical syndrome occurs primarily in females with onset most often during adolescence. There is often an intense fear of losing control of eating and becoming fat. Unless there is intervention, anorexia nervosa results in **emaciation,** excessive leanness caused by disease or lack of nutrition.

Additional terms associated with eating disorders or problems with absorption of nutrients include:

adipsia Absence of thirst.

bulimia* Eating disorder that occurs predominantly in females with onset usually in adolescence or early adulthood; characterized by episodes of binge eating that often end in purging (self-induced vomiting or the use of laxatives) and depression.

celiac disease an inborn error of metabolism characterized by the inability to digest gluten, resulting in abdominal distension, vomiting, diarrhea, extreme lethargy, and sometimes lactose intolerance. **Gluten** is an insoluble protein found in wheat and other grains. Some individuals have gluten sensitivity or intolerance, but do not have celiac disease.

dyspepsia Faulty or painful digestion, and symptomatic of other diseases or disorders; indigestion.

dysphagia Difficulty or inability to swallow. (Caution: Its literal translation is difficult eating.)

eructation[†] Belching; results from drawing up air from the stomach and expelling it through the mouth. Differs from a hiccup, produced by involuntary contraction of the diaphragm, followed by rapid closure of the glottis.

hematemesis Vomiting of blood; indicates upper GI bleeding. **Emesis** means vomiting.

hyperemesis Excessive vomiting, usually accompanied by nausea.

malabsorption syndrome Subnormal absorption of dietary constituents characterized by anorexia, weight loss, abdominal bloating, muscle cramps, and the presence of fat in stool samples; can be caused by a number of disorders, including several inborn errors of metabolism, such as celiac disease.

malnutrition Improper or poor nutrition.

polydipsia Excessive thirst, characteristic of several conditions, including diabetes mellitus (see Chapter 12).

polyphagia Excessive eating; if it occurs over a long period, it generally leads to weight gain.

obesity

6-55 Obesity is an abnormal increase in the proportion of fat cells of the body, and a person is regarded as medically obese if he or she is 20% above desirable body weight for the person's age, sex, height, and body build. The calculated body mass index (BMI) using weight-to-height ratios is an index of obesity or altered body fat distribution. An abnormal increase in the proportion of fat cells of the body is called _____.

Exo/gen/ous obesity is caused by a greater caloric intake than that needed to meet the metabolic needs of the body. **Endo/gen/ous obesity** originates from within the body, as seen in hormonal disorders such as uncontrolled diabetes. Want more information? Go to *www.eatright.org.*

Statistics show that approximately two-thirds of adults and one-fifth of children in the United States are either overweight or obese, placing them at high absolute risk for mortality from numerous chronic diseases. Obesity is defined as a BMI of 30 or greater. BMI is calculated by dividing a person's weight in kilograms by the square of the person's height in meters. To calculate your BMI, visit *http://www.nhlbi.nih.gov/guidelines/obesity/BMI/bmicalc.htm.*

---

*Bulimia *(G.): bous,* ox; *limos,* hunger.
[†]Eructation *(L.): eructare,* to belch.

BUILD IT!
EXERCISE 19

Use the following word parts to build terms. (Some word parts will be used more than once.)

a-, an-, eu-, exo-, hyper-, gen(o), -emesis, -dipsia, -orexia, -ous, -pepsia

1. lack of appetite _____/_____

2. excessive vomiting _____/_____

3. normal digestion _____/_____

4. pertaining to development outside the body _____/_____/_____

5. condition of the absence of thirst _____/_____

Upper Digestive Tract

eating

6-56 Diseases of the upper digestive tract include those diseases or disorders that affect the mouth, the esophagus, and the stomach.

Literal translation of a/phag/ia is absence of _____, but you will need to remember that **aphagia** means an inability to swallow as a result of an organic or psychological cause. This differs from anorexia nervosa, a disorder characterized by self-imposed starvation.

mouth

6-57 Any oral disease caused by a fungus is stomatomycosis. **Stomato/myc/osis** is a fungal condition of the _____.

Candida albicans is a yeast type of fungus that is part of the normal flora of the oral cavity (see Fig. 2.8, B). Because antibiotic therapy destroys the normal bacteria that usually prevent fungal infections, candidiasis (an infection caused by *Candida*, usually *C. albicans*) can result. Also, patients receiving chemo/therapy often develop candidiasis, because chemotherapy diminishes the ability of the immune system to prevent infection.

FIND IT!
EXERCISE 20

Draw a slash between the word parts in the following list. Then find the meanings of the word parts within the definitions. (Draw the slash, and then perform the remainder of the activity as a mental exercise.)

1. cheilitis inflammation of the lip, often causing pain when one attempts to eat

2. gingivalgia painful gums

3. gingivitis inflammation of the gum

4. gingivoglossitis inflammation of the tongue and gums

5. gingivostomatitis inflammation of the gums and mouth

6. glossitis inflammation of the tongue

7. glossopathy any disease of the tongue

8. glossoplegia paralysis of the tongue

tongue

6-58 **Glosso/pyr/osis** is an abnormal sensation of pain, burning, and stinging of the tongue without apparent lesions or cause. The combining form pyr(o), which means fire, in glosso/pyr/osis refers to the stinging sensation of the _____.

inflammation

6-59 Stomat/itis makes eating difficult because the mouth is painful. **Stomatitis** is _____ of the mouth.

Stomato/dynia means painful mouth. Ulcers are defined, craterlike lesions. Ulcerations on the lips are often called *cold sores* or *fever blisters* (usually caused by the herpes simplex virus [HSV] type 1) (see Fig. 13.15).

lips

6-60 **Cheil/osis** is a condition of the _____. In cheilosis there is splitting of the lips and angles of the mouth. Cheilosis is a characteristic of riboflavin deficiency in the diet.

WORD ORIGIN
caries *(L.)*
decay

pulp

6-61 **Dent/algia** means a toothache. Dentalgia is often caused by caries that have extended into the tooth pulp. **Caries** means decay. Neglected dental caries, over time, invade and inflame pulpal tissues. **End/odont/itis** means inflammation of the endodontium, or the tooth _____.

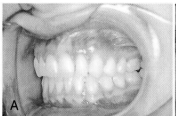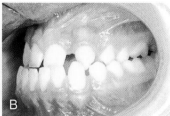

Figure 6.14 Malocclusion. Such malposition and contact of the maxillary and mandibular teeth interfere most during chewing. **A,** Protrusion of the upper front teeth (overbite). **B,** Positioning of the lower front teeth outside the upper front teeth (underbite).

<table>
<tr><td>

WORD ORIGIN
halitosis *(L.)*
halitus, breath

halitosis

straighten

periodontium

pus

temporomandibular

</td><td>

6-62 Halitosis is an offensive breath resulting from poor oral hygiene, dental or oral infections, use of tobacco, ingestion of certain foods (such as, garlic), or some systemic diseases (such as, the odor of acetone in diabetes or ammonia in liver disease). Write the term that means bad breath: _____.

6-63 An impacted tooth is one that is unable to erupt because of crowding by adjacent teeth or mal/position of the tooth.

   Mal/occlusion, or improper bite, is abnormal contact of the teeth of the upper jaw, the maxilla, with the teeth of the lower jaw, the mandible (Fig. 6.14). Ortho/dontic braces are used to move the teeth into alignment—in other words, to _____ the teeth.

6-64 Peri/odont/itis is inflammation of the _____, the structure that supports the tooth.

   Pyorrhea is one type of periodontal disease. Pyorrhea is an inflammation of the gingiva and the periodontal ligament, the fibrous connective tissue that anchors the tooth to the base. Literal interpretation of pyo/rrhea is discharge of _____.

6-65 TMJ pain dysfunction syndrome is an abnormal condition that interferes with eating and is believed to be caused by a defective or dislocated **temporo/mandibular joint** (TMJ), one of a pair of joints connecting the mandible to the skull.

   Often called *TMJ syndrome,* this condition is characterized by facial pain and clicking sounds while chewing. Malocclusion, ill-fitting dentures, and a variety of conditions can cause TMJ syndrome. TMJ refers to the _____ joint.

</td></tr>
</table>

ANALYZE IT! EXERCISE 21

Divide these words into their component parts, and write the meaning of each term.

1. cheilosis _____

2. gingivalgia _____

3. endodontitis _____

4. glossopyrosis _____

5. pyorrhea _____

6. stomatomycosis _____

6-66 The mouth is examined for oral cancer during a routine dental examination. Tumors of the oral cavity can cause pain and change aspects of talking, swallowing, or chewing. Oral tumors can be classified as pre/malignant, malignant, or benign (see Chapter 14).

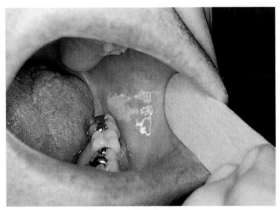

Figure 6.15 Leukoplakia. This slowly developing change in the buccal mucosa, characterized by white, sharply circumscribed patches, is a precancerous lesion.

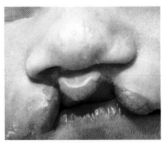

Figure 6.16 Cleft lip. This particular cleft in the upper lip is bilateral, but the congenital defect may be unilateral, median, or bilateral and may be accompanied by cleft palate.

Leuko/plakia is a precancerous, slowly developing change in a mucous membrane characterized by white patches with sharply defined edges that are slightly raised. Leukoplakia may occur on the genitals or the lips and buccal mucosa (Fig. 6.15). The **buccal mucosa** is the mucous membrane that lines the insides of the _____.

cheeks

6-67 Parot/itis is inflammation of the parotid gland. Epidemic or infectious parotitis is another name for mumps, which is a contagious viral disease that can generally be prevented by immunization.

Mumps is an acute viral infection that is characterized by swelling of the parotid glands and may affect one or both glands. The parotid gland is a salivary gland located _____ the ear.

near

6-68 Cleft palate, often associated with cleft lip, is a congenital defect in which there is a division of the palate, resulting from the failure of the two sides of the palate to fuse during development. Cleft lip is one or more clefts in the upper lip (Fig. 6.16). Surgical repair beginning in infancy is generally recommended for both of these congenital defects. Failure of the two sides of the palate to fuse during development results in _____ palate.

cleft

WORD ORIGIN
achalasia *(G.)*
chalasis, relaxation

6-69 The esophagus is susceptible to a variety of inflammatory, structural, and neoplastic disorders. **Esophageal achalasia** is an abnormal condition in which the lower esophageal sphincter fails to relax properly. It is characterized by dysphagia. Regurgitation, the return of swallowed food into the mouth, may also occur. Changes in diet and certain drugs may be helpful, but dilation of the esophagus with progressively larger sizes of dilators is also used. Write the name of the condition in which the lower esophageal sphincter fails to relax appropriately in response to swallowing: esophageal _____.

achalasia

WORD ORIGIN
atresia *(G.)*
tresis, hole

6-70 Esophageal atresia, usually a congenital abnormality, is an esophagus that ends in a blind pouch or narrows so much that it obstructs continuous passage of food to the stomach. Write this term that is a congenital abnormality that results in a blind pouch or narrowing of the esophagus: esophageal _____. Narrowing may be improved by progressively larger dilators, or corrective surgery may be necessary.

atresia

6-71 Esophageal varices (singular, varix) are enlarged and swollen veins at the lower end of the esophagus, which are especially susceptible to hemorrhage (Fig. 6.17). These large and swollen veins are called _____.

varices

Upper gastrointestinal bleeding is usually caused by esophageal varices, gastritis, ulcerations, or cancer of either the esophagus or stomach (Fig. 6.18).

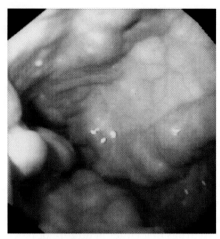

Figure 6.17 **Esophageal varices.**

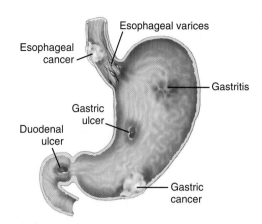

Figure 6.18 **Common causes of upper gastrointestinal bleeding.**

esophagus

6-72 Gastroesophageal reflux disease (GERD) is a dysfunction that involves a backflow of the contents of the stomach into the _____. The cause is often a weak cardiac sphincter. Repeated episodes of reflux can result in esophagitis, stricture (narrowing) of the esophagus, or an esophageal ulcer (craterlike lesion). Treatment of the disorder in its early stages is elevation of the head of the bed, avoidance of acid-stimulating foods, and use of ant/acids or anti/ulcer medications.

6-73 GERD is one of the major symptoms of a **hiatal hernia,** protrusion of a portion of the stomach upward through a defect in the diaphragm. Fig. 6.19 shows two types of hiatal hernias.

    As much as 40% of the population may have hiatal hernia, but most are asymptomatic. Diagnosis is generally confirmed by radiology, and surgery is seldom necessary. This type of herniation is

hiatal

called a _____ hernia. (See Chapter 3, Frame 3-28, for information about other types of hernias.)

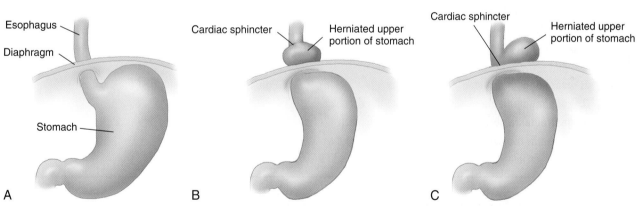

Figure 6.19 **The normal position of the stomach versus two types of hiatal hernias. A,** Normal position of the stomach. **B,** The sliding type of hiatal hernia accounts for 85% to 90% of hiatal hernias. The upper portion of the stomach slides up and down through the opening in the diaphragm. **C,** The rolling type of hiatal hernia accounts for 10% to 15% of hiatal hernias. The upper portion of the stomach is found above the diaphragm, alongside the esophagus.

6-74 Gastr/itis, one of the most common stomach disorders, is inflammation of the lining of the stomach. Causes of gastritis include medicines, food allergies, and toxins of microorganisms. Chronic gastritis can be a sign of another disease, such as cancer of the stomach or peptic ulcer.

    Peptic ulcers occur in the stomach, the duodenum, and occasionally the esophagus, and are sometimes caused by a bacterium, *Helicobacter pylori.* The ulcerations are breaks in the continuity

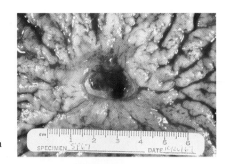

Figure 6.20 Photograph of a peptic ulcer. This peptic ulcer is located in the lesser curvature of the stomach.

of the mucous membrane that comes in contact with the acids of the stomach. They usually occur near the pyloric opening (Fig. 6.20). These types of ulcers cause stomachache, also called **gastr/algia.** The literal interpretation of gastralgia is _____ of the stomach. Most peptic ulcers eventually heal, and the pain is controlled with drugs that either neutralize or block secretion of acid. The immediate cause of peptic ulcers remains unknown.

A small percentage of patients with ulcers need surgery to remove the affected part of the stomach or to sever a branch of the vagus nerve to reduce the amount of gastric acid produced.

6-75 Pyloric stenosis is narrowing of the pyloric sphincter. The condition is a congenital defect, and it interferes with the flow of food into the small intestine. This condition in which there is narrowing of the pyloric sphincter is pyloric _____.

6-76 Some prominent signs and symptoms of gastric dysfunction are pain, excessive belching, flatulence, nausea, vomiting, blood in the stool, and diarrhea. Flatulence is excessive gas in the stomach or intestines. Diarrhea is frequent passage of watery bowel movements, often accompanied by cramping. Write the term that means excessive gas in the stomach or intestines: _____.

pain

stenosis

flatulence

FIND IT!   EXERCISE 22

Draw a slash between the word parts in the following list. Then find the meanings of the word parts within the definitions. (Draw the slash, and then perform the remainder of the activity as a mental exercise.)

1. **esophagitis** inflammation of the mucosal lining of the esophagus caused by infection, backflow of gastric juice from the stomach, or irritation from a nasogastric tube
2. **esophagodynia** pain of the esophagus
3. **esophagomalacia** morbid softening of the esophagus
4. **gastrectasia** abnormal stretching of the stomach, caused by overeating, a hernia, or obstruction of the pyloric opening

5. **gastric carcinoma** cancer of the stomach
6. **gastromalacia** morbid softening of the stomach
7. **gastromegaly** abnormal enlargement of the stomach or abdomen
8. **gastropathy** any disease of the stomach

BUILD IT!   EXERCISE 23

Use the following word parts to build terms. (Some word parts will be used more than once.)
esophag(o), gastr(o), -algia, -dynia, -eal, -malacia, -pathy

1. pain in the stomach   _____/_____
2. any disease of the stomach   _____/_____
3. pertaining to the stomach and the esophagus   _____/_____/_____
4. morbid softening of the esophagus   _____/_____
5. pain in the esophagus   _____/_____

Match pathologies of the upper digestive tract in the left column with their meanings or characteristics in the right column.

___	**1.** dyspepsia	**A.** enlarged and swollen veins of the esophagus
___	**2.** esophageal achalasia	**B.** esophageal sphincter fails to relax properly
___	**3.** esophageal atresia	**C.** esophagus ends in a blind pouch or narrows
___	**4.** esophageal varices	**D.** excessive eating
___	**5.** gastritis	**E.** excessive thirst
___	**6.** gingivitis	**F.** indigestion
___	**7.** glossitis	**G.** inflammation of the stomach
___	**8.** hematemesis	**H.** inflammation of a salivary gland
___	**9.** leukoplakia	**I.** inflammation of the gums
___	**10.** polydipsia	**J.** inflammation of the tongue
___	**11.** polyphagia	**K.** painful mouth
___	**12.** sialadenitis	**L.** precancerous change in a mucous membrane
___	**13.** stomatodynia	**M.** vomiting of blood

Lower Digestive Tract

6-77 Intestinal disorders can be classified as inflammatory or noninflammatory.

Periton/itis (the "e" in peritone[o] is dropped to facilitate pronunciation) is an acute inflammation of the peritoneum (the lining of the abdominal cavity). Causes of peritonitis include rupture of abdominal organs, such as the appendix, peptic ulcers, or perforations of an organ in the GI tract. Without treatment, it becomes a life-threatening illness.

peritonitis

A rupture or perforation of an organ in the GI tract may lead to _____.

6-78 Three examples of acute inflammatory bowel problems are appendicitis, gastroenteritis, and dysentery. **Appendic/itis** (Fig. 6.21) is acute inflammation of the vermiform

appendix
intestine

_____.

Gastro/enteritis means inflammation of the stomach and _____. It primarily affects the small intestine and can be either viral or bacterial. Intestinal flu (or influenza) is a viral gastroenteritis.

Symptoms of gastroenteritis are anorexia, nausea, vomiting, abdominal discomfort, diarrhea, and possibly fever. The feces may contain blood, mucus, pus, or excessive amounts of fat. Untreated severe diarrhea may lead to rapid dehydration. Dehydration is excessive loss of _____ from body tissues.

water

Dysentery (dys-, bad, + enter(o), intestine, + -y, condition) is inflammation of the intestine, especially the colon. The most common types are caused by bacteria or ameba (parasitic organisms), characterized by frequent and blood feces. Diarrhea, the frequent passage of loose, watery stools, is an important symptom of dysentery as well as several other disorders.

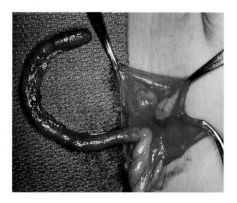

Figure 6.21 Appendicitis. Note the pink color (indicating inflammation). Pain usually develops rapidly and becomes localized in the right abdominal quadrant.

Figure 6.22 Two disorders of the anorectal area.
A, Anal fissures. An ulceration or tear of the lining of the anal canal may be caused by excessive tissue stretching. These tears are very tender and tend to reopen when stool is passed. **B,** Hemorrhoids. Three types of hemorrhoids are shown: internal, external, and prolapsed. Internal hemorrhoids lie above the anal sphincter and cannot be seen on inspection of the anal area. External hemorrhoids lie below the anal sphincter and can be seen on inspection of the anal region. Hemorrhoids that enlarge, fall down, and protrude through the anus are called *prolapsed hemorrhoids.*

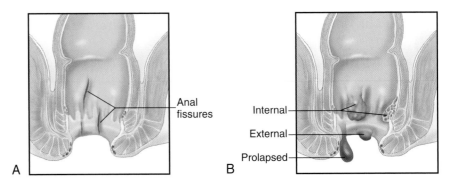

6-79 Literal translation of **col/itis** is inflammation of the large intestine. Ulcerative col/itis, irritable bowel syndrome (IBS), and Crohn disease are three of the more common chronic inflammatory bowel diseases (IBDs). Ulcerative colitis is a chronic inflammatory disorder of the colon or rectum, characterized by profuse, watery diarrhea containing mucus, blood, and pus. The chronic inflammation results in a loss of the mucosal lining and ulceration or abscess formation.

colitis

This type of chronic IBD is called ulcerative _____.

6-80 Crohn disease is another IBD that can affect any part of the GI tract, from the mouth to the anus. As with ulcerative colitis, the cause is unknown. The lesions of Crohn disease are patchy and often extend through all bowel layers.

> **WORD ORIGIN**
> fistula *(L.)*
> *fistula,* pipe

Abnormal passages between internal organs or abnormal communications leading from internal organs to the body surface are called **fistulas.** Fistulas can occur between the bowel and almost any adjacent structures. An anal fistula is an abnormal opening near the _____.

anus

6-81 A **fissure** is a cleft or a groove or a cracklike lesion of the skin. A painful linear ulceration or tear at the anal opening is called an anal _____.
Fissures are sometimes associated with constipation, diarrhea, or Crohn disease (Fig. 6.22, A).

fissure

6-82 Rectal bleeding may be indicative of an intestinal disorder. **Hemorrhoids,** a common cause of rectal bleeding, are masses of dilated veins of the anal canal that lie just inside or outside the rectum. Commonly called piles, hemorrhoids are often accompanied by pain and itching (Fig. 6.22, B). Constipation, straining to **defecate** (evacuate feces), and prolonged sitting contribute to their development. Masses of dilated veins of the anal canal are called _____.

hemorrhoids

6-83 Parasites and pathogenic bacteria or viruses can invade the GI tract. Food poisoning results when a person ingests toxic substances or infectious organisms in food, but unlike gastroenteritis, food poisoning cannot be passed directly to another person. Mushroom poisoning is a type of _____ poisoning.
Common types of bacterial food poisoning include staphylococcal infection, *Escherichia coli* (often called *E. coli*) infection, botulism, and **salmonell/osis,** caused by the bacterium, *Salmonella.*

food

6-84 A duodenal ulcer, the most common type of peptic ulcer, is one that occurs in the _____. Inflammation of the duodenum is **duodenitis.** Inflammation of the ileum is **ileitis. Gastro/duoden/itis** is inflammation of the _____ and duodenum.

duodenum
stomach

6-85 Common causes of lower gastrointestinal bleeding are shown in Fig. 6.23. Colonic polyps, small, tumor-like growths, can arise from the mucosal surface of the colon, are best considered as premalignant, and are thus removed (Fig. 6.24). Some types of colonic polyps are closely linked to colorectal cancer and, for this reason, should be removed when observed during coloscopy. **Polyp/ectomy,** removal of a polyp, can be performed during a colonoscopy. Small, tumor-like growths on the colon's mucosal surface are called colonic _____.

polyps

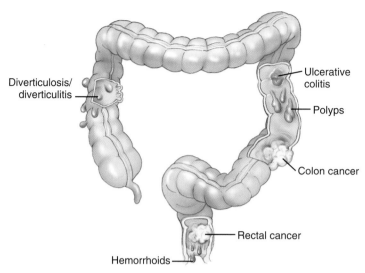

Diverticulosis/
diverticulitis

Ulcerative
colitis

Polyps

Colon cancer

Rectal cancer

Hemorrhoids

Figure 6.23 **Common causes of lower gastrointestinal bleeding.**

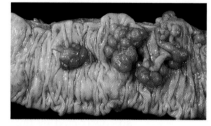

Figure 6.24 **Colonic polyps.** Multiple polyps of the colon.

6-86 Noninflammatory intestinal disorders include malignant diverticulosis, tumors, obstructions, malabsorption, and trauma. Irritable bowel syndrome (IBS), also called *spastic colon, spastic bowel,* and *mucous colitis,* is a common chronic noninflammatory intestinal disorder. The cause is unknown, and it primarily involves increased motility of the intestines, diarrhea, and pain in the lower abdomen. Women are affected more than men. IBS is a noninflammatory condition and no specific treatment is required; however, more serious conditions such as dysentery, lactose intolerance (sensitivity disorder resulting in the inability to digest lactose from milk products), and the inflammatory bowel diseases (for example, Crohn disease) must be ruled out.

This noninflammatory intestinal disorder is called _____ bowel syndrome.

6-87 Diverticular disease includes divercul/itis and diverticu/losis. A **diverticulum** is a pouchlike herniation through the muscular wall of a tubular organ. A diverticulum (plural is diverticula) is most commonly present in the colon but also can occur in the esophagus, stomach, or small intestine (Fig. 6.25, A).

If diverticula are present in the colon without inflammation or symptoms, the condition is called **diverticulosis.** Diverticula generally do not cause a problem. **Diverticul/itis** is _____ of one or more diverticula (Fig. 6.25, B).

irritable

inflammation

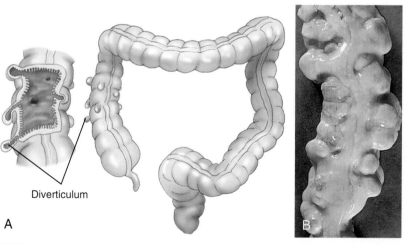

Diverticulum

A

B

Figure 6.25 **Diverticulosis. A,** Several abnormal outpouchings (diverticula) in the wall of the intestine. **B,** Diverticulitis that occurred secondary to diverticulosis (photo of a removed section of large intestine).

6-88 An accumulation of hardened feces in the rectum or sigmoid colon that the individual cannot expel is **impaction.** Write the term that means the presence of a large or hard fecal mass in the rectum or colon: _____. Impaction leads to colonic stasis, also called **entero/stasis.** When enterostasis occurs, there is a delay or a stopping of the movement of food in the intestinal tract.

impaction

6-89 Intestinal obstruction occurs when intestinal contents cannot pass through the GI tract. The obstruction may be partial or complete and can occur anywhere in the intestinal tract. Fig. 6.26 shows several causes of intestinal obstruction. Look closely at the illustration as you read about the different types of bowel obstructions.

    Adhesions are bands of scar tissue that bind surfaces that normally are separated. They most commonly form in the abdomen after abdominal surgery, inflammation, or injury. Write the term that means scar tissue that binds surfaces together that are normally separate: _____.

adhesion

6-90 Inguinal hernias develop because of a weakness in the abdominal muscle wall or a widened space at the inguinal ligament (see Fig. 3.28, B). In a strangulated hernia, the blood vessels become so constricted by the neck of the hernial sac that circulation is stopped in the constricted area. Surgical intervention is necessary. A hernia in which the blood vessels are constricted by the neck of the hernial sac is called a _____ hernia.

strangulated

6-91 Intussusception is a telescopic folding back of the bowel into itself. Mesenteric occlusion is a binding or closing off of a segment of the intestine by the mesentery, the peritoneum that suspends the intestine from the abdominal wall. A twisting of the bowel is called **volvulus,** and a folding back of the bowel onto itself is called _____.

    Neoplasms or tumors are the most common cause of obstruction of the large intestine. Surgery is usually necessary to correct obstructions of the bowel.

intussusception

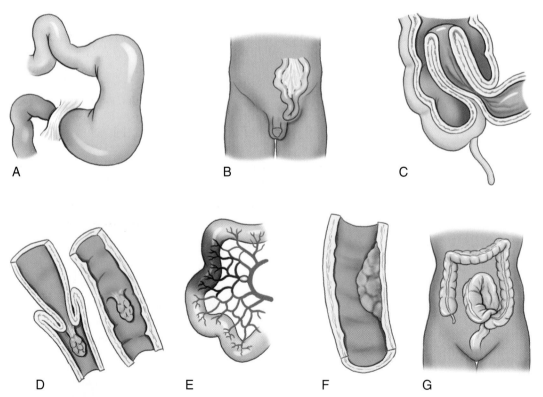

       A   B   C

       D   E   F   G

Figure 6.26 Bowel obstructions. A, Adhesion. **B,** Strangulated inguinal hernia. **C,** Ileocecal intussusception. **D,** Polyp and intussusception. **E,** Mesenteric occlusion. **F,** Neoplasm. **G,** Volvulus of the sigmoid colon.

6-92 Mal/absorption syndrome is a disorder in which one or multiple nutrients are not digested or absorbed. The nutrient that is not absorbed well depends on which abnormality exists. Various deficiencies can lead to malabsorption of fats, various vitamins, lactose, or iron. **Lipo/penia** is a

fats

deficiency of _____.

BUILD IT!

EXERCISE 25

Use the following word parts to build terms. (Some word parts will be used more than once.)

appendic(o), duoden(o), enter(o), gastr(o), lip(o), -itis, -penia, -stasis

1. delay or stopping of movement of food in the intestinal tract _____/_____
2. inflammation of the vermiform appendix _____/_____
3. inflammation of the stomach and duodenum _____/_____/_____
4. deficiency of fats _____/_____

WRITE IT!

EXERCISE 26

Write a word in each blank to complete these sentences. The first letter of the word is given as a clue.

1. Inflammation of the stomach and intestines is g_____.
2. Inflammation of the colon that is characterized by abdominal pain and frequent, bloody stools is
   d_____.
3. An abnormal passage between two internal organs is a f_____.
4. The presence of diverticula in the colon without inflammation is called d_____.
5. A painful linear ulceration or tear at the anal opening is an anal f_____.
6. A common noninflammatory intestinal disorder has many names, including spastic bowel, mucous colitis, spastic colon, and i_____ bowel syndrome.
7. Masses of dilated veins that are varicose and lie just inside or outside the rectum are h_____.
8. An accumulation of feces that the individual cannot expel is called an i_____.
9. A telescopic folding back of one part of the intestine into itself is i_____.
10. A twisting of the bowel is called v_____.

Accessory Organs of Digestion

liver

6-93 The liver is one of the most vital internal organs. Degeneration of the liver may lead to severe consequences, including ascites (accumulation of abdominal fluid), defects in coagulation of the blood, jaundice, neurologic symptoms, and hepatic and renal failure.

Hepato/renal syndrome is a type of kidney failure that is associated with hepatic failure. In hepat/ic failure, the _____ cannot perform its vital functions for the body. Hepatorenal syndrome has a poor prognosis because both the kidneys and liver fail.

enlargement

6-94 Any disease of the liver is **hepato/pathy. Hepato/spleno/megaly** is _____ of the liver and spleen.

6-95 A tumor of the liver is a **hepatoma.** This term is usually reserved for a specific type of primary liver carcinoma.

carcinoma

Tumors of the liver may be benign or malignant. Cancer of the liver is called hepatic _____. Malignancy in the liver that is spread from another source (metastasis) is many times more common than primary tumor of the liver.

inflammation

enlarged

6-96 **Hepat/itis** is _____ of the liver. It is characterized by jaundice, **hepatomegaly,** anorexia, abnormal liver function, clay-colored stools, and tea-colored urine. Hepato/megaly means an _____ liver.

Jaundice is a yellow discoloration of the skin, the mucous membranes, and the whites of the eyes, caused by greater than normal amounts of bilirubin (a yellow-orange pigment of bile) in the blood (Fig. 6.27).

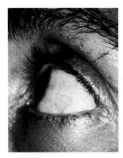

Figure 6.27 Jaundice. This yellow discoloration of the skin, mucous membranes, and sclera (white parts) of the eyes is characteristic of hepatitis.

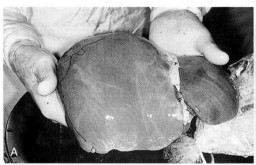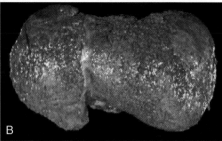

Figure 6.28 Comparison of a normal liver and a cirrhotic liver. A, A normal liver removed in autopsy. **B,** Cirrhosis of the liver. Note the nodelike structures on the liver's surface.

6-97 Hepatitis may result from bacterial or viral infections or other causes, such as medications, toxins, or alcohol. Viral hepatitis is generally one of five major types. Other types of hepatitis are less common or generally have mild symptoms.

virus

Hepatitis A is caused by HAV, the abbreviation for hepatitis A _____.

🔑 **KEY** POINT **Five major types of viral hepatitis and their associated viruses are:**
- Hepatitis A (hepatitis A virus [HAV])
- Hepatitis B (hepatitis B virus [HBV])
- Hepatitis C (hepatitis C virus [HCV])
- Hepatitis D (hepatitis D virus [HDV])
- Hepatitis E (hepatitis E virus [HEV])

Hepatitis A and hepatitis E can be acquired by ingestion of contaminated food, but the other types are acquired only by contact with an infected person or infected materials. Most of the latter types can be acquired by contaminated blood, sexual contact, or the use of contaminated needles and instruments. Immunization is available for some types of hepatitis. Read more about viral hepatitis in the Sexually Transmitted Diseases section of Chapter 8.

6-98 Severe hepatitis may lead to **cirrhosis,** a chronic, progressive liver disease that is characterized by degeneration of liver cells with eventual increased resistance to flow of blood through the liver (Fig. 6.28). Cirrhosis is a disease of what organ? _____

liver

Alcoholic cirrhosis occurs in approximately 20% of chronic alcoholics. Unless alcohol is avoided, coma, gastrointestinal hemorrhage, and kidney failure may occur. Nutritional deficiencies, poisons, toxic drugs, some types of heart disease, and prior viral hepatitis can also lead to cirrhosis.

6-99 Bile is produced by the liver, stored in the gallbladder, and released into the duodenum via the common bile duct when needed for digestion. Anything that interferes with the flow of bile interferes with digestion. **Chole/stasis** is stoppage or suppression of bile flow. Obstruction of bile flow can cause inflammation of the gallbladder, the liver, or the pancreas.

bile

Chol/angitis is inflammation of a _____ vessel or duct. (Note that the "e" is dropped from chol[e] when it is combined with angi[o].) Cholangitis can be caused by bacterial infection or by obstruction of the ducts by calculi or a tumor.

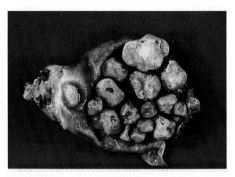

Figure 6.29 Cholelithiasis, the presence of gallstones. After cholecystectomy, this photograph of an opened gallbladder shows several stones of different sizes. In general, gallstones vary from very small to 4 to 5 cm in diameter.

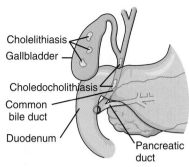

Figure 6.30 Common locations of biliary calculi. Tiny stones may pass spontaneously into the duodenum. Very large stones remain in the gallbladder (cholelithiasis). Smaller stones can become lodged in the common bile duct (choledocholithiasis).

gallstones (or calculi)	**6-100 Chole/lith/iasis** is the presence of _____ in the gallbladder (Fig. 6.29). Acute **cholecyst/itis,** inflammation of the gallbladder, is usually caused by a gallstone. If surgery is not performed to remove the gallbladder, a perforation (opening or hole) in its wall may occur. An abscess may form, or peritonitis may result if the perforation is large. Acute cholecystitis may occur in the absence of gallstones, possibly because of bacterial invasion.
calculus (stone)	**6-101 Choledoch/itis** is inflammation of the common bile duct. **Choledocho/lith/iasis** is the presence of a _____ in the common bile duct. Stones may remain in the gallbladder, may pass into the common bile duct, or may pass into the duodenum (Fig. 6.30).
pancreas	**6-102** Both cholangitis and pancreatitis can occur as complications of cholecystitis, resulting from the backup of bile through the biliary tract. **Pancreat/itis** is inflammation of the _____. Acute pancreatitis can be life-threatening, resulting in destruction of the organ by its own enzymes. Destruction of pancreatic tissue is **pancreatolysis.** Several factors that contribute to acute pancreatitis include alcoholism, gallstones, trauma, tumors, peritonitis, viral infections, and drug toxicity. Chronic pancreatitis may develop after repeated episodes of acute pancreatitis or chronic obstruction of the common bile duct. A pancreatic
pus	abscess, a collection of _____ in or around the pancreas, is a serious complication of pancreatitis.
calculus (stone)	**6-103** Stones, tumors, or cysts can cause pancreatic obstructions. **Pancreato/lithiasis** is the presence of calculi in the pancreas or pancreatic duct. **Pancreato/lith** means a pancreatic _____. Pancreatic carcinoma is one of the most deadly malignancies. The cancer is usually discovered in the late stages, and the prognosis is poor. Like pancreatic carcinoma, the prognosis for cancer of the gallbladder is poor. However, cancer of the gallbladder is rare.
inflammation	**6-104** Two of the more likely disorders of the salivary glands are sialadenitis and sialolithiasis. Tumors of the salivary glands are not common. **Sial/aden/itis,** _____ of the salivary glands, can be caused by an infectious microorganism, an allergic reaction, or radiation therapy. **Sialo/lithiasis,** the presence of salivary stones either within the gland itself or in the salivary ducts, may cause few symptoms unless the duct becomes obstructed.

MATCH IT!   EXERCISE 27

Match terms in the left column with their meaning or characteristics in the right column. (Use all choices once.)

___ **1.** ascites
___ **2.** cholangitis
___ **3.** cholecystitis
___ **4.** choledochitis
___ **5.** choledocholithiasis
___ **6.** cirrhosis
___ **7.** hepatoma
___ **8.** jaundice

A. accumulation of abdominal fluid
B. calculus in the common bile duct
C. chronic degeneration of liver cells
D. inflammation of a bile duct
E. inflammation of the common bile duct
F. inflammation of the gallbladder
G. tumor of the liver
H. yellow discoloration of the skin and increased bilirubin

BUILD IT!   EXERCISE 28

Use the following word parts to build terms. (Some word parts will be used more than once.)

chol(e), hepat(o), pancreat(o), ren(o), -al, -lith, -lysis, -megaly, -stasis

1. enlargement of the liver _____/_____
2. suppression of bile flow _____/_____
3. pertaining to the liver and the kidney _____/_____/_____
4. destruction of pancreatic tissue _____/_____
5. a pancreatic calculus _____/_____

WRITE IT!   EXERCISE 29

Case Study. *Define the underlined terms.*

Gregory Harper is examined by Dr. Harry Malone, a <u>gastroenterologist</u>. Mr. Harper underwent an endoscopy last May that showed active <u>colitis</u>. His mother, deceased, had hemorrhoids, <u>gastrocele</u>, and <u>diabetes mellitus</u>. Rectal exam: Good tone, but painful. Assessment: Toxic colitis.

1. gastroenterologist _____
2. colitis _____
3. gastrocele _____
4. diabetes mellitus _____

SURGICAL AND THERAPEUTIC INTERVENTIONS

Digestive Tract

gingival

6-105 You may already be familiar with some dental surgeries, such as extraction of wisdom teeth. **Gingivectomy,** surgical removal of all loose and diseased _____ tissue, is performed by a dentist or periodontist to arrest the progress of periodontal disease.

Cancer or trauma can affect any structure of the digestive system and may require plastic surgery if there is extensive damage. Learn several new surgical terms pertaining to the mouth in the next exercise.

FIND IT!   EXERCISE 30

Draw a slash between the word parts in the following list. Then find the meanings of the word parts within the definitions. (Draw the slash, and then perform the remainder of the activity as a mental exercise.)

1. cheiloplasty surgical repair of the lip
2. cheilorrhaphy suture of the lip
3. glossectomy excision of the tongue
4. glossoplasty surgical repair of the tongue

5. glossorrhaphy suture of the tongue
6. stomatoplasty surgical repair of the mouth
7. cheilostomatoplasty surgical repair of the lips and mouth

esophagectomy

6-106 Write a term that means surgical excision of all or part of the esophagus: _____. This surgical procedure may be required to treat severe bleeding of the esophagus or esophageal cancer.

Esophago/myo/tomy is an incision into the muscle of the lower part of the esophagus, performed to expedite the passage of food in esophageal achalasia, an abnormal condition characterized by the inability of the muscle to relax.

stomach

6-107 Patients who can digest and absorb nutrients but need nutritional support may receive enteral nutrition (provision of liquid nutrients through the GI tract when the patient cannot ingest, chew, or swallow food but can digest and absorb nutrients; it is accomplished using an enteral feeding tube). Naso/gastric (NG) means pertaining to the nose and stomach, and nasogastric enteral feeding uses a **naso/gastric tube** (NG tube) that is inserted through the nose into the _____.

opening

Terms for surgical procedures to establish this means of feeding by placement of the enteral tube directly into the esophagus, stomach, or jejunum are **esophago/stomy, gastro/stomy,** and **jejuno/stomy,** respectively, which mean formation of a new _____ into these structures. Locations for enteral feeding tubes are shown in Fig. 6.31.

6-108 Par/enteral means not through the alimentary tract but through some other route; in other words, by injection. **Total parenteral nutrition** (TPN) is the administration of all nutrition through an indwelling catheter into the vena cava or other main vein. This method of feeding has several names, including intravenous alimentation and **hyperalimentation.**

parenteral

TPN is the abbreviation for total _____ nutrition.

Translated literally, hyper/alimentation means excessive nutrition. Hyperalimentation has a second meaning of overfeeding, or the ingestion or administration of an amount of nutrients that exceeds the demands of the body. Overfeeding on one's own can lead to obesity.

6-109 Bariatrics is the field of medicine that focuses on the treatment and control of obesity. There are broadly three options available for managing obesity: lifestyle modification (alterations in diet and physical activity), pharmacotherapy, (**anorexiants** are drugs or other agents that suppress the appetite), and finally bariatric surgery. Lifestyle modification is a necessary component to any obesity management to losing weight and keeping it off. Write the name of the field that focuses on obesity: _____.

WORD ORIGIN
bariatrics *(G.)*
baros, weight

bariatrics

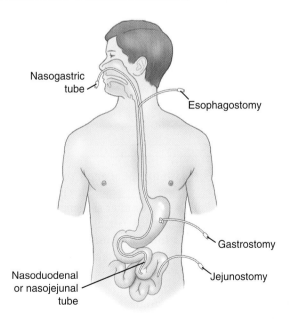

Nasogastric tube

Esophagostomy

Gastrostomy

Nasoduodenal or nasojejunal tube

Jejunostomy

Figure 6.31 **Common placement locations for enteral feeding tubes.**

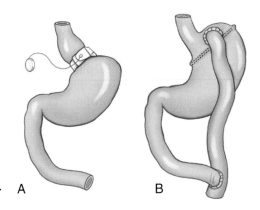

Figure 6.32 Surgical procedures for limiting nutrient intake. **A,** Adjustable gastric band system. **B,** Gastric bypass surgery. **A** **B**

6-110 The surgical options that are commonly offered in the United States include limiting the food intake (for example, adjustable gastric band or gastric bypass [Fig. 6.32]) or a complex bariatric surgery: removing much of the stomach (creating a smaller "gastric sleeve") and linking it to a very short part of the duodenum. In some bariatric surgeries, the duodenum is directly linked to a lower part of the small intestine. However, the decrease in the amount of food, vitamins, and minerals absorbed creates chances for long-term problems, such as malnutrition and osteoporosis.

The term **gastroplasty** means any surgery performed to reshape or repair the

_____.

stomach

6-111 Two procedures that are performed to remove unsightly flabby folds of fat tissue or to improve body contours are **lipectomy** and **liposuction.** Both procedures are performed for cosmetic reasons rather than weight reduction. Lip/ectomy is excision of subcutaneous _____, and lipo/suction removes fat with a suction pump device.

fat

ANALYZE IT! **EXERCISE 31**

Divide these words into their component parts, and define each term.

1. cheilorrhaphy _____
2. cheilostomatoplasty _____
3. esophagomyotomy _____
4. esophagostomy _____
5. gingivectomy _____
6. glossorrhaphy _____
7. jejunostomy _____
8. lipectomy _____
9. nasogastric _____
10. stomatoplasty _____

6-112 Lavage is irrigation or washing out of an organ, such as the stomach or bowel. Washing out of the stomach is _____ lavage, which is performed to remove irritants or toxic substances, and is done before or after surgery on the stomach.

gastric

Flushing of the inside of the colon is called _colonic irrigation;_ this is not the same as an enema. Colonic irrigation may be used to remove any material high in the colon, whereas an enema is introduction of a solution into the rectum either for cleansing the rectum or as a treatment for constipation.

6-113 Some types of ulcers of the stomach, esophagus, and duodenum are caused by a particular bacterium called _Helicobacter pylori_ and can be treated with antibiotics. Certain medications can also cause ulcers. Treatment of gastric ulcers can include any of the following: antibiotics, change of a suspected medication, dietary management, and antacids to counteract the acidic gastric contents. Treatment is necessary for **hyper/acidity,** _____ acid in the stomach. Gastric hyperacidity may lead to ulcers. (Note the omission of the "i" in antacid.)

excessive

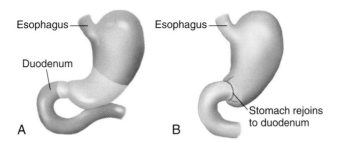

Esophagus —

Duodenum

A

Esophagus —

Stomach rejoins
to duodenum

B

Figure 6.33 Partial gastrectomy. A, The stomach before surgery, showing the distal acid-secreting portion *(tan).* **B,** The stomach after surgery: A new opening has been made between the stomach and the duodenum, the first part of the small intestine. This type of surgery, gastroduodenostomy, might be performed for severe chronic gastric ulcers.

excision (removal)

6-114 Persons with ulcers who do not respond to medical treatment or who develop complications (perforation or hemorrhage) may require partial **gastr/ectomy,** which is _____ of part of the stomach (Fig. 6.33). Severing of certain branches of the vagus nerve, **vagotomy,** is sometimes done to reduce the amount of gastric secretion and lessen the chance of recurrence of a gastric ulcer.

A gastrectomy, removal of part or all of the stomach, is done also to remove a malignancy.

WORD ORIGIN
anastomose *(G.)*
anastomoien, to
    provide a mouth

esophagus

duodenum

ileum

6-115 Anastomosis means a connection between two vessels. It may be created by surgical, traumatic, or pathologic means between two normally distinct organs or spaces. The communication (union) itself is also called an anastomosis. The verb that means to join the structures is **anastomose.**

A total gastrectomy requires anastomosis of the esophagus to the small intestine. **Esophagoje-junostomy** means surgical anastomosis of the _____ to the jejunum.

In an **esophago/duodeno/stomy,** the anastomosis is between the esophagus and the _____.

6-116 Trauma or a tumor in the cardiac region of the stomach may necessitate creation of a new opening between the esophagus and stomach, **esophagogastrostomy.** Likewise, trauma or tumor of the jejunum or ileum may require anastomosis. **Jejuno/ileo/stomy** is formation of an opening between the jejunum and the _____.

6-117 Trauma or cancer may require making a new opening between the stomach and small intestine. Study the three types of anastomoses in Fig. 6.34. Note that in writing terms pertaining to anastomoses, the term begins with the proximal organ (organ nearest the place where nutrition begins):
- **gastro/entero/stomy** The body of the stomach is joined with some part of the small intestine. This is the simplest of these three procedures.
- **gastro/duodeno/stomy** Anastomosis of the gastric stump with the duodenum; same as **gastro-duodenal anastomosis.**
- **gastro/jejuno/stomy** Anastomosis of the gastric stump with the jejunum; same as **gastrojejunal anastomosis.**

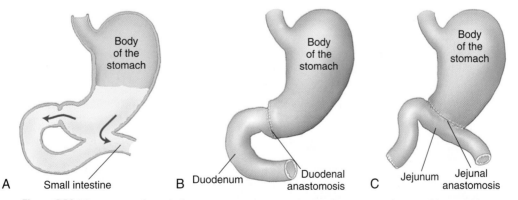

A   Small intestine

Body
of the
stomach

B   Duodenum   Duodenal
anastomosis

Body
of the
stomach

C   Jejunum   Jejunal
anastomosis

Body
of the
stomach

Figure 6.34 Three types of surgical anastomoses. A, Gastroenterostomy. A passage is created between the stomach and some part of the small intestine, often the jejunum. **B,** Gastroduodenostomy. The lower portion of the stomach is removed, and the remainder is anastomosed to the duodenum. **C,** Gastrojejunostomy. The lower portion of the stomach is removed and the remainder is anastomosed to the jejunum. The remaining duodenal stump is closed.

stomach

Note that in both gastroduodenal and gastrojejunal anastomoses, the lower portion of the _____ is removed before the gastric stump is joined to some part of the small intestine.

6-118 Pyloro/plasty is surgical repair of the pyloric sphincter. It may be done when other methods of treating peptic ulcers have not been effective. Pyloroplasty consists of surgical enlargement of the pyloric sphincter to facilitate the easy passage of the stomach contents to the duodenum. (Pyloroplasty may be necessary when there is pyloric stenosis, a narrowing of the pyloric sphincter at the outlet of the stomach.) Learn additional surgical terms in Exercise 32.

FIND IT!
EXERCISE 32

Draw a slash between the word parts in the following list. Then find the meanings of the word parts within the definitions. (Draw the slash, and then perform the remainder of the activity as a mental exercise.)

1. **esophagogastroplasty** surgical repair of the esophagus and stomach in the area of the cardiac sphincter
2. **gastropexy** surgical fixation of the stomach that involves suturing the stomach to the abdominal wall to prevent displacement
3. **gastrorrhaphy** suture of the stomach
4. **pylorotomy** incision of the pylorus; often called **pyloromyotomy,** which is incision of the muscles of the pylorus and is done to expedite the passage of food from the stomach

BUILD IT!
EXERCISE 33

Use the following word parts to build terms. (Some word parts will be used more than once.)
duoden(o), gastr(o), ile(o), jejun(o), pylor(o), vag(o), -pexy, -stomy, -tomy

1. incision of the pylorus _____/_____
2. surgical fixation of the stomach _____/_____
3. formation of an opening between the jejunum and the ileum _____/_____/_____
4. severing of vagus nerve branches to reduce stomach acid _____/_____
5. anastomosis of the stomach and the duodenum _____/_____/_____

colon

6-119 A **colo/stomy** is generally performed after partial colectomy. A colostomy is surgical creation of an artificial anus on the abdominal wall by drawing the colon out to the surface or, in other words, creating an artificial opening (stoma) from the _____ on the abdominal surface. Colostomies may be permanent or temporary, perhaps to divert feces after surgery (see Fig. 2.47). Colostomy irrigation is used to clear the bowel of fecal matter (Fig. 6.35).

removal (excision)

6-120 In cases of acute appendic/itis (Fig. 6.36), an append/ectomy is usually performed. An **append/ectomy** is _____ of the appendix. A laparoscopic appendectomy may be performed at the time of laparoscopy for some patients (Fig. 6.37). The next exercise includes selected surgeries of the intestinal tract.

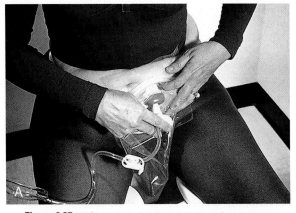
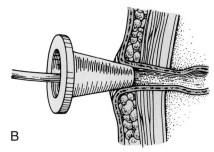

Figure 6.35 Colostomy irrigation. A, Patient places irrigation cone in the stomal opening. **B,** Cone with irrigation tubing in place and instillation of fluid to promote evacuation of feces.

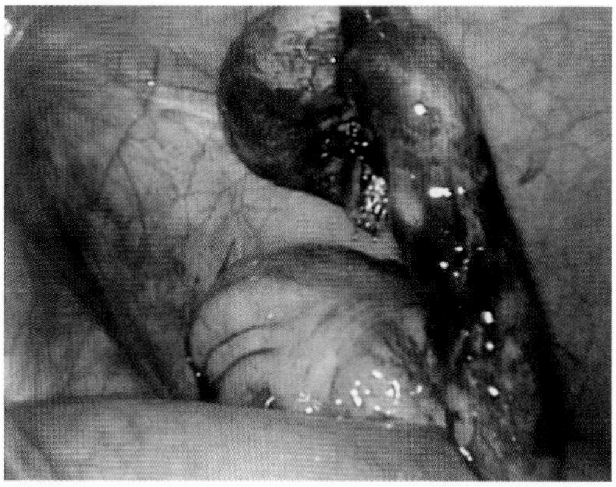

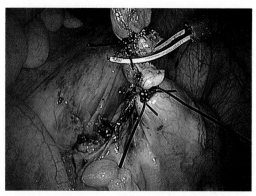

Figure 6.36 Laparoscopic view of appendicitis. Pain in the right lower quadrant prompted this patient to see the physician. Laparoscopy revealed acute appendicitis, which was easily removed laparoscopically.

Figure 6.37 Robotic laparoscopic appendectomy. While viewing through a laparoscope, the surgeon ties off the appendix at the proximal and distal ends, excises it with scissors or cautery, and then removes it through an umbilical port.

FIND IT!

EXERCISE 34

Draw a slash between the word parts in the following list. Then find the meanings of the word parts within the definitions. (Draw the slash, and then perform the remainder of the activity as a mental exercise.)

1. **cecoileostomy** formation of a new opening between the cecum and the ileum

2. **colectomy** excision of all, or a part, of the colon; a **hemicolectomy** is excision of approximately half of the colon and is sometimes referred to as either left hemicolectomy or right hemicolectomy

3. **diverticulectomy** surgical excision of a diverticulum; it may be performed if repeated bouts of diverticulitis result in obstruction of the colon

4. **duodenotomy** surgical incision of the duodenum. Formation of a new opening into the duodenum is **duodenostomy**

5. **ileostomy** forming an ileal stoma onto the surface of the abdomen—this is necessary if all of the colon is

removed; fecal material drains from the ileum into a bag worn on the abdomen

6. **jejunotomy** surgical incision of the jejunum

7. **laparoenterostomy** formation of an opening through the abdominal wall into the small intestine; sometimes done to install a tube to drain the bowel

8. **palatopharyngoplasty** surgical excision of palatal and oropharyngeal tissues; may be performed to remove obstructions thought to be causing snoring or sleep apnea; also called **uvulopalatopharyngoplasty**

9. **proctoplasty** surgical repair of the rectum and anus

WORD ORIGIN
ligation *(L.)*
ligare, to bind

pain

hemorrhoids

6-121 Stool softeners are used to prevent constipation, which can lead to hemorrhoids.

Nonsurgical management of hemorrhoids is aimed at reducing symptoms without surgery and decreasing the likelihood that the symptoms will recur. Topical anesthetics, application of cold packs, and soaks are used to alleviate hemorrhoidal pain. **Topi/cal** (top[o], place + -ical, pertaining to) means pertaining to a particular place on the surface area. You have learned that an anesthetic is used to produce a loss of sensation or feeling. The purpose of a topical an/esthetic is to alleviate _____ on a particular area of the skin.

Several surgical methods are available if symptoms persist, and treatment is determined by the type of hemorrhoid. Treatments include elastic band ligation and a **hemorrhoidectomy.** In elastic band ligation, the hemorrhoids are bound with rubber bands, become necrotic, and eventually slough off. A hemorrhoid/ectomy is excision of _____.

BUILD IT!
EXERCISE 35

Use the following word parts to build terms. (Some word parts will be used more than once.)

hemi-, cec(o), col(o), diverticul(o), enter(o), ile(o), lapar(o), -ectomy, -stomy

1. excision of approximately half of the colon   _____/_____/_____

2. formation of a new opening between the cecum and the ileum   _____/_____/_____

3. forming an ileal stoma   _____/_____

4. formation of an opening through the abdominal wall into the small intestine

    _____/_____/_____

5. surgical excision of a diverticulum   _____/_____

Accessory Organs of Digestion

insulin

6-122 Diabetes mellitus results primarily from either a deficiency or lack of insulin secretion by the pancreas or a resistance to insulin. Some forms of diabetes are treated with diet, exercise, and weight control; other forms require glucose-lowering agents (oral agents or insulin by injection). Diabetes mellitus results primarily from a lack of _____ secretion by the pancreas or resistance to insulin.

6-123 Gallstones are a common disorder of the gallbladder and bile ducts and are usually associated with cholecystitis. Several nonsurgical approaches are available, including oral drugs that dissolve stones, **laser lithotripsy,** and **extracorporeal shock wave lithotripsy** (ESWL).

lithotripsy

   In ESWL, extracorporeal (outside the body) shock wave _____, a lithotriptor uses high-energy shock waves to disintegrate the stone. The patient is positioned over a shock wave generator (lithotriptor) by means of a table that moves upward and downward, forward and backward, and side to side. Particles slough off the gallstone as the lithotriptor is fired, and the particles pass through the biliary ducts and are eliminated. The name of the shock wave generator

lithotriptor

in biliary lithotripsy is a _____ (Fig. 6.38).

6-124 **Litho/tripsy** is nonsurgical management of gallstones and can sometimes be an alternative to **cholecyst/ectomy,** surgical removal of the gallbladder. The gallbladder stores bile but is not essential for life, because bile is produced continuously.

   Endoscopic removal of biliary stones is called **endoscopic sphinctero/tomy** because the endoscope is passed to the duodenum, and then the sphincter muscle is incised to reach and retrieve the stone.

   Laparo/scopic cholecystectomy, removal of the gallbladder through four small incisions in the

abdominal

_____ wall, is currently preferred to open cholecystectomy whenever possible. Laparoscopic cholecystectomy is commonly done as an outpatient surgery. The surgical site is exposed through four small portals inserted into the abdominal wall, allowing the gallbladder to be excised and removed easily. The tissue removed is then sent to pathology for histologic examination.

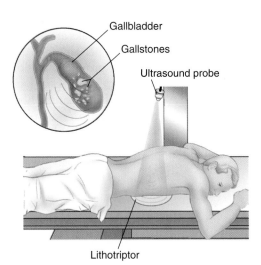

Figure 6.38 Biliary lithotripsy. The gallbladder is positioned over the lithotriptor; then the lithotriptor is fired and particles slough off the gallstones until they are fragmented and can pass through the biliary ducts.

cholecystotomy

6-125 Write a term that means surgical incision of the gallbladder: _____. This new term means incision of the gallbladder for the purpose of exploration, drainage, or removal of stones.

Laparo/cholecysto/tomy means incision into the gallbladder through the abdominal wall.

opening

6-126 Choledocho/litho/tripsy means the mechanical crushing of gallstones in the common bile duct. **Choledocho/stomy** is surgical formation of an _____ into the common bile duct through the abdominal wall. This is commonly done for temporary drainage of the duct after cholecystectomy.

jejunum

Choledocho/jejuno/stomy is surgical formation of a new opening between the common bile duct and the _____.

liver

6-127 Carcinoma that has spread from another site to the liver (metastasized) is more common than primary liver cancer. If the tumor is localized in one portion of the liver, **hepatic lob/ectomy,** excision of a lobe of the _____, may be performed. Other surgeries and chemotherapy are also used, depending on the type of liver cancer.

hepatectomy

6-128 Surgical incision of the liver is **hepato/tomy.** Excision of part of the liver is _____. Liver transplantation may be performed in some cases, usually for liver disease related to chronic viral hepatitis.

pancreatectomy

6-129 Pancreato/tomy is incision of the pancreas. Removal of all or part of the pancreas is a _____. **Pancreato/lith/ectomy** is removal of pancreatic stones.

6-130 Treatment of infected salivary glands includes antibiotics and warm compresses. If the flow of saliva is obstructed by a stone, the duct's opening may be dilated and massaged. If these measures fail, surgery may be necessary to remove the stone.

Tumors of the salivary glands, either benign or malignant, are excised. However, radiation therapy may be used for highly malignant or very large tumors or for recurrence of a tumor after surgery.

BUILD IT! EXERCISE 36

Use the following word parts to build terms. (Some word parts will be used more than once.)

choledoch(o), hepat(o), lith(o), pancreat(o), -ectomy, -stomy, -tomy, -tripsy

1. surgical crushing of a stone   _____/_____
2. incision of the pancreas   _____/_____
3. surgical removal of a stone from the pancreas   _____/_____/_____
4. surgical incision of the liver   _____/_____
5. formation of an opening into the common bile duct   _____/_____

MATCH IT! EXERCISE 37

Match terms in the left column with their descriptions in the right column.

____ **1.** anastomosis
____ **2.** antidiarrheals
____ **3.** diabetes mellitus
____ **4.** total parenteral nutrition
____ **5.** gastric bypass
____ **6.** hyperalimentation
____ **7.** lavage
____ **8.** liposuction
____ **9.** parenteral
____ **10.** topical anesthetics

A. a type of gastroplasty
B. administration of all nutrition through an indwelling catheter
C. agents to reduce feeling, applied to the mucous membranes or skin
D. connection between two organs
E. results primarily from deficiency or lack of insulin
F. irrigation or washing out of an organ
G. medications to treat diarrhea
H. not through the alimentary canal
I. overfeeding
J. removal of fat with a suction pump device

PHARMACOLOGY

Several pharmaceutics are helpful in the treatment of gastrointestinal problems. Various antibiotics are used, depending on the type of infectious microorganisms that are present.

Drug Class: Effects and Uses

Antacids: Neutralize stomach acid

calcium carbonate (Rolaids)

aluminum hydroxide and magnesium hydroxide (Mylanta)

Antidiabetic Drugs: Control blood sugar levels in patients with diabetes mellitus

acarbose (Precose)

glipizide (Glucotrol)

glyburide (DiaBeta)

insulin recombinant human (Humulin R)

insulin glargine (Lantus)

liraglutide (Victoza)

metformin (Glucophage)

miglitol (Glyset)

pioglitazone (Actos)

repaglinide (Prandin)

rosiglitazone (Avandia)

Antidiarrheals: Relieve symptoms of diarrhea

bismuth subsalicylate (Pepto-Bismol)

diphenoxylate with atropine (Lomotil)

loperamide (Imodium)

Antiemetics: Prevent or alleviate nausea and vomiting

Various anticholinergics, antihistamines, dopamine antagonists, serotonin antagonists, or benzodiazepines are used for their antiemetic effects.

dimenhydrinate (Dramamine)

meclizine (Antivert)

ondansetron (Zofran)

prochlorperazine (Compro)

trimethobenzamide (Tigan)

Antiobesity Drugs: Aid in weight loss

Anorexiants: Suppress the appetite

benzphetamine (Didrex)

phentermine (Adipex-P)

Lipase Inhibitors: Block absorption of fat from food

orlistat (Alli)

> **BEYOND** THE BLUEPRINT Alli, an over-the-counter drug, is not an anorexiant, but causes weight loss by preventing the body from breaking down excessive fats in the diet. The treatment effects of excess undigested fat passing out of the body are gas, loose stools, and sometimes diarrhea.

Antispasmodics: Relax smooth muscle of GI tract

dicyclomine (Bentyl)

hyoscyamine (Levbid)

Antiflatulents: Relieve or prevent excessive gas in the stomach and intestinal tract

lactase (Lactaid)

simethicone (Gas-X)

Emetics: Induce vomiting

*ipecac (*no brand name)*

Histamine-2 Receptor Antagonists (H2RAs): Block histamine-2 receptors to decrease gastric acid production

cimetidine (Tagamet)

famotidine (Pepcid)

ranitidine (Zantac)

Laxatives: Promote bowel evacuation; treat constipation

Multiple therapy types: increase the bulk of the feces, soften the stool, lubricate the intestinal wall, or stimulate contraction of the bowels

bisacodyl (Dulcolax)

docusate (Colace)

magnesium hydroxide (Milk of Magnesia)

mineral oil (Fleet Mineral Oil Enema)

psyllium (Metamucil)

senna (Senokot)

sennosides (Ex-Lax)

Purgatives or Cathartics: Cause full evacuation of the bowel, as in preparation for diagnostic studies or surgery of the digestive tract

PHARMACOLOGY, cont'd

Proton Pump Inhibitors (PPIs): Block final step of gastric acid production for long-lasting stomach acid suppression

esomeprazol (Nexium)
lansoprazole (Prevacid)

omeprazole (Prilosec)

Miscellaneous
activated charcoal (Actidose-Aqua): Bind toxins in stomach to prevent absorption in poison situations
mesalamine (Asacol): Antiinflammatory that works topically in the colon to treat ulcerative colitis

WRITE IT! EXERCISE 38

Write a word in the blank to complete these sentences.

1. The general class of pharmaceutics that neutralize stomach acid is _____.
2. The general class of pharmaceutics that prevent or alleviate nausea is _____.
3. The general class of pharmaceutics that relax the smooth muscle of the GI tract is _____.
4. The general class of pharmaceutics that suppress the appetite is _____ drugs.
5. The general class of pharmaceutics that induce vomiting is _____.

CHAPTER ABBREVIATIONS*

ALT	alanine aminotransferase
AST	aspartate aminotransferase
BMI	body mass index
DM	diabetes mellitus
DRI	dietary reference intake
EGD	esophagogastroduodenoscopy
ESWL	extracorporeal shock wave lithotripsy
GERD	gastroesophageal reflux disease
GI	gastrointestinal
HAV	hepatitis A virus
HBV	hepatitis B virus
HCV	hepatitis C virus
HDV	hepatitis D virus
HEV	hepatitis E virus
HSV	herpes simplex virus
H2RA	histamine-2 receptor antagonist

IBD	inflammatory bowel disease
IBS	irritable bowel syndrome
LFT	liver function test
N&V	nausea and vomiting
NG	nasogastric
PPI	proton pump inhibitor
SGOT	serum glutamate-oxaloacetic transaminase (enzyme test of heart and liver function, now called AST)
SGPT	serum glutamate-pyruvate transaminase (enzyme test of liver function, now called ALT)
TMJ	temporomandibular joint
TPN	total parenteral nutrition
UGI	upper gastrointestinal (or upper GI)

*Many of these abbreviations share their meanings with other terms.

A Career as a Registered Dietician

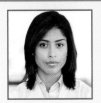

Maggie Sage is a registered dietician who works in a hospital. Maggie counsels patients about how the foods they eat affect disease processes, such as diabetes and heart disease. She worked in food service management previously but decided that she prefers the higher level of patient contact in clinical dietetics. Some of her friends work in sports dietetics; others counsel patients online. Maggie knows her work is vital to management of patients' conditions and that eating right is its own reward. For more information, visit the American Dietetic Association's website: *www.eatright.org*.

CHAPTER 6 SELF-TEST

BASIC UNDERSTANDING

Review the new word parts for this chapter. Work all of the following exercises to test your understanding of the material before checking your answers against those in Appendix IV.

Labeling

I.   Label the structures (1 through 13) in the diagram with the corresponding combining form. (Write two combining forms for numbers 2 and 6.)

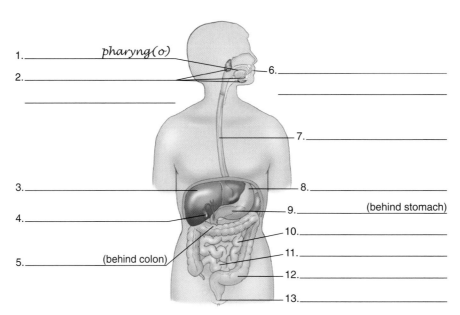

Matching

II.   Match the major functions of the digestive tract in the left column with their descriptions in the right column.

_____ **1.** absorption   **A.** eating food
_____ **2.** digestion   **B.** mechanically and chemically breaking down food
_____ **3.** elimination   **C.** passing nutrient molecules into blood or lymph
_____ **4.** ingestion   **D.** removing wastes

III.   Match structures of the digestive system in the left column with their descriptions in the right column.

_____ **1.** duodenum   **A.** connects with the cecum
_____ **2.** esophagus   **B.** first major site of digestion
_____ **3.** gallbladder   **C.** its lower end connects with the stomach
_____ **4.** ileum   **D.** its upper end connects with the stomach
_____ **5.** jejunum   **E.** midsection of the three parts of the small intestine
_____ **6.** liver   **F.** part of the large intestine
_____ **7.** mouth   **G.** produces bile
_____ **8.** pancreas   **H.** produces insulin
_____ **9.** stomach   **I.** stores bile
_____ **10.** transverse colon   **J.** where the buccal cavity is located

Listing

IV.   List the three classes of nutrients and explain their functions.

1. _____

2. _____

3. _____

V. List the four accessory organs of digestion and write their combining form(s).

1. _____ = _____

2. _____ = _____

3. _____ = _____

4. _____ = _____

Identifying Illustrations

VI. Label these illustrations using one of the following: bulimia, cholecystogram, cheilosis, diverticulitis, esophagojejunostomy, gastroscopy, lithotripsy, palatopharyngoplasty, polypectomy

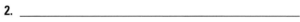

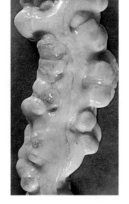

1. _____

2. _____

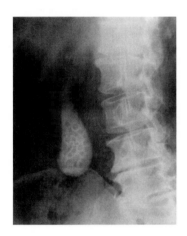

Gallbladder

Gallstones

Ultrasound probe

Lithotriptor

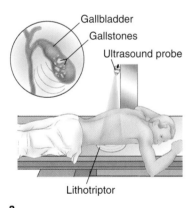

3. _____

4. _____

Deconstructing Words

VII. Divide these words into their component parts, and write the meanings of the terms.

1. ileocecal _____

2. choledocholithotripsy _____

3. cholestasis _____

4. esophagomyotomy _____

5. gastroduodenostomy _____

Using Vocabulary

VIII. Circle the correct answer for each of the following multiple choice questions.

1. Mrs. Vogel's physician tells her that she needs to see a specialist for the problem that she's been having with her colon. What is the name of the specialty practiced by the physician Mrs. Vogel should see? (cardiology, gastroenterology, gynecology, urology)

2. Cal Stone undergoes radiography of the gallbladder. What is the name of this diagnostic test? (barium enema, barium meal, cholecystography, esophagogastroscopy)

3. Tests show that Cal Stone has a gallstone in the common bile duct. Which of the following is a noninvasive conservative procedure to alleviate Cal's problem? (cholecystostomy, choledochostomy, choledochojejunostomy, extracorporeal shock wave lithotripsy)

4. Linda M., a 16-year-old girl, is diagnosed as having self-induced starvation. Which of the following is the name of the disorder associated with Linda's problem? (anorexia nervosa, aphagia, malaise, polyphagia)

5. Unless there is intervention for Linda's self-induced starvation, which condition is likely to result? (adipsia, atresia, emaciation, volvulus)

6. Mr. Gibson is diagnosed with cancer of the colon. Which term indicates a surgical intervention for this condition? (colectomy, colonoscopy, colonic irrigation, colonic stasis)

7. Baby Jake is born with a narrowing of the muscular ring that controls the outflow of food from the stomach. What is the name of this disorder? (pyloric sphincter, pyloric stenosis, pyloroplasty, pyloromyotomy)

8. Mary suffers from GERD. The physician explains to her that radiography indicates that a portion of the stomach is protruding upward through the diaphragm. What is the name of this disorder? (caries, cholelith, hiatal hernia, varices)

9. Jane is scheduled for a cheilostomatoplasty. What structures are involved in her surgery? (gums and mouth, lips and mouth, mouth and stomach, tongue and mouth)

10. A 70-year-old woman has an obstruction that has led to stagnation of the normal movement of food in the intestinal tract. What is the name of this condition? (duodenitis, enterostasis, peptic ulcer, peristalsis)

Writing Terms

IX.   Write a term for each of the following.

1. absence of thirst   _____
2. any disease of the stomach   _____
3. enzyme that breaks down starch   _____
4. excessive vomiting   _____
5. excision of the gallbladder   _____
6. incision of the vagus nerve   _____
7. inflammation of the stomach   _____
8. pertaining to the throat   _____
9. poor digestion   _____
10. visual inspection of the duodenum   _____

Making Connections

X.   Describe the relationship of these terms.

1. ingestion and digestion _____
_____

2. amylase and starch _____
_____

Finetuning Terms

XI.   In addition to spelling, describe at least one difference in the following:

1. fistula and fissure _____
_____

2. polydipsia and polyphagia _____
_____

3. gastralgia and gastritis _____
_____

Opting for Opposites

XII.   Write a term that you learned that means opposite of these words.

1. dyspepsia _____   2. hyperglycemia _____

GREATER COMPREHENSION

Health Care Reporting

XIII. Read this operative report, and answer the questions that follow it. Although you may be unfamiliar with some of the terms, you should be able to decide their meaning by determining the word parts.

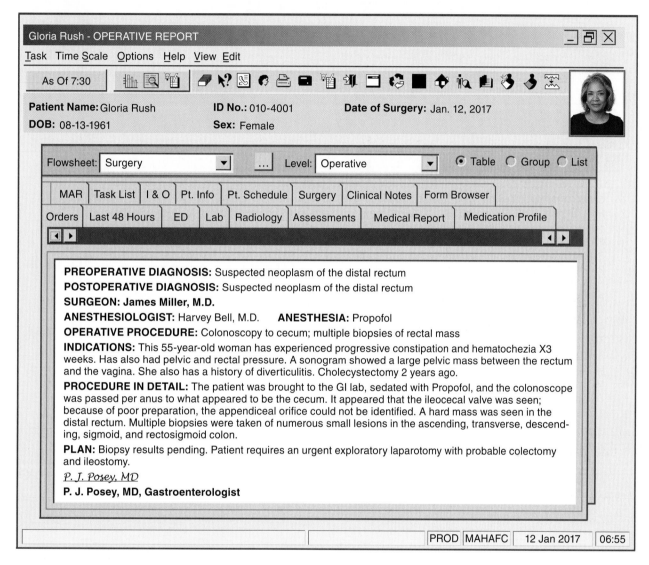

Gloria Rush - OPERATIVE REPORT

Task Time Scale Options Help View Edit

As Of 7:30

Patient Name: Gloria Rush   **ID No.:** 010-4001   **Date of Surgery:** Jan. 12, 2017
DOB: 08-13-1961   **Sex:** Female

Flowsheet: Surgery   Level: Operative   ● Table ○ Group ○ List

MAR | Task List | I & O | Pt. Info | Pt. Schedule | Surgery | Clinical Notes | Form Browser

Orders | Last 48 Hours | ED | Lab | Radiology | Assessments | Medical Report | Medication Profile

PREOPERATIVE DIAGNOSIS: Suspected neoplasm of the distal rectum
POSTOPERATIVE DIAGNOSIS: Suspected neoplasm of the distal rectum
SURGEON: James Miller, M.D.
ANESTHESIOLOGIST: Harvey Bell, M.D.   **ANESTHESIA:** Propofol
OPERATIVE PROCEDURE: Colonoscopy to cecum; multiple biopsies of rectal mass
INDICATIONS: This 55-year-old woman has experienced progressive constipation and hematochezia X3 weeks. Has also had pelvic and rectal pressure. A sonogram showed a large pelvic mass between the rectum and the vagina. She also has a history of diverticulitis. Cholecystectomy 2 years ago.
PROCEDURE IN DETAIL: The patient was brought to the GI lab, sedated with Propofol, and the colonoscope was passed per anus to what appeared to be the cecum. It appeared that the ileocecal valve was seen; because of poor preparation, the appendiceal orifice could not be identified. A hard mass was seen in the distal rectum. Multiple biopsies were taken of numerous small lesions in the ascending, transverse, descending, sigmoid, and rectosigmoid colon.
PLAN: Biopsy results pending. Patient requires an urgent exploratory laparotomy with probable colectomy and ileostomy.
P. J. Posey, MD
P. J. Posey, MD, Gastroenterologist

PROD | MAHAFC | 12 Jan 2017 | 06:55

Circle one answer for each of these questions.

1. To which body structure does the diagnosis pertain? (gallbladder, large intestine, small intestine, stomach)
2. Which of the following describes the rectum in the preoperative diagnosis? (abnormal new growth, enlarged, inflamed, impacted with feces)
3. The patient has a history of cholecystectomy. Which organ is removed in a cholecystectomy? (colon, gallbladder, liver, small intestine)
4. What structure is incised in a laparotomy? (abdominal wall, cecum, ileum, umbilicus)
5. All or part of which structure is excised in a colectomy? (large intestine, small intestine, stomach, umbilicus)
6. Where is the stoma created in an ileostomy? (abdomen, anus, colon, umbilicus)
   Write T *for True or* F *for False for each of these statements.*
7. The procedure involved a visual inspection of the large intestine. _____
8. The procedure involved excising tissue from a visible hard mass. _____
9. The patient has a history of hematochezia, which means she experienced bloody vomitus. _____
10. The patient has a history of diverticula with accompanying inflammation. _____
11. The surgeon identified the opening to the appendix. _____
12. The surgeon examined most of the small intestine. _____

XIV. Read the gastrointestinal consult and circle the correct answer in Questions 1-5.

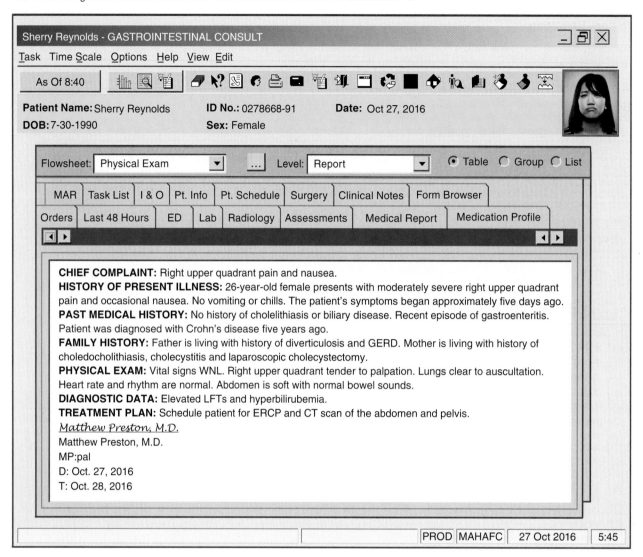

Circle the correct answer.

1. GERD indicates the patient's father suffered from a backflow of contents from the
   (esophagus, small intestine, stomach, colon).
2. The "L" in the abbreviation "LFT" refers to (lactose, lavage, lip, liver).
3. The term in the report which refers to a stone in the gallbladder is (cholecystectomy, cholecystitis, choledocholithiasis, cholelithiasis).
4. The term gastroenteritis indicates a disease involving the stomach and the (esophagus, liver, mouth, small intestine).
5. Which type of term is the abbreviation "LFT"? (anatomic, diagnostic, pathology, therapeutic)

XV. Read this consultation report. Although you may be unfamiliar with some of the terms, you should be able to decide their meanings by determining the word parts.

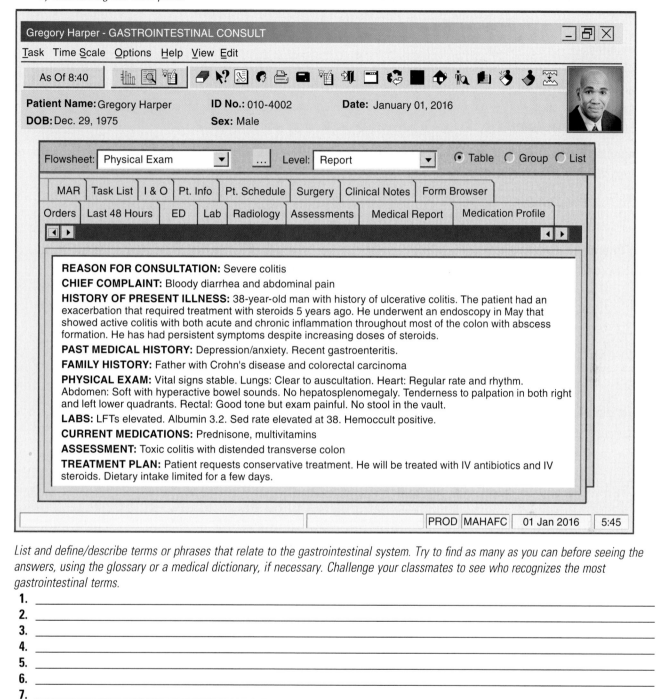

List and define/describe terms or phrases that relate to the gastrointestinal system. Try to find as many as you can before seeing the answers, using the glossary or a medical dictionary, if necessary. Challenge your classmates to see who recognizes the most gastrointestinal terms.

1. _____
2. _____
3. _____
4. _____
5. _____
6. _____
7. _____
8. _____
9. _____
10. _____

Spelling

XVI. Circle all misspelled terms, and write their correct spelling.

emaciation   enteral   glossorhaphy   nasogastrik   varaces

Abbreviating

XVII. Write a letter in each blank that corresponds to the clue.

1. aspartate aminotransferase ___ ___ ___

2. calculated index of obesity ___ ___ ___

3. esophagogastroduodenostomy ___ ___ ___

4. temporomandibular joint ___ ___ ___

5. virus associated with hepatitis B ___ ___ ___

6. upper gastrointestinal ___ ___ ___

Pronouncing Terms

XVIII. Write the correct term for the following phonetic spellings.

1. uh-**met**-ik _____

2. pal-uh-tō-fuh-**ring**-gō-plas-tē _____

3. stō-muh-tō-mī-**kō**-sis _____

4. uh-nas-tuh-**mō**-sis _____

5. uh-ruk-**tā**-shun _____

6. uh-**trē**-zhuh _____

Using Pharmacologic Terms

XIX. Use all selections to match terms in the left column with their descriptions in the right column.

_____ **1.** antidiabetic drugs

_____ **2.** antiflatulents

_____ **3.** antiobesity drugs

_____ **4.** laxatives

_____ **5.** emetics

_____ **6.** lipase inhibitors

A. block absorption of fats in foods

B. cause evacuation of the bowels

C. control blood sugar levels

D. induce vomiting

E. relieve or prevent excessive GI gas

F. suppress the appetite or block absorption of fats

Categorizing Terms and Practicing Pronunciation

XX. Categorize the terms in the left column by selecting A, B, C, D, or E.

_____ **1.** achalasia

_____ **2.** antiemetics

_____ **3.** cholecystogram

_____ **4.** choledochal

_____ **5.** diverticulosis

_____ **6.** esophagogram

_____ **7.** esophagoduodenostomy

_____ **8.** gingivoglossitis

_____ **9.** jaundice

_____ **10.** sialolithiasis

A. anatomy

B. diagnostic test or procedure

C. pathology

D. surgery

E. nonsurgical therapy

Be prepared to pronounce terms 1-10 in class after listening to the Chapter 6 terms at *http://evolve.elsevier.com/Leonard/building*. In addition, practice categorizing all boldface terms in this chapter.

New Construction

XXI. Break these words into their component parts, and write their meanings. Even if you have not seen these terms before, you may be able to break them apart and determine their meanings.

1. cecocolostomy _____

2. esophagogastrectomy _____

3. hemigastrectomy _____

4. sialogenous _____

5. sigmoidosigmoidostomy _____

(Use Appendix IV to check your answers to the exercises.)

BMV LIST

Visit *http://evolve.elsevier.com/Leonard/building/* to listen to the boldface terms in Chapter 6. Look closely at the spelling of each term as it is pronounced.

absorption (ab-**sorp**-shun)
adipsia (uh-**dip**-sē-uh)
alimentary tract (al-uh-**men**-tur-ē trakt)
alimentation (al-uh-men-**tā**-shun)
amylase (**am**-uh-lās)
amylolysis (am-uh-**lol**-uh-sis)
anal (**ā**-nul)
anastomose (uh-**nas**-tuh-mōs)
anastomosis (uh-nas-tuh-**mō**-sis)
anorexia (an-ō-**rek**-sē-uh)
anorexia nervosa (an-ō-**rek**-sē-uh ner-**vō**-suh)
anorexiant (an-ō-**rek**-sē-unt)
antacid (ant-**as**-id)
antidiabetic drugs (an-tē-dī-uh-**bet**-ik drugz)
antidiarrheal (an-tē-dī-uh-**rē**-ul)
antiemetics (an-tē-uh-**met**-iks)
antiflatulents (an-tē-**flat**-ū-lunts)
antiobesity drugs (an-tē-ō-**bēs**-i-tē drugz)
antispasmotics (an-tē-spaz-**mod**-iks)
anus (**ā**-nus)
aphagia (uh-**fā**-juh)
appendectomy (ap-en-**dek**-tuh-mē)
appendicitis (uh-pen-di-**sī**-tis)
appendicular (ap-en-**dik**-ū-lur)
bariatrics (bar-ē-**at**-riks)
bicuspids (bī-**kus**-pidz)
biliary (**bil**-ē-ar-ē)
bolus (**bō**-lus)
buccal cavity (**buk**-ul **kav**-i-tē)
buccal mucosa (**buk**-ul mū-**kō**-suh)
bulimia (bōō-**lē**-mē-uh)
cardiac region (**kahr**-dē-ak **rē**-jun)
caries (**kar**-ēz)
cecoileostomy (sē-kō-il-ē-**os**-tuh-mē)
cecum (**sē**-kum)
celiac disease (**sē**-lē-ak di-**zēz**)
cheilitis (kī-**lī**-tis)
cheiloplasty (**kī**-lō-plas-tē)
cheilorrhaphy (kī-**lor**-uh-fē)
cheilosis (kī-**lō**-sis)
cheilostomatoplasty (kī-lō-stō-**mat**-ō-plas-tē)
cholangiography (kō-lan-jē-**og**-ruh-fē)
cholangitis (kō-lan-**jī**-tis)
cholecystectomy (kō-luh-sis-**tek**-tuh-mē)
cholecystic (kō-luh-**sis**-tik)
cholecystitis (kō-luh-sis-**tī**-tis)
cholecystogastric (kō-luh-sis-tō-**gas**-trik)
cholecystogram (kō-luh-**sis**-tō-gram)
cholecystography (kō-luh-sis-**tog**-ruh-fē)
cholecystotomy (kō-luh-sis-**tot**-uh-mē)
choledochal (kō-**led**-uh-kul)

choledochitis (kō-luh-dō-**kī**-tis)
choledochojejunostomy (kō-led-uh-kō-juh-jōō-**nos**-tuh-mē)
choledocholithiasis (kō-led-uh-kō-li-**thī**-uh-sis)
choledocholithotripsy (kō-led-uh-kō-**lith**-ō-trip-sē)
choledochostomy (kō-led-uh-**kos**-tuh-mē)
cholelithiasis (kō-luh-li-**thī**-uh-sis)
cholestasis (kō-luh-**stā**-sis)
chyme (kīm)
cirrhosis (si-**rō**-sis)
colectomy (kō-**lek**-tuh-mē)
colic (**kol**-ik)
colitis (kō-**lī**-tis)
colon (**kō**-lun)
colonic (kō-**lon**-ik)
colonoscope (kō-**lon**-ō-skōp)
colonoscopy (kō-lun-**os**-kuh-pē)
colorectal (kō-lō-**rek**-tul)
coloscopy (kō-**los**-kō-pē)
colostomy (kuh-**los**-tuh-mē)
cuspids (**kus**-pidz)
defecate (**def**-uh-kāt)
defecation (def-uh-**kā**-shun)
dental (**den**-tul)
dentalgia (den-**tal**-juh)
dentilingual (den-ti-**ling**-wul)
denture (**den**-chur)
diabetes mellitus (dī-uh-**bē**-tēz **mel**-luh-tus, muh-**lī**-tis)
digestion (dī-**jes**-chun)
diverticulectomy (dī-vur-tik-ū-**lek**-tuh-mē)
diverticulitis (dī-vur-tik-ū-**lī**-tis)
diverticulosis (dī-vur-tik-ū-**lō**-sis)
diverticulum (dī-vur-**tik**-ū-lum)
duodenal (dōō-ō-**dē**-nul, dōō-**od**-uh-nul)
duodenitis (dōō-od-uh-**nī**-tis)
duodenoscope (dōō-ō-**dē**-no-skōp)
duodenoscopy (dōō-ō-duh-**nos**-kuh-pē)
duodenostomy (dōō-ō-duh-**nos**-tuh-mē)
duodenotomy (dōō-ō-duh-**not**-uh-mē)
duodenum (dōō-ō-**dē**-num, dōō-**od**-uh-num)
dysentery (**dis**-un-ter-ē)
dyspepsia (dis-**pep**-sē-uh)
dysphagia (dis-**fā**-jē-uh)
elimination (ē-lim-i-**nā**-shun)
emaciation (ē-mā-shē-**ā**-shun)
emesis (**em**-uh-sis)
emetic (uh-**met**-ik)
endodontics (en-dō-**don**-tiks)
endodontist (en-dō-**don**-tist)
endodontitis (en-dō-don-**tī**-tis)
endodontium (en-dō-**don**-shē-um)
endogastric (en-dō-**gas**-trik)

endogenous obesity (en-**doj**-uh-nus ō-**bēs**-i-tē)
endoscopic sphincterotomy (en-dō-**skop**-ik
  sfingk-tur-**ot**-uh-mē)
enteral (**en**-tur-ul)
enteric (en-**ter**-ik)
enteritis (en-ter-ī-tis)
enterostasis (en-ter-ō-**stā**-sis)
eructation (uh-ruk-**tā**-shun)
esophageal (uh-sof-uh-**jē**-ul)
esophageal achalasia (uh-sof-uh-**jē**-ul ak-uh-**lā**-zhuh)
esophageal atresia (uh-sof-uh-**jē**-ul uh-**trē**-zhuh)
esophageal varices (uh-sof-uh-**jē**-ul **vār**-i-sēz)
esophagectomy (uh-sof-uh-**jek**-tuh-mē)
esophagitis (uh-sof-uh-**jī**-tis)
esophagoduodenostomy (uh-sof-uh-gō-doo-ō-duh-**nos**-tuh-mē)
esophagodynia (uh-sof-uh-gō-**din**-ē-uh)
esophagogastroduodenoscopy (uh-sof-uh-gō-gas-trō-doo-
  od-uh-**nos**-kuh-pē)
esophagogastroplasty (uh-sof-uh-gō-**gas**-trō-plas-tē)
esophagogastroscopy (uh-sof-uh-gō-gas-**tros**-kuh-pē)
esophagogastrostomy (uh-sof-uh-gō-gas-**tros**-tuh-mē)
esophagogram (uh-**sof**-uh-gō-gram)
esophagojejunostomy (uh-sof-uh-gō-juh-joo-**nos**-tuh-mē)
esophagomalacia (uh-sof-uh-gō-muh-**lā**-shuh)
esophagomyotomy (uh-sof-uh-gō-mī-**ot**-uh-mē)
esophagoscopy (uh-sof-uh-**gos**-kuh-pē)
esophagostomy (uh-sof-uh-**gos**-tuh-mē)
esophagram (uh-**sof**-uh-gram)
esophagus (uh-**sof**-uh-gus)
eupepsia (ū-**pep**-sē-uh)
exogenous obesity (ek-**soj**-uh-nus ō-**bēs**-i-tē)
extracorporeal shock wave lithotripsy (eks-truh-kor-**por**-ē-ul
  shok wāv **lith**-ō-trip-sē)
extrahepatic (eks-truh-huh-**pat**-ik)
feces (**fē**-sēz)
fissure (**fish**-ur)
fistula (**fis**-tū-luh)
fundus (**fun**-dus)
gastralgia (gas-**tral**-juh)
gastrectasia (gas-trek-**tā**-zhuh)
gastrectomy (gas-**trek**-tuh-mē)
gastric (**gas**-trik)
gastric carcinoma (**gas**-trik kahr-si-**nō**-muh)
gastritis (gas-**trī**-tis)
gastroduodenal anastomosis (gas-trō-doo-ō-**dē**-dul
  uh-nas-tuh-**mō**-sis)
gastroduodenitis (gas-trō-doo-ō-duh-**nī**-tis)
gastroduodenostomy (gas-trō-doo-ō-duh-**nos**-tuh-mē)
gastroenteritis (gas-trō-en-tur-ī-tis)
gastroenterology (gas-trō-en-tur-**ol**-uh-jē)
gastroenterostomy (gas-trō-en-tur-**os**-tuh-mē)
gastrointestinal (gas-trō-in-**tes**-ti-nul)
gastrojejunal anastomosis (gas-trō-juh-**joo**-nul
  uh-nas-tuh-**mō**-sis)
gastrojejunostomy (gas-trō-juh-joo-**nos**-tuh-mē)
gastromalacia (gas-trō-muh-**lā**-shuh)
gastromegaly (gas-trō-**meg**-uh-lē)

gastropathy (gas-**trop**-uh-thē)
gastropexy (gas-trō-pek-sē)
gastroplasty (**gas**-trō-plas-tē)
gastrorrhaphy (gas-**tror**-uh-fē)
gastroscope (**gas**-trō-skōp)
gastroscopy (gas-**tros**-kuh-pē)
gastrostomy (gas-**tros**-tuh-mē)
gerodontics (jer-ō-**don**-tiks)
gerodontist (jer-ō-**don**-tist)
gingiva (**jin**-ji-vuh)
gingival (**jin**-ji-vul)
gingivalgia (jin-ji-**val**-juh)
gingivectomy (jin-ji-**vek**-tuh-mē)
gingivitis (jin-ji-**vī**-tis)
gingivoglossitis (jin-ji-vō-glos-ī-tis)
gingivostomatitis (jin-ji-vō-stō-muh-**tī**-tis)
glossal (**glos**-ul)
glossectomy (glos-**ek**-tuh-mē)
glossitis (glos-ī-tis)
glossopathy (glos-**op**-uh-thē)
glossopharyngeal (glos-ō-fuh-**rin**-jē-ul)
glossoplasty (**glos**-ō-plas-tē)
glossoplegia (glos-ō-**plē**-juh)
glossopyrosis (glos-ō-pī-**rō**-sis)
glossorrhaphy (glos-**or**-uh-fē)
glucagon (**gloo**-kuh-gon)
glucose (**gloo**-kōs)
gluten (**gloo**-tun)
glycolysis (glī-**kol**-uh-sis)
halitosis (hal-i-**tō**-sis)
hematemesis (hē-muh-**tem**-uh-sis)
hematochezia (hē-muh-tō, hem-uh-tō-**kē**-zhuh)
hemicolectomy (hem-ē-kō-**lek**-tuh-mē)
hemorrhoid (**hem**-uh-roid)
hemorrhoidectomy (hem-uh-roid-**ek**-tuh-mē)
hepatectomy (hep-uh-**tek**-tuh-mē)
hepatic (huh-**pat**-ik)
hepatic lobectomy (huh-**pat**-ik lō-**bek**-tuh-mē)
hepatitis (hep-uh-**tī**-tis)
hepatolytic (hep-uh-tō-**lit**-ik)
hepatoma (hep-uh-**tō**-muh)
hepatomegaly (hep-uh-tō-**meg**-uh-lē)
hepatopathy (hep-uh-**top**-uh-thē)
hepatorenal syndrome (hep-uh-tō-**rē**-nul **sin**-drōm)
hepatosplenomegaly (hep-uh-tō-splē-nō-**meg**-uh-lē)
hepatotomy (hep-uh-**tot**-uh-mē)
hepatotoxic (**hep**-uh-tō-tok-sik)
hiatal hernia (hī-**ā**-tul **hur**-nē-uh)
histamine-2 receptor antagonists (**his**-tuh-mēn-2 rē-**sep**-tur
  an-**tag**-uh-nists)
hyperacidity (hī-pur-uh-**sid**-i-tē)
hyperalimentation (hī-pur-al-uh-men-**tā**-shun)
hyperemesis (hī-pur-**em**-uh-sis)
hyperglycemia (hī-pur-glī-**sē**-mē-uh)
hypoglossal (hī-pō-**glos**-ul)
hypoglycemia (hī-pō-glī-**sē**-mē-uh)
ileac (**il**-ē-ak)

ileal (**il**-ē-ul)
ileitis (il-ē-**ī**-tis)
ileocecal valve (il-ē-ō-**sē**-kul valv)
ileostomy (il-ē-**os**-tuh-mē)
ileum (**il**-ē-um)
impaction (im-**pak**-shun)
incisors (in-**sī**-zurs)
ingestion (in-**jes**-chun)
insulin (**in**-suh-lin)
interdental (in-tur-**den**-tul)
intestinal (in-**tes**-ti-nul)
intussusception (in-tuh-suh-**sep**-shun)
jaundice (**jawn**-dis)
jejunal (juh-**joo**-nul)
jejunoileostomy (juh-joo-nō-il-ē-**os**-tuh-mē)
jejunostomy (juh-joo-**nos**-tuh-mē)
jejunotomy (juh-joo-**not**-uh-mē)
jejunum (juh-**joo**-num)
laparocholecystotomy (lap-uh-rō-kō-luh-sis-**tot**-uh-mē)
laparoenterostomy (lap-uh-rō-en-tur-**os**-tuh-mē)
laparoscopic cholecystectomy (lap-uh-rō-**skop**-ik
   kō-luh-sis-**tek**-tuh-mē)
laser lithotripsy (**lā**-zur **lith**-ō-trip-sē)
lavage (lah-**vahzh**)
laxative (**lak**-suh-tiv)
leukoplakia (loo-kō-**plā**-kē-uh)
lingual (**ling**-gwul)
lipase (**lip**-ās, **lī**-pās)
lipectomy (li-**pek**-tuh-mē)
lipids (**lip**-idz)
lipoid (**lip**-oid)
lipopenia (lip-ō-**pē**-nē-uh)
liposuction (lip-ō-**suk**-shun)
lithotripsy (**lith**-ō-trip-sē)
lithotriptor (**lith**-ō-trip-tur)
lower gastrointestinal series (**lō**-ur gas-trō-in-**tes**-ti-nul
   sēr-ēz)
malabsorption syndrome (mal-ub-**sorp**-shun **sin**-drōm)
malnutrition (mal-noo-**trish**-un)
malocclusion (mal-uh-**kloo**-zhun)
mandible (**man**-di-bul)
mandibular (man-**dib**-ū-lur)
maxilla (mak-**sil**-uh)
maxillary (**mak**-si-lar-ē)
metabolism (muh-**tab**-uh-liz-um)
molars (**mō**-lurz)
mucoid (**mū**-koid)
mucosa (mū-**kō**-suh)
mucous (**mū**-kus)
nasogastric tube (nā-zō-**gas**-trik toob)
obesity (ō-**bēs**-i-tē)
oral cavity (**or**-ul **kav**-i-tē)
oropharyngeal (or-ō-fuh-**rin**-jē-ul)
orthodontics (or-thō-**don**-tiks)
orthodontist (or-thō-**don**-tist)
palatine (**pal**-uh-tīn)
palatopharyngoplasty (pal-uh-tō-fuh-**ring**-gō-plas-tē)

pancreatectomy (pan-krē-uh-**tek**-tuh-mē)
pancreatic (pan-krē-**at**-ik)
pancreatitis (pan-krē-uh-**tī**-tis)
pancreatography (pan-krē-uh-**tog**-ruh-fē)
pancreatolith (pan-krē-**at**-ō-lith)
pancreatolithectomy (pan-krē-uh-tō-li-**thek**-tuh-mē)
pancreatolithiasis (pan-krē-uh-tō-li-**thī**-uh-sis)
pancreatolysis (pan-krē-uh-**tol**-i-sis)
pancreatotomy (pan-krē-uh-**tot**-uh-mē)
parenteral (puh-**ren**-tur-ul)
parotid gland (puh-**rot**-id gland)
parotitis (par-ō-**tī**-tis)
pedodontics (pē-dō-**don**-tiks)
pedodontist (pē-dō-**don**-tist)
percutaneous transhepatic cholangiography (pur-kū-**tā**-nē-us
   trans-he-**pat**-ik kō-lan-jē-**og**-ruh-fē)
pericolic (per-ē-**kol**-ik)
periodontal (per-ē-ō-**don**-tul)
periodontics (per-ē-ō-**don**-tiks)
periodontist (per-ē-ō-**don**-tist)
periodontitis (per-ē-ō-don-**tī**-tis)
periodontium (per-ē-ō-**don**-shē-um)
peristalsis (per-i-**stawl**-sis)
pharyngeal (fuh-**rin**-jē-ul)
pharynx (**far**-inks)
polydipsia (pol-ē-**dip**-sē-uh)
polypectomy (pol-i-**pek**-tuh-mē)
polyphagia (pol-ē-**fā**-juh)
postesophageal (pōst-uh-sof-uh-**jē**-ul)
proctologist (prok-**tol**-uh-jist)
proctoplasty (**prok**-tō-plas-tē)
proctosigmoidoscopy (prok-tō-sig-moi-**dos**-kuh-pē)
protease (**prō**-tē-ās)
proteinase (**prō**-tēn-ās)
proteolysis (prō-tē-**ol**-i-sis)
proton pump inhibitor (**prō**-ton pump in-**hib**-i-tur)
pyloric region (pī-**lor**-ik **rē**-jun)
pyloromyotomy (pī-lor-ō-mī-**ot**-uh-mē)
pyloroplasty (pī-**lor**-ō-plas-tē)
pyloroscopy (pī-lor-**os**-kuh-pē)
pylorotomy (pī-lor-**ot**-uh-mē)
pylorus (pī-**lor**-us)
pyorrhea (pī-ō-**rē**-uh)
rectal (**rek**-tul)
rectum (**rek**-tum)
retrocecal (ret-rō-**sē**-kul)
retrocolic (ret-rō-**kol**-ik)
rugae (**roo**-jē)
salmonellosis (sal-mō-nul-**ō**-sis)
serosa (sēr-**ō**-suh, sēr-**ō**-zuh)
sialadenitis (sī-ul-ad-uh-**nī**-tis)
sialography (sī-uh-**log**-ruh-fē)
sialolithiasis (sī-al-ō-li-**thī**-uh-sis)
sigmoid colon (**sig**-moid)
sigmoidoscope (sig-**moi**-dō-skōp)
sigmoidoscopy (sig-moi-**dos**-kuh-pē)
sphincter (**sfingk**-tur)

stomatitis (stō-muh-**tī**-tis)
stomatodynia (stō-muh-tō-**din**-ē-uh)
stomatomycosis (stō-muh-tō-mī-**kō**-sis)
stomatoplasty (**stō**-muh-tō-plas-tē)
sublingual (sub-**ling**-gwul)
sublingual gland (sub-**ling**-gwul gland)
submandibular glands (sub-man-**dib**-ū-lur glandz)
suprahepatic (soo-pruh-huh-**pat**-ik)
temporomandibular joint (tem-puh-rō-man-**dib**-ū-lur joint)
topical (**top**-i-kul)

total parenteral nutrition (**tō**-tul puh-**ren**-tur-ul noo-**trish**-un)
upper gastrointestinal series (**up**-ur gas-trō-in-**tes**-ti-nul
      sēr-ēz)
uvulopalatopharyngoplasty
      (ū-vū-lō-pal-uh-tō-fuh-**ring**-gō-plas-tē)
vagotomy (vā-**got**-uh-mē)
vermiform appendix (**vur**-mi-form uh-**pen**-diks)
villi (**vil**-ī)
volvulus (**vol**-vū-lus)

Español ENHANCING SPANISH COMMUNICATION

English	Spanish (Pronunciation)
appetite	apetito (ah-pay-TEE-to)
belch	eructo (ay-ROOK-to)
chew, to	masticar (mas-te-KAR)
constipation	estreñimiento (es-tray-nye-me-EN-to)
defecate	evacuar (ay-vah-koo-AR)
dentist	dentista (den-TEES-tah)
diabetes	diabetes (de-ah-BAY-tes)
digestion	digestión (de-hes-te-ON)
enzyme	enzima (en-SEE-mah)
esophagus	esófago (ay-SO-fah-go)
excretion	excreción (ex-kray-se-ON)
feces	excremento (ex-kray-MEN-to)
gallbladder	vesícula biliar (vay-SEE-koo-la be-le-AR)
gallstone	cálculo biliar (KAHL-koo-lo be-le-AR)
glucose	glucosa (gloo-KO-sah)
gum, gingiva	encía (en-SEE-ah)
hunger	hambre (AHM-bray)
insulin	insulina (in-soo-LEE-nah)
laxative	purgante (poor-GAHN-tay)
lips	labios (LAH-be-os)
milk	leche (LAY-chay)
mouth	boca (BO-kah)
orthodontist	ortodóntico (or-to-DON-te-ko)
pancreas	páncreas (PAHN-kray-as)
rectum	recto (REK-to)
saliva	saliva (sah-LEE-vah)
starch	almidón (al-me-DON)
swallow	tragar (trah-GAR)
teeth	dientes (de-AYN-tays)
thirst	sed (sayd)
tongue	lingua (LEN-goo-ah)

Urinary System

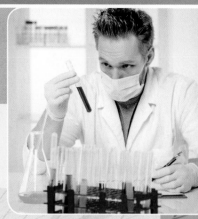

Urology is the specialized knowledge and skill regarding problems of the male and female urinary tract and the male reproductive organs. Urine is liquid waste that is produced by the kidneys and eliminated through urination. A number of diseases and conditions can be detected in the urine, thus urinalysis is often part of a health check-up. Because many drugs are excreted in the urine, toxicology screening is routine in some occupations to detect illegal drug use.

CONTENTS

Basic Understanding

In this chapter, you will learn to do the following:

1. State the function of the urinary system, and analyze associated terms.
2. Write the names of the structures of the urinary system, define the terms associated with these structures, and label the structures.
3. Write the meanings of the word parts associated with the urinary system, and use them to build and analyze terms.
4. Identify the major structures of the nephron and their functions.
5. Sequence the formation and excretion of urine.
6. Write the names of the diagnostic tests and procedures for assessment of the urinary system when given descriptions of the tests and procedures, or match the names with their descriptions.
7. Distinguish between normal and abnormal components of urine.
8. Match the terms for urinary system pathologies with their meanings, or write the names of the pathologies when given their descriptions.
9. Describe the significance of genitourinary infections and their association with sexually transmitted diseases.
10. Match terms for surgical and other therapeutic interventions for urinary system pathologies with descriptions of the interventions, or write the names of the interventions when given their descriptions.
11. Build terms from word parts to label illustrations.

Greater Comprehension

12. Select the correct meanings of terms and write the meanings of abbreviations in a health care report pertaining to the urinary system.
13. Spell the terms accurately.
14. Pronounce the terms correctly.
15. Write the meanings of the abbreviations.
16. Categorize terms as anatomy, diagnostic test or procedure, pathology, surgery, or nonsurgical therapy.
17. Recognize the meanings of general pharmacological terms from this chapter as well as the drug classes and their uses.

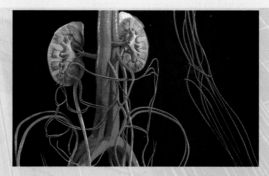

FUNCTION FIRST

The urinary system plays an important role in maintaining homeostasis by constantly filtering the blood to remove urea and other waste products, maintaining the proper balance of water, salts, and other substances by removing or reabsorbing them as needed, maintaining the blood pH, and excreting the waste products via the urine. Less known roles are production of renin, erythropoietin, and prostaglandins, as well as degradation of insulin and metabolism of vitamin D to its active form.

WRITE IT!   EXERCISE 1

List the five functions of the urinary system.

1. _____   4. _____
2. _____   5. _____
3. _____

ANATOMY AND PHYSIOLOGY

7-1 There are several **excretory** routes through which the body eliminates wastes. The lungs eliminate carbon dioxide. The digestive system provides a means of expelling solid wastes. The skin serves as an excretory organ by eliminating wastes in the form of perspiration. Another important mode of **excretion** is performed by the kidneys, which are part of the urinary system.

urine

The combining form urin(o) means urine. **Urin/ary** means pertaining to _____. The organs and ducts that are involved in the secretion and excretion (elimination) of urine from the body are referred to as the **urinary tract**.

Anatomy of Major Urinary Structures

7-2 You learned in an earlier chapter that ur(o) means urinary system or urine. In terms that use the combining form ur(o), you will use your critical thinking skills to decide which meaning is intended.

The urinary system consists of paired kidneys, one on each side of the spinal column, a ureter for each kidney, a bladder, and a urethra. The terms *ureter* and *urethra* are often confused, but note the difference in their spelling. Remember, the body has two kidneys, two ureters, one bladder, and only one _____.

urethra

7-3 The kidneys are located in the dorsal part of the abdomen. Fig. 7.1 shows the location of these structures. Read all the information that accompanies Fig. 7.1. Complete the blank lines 1 through 4 by reading the following information.

Urine is formed in the kidneys. Label the left kidney *(1)*. The **ureters** carry the urine to the urinary bladder. Label the left ureter *(2)*. The **bladder** *(3)* is a temporary reservoir for the urine until it is excreted via the **urethra** *(4)*. The external opening of the urethra is called the **urinary meatus.**

The information that accompanies Fig. 7.1 explains that blood is transported to the kidneys by vessels of the cardio/vascular (cardi[o], heart + vascul[o], vessel + -ar, pertaining to) system. These vessels that carry blood to the kidneys are **renal** _____. The notch or depression on the inner border of the kidney, called the **hilum,** is where blood vessels, lymphatics, and nerves enter or leave the kidney.

arteries

➤ **BEYOND** THE BLUEPRINT Perhaps thinking of a kidney bean, which is so named because it is shaped like a kidney, will help your understanding of the kidney's anatomy.

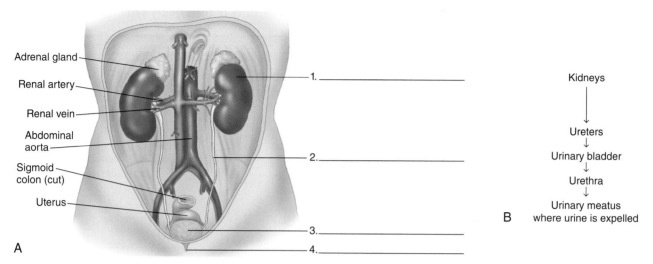

Figure 7.1 The urinary system and flow of urine. A, Major urinary structures. Adjacent vessels of the cardiovascular system are also shown. The right and left renal arteries branch off the abdominal aorta to transport blood to the kidneys. Urine, formed in the kidneys, leaves by way of the ureters and passes to the bladder, where it is stored. When voluntary control is removed, urine is expelled through the urethra. When blood is filtered by the kidneys, wastes are removed, but much of the water and other substances are reabsorbed. They enter the renal vein and are returned to the bloodstream via the inferior vena cava. **B,** The flow of urine from where it is formed in the kidney to where it is expelled.

---

ureter

7-4 The funnel-shaped structure where a kidney joins the ureter is called the *renal pelvis,* and it drains urine from the kidney to the _____.

Anatomic features of the kidney are shown in Fig. 7.2. Each kidney is encased in a fibrous capsule, which provides protection for the delicate internal parts. The ribs and muscle near the kidneys are added protection.

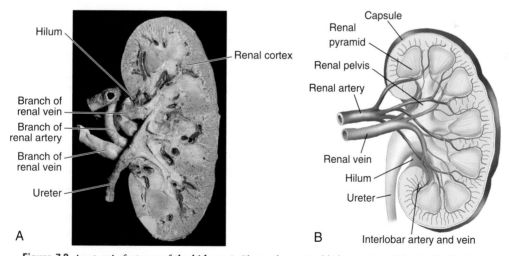

Figure 7.2 Anatomic features of the kidney. A, Photo of an excised kidney, sectioned longitudinally shows the renal cortex, the thick outer part as well as the major vessels. **B,** Illustration of the internal structure of the kidney. Looking at both **A** and **B,** try to locate the capsule and renal pyramids in **A.**

WRITE IT!
EXERCISE 2

Write a word in each blank to complete this paragraph.

Filtering occurs in the paired structures, the (1) _____. Urine is carried to the urinary bladder by the two (2) _____, where it is temporarily stored until it is excreted via the (3) _____.

Learn the following word parts for major structures of the urinary system.

Word Parts: Urinary Structures

Word Part	Meaning	Combining Form	Meaning
ur(o)	urine, urinary tract	**Internal Structures of the Kidneys**	
urin(o)	urine	glomerul(o)	glomerulus
-uria	urine or urination	pyel(o)	renal pelvis
Major Urinary Structures		**Other**	
cyst(o)	bladder (also cyst or fluid-filled sac)	genit(o)	organs of reproduction
nephr(o), ren(o)	kidney	gon(o)	genitals or reproduction
ureter(o)	ureter	rect(o)	rectum
urethr(o)	urethra		
vesic(o)	bladder or blister		

WRITE IT!   EXERCISE 3

Write combining forms for the following.

1. bladder or cyst _____
2. bladder or blister _____
3. genitals or reproduction _____

4. renal pelvis _____
5. ureter _____
6. urine or urinary tract _____

7-5 Most of the work of the urinary system takes place in the **kidneys.** The average adult kidney is about 11 cm long by 6 cm wide (about 4½ by 2⅓ inches) and weighs about 145 grams (less than half a pound). Playing a major role in homeostasis of the body, the kidneys are the major regulators of the water and pH ("potential" hydrogen; hydrogen ion concentration) of the blood and, indirectly, all body fluids.

red

Lesser known kidney functions are production of **erythropoietin** (causes the production of red blood cells [RBCs]), renin (helps regulate blood pressure), and prostaglandins (act in several target organs with a variety of effects). Erythr(o) means _____, and -poietin means that which causes production. In addition, the kidneys help degrade insulin and metabolize vitamin D.

7-6 Urine leaves the kidney by way of the right and left ureters, which take it to the bladder. **Vesic/al** means pertaining to a fluid-filled sac, usually the urinary bladder. **Vesico/ureter/al**

ureter

or **ureterovesical** means pertaining to the urinary bladder and a _____. **Vesico/vaginal** means pertaining to the urinary bladder and the vagina.

7-7 Urine leaves the bladder by way of the urethra and is expelled from the body. **Urethr/al** means

urethra

pertaining to the _____.

The urethra is about 3 cm long in women and lies anterior to the vagina. In men the urethra is about 20 cm long and serves as a passageway for semen and as a canal for urine.

FIND IT!   EXERCISE 4

Draw a slash between the word parts in the following list. Then find the meanings of the word parts within the definitions. Think! (Draw the slash, and then perform the remainder of the activity as a mental exercise.)

1. **cystic** pertaining to a cyst, the gallbladder, or the urinary bladder (Note: When reading, look at how the word is used in a sentence to determine which meaning is intended.)
2. **abdominocystic** pertaining to the abdomen and the urinary bladder; same as **abdominovesical**
3. **extracystic** outside a cyst or outside the bladder
4. **interrenal** between the kidneys

5. **genitourinary** (GU) pertaining to the genitals as well as the urinary organs; same as **urogenital**
6. **rectourethral** pertaining to the rectum and the urethra; same as **urethrorectal**
7. **renal** pertaining to the kidney
8. **suprarenal** above a kidney
9. **ureteral** pertaining to a ureter
10. **urethrovaginal** pertaining to the urethra and the vagina

Use the following word parts to build terms. (Some word parts will be used more than once.)

ureter(o), urethr(o), urin(o), vesic(o), -al, -ary

1. pertaining to the urethra   _____/_____

2. pertaining to urine   _____/_____

3. pertaining to a fluid-filled sac   _____/_____

4. pertaining to the bladder and the ureters   _____/_____/_____

Formation and Excretion of Urine

nephr(o)

7-8 About 1 million **nephrons** serve as the functional units of each kidney. The nephron is named for the combining form _____, which means kidney. A nephron is shown in Fig. 7.3. Its components are a **glomerulus** and **tubules.**

7-9 Nephrons have three important functions:

- **glomerular filtration:** The glomerulus allows water, salts, wastes, and practically everything except blood cells and proteins to pass through the filter. **Bowman capsule** collects the filtrate and passes it to the tubules.
- **tubular reabsorption:** As fluid passes through the tubules, substances that the body conserves, such as sugar and much of the water, are reabsorbed into blood vessels surrounding the tubules.
- **tubular secretion:** As fluid passes through the renal tubule, some substances from the bloodstream (waste products of metabolism and certain drugs, such as penicillin) are secreted into the tubule to be expelled in urine.

urine

These functions depend on a healthy blood pressure, and the ultimate goal is to filter the blood and excrete water and wastes in the _____.

near

7-10 Each tubule consists of a proximal tubule, a loop of Henle, and a distal tubule. The **proxim/al tubule** is that part of the tubule _____ the glomerulus. The **distal tubule** is that part of the tubule that is farther from the glomerulus than the proximal tubule.

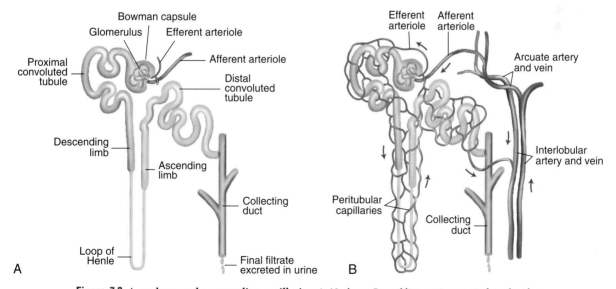

Figure 7.3 A nephron and surrounding capillaries. A, Nephron. Resembling a microscopic funnel with a long stem and tubular sections, a nephron consists of a renal corpuscle (nephron and Bowman capsule) and renal tubules. **B,** Nephron shown with peritubular capillaries.

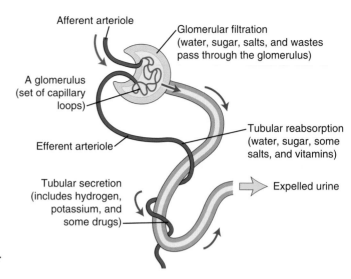

Afferent arteriole

Glomerular filtration
(water, sugar, salts, and wastes
pass through the glomerulus)

A glomerulus
(set of capillary
loops)

Tubular reabsorption
(water, sugar, some
salts, and vitamins)

Efferent arteriole

Tubular secretion
(includes hydrogen,
potassium, and
some drugs)

Expelled urine

Figure 7.4 Functions of the nephron: glomerular filtration, tubular reabsorption, and tubular secretion.

7-11 Follow the arrows in Fig. 7.4, and try to visualize how a nephron carries out these three functions.

glomerulus

Filtering occurs in what part of the nephron? _____

tubule

In what part of the nephron does reabsorption occur? _____

The third process in urine formation, called *tubular secretion,* is the secretion of some substances from the bloodstream into the renal tubule (waste products of metabolism that become toxic if they are not excreted and certain drugs, such as penicillin).

KEY POINT What does urine have to do with math?
Substances that are filtered by the glomerulus
− substances that are reabsorbed
+ substances that are added by tubular secretion
= URINE

Anti/diuretic hormone (ADH) increases the reabsorption of water by the renal tubules, thus decreasing the amount of urine produced. ADH is secreted by the brain and released as needed. A schematic diagram of the forming and expelling of urine is included in Fig. 7.5.

7-12 Waste products and some of the water remaining in the tubules after reabsorption combine to become **urine,** which passes to the collecting duct. Thousands of collecting ducts deposit urine in the renal pelvis, the large central reservoir of the kidney.

After urine collects in the **renal pelvis,** it drains to the bladder by passing through a tube called

ureter

the _____.

The urinary bladder is a collapsible muscular bag that serves as a reservoir for urine until it is expelled. It has a storage capacity in health of about 500 mL (1 pint) or more. **Micturition,** or **voiding,** means **urination,** expelling urine from the bladder.

Filling of the bladder with urine stimulates receptors, producing the desire to urinate. Voluntary control prevents urine from being released. When the control is removed, urine is expelled through the urethra.

7-13 The **glomerular filtration rate** (GFR) is a calculated volume of fluid filtered by the glomeruli. GFR decreases with advancing age, and the decline in the filtration rate is more rapid in persons with diabetes or hypertension (elevated blood pressure). GFR forms the basis of a test for how well the kidneys are functioning.

glomerular

This calculated volume of fluid filtered by the glomeruli is called the _____ filtration rate.

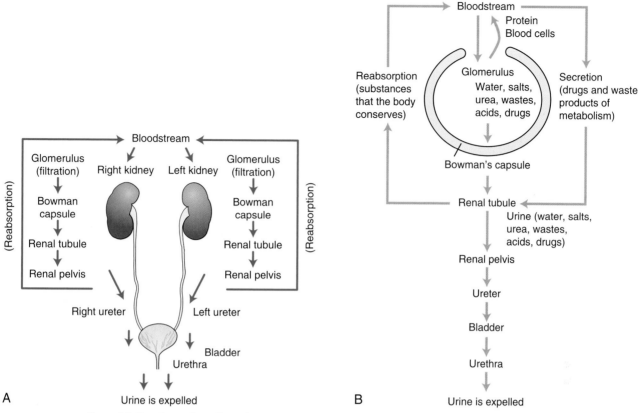

Figure 7.5 Forming and expelling of urine. A, Diagram of forming and expelling urine. **B,** Schematic of filtration of the blood, the processes of reabsorption and secretion, and expelling urine.

WRITE IT! **EXERCISE 6**

Write the names of the structures to complete these sentences.

1. The cavity in the kidney that collects urine from many collecting ducts is the renal _____.

2. A tube that carries urine to the bladder is a/an _____.

3. The tube that carries urine from the bladder is the _____.

4. The _____ is the functional unit of the kidney.

5. The _____ is the reservoir for urine until it is expelled.

6. The filtering structure of the kidney is the _____.

7. Reabsorption occurs in structures called the _____.

8. The external opening of the urethra is the urinary _____.

WRITE IT! **EXERCISE 7**

List the three functions of the nephron.

1. _____

2. _____

3. _____

DIAGNOSTIC TESTS AND PROCEDURES

output

7-14 Physical assessment of the kidneys, ureters, and bladder (KUB) includes abdominal inspection, auscultation, palpation, and percussion (see Fig. 2.29). Laboratory tests, biopsies, radiography, and endoscopy are helpful in diagnostic assessment of the urinary system.

A 24-hour record of **intake and output** (I&O) often provides valuable information regarding fluid and/or electrolyte problems. Intake should include oral, intravenous, and tube feedings. A major source of fluid output is urine, but other output to record includes excess perspiration, vomitus, and diarrhea. I&O is the abbreviation for intake and _____.

Laboratory Tests

urinalysis

7-15 Several urine tests are used to evaluate the status of the urinary system. A **urinalysis** is usually part of a physical examination but is particularly useful for patients with suspected urologic disorders. The urin/alysis is an examination of urine. Urinalysis was originally called *urine analysis*. It is often abbreviated UA or U/A. Examination of the urine is called _____.

Learn the meanings of the following word parts.

Word Parts: Urine

Combining Form	Meaning	Combining Form	Meaning
urin(o)	urine	**Substances Generally Not Detected in Urine**	
Other		albumin(o)	albumin
noct(i), nyct(o)	night	glyc(o), glycos(o)	sugar
olig(o)	few, scanty	ket(o), keton(o)	ketone bodies
		prote(o), protein(o)	protein

WRITE IT EXERCISE 8

Write the meaning of these word parts.

1. glyc(o) _____
2. glycos(o) _____
3. ket(o) _____
4. noct(i) _____
5. nyct(o) _____
6. olig(o) _____

high

7-16 The complete urinalysis (ideally collected at the first morning's voiding) generally includes these types of examinations:
- Physical (color, turbidity, and specific gravity)
- Chemical (pH, sugar, ketones, protein, and blood)
- Microscopic (for example, epithelial cells, erythrocytes, leukocytes)

Changes in the color may result from diet or medication; dark red or brown urine may indicate blood. In a urinalysis the **specific gravity** is the density of urine compared with the density of water (1.0). Dilute urine has a low specific gravity, and concentrated urine has a _____ specific gravity. Specific gravity can be measured using a **urino/meter** (Fig. 7.6, A).

7-17 Chemical analysis of urine may include pH (potential of hydrogen; the numeric pH value indicates the relative concentration of hydrogen ions in a solution) and other chemicals (see Fig. 7.6, B). Glucose test strips, such as Diastix (R), test only for glucose in the urine (Fig. 7.6, C).

These waste products <u>are</u> normally excreted in urine:
- **urea**, a nitrogen compound that is the final product of protein metabolism
- ammonia
- **creatinine**, a nitrogen product produced by the body's normal metabolism
- various salts

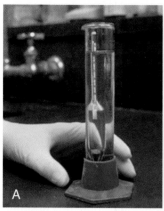
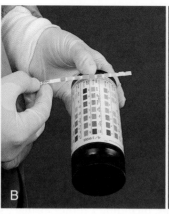
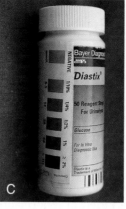

Figure 7.6 Simple Urine Tests. A, A urinometer is used to determine the specific gravity (density) of a sample of urine. **B,** Testing urine with a Multistix, a plastic strip with reagent areas for testing various chemical constituents that may be present in the urine. These reagent strips are considered qualitative tests, and a positive result for an abnormal substance in the urine generally requires further testing. **C,** Glucose test strips screen for the presence of glucose in the urine.

7-18 These substances are <u>not</u> found in normal urine specimens: sugar, ketones, albumin, and hemolyzed blood (must rule out menstrual contamination).

When present in urine, protein is generally **albumin. Ketones** are end products of the body's normal lipid (fat) metabolism; however, excessive production of ketones leads to excretion of ketones in the urine (abnormal). Ketone excretion in urine sometimes indicates **keto/acid/osis,** acidosis resulting from faulty carbohydrate metabolism and accumulation of ketones in the body, primarily a complication of diabetes mellitus. Write this new term that means an accumulation of ketones in the body: _____.

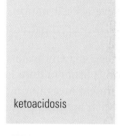
ketoacidosis

Terms in the following exercise represent abnormal findings in urine.

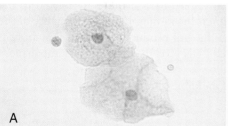

Draw a slash between the word parts in the following list. Then find the meanings of the word parts within the definitions. (Draw the slash, and then perform the remainder of the activity as a mental exercise.)

1. albuminuria albumin in the urine

2. glycosuria sugar in the urine

3. hematuria blood in the urine

4. ketonuria ketones in the urine

5. proteinuria protein in the urine, which is usually albumin

7-19 You learned that glucose is reabsorbed in the tubules; therefore, glucose is not normally present in urine. When the blood glucose rises above a certain level, the **renal threshold** for reabsorption is exceeded, and glucose is excreted in the urine. Glycosuria may indicate diabetes and requires further testing. Glycosuria means _____ in the urine.

sugar

7-20 A microscopic study is generally part of a complete urinalysis. Body cells (for example, squamous epithelial cells, blood cells), crystals, and bacteria are some of the particles present in a microscopic study (Fig. 7.7). These are generally reported as number/high-power field (HPF).

A healthy urine sample contains a few squamous epithelial cells (Fig. 7.7, A), and very few white blood cells (WBCs) (Fig. 7.7, B). The presence of a large number of WBCs may be indicative of an infectious or inflammatory process somewhere in the urinary tract. For example, there is usually a large number of WBCs/HPF in most urinary tract infections.

Pus cells, necrotic WBCs, are a major component of pus. **Py/uria** means the presence of pus in the _____.

urine

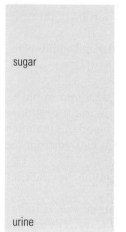
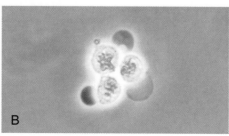

Figure 7.7 Structures seen in a microscopic examination of urine. A, Squamous epithelial cells. **B,** White blood cells (WBCs) (the nucleated cells shown).

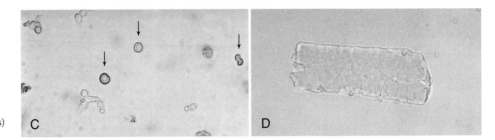

Figure 7.7, cont. **C,** Red blood cells (RBCs) *(arrows).* **D,** Waxy cast.

7-21 Only a few RBCs are normally present in urine. If several RBCs/HPF are present (Fig. 7.7, C), it may indicate a variety of abnormalities, including a tumor, urinary stones, infection, or a bleeding disorder.

Urinary casts are gelatinous structures that take the shape of the renal tubules (Fig. 7.7, D). Casts are described by the type of element in the structure (for example, WBC cast, RBC cast, granular cast, waxy cast). There are usually few to no casts, so the presence of several casts in urine generally indicates renal disease or urinary calculi. Renal disease means disease of a _____.

kidney

7-22 Few bacteria reside in freshly collected urine. The presence of many bacteria may indicate a urinary tract infection. If the patient has symptoms of a urinary tract infection, a **urine culture** is used to determine the types of pathogenic bacteria present. When bacteria are present in significant numbers, another test (an **antibiotic sensitivity test**) is used to determine which antibiotics are effective against that particular pathogen.

The test is ordered as a culture and sensitivity (C&S). The cultivation of microorganisms in the laboratory on special culture medium is called a _____.

culture

7-23 Urine specimens are collected according to the laboratory or physician's instructions. A **voided specimen** is one in which the patient _____ into a container supplied by the laboratory or physician's office. Because improperly collected urine may yield incorrect test results, voided urine should always be collected using the clean-catch midstream technique. This technique is based on the concept that the tissues adjacent to the urethral meatus must be cleansed before collection to avoid contamination of the specimen, and only the middle portion of the urine stream (**clean-catch specimen**) is collected.

voids (or urinates)

A **catheterized urine specimen** is obtained by placing a catheter into the bladder and withdrawing urine. This may be necessary to obtain an uncontaminated urine specimen.

7-24 Creatinine is a substance formed in normal metabolism and is commonly found in blood, urine, and muscle tissue. Creatinine is measured in blood and urine as an indicator of kidney function. A serum creatinine test is a measurement of the creatinine level in the blood. A **creatinine clearance test** is a diagnostic test that measures the rate at which creatinine is cleared from the blood by the kidney. This kidney function test is called a _____ clearance test, one example of a renal clearance test. **Renal clearance tests** determine the efficiency with which the kidneys excrete particular substances.

creatinine

A 24-hour urine collection is collection of all of the urine voided in a 24-hour period. This type of collection may be ordered to measure levels of various substances in the urine, such as calcium or creatinine.

7-25 In addition to blood creatinine levels, **blood urea nitrogen** (BUN) is directly related to the metabolic function of the liver and the excretory function of the kidney. BUN is a measure of the amount of urea in the blood. Urea forms in the liver as the end product of protein metabolism and is excreted by the kidneys in urine. A critically elevated BUN level indicates serious impairment of renal function.

urea

BUN, a blood test that measures the excretory function of the kidney, means blood _____ nitrogen.

BUILD IT!

EXERCISE 10

Use the following word parts to build terms. (Some word parts will be used more than once.)

glycos(o), keton(o), protein(o), py(o), urin(o), -meter, -uria

1. protein in the urine   _____/_____
2. sugar in the urine   _____/_____
3. instrument to measure the specific gravity of urine   _____/_____
4. pus in the urine   _____/_____
5. presence of the end products of fat metabolism in the urine   _____/_____

Urinary Catheterization

catheter

7-26 In **urinary catheterization,** a catheter is inserted through the urethra and into the bladder for temporary or permanent drainage of urine. Urinary catheterization may be done to collect a urine specimen and for other reasons, including urinary testing, instillation of medications into the bladder, and drainage of the bladder during many types of surgeries or in cases of urinary obstruction or paralysis. The hollow tube that is used in catheterization is a _____.

7-27 An **indwelling catheter** is designed to be left in place for a prolonged period. A **Foley catheter** is held securely in place by a balloon tip that is filled with a sterile liquid after the catheter has been placed in the bladder (Fig. 7.8). This type of catheter is used when continuous drainage of the bladder is desired, such as in surgery, or when repeated urinary catheterization would be necessary if an indwelling catheter were not used.

Foley

An indwelling catheter that has a balloon tip and is left in place in the bladder is a _____ catheter.

7-28 Ureteral catheters are usually passed into the distal ends of the ureters from the bladder via a cystoscope and may be threaded up the ureters into the renal pelves (plural for pelvis). A ureteral catheter may also be surgically inserted through the abdominal wall into a ureter. Placement of catheters through the urethra into a ureter is _____ catheterization.

ureteral

Ureteral catheters may be placed temporarily as part of a diagnostic procedure called a *retrograde urogram* or *retrograde pyelogram,* which permits visualization of the renal collecting system in patients whose renal function is too limited for adequate visualization with intravenous urography.

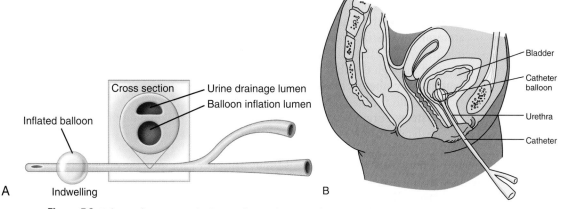

Figure 7.8 Foley catheter. A, Indwelling catheter. This type of catheter has a balloon tip to be filled with a sterile liquid after it has been placed in the bladder. This is a type of indwelling catheter and is used when continuous drainage is desired. **B,** Placement of a Foley catheter in an adult female.

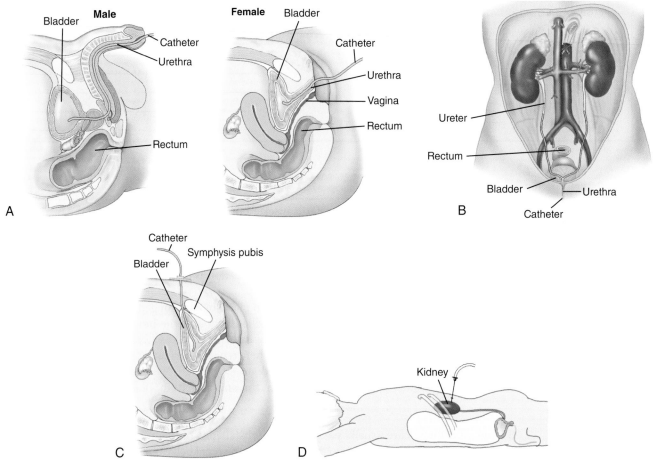

Figure 7.9 Urinary diversion. A, Urethral catheterization. Compare the length of the male vs. the female urethra: approximately 20 cm (8 inches) vs. 3.7 cm (1.5 inches). **B,** Ureteral catheterization. **C,** Suprapubic catheterization. **D,** Percutaneous nephrostomy.

7-29 Four methods are used to divert the regular flow of urine. They are urethral, ureteral, suprapubic catheterization, and nephrostomy. The four types of urinary catheterization are shown in Fig. 7.9.
- **urethral catheterization** Insertion of a catheter via the urethra into the bladder (**A**).
- **ureteral catheterization** Insertion of a catheter into the distal ends of the ureters, usually via the urethra into the bladder, then into the ureters using a cystoscope; may also be surgically inserted through the abdominal wall (**B**).
- **suprapubic catheterization** Surgical insertion of a catheter through the skin above the pubic arch and into the bladder (**C**).
- **nephrostomy** Surgical insertion of a catheter via a new opening into the renal pelvis through the overlying skin (**D**).

7-30 Urodynamic studies measure various aspects of the process of voiding and are used along with other procedures to evaluate problems with urine flow. Types of urodynamic studies include cystometrography, electromyography, and urethral pressure profile.

Cysto/metro/graphy (cyst[o], bladder + metr[o], to measure + -graphy, process of recording) provides information about the amount of pressure exerted on the bladder wall. This procedure may incorporate the use of a urinary catheter with an attached **cysto/meter** that measures bladder capacity in relation to changing urine pressure. Looking at its word parts, it is noted that a cysto/meter is an instrument that measures aspects of the _____.

bladder

muscle

Electro/myo/graphy (electr[o], electricity + my[o], muscle + -graphy) (EMG) can be used to evaluate the strength of the muscles (the **perineal muscles**) used in voiding. The **perineum** supports and surrounds the distal parts of the uro/genital and gastro/intestinal tracts of the body. Electro-myography is the electric recording of _____ action, in this case, the strength of the perineal muscles. This test can be used to evaluate urinary incontinence, the inability to control urination.

A urethral pressure profile provides information about the nature of urinary incontinence or retention (accumulation of urine in the bladder that results from inability to urinate).

Divide these words into their component parts, and write the meaning of each term.
1. cystometrography _____
2. nephrostomy _____
3. cystometer _____
4. electromyography _____

Urinary Radiography

7-31 Abdominal x-ray images and special radiologic procedures are helpful in diagnosing many abnormalities of the kidneys, ureters, and bladder (KUB) (Table 7.1). A KUB radiographic study determines the size and location of the kidneys, ureters, and bladder.

🔑 **KEY POINT Many noninvasive radiologic tests are available.** Plain x-ray images, nephrosonography, nephrotomography, and magnetic resonance imaging (MRI) along with urine and blood studies provide a great deal of diagnostic information about the urinary system. Bladder scans are particularly useful in determining bladder volume as well as postvoiding residual volume.

Table 7.1 Common Renal and Urinary Diagnostic Tests

Noninvasive	Others
Plain radiography of the kidneys, ureters, and bladder	Cystography and cystoscopy
Magnetic resonance imaging (MRI)	Intravenous urography
Nephrotomography	Renal arteriography
Ultrasonography	Renal scan
	Nephroscopy (not as common)

Radiographic procedures include the following:

cystography Radiography of the bladder using radiopaque contrast medium.

cystourethrography Radiography of the bladder and urethra after using a urinary catheter to instill the contrast medium. **Voiding cystourethrograms** (VCUGs) are radiographs made before, during, and after voiding (urination). This procedure checks for reflux (abnormal backward flow) of urine.

intravenous urography (IVU) X-ray images of the entire urinary system or part of it after the urine has been rendered opaque by an intavenously injected contrast medium. Both structural and functional abnormalities may be detected. The renal pelvis and ureters are clearly visible in the normal **urogram** (Fig. 7.10); formerly called **intravenous pyelography** (IVP), with the resulting image called a **pyelogram.**

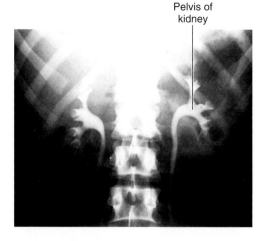

Pelvis of kidney

Figure 7.10 Intravenous urogram. The x-ray image was taken as the contrast medium was cleared from the blood by the kidneys. The renal pelvis and ureters are clearly visible and indicate normal findings.

nephrosonography Ultrasonic scanning of the kidney.

nephrotomography Tomography of the kidney, resulting in an image called a **nephrotomogram** (Fig. 7.11).

renal angiography Radiographic study to assess the arterial blood supply to the kidneys; also called *renal arteriography,* and the record produced is a **renal arteriogram** (Fig. 7.12).

renal scan Scanning of the kidney for radioactivity after intravenous injection of radioactive material; also called **renography.** Special equipment measures, records, and produces an image of the low-level radioactivity that is emitted.

urethrography Radiography of the urethra using radiopaque contrast medium.

Kidney

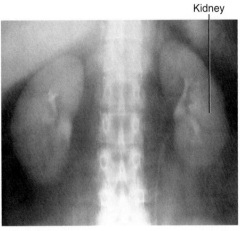

Figure 7.11 Nephrotomogram. The procedure, nephrotomography, is helpful in assessing various planes of kidney tissue for tumors, cysts, or stones.

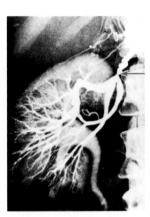

Figure 7.12 Renal arteriogram showing stenosis *(arrow)* **of the right renal artery.**

MATCH IT!

EXERCISE 12

Match descriptions in the left column with the names of the procedures in the right column.

___ **1.** assessing the arterial blood supply to the kidneys

___ **2.** radiographic image of the urinary system

___ **3.** radiography of the bladder

___ **4.** radiography of the urethra

___ **5.** renal test that involves scanning for radioactivity

___ **6.** ultrasonic scanning of the kidney

A. cystography

B. nephrosonography

C. renal angiography

D. renography

E. urogram

F. urethrography

Endoscopy

A number of endoscopic procedures are helpful in diagnosing abnormalities of urinary structures:

cystoscopy A **cystoscope** is passed through the urethra and into the bladder. The bladder mucosa is examined, sometimes biopsy specimens are obtained, polyps (growths protruding from the lining) or stones may be removed, or the distal ends of the ureters are examined (Fig. 7.13).

nephroscopy Visualization of the kidney using a **nephroscope** inserted through the skin into a small incision in the renal pelvis (Fig. 7.14).

ureteroscopy Visual examination within a ureter.

urethroscopy Visual examination within the urethra. If the examination uses a cystoscope to also examine the bladder, it is called a **cystourethroscopy.**

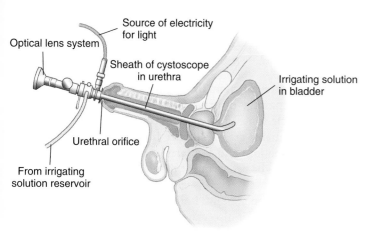

Figure 7.13 **A cystoscope in place inside the male bladder.**

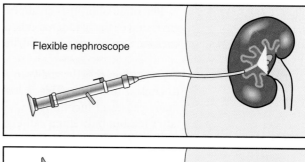
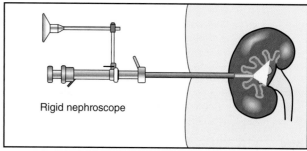

Figure 7.14 **Two types of nephroscopes.** The nephroscope, a fiberoptic instrument, is inserted percutaneously into the kidney. Additional instruments can be introduced through the scope, for example, to remove or break up calculi.

WRITE IT! **EXERCISE 13**

Write a term for each meaning.
1. direct visualization of the bladder _____
2. direct visualization of the urethra and bladder _____
3. instrument used in nephroscopy _____

PATHOLOGIES

7-32 An overactive bladder is characterized by a nearly constant urge to urinate, sometimes called an irritable bladder. Discomfort during urination and unexplained change in the volume of urine are sometimes the earliest indications of a urinary problem. **Dys/uria** is _____ or painful urination and can be caused by a bacterial infection or an obstruction of the urinary tract.

Poly/uria also called **diuresis**, is excretion of an abnormally large quantity of urine. Literal translation of polyuria is _____ urines or urinations. You will need to remember that polyuria means excretion of an abnormally large quantity of urine. This can be brought about by excessive intake of fluids or the use of medications. Two pathologies in which polyuria is common are diabetes insipidus and diabetes mellitus. Both are described later in this section.

7-33 Literal translation of an/uria is absence of _____. The full meaning of **anuria** is a urinary output of less than 100 mL per day. The patient who has less than 100 mL of urine output per day is described as **anur/ic.**

Compare anuria and **olig/uria,** which means diminished capacity to form urine, excreting less than 500 mL of urine per day. The combining form olig(o) means few or scanty. Write this term that means diminished urine production of less than 500 mL per day: _____.

KEY POINT Be sure you can distinguish these terms ending in -uria:
• *Polyuria* is excretion of an abnormally large quantity of urine.
• *Dysuria* is difficult or painful urination.
• *Oliguria* is excreting less than 500 mL of urine per day.
• *Anuria* is excreting less than 100 mL of urine per day.

7-34 *Urgency, frequency,* and *hesitancy* are terms that are often used to describe urination patterns. **Urgency** is a sudden onset of the need to urinate immediately. Increased **frequency** is a greater number of urinations than expected in a given time. (Uterine prolapse, the loss of support that anchors the uterus, can result in pressure on the bladder and lead to urinary frequency.) **Hesitancy** is difficulty in beginning the flow, often with a decrease in the force of the urine stream.

retention

WORD ORIGIN
continence (L.)
continere, to contain

Retention of urine is an abnormal, involuntary accumulation of urine in the bladder. Incomplete emptying of the bladder is called **urinary** _____. **Urinary reflux** is an abnormal backward or return flow of urine from the bladder into the ureters.

7-35 Continence is the ability to control bladder or bowel function. **Urinary incontinence** is inability to control urination. This is loss of control of the passage of urine from the bladder. There are many causes of incontinence, such as loss of muscle tone, obesity, or unconsciousness. For the latter reason, indwelling catheters are used when patients are anesthetized.

Enuresis also means the inability to control urination, and the term is applied especially to nocturnal bedwetting. Nocturnal means pertaining to or occurring at night.

7-36 Noct/uria, also called **nyct/uria,** is excessive urination at night. Both noct(i) and nyct(o) mean night. Although nocturia may be a symptom of disease, it also can occur in people who drink excessive amounts of fluids before bedtime or when nearby structures put pressure on the bladder. An example of the latter is pressure on the bladder by a prolapsed uterus.

night

Both nocturia and nycturia mean excessive urination at _____, sometimes interfering with sleep because of the need to urinate several times during the night.

MATCH IT! **EXERCISE 14**

Match terms in the left column with their descriptions in the right column.

___ **1.** anuria
___ **2.** dysuria
___ **3.** hesitancy
___ **4.** nycturia
___ **5.** oliguria
___ **6.** polyuria
___ **7.** urgency
___ **8.** urinary incontinence
___ **9.** urinary reflux
___ **10.** urinary retention

A. a decrease in the force of the urine stream
B. backward flow of urine from the bladder
C. difficult or painful urination
D. excessive urination at night
E. excretion of an abnormally large volume of urine
F. excretion of less than 100 mL of urine a day
G. excretion of less than 500 mL of urine a day
H. incomplete emptying of the bladder
I. loss of control of the passage of urine from the bladder
J. the sense of the need to urinate immediately

urinary

7-37 A **uro/pathy** is any disease or abnormal condition of the _____ tract. Uropathies include inflammatory, hereditary, obstructive, and renovascular disorders. In addition, some uropathies are the result of metabolic disease processes that affect renal function.

Kidney cancer is a malignant neoplasm of the renal parenchyma (Fig. 7.15) or the renal pelvis. **Wilms tumor** is a malignant neoplasm of the kidney occurring in young children.

7-38 Because the urinary system is responsible for removing harmful waste products from the blood, anything that interferes with excretion of wastes can be dangerous. **Uremia** is an accumulation of toxic products in the blood. This occurs when the kidneys fail to function properly. The meaning of ur/emia (ur[o], urine + -emia, blood) is implied.

uremia

Write this term that means an accumulation of waste products in the blood resulting from inadequate functioning of the urinary system: _____.

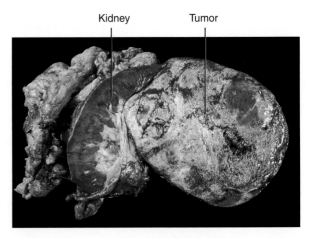

Kidney   Tumor

Figure 7.15 Kidney cancer. Note the large tumor in this adult kidney that has been excised.

🔑 **KEY** POINT **Note the difference in uremia and hematuria.** Uremia is an accumulation of waste products in the blood. Hematuria is the presence of blood in urine.

chronic

7-39 Inability of the kidneys to excrete waste, concentrate urine, and function properly is **renal failure.** It may be acute or chronic. Acute renal failure (ARF) has symptoms that are more severe than those of _____ renal failure (CRF).

ARF is characterized by oliguria and by the rapid accumulation of nitrogenous wastes in the blood, indicated by a higher than normal amount of blood urea nitrogen. ARF may be caused by nephr/itis (inflammation and abnormal functioning of the kidney), interference in blood flow to the kidney, or conditions that disrupt urinary output.

ARF can often be reversed after the cause has been identified (for example, removal of an obstruction in the urinary tract). However, CRF may lead to the need for dialysis if all other medical measures have not alleviated the problem.

7-40 Poly/cyst/ic kidney disease, one of the more common hereditary renal disorders, is characterized by enlarged kidneys containing many cysts. Poly/cystic means containing many cysts. See Fig. 7.16 for comparison of a polycystic kidney and a normal kidney.

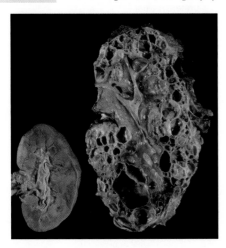

Figure 7.16 Comparison of polycystic kidney with a normal kidney. Note the diseased kidney's enlargement and the replacement of normal tissue by numerous fluid-filled cysts.

inflammation

7-41 Nephr/itis is one of a large group of kidney diseases that is characterized by _____ and abnormal function. The most usual form is **glomerulo/nephritis,** in which glomeruli within the kidney are inflamed. Glomeruli are clusters of capillaries that act as filters. In glomerulonephritis there is impairment of the filtering process. Inflammation of the kidney may be caused by microorganisms or their toxins or even by toxic drugs or alcohol. **Glomerulopathy** means any disease of the glomeruli.

7-42 Interstitial nephritis is inflammation of the interstitial tissue of the kidney, including the tubules. This type of nephritis can be acute or chronic. When acute interstitial nephritis is an adverse immunologic reaction to a drug, normal kidney function is generally regained when the offending drug is discontinued. In interstitial nephritis, there is inflammation of the _____ tissue of the kidney.

interstitial

7-43 Nephrotic syndrome is an abnormal condition of the kidney characterized by marked proteinuria and edema. It occurs as a complication of many systemic diseases, such as diabetes mellitus.

Diabetes mellitus is a complex disorder of carbohydrate, fat, and protein metabolism that is primarily a result of a deficiency or lack of insulin secretion by the pancreas or a resistance to insulin (See Chapter 12).

WRITE IT! EXERCISE 15

Case Study. *Define the terms as indicated.* Prem Chadry's catheterized urine specimen was tested and he is found to have glycosuria, proteinuria, and hematuria. Ketones were not detected. He has been tested and treated in the past for diabetes mellitus.

1. glycosuria _____

2. proteinuria _____

3. hematuria _____

4. ketones _____

5. diabetes mellitus _____

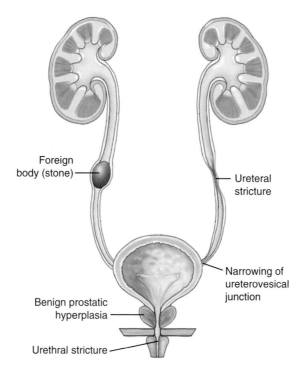

Figure 7.17 Five common causes of urinary tract obstruction are illustrated.

🔑 **KEY** POINT **Another disorder that shares the name diabetes is diabetes insipidus.** The disorder is not related to diabetes mellitus but was so named because of the large quantity of urine excreted.

Unlike diabetes mellitus, **diabetes insipidus** is not related to the body's use of insulin. Its cause may be hormonal or renal, and the disorder refers to several types of polyuria in which the urinary output exceeds 3000 mL a day.

kidneys

blood

7-44 Diabetic nephro/pathy is a disease of the _____ resulting from diabetes mellitus. Chronic hyperglycemia and increased blood pressure accelerate the progression of the disorder. **Hyper/glycemia** means excessive glucose in the _____.

Diabetes mellitus is a major cause of end-stage renal disease in the United States and can result from either type 1 or type 2 diabetes mellitus.

7-45 Obstructive nephropathies are conditions that block or interfere with the flow of urine. Several causes are illustrated in Fig. 7.17 and include prolapsed adjacent structures, tumors (benign or malignant), stones, narrowing of the ureters or urethra, and dysfunctions of the bladder that result from spinal cord injury or a lesion of the nervous system (neurogenic bladder).

Try to remember that **neuro/genic bladder** is a dysfunction of the bladder caused by a lesion

nervous

of the _____ system.

FIND IT! **EXERCISE 16**

Draw a slash between the word parts in the following list. Then find the meanings of the word parts within the definitions. (Draw the slash, and then perform the remainder of the activity as a mental exercise.)

1. **nephrolysis** destruction of kidney substance; a second meaning is freeing of a kidney from adhesions, bands of scar tissue that bind together surfaces that normally are separate

2. **nephromalacia** abnormal softening of the kidney

3. **nephromegaly** enlargement of a kidney, especially hypertrophy of a kidney after removal of the other kidney; bilateral nephromegaly involves both kidneys

4. **nephropathy** any disease of the kidney, including inflammatory, degenerative, or sclerotic conditions

5. **nephrotoxic** toxic or destructive to kidney cells

7-46 Bacterial infection is the most common cause of inflammation of the urinary tract, but inflammation may be attributed to other disorders, such as the presence of a stone.

A **urinary tract infection** (UTI), an infection of one or more structures in the urinary system, is one of the more common disorders of the urinary tract. A UTI may be asymptomatic but is usually characterized by urinary frequency and possibly discomfort during urination. Other signs and symptoms, particularly in severe infections, include backache, fever, and blood and/or pus in the urine. It is important to diagnose and treat urinary tract infections to prevent their spreading to another part of the body, such as the blood. **Septic/emia** (sept[o], infection + -emia, blood) is a systemic infection in which pathogens are present in the circulating blood, having spread from an infection in another part of the body, such as the urinary tract.

infection

UTI means urinary tract _____.

7-47 UTIs can include cyst/itis, urethritis, and pyelonephritis. Most urinary infections are caused by bacteria (especially *Escherichia coli*), but certain fungi *(Candida)* can also cause infection. When UTIs are caused by bacteria, they are treated with an antibiotic.

KEY POINT **Most of the time, UTIs are caused by ascending infection.** The anus serves as a reservoir for bacteria, and organisms spread directly from the anal area (occasionally the vagina) to the urethral meatus, where they multiply and can ascend throughout the urethra to the bladder and eventually the kidney in some cases. Infection is more likely in females than in males because of the short distance separating the anus and the urethra, as well as a shorter urethra. Both catheterization and sexual intercourse promote the ascent of bacteria. Urinary tract infections are also more common in persons with structural abnormalities or lowered immunity and are a major type of hospital-acquired infections.

water

ureter

7-48 **Hydro/nephrosis** is distension (or distention) of the renal pelvis and kidney by urine that cannot flow past an obstruction in a ureter. The literal translation of hydronephrosis is a condition of _____ in the kidney. Remember that hydronephrosis means distension of the renal pelvis with urine as a result of an obstruction in the upper part of a ureter.

If a stone or another obstruction occurs in the lower part of the ureter, the condition that results is called **hydroureter,** abnormal distension of a _____ with urine or watery fluid. See Fig. 7.18 for comparison of hydronephrosis and hydroureter.

7-49 A polyp is any growth or mass protruding from a mucous membrane. A **bladder polyp** is a growth protruding from the lining of the bladder. This abnormality is one of the conditions that may be detected during cystoscopy. Polyps may occur anywhere there is mucous membrane, such as the urethra.

Polyps are removed and the tissue is studied microscopically, even though cancer may not be suspected.

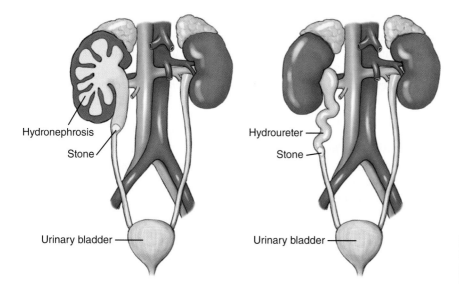

Hydronephrosis
Stone
Urinary bladder

Hydroureter
Stone
Urinary bladder

Figure 7.18 Hydronephrosis and hydroureter. Hydronephrosis is caused by obstruction in the upper part of the ureter. Hydroureter is caused by obstruction in the lower part of the ureter.

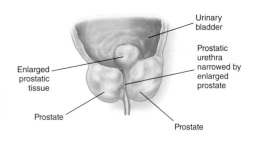

Figure 7.19 Benign prostatic hyperplasia. This nonmalignant enlargement of the prostate is common among men older than 50 years. As the prostate enlarges, it extends upward into the bladder and inward, obstructing the outflow of urine from the bladder.

bladder

7-50 Bladder cancer is the most common malignancy of the urinary tract and occurs more than twice as frequently in men than women. Bladder-wash specimens and bladder biopsies (obtained during cystoscopy) are often used to diagnose cancer of the bladder. The most common malignancy of the urinary tract is _____ cancer.

7-51 Enlargement of a nearby structure (for example, the prostate) also puts pressure on urinary structures. The prostate is a gland in men that surrounds the neck of the bladder. **Benign prostatic hyperplasia** (BPH) is a nonmalignant, noninflammatory enlargement of the prostate that is common among men older than 50 years. It may lead to urethral obstruction and interference with urine flow, causing frequency, dysuria, nocturia, and urinary tract infections (Fig. 7.19).

benign

Prostatic hyperplasia results in enlargement of the prostate. This is not a malignant disease, as noted by its name, _____ prostatic hyperplasia.

🔑 **KEY** POINT **Nephro/sclerosis is hardening of the small arteries of the kidney and results in decreased blood flow and eventually necrosis of kidney cells.** This condition occurs in a small number of persons with hypertension (elevated blood pressure). Treatment of nephrosclerosis is the use of medications to lower the blood pressure.

vessels

7-52 Reno/vascular disorders are those affecting the blood _____ of the kidneys and include nephrosclerosis, stenosis of the renal artery, and thrombosis of the renal vein.

7-53 Renal artery stenosis is partial or complete blocking of one or both renal arteries. The pathologic changes to the renal arteries result in drastically reduced blood flow through the kidneys and lead to hypertension and damage to the kidneys. Hypertension resulting from renal artery stenosis (see Fig. 7.12) or other kidney disorders is called **renal hypertension.**

A blood clot in the renal vein is called **renal vein thrombosis.** The cause of the blood clot (the thrombus) includes compression by a nearby tumor, renal carcinoma, or renal trauma. The presence of a thrombus in the renal vein is called renal vein _____.

thrombosis

urinary

7-54 Genitourinary infections are those affecting both the genital and _____ structures. *E. coli,* normally present and the most abundant bacteria in the intestinal tract, is a frequent cause of female urinary tract infections. These microorganisms as well as other intestinal bacteria normally colonize the anus and surrounding area, sometimes causing cross contamination to the nearby urethra. Both chlamydia and gonorrhea can affect the urinary system as well as the genitals.

A **sexually transmitted disease** (STD), also called *sexually transmitted infection (STI),* is one that may be acquired as a result of sexual contact with a person who has the disease or with secretions containing the suspected organism. Sexually transmitted diseases were formerly called **venereal diseases** (VDs).

Chlamydial infections, caused by *Chlamydia trachomatis,* can be transmitted during vaginal, anal, or oral sex. Many people with the disease are asymptomatic, but male signs and symptoms include dysuria and urethral discharge. Females may experience discharge from the cervix, urethritis, dysuria, polyuria and pyuria, or the infection may spread.

7-55 You have learned that -rrhea means flow or discharge, and you probably have heard of **gono/rrhea,** a sexually transmitted disease. Gonorrhea is derived from gon(o), which means the genitals or reproduction. This sexually transmitted disease, caused by the bacterium *Neisseria gonorrhoeae,* is characterized by a heavy discharge from the vagina in females or from the urethra in either males or females. The discharge may be accompanied by urethritis and dysuria. See Chapter 9 for more information about gonorrhea.

gonorrhea

Write the name of the sexually transmitted disease that can cause urethritis: _____.

7-56 The absence of both kidneys in a developing fetus is not compatible with life outside the uterus, but less severe congenital defects of the urinary system do occur. Hypo/plasia may affect only one kidney or both kidneys and is a common cause of hypertension in the first decade of life. High blood pressure resulting from any type of renal disorder is called _____ hypertension.

renal

7-57 Two anomalies of the urethra are hypospadias and epispadias. **Hypo/spadias** is a congenital defect in which the urinary meatus is located below its usual location (usually seen in males with the opening on the underside of the penis). **Epi/spadias** is a developmental defect in which the urinary meatus is located above its usual location (usually seen in males with the opening on the upper surface of the penis). Epispadias occurs as a groove or cleft without a covering and not in its usual location. Remember that in hypo/spadias the urinary meatus is usually located _____ its normal location and above its normal location in epispadias. Compare these two anomalies (Fig. 7.20).

below

> **WORD ORIGIN**
> hypospadias *(G.)*
> *hypo*, under; *spădon*, a cleft or rent

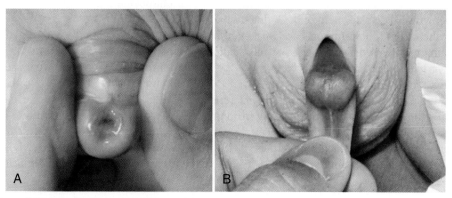

Figure 7.20 Two developmental defects of the urinary meatus in male infants. A, Hypospadias. Note the location of the urinary meatus below its usual location. **B,** Epispadias. Note the urethral opening on the upper side of the penis.

BUILD IT!
EXERCISE 17

Use the following word parts to build terms. (Some word parts will be used more than once.)
hydr(o), nephr(o), ren(o), vascul(o), -ar, -malacia, -megaly, -pathy, -osis

1. distension of the renal pelvis and kidney _____/_____/_____

2. softening of the kidney _____/_____

3. pertaining to the blood vessels of the kidney _____/_____/_____

4. any disease of the kidney _____/_____

5. enlargement of a kidney _____/_____

Read about additional urinary pathologies.

cystitis Inflammation of the bladder.

cystocele Herniation of the bladder (Fig. 7.21).

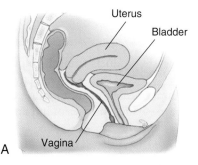

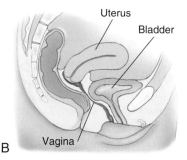

Figure 7.21 Normal bladder compared with cystocele.
A, Normal position of the bladder in relation to other pelvic structures. **B,** A cystocele, herniation of the bladder. Note how the bladder sags and protrudes into the vagina.

cystolithiasis The presence of a **cystolith,** a calculus in the urinary bladder (Fig. 7.22).

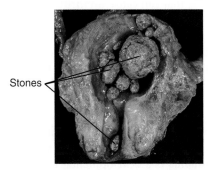

Stones

Figure 7.22 Dissected bladder showing cystolithiasis. Note the thickening of the bladder wall (signifying inflammation) and the presence of numerous stones in the urinary bladder; one stone has moved to the urethra.

nephrolithiasis A condition marked by the presence of kidney stones, also called a *renal calculus* or **nephrolith.**

nephroptosis Downward displacement of the kidney, which can occur when the kidney supports are weakened by sudden strain or blow, or may be congenital; also called *floating, hypermobile,* or *wandering kidney.*

pyelitis Inflammation of the renal pelvis.

pyelonephritis Inflammation of the kidney and its renal pelvis, usually the result of infection spreading from the lower urinary tract. Chronic pyelonephritis can develop after bacterial infection of the kidney that is either untreated or resistant to treatment.

ureteral dysfunction A disturbance of the normal flow of urine through one or both ureters.

ureteritis Inflammation of a ureter that may be caused by mechanical irritation of a stone.

ureterocele Prolapse or herniation of a ureter, which may lead to obstruction of the flow of urine and hydronephrosis.

ureterolithiasis Presence of a **ureterolith,** a ureteral stone.

ureteropathy Any disease of a ureter.

ureteropyelonephritis Inflammation of a ureter, renal pelvis, and kidney.

ureterostenosis Stricture (narrowing of the lumen) of a ureter.

urethritis Inflammation of the urethra, characterized by dysuria; may result from minor trauma or infection.

urethrocele Urethral herniation, characterized by protrusion of the female urethra through the urethral opening or encroachment of a segment of the urethral wall upon the vaginal canal. Compare with cystocele.

urethrocystitis Inflammation of the urethra and bladder; **cystourethritis.**

urethrorrhagia Urethral hemorrhage.

urethrorrhea Discharge from the urethra.

urethrospasm Spasm of the muscular tissue of the urethra.

urethrostenosis A stricture of the urethra.

urolithiasis Formation of urinary calculi, often named according to their location; vary greatly in size, from small enough to pass in urination to large stones that occupy the entire renal pelvis and have roughly the shape of a deer antler (staghorn calculi).

WRITE IT!

EXERCISE 18

Write a word in each blank to complete these sentences. The first letter of each answer is given as a clue.

1. Distension of a ureter with urine or a watery fluid is *h*_____.
2. Hernial protrusion of the bladder into the vagina is a *c*_____.
3. A nonmalignant, noninflammatory enlargement of the prostate is called benign prostatic *h*_____.
4. A condition marked by the presence of kidney stones is *n*_____.
5. A hormonal or renal disorder in which the urinary output exceeds 3000 mL a day is diabetes *i*_____.
6. A congenital defect in which the urinary meatus is located *below* its usual location is *h*_____.
7. A congenital defect in which the urinary meatus is located *above* its usual location is *e*_____.
8. Inflammation of the kidney and its renal pelvis is *p*_____.
9. Stricture of the urethra is *u*_____.
10. Discharge from the urethra is *u*_____.

SURGICAL AND THERAPEUTIC INTERVENTIONS

blood

7-58 Kidney dialysis is required when the kidneys fail to remove waste products from the blood. This is also called **hemo/dialysis,** which means dialysis of the _____. Kidney dialysis or hemodialysis is the process of diffusing blood through a semipermeable membrane for the purpose of removing toxic materials and maintaining the acid–base balance in cases of impaired kidney function (Fig. 7.23).

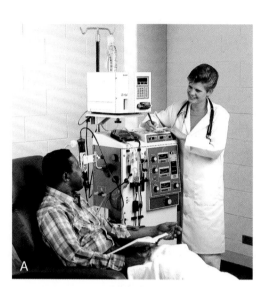

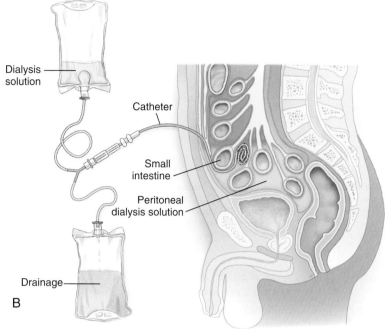

Dialysis solution

Catheter

Small intestine

Peritoneal dialysis solution

Drainage

A

B

Figure 7.23 Dialysis. Hemodialysis, also called kidney dialysis. **A,** Patient receiving hemodialysis. Blood is shunted from the patient, and impurities or wastes are removed before returning it to the patient's bloodstream. **B,** Peritoneal dialysis. Instead of diffusing the blood, the perineum is used as a diffusible membrane; it may be performed at home while the patient sleeps.

Peritoneal dialysis is dialysis through the peritoneum, with the solution introduced into and removed from the peritoneal cavity. This type of dialysis is done as an alternative to hemodialysis.

7-59 In a **renal transplant** the patient (recipient) receives a kidney from a suitable donor (Fig. 7.24). The donated kidney is surgically removed from the donor. Build a word that means surgical excision of a kidney, using nephr(o) and the suffix for excision: _____.

nephrectomy

In addition to donation of a kidney, nephrectomies are performed to remove tumors or certain diseased kidneys, for example, when the kidneys are the cause of extremely high blood pressure. A flank incision, on either side of the body, below the ribs and superior to the hip bone, is often used to remove a kidney (Fig. 7.25). The kidney may be removed by other means (abdominally, transabdominally, as well as laparoscopically).

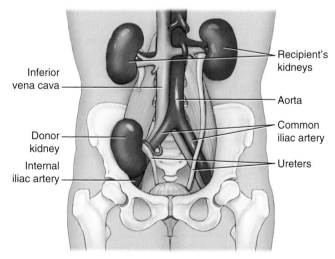

Inferior vena cava

Donor kidney

Internal iliac artery

Recipient's kidneys

Aorta

Common iliac artery

Ureters

Figure 7.24 Renal transplantation (anterior view of the body). In kidney transplants, a complete kidney from a donor is transferred to a recipient whose kidneys have failed. Note the location of the donated kidney, leaving the diseased kidneys in place.

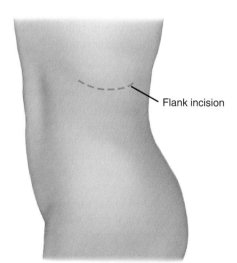

Flank incision

Figure 7.25 One common incision for a nephrectomy, left kidney. This is called a *flank incision,* either side of the body superior to the ilium (upper hip bone).

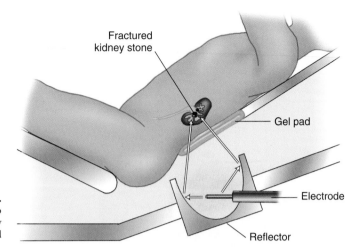

Figure 7.26 Lithotripsy, crushing of a kidney stone (calculus). Extracorporeal shock wave lithotripsy (ESWL), illustrated here, is used to crush certain types of urinary stones. The reflector focuses a high-energy shock wave on the stone. The stone disintegrates into particles and is passed in the urine.

7-60 Stones in the urinary tract are sometimes passed out through the urethra, but many are either too large or do not dissolve. Stones can cause urinary obstruction, which interferes with function and can be very painful. There are several methods of dealing with stones, including lithotripsy and open surgery to remove a large stone if it cannot be broken up or removed by other means.

    Litho/tomy is the incision of an organ or duct for removal of a calculus, especially one from the urinary tract. The suffix -tomy means incision, so the meaning of lithotomy is implied. Write this term that means an incision of an organ or duct for removal of a calculus: _____. Be aware that the term *lithotomy* is also used to mean the lithotomy position, often used in obstetrics and gynecology. In the lithotomy position, the patient lies on the back with the hips and the knees flexed and the thighs rotated outward.

lithotomy

7-61 Litho/tripsy is the crushing of a _____ within the body, followed by the washing out of the fragments. This was originally done by surgical removal, but noninvasive methods, such as high-energy shock waves or lasers, often eliminate the need for surgery. This is called **extracorporeal shock wave lithotripsy** (ESWL). Extra/corpor/eal means outside the body. ESWL uses ultrasonic energy from a source outside the body (Fig. 7.26). This technique is used on stones that resist passage and is far less incapacitating than a full-scale operation, even laparoscopic surgery.

    Write the name of the procedure that uses ultrasonic energy from a source outside the body to break up a stone: _____ shock wave lithotripsy.

stone

extracorporeal

7-62 Invasive lithotripsy may be successful with small stones in the bladder. This type of lithotripsy is accomplished by inserting a catheter through the urethra. The stone is then crushed with an instrument called a **lithotrite.** The fragments may then be expelled or washed out. Write the name of the instrument that is used in conjunction with a catheter to crush stones in the bladder: _____.

lithotrite

ureter

7-63 Nephroureterectomy means surgical excision of a kidney with the _____. Selected situations may allow **laparo/scopic nephrectomy,** removal of the kidney through several small incisions in the abdominal wall, rather than an open surgical excision.

    Immuno/suppressive therapy, the administration of agents that significantly interfere with the immune response of the recipient, are provided after renal transplantation to prevent rejection of the donor kidney.

7-64 Either removal of the diseased kidney or radiation therapy can be used to treat renal carcinoma. **Ren/al carcinoma** is cancer of a _____.

kidney

    Treatment for bladder cancer depends on several factors, including the size of the lesion. Tests of the urine may show atypical cells or the presence of factors associated with cancer, but cystoscopy and biopsy are generally used for confirmation. Radiation therapy, laser eradication of small lesions, chemotherapy, and cystectomy may be used. Chemotherapy can be given systemically, or in some cases, the chemical treatment is instilled directly into the bladder through a catheter.

bladder

Cyst/ectomy is surgical excision of the _____. It may be a partial cystectomy, in which only a portion of the bladder is removed, or the cystectomy may be radical, in which all of the bladder is removed along with selected adjacent organs (the prostate and seminal vesicles in males; the uterus, cervix, ovaries, and urethra in females).

7-65 Various surgical procedures may be performed for urinary diversion if the bladder is removed. The ureters must be diverted into some type of collecting reservoir, opening either onto the abdomen or into the large intestine so that urine is expelled with bowel movements.

Formation of a new opening through which a ureter empties is called a **ureterostomy**. In a bilateral or double ureterostomy, there are two pouches on the abdominal surface, one for each ureter, to receive drainage of the urine (Fig. 7.27, A). Surgical connection of one ureter to another is called **trans/ureteroureterostomy.** In other words, one ureter is brought across and joined to the

ureter

other _____. The latter results in only one opening on the abdominal surface that serves both ureters (Fig. 7.27, B).

A nephrostomy, formation of a new opening into the renal pelvis, may be performed on one or both kidneys and may be temporary or permanent. If both ureters are removed, a bilateral nephrostomy is necessary. Compare bilateral nephrostomy and the two types of ureterostomies just described (Fig. 7.27, C).

Cancer is one reason for urinary diversion. An obstruction lower in the urinary tract could also require formation of a new opening through which the ureter could discharge its contents.

calculi

7-66 Nephro/litho/tomy is removal of renal _____ by cutting through the body of the kidney. Notice that -tomy is used rather than -ectomy, because -tomy refers to incision of the kidney, and removal of the stone is only implied. Nephrolithotomy is necessary if the stone is too large to pass or break up or if it will not dissolve.

pelvis

Pyelo/litho/tomy is surgical removal of a stone from the renal _____. Literal translation of this term is incision of the renal pelvis for stones, and it is understood that the

pyelolithotomy

procedure is done for this purpose. Write the term: _____.

bladder

Ureterolithotomy and **cysto/litho/tomy** are procedures for surgical removal of a stone or stones from the ureter and the _____, respectively. It is important that the patient have a high fluid intake after a stone is removed to prevent the formation of another stone. Stones are routinely analyzed in the laboratory to determine their chemical makeup.

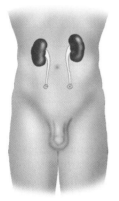 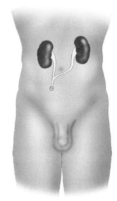 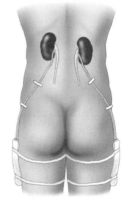
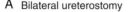

A Bilateral ureterostomy   B Transureteroureterostomy   C Bilateral nephrostomy

Figure 7.27 Comparing two ureterostomies and a bilateral nephrostomy. A, Bilateral ureterostomy (anterior view). Both ureters are brought out onto the skin for drainage of urine into bags. **B,** Transureteroureterostomy. One ureter is surgically attached to the other ureter, which is brought out onto the skin for drainage of urine into a bag. **C,** Bilateral nephrostomy (posterior view). The skin is punctured, and openings are made into the renal pelves. Urine is diverted to bags.

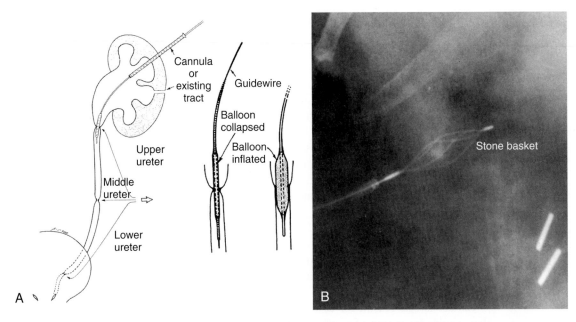

Figure 7.28 Two procedures that can be performed after percutaneous nephrostomy. A, Dilation of a stenosed ureter. After percutaneous nephrostomy, a collapsed balloon catheter is introduced. After reaching the area of stenosis, the balloon is inflated to stretch the stenosed area, and then the balloon catheter is withdrawn. **B,** Removal of a kidney stone. This radiograph shows a renal calculus that has been caught in a stone basket and is ready for removal. After percutaneous nephrostomy, the stone basket is maneuvered to engage the renal calculus, and then both are removed through the cannula.

7-67 **Percutaneous nephro/stomy** is a surgical procedure in which the skin of the flank (or side) is punctured so that a catheter can be inserted into the renal pelvis. Literal translation of nephro/stomy is formation of a new opening into the kidney. Percutaneous tells us that the _____ is punctured to gain access to the renal pelvis. This procedure allows for drainage, drug instillation, and selected surgical procedures, including dilation of a stenosed ureter (Fig. 7.28, A) or removal of calculi (see Fig. 7.28, B).

skin

BUILD IT!

EXERCISE 19

Use the following word parts to build terms. (Some word parts will be used more than once.)

trans-, cyst(o), lith(o), nephr(o), ureter(o), -ectomy, -stomy, -tomy, -tripsy

1. surgical connection of one ureter to another

_____/_____/_____/_____

2. surgical crushing of a stone _____/_____

3. excision of the bladder _____/_____

4. excision of a kidney with its ureter _____/_____/_____

5. incision of an organ for removal of a calculus (or stones) _____/_____

7-68 Renal artery stenosis, partial blocking of one or both renal arteries, is treated by **percutaneous transluminal renal angio/plasty** or by using another major artery to route blood to the kidney. In percutaneous angio/plasty, the repair of the renal artery is via an incision of the _____.

skin

Anticoagulant therapy is used in renal vein thrombosis, a blood clot in the renal vein. A thromb/ectomy may also be performed, which means surgical excision of the _____.

thrombus

7-69 **Catheter dilation** is useful in treating strictures of the ureter (see Figure 7.28, A) or urethra. Severe stricture that does not respond to dilation may require **ureter/ectomy,** partial or complete surgical excision of the ureter.

The section of the ureter that remains after ureterectomy is attached to a different site on the bladder. This surgical procedure is called **ureterocystostomy.** This involves surgical transplantation of the ureter to a different site on the bladder and is called **uretero/cysto/neo/stomy.**

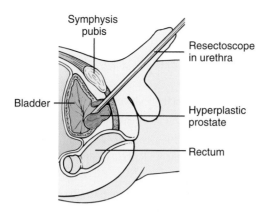

Symphysis
pubis

Resectoscope
in urethra

Bladder

Hyperplastic
prostate

Rectum

Figure 7.29 Transurethral resection of the prostate. This surgical procedure involves passing a resectoscope through the urethra and then excising pieces of the obstructing prostatic tissue.

pyeloplasty

7-70 Ureteroplasty means surgical repair of a ureter. Write a term that means surgical repair of the renal pelvis: _____.

cystoplasty

bladder

7-71 Write another term that means surgical repair of the bladder: _____.
Cystostomy means formation of a new opening into the bladder. **Suprapubic cystotomy** is surgical incision of the _____ via an incision just above the symphysis pubis. **Cystotomy** means incision of the bladder.

urethrotomy

urethra

7-72 Surgical incision of the urethra is _____.
Remembering that trans- means through or across, **trans/urethral** means through the _____. Transurethral surgery is performed by inserting an instrument through or across the wall of the urethra and makes it possible to perform surgery on certain organs that lie near the urethra without having an abdominal incision. In **transurethral resection** (TUR), small pieces of tissue from a nearby structure are removed through the wall of the urethra.

7-73 One surgery of this type is a **transurethral resection of the prostate** (TURP). In a TURP, surgery is performed on the prostate gland by means of an instrument passed through the wall of the urethra and is sometimes done to alleviate the problems of benign prostatic hyperplasia.
In a TURP (Fig. 7.29), an abdominal incision is not involved, because the surgeon approaches the prostate through the urethra. Small pieces of the prostate are removed with a special instrument called a *resectoscope*. Because this surgery is performed by passing the instrument through the

transurethral

urethra, it is called _____ resection of the prostate. In some cases, TURP is replaced by a less invasive laser TURP.

nephropexy

7-74 Use nephr(o) and -pexy to write a word that means surgical fixation of the kidney: _____. This type of surgery is often used to correct nephroptosis.

7-75 There are several types of urinary incontinence, and treatment depends on the cause. One of the more common types, stress incontinence (leakage of urine when coughing, sneezing, or straining), is sometimes helped with the use of **Kegel exercises** to strengthen the pelvic muscles. Also, weight loss in overweight persons, drug therapy, and/or surgery can be helpful. Incontinence resulting from spinal cord injury necessitates use of an indwelling catheter. Urinary incontinence means

urination

the inability to control _____.
Urinary retention may require catheterization, either intermittent or indwelling. Certain medications are also helpful.
Want more information? Go to *http://www.kidney.org*.

SELECT IT!
EXERCISE 20

Circle the correct answer for the following questions.
1. Which term means excision of a kidney? (nephrectomy, nephroscopy, nephrostomy, nephrotomy)
2. Which of the following terms is a type of urinary diversion? (cystometrography, glomerular filtration, hemodialysis, ureterostomy)
3. Which of the following is least likely to cause a urinary obstruction? (infection, stone, tumor, ureterolith)
4. Which of the following is not a likely treatment of a stone located in the bladder? (cystolithotomy, ESWL, lithotripsy, pyelolithotomy)
5. Which of the following may be used to treat renal vein thrombosis? (anticoagulant therapy, cystoplasty, nephropexy, shock wave lithotripsy)
6. Which term means a procedure that is performed by inserting an instrument through or across the wall of the urethra? (nephroptosis, transurethral resection, ureterocystostomy, urinary retention)

PHARMACOLOGY

Treatment of urinary tract infections includes antibiotics, analgesics, and increased intake of water.

Drug Class: Effect and Uses

Antidiuretics: Suppress urine formation
desmopressin (DDAVP) vasopressin (Vasostrict)

Antihypertensives: Reduce blood pressure in the kidneys
See Chapter 4 pharmacology section

Antiinfectives: Fight microorganisms to treat urinary tract infections (UTIs)
Various antibiotics (antibacterials and antifungals) are used for UTIs
nitrofurantoin (Macrobid)
See Chapter 3 for examples of antibacterials and antifungals.

Antispasmodics: Relax smooth muscle of bladder to treat overactive bladder
fesoterodine (Toviaz) oxybutynin (Ditropan)
flavoxate (Urispas) tolterodine (Detrol)

Diuretics: Increase formation of urine
bumetanide (Bumex) metolazone (Zaroxolyn) triamterene (Dyrenium)
furosemide (Lasix) spironolactone (Aldactone)
hydrochlorothiazide (Microzide) torsemide (Demadex)

Urinary pH Modifiers: Alkalinize or acidify the urine to prevent kidney stones, treat acidosis or metabolic alkylosis or promote excretion of drugs and toxins
ammonium chloride (*no brand name) potassium citrate (Urocit-K) sodium bicarbonate (Neut)

CIRCLE IT!
EXERCISE 21

Write the correct term to complete these sentences.
1. A drug class that treats an overactive bladder is _____.
2. Drugs that reduce blood pressure in the kidneys are _____.
3. Drugs that suppress urine formation are called _____.
4. Various antibacterials and antifungals are in a general class called _____.

Be Careful With These!

Prostate is a frequently misspelled term.
Note the difference in spelling of prostate and prostrate, which means lying in a facedown, horizontal position.

CHAPTER ABBREVIATIONS*

ADH	antidiuretic hormone
ARF	acute renal failure
BPH	benign prostatic hyperplasia
BUN	blood urea nitrogen
C&S	culture and sensitivity
CRF	chronic renal failure
EMG	electromyography
ESWL	extracorporeal shock wave lithotripsy
GFR	glomerular filtration rate
GU	genitourinary
I&O	intake and output
IVP	intravenous pyelography
IVU	intravenous urography
KUB	kidneys, ureters, and bladder

pH	potential of hydrogen; symbol for hydrogen ion concentration
PVP	photoselective vaporization of the prostate; Green Light PVP
STD	sexually transmitted disease
STI	sexually transmitted infection
TUR	transurethral resection
TURP	transurethral resection of the prostate
UA, U/A	urinalysis
UTI	urinary tract infection
VCUG	voiding cystourethrogram
VD	venereal disease

*Many of these abbreviations share their meanings with other terms.

A Career as a Radiologist Assistant

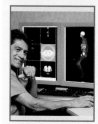

Thomas Clark, a radiologist assistant (RA), is an experienced, registered radiographer who has obtained additional education and certification that qualifies him to serve as a radiology extender, working under the supervision of a radiologist to provide patient care in the diagnostic imaging environment. Radiologist assistants take a leading role in patient management and assessment and perform selected radiology examinations and procedures. The RA also may be responsible for evaluating image quality, making initial image observations and forwarding those observations to the supervising radiologist. Radiologist assistants complete an academic program and a radiologist-supervised clinical internship and must be certified by the American Registry of Radiologic Technologists. For more information, visit *www.arrt.org*.

CHAPTER 7 SELF-TEST

Review the new word parts for this chapter. Work all of the following exercises to test your understanding of the material before checking your answers against those in Appendix IV.

BASIC UNDERSTANDING

Labeling

I. Label the numbered structures with their corresponding combining form. Numbers 1 and 3 have two answers.

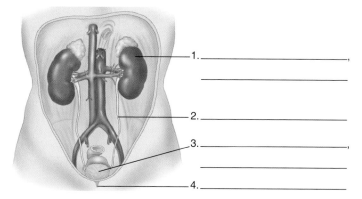

Matching

II.   Match structures in the left column with their functions in the right column.

___ **1.** bladder
___ **2.** nephron
___ **3.** renal pelvis
___ **4.** ureter
___ **5.** urethra

A. cavity in the kidney that collects urine from many collecting ducts
B. carries urine from the bladder
C. carries urine to the bladder
D. functional unit of the kidney
E. reservoir for urine until it is expelled

Listing

III.   List three major functions of the urinary system.

1. _____
2. _____
3. _____

True or False

IV.   Several urinary substances are listed. Write T for those substances that are normally detected in urine and F for those substances that are not normally detected.

1. albumin   _____
2. blood   _____
3. creatinine   _____
4. glucose   _____

5. ketones   _____
6. protein   _____
7. sugar   _____
8. urea   _____

Deconstructing Words

V.   Divide these terms into their component parts, and define the terms.

1. anuric   _____
2. lithotomy   _____
3. nocturia   _____
4. oliguria   _____
5. transurethral   _____   _____

Identifying Illustrations

VI.   Label these illustrations using one of the following terms: cystometry, cystoscopy, micturition, nephrostomy, nephrotomogram, renography, urinometer.

Source of electricity for light
Optical lens system
Sheath of cystoscope in urethra
Irrigating solution in bladder
Urethral orifice
From irrigating solution reservoir

1. _____   2. _____

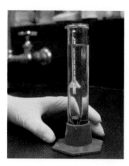

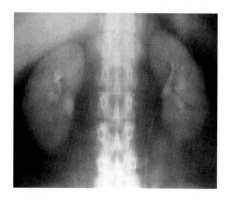

3. _____   **4.** _____

Using Vocabulary

VII. Circle the correct answer for each of the following multiple choice questions.

1. Raoul's physician is trying to explain that the filtering units of his kidneys are inflamed and not functioning properly. Which structures are inflamed? (Bowman capsules, glomeruli, tubules, ureters)

2. Which surgical procedure would remove a large calculus from Richard's renal pelvis? (cystolithectomy, lithotripsy, pyelolithotomy, pyelostomy)

3. Gayle has renal enlargement. Which term describes this condition? (floating kidney, kidney dialysis, nephromegaly, renal stone)

4. The nursing instructor is teaching different methods of collecting a urine sample. Which of the following is not a method for collecting urine? (catheterization, lithotripsy, urinating, voiding)

5. Prem's physician orders a test in which radiographic images of the urinary system are taken after the urine has been rendered opaque by a contrast medium. What is the name of this test? (cystoscopy, cystoureteroscopy, intravenous urography, nephrotomography)

6. Carl's laboratory results show a greatly elevated blood urea nitrogen. Which disorder is indicated? (pyelostomy, pyuria, renal clearance, renal failure)

7. Mr. Smith is catheterized because he is unable to control his urination. Which term indicates his inability to control urination? (frequency, hesitancy, incontinence, retention)

8. Which of the following symptoms of untreated diabetes is most frequently noted by the patient? (anuria, dysuria, oliguria, polyuria)

9. Nursing students are studying various means of urinary tract catheterization. Which of the following procedures is not included? (endoscopy, nephrostomy, suprapubic catheterization, ureteral catheterization, urethral catheterization)

10. Which of the following is a toxic condition of the body that occurs when the kidneys fail to function properly? (nephromalacia, nephrolithiasis, uremia, urography)

Writing Terms

VIII. Write a term for each of the following:

1. any disease of the urinary tract _____

2. between the kidneys _____

3. blood in the urine _____

4. herniation of the urethra _____

5. inflammation of the renal glomeruli _____

6. Inflammation of the renal pelvis _____

7. kidney dialysis _____

8. outside the urinary bladder _____

9. radiography of the bladder _____

10. surgical crushing of a stone _____

Making Connections

IX.   Describe the relationship of these terms.

1. hilum, renal artery, renal vein _____
_____

2. kidneys and blood pressure _____
_____

3. micturition and urination _____
_____

4. specific gravity and urinometer _____
_____

Finetuning Terms

X.   In addition to spelling, describe at least one difference in the following:

1. hypospadias and epispadias _____
_____

2. tubular reabsorption and tubular secretion _____
_____

3. anuria and oliguria _____
_____

4. diabetes insipidus and diabetes mellitus _____
_____

5. hydroureter and hydronephrosis _____
_____

Opting For Opposites

XI.   Write a term that you learned that means the opposite of these words.

1. anuria _____

2. diuretic _____

GREATER COMPREHENSION

Labeling

XII.   Choose from the following list to label parts of the nephron shown (1 to 5):

distal convoluted tubule, glomerulus, Bowman capsule, proximal convoluted tubule, collecting duct

1. _____

2. _____

3. _____

4. _____

5. _____

Loop of Henle

Final filtrate excreted in urine

Health Care Reporting

XIII. Read the urology clinic note, and answer the questions that follow. Although some of the terms are new, you should be able to determine their meanings by analyzing the word parts.

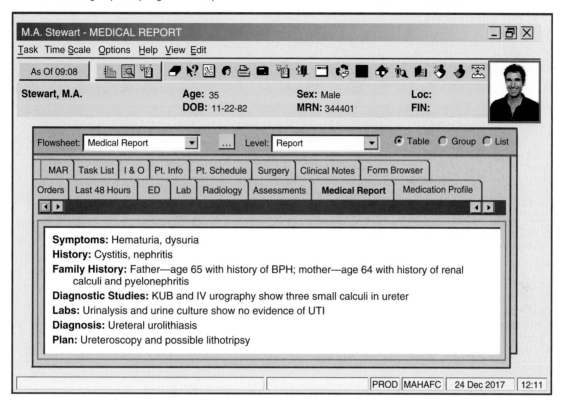

M.A. Stewart - MEDICAL REPORT

Task Time Scale Options Help View Edit

As Of 09:08

Stewart, M.A.   Age: 35   Sex: Male   Loc:
                       DOB: 11-22-82   MRN: 344401   FIN:

Flowsheet: Medical Report   Level: Report   ○ Table ○ Group ○ List

MAR | Task List | I & O | Pt. Info | Pt. Schedule | Surgery | Clinical Notes | Form Browser

Orders | Last 48 Hours | ED | Lab | Radiology | Assessments | **Medical Report** | Medication Profile

Symptoms: Hematuria, dysuria
History: Cystitis, nephritis
Family History: Father—age 65 with history of BPH; mother—age 64 with history of renal calculi and pyelonephritis
Diagnostic Studies: KUB and IV urography show three small calculi in ureter
Labs: Urinalysis and urine culture show no evidence of UTI
Diagnosis: Ureteral urolithiasis
Plan: Ureteroscopy and possible lithotripsy

PROD | MAHAFC | 24 Dec 2017 | 12:11

Circle the correct answer (A, B, C, or D) for each question.

1. Mr. Stewart's symptom of dysuria indicates which characteristic of urine or urination?
(A) blood (B) decreased output (C) difficult or painful (D) protein

2. Which of the following conditions does his history indicate?
(A) bladder and kidney stones (B) inflammation of the bladder and kidney (C) inflammation caused by trauma
(D) frequent urinary infections

3. Which of the following is indicated in his mother's history?
(A) kidney stones (B) polycystic kidney (C) renal stenosis (D) uremia

4. Which of the following is M. A. Stewart's diagnosis?
(A) narrowing of the ureter (B) obstruction of the ureter (C) stone in the ureter (D) urinary infection

5. Which procedure is indicated by a ureteroscopy?
(A) surgical fixation (B) renal angiography (C) ureteral resection (D) visual examination

Categorizing Terms

XIV. Classify the terms in the left columns (1 to 10) by selecting A, B, C, D, or E from the right column.

_____ **1.** cystourethrography	_____ **6.** nephrectomy	**A.** anatomy
_____ **2.** diuretics	_____ **7.** nephrosclerosis	**B.** diagnostic test or procedure
_____ **3.** genitourinary	_____ **8.** nephrosonography	**C.** pathology
_____ **4.** glycosuria	_____ **9.** tubule	**D.** surgery
_____ **5.** hemodialysis	_____ **10.** ureterocele	**E.** nonsurgical therapy

Be prepared to pronounce terms 1-10 in class after listening to the Chapter 7 terms at *http://evolve.elsevier.com/Leonard/building*. In addition, practice categorizing all boldface terms in this chapter.

XV. Read the following report and circle an answer to the multiple-choice questions.

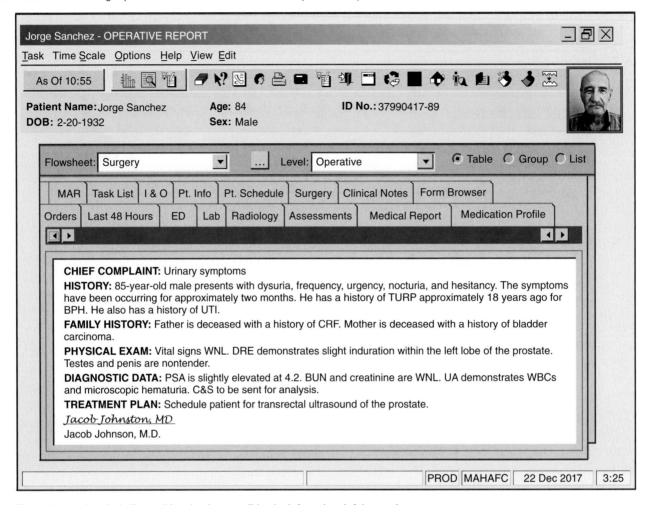

1. The patient's dysuria indicates his urination was (bloody, infected, painful, scant)

2. The term in the report which indicates urination at night is (frequency, hesitancy, nocturia, urgency)

3. The abbreviation which describes testing of the patient's urine sample is (BUN, DRE, PSA, UA)

4. The patient's father suffered from a disease which primarily affected the (kidneys, ureters, urethra, urinary bladder)

5. The abbreviation which describes nonmalignant enlargement of the prostate gland is (BPH, C&S, TURP, UTI)

Pronouncing Terms

XVI. Write the correct term for the following phonetic spellings.

1. dī-ū-**rē**-sis   _____

2. **lith**-ō-trip-sē   _____

3. nef-rō-li-**thī**-uh-sis   _____

4. **pī**-uh-lō-gram   _____

5. ū-**rē**-tur-ō-plas-tē   _____

6. ū-**rop**-uh-thē   _____

Using Pharmacologic Terms

XVII. Match terms in the right column with those in the left column.

___ **1.** reduce blood pressure   **A.** antidiuretics

___ **2.** suppress urine formation   **B.** antihypertensives

___ **3.** treat urinary tract infections   **C.** antiinfectives

___ **4.** treat overactive bladder   **D.** antispasmodics

XVIII. Read the following partial operative report and answer the questions that follow.

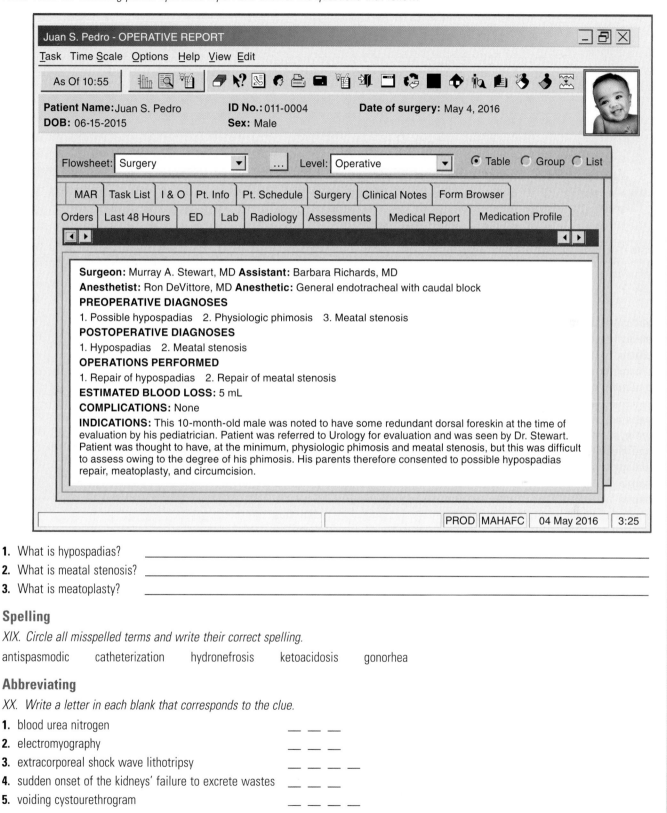

Juan S. Pedro - OPERATIVE REPORT

Task   Time Scale   Options   Help   View   Edit

As Of 10:55

Patient Name: Juan S. Pedro   **ID No.:** 011-0004   **Date of surgery:** May 4, 2016
DOB: 06-15-2015   **Sex:** Male

Flowsheet: Surgery   ...   Level: Operative   ⦿ Table   ○ Group   ○ List

MAR | Task List | I & O | Pt. Info | Pt. Schedule | Surgery | Clinical Notes | Form Browser

Orders | Last 48 Hours | ED | Lab | Radiology | Assessments | Medical Report | Medication Profile

Surgeon: Murray A. Stewart, MD **Assistant:** Barbara Richards, MD
Anesthetist: Ron DeVittore, MD **Anesthetic:** General endotracheal with caudal block
PREOPERATIVE DIAGNOSES
1. Possible hypospadias   2. Physiologic phimosis   3. Meatal stenosis
POSTOPERATIVE DIAGNOSES
1. Hypospadias   2. Meatal stenosis
OPERATIONS PERFORMED
1. Repair of hypospadias   2. Repair of meatal stenosis
ESTIMATED BLOOD LOSS: 5 mL
COMPLICATIONS: None
INDICATIONS: This 10-month-old male was noted to have some redundant dorsal foreskin at the time of evaluation by his pediatrician. Patient was referred to Urology for evaluation and was seen by Dr. Stewart. Patient was thought to have, at the minimum, physiologic phimosis and meatal stenosis, but this was difficult to assess owing to the degree of his phimosis. His parents therefore consented to possible hypospadias repair, meatoplasty, and circumcision.

PROD | MAHAFC | 04 May 2016 | 3:25

1. What is hypospadias?   _____
2. What is meatal stenosis?   _____
3. What is meatoplasty?   _____

Spelling

XIX. Circle all misspelled terms and write their correct spelling.

antispasmodic   catheterization   hydronefrosis   ketoacidosis   gonorhea

Abbreviating

XX. Write a letter in each blank that corresponds to the clue.

1. blood urea nitrogen   — — —
2. electromyography   — — —
3. extracorporeal shock wave lithotripsy   — — — —
4. sudden onset of the kidneys' failure to excrete wastes   — — —
5. voiding cystourethrogram   — — — —

New Constructions

XXI. Break these words into their component parts, and write their meanings. Even if you have not seen these terms before, you may be able to break them apart and determine their meanings.

1. cystorrhagia _____

2. ketonemia _____

3. nephrotoxic _____

4. perineocele _____

5. urogenital _____
(Use Appendix IV to check your answers to the exercises.)

> **TOOL TIP!** *Pay attention to spelling.*

BMV LIST

Visit *http://evolve.elsevier.com/Leonard/building* to listen to the boldface terms in Chapter 7. Look closely at the spelling of each term as it is pronounced.

abdominocystic (ab-dom-i-nō-**sis**-tik)
abdominovesical (ab-dom-i-nō-**ves**-i-kul)
albumin (al-**bū**-min)
albuminuria (al-bū-mi-**nū**-rē-uh)
antibiotic sensitivity test (an-tē-bī-**ot**-ik sen-si-**tiv**-i-tē test)
antidiuretic hormone (an-tē-dī-ū-**ret**-ik **hor**-mōn)
antidiuretics (an-tē-dī-ū-**ret**-iks)
antihypertensives (an-tē-hī-pur-**ten**-sivz)
antiinfectives (an-tē-in-**fek**-tivz)
antispasmodics (an-tē-spaz-**mod**-ikz)
anuria (an-**ū**-rē-uh)
anuric (an-**ū**-rik)
benign prostatic hyperplasia (buh-**nīn** pros-**tat**-ik hī-pur-**plā**-zhuh)
bladder (**blad**-ur)
bladder cancer (**blad**-ur **kan**-sur)
bladder polyp (**blad**-ur **pol**-ip)
blood urea nitrogen (blud ū-**rē**-uh **nī**-trō-jun)
Bowman capsule (**bō**-mun **cap**-sul)
catheter dilation (**kath**-uh-tur dī-**lā**-shun)
catheterized urine specimen (**kath**-uh-ter-īzd **ū**-rin **spes**-i-mun)
chlamydial infection (kluh-**mid**-ē-ul in-**fek**-shun)
clean-catch specimen (klēn kach **spes**-i-mun)
creatinine (krē-**at**-i-nin)
creatinine clearance test (krē-**at**-i-nin **klēr**-uns test)
cystectomy (sis-**tek**-tuh-mē)
cystic (**sis**-tik)
cystitis (sis-**tī**-tis)
cystocele (**sis**-tō-sēl)
cystography (sis-**tog**-ruh-fē)
cystolith (**sis**-tō-lith)
cystolithiasis (sis-tō-li-**thī**-uh-sis)
cystolithotomy (sis-tō-li-**thot**-uh-mē)
cystometer (sis-**tom**-uh-tur)
cystometrography (sis-tō-muh-**trog**-ruh-fē)
cystoplasty (**sis**-tō-plas-tē)

cystoscope (**sis**-tō-skōp)
cystoscopy (sis-**tos**-kuh-pē)
cystostomy (sis-**tos**-tuh-mē)
cystotomy (sis-**tot**-uh-mē)
cystourethritis (sis-tō-ū-rē-**thrī**-tis)
cystourethrography (sis-tō-ū-ruh-**throg**-ruh-fē)
cystourethroscopy (sis-tō-ū-rē-**thros**-kuh-pē)
diabetes insipidus (dī-uh-**bē**-tēz in-**sip**-i-dus)
diabetes mellitus (dī-uh-**bē**-tēz **mel**-luh-tus, muh-**lī**-tis)
diabetic nephropathy (dī-uh-**bet**-ik nuh-**frop**-uh-thē)
distal tubule (**dis**-tul **tōō**-būl)
diuresis (dī-ū-**rē**-sis)
diuretics (dī-ū-**ret**-iks)
dysuria (dis-**ū**-rē-uh)
electromyography (ē-lek-trō-mī-**og**-ruh-fē)
enuresis (en-ū-**rē**-sis)
epispadias (ep-i-**spā**-dē-us)
erythropoietin (uh-rith-rō-**poi**-uh-tin)
excretion (eks-**krē**-shun)
excretory (**eks**-kruh-tor-ē)
extracorporeal shock wave lithotripsy (eks-truh-kor-**por**-ē-ul shok wāv **lith**-ō-trip-sē)
extracystic (eks-truh-**sis**-tik)
Foley catheter (**fō**-lē **kath**-uh-tur)
frequency (**frē**-kwun-sē)
genitourinary (jen-i-tō-**ū**-ri-nar-ē)
genitourinary infections (jen-i-tō-**ū**-ri-nar-ē in-**fek**-shunz)
glomerular filtration (glō-**mer**-ū-lur fil-**trā**-shun)
glomerular filtration rate (glō-**mer**-ū-lur fil-**trā**-shun rāt)
glomerulonephritis (glō-mer-ū-lō-nuh-**frī**-tis)
glomerulopathy (glō-mer-ū-**lop**-uh-thē)
glomerulus (glō-**mer**-ū-lus)
glycosuria (glī-kō-**sū**-rē-uh)
gonorrhea (gon-ō-**rē**-uh)
hematuria (hē-muh-, hem-uh-**tū**-rē-uh)
hemodialysis (hē-mō-dī-**al**-uh-sis)

hesitancy (**hez**-uh-tun-sē)
hilum (**hī**-lum)
hydronephrosis (hī-drō-nuh-**frō**-sis)
hydroureter (hī-drō-ū-**rē**-tur)
hyperglycemia (hī-pur-glī-**sē**-mē-uh)
hypospadias (hī-pō-**spā**-dē-us)
indwelling catheter (**in**-dwel-ing **kath**-uh-tur)
intake and output (**in**-tāk and **out**-poot)
interrenal (in-tur-**rē**-nul)
interstitial nephritis (in-tur-**stish**-ul nuh-**frī**-tis)
intravenous pyelography (in-truh-**vē**-nus pī-uh-**log**-ruh-fē)
intravenous urography (in-truh-**vē**-nus ū-**rog**-ruh-fē)
Kegel exercises (**kā**-gul **ek**-sur-sīz-uz)
ketoacidosis (kē-tō-as-i-**dō**-sis)
ketone (**kē**-tōn)
ketonuria (kē-tō-**nū**-rē-uh)
kidney dialysis (**kid**-nē dī-**al**-uh-sis)
kidneys (**kid**-nēz)
laparoscopic nephrectomy (lap-uh-rō-**skop**-ik nuh-**frek**-tuh-mē)
lithotomy (li-**thot**-uh-mē)
lithotripsy (**lith**-ō-trip-sē)
lithotrite (**lith**-ō-trīt)
micturition (mik-tū-**ri**-shun)
nephrectomy (nuh-**frek**-tuh-mē)
nephritis (nuh-**frī**-tis)
nephrolith (**nef**-rō-lith)
nephrolithiasis (nef-rō-li-**thī**-uh-sis)
nephrolithotomy (nef-rō-li-**thot**-uh-mē)
nephrolysis (nuh-**frol**-uh-sis)
nephromalacia (nef-rō-muh-**lā**-shuh)
nephromegaly (nef-rō-**meg**-uh-lē)
nephrons (**nef**-ronz)
nephropathy (nuh-**frop**-uh-thē)
nephropexy (**nef**-rō-pek-sē)
nephroptosis (nef-rop-**tō**-sis, nef-rō-**tō**-sis)
nephrosclerosis (nef-rō-skluh-**rō**-sis)
nephroscope (**nef**-rō-skōp)
nephroscopy (nuh-**fros**-kuh-pē)
nephrosonography (nef-rō-sō-**nog**-ruh-fē)
nephrostomy (nuh-**fros**-tuh-mē)
nephrotic syndrome (nuh-**frot**-ik **sin**-drōm)
nephrotomogram (nef-rō-**tō**-mō-gram)
nephrotomography (nef-rō-tō-**mog**-ruh-fē)
nephrotoxic (**nef**-rō-tok-sik)
nephroureterectomy (nef-rō-ū-rē-tur-**ek**-tuh-mē)
neurogenic bladder (noor-ō-**jen**-ik **blad**-ur)
nocturia (nok-**tū**-rē-uh)
nycturia (nik-**tū**-rē-uh)
obstructive nephropathies (ob-**struk**-tiv nuh-**frop**-uh-thēz)
oliguria (ol-i-**gū**-rē-uh)
percutaneous nephrostomy (pur-kū-**tā**-nē-us nuh-**fros**-tuh-mē)
percutaneous transluminal renal angioplasty (pur-kū-**tā**-nē-us trans-**loo**-mi-nul **rē**-nul **an**-je-ō-plas-tē)
perineal muscles (per-i-**nē**-ul **mus**-ulz)
perineum (per-i-**nē**-um)
peritoneal dialysis (per-i-tō-**nē**-uhl dī-**al**-uh-sis)
polycystic kidney disease (pol-ē-**sis**-tik **kid**-nē di-**zēz**)

polyuria (pol-ē-**ū**-rē-uh)
proteinuria (prō-tē-**nū**-rē-uh)
proximal tubule (**prok**-si-mul **too**-būl)
pus cells (pus selz)
pyelitis (pī-uh-**lī**-tis)
pyelogram (**pī**-uh-lō-gram)
pyelolithotomy (pī-uh-lō-li-**thot**-uh-mē)
pyelonephritis (pī-uh-lō-nuh-**frī**-tis)
pyeloplasty (**pī**-uh-lō-plas-tē)
pyuria (pī-**ū**-rē-uh)
rectourethral (rek-tō-ū-**rē**-thrul)
renal (**rē**-nul)
renal angiography (**rē**-nul an-jē-**og**-ruh-fē)
renal arteries (**rē**-nul **ahr**-tuh-rēz)
renal arteriogram (**rē**-nul ahr-**tēr**-e-ō-gram)
renal artery stenosis (**rē**-nul **ahr**-tuh-rē stuh-**nō**-sis)
renal carcinoma (**rē**-nul kahr-si-**nō**-muh)
renal clearance tests (**rē**-nul **klēr**-uns tests)
renal failure (**rē**-nul **fāl**-yur)
renal hypertension (**rē**-nul hī-pur-**ten**-shun)
renal pelvis (**rē**-nul **pel**-vis)
renal scan (**rē**-nul skan)
renal threshold (**rē**-nul **thresh**-ōld)
renal transplant (**rē**-nul **trans**-plant)
renal vein thrombosis (**rē**-nul vān throm-**bō**-sis)
renography (rē-**nog**-ruh-fē)
renovascular disorders (rē-nō-**vas**-kū-lur dis-**or**-durz)
septicemia (sep-ti-**sē**-mē-uh)
sexually transmitted disease (**sek**-shoo-uh-lē trans-**mit**-ud di-**zēz**)
specific gravity (spuh-**sif**-ik **grav**-i-tē)
suprapubic catheterization (soo-pruh-**pū**-bik kath-uh-tur-i-**zā**-shun)
suprapubic cystotomy (soo-pruh-**pū**-bik sis-**tot**-uh-mē)
suprarenal (soo-pruh-**rē**-nul)
transureteroureterostomy (trans-ū-rē-tur-ō-ū-rē-tur-**os**-tuh-mē)
transurethral (trans-ū-**rē**-thrul)
transurethral resection (trans-ū-**rē**-thrul rē-**sek**-shun)
transurethral resection of the prostate (trans-ū-**rē**-thrul rē-**sek**-shun ov thuh **pros**-tāt)
tubular reabsorption (**too**-bū-lur rē-ab-**sorp**-shun)
tubular secretion (**too**-bū-lur sē-**krē**-shun)
tubules (**too**-būlz)
urea (ū-**rē**-uh)
uremia (ū-**rē**-mē-uh)
ureter (ū-**rē**-tur, **ū**-ruh-tur)
ureteral (ū-**rē**-tur-ul)
ureteral catheterization (ū-**rē**-tur-ul kath-uh-tur-i-**zā**-shun)
ureteral dysfunction (ū-**rē**-tur-ul dis-**funk**-shun)
ureterectomy (ū-rē-tur-**ek**-tuh-mē)
ureteritis (ū-rē-tur-**ī**-tis)
ureterocele (ū-**rē**-tur-o-sēl)
ureterocystoneostomy (ū-rē-tur-ō-sis-tō-nē-**os**-tuh-mē)
ureterocystostomy (ū-rē-tur-ō-sis-**tos**-tuh-mē)
ureterolith (ū-**rē**-tur-ō-lith)
ureterolithiasis (ū-rē-tur-ō-li-**thī**-uh-sis)
ureterolithotomy (ū-rē-tur-ō-li-**thot**-uh-mē)

ureteropathy (ū-rē-tur-**op**-uh-thē)
ureteroplasty (ū-**rē**-tur-ō-plas-tē)
ureteropyelonephritis (ū-rē-tur-ō-pī-uh-lō-nuh-**frī**-tis)
ureteroscopy (ū-rē-tur-**ōs**-kuh-pē)
ureterostenosis (ū-rē-tur-ō-stuh-**nō**-sis)
ureterostomy (ū-rē-tur-**ōs**-tuh-mē)
ureterovesical (ū-rē-tur-ō-**ves**-i-kul)
urethra (ū-**rē**-thruh)
urethral (ū-**rē**-thrul)
urethral catheterization (ū-**rē**-thrul kath-uh-tur-i-**zā**-shun)
urethritis (ū-ruh-**thrī**-tis)
urethrocele (ū-**rē**-thrō-sēl)
urethrocystitis (ū-rē-thrō-sis-**tī**-tis)
urethrography (ū-ruh-**throg**-ruh-fē)
urethrorectal (ū-rē-thrō-**rek**-tul)
urethrorrhagia (ū-rē-thrō-**rā**-juh)
urethrorrhea (ū-rē-thrō-**rē**-uh)
urethroscopy (ū-ruh-**thros**-kuh-pē)
urethrospasm (ū-**rē**-thrō-spaz-um)
urethrostenosis (ū-rē-thrō-stuh-**nō**-sis)
urethrotomy (ū-ruh-**throt**-uh-mē)
urethrovaginal (ū-rē-thrō-**vaj**-i-nul)
urgency (**ur**-jun-sē)
urinalysis (ū-ri-**nal**-i-sis)
urinary (**ū**-ri-nar-ē)
urinary casts (**ū**-ri-nar-ē kasts)

urinary catheterization (**ū**-ri-nar-ē kath-uh-tur-i-**zā**-shun)
urinary incontinence (**ū**-ri-nar-ē in-**kon**-ti-nuns)
urinary meatus (**ū**-ri-nar-ē mē-**ā**-tus)
urinary pH modifiers (**ū**-ri-nar-ē pH **mod**-i-fī-urz)
urinary reflux (**ū**-ri-nar-ē **rē**-fluks)
urinary retention (**ū**-ri-nar-ē rē-**ten**-shun)
urinary tract (**ū**-ri-nar-ē trakt)
urinary tract infection (**ū**-ri-nar-ē trakt in-**fek**-shun)
urination (ū-ri-**nā**-shun)
urine (**ū**-rin)
urine culture (**ū**-rin **kul**-chur)
urinometer (ū-ri-**nom**-uh-tur)
urodynamic studies (ū-rō-dī-**nam**-ik **stud**-ēz)
urogenital (ū-rō-**jen**-i-tul)
urogram (**ū**-rō-gram)
urolithiasis (ū-rō-li-**thī**-uh-sis)
uropathy (ū-**rop**-uh-thē)
venereal diseases (vuh-**nēr**-ē-ul di-**zēz**-uz)
vesical (**ves**-i-kul)
vesicoureteral (ves-i-kō-ū-**rē**-tur-ul)
vesicovaginal (ves-i-kō-**vaj**-i-nul)
voided specimen (**voi**-dud **spes**-i-mun)
voiding (**void**-ing)
voiding cystourethrogram (**void**-ing sis-tō-ū-**rē**-thrō-gram)
voids (voidz)
Wilms tumor (wilmz **too**-mur)

Español ENHANCING SPANISH COMMUNICATION

English	Spanish (pronunciation)
acidity	acidez (ah-se-DES)
albumin	albúmina (al-BOO-me-nah)
catheter	catéter (kah-TAY-ter)
cystitis	cystitis (sis-TEE-tis)
dialysis	diálisis (de-AH-le-sis)
excretion	excreción (ex-kray-se-ON)
incontinence	incontinencia (in-kon-te-NEN-se-ah)
lithotripsy	litotricia (le-to-TREE-see-ah)
lithotriptor	lithotritor (le-to-tre-TOR)
nephrectomy	nefrectomia (nay-fra-to-MEE-ah)
nephritis	nefritis (nay-FREE-tis)
nephrotomy	nefrotomia (nay-fro-to-MEE-ah)
perineum	perineo (pay-re-NAY-o)
renal artery	arteria renal (ar-TAY-re-ah ray-NAHL)
renal calculus	cálculo renal (KAHL-koo-lo ray-NAHL)
specimen	muestra (moo-AYS-trah)
urea	urea (oo-RAY-ah)
urinalysis	urinálisis (oo-re-NAH-le-sis)
urinary	urinario (oo-re-NAH-re-o)
urinate	orinar (o-re-NAR)
urination	urinación (oo-re-nah-se-ON)
voided specimen	orinado (o-re-NAH-do)
voiding	urinar (oo-re-NAR)

Reproductive System

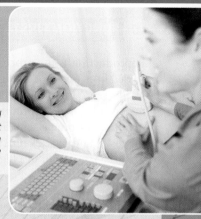

This sonographer has special training in the use of ultrasound equipment and works mainly with obstetric patients throughout their pregnancies. She occasionally works in the delivery room with an obstetrician. Her talent for visualizing objects in three dimensions is very helpful in her ultrasonography career.

Basic Understanding

In this chapter, you will learn to do the following:

1. State the functions of the reproductive systems, and analyze associated terms.
2. Write, define, and label the reproductive structures.
3. Write the meanings of the word parts associated with the reproductive systems, and use the word parts to build and analyze terms.
4. Select the correct terms to match descriptions of fertilization, implantation, and growth of the embryo, and label the structures of the embryo.
5. Define or select the correct meaning of terms related to pregnancy, labor, and the newborn.
6. Write the names of the diagnostic tests and procedures for assessment of the reproductive systems when given descriptions of the procedures, or match the procedures with their descriptions.
7. Write the names of pathologies of the reproductive systems when given their descriptions, or match them with their descriptions.
8. Match surgical and therapeutic interventions for reproductive system pathologies with descriptions of the interventions, or write the names of the interventions when given their descriptions.
9. Match sexually transmitted diseases with their characteristics, or write the names of the diseases when given their descriptions.
10. Build terms from word parts to label illustrations.

Greater Comprehension

11. Use word parts from this chapter to determine the meaning of terms in a health care report.
12. Spell the terms accurately.
13. Pronounce the terms correctly.
14. Write the meanings of the abbreviations.
15. Categorize terms as anatomy, diagnostic test or procedure, pathology, surgery or nonsurgical therapy.
16. Recognize the meanings of general pharmacological terms from this chapter as well as the drug classes and their uses.

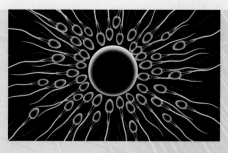

FUNCTION FIRST

Reproduction is the process by which genetic material is passed from one generation to the next. The major function of the reproductive system is to produce offspring. The male and female reproductive systems can be broadly organized by organs with different functions. For example, the testes and ovaries function in the production of spermatozoa (sperm) or ova (eggs), and they secrete important hormones. Ducts transport and receive eggs or sperm and important fluids. Still other reproductive organs produce materials that support the sperm and ova.

Sexually transmitted diseases (STDs) are passed from one person to another by anal, oral, or vaginal contact, but some are transmitted by contact with contaminated materials. STDs may infect the fetus or the infant at birth.

FEMALE REPRODUCTIVE SYSTEM
ANATOMY AND PHYSIOLOGY

8-1 The female reproductive system aids in the creation of new life and provides an environment and support for the developing child. After birth, the female breasts produce milk to feed the child. Information about the breasts, often considered a part of this system, is found in Chapter 12, which covers hormones and the endocrine system.

The female reproductive system includes the ovaries, fallopian tubes, uterus, vagina, accessory glands, and external genital structures. The ovaries are the female gonads. A **gonad** produces the reproductive cells.

The reproductive organs, whether male or female, are called the *genitals* or **genitalia.** The combining form genit(o) refers to organs of reproduction. The genitalia include both external and internal organs. Another name for genitals is _____.

genitalia

8-2 The combining form that means woman or female is gynec(o). **Gynecology** is the medical specialty that treats diseases of the female reproductive organs. **Gyneco/logic** means pertaining to gynecology (Gyn) or study of diseases that occur only in _____.

females

Vulva refers to the external genitalia in the female, and the combining form is vulv(o). **Vulv/ar** and **vulv/al** mean pertaining to the _____.

vulva

The structures that comprise the vulva are external to the vagina. Label the structures as you read the material that accompanies Fig. 8.1.

8-3 The **mons pubis** is a pad of fatty tissue and thick skin that overlies a bone called the *symphysis pubis.* The pubis is the anterior portion of the hipbones. After puberty, the mons pubis is covered with hair.

WORD ORIGIN
mons *(L.)*
mons, mountain

The **clitoris** is a small mass of erectile tissue and nerves that has similarities to the male penis. This small mass of erectile tissue becomes erect in response to sexual stimulation.

Two pairs of skin folds, the **labia majora** and the **labia minora,** protect the vaginal opening. (The singular forms are labium majus and labium minus.) The larger pair of skin folds is called the labia _____. The smaller pair of skin folds, the labia minora, merge and form a hood over the clitoris. This fold of skin that forms a retractable cover is called the **prepuce.**

majora

The name of the **para/urethral glands** tells us they are located _____ the urethra.

near

Other glands, the **vestibular glands,** lie adjacent to the vaginal opening.

8-4 **Vestibule** is any space or cavity at the entrance to a canal. The vaginal vestibule is the space between the two labia minora into which the urethra and vagina open. The greater vestibular glands **(Bartholin glands)** produce a mucuslike secretion for lubrication during sexual intercourse.

Another important locational term is **perineum,** the area between the vaginal opening and the anus. **Perine/al** means pertaining to the _____.

perineum

Knowing that ur(o) means pertaining to urine or the urinary system, **uro/genit/al** or **genito/urinary** (GU) means pertaining to the urinary and the reproductive systems.

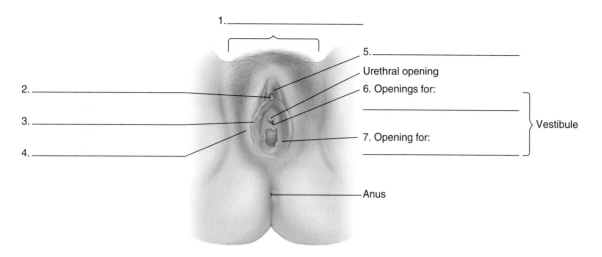

1. _____

5. _____

Urethral opening

6. Openings for:

_____

7. Opening for:

_____

Vestibule

2. _____

3. _____

4. _____

Anus

Figure 8.1 Female external genitalia. These structures are external to the vagina and are called the *vulva*. The mons pubis *(1)* is a pad of fatty tissue and thick skin that overlies the front of the pubic bone. The clitoris *(2)* is a small mass of erectile tissue and nerves. Two pairs of skin folds protect the vaginal opening. The smaller pair is called the *labia minora (3)*, and the larger pair is called the *labia majora (4)*. The retractable cover around the clitoris is the prepuce *(5)*. The paraurethral glands *(6)* and the vestibular glands *(7)* are also shown.

WRITE IT!   EXERCISE 1

Write a word in each blank.

1. The purpose of reproduction is to produce _____.
2. The term for reproductive organs, whether male or female, is _____.
3. The general term for a structure that produces reproductive cells is _____.
4. Vulva refers to the _____ female genitalia.
5. The smaller pair of skin folds that protect the vaginal opening is the labia _____

8-5 Label the internal structures as you read the material that accompanies Fig. 8.2. The right **ovary** and left ovary are the primary reproductive structures, because they produce **ova** (eggs) and hormones. The singular form of ova is ovum. The drawing in Fig. 8.2 is a midsagittal view of the internal genitalia, so only one ovary is shown. An ovary is about the size and shape of an almond.

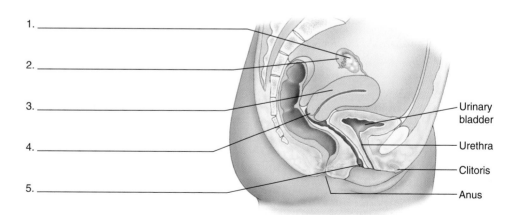

1. _____

2. _____

3. _____

4. _____

5. _____

Urinary bladder

Urethra

Clitoris

Anus

Figure 8.2 Female genitalia, midsagittal section. Write the names of the structures on the numbered lines as you read the following. Each ovary *(1)* produces ova and hormones. One uterine tube *(2)* is associated with each ovary. The uterus *(3)* is the muscular organ that prepares to receive and nurture the fertilized ovum. The lower and narrower part that has the outlet from the uterus is the cervix uteri *(4)*. The vagina *(5)* is the connection between the internal genitalia and the outside.

uterus

8-6 Examine Table 8.1, which lists the internal and external structures of the female genitalia. Note that the ovaries, uterus, vagina, and several glands make up the internal structures of the female genitalia.

8-7 One **fallopian tube** is associated with each ovary (Fig. 8.3). These tubes are also called **uterine tubes,** because they extend laterally from the upper portion of the _____ to the region of the ovary. There is no direct connection between the ovary and the fingerlike projections of the fallopian tube, the **fimbriae.** When an ovum is produced, the fimbriae create currents that sweep the ovum into the tube, and it is then carried along toward the uterus over the next 5 to 7 days. The fallopian tube is the most common site of fertilization of the ovum, which disintegrates or dies within 24 to 48 hours if it is not fertilized.

🔑 **KEY** POINT The **uterus is a muscular organ that prepares to receive and nurture the fertilized ovum.** The uterus is hollow and pear shaped. The lower and narrower part that has the outlet from the uterus is the cervix uteri, commonly called the *uterine cervix* (Cx). When used alone, the term *cervix* often means the cervix uteri.

Table 8.1	Female Genitalia	
Internal Structures		**External Structures**
Left ovary and associated left uterine tube		Mons pubis
Right ovary and associated left uterine tube		Labia majora
Uterus		Labia minora
Vagina		Clitoris
Special glands		Prepuce
		Openings for glands

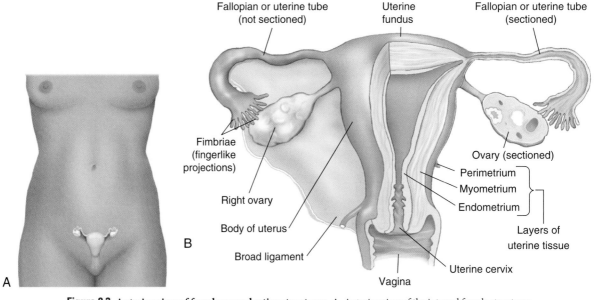

Figure 8.3 **Anterior view of female reproductive structures. A,** Anterior view of the internal female structures in reference to location. **B,** Anterior view of the internal organs of the female reproductive system. The left ovary, the left uterine tube, and the left side of the uterus are sectioned to show their internal structure.

The **vagina,** commonly called the *birth canal*, is muscular and capable of sufficient expansion for passage of the child during childbirth. It also serves as the repository for sperm during intercourse and the passageway for menstrual flow. The vagina is the connection between the internal genitalia and the outside through its opening called the *vaginal orifice* (opening). Note that there is one uterus but two ovaries and two _____ tubes.

uterine (or fallopian)

MATCH IT! EXERCISE 2

Match terms in the left column with definitions or descriptions in the right column.

_____ **1.** ovary
_____ **2.** uterine cervix
_____ **3.** uterine tube
_____ **4.** uterus
_____ **5.** vagina

A. birth canal
B. most common site of fertilization
C. outlet from the uterus
D. produces ova
E. receives and nurtures a fertilized ovum

Learn the following word parts that are used to write terms about the female genitalia.

Word Parts: Female Genitalia

Combining Form	Meaning	Other Word Parts	Meaning
cervic(o)	neck; uterine cervix	-an, -ile	belonging to or pertaining to
colp(o), vagin(o)	vagina	lapar(o)	abdominal wall
genit(o)	organs of reproduction	men(o)	month
hyster(o), uter(o)	uterus	o(o)	egg (ovum)
metr(o)	measure; uterine tissue	top(o)	place or position
oophor(o), ovari(o)	ovary	-tropin	that which stimulates
perine(o)	perineum		
salping(o)	fallopian tube		
vulv(o)	vulva		

WRITE IT! EXERCISE 3

Write word parts or meanings as indicated in the following blanks.

Combining Form   Meaning

1. colp(o) _____
2. genit(o) _____
3. hyster(o) _____
4. men(o) _____
5. metr(o) _____
6. o(o) _____
7. oophor(o) _____

8. ovari(o) _____
9. uter(o) _____
10. vagin(o) _____
11. _____ perineum
12. _____ cervix uteri or neck
13. _____ fallopian tube
14. _____ vulva

8-8 Two combining forms that mean uterus are uter(o) and hyster(o). You may wonder about the connection between *hysterical* and the word part that means uterus.

➤ **BEYOND** THE BLUEPRINT Hysterics, hysterical, or hysterectomy use the combining form hyster(o), which means uterus. The use of hyster(o) as a combining form may have originated with the ancient Greeks who believed that women were especially susceptible to emotional disorders that arose from the womb. The Greeks used the word *hysterikos* to refer to suffering in the womb and the emotional upheaval caused by this suffering.

A third combining form, metr(o), also means the uterus, and occasionally metr(o) means measure. Whenever you see metr(o) used in a word, use your critical thinking skills to decide if it means measure or _____ tissue. It is not as difficult as it might seem. For example, **metr/itis** could only refer to inflammation of _____ tissue.

uterine
uterine

uterine

8-9 The uterus consists of three layers of tissue. From the outermost layer to the innermost layer, the layers are called *perimetrium, myometrium,* and *endometrium.* Find these three layers of uterine tissue in Fig. 8.3.

The outer layer is **visceral peritoneum** and is called **peri/metr/ium.** When you analyze its word parts, peri- means around, metr(o) means _____ tissue, and -ium means membrane. In other words, perimetrium is a membrane that surrounds the uterus.

endometrium

The **myo/metr/ium** (my[o] means muscle) is the thick muscular wall of the uterus. The inner layer, the **endo/metr/ium,** is a mucous membrane. Write the name of this mucous membrane that lines the uterus: _____.

8-10 The uterus is the normal site where a fertilized ovum implants and develops. Examine the anterior view of the female genitalia in Fig. 8.3.

fundus

The uterus consists of an upper portion, a large main portion, and a narrow region that connects with the vagina. The upper, bulging surface of the uterus, above the entrance of the uterine tubes, is called the uterine _____. The large, main portion is called the *body of the uterus,* and the narrow region is the uterine cervix.

8-11 The word **cervix** refers to the neck itself or part of an organ that resembles a neck. The **cervix uteri** specifically means the lower, necklike portion of the uterus, although it is common to see cervix written alone and meaning the cervix uteri. The proper name of the uterine cervix is the

uteri

cervix _____. The combining form cervic(o) means neck or cervix uteri. Look at other parts of a term to decide which meaning of cervic(o) is intended. **Cervico/colp/itis** is

uteri

inflammation of the cervix _____ and the vagina.

FIND IT!
EXERCISE 4

Draw a slash between the word parts in the following list. Then find the meanings of the word parts within the definitions. (Draw the slash, and then perform the remainder of the activity as a mental exercise.)

1. **colpocystitis** inflammation of the vagina and the urinary bladder
2. **ovarian** pertaining to the ovary
3. **uterine** pertaining to the uterus
4. **vaginal** pertaining to the vagina

BUILD IT!
EXERCISE 5

Use the following word parts to build terms. (Some word parts will be used more than once.)

endo-, intra-, peri-, cervic(o), metr(o), my(o), ovari(o), uter(o), -al, -an, -ine, -ium

1. pertaining to the cervix   _____/_____
2. pertaining to the ovary   _____/_____
3. pertaining to within the uterus   _____/_____/_____
4. a membrane that surrounds the uterus _____/_____/_____
5. thick muscular wall of the uterus   _____/_____/_____
6. inner layer of the uterus   _____/_____/_____

Ovarian and Uterine Cycles

8-12 During much of a woman's life, the endometrium goes through a monthly cycle of growth and discharge known as the **menstrual cycle.** Reproductive cycles normally occur in females from shortly after the onset of menstruation to menopause.

menstrual

The monthly cycle of growth and discharge of the endometrium is called the _____ cycle.

8-13 The hypothalamus (part of the brain) and the pituitary gland, located just beneath the brain, have significant roles in the control of reproductive functions.

KEY POINT The hormones produced by these structures act on the ovaries to bring about two important functions: The production of ova and additional hormones, **estrogen** and **progesterone**.

8-14 Female reproductive cycles begin at puberty and continue for about 40 years until menopause. Remember the meaning of these important stages in a female's life:

- **puberty:** Stage of development when genitalia reach maturity and secondary sex characteristics appear. The external characteristics of sexual maturity include adult distribution of hair and development of the breasts and menarche, usually between 9 and 13 years of age. **Menarche** is the first occurrence of **menstruation,** the periodic bloody discharge caused by the shedding of the endometrium from the nonpregnant uterus. The date of the last menstrual period (LMP) is important, particularly when pregnancy is suspected or menopause is being investigated.
- **menopause,** also called the **climacteric:** the natural cessation of reproductive cycles and menstruation with the decline of reproductive hormones in later years. Menopause may occur earlier as a result of illness or surgical removal of the uterus or both ovaries.

WRITE IT! EXERCISE 6

Write a word in each blank.

1. The stage of development when genitalia reach maturity is _____.
2. The periodic bloody discharge caused by shedding of the endometrium is _____.
3. The term for the first occurrence of menstruation _____.
4. Another term for menopause is _____.

ovaries
uterus

8-15 The secretion of female reproductive hormones follows monthly cyclic patterns that affect the ovaries and uterus. Together, these cycles, called the *ovarian cycle* and the *menstrual (uterine) cycle,* make up the female reproductive cycle (having an average of 28 days). The ovarian cycle reflects the changes that occur within the _____. The uterine (menstrual) cycle reflects the changes that take place in the _____.

follicle

8-16 The ovarian and uterine cycles begin at puberty when certain unknown stimuli cause the hypothalamus to start secreting a hormone that acts on the pituitary gland. The pituitary gland then begins to secrete two hormones, **follicle-stimulating hormone** (FSH) and **luteinizing hormone** (LH), that act on follicles in the ovaries. By its name, it is evident that follicle-stimulating hormone stimulates a _____ (in this particular case, a graafian follicle).

The **graafian follicle** is a small ovarian recess or pit that contains fluid and surrounds an ovum (egg). Generally one ovum is released each month. The follicle produces hormones and grows in preparation for release of the ovum. These changes in the follicle are classified as the follicular phase, which is followed by the luteal phase. Find these two phases in Fig. 8.4.

🔑 **KEY** POINT **Ovulation is the release of the ovum from the follicle.** After the ovum is released, the ruptured follicle enlarges, takes on a yellow appearance, and is called the **corpus luteum,** meaning yellow body.

ovulation

The follicular changes are represented by follicle development, _____, and corpus luteum.

8-17 Looking at Fig. 8.4, you see that FSH acts on the graafian follicle and undergoes changes, which result in release of the ovum.

luteum

The luteal phase is named after the yellowish structure called the corpus _____.

8-18 Two important hormones that are secreted by the follicles influence the uterine cycle. During the follicular phase, increasing amounts of estrogen are secreted and stimulate repair of the endometrium. Estrogen reaches its peak near the middle of the cycle, and then decreases until the next month. The corpus luteum secretes another important hormone, progesterone, which causes continued growth and thickening of the endometrium with additional preparatory activities to support a potential embryo. If fertilization (union of the ovum and sperm) does not occur, the corpus luteum begins to degenerate and the cycle starts again.

The initial hormone, estrogen, is the same hormone that brings about development of the female secondary sex characteristics, the external physical signs of sexual maturity, such as the development of breasts and pubic hair.

A second hormone is secreted by the corpus luteum. That hormone is called

progesterone

_____.

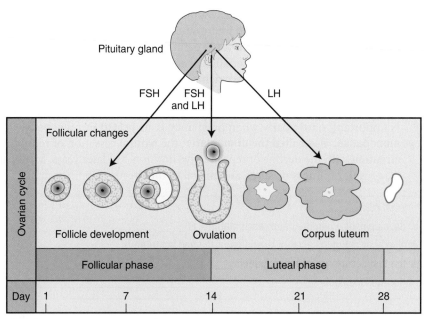

Figure 8.4 The ovarian cycle. This portion of the menstrual cycle has two important phases. The follicular phase is represented by changes in the follicle and results in ovulation (release of the ovum). The luteal phase is represented by changes in the follicle that results in secretion of progesterone by the matured follicle.

8-19 The uterine cycle occurs simultaneously with the ovarian cycle and is the result of estrogen and progesterone secretion by the ovaries. The uterine cycle begins with menstruation (which occurs on day 1 of the cycle and continues for 3 to 5 days), followed by thickening of the endometrium along with secretion of glycogen, which will nourish a developing embryo if fertilization occurs.

The term **menses** means the normal flow of blood during menstruation when fertilization has not occurred. Menses and menstruation are often used interchangeably. Write the second term that means the same as menses: _____.

menstruation

8-20 Estrogen and progesterone (secreted by the ovarian follicle) prepare the uterus for pregnancy. Write a word that means formation of ova, using the combining form for ovum, o(o), and the suffix -genesis, which means origin or beginning: _____.

oogenesis

WRITE IT! EXERCISE 7

Write a term for each description or definition.
1. another term for menses _____
2. what FSH represents _____
3. what LH represents _____
4. release of an ovum from the ovarian follicle _____
5. initial hormone that causes thickening of the endometrium _____
6. the second hormone secreted by the corpus luteum _____

DIAGNOSTIC TESTS AND PROCEDURES

8-21 Gynecologic problems and obstetric care account for one fifth of all visits by females to physicians. Many diagnostic procedures and treatments are available to females with gynecologic disorders.

The physical assessment of the female reproductive system includes examination of the breasts, the external genitalia, and the pelvis. A **vaginal speculum** is an instrument that can be pushed apart after it is inserted into the vagina to allow examination of the cervix and the walls of the vagina (Fig. 8.5).

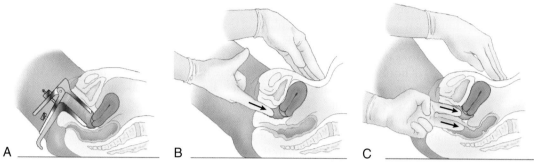

A

B

C

Figure 8.5 **The gynecologic examination. A,** Proper position of inserted speculum. **B,** The bimanual examination. The abdominal hand presses the pelvic organs toward the intravaginal hand. **C,** Rectovaginal examination. The examiner's index finger is placed in the vagina and the middle finger is inserted into the rectum. The gynecologic inspection consists of four parts: *(1)* Inspection of the external genitalia. *(2)* The speculum examination. The vaginal walls and cervix are inspected. Smears (Pap smear for cytologic examination) are obtained. *(3)* Bimanual examination assesses the location, size, and mobility of the pelvic organs. *(4)* The rectovaginal examination is not always performed. In this examination, the posterior aspect of the genital organs and rectal tissue can be evaluated.

cells

8-22 Specimens (scrapings) for cytology can be collected during the pelvic examination. **Cyto/logy** means the study of _____. Both Pap smears and endo/metrial biopsies are performed to detect cancer of the cervix.

Pap smear is an abbreviated way of saying **Papanicolaou test** or smear. In a Pap smear, material is collected from areas of the body that shed cells. The cells are then studied microscopically.

8-23 The term *Pap smear* may refer to collection of material from other surfaces that shed cells, but it usually refers to collection and examination of cells from the vagina and cervix (Fig. 8.6). Early diagnosis of **cervical cancer,** cancer of the uterine cervix, is possible with the Pap test. When the Pap smear is examined microscopically, malignant cells have a characteristic appearance that indicates cancer, sometimes before symptoms appear.

Cancer of the uterus may begin with a change in shape, growth, and number of cells, called **dysplasia.** The dysplasia (dys-, bad + -plasia, development) is not cancer, but cells of this type tend to become malignant. This abnormality, which can be detected before cancer occurs, is called

dysplasia

_____.

It is standard practice to grade Pap smears as class I, II, III, IV, or V. Class I is normal, and class V is definitely cancer. Most physicians recommend having Pap smears done on a routine basis. Regular Pap smears are an excellent method for early detection of cervical cancer, when it is possible that the lesion can be excised, thus preventing spread of cancer to other organs.

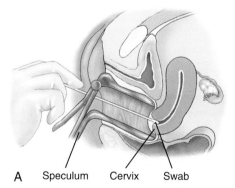

A   Speculum   Cervix   Swab

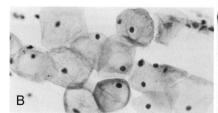

B

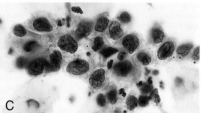

C

Figure 8.6 **Papanicolaou (Pap) smear. A,** Obtaining a Pap smear. **B,** Appearance of normal cervical cells in a Pap smear. **C,** Appearance of cervical cancer cells in a Pap smear.

8-24 Specimens of vaginal or cervical discharge are collected and tested for the presence of mico-organisms using several techniques. Wet mounts, the direct microscopic examination of the fluid, aid in diagnosis of infections with yeast or **Trichomonas,** a vaginal and urethral parasite. Gram stain, a slide-staining technique that aids in classification and identification of bacteria, is especially useful for vaginal smears if **gonorrhea** or **chlamydial infection** is suspected. Bacterial or fungal cultures may also be helpful in identifying the cause of infections.

The Venereal Disease Research Laboratories (VDRL) test and the **rapid plasma reagin** (RPR) **test** are blood tests to detect and monitor **syphilis.** (More about STDs is presented later in this chapter.)

Levels of hormones in the blood and urine are helpful in determining the function of the ovaries, particularly in fertility studies and pregnancy. **Human chorionic gonadotropin** (HCG) is present in body fluids of pregnant females, and blood or urine is tested to determine whether pregnancy exists. Chorion/ic pertains to the chorion, a membrane that develops around a fertilized embryo. **Gonado/tropin** (gonad[o] + -tropin, that which stimulates) is a hormonal substance that stimulates the _____ in this case, the ovaries.

| gonads |

HCG can be detected long before other signs of pregnancy appear. This test may also be used to detect rare forms of tumors in either men or women, but more often the test is performed to ascertain pregnancy. Write the name of the hormone that is tested for in pregnancy tests: human chorionic _____.

| gonadotropin |

8-25 Colposcopy involves the use of a low-powered microscope to magnify the mucosa of the vagina and the cervix. The instrument used is a _____ (Fig. 8.7).

| **colposcope** |

Suspicious cervical or vaginal lesions may be seen during colposcopy. Some findings indicate the need for a cervical or endometrial biopsy. A **cervical biopsy** is removal of tissue from the _____. An **endometrial biopsy** requires collection of tissue from the lining of the _____.

| cervix |
| uterus |

8-26 Hysteroscopy is direct visual inspection of the cervical canal and uterine cavity, using an endoscope passed through the vagina (Fig. 8.8). Change the suffix of hysteroscopy to write the name of the endoscope: _____.

| **hysteroscope** |

8-27 Pelvic sonography may be helpful in detecting masses, such as ovarian cysts. Computed tomography (CT) may be used to detect a tumor within the pelvis.

Hystero/salpingo/graphy is radiologic examination of the uterus and the _____ tubes after an injection of radiopaque material into those organs (Fig. 8.9). It allows evaluation of the size, shape, and position of the organs, including tumors and certain other abnormalities, as well as obstruction of a uterine tube.

| uterine (or fallopian) |

A **hysterosalpingogram** is the _____ that is produced in hysterosalpingography.

| record |

8-28 Laparo/scopy is the examination of the abdominal cavity with a **laparoscope** through one or more small incisions in the abdominal wall. This surgical procedure is especially useful for inspection of the ovaries and other structures within the pelvic cavity, as well as collection of biopsy specimens or performance of tubal ligation to prevent pregnancy (Fig. 8.10). Write the name of the instrument used in laparoscopy: _____.

| laparoscope |

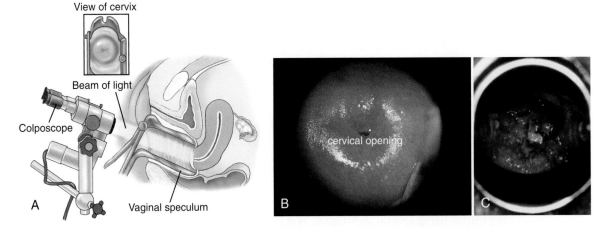

Figure 8.7 Colposcopy. A, The vagina and cervix are examined with a colposcope. **B,** The appearance of a normal uterine cervix using a speculum. **C,** The colposcopic appearance of an abnormal nonsmooth surface and a crater-like ulceration of the cervix that was followed up with a biopsy and determined to be cervical cancer.

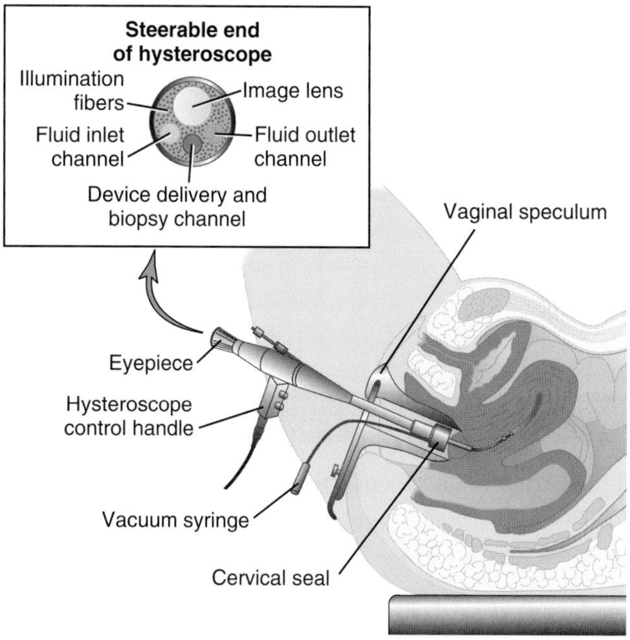

Steerable end of hysteroscope

Illumination fibers
Image lens
Fluid inlet channel
Fluid outlet channel
Device delivery and biopsy channel

Vaginal speculum

Eyepiece

Hysteroscope control handle

Vacuum syringe

Cervical seal

Figure 8.8 Hysteroscopy. Direct visual examination of the cervical canal and uterine cavity using a hysteroscope is performed to examine the endometrium to obtain a specimen for biopsy, to excise cervical polyps, or to remove an intrauterine device.

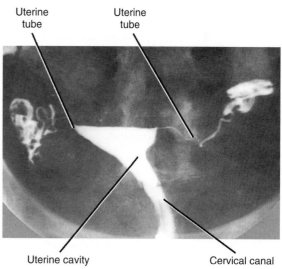

Uterine tube
Uterine tube

Uterine cavity
Cervical canal

Figure 8.9 Hysterosalpingogram. This x-ray image of the uterus and uterine tubes was made after the introduction of a radiopaque substance through the cervix.

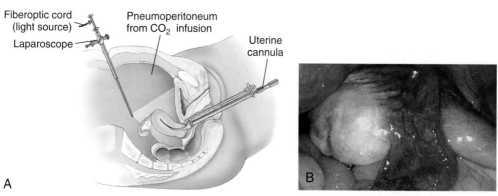

Fiberoptic cord (light source)
Pneumoperitoneum from CO_2 infusion
Laparoscope
Uterine cannula

A

B

Figure 8.10 Laparoscopy. A, Drawing of laparoscopy. Using the laparoscope with a fiberoptic light source, the surgeon can view the pelvic cavity and the reproductive organs. The purpose of the uterine cannula is to allow movement of the uterus during laparoscopy. **B,** Laparoscopic view of the right uterine tube and the right ovary (suspended by mesovarium, which is a type of peritoneum). The rich vascular supply of oxygen and nutrients to the ovary is shown by the many arteries visible in the mesovarium.

WRITE IT!   EXERCISE 8

Write a term in each of the blanks to complete the sentences. The first letter of each term is given as a clue.

1. An instrument used to examine the vagina and cervix walls is a s_____.
2. The study of cells in a Pap test is called c_____.
3. In a Pap smear, an alteration in the shape, growth, or number of cells that is not a sign of cancer but indicates a tendency of the cells to become malignant is called d_____.
4. A hormone that is tested to ascertain pregnancy is human chorionic g_____.
5. Using low-powered microscopy to examine the vaginal mucosa and cervix is called c_____.
6. Direct visualization of the uterus with a hysteroscope is h_____.
7. A radiographic examination of the uterus and the uterine tubes after an injection of a radiopaque contrast medium is called h_____.
8. Examining the pelvic cavity after making one or more small abdominal incisions is l_____.

MATCH IT!
EXERCISE 9

Match descriptions in the left column with the correct terms in the right column.

____ **1.** membrane that develops around the fertilized embryo

____ **2.** blood test to detect and monitor syphilis

____ **3.** slide-staining technique that helps identify bacteria

____ **4.** collection and examination of cells from the vagina and cervix

____ **5.** direct microscopic examination of fluid

A. Pap smear

B. rapid plasma reagin

C. wet mounts

D. Gram stain

E. chorion

 PATHOLOGIES

8-29 Menstrual disorders include painful menstruation, heavy or irregular flow, spotting, absence of or skipping periods, and premenstrual syndrome.

FIND IT!
EXERCISE 10

Draw a slash between the word parts in the following list. Then find the meanings of the word parts within the definitions. (Draw the slash, and then perform the remainder of the activity as a mental exercise.)

1. amenorrhea absence of menstruation, such as absence of menstruation due to underdevelopment of the reproductive organs or hormonal disturbances. Amenorrhea is normal before puberty, after menopause, and during pregnancy.

2. dysmenorrhea painful or difficult menstruation

3. menorrhagia heavy or long menstrual periods

4. menorrhea normal menstruation; sometimes too profuse menstruation

5. metrorrhagia uterine bleeding other than that caused by menstruation; may occur as spotting or outright bleeding and is caused by cervical cancer or uterine tumors

8-30 Premenstrual syndrome (PMS) is nervous tension, irritability, edema, headache, and painful breasts that can occur the last few days before the onset of menstruation. Various studies indicate that many females experience some degree of PMS, but fewer than half experience symptoms that disrupt their lives. PMS means _____ syndrome.

premenstrual

WORD ORIGIN
mittelschmerz *(D.)*
mittel, mid, middle;
schmerz, pain, suffering

Mittelschmerz means abdominal pain in the region of an ovary during ovulation. It is helpful in pinpointing the fertile period of the ovarian cycle.

8-31 Vagin/itis is inflammation of the vaginal tissues. This may be accompanied by itching, burning or discomfort during urination, and vaginal discharge; however, some infections are asymptomatic. Many of these lower genital tract infections are related to sexual intercourse, which can irritate vaginal tissues and transmit microorganisms. Vaginal infections are sometimes considered a STD, but infection can also occur after childbirth or after taking antibiotics that produce changes in the vaginal tissues that allow overgrowth of normal flora, such as *C. albicans,* which can cause a yeast infection (see Frames 8-33 and 8-155).

vaginitis

Write this term that means infection of the vagina: _____. This is the same as **colp/itis.**

vulva

8-32 Vulv/itis is inflammation of the _____ and is associated with itching and burning. This can be caused by infection, contact with irritants, or systemic conditions.

8-33 Vulvo/vaginitis is inflammation of the vulva and vagina. Vulvar infections can be extensions of vaginal infections. Vulvo/vagin/al candidiasis is infection of the vagina and vulva with *C. albicans.* An infection caused by *Candida* is called **candidiasis.** Remembering that -iasis means condition, write this term that means a condition caused by *C. albicans:* _____.

candidiasis

8-34 An/ovulation, absence of ovulation, is failure of the ovaries to produce, mature, or release ova. Its causes include altered ovarian function or dysfunction, side effects of medications, and stress or disease. Write this term that means lack of ovulation: _____.

anovulation

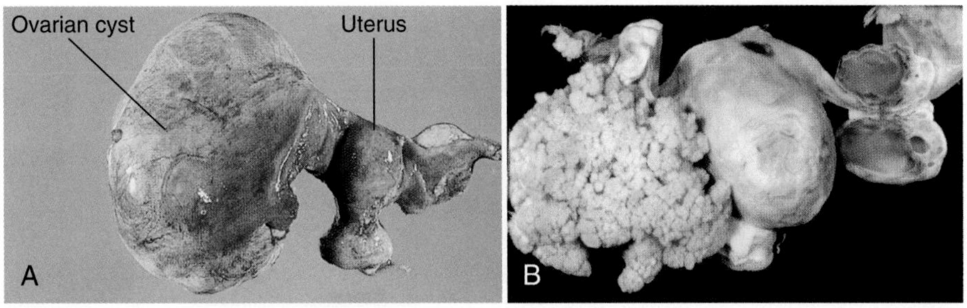

Figure 8.11 An ovarian cyst vs. ovarian carcinoma. A, Ovarian cyst. This very large benign cyst is soft and surrounded by a thin capsule. Ovarian masses are often asymptomatic until they are large enough to cause pressure in the pelvis. **B,** Carcinoma of the ovary. The ovary is enormously enlarged by the tumor. Ovarian cancer is often far advanced when diagnosed.

8-35 Polycystic ovary syndrome is a hormonal disturbance characterized by anovulation, amenorrhea, and infertility. It is caused by increased levels of testosterone (a hormone that is secreted in large quantities in males, in smaller quantities in females), estrogen, and LH and decreased secretion of FSH. Numerous cysts may develop, and the affected ovary sometimes doubles in size.

Polycystic ovary syndrome differs from what is usually meant by the term **ovarian cyst,** which is a globular sac filled with fluid or semisolid material that develops in or on the ovary. This type of ovarian cyst may be transient or pathologic. Benign cysts are common and may be asymptomatic, or they may cause pelvic pain and menstrual irregularities. If a female is a/symptomatic, this means

without

that she is _____ symptoms.

Ovarian cancer is the leading cause of death from reproductive cancers, because the disease has usually spread to other organs by the time it is discovered. Sonography and CT may detect the ovarian mass, but diagnosis generally requires surgical exploration and pathologic confirmation of the diagnosis. Compare a benign ovarian cyst and a malignant ovarian tumor (Fig. 8.11).

FIND IT! EXERCISE 11

Draw a slash between the word parts in the following list. Then find the meanings of the word parts within the definitions. (Draw the slash, and then perform the remainder of the activity as a mental exercise.)

1. **oophoralgia** ovarian pain
2. **oophoritis** inflammation of an ovary
3. **oophoropathy** any disease of an ovary
4. **oophorosalpingitis** inflammation of an ovary and a uterine tube
5. **salpingitis** inflammation of a uterine tube
6. **salpingocele** hernial protrusion of a uterine tube

8-36 Sometimes a fertilized ovum implants in a site other than within the uterine wall. The abnormal implantation site is usually in the uterine tube, and this is called a *tubal pregnancy.* Treatment is removal of the pregnancy, sometimes with removal of the uterine tube.

KEY POINT An ectopic pregnancy is one in which a fertilized ovum implants somewhere outside the uterine cavity. Ectopic (ect[o], outside + top[o], position + -ic, pertaining to) means situated in an unusual place, away from its normal location.

8-37 The uterine tubes are usually infected in **pelvic inflammatory disease** (PID). Without treatment, the tubes can become obstructed and cause infertility. PID is any infection that involves the upper genital tract beyond the cervix. Untreated gonococcal or staphylococcal infections, for example, can spread along the endometrium to the uterine tubes and cause an acute salpingitis. If untreated or treated inadequately, the tubes can become obstructed. PID stands for _____

pelvic

inflammatory disease.

Septicemia (sept[o], infection + -emia, blood) and other severe complications rarely occur in PID as they do in **toxic shock syndrome** (TSS). A sudden high fever, headache, confusion, acute renal failure, and abnormal liver function are characteristic of TSS. This acute disease is caused by a type of *Staphylococcus* species and is most common in menstruating women who use tampons.

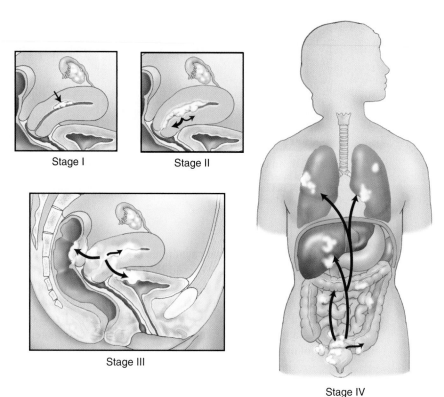

Figure 8.12 Staging uterine cancer. Stage I: Tumor is confined to the uterine corpus. Stage II: The cancer has also invaded the cervix. Stage III: The cancer has spread beyond the uterus but remains confined to the pelvis, such as in the bladder or rectum. Stage IV: The highest level of invasiveness; the cancer has spread beyond the pelvis, causing metastatic disease and large masses, such as in the liver or lungs.

Stage I

Stage II

Stage III

Stage IV

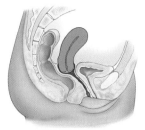
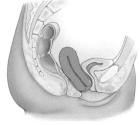
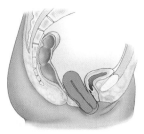

Figure 8.13 Hysteroptosis. Three stages of uterine prolapse. **A,** Grade I: Uterus bulges into the vagina but does not protrude through the entrance. **B,** Grade II: Cervix is visible within the vagina. **C,** Grade III: Body of the uterus and the cervix protrude through the vaginal orifice.

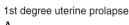

1st degree uterine prolapse
A

2nd degree uterine prolapse
B

3rd degree uterine prolapse
C

8-38 You learned in Chapter 2 that cervical cancers are often caused by the human papillomavirus (HPV) for which a vaccine is available. Cervical cancer can be detected in the early, curable stage by the Pap test. Cancer of the cervix or other reproductive structures can spread to other organs. The stage of **uterine cancer** is identified by the extent to which it has spread to other organs (Fig. 8.12). Early removal of cancerous tissue is vital for preventing the spread of cancer.

hysteropathy

Write a word that means any disease of the uterus: _____.

8-39 The uterus is normally held in its proper alignment with the vagina and the uterine tubes by ligaments that hold each structure in its proper place. Weakening of the ligaments causes a prolapsed uterus. Using -ptosis, write a word that means uterine prolapse: _____.

hysteroptosis

A prolapsed uterus can be congenital or caused by heavy physical exertion. It is classified according to its severity (Fig. 8.13).

8-40 The uterus normally lies midline in the pelvis; however, some variations, called **uterine displacements,** occur (Fig. 8.14). Mild degrees of these four types of displacements are common, may or may not cause symptoms, and may be determined by the position of the cervix when the pelvic examination is performed. Use the information in Fig. 8.14 to complete these sentences.

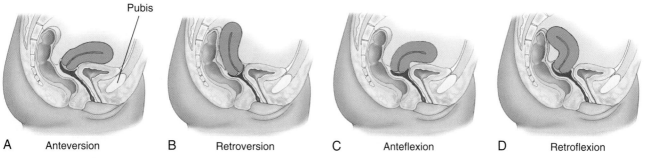

Figure 8.14 Abnormal (forward or backward) displacements of the uterus. A, Anteversion, forward displacement of the body of the uterus toward the pubis with the cervix tilted up. **B,** Retroversion, tipped backward (the opposite of anteversion). **C,** Anteflexion, bending forward. **D,** Retroflexion, bending backward.

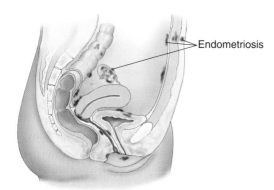

Figure 8.15 Common sites of endometriosis. Dark spots in the drawing indicate sites of endometriosis. The abnormal location of endometrial tissue is often the ovaries and less commonly other pelvic structures.

anteversion backward	A forward displacement of the body of the uterus toward the pubis, the anterior portion of the hipbone, is _____. **Retro/version** is a common condition in which the uterus is tipped _____ and is the opposite of anteversion.
anteflexion	A bending forward of the uterus is called _____, and a bending backward of the uterus is **retroflexion.**
myometritis	8-41 Write a term that means inflammation of the myometrium: _____.
	8-42 **Endometritis** is inflammation of the endometrium and is generally produced by bacterial invasion of the endometrium. **Endometriosis,** however, is an abnormal condition in which tissue that contains typical endometrial elements is present outside the uterus, usually within the pelvic cavity. See the common sites of endometriosis in Fig. 8.15.
endometriosis	Endometrial tissue that is located outside the uterine lining responds to hormonal changes and goes through cyclic changes of bleeding and proliferation. Scarring and adhesions result. (An adhesion is an abnormal adherence of structures that are not normally joined.) A condition in which endometrium occurs in other places besides the uterus is called _____.
adhesion	8-43 The formation of adhesions (scar tissue that binds anatomic surfaces that normally are separate) is the body's response to peritoneal trauma. For example, adhesions commonly form in the abdomen after abdominal surgery, inflammation, or injury, and may cause amenorrhea or infertility. Adhesions are frequently seen during laparoscopic procedures. For example, scar tissue that has formed within the abdomen after repeated surgeries is a type of abdominal _____.

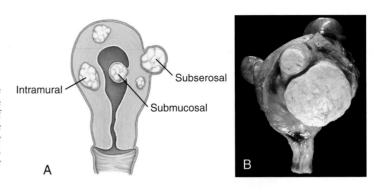

Figure 8.16 Leiomyomas, also called *uterine fibroids.* **A,** This uterine section shows the locations of the most common leiomyomas. The tumors develop from the myometrium and stay attached by means of a pedicle. Subserosal, submucosal, and intramural leiomyomas protrude through the outer surface of the uterine wall, protrude into the cavity of the uterus, or are contained within the uterine wall, respectively. **B,** Surgical removal of this uterus was necessary because of the very large myoma.

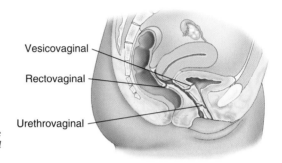

Figure 8.17 Sites of vaginal fistulas. Abnormal openings between the vagina and the bladder, rectum, and urethra are shown. These abnormal openings are called *vesicovaginal fistula, rectovaginal fistula,* and *urethrovaginal fistula,* respectively.

leiomyoma	**8-44** A **leiomyoma** (leio-, smooth + my[o], muscle + -oma, tumor) is the most common benign tumor occurring within the uterus and is also called a **uterine fibroid** (Fig. 8.16). Leiomyomas can occur in other smooth muscle, and large tumors may cause a general enlargement of the lower abdomen. The term that means the same as a uterine fibroid is uterine _____.

cervicitis	**8-45 Cervical polyps** are benign lesions attached to the cervix, often by a stalk, and can sometimes be seen in a gynecologic examination.
	    Cervic/itis refers specifically to inflammation of the cervix uteri. Acute cervicitis is infection of the cervix marked by redness, bleeding on contact, a foul-smelling discharge from the vagina, and often pain, itching, or burning. Acute cervicitis may be caused by several species of bacteria, *Chlamydia* (specialized bacteria), *Candida albicans* (yeast), or the parasite *Trichomonas vaginalis.* Some STDs—for example, gonorrhea—cause cervicitis. Diagnosis of gonorrhea can often be made by examination of a stained smear and is confirmed by culture.
	    Persistent inflammation of the cervix is called chronic _____.

white	**8-46 Leuko/rrhea** normally occurs in the adult female and is somewhat increased before and after the menstrual period. It may be abnormal if there is either an increase in amount or a change in color or odor. Literal translation of leuko/rrhea is _____ discharge. This new term specifically refers to a white, viscid discharge from the vagina and the uterine cavity.
vagina **colporrhagia**	**8-47 Colpo/dynia** is pain of the _____. Use colp(o) to write a word that means hemorrhage from the vagina: _____.
urethra bladder	**8-48** Vaginal **fistulas** are abnormal openings between the vagina and the urethra, the bladder, or the rectum. **Urethro/vaginal** fistulas occur between the _____ and the vagina. A **rectovaginal** fistula is one that occurs between the rectum and the vagina. Knowing that vesic(o) means bladder, a **vesicovaginal** fistula occurs between the urinary _____ and the vagina. (See the locations of these types of fistulas in Fig. 8.17.)
	8-49 A **cysto/cele** (cyst[o], bladder + -cele, herniation), protrusion of the urinary bladder through the wall of the vagina, occurs when support is weakened between the two structures. A **recto/cele** (rect[o], rectum) occurs from a weakening between the vagina and rectum. Both problems are

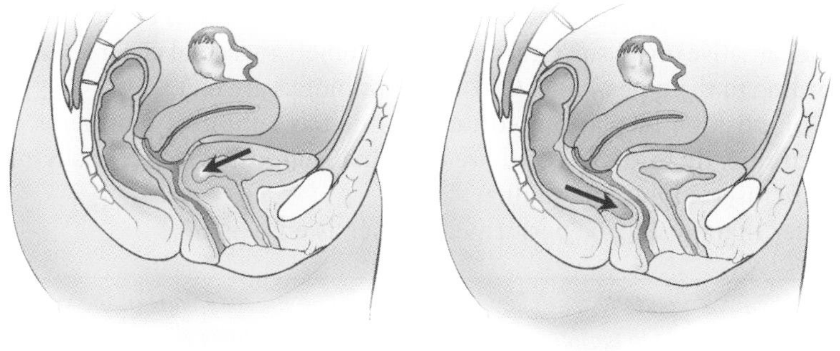

Figure 8.18 Comparison of a cystocele and a rectocele. A, Cystocele. The urinary bladder is displaced downward, causing bulging of the anterior vaginal wall. **B,** Rectocele. The rectum is displaced, causing bulging of the posterior vaginal wall.

common and often asymptomatic. A large cystocele can interfere with emptying the bladder, and a large rectocele can interfere with emptying the rectum. (Compare these two types of herniations in Fig. 8.18.)

cystocele   Herniation of the urinary bladder through the wall of the vagina is called a _____. See the Sexually Transmitted Diseases section for additional pathologies.

WRITE IT! EXERCISE 12

Write words in the blanks to complete these sentences.

1. PMS means _____ syndrome.
2. Mittelschmerz means pain in the region of the ovary during _____.
3. Failure of the ovaries to produce, mature, or release ova is _____.
4. The leading cause of death from reproductive cancer is _____ carcinoma.
5. PID means _____ inflammatory disease.
6. Weakening of the ligaments that hold the uterus in place is uterine _____.
7. A common uterine condition in which it is tipped backward _____.
8. A uterine fibroid is also called a/an _____.
9. An abnormal opening between the rectum and the vagina is called a rectovaginal _____.
10. Herniation of the urinary bladder through the wall of the vagina is a/an _____.

SURGICAL AND THERAPEUTIC INTERVENTIONS

menstrual   **8-50** Some of the most common gynecologic problems for which females seek treatment are vaginal discharge, bleeding, and pain. Dysmenorrhea, painful _____ flow, is caused by uterine cramping and can usually be alleviated with aspirin or antiinflammatory drugs, such as ibuprofen. Other medications and changes in diet may be recommended for premenstrual syndrome.

8-51 After the cause of amenorrhea is established, it can be treated by surgical and pharmaceutical means (for example, hormone replacement and stimulation of the ovaries).

Menopause, though, is a natural termination of menstruation, and many women experience few if any unpleasant symptoms of hot flashes and night sweats. Hormone replacement therapy (HRT), a combination of estrogen and progesterone, is the primary intervention for women who experience the symptoms of transition or those at high risk for osteoporosis (abnormal loss of bone density) and deterioration of bone tissue. There is no agreement on the value versus risk of HRT (that is, prevention of osteoporosis, heart disease, and Alzheimer disease [progressive mental hormone   deterioration]) versus the risks of breast and endometrial cancer. HRT means _____ replacement therapy.

mouth

8-52 Treatment of vulvitis can sometimes be as simple as avoiding contact with irritants, such as soaps or detergents. Therapeutic interventions for infections of the vulva, vagina, and cervix depend on the causative organism. Oral or topical antibiotics, vaginal creams, and suppositories are prescribed according to the type of infection. Oral antibiotics are taken by _____. Topical (top[o], position or place) medications, such as antibiotic ointments or gynecologic creams, are applied directly to the affected area. Vaginal suppositories are easily melted medicated materials that are inserted into the vagina.

Laser therapy may be performed for persistent vulvitis.

FIND IT! **EXERCISE 13**

Draw a slash between the word parts in the following list. Then find the meanings of the word parts within the definitions. (Draw the slash, and then perform the remainder of the activity as a mental exercise.)

1. **colpoplasty** surgical repair of the vagina
2. **colporrhaphy** suture of the vagina
3. **hysterectomy** removal of the uterus; removal of the uterus through the abdominal wall is an **abdominal hysterectomy**. A **vaginal hysterectomy,** also called a **colpohysterectomy,** is removal of the uterus by way of the vagina. A **laparohysterectomy** is laparoscopic removal of the uterus.
4. **hysteropexy** surgical fixation of a displaced uterus
5. **oophorectomy** surgical excision of one ovary (for example, **laparoscopic oophorectomy** of a polycystic ovary) or both ovaries (for example, ovarian cancer) is performed when possible. Removal of both ovaries prohibits reproduction.
6. **oophorohysterectomy** is removal of the uterus and the ovaries

7. **oophoropexy** surgical fixation to correct an ovary that has lost its normal support
8. **oophorosalpingectomy** removal of an ovary and its uterine tube; **salpingo-oophorectomy**
9. **ovarian cystectomy** removal of a benign ovarian cyst, using either laparoscopy (Fig. 8.19) or open (abdominal) surgery
10. **radical hysterectomy** removal of ovaries, fallopian tubes, lymph nodes, and lymph channels, as well as the uterus and cervix
11. **salpingopexy** surgical fixation of a uterine tube
12. **salpingorrhaphy** suture of a fallopian tube
13. **vaginectomy** removal of all or part of the vagina, used to treat vaginal cancer; **colpectomy**
14. **vulvectomy** excision of the vulva, characteristically used to treat vulval cancer (Fig. 8.20).

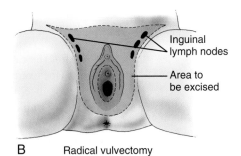

Figure 8.19 An excised ovarian cyst is being bagged during laparoscopic surgery. Bagging the specimen avoids contamination of the peritoneal cavity or the incision. Once the specimen is completely within the bag, the drawstring is closed.

Figure 8.20 Vulvectomy. A, Simple vulvectomy includes the removal of the skin of the labia minora, labia majora, and clitoris. **B,** Radical vulvectomy is excision of the labia majora, labia minora, clitoris, surrounding tissues, and pelvic lymph nodes.

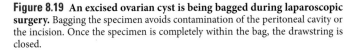

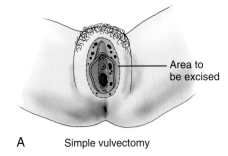

A Simple vulvectomy

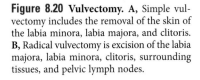

B Radical vulvectomy

Inguinal lymph nodes

Area to be excised

Area to be excised

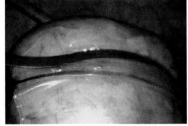
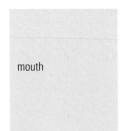

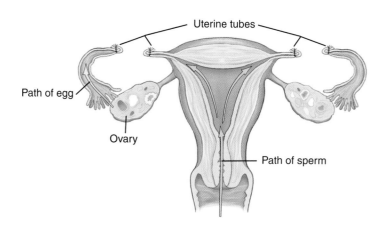

Uterine tubes

Path of egg

Ovary

Path of sperm

Figure 8.21 **Tubal ligation.** Note the ligation (tying) of both uterine tubes in this diagram.

uterine

8-53 Salpingectomy is surgical removal of one or both _____ tubes, and one must state which uterine tube is removed or if it is bilateral removal. It is performed for removal of a tumor or cyst or as a method of sterilization and is included in a hysterectomy and oophorectomy.

A **tubal ligation** is one of several sterilization procedures in which both uterine tubes are constricted, severed, or crushed to prevent conception. The procedure originally involved the use of a ligature (a substance that tied or constricted), hence its name (Fig. 8.21). This is now most often performed laparoscopically. Tubal ligation can be reversed in some cases by making a new opening to restore patency (condition of being open), but this is not always successful. **Salpingostomy,**

opening

making a new _____ into a uterine tube, may be performed also for the purpose of drainage if a uterine tube is obstructed by infection or scar tissue.

8-54 A common surgical procedure that is performed for either diagnosis or treatment is **dilation and curettage** (D&C). In this procedure, the cervix is dilated to allow the insertion of a curet into the uterus. The **curet** is a surgical instrument shaped like a spoon or scoop and is used for scraping

cervix
endometrium

and removal of material from the endometrium. In a D&C, the _____ is dilated, and the _____ is scraped.

This surgical procedure is done to assess disease of the uterus, to correct heavy or prolonged vaginal bleeding, to empty the uterus of residue after childbirth, and/or to remove the products of conception.

8-55 Dysfunctional uterine bleeding is that which is excessive or abnormal without known anatomic or systemic cause. Nonsurgical management includes the use of hormones or, in some cases, surgical management, for example, D&C or **endometrial ablation,** laser removal of the endometrium. Write

ablation

this term that means destruction of the endometrium: endometrial _____.

8-56 Lysis of adhesions is **adhesiolysis** (Fig. 8.22). Write this term that means destruction of

adhesiolysis

adhesions: _____.

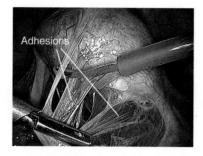

Adhesions

Figure 8.22 **Laparoscopic view of uterine adhesions.** This 31-year-old patient has had numerous laparoscopic treatments for endometriosis and suffers from infertility and chronic pelvic pain. Numerous small bowel and uterine adhesions (shown here), were excised.

8-57 Cryo/therapy, also called **cryosurgery,** is a treatment that uses a subfreezing temperature to destroy tissue. Cryosurgery and laser surgery are especially useful in the treatment of lesions of genital warts (see the Sexually Transmitted Diseases section). In cryotherapy, cry(o) means cold, and -therapy is a suffix that means treatment. The literal interpretation of cryotherapy is treatment

cold

using _____ temperatures.

To burn tissues by laser, hot metal, electricity, or another agent with the objective of destroying tissue is **cauterization.** The verb is **cauterize.** For example, tissue is cauterized in cauterization.

pelvic

8-58 Pelvic exenteration, removal of all _____ organs, is done when other forms of therapy are ineffective in controlling the spread of cancer and no metastases have been found outside the pelvis. This radical surgery usually involves removal of the uterus, ovaries, uterine tubes, vagina, bladder, urethra, and pelvic lymph nodes.

WRITE IT! EXERCISE 14

Write a word in each blank to complete these sentences.

1. A pharmaceutical intervention for treating the symptoms of menopause is _____ replacement therapy.
2. Excision of the vulva is _____.
3. Surgical fixation of an ovary is _____.
4. When the ovaries, uterus, and fallopian tubes are removed, this surgery is called a total abdominal _____.
5. Removal of the uterus through a small opening in the abdominal wall is _____.
6. Removal of a fallopian tube is _____.
7. The sterilization procedure in which both fallopian tubes are constricted, severed, or crushed is called tubal _____.
8. Forming a new opening into a fallopian tube is _____.
9. Dilation of the cervix and removal of material from the endometrium is called dilation and _____.
10. Treatment using subfreezing temperature to destroy tissue is _____.

BUILD IT! EXERCISE 15

Use the following word parts to build terms. (Some word parts will be used more than once.)
colp(o), hyster(o), lapar(o), oophor(o), salping(o), -ectomy, -pexy, -rrhaphy, -scope

1. suture of the vagina _____/_____
2. surgical fixation of a fallopian tube _____/_____
3. surgical removal of the ovaries and uterus _____/_____/_____
4. surgical fixation of the uterus to the abdominal wall _____/_____
5. instrument to visualize the abdominal cavity _____/_____

WRITE IT! EXERCISE 16

Case Study. *Define the terms as indicated.*
Mary Lou Garcia is experiencing pelvic pressure. She is <u>postmenopausal</u> and had <u>bilateral salpingo-oophorectomy</u> one year ago. A <u>pelvic examination</u> reveals a <u>cystocele</u>. She is scheduled for repair one week from today.

1. postmenopausal _____
2. bilateral salpingo-oophorectomy _____
3. pelvic examination _____
4. cystocele _____

MALE REPRODUCTIVE SYSTEM
ANATOMY AND PHYSIOLOGY

8-59 The male reproductive system produces, sustains, and transports spermatozoa; introduces them into the female vagina; and produces hormones. The testes are responsible for production of both spermatozoa and hormones. Testes is the plural form of testis, which means the same as testicle.

All other organs, ducts, and glands in this system transport and sustain the spermatozoa, the male sex cells, often shortened to sperm (singular, spermatozoon or sperm).

testes

The male gonads are the testes, the primary organs of the male reproductive system. The _____ are the male gonads. Learn the following word parts that pertain to the male reproductive system.

Word Parts: Male Reproductive System

Combining Form	Meaning	Other Word Parts	Meaning
Male Reproductive Structures		rect(o)	rectum
balan(o)	glans penis	semin(o)	semen
epididym(o)	epididymis	sperm(o), spermat(o)	spermatozoa
orchi(o), orchid(o),* test(o), testicul(o)	testicle	urethr(o)	urethra
pen(o)	penis	**Suffix**	
prostat(o)	prostate	-ile	pertaining to
scrot(o)	scrotum		
vas(o)	vessel; ductus deferens		

*Do you wonder why orchid(o) means testicle and a flower is named orchid? Answer: Orchis (G.) is a genus of orchids; it is so named because the roots or rhizomes of certain species resemble testicles.

WRITE IT!
EXERCISE 17

Write the meaning of the following combining forms.

1. balan(o) _____
2. epididym(o) _____
3. orchi(o) _____
4. rect(o) _____

5. scrot(o) _____
6. semin(o) _____
7. urethr(o) _____
8. vas(o) _____

8-60 Study Fig. 8.23, and write the names of the structures in the blank lines as you read the following information. Label the penis on line l. A loose fold of skin, the **prepuce** (foreskin, line 2), covers the glans penis (line 3).

Fig. 8.23 is a midsagittal section, so only one testis is shown. Label the **testis** (line 4). Sperm leave the testes through ducts that enter the **epididymis,** a tightly coiled comma-shaped organ located along the superior and posterior margins of the testes. Label the epididymis (line 5). The testes and epididymides are contained in a pouch of skin that is posterior to the penis. This pouch of skin is called the **scrotum.** Label the scrotum (line 6).

Each **ductus deferens** (line 7), also called the **vas deferens,** begins at the epididymis, continues upward, and then enters the abdominopelvic cavity. Each ductus deferens joins a duct from the seminal vesicle (line 8) to form a short **ejaculatory duct.** Label the ejaculatory duct (line 9), which passes through the prostate gland and empties into the urethra. Label the **prostate** (line 10) and urethra (line 11). Paired **bulbourethral glands** contribute an alkaline mucuslike fluid to the semen. Label the bulbourethral gland (line 12). **Ejaculation** is expulsion of semen from the urethra.

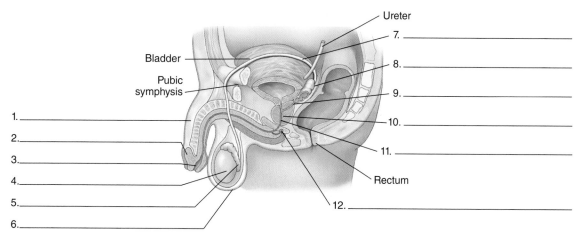

Figure 8.23 Structures of the male reproductive system. Lateral view of the internal structures. The structures that are already labeled lie near, but are not part of, the male reproductive system.

8-61 The **penis,** the male organ for copulation, transfers sperm to the vagina. The combining form pen(o) means penis. The conical tip of the penis is the **glans penis.**

Sexual intercourse refers to physical contact involving stimulation of the genitals between persons of the same or opposite gender. However, the medical definition of **copulation,** also called **coitus,** is sexual union between male and female during which the penis is inserted into the vagina.

Write this word that means the same as copulation: _____.

WORD ORIGIN
coitus *(L.)*
coitio, a coming together

coitus

8-62 The ductus deferens is a long duct that begins at the epididymis, enters the abdominal cavity, and connects with other structures of the internal reproductive tract. The combining form for ductus deferens is vas(o), which also means vessel. It will mean the ductus deferens most of the time in this chapter.

The prostate, the **seminal vesicles,** and the bulbourethral glands produce fluids that contribute to the semen and are necessary for the survival of the sperm. Semen is the secretion of the male reproductive organs that is discharged from the **urethra** during ejaculation. Combine semin(o) and -al to write a word that means pertaining to semen: _____.

seminal

FIND IT! EXERCISE 18

Draw a slash between the word parts in the following list. Then find the meanings of the word parts within the definitions. (Draw the slash, and then perform the remainder of the activity as a mental exercise.)

1. **penile** pertaining to the penis
2. **prostatic** pertaining to the prostate
3. **scrotal** pertaining to the scrotum
4. **spermatic** pertaining to sperm or pertaining to semen
5. **testicular** pertaining to a testicle

➤ **BEYOND** THE BLUEPRINT Do not confuse penile (pronounced with a long i), which means pertaining to the penis, with penal, which means relating to or involving punishment, penalties, or punitive institutions.

Spermatogenesis

production
(or formation)

8-63 Each testis is capable of producing sperm and male hormones. **Spermato/genesis** is the _____ of mature, functional sperm capable of participating in conception, the union of a sperm with an ovum.

8-64 Sperm production requires a temperature slightly lower than normal body temperature. Because the scrotum is outside the body cavity, it provides the proper environment.

The testes are paired oval glands. In Fig. 8.24, A, note that a testis is divided into several compartments called *lobules,* and each lobule contains convoluted **seminiferous tubules.** Sperm are produced in these tubules. Lying just posterior to the testis is the epididymis, where sperm are stored until they are released. The duct leading from the epididymis is the vas _____.

deferens

A cross-section of a seminiferous tubule (see Fig. 8.24, B) shows that seminiferous tubules are surrounded by cells called **interstitial cells of Leydig.** These cells produce a major male sex hormone, **testosterone.**

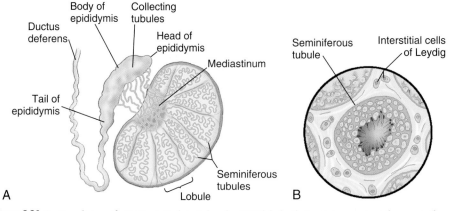

Figure 8.24 Sectional view of a testis. A, Each testis has about 250 lobules that contain as many as four seminiferous tubules where sperm are produced. **B,** Cross-section of a seminiferous tubule. The tubule is surrounded by interstitial cells, which are responsible for the production of testosterone.

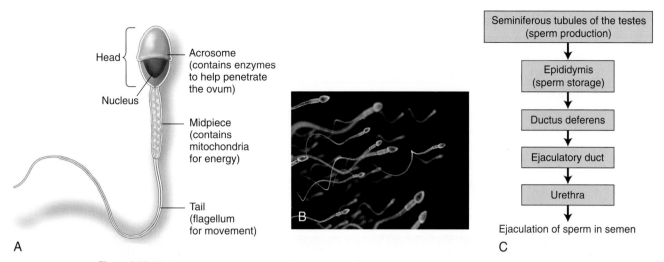

Figure 8.25 **The human spermatozoon and passageway of sperm. A,** A sperm in cross-section. The nucleus contains the chromosomes and is located in the head. The tip of the head is covered by an acrosome, which contains enzymes that help the sperm penetrate the ovum. The midpiece contains mitochondria that provide energy, and the tail is a typical flagellum. **B,** 3-D depiction of spermatozoa. **C,** The passage of sperm from where they are produced in the testes to ejaculation in semen.

spermatozoon

8-65 Sperm are produced within the seminiferous tubules. In the development of mature sperm, early spermatocytes undergo a process called *meiosis,* which eventually results in mature, functional spermatozoa (Fig. 8.25, A and B). Write the singular form of spermatozoa: _____.

There are usually millions of sperm each time semen is ejaculated, and although only one sperm fertilizes an ovum, it takes millions of sperm to ensure that fertilization will take place. Be sure you understand the route of sperm from the time of production to when they are ejaculated in semen (see Fig. 8.25, C).

8-66 The hypothalamus in the brain, the pituitary gland, and the testes produce hormones that influence spermatogenesis.

FSH and testosterone produced by the testes stimulate spermatogenesis. LH acts on interstitial cells in the testes to produce testosterone. Testosterone also brings about male secondary sex characteristics—for example, enlarging of the sex organs, distribution of hair, deepening of the voice, and increased muscular development. Write the name of this hormone, which is often called the masculinizing hormone: _____.

testosterone

8-67 Spermatogenesis begins at puberty and normally continues throughout life, showing a decline in later years. **Semen,** also called *seminal fluid,* is a mixture of sperm cells and secretions from the accessory glands (prostate, seminal vesicles, and bulbourethral glands). The combining form semin(o) means semen. Write the other name for semen that uses this combining form: _____ fluid.

seminal

Erection is the condition of swelling, rigidity, and elevation of the penis, and to a lesser degree in the clitoris of the female, caused by sexual arousal. It can also occur during sleep. Erection is necessary for the introduction of the penis into the vagina and for the emission of semen.

Write a term in each blank.

1. The production of sperm is called _____ .

2. The structure that is responsible for sperm production is the _____ .

3. Sperm are produced within the _____ tubules.

4. The major male sex hormone produced by the testicles is _____ .

5. Two important hormones that stimulate sperm production are FSH and _____ hormone.

DIAGNOSTIC TESTS AND PROCEDURES

8-68 Three important parts of a routine examination of the male genitalia are inspection of the external genitalia, palpation for inguinal hernias, and examination of the rectum digitally.

The external genitalia are examined for the descent and size of the testicles, abnormalities of the scrotum and penis, and the presence of urethral discharge. **Urethr/al discharge** means secretions

urethra

from the _____ . Smears of the secretions are stained and examined microscopically if gonorrhea is suspected. Material may be collected for bacterial or fungal culture.

Lesions or ulcers on the penis may indicate a STD (such as, genital herpes that produces blisters) or a chancre, which is a lesion that indicates the first stage of syphilis. The VDRL and the RPR tests (see Frames 8-24 and 8-147) are blood tests to detect and monitor syphilis.

8-69 Palpation may reveal an inguinal hernia, one in which a loop of intestine enters the inguinal canal, which is the passageway in the lower muscular layers of the abdominal wall that is a common

inguinal

site for hernias. This type of hernia, an _____ hernia, sometimes fills the entire scrotal sac.

8-70 The digital rectal examination (Fig. 8.26) is an assessment of the prostate gland and the

rectum

_____ . The examiner inserts a lubricated, gloved finger (a digit—hence, the name of the procedure) into the rectum, and the size and consistency of the prostate gland are assessed.

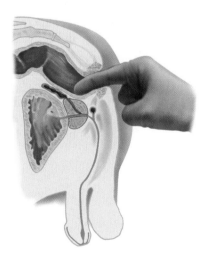

Figure 8.26 Digital rectal examination. Palpation of the posterior surface of the reprostate gland.

prostate

8-71 Testicular self-examination is a procedure recommended by the National Institutes of Health (NIH) for detecting tumors or other abnormalities of the testicles. The presence of swelling or a small lump on either testicle should be reported to one's physician.

The **prostate-specific antigen** (PSA) test is a blood test used to screen for prostatic cancer and to monitor the patient's response to treatment. Elevated PSA levels are associated with prostatic cancer.

The antigen that is a tumor marker for prostatic cancer is called _____ -specific antigen.

cells

8-72 Needle biopsy of the prostate is generally performed if cancer of the prostate is suspected. In a needle biopsy, a small amount of tissue is removed using a needle inserted from the outside. In this case the needle is inserted through the rectal mucosa to the prostate. Cyto/logy is performed on the tissue, examining the cells microscopically for the presence of cancer cells. Cyto/logy is the study of _____.

sperm

8-73 Semen analysis, one of the most important aspects of a fertility study, involves measuring freshly collected semen for volume and sperm count, as well as motility and morphology. The sperm count is a test for male fertility. In a sperm count, the number, appearance, and motility of the sperm in a collected sample of semen are examined. The test that evaluates the number and health of spermatozoa is called a _____ count.

MATCH IT! EXERCISE 20

Match the diagnostic tests in the left column with their descriptions in the right column.

_____ **1.** needle biopsy	**A.** blood test for prostatic cancer
_____ **2.** PSA	**B.** blood test for syphilis
_____ **3.** RPR	**C.** removal of tissue for microscopic study
_____ **4.** sperm count	**D.** test of semen

PATHOLOGIES

testicular

8-74 Uro/logy is the branch of medicine that specializes in the male and female urinary tract and also includes male reproductive structures.

Statistically testicular cancer occurs most often in younger men, and prostatic cancer is common in older men. Which type of cancer is more common in younger men? _____ cancer

Learn these word parts that are used to describe pathologies of the male reproductive system.

Word Parts: Male Reproductive Pathologies

Combining Form	Meaning
crypt(o)	hidden
olig(o)	few
varic(o)	twisted and swollen

WRITE IT! EXERCISE 21

Write combining forms for the following.

1. few _____

2. hidden _____

3. twisted and swollen _____

8-75 The inability to achieve penile erection, alternating periods of normal function and dysfunction, or inability to ejaculate after achieving an erection is called **erectile dysfunction,** also known as *male impotence.*

dysfunction

Poor health, certain drugs, fatigue, and vascular problems can cause sexual dysfunction. Males can often be treated medically or by changing the drugs that are causing erectile _____.

8-76 An **orchio/pathy** is any disease of the testes. The production of sperm outside the body cavity is necessary for the production of viable sperm. The testes develop in the abdominal cavity of the fetus and normally descend through the inguinal canal into the scrotum shortly before birth (sometimes shortly after birth). This provides a temperature about 3° F below normal body temperature.

Crypt/orchid/ism is a developmental defect characterized by the failure of one or both testes to descend into the scrotum (Fig. 8.27). The combining form crypt(o) means hidden. The "o" in crypt(o) is usually omitted when the word part is joined to a combining form that begins with a

hidden

vowel. Translated literally, crypt/orchid/ism means a condition of _____ testicle or testes.

Cryptorchidism is the same as undescended testicle. If the testes do not descend spontaneously or with hormonal injections, surgery is usually performed. Write the word that means the same

cryptorchidism

as undescended testicle: _____.

8-77 Hermaphroditism is a rare chromosomal abnormality in which both testicular and ovarian elements exist in the same person. Abnormal genitalia may result (Fig. 8.28). The word *intersex* has become the preferred usage for humans. An individual who has both testicular and ovarian tissue is referred to as intersex.

> **BEYOND** THE BLUEPRINT In Greek mythology, Hermaphroditus was the child of the goddess Aphrodite and the god, Hermes. Hermaphroditus was bisexual, and his name is the basis for the term *hermaphrodite.*

Human genitalia are identical in both genders early in development, beginning as undifferentiated structures. Genetics, hormones, and fetal environment modify the structure and function of the genitalia and usually produce genital structures appropriate to the individual's gender. Abnormal development sometimes occurs, resulting in genitalia of a nature that is not precisely determined (for example, there may be both a penis and a vagina or the external organs may be difficult to differentiate). A complete external evaluation and radiology, genetic, and endocrine evaluations are important in this diagnosis.

8-78 Testicular cancer is a malignant neoplasm of the testis, occurring most frequently in men between 20 and 35 years of age. Fortunately, testicular cancers are often curable.

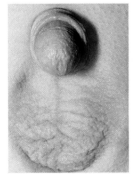

Figure 8.27 Cryptorchidism. In this photograph, both testes have failed to descend into the scrotum. If the testes do not descend spontaneously, hormonal injections may be given. If injections are unsuccessful, surgery is usually performed before age 3.

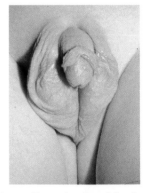

Figure 8.28 Intersex. External male and female genitalia are present. The existence of both ovaries and testes were revealed by ultrasound and other radiologic procedures.

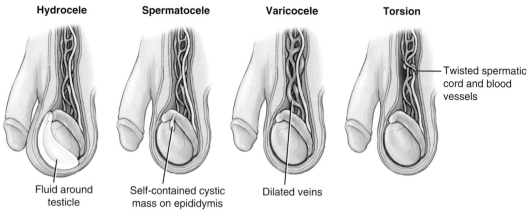

Figure 8.29 **Comparison of four common problems that affect the testes and adjacent structures.**

torsion

Testicular torsion is twisting of the testis. Axial rotation of the spermatic cord cuts off blood supply and can lead to loss of the testicle unless corrective surgery is performed. Twisting of the testicle is called testicular _____.

8-79 Several less severe problems occur within the scrotum, including hydrocele, spermatocele, and varicocele. You have learned that -cele means hernia, but in these three terms -cele is used to mean a swelling. Fig. 8.29 illustrates these three disorders as well as testicular torsion.

water

A **hydro/cele** is a mass, usually filled with a straw-colored fluid. For this reason, its name incorporates the combining form hydr(o), which means _____. In this term, hydr(o) may help you remember that the swelling contains a straw-colored fluid. A hydrocele in the scrotum may be the result of orchitis, epididymitis, or venous or lymphatic obstruction.

sperm

A **spermato/cele** is a mass that contains _____. This develops on the epididymis. A spermatocele is often painless and may need no intervention.

A **varico/cele** is a cluster of dilated veins that occurs above the testis. The combining form varic(o) means twisted and swollen. In many cases, varicoceles are asymptomatic but may contribute to infertility.

WORD ORIGIN
phimosis *(G.)*
phimgsis, a muzzling or closure

phimosis

8-80 Phimosis and balanitis are disorders of the penis. **Phimosis** occurs when the prepuce is constricted at the opening so that it cannot be retracted back over the glans penis. It is caused by inflammation or edema. It is sometimes accompanied by **balan/itis** (balan[o], glans penis + -itis, inflammation), inflammation of the glans penis.

When the prepuce is constricted so that it cannot be retracted, the disorder is called _____.

Two congenital anomalies (epispadius and hypospadius) in which the urinary meatus is abnormally located above or below its usual location are described in Chapter 7.

8-81 Hyperplasia is an increase in the size of an organ from an increase in the number of cells.

🔑 **KEY POINT Benign prostatic hyperplasia** (BPH) is a common disorder, particularly in men older than 50 years. BPH is not malignant; however, it is usually progressive and may lead to obstruction of the urethra and to interference with urination (see Fig. 7.19). The increase in the number of cells (hyperplasia) results in prostatic enlargement (hypertrophy).

hyperplasia

The common name of the disorder that is nonmalignant and results in an enlarged prostate is benign prostatic _____.

Urinary frequency, pain, and urinary tract infections are characteristic of BPH. Inflammation of the prostate may also occur.

prostate

8-82 Prostatic carcinoma usually occurs after 50 years of age and is the most common cancer among men, excluding skin cancer. **Prostatic carcinoma** is cancer of the _____. See the Sexually Transmitted Diseases section for additional pathologies.

Additional disorders of the male reproductive system include the following:

anorchidism Congenital absence of one or both testicles; same as **anorchism.**

aspermia absence of formation or ejaculation of semen.

aspermatogenesis Absence of sperm in semen. **Azoospermia** is absence of living sperm. **Oligospermia** is an insufficient number of sperm in the semen.

epididymitis Inflammation of the epididymis.

orchiditis Inflammation of a testis, marked by pain, swelling, and a feeling of weight; same as **orchitis.**

orchiepididymitis Inflammation of a testicle and its epididymis.

prostatitis Inflammation of the prostate; can be acute or chronic, bacterial or abacterial.

testalgia Testicular pain; same as **orchialgia** and **orchidalgia.**

BUILD IT! EXERCISE 22

Use the following word parts to build terms.

crypt(o), epididym(o), hydr(o), olig(o), orchid(o), sperm(o), ur(o), -ia, -cele, -ism, -itis, -logy

1. specialty for the urinary tract and male reproductive system   _____ / _____
2. insufficient number of sperm in the semen   _____ / _____ / _____
3. failure of testes to descend into the scrotum   _____ / _____ / _____
4. inflammation of the epididymis   _____ / _____
5. scrotal mass containing straw-colored fluid   _____ / _____

WRITE IT! EXERCISE 23

Write a word in each blank to complete the sentences.

1. Axial rotation of the spermatic cord is testicular _____.
2. A cluster of dilated veins above the testis is _____.
3. Tightness of the prepuce that prevents the retraction of the foreskin over the glans penis is _____.
4. Inflammation of the glans penis is _____.
5. A nonmalignant increase in the size of the prostate is benign prostatic _____.

ANALYZE IT! EXERCISE 24

Break these words into their component parts by placing a slash between the word parts. Write the meaning of each term.

1. azoospermia _____
2. orchidalgia _____
3. prostatitis _____
4. anorchism _____
5. hypertrophy _____

SURGICAL AND THERAPEUTIC INTERVENTIONS

excision

8-83 Testicular cancer is often curable. Some men choose semen storage as soon as possible after diagnosis. Semen storage is a special processing, freezing, and storage of sperm by a sperm bank for future use. Depending on the type of cancer, chemo/therapeutic agents may save the testis. Otherwise, orchi/ectomy may be necessary. **Orchi/ectomy** is _____ of the testis. Removal of both testes results in infertility. Radiation therapy is sometimes used after surgery.

Stem-cell transplantation is sometimes used after high-dose chemotherapy. In stem-cell transplantation, the patient's stem cells are removed from the bone marrow and preserved by freezing for later transplantation.

8-84 When torsion, twisting of the spermatic cord, has occurred, loss of blood supply to a testicle for more than a few hours will result in deterioration of the testicle. Surgical correction soon after the injury is important to prevent loss of the testicle. Write a term using orchi(o) that means surgical

orchioplasty   repair of a testicle: _____.

     Orchio/tomy is incision (and drainage) of a testis. **Orchio/rrhaphy** is suture of a testicle.

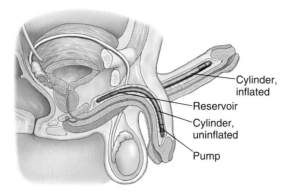

Figure 8.30 A penile prosthesis. One of several types of prostheses, this self-contained type consists of a pump, a cylinder filled with fluid, and a reservoir, all in one unit. The patient squeezes the pump just below the head of the penis to fill the cylinder and achieve erection. When an erection is no longer desired, the patient presses a release valve located behind the pump.

Cylinder, inflated

Reservoir

Cylinder, uninflated

Pump

8-85 Drugs, such as sildenafil (Viagra) or tadalafil (Cialis), are used to treat erectile dysfunction, particularly when the problem is inability to sustain an erection.

In some cases, treatment may include correction of the cause of the problem, such as restoration of the flow of blood to the penis or modification of medications that interfere with sexual activity. Surgical treatment includes injections and surgical implantation of a **penile prosthesis.** The term *prosthesis* means an artificial replacement for a body part (for example, an artificial arm or leg) or a device designed to improve function (for example, a hearing aid). The prosthesis that is designed to treat an erectile dysfunction is called a _____ prosthesis (Fig. 8.30).

penile

8-86 Orchio/pexy is corrective surgery for cryptorchidism. Orchiopexy, sometimes called **orchidopexy,** is the attachment of the previously undescended testis to the wall of the scrotum.

8-87 A hydrocele in a newborn may resolve spontaneously. In an adult a hydrocele may become large and uncomfortable and require surgical incision of the scrotum and removal of the hydrocele, because aspiration of the fluid with a needle is a temporary measure and may induce infection.

A **hydrocel/ectomy** is surgical removal of a _____.

hydrocele

8-88 The tightness of the prepuce in phimosis can usually be corrected by circumcision. **Circumcision** is surgical removal of the end of the prepuce and is commonly performed on the male infant at birth. Write this term that means surgical removal of the end of the prepuce:

_____.

circumcision

> **BEYOND** THE BLUEPRINT The extended meaning of circumcision includes ritual female circumcision (excision of the prepuce of the clitoris) performed in some parts of the world and may include largely closing up the vagina with clips or stitches. The World Health Organization (WHO) adopted the term *female genital mutilation* in 1991 *(http://www.who.int/mediacentre/factsheets/fs241/en/).*

8-89 In prostatitis, inflammation is often the result of infection and is treated with antibiotics. When the prostate gland is so enlarged (BPH) that it interferes with urination or causes frequent infection, a **transurethral resection prostatectomy** or transurethral resection of the prostate (TURP) may be necessary. A trans/urethral resection is a surgical procedure that is performed through the _____. In a TURP, small pieces of the enlarged prostate are excised (see Fig. 7.29). This procedure has been replaced in selected cases by photoselective vaporization of the prostate (Green Light PVP).

urethra

Several less invasive technologies are available for treatment of obstructive BPH, particularly in the early stages of the disease. **Transurethral microwave thermo/therapy** (TUMT) uses microwave energy to raise the temperature of the prostatic tissue, and **transurethral needle ablation** (TUNA) uses low-level radiofrequency energy. **Ablation** means removal or excision of a growth on any part of the body. In both of these procedures, the heat causes necrosis and death of the prostatic tissue, thus relieving the obstruction. Because trans/urethral is part of their names, you know that the procedures are performed through the _____.

urethra

A variety of laser procedures are available, sometimes referred to as *laser prostatectomy.*

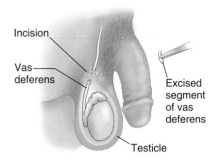

Figure 8.31 **Vasectomy.** This elective surgical procedure is performed as a permanent method of contraception (although it sometimes can be surgically reversed). It can be performed under local anesthesia. A small incision is made in the scrotum, and a piece of the vas deferens is removed.

excision

8-90 There are several treatments for prostatic carcinoma, including radiation (especially radioactive seed implants), hormonal therapy, and prostatectomy. A **prostat/ectomy** is _____ of all or part of the prostate gland.

Castration, surgical excision of one or both testicles (or ovaries in females), is performed most frequently to reduce the production and secretion of hormones that may stimulate the proliferation of malignant cells and results in sterility. If a boy is castrated before puberty, male secondary sex characteristics do not develop and he becomes a eunuch.

excision

incision

8-91 A **vas/ectomy** is _____ of a portion of the vas deferens (Fig. 8.31). Bilateral vasectomy results in sterility.

Vaso/tomy is _____ of the vas deferens. A **vasostomy** is surgical formation of a new opening into the vas deferens, but the term is sometimes used as a synonym for vasotomy.

8-92 A **vaso/vaso/stomy** can sometimes be used to correct an obstruction or to restore the severed ends of the vas deferens. The latter procedure is used to reverse a vasectomy.

Want more information? Go to *www.nih.gov*.

MATCH IT! **EXERCISE 25**

Match the procedures listed in the left column with their descriptions in the right column.

_____ **1.** chemotherapy
_____ **2.** circumcision
_____ **3.** orchiectomy
_____ **4.** orchiopexy
_____ **5.** orchioplasty
_____ **6.** penile prosthesis
_____ **7.** TURP
_____ **8.** vasectomy

A. chemical treatment for cancer
B. removal of small pieces of the prostate via the urethra
C. surgical repair of a testicle
D. surgical excision of a testicle
E. surgical fixation of a testicle
F. surgical implantation to correct erectile dysfunction
G. surgical removal of the end of the prepuce
H. surgical excision of a portion of the vas deferens

BUILD IT! **EXERCISE 26**

Use the following word parts to build terms.
trans-, orchi(o), prostat(o), urethr(o), vas(o), -al, -ectomy, -stomy, -tomy

1. incision of a testis _____/_____
2. creation of a new opening in the vas deferens _____/_____
3. pertaining to through the urethra _____/_____/_____
4. surgical excision of the prostate gland _____/_____

REPRODUCTION

gonad

8-93 The **gonads,** ovaries and testes, produce ova and sperm as well as the hormones necessary for proper functioning of the reproductive organs. Write this term that means an organ that produces ova or sperm: _____.

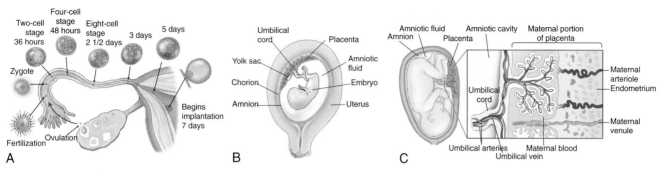

Figure 8.32 Fertilization implantation, and growth of the embryo and fetus. A, A mature ovum is fertilized by a sperm and the product of fertilization, the zygote, undergoes rapid cell division, finally implanting in the endometrium at approximately day 7. **B,** The embryo in utero at approximately 7 weeks. The placenta and extraembryonic membranes (the amnion and the chorion) form and surround the embryo, providing nourishment and protection. **C,** Drawing of fetus at several months to show the interface between maternal and fetal circulation.

🔑 **KEY** POINT **The union of the ovum and the sperm in sexual reproduction initiates development of a new individual.** Remember these terms:
- **Gamete** is a reproductive cell (ovum or spermatozoon).
- **Ovum** (plural, ova) is also called the *egg* and lives only a few days.
- **Spermatozoon** is singular for **spermatozoa** or sperm, which also live only a few days before they die after being discharged into the vagina.

8-94 Ovulation is the release of an ovum from the ovary. Fertilization, or **conception,** is the union of the sperm cell nucleus with an egg cell nucleus. This usually occurs in the uterine tube.

The fertilized ovum undergoes a series of cell divisions as it moves along the uterine tube and then enters into the uterine cavity. About the seventh day after ovulation, the fertilized ovum attaches to the endometrium. This is called **implantation.**

uterus

The endo/metr/ium is the inner lining of the _____.

8-95 The product of fertilization is the **zygote,** which undergoes rapid cell divisions. The zygote is known by different names at various stages. Some of these stages between fertilization and implantation are shown in Fig. 8.32A. The product of fertilization is called a _____.

zygote

8-96 It is usually at the beginning of the third week that the developing offspring is called an **embryo.** It is during the embryonic stage that all the organ systems form, making this the most critical time in development. This is also when the extraembryonic membranes form. Knowing that embryonic refers to the embryo, extra/embryonic means located _____ the embryo. Look at Fig. 8.32, B and locate two **extraembryonic membranes,** the **amnion** and the **chorion,** that surround the embryo. The amnion and chorion are membranes that provide protection by surrounding the embryo with amniotic fluid. Although **amnion/ic** has the same meaning as **amniotic,** the latter is more commonly used. The embryo is called a **fetus** after the eighth week. The combining form fet(o) means fetus, so **fet/al** means pertaining to the _____.

outside

fetus

8-97 The **placenta,** formed in the embryonic stage, is a highly vascular structure that nourishes the fetus. It secretes large amounts of progesterone, which is necessary for maintaining the uterus during pregnancy. The hormone that is responsible for maintaining the uterus throughout pregnancy is _____. Along with the placenta, the amnion and chorion are called the *afterbirth* and are shed shortly after birth.

progesterone

The maternal blood vessels of the placenta are in close contact with the fetal blood vessels from the cord but do not directly mix. Rather, the nutrients from the mother pass across the vessel walls into the blood of the unborn and the waste products from the unborn pass across to the mother (Fig. 8.32, C).

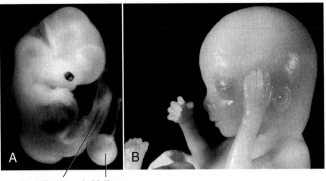

Umbilical cord   Yolk sac

Figure 8.33 Human embryo (A), and fetus (B).

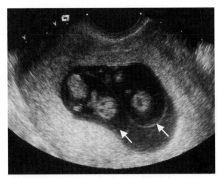

Figure 8.34 **Determination of identical twins on the first trimester ultrasound scan.** Only two thin amniotic membranes *(arrows)* separate the two fetuses.

🔑 **KEY** POINT **Remember these early stages of human development and their approximate length:**
- zygote: Begins with the fertilization of the ovum and implantation, through approximately the first 2 weeks.
- embryo: Begins about the beginning of the third week. Organ systems and extraembryonic membranes form. Lasts through approximately the eighth week.
- fetus: Begins after the eighth week and lasts until birth. Major structures have been outlined in the embryo, and body structures continue to define during the fetal stage until birth (Fig. 8.33). Note the definition of structures in the pelvic sonography of twins during the first trimester of pregnancy (Fig. 8.34).

Learn the following word parts and their meanings.

Principal Word Parts: Reproduction

Combining Form	Meaning	Prefix	Meaning
amni(o)	amnion	secundi-*	second
chori(o)	chorion	**Suffix**	
fet(o)	fetus	-blast	embryonic or immature
gonad(o)	gonad		
o(o)	ovum	*Secundus, second or following	
spermat(o)	sperm		

WRITE IT!
EXERCISE 27

Write combining forms for these terms.

1. amnion _____   4. gonad _____
2. chorion _____   5. ovum _____
3. fetus _____   6. spermatozoa _____

8-98 Infertility is the condition of being unable to produce offspring. It may be present in one or both sex partners and may be temporary and reversible, such as in the performance of a vasovasostomy. Administration of hormones, use of vaginal medications, surgery, and counseling are some of the treatments used in correcting infertility, depending on the cause. In/fertility is the condition of _____ being able to produce offspring.

not

In vitro fertilization (IVF) is a complex series of procedures used to treat fertility or genetic problems and assist with conception (Fig. 8.35). After mature ova are collected from a female's ovaries and artificially fertilized by sperm in a laboratory, the fertilized egg or eggs are implanted in the uterus. In some cases, a gestational carrier, another woman who has an embryo implanted in her uterus, might be used. IVF is expensive and invasive; in addition, IVF can result in multiple fetuses or may not be effective.

ovum

8-99 The combining form o(o) means ovum. An **ooblast** is an immature _____. A **spermato/blast** is an immature stage in the development of a mature sperm.

chorionic

8-100 Use chori(o) to write words about the chorion. Join chorion and -ic to write a word that means pertaining to the chorion: _____.

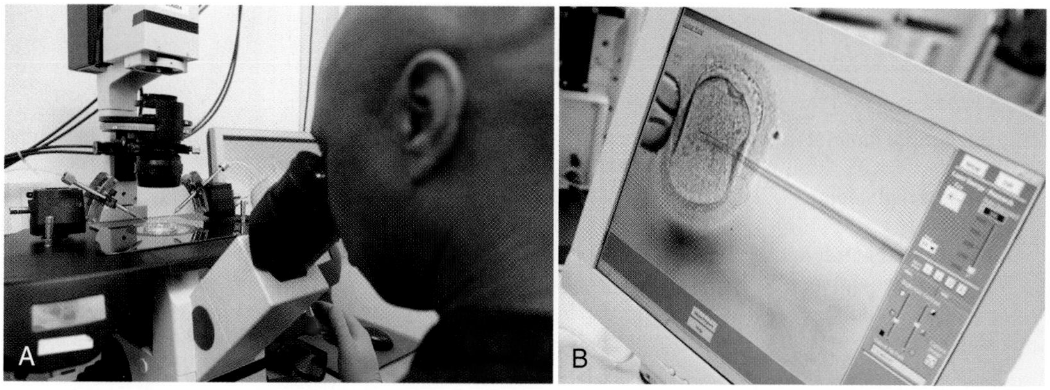

Figure 8.35 In vitro fertilization. A, Medical personnel monitors fertilization of the eggs. **B,** Monitor shows intracytoplasmic sperm injection.

amnion

Amnio/chorionic pertains to two membranes, the _____ and the chorion. **Amnio/chorial** is another word that means pertaining to the amnion and chorion.

WRITE IT! EXERCISE 28

Write a word in each blank space to complete these sentences.

1. An organ that produces ova or sperm is called a/an _____.

2. An ovum or sperm is called a/an _____.

3. The product of fertilization is called a/an _____.

4. The release of an ovum from the ovary is called _____.

5. Another name for fertilization is _____.

6. Attachment of the fertilized ovum to the endometrium is called _____.

7. After the eighth week, the developing individual is called a/an _____.

8. Two extraembryonic membranes are the amnion and the _____.

9. An embryonic sperm is called a/an _____.

10. The placenta secretes large amounts of the hormone _____, which is necessary for maintaining the uterus during pregnancy.

CONTRACEPTION

against

8-101 Knowledge of the interaction of hormones that prevent ovulation forms the basis of some types of contraception. Literal translation of contra/ception is _____ conception. In other words, **contraception** is birth control, which is a process or technique for preventing pregnancy. **Contra/ceptives** diminish the likelihood of or prevent pregnancy.

A **postcoital contraceptive** is a pill that blocks or terminates pregnancy and must be taken within 72 hours after unprotected intercourse. **Abstinence,** refraining from sexual intercourse, is the only means of contraception that is 100% effective. Note that **coitus interruptus,** withdrawal of the penis before ejaculation, and douching, washing out the vagina immediately after intercourse, are *not* recommended as contraceptives because of high failure rates.

Other means of contraception (grouped by their effectiveness) are described in Table 8.2. Condoms (male or female) are the only contraceptives that also offer any protection from STDs. For more information, see the Birth Control Methods fact sheet at *www.womenshealth.gov*.

➤ **BEYOND** THE BLUEPRINT Precursor to the first IUD for humans was marketed in 1902. The developers of IUDs may have gotten their idea from the legend that Arab traders inserted small stones in the camel's uterus to prevent pregnancy, but early devices were associated with high infection rates. The first poorly-designed plastic IUD was introduced in 1958. Copper IUDs with an effectiveness rate of 99% were introduced in the 1970s, followed by the popular hormonally-based devices that are now available.

TABLE 8.2   Selected Contraceptive Methods and Their Effectiveness

	Method	Action
Most Effective ↑	**Subdermal implant**	capsule implanted under the skin slowly releases a hormone that blocks the release of ova; surgical implant considered permanent
	Intrauterine device (IUD)	small plastic or metal device placed in the uterus (some release hormones); mode of action is not known but is believed to prevent fertilization or implantation (Fig. 8.36)
	Injectable contraceptive	hormonal injection on a specific schedule prevents ovulation
	Oral contraceptive	"pill" that contains hormones, usually progestin and estrogen, which prevent ovulation (Fig. 8.37)
	Contraceptive patch	skin patch that releases the hormones progestin and estrogen in the bloodstream; one patch weekly for three weeks, then one week without a patch.
	Vaginal contraceptive ring	ring that is inserted into the vagina and releases progestin and estrogen; worn 3 weeks out of every 4 weeks
	Diaphragm (with spermicide)	soft rubber cup that covers the uterine cervix, designed to prevent sperm from entering the cervical canal
	Sponge (with spermicide)*	acts as a vaginal barrier to the sperm; also releases spermicide
	Cervical cap (with spermicide)*	small cup that fits over the cervix to prevent sperm from entering the cervical canal
	Male condom	thin sheath (usually latex) worn over the penis to collect the semen; informally called rubbers. *Other than abstinence, latex condoms are the best protection against STDs.*
	Female condom	thin sheath (usually latex) worn in the vagina to collect the semen
	Vaginal spermicide	foam, cream, or jelly that is inserted into the vagina before intercourse to destroy sperm
	Natural family planning methods	any of several methods of conception control that do not rely on a medication or a physical device for effectiveness. The **calendar** or **rhythm method** of natural family planning relies on determining the fertile period and practicing abstinence during "unsafe" days. The **basal body temperature** method determines ovulation by a drop and subsequent rise in the basal body temperature. The **ovulation method** uses observation of changes in the cervical mucus to determine ovulation. The **symptothermal method** incorporates ovulation and basal body temperature methods.
Least Effective		

Data from www.fda.gov and www.emedicinehealth.com.
*The cap and sponge with spermicide are more effective in females who have not given birth than in those who have given birth.

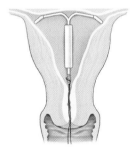

Figure 8.36 Intrauterine device that releases hormone. A T-shaped flexible plastic device inserted by a physician releases hormone on a regular schedule.

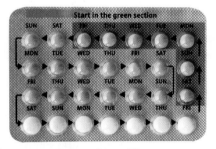

Figure 8.37 Oral contraceptive, "the pill." An oral contraceptive contains estrogen and progestin. The hormones can cause lighter periods. Skipping a day increases risk of pregnancy.

MATCH IT!   EXERCISE 29

Match the terms in the left columns with their descriptions in the right column.

_____ **1.** coitus interruptus   **A.** rubber cup that covers the uterine cervix

_____ **2.** condom   **B.** thin sheath that collects semen

_____ **3.** diaphragm   **C.** substance placed in the vagina to destroy the sperm

_____ **4.** subdermal implant   **D.** surgically implanted capsules that prevent ovulation

_____ **5.** spermicide   **E.** withdrawal of the penis before ejaculation

WRITE IT!   EXERCISE 30

Write a word in each blank to complete the sentences.

1. A pill that blocks or terminates pregnancy after intercourse is a _____ contraceptive.
2. A term for refraining from sexual intercourse is _____.
3. The abbreviation IUD means _____ device.
4. The "pill" that prevents ovulation is called an oral _____.

---

vasectomy

8-102 Vasectomy is a surgical procedure for male sterilization that involves bilateral removal of a part of the vas deferens (see Fig. 8.31). A vaso/vasostomy is sometimes able to restore the cuts ends of the vas deferens, thereby reversing a _____.

8-103 Conception cannot occur after a hysterectomy (removal of the uterus); however, hysterectomy is performed for disease, not for contraceptive purposes.

Tubal ligation is one of several sterilization procedures in which both uterine tubes are blocked to prevent conception, accomplished by constricting, severing, or crushing the uterine tubes. In

uterine

tubal ligation, tubal refers to the _____ tubes.

Adhesions are not an unusual finding during laparoscopy or open surgery. Adhesio/lysis is destruction of adhesions, often by laser (or excision during open surgery).

KEY POINT Tubal ligation is generally done laparoscopically. Many techniques are used for tubal ligation, all for the purpose of interrupting the continuity of the uterine tubes. A method of tying off a loop of uterine tube, cutting the loop in half, and burning, using clips, or tying off the ends is sometimes done after a cesarean section when no more pregnancies are wanted. Burning to seal the cut ends of the tube is accomplished by several means, including laser and cauterization. Most tubal ligations are done laparoscopically, which is sometimes called the "belly button" surgery (Fig. 8.38).

8-104 All methods of tubal ligation should be considered permanent means of sterilization, but **tubal ligation reversal** (often referred to as *tubal anastomosis*) may be possible, especially in younger women with no other infertility factors. The surgery may be laparoscopic or conventional surgery.

WRITE IT!   EXERCISE 31

Write a word in each blank to complete these sentences.

1. Bilateral excision of the vas deferens is a/an _____.
2. Constricting, severing, or crushing the fallopian tubes is called a tubal _____.
3. In vitro _____ is a method of fertilizing the ova outside the body and then placing them in the uterus for implantation.
4. Birth control is also called _____.

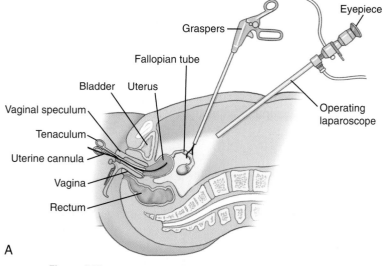
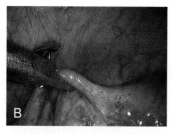

Figure 8.38 Laparoscopic tubal ligation. A, Drawing of laparoscopic tubal ligation. A laparoscope is an illuminated tube with an optical system. Graspers or forceps are used to grasp the uterine tubes or other tissue. The vaginal speculum keeps the vaginal cavity open; the tenaculum and cannula hold and manipulate the uterine cervix. **B,** Laparoscopic view of a clip being applied to one of the uterine tubes; the procedure is repeated for the second uterine tube.

PREGNANCY AND CHILDBIRTH

parturition

8-105 Pregnancy is the process of growth and development of a new individual from conception through the embryonic and fetal periods to birth. The birth of the baby is **parturition.** Write this term that means childbirth: _____.

obstetrics

8-106 An **obstetrician** specializes in _____, the medical specialty that is concerned with the care of the mother and fetus throughout pregnancy, childbirth, and the time immediately after childbirth. OB is the abbreviation for obstetrics.

A nurse midwife has advanced education and clinical experience in obstetric care and care of the newborn. The nurse midwife manages care of women having a normal pregnancy, labor, and childbirth. A midwife is a person who assists women in childbirth.

Learn the meanings of the following terms.

Word Parts: Pregnancy and Childbirth

Combining Form	Meaning	Suffix	Meaning
nat(o)	birth	-cyesis	pregnancy
par(o)	bearing offspring	-gravida	pregnant female
tert(i)	third	-para	woman who has given birth
Prefix		-tropin	that which stimulates
pseudo-	false		

WRITE IT! **EXERCISE 32**

Write suffixes for these terms.
1. pregnancy _____
2. pregnant female _____
3. that which stimulates _____
4. woman who has given birth _____

before

8-107 Gestation is another name for pregnancy. This is also called the *prenatal period.* Knowing that nat(o) means birth, **pre/natal** is that time _____ birth. **Quickening,** the first recognizable movements of the fetus in the uterus, occurs at about 18 to 20 weeks in a first pregnancy and slightly sooner in later pregnancies.

8-108 The average period of gestation is about 266 days from the date of fertilization, but it is clinically considered to last 280 days from the first day of the LMP. The expected date of delivery (EDD), commonly called the *due date,* is usually calculated on the latter basis.

➤ **BEYOND THE BLUEPRINT** Fewer than 5% of births occur on the EDD (50% are within the first week, and 90% are within 2 weeks).

abortion

8-109 Termination of pregnancy before the fetus is capable of survival outside the uterus is an **abortion.** In lay language, a spontaneous or natural loss of the fetus is called a *miscarriage,* and abortion most often refers to a deliberate interruption of pregnancy. In the medical sense, both spontaneous loss and deliberate interruption of pregnancy are called *abortion.* A miscarriage is a spontaneous _____.

8-110 In many medical or legal definitions, human pregnancy is arbitrarily divided into three trimester periods as a means to simplify reference to the stages of prenatal development.

🔑 **KEY POINT** **A trimester is one of the three periods of approximately 3 months into which pregnancy is divided:**
- First trimester: Time from the first day of the LMP to the end of 12 weeks (carries the greatest risk of miscarriage)
- Second trimester: Extends from the twelfth to the twenty-eighth week (The fetus and pregnancy are now easier to monitor. A **viable offspring,** one that is able to survive outside the uterus, with or without medical help, occurs at about the twenty-fourth week.)
- Third trimester: Begins at the twenty-eighth week and extends to the time of delivery (The body systems that formed earlier develop further, especially the respiratory and nervous systems.)

trimester

The time from the first day of the LMP to the end of 12 weeks is the first _____.

first

8-111 The suffix -gravida refers to a pregnant female and is combined with various prefixes that designate the number of pregnancies. Because the prefix primi- means first, a **primi/gravida** is a female during her _____ pregnancy. This is the same as gravida 1. The prefix multi- means many, and **multi/gravida** means a female who has been pregnant more than one time.

offspring

8-112 Para is a term used with numerals to indicate the number of pregnancies carried to more than 20 weeks' gestation, such as para III or 3, indicating three pregnancies, regardless of the number of offspring produced in a single pregnancy or the number of stillbirths after 20 weeks. **Par/ous** is a general term that refers to having borne one or more _____.

8-113 There are several methods that are used to provide an overview of a female's obstetric history; the methods use terms for pregnancy (**gravid**) and the number of previous successful live births **(parity)**. **Gravida** refers to a pregnant female. Likewise, if a female is gravid, she is pregnant.

One designation, gravida/para or simply the designation G/P shows the number of pregnancies and the number of viable births. For example, $G_2 P_2$ indicates a woman who has had two pregnancies and two viable births.

A second designation, GPA means gravid/para/abortus, or the number of pregnancies, the number of viable births, and the number of abortions. So $G_4 P_3 A_1$ designates four pregnancies, three viable births, and one abortion. If the designation were $G_4 P_4 A_0$, this designates four preg-

four

nancies, _____ viable births, and no abortions.

A third designation, TPAL, gives more information:
- *T* refers to term births (after 37 weeks' gestation)
- *P* refers to premature births
- *A* refers to abortions (includes induced abortions and miscarriages or ectopic pregnancies)
- *L* refers to living children

> **BEYOND** THE BLUEPRINT Here's an example of the TPAL designating system: Jan (3 months pregnant) is visiting her gynecologist/obstetrician, who makes this annotation: para 1-1-1-3. Try to discern what each number tells us about Jan's obstetric history. Then look at the following answer:
> - Jan has one childbirth carried to term, T1.
> - She has had one premature birth, P1.
> - She has had one abortion, A1.
> - She has 3 living children, L3.
>
> Jan's history shows that she had one pregnancy to term with a surviving infant; carried one pregnancy to 35 weeks with surviving twins; carried one pregnancy to 9 weeks as an ectopic (tubal) pregnancy, and has three living children: Zach, age 9, and Marta and Mariam, 3 years old. Since she is currently pregnant, we could use the annotation GTPAL, with the G meaning gravid.

para I or 1

8-114 The suffix -para refers to a female who has given birth, specifically one who has produced viable offspring.

Determine the designation, para I or 1, para II or 2, or para III or 3, for the following females. In each case, the pregnancies lasted more than 20 weeks.

What is the para designation for a female who has one living child and has had no other pregnancies? _____

para III or 3

The para status of a female who has twins and has had no other pregnancies is para 1. What is the para status of a female who has four children that resulted from three pregnancies and has had no additional pregnancies? _____

one

8-115 A female who is designated as para 1 is also called a **primi/para,** which means that she has produced _____ viable offspring. (The number is implied from the prefix primi-, which means first.)

Because the number or prefix indicates how many pregnancies, a multiple birth counts as just one in the calculation. Translated literally, a **multi/para** has produced many viable offspring, but the term is used to indicate a woman who has delivered more than one viable offspring.

Draw a slash between the word parts in the following list of new terms. Then find the meanings of the word parts within the definitions. (Draw the slash, and then perform the remainder of the activity as a mental exercise.)

1. **nullipara** a woman who has not given birth to a viable infant; para 0.
2. **quadripara** a woman who has had four successful pregnancies; para 4.
3. **secundipara** a woman who has had two pregnancies that resulted in viable offspring; para 2. *Bipara* is not as common.
4. **tripara** a woman who has had three pregnancies that resulted in viable offspring; **tertipara**; para 3.

amniorrhexis

8-116 Using -rrhexis, write a new word that means rupture of the amnion: _____.
Amniorrhexis ("water breaks") occurs before the child is born and sometimes is the mother's first sign of impending labor. The "water breaks" or the "bag of water breaks" are common sayings.

8-117 **Labor,** the process by which the child is expelled from the uterus, is that time from the beginning of cervical dilation to the delivery of the placenta. A synonym for dilation is **dilatation.**
Cervical dilation is enlargement of the diameter of the opening of the uterine cervix in labor. The

uterus

uterine cervix is the neck of the _____.
   Dilatation is the condition of being dilated or stretched beyond the normal dimensions. Cervical dilatation is the dilation or stretching of the cervical opening. The shortening and thinning of the cervix during labor is called **effacement.** This term describes how the constrictive neck of the uterus is obliterated or effaced.

effacement

   Shortening and thinning of the cervix during labor is called _____.
When this occurs, the mucous plug that fills the cervical canal dislodges.

8-118 Labor may be divided into three (or sometimes four) stages: cervical dilatation, expulsion, placental, and postpartum stages (Fig. 8.40). Not everyone recognizes the postpartum stage as a stage of labor, because it occurs after childbirth. The first stage (cervical dilatation) begins with

cervical

the onset of regular uterine contractions and ends when the _____ opening is completely dilated.

   The second stage **(expulsion)** extends from the end of the first stage until complete

expulsion

_____ of the infant. During this stage the amniotic sac ruptures if that has not occurred already.

   The third stage, the **placental stage,** extends from the expulsion of the child until what structure

placenta

and the membranes are expelled? _____

WORD ORIGIN
puerpus, L
childbirth

   The fourth stage **(postpartum)** is the hour or two after delivery, when uterine tone is established. Study Fig. 8.39, and try to determine the stage of labor for each drawing. Notice how the fetal head turns in order to pass through the vaginal opening. The fourth and final stage of labor is not shown. **Puerpera** means a woman who has just given birth.

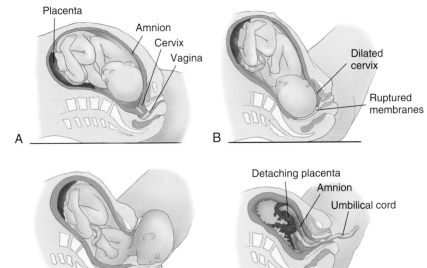

Placenta
Amnion
Cervix
Vagina

A _____

Dilated cervix
Ruptured membranes

B _____

C _____

Detaching placenta
Amnion
Umbilical cord

D _____

Figure 8.39 The fetus in utero before labor compared with three stages of labor. A, The normal position of the fetus shortly before labor begins. **B,** The first stage of labor (cervical dilatation) begins with the onset of regular uterine contractions and ends when the cervical opening is completely dilated. **C,** The second stage (expulsion) results in expulsion of the infant. **D,** The third stage (placental) ends when the placenta and membranes are expelled. A fourth stage (not shown) is sometimes identified as the hour or two after delivery when uterine tone is established.

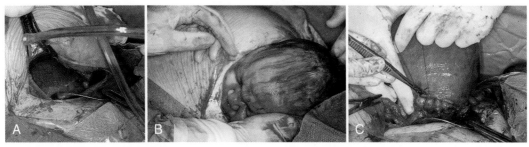

Figure 8.40 Cesarean section. A, The uterus is entered through a transverse incision. **B,** The fetal head is brought through the incision. **C,** The final step involves the use of heavy sutures to close the uterus.

8-119 The events just described are the stages of a vaginal delivery. A cesarean section or cesarean birth is performed when abnormal fetal or maternal conditions make vaginal delivery hazardous. A **cesarean section,** which is sometime abbreviated as CS or C-section, is a surgical procedure in which the abdomen and uterus are incised, and the baby is removed from the uterus (Fig. 8.40). Write this term that means removing the baby from the uterus after incision of the abdomen and uterus: _____ birth.

cesarean

> **BEYOND** THE BLUEPRINT The Apgar scoring system is an evaluation of a newborn's physical condition and is based on a rating of five factors (heart rate, respiratory effort, muscle tone, reflex irritability, and color) that reflect the infant's ability to adjust to extrauterine life. The Apgar score (0 to a normal value of 2 for each factor) rapidly identifies infants who require intervention or transfer to a neonatal intensive care unit.

after

8-120 Post/partum means after childbirth, because the prefix post- means _____. *Partum* is a term that refers to the mother.

Changes in the mammary glands prepare the breasts of a pregnant female for the production of milk. The mammary glands secrete a cloudy fluid called **colostrum** during the first few days after a female gives birth. This fluid serves adequately as food for the infant until milk production begins 2 to 3 days after birth. See Chapter 12 for more information about **lacto/genesis,** the production of _____.

milk

8-121 You have learned that the prefixes ante- and pre- mean before. Prenatal and **ante/natal** both refer to the time _____ birth, but often are replaced by **preterm.**

The prefix ante- is not always joined to the word, and sometimes there are two acceptable ways to write the same word. Either **antepartum** or ante partum is acceptable and means before _____.

before

parturition (childbirth)

birth

8-122 Postnatal means the time after _____, with reference to the newborn and extends for about 6 weeks. A **neonate** is a newborn child. **Neo/natal** is a specific term that refers to the period covering the first 28 days after birth. Neonatal also means pertaining to the newborn child. **Neonatology** is the branch of medicine that specializes in the care of the newborn, and the specialist is a **neonatologist.**

MATCH IT!   EXERCISE 34

Match the terms in the left column with the descriptions in the right column.

_____	**1.** antepartum	**A.** a female who has had one successful pregnancy
_____	**2.** cervical dilation	**B.** a female who is pregnant for the first time
_____	**3.** expulsion	**C.** a woman who has had two children who aren't twins
_____	**4.** neonate	**D.** before childbirth
_____	**5.** para 1	**E.** newborn child
_____	**6.** primigravida	**F.** the first stage of labor
_____	**7.** placental stage	**G.** the second stage of labor
_____	**8.** postnatal	**H.** the time after childbirth with reference to the newborn
_____	**9.** postpartum	**I.** the third stage of labor
_____	**10.** secundipara	**J.** the time after birth with reference to the mother

Break these words into their component parts, and write the meaning of each term.

1. postnatal _____

2. amniorrhexis _____

3. primigravida _____

4. antepartum _____

5. neonatologist _____

DIAGNOSTIC TESTS AND PROCEDURES

stimulates

gonadotropin

amniocentesis

chorionic

fetoscope

8-123 Within a few days after conception, the chorion starts producing a hormone, **human chorionic gonadotropin** (HCG). Gonado/tropin means a substance (hormone) that _____ the gonads. HCG is present in body fluids (urine, blood) of pregnant females, and blood or urine is tested to determine whether pregnancy exists (Fig. 8.41). HCG can be detected long before other signs of pregnancy appear. The hormone that is tested for in pregnancy tests is HCG, or human chorionic _____.

8-124 **Amnio/centesis** (amni[o], amnion + -centesis, surgical puncture) is a surgical procedure in which a needle is passed through the abdominal and uterine walls to obtain a small amount of amniotic fluid for laboratory analysis (Fig. 8.42). The procedure is usually performed to aid in the assessment of fetal health and diagnosis of genetic defects or other abnormalities. Fetal cells in the fluid can be cultured (grown in the laboratory), and biochemical and cytologic studies may be performed. Write the name of this procedure in which a needle is passed trans/abdominally to collect amniotic fluid: _____.

8-125 **Chorionic villi** are the tiny fingerlike projections of the chorion that infiltrate the endometrium and help form the placenta. **Chorionic villus sampling** is sampling of these villi (placental tissue) for prenatal diagnosis of potential genetic defects and is usually performed between the eighth and twelfth weeks of pregnancy (Fig. 8.43). This test is called _____ villus sampling.

8-126 The fetal heart begins beating around day 22. A **feto/scope** is a stethoscope for assessing the fetal heart rate (FHR) through the mother's abdomen (Fig. 8.44). It may be used during prenatal visits to the doctor and during labor when it also gives information about uterine contractions. Write the name of this special type of stethoscope that is used to monitor the fetal heartbeat: _____.

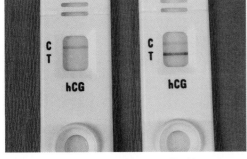

Negative   Positive

Figure 8.41 Urine pregnancy test. The positive test has a red line near the label *HCG* (human chorionic gonadotropin) and a light blue line. The negative test lacks the red band of color near the HCG.

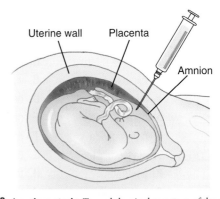

Uterine wall   Placenta   Amnion

Figure 8.42 Amniocentesis. Transabdominal puncture of the amniotic sac is done to remove fluid for diagnostic study after the ultrasound indicates the position of the fetus and the location of the placenta.

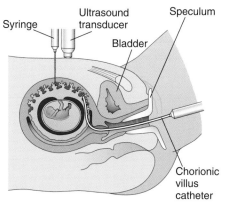

Figure 8.43 **Chorionic villus sampling.** Two types of chorionic tissue sampling are illustrated. One type of villus sample is obtained by insertion of a needle through the mother's abdominal and uterine walls. Another method is aspiration by catheter through the cervix. Both methods are performed using ultrasonic guidance.

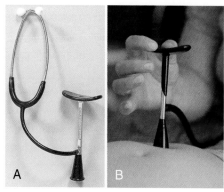

Figure 8.44 **Fetoscope. A,** A fetoscope is a special stethoscope for monitoring the fetal heartbeat. **B,** Fetoscope in use.

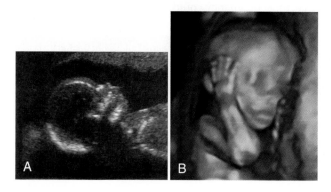

Figure 8.45 **Fetal ultrasound imaging. A,** Two-dimensional ultrasound image of a fetus in the second trimester. **B,** Three-dimensional ultrasound image of a fetus. 3D ultrasounds allow the examiner to see width, height, and depth.

fetal

8-127 An electronic fetal monitor (EFM) may be used during labor to monitor the fetal heart and record the FHR and the maternal uterine contractions. The EFM may be applied either internally or externally. EFM means an electronic _____ monitor.

measurement

8-128 Literal translation of pelvi/metry is _____ of the pelvis. This procedure is usually performed by the obstetrician during the first prenatal examination of a pregnant woman or may be used if problems arise during labor. Clinical **pelvimetry** is vaginal palpation of specific bony landmarks and is used to estimate the size of the birth canal.

    Cephalo/pelvic disproportion (CPD) is a condition in which a baby's head is too large or the mother's birth canal is too small to permit normal labor or birth. If the disproportion is too great, a cesarean delivery will be necessary. X-ray pelvimetry can be performed but is not generally used because of the risk of radiation exposure to the fetus.

fetus

8-129 Other diagnostic tools, such as sonography, provide a great deal of information about the fetus with less apparent risk. Fetal sonography is a noninvasive procedure that is used to assess structural abnormalities and monitor development of the _____.

    Compare the standard two-dimensional (2D) obstetric scanning with three-dimensional (3D) scanning (3D fetal ultrasound), which provides a much clearer 3D image of the fetus (Fig. 8.45). 3D scanning is used in monitoring known fetal abnormalities, but it also may improve the fetal–maternal bonding.

> **BEYOND** THE BLUEPRINT Four-dimensional (4D) baby scans provide a video clip and are similar to 3D scans except that they show fetal movement. Expectant parents often pay for the cost of the videos; their expense generally prohibits routine use.

Write a word in each blank to complete these sentences.

1. HCG is the hormone that is tested for in _____ tests.

2. An estimation of the size of the birth canal to determine whether the baby's head is too large to permit normal birth is called _____.

3. Surgical puncture of the amnion to obtain amniotic fluid for testing is _____.

4. A sampling of placental tissue early in pregnancy to determine potential genetic defects is called _____ villus sampling.

5. A stethoscope for assessing the fetal heart rate is a/an _____.

PATHOLOGIES

ectopic

8-130 Whenever a fertilized ovum implants anywhere other than the uterus, this is an ectopic pregnancy. The prefix ecto- means situated on or outside. The combining form top(o) refers to place. When ecto- and top(o) are combined, such as in ectopic, it means outside the usual place. If the ovum implants in a fallopian tube, this is called a *tubal pregnancy* (Fig. 8.46) or an _____ pregnancy. An ectopic pregnancy could also be called an **extrauterine pregnancy,** because extra- means outside.

> **BEYOND** THE BLUEPRINT The most common ectopic pregnancy site is one of the uterine tubes, but implantation can occur in an ovary, in the abdomen, or an abnormal implantation site in the uterus (the cervix or one of the uterine horns). The embryo is not viable, and removal is essential, because rupture of an ectopic pregnancy can jeopardize the mother's life.

pregnancy

8-131 The prefix pseudo- means false, and -cyesis means pregnancy. **Pseudo/cyesis** is a term for false _____. This is also called **pseudopregnancy,** in which certain signs and symptoms suggest pregnancy, such as the absence of menstruation. Pseudocyesis is the presence of one or more of these signs or symptoms when conception has not occurred. The condition may be psycho/genic, or it may be caused by a physical disorder.

preeclampsia

8-132 **Pre/eclampsia** is one of several complications of pregnancy. This condition is characterized by the onset of acute high blood pressure after the twenty-fourth week of gestation. **Protein/uria,** protein in the urine, and edema may also be present. Write the name of this complication of pregnancy characterized by acute high blood pressure: _____.

Preeclampsia may progress to **eclampsia,** which is the gravest form of pregnancy-induced high blood pressure. The latter, characterized by seizures, coma, high blood pressure, proteinuria, and edema, leads to convulsions and death if untreated.

WORD ORIGIN
abruptio *(L.)*
ab, away from;
rumpere, to rupture

abruptio

8-133 A second complication of pregnancy is **abruptio placentae.** This condition is a premature separation of the placenta from the uterine wall (implanted in normal position) after 20 weeks or more or during labor, and it often results in severe hemorrhage. Fetal death results if there is complete separation of the placenta from the uterine wall, so cesarean sections are performed in severe cases. Labor and normal delivery may be possible if only partial separation exists. This complication of separation of the placenta from the uterine wall is called _____ placentae.

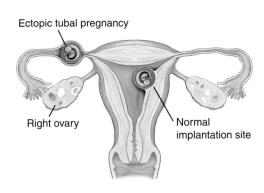

Figure 8.46 Tubal pregnancy, the most common type of ectopic pregnancy. Note that normal implantation is in the upper portion of the uterus.

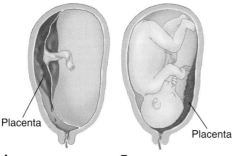

Placenta

Placenta

A Abruptio placentae   **B** Placenta previa

Figure 8.47 Comparison of two complications of pregnancy. **A,** Abruptio placentae. Separation of the placenta implanted in a normal position in a pregnancy of 20 weeks or more, or during labor before delivery of the fetus. This causes severe maternal hemorrhage that may be evident externally (as shown in this example), or the hemorrhage may be concealed within the uterus. **B,** Placenta previa. Abnormal implantation of the placenta too low in the uterus. Even slight dilation of the cervical opening can cause separation of an abnormally implanted placenta.

previa

8-134 Placenta previa is a condition in which the placenta is implanted abnormally in the uterus so that it impinges on or covers the **internal os** (opening at the upper end of the uterine cervix). This is one of the most common reasons for painless bleeding in the last trimester. Cesarean section is required if severe hemorrhage occurs. This condition in which the placenta is implanted abnormally in the uterus is called placenta _____.

Study Fig. 8.47, and compare placenta previa with abruptio placentae, which was described in the previous frame.

stillbirth

8-135 Stillbirth is the birth of a fetus that died before or during delivery. A fetus that is born dead is also called a _____.

WORD ORIGIN
dystocia *(G.)*
dys-, abnormal; *tokos,*
   birth
difficult

8-136 Abnormal or difficult labor is called **dystocia.** It may be caused either by an obstruction or constriction of the birth passage or by an abnormal shape, size, position, or condition of the fetus. Literal translation of dys/tocia is _____ labor.

MATCH IT!
EXERCISE 37

Match terms in the left columns with their descriptions in the right column.

_____ **1.** abruptio placentae   **A.** abnormal or difficult labor
_____ **2.** dystocia   **B.** false pregnancy
_____ **3.** ectopic pregnancy   **C.** fertilized egg implants outside the uterus
_____ **4.** placenta previa   **D.** placenta covers the internal os
_____ **5.** pseudocyesis   **E.** separation of the placenta from the uterine wall

Down

8-137 One of the genetic disorders that can be detected by study of the amniotic fluid is **Down syndrome.** Patients with Down syndrome have an extra chromosome, usually number 21, and have moderate to severe mental retardation. This chromosomal aberration, also called *trisomy 21* (tri- means three), is often associated with late maternal age (Fig. 8.48). The name of this genetic disorder, usually associated with trisomy of chromosome number 21, is _____ syndrome.

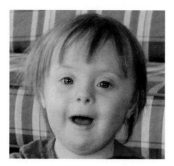

Figure 8.48 Typical facial characteristics of Down syndrome. This congenital condition, usually caused by an extra chromosome 21, is characterized by varying degrees of mental retardation and multiple defects. It can be diagnosed prenatally by amniocentesis. Infants with the syndrome generally have a small, flattened skull, flat-bridge nose, and eyes with the mongoloid slant shown here. Down syndrome was formerly called *mongolism.*

8-138 Another condition that may be diagnosed by means of amniocentesis is **hemolytic disease of the newborn,** which is an anemia of newborns characterized by premature destruction of red blood cells and resulting from maternal–fetal blood group incompatibility, especially involving the Rh factor and the ABO blood groups. Severity of the latter is usually mild.

> **KEY** POINT In Rh incompatibility, the hemolytic reaction occurs because the mother is Rh negative and the infant is Rh positive. The name of the disease, *hemolytic disease of the newborn,* describes the destruction of the red blood cells. This is also called **erythro/blast/osis fetalis** (Fig. 8.49). An erythro/blast is an immature form of a red blood cell that is present in the blood of newborns with this type of anemia. The first pregnancy usually does not present a serious problem, and complications in a future pregnancy can generally be prevented by injection of the mother shortly after delivery with RhoGAM or a similar immune globulin. Otherwise, future spontaneous abortion of an Rh-positive fetus may occur.

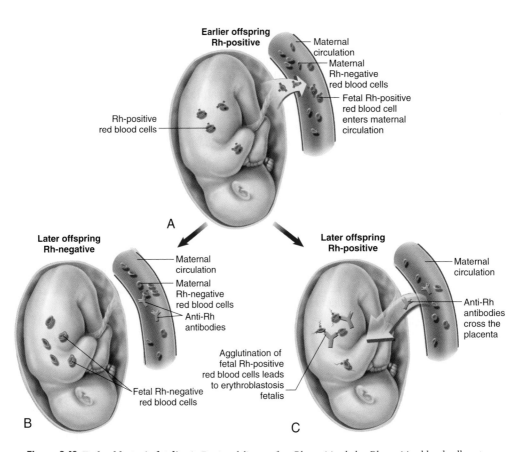

Figure 8.49 Eythroblastosis fetalis. A, During delivery of an Rh-positive baby, Rh-positive blood cells enter the mother's bloodstream. **B,** A later pregnancy involving an Rh-negative baby does not present a problem with Rh incompatibility. **C,** A later pregnancy involving another Rh-positive baby may result in erythroblastosis fetalis. Anti-Rh antibodies enter the baby's blood supply and cause agglutination of RBCs that have the Rh antigen. This complication is usually avoided by the use of RhoGam or a similar immune globulin.

When hemolytic disease of the newborn is suspected, prenatal diagnosis of the disease is confirmed by high levels of bilirubin (a product of red blood cell destruction) in the amniotic fluid, which is obtained by amniocentesis. Intra/uterine transfusion or immediate exchange transfusions after birth may be necessary. Intra/uterine transfusion is transfusion of the fetus while it is still within the uterus. Another name for hemolytic disease of the newborn is

erythroblastosis

_____ fetalis.

8-139 Fetal presentation describes the part of the fetus that is touched by the examining finger through the cervix or has entered the mother's lesser pelvis (lower part of the pelvis) during labor. Positions of the fetus are defined as follows:
- **cephalic presentation:** The top of the head (cephal[o]), the brow, the face, or the chin presents itself at the cervical opening during labor.

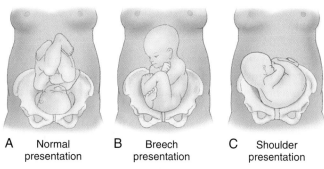

A Normal
presentation

B Breech
presentation

C Shoulder
presentation

Figure 8.50 Fetal presentation. A, Cephalic presentation, the normal presentation of the top of the head, the brow, the face, or the chin at the cervical opening. **B,** Breech presentation. **C,** Shoulder presentation.

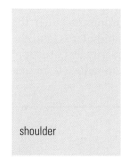

shoulder

- **breech presentation:** The buttocks, knees, or feet are presented (occurs in approximately 3% of labors).
- **shoulder presentation:** One in which the long axis of the baby's body is across the long axis of the mother's body, and the shoulder is presented at the cervical opening; also called **transverse presentation.** Vaginal delivery is impossible unless the baby turns spontaneously or is turned in utero.

Shoulder and transverse presentations are the same type of presentation because the _____ is presented at the cervical opening. Compare the different types of presentations shown in Fig. 8.50.

MATCH IT!

EXERCISE 38

Match terms in the left column with the descriptions in the right column.

_____ **1.** breech presentation
_____ **2.** cephalic presentation
_____ **3.** Down syndrome
_____ **4.** erythroblastosis fetalis
_____ **5.** transverse presentation

A. genetic disorder of extra chromosome 21
B. hemolytic disease of the newborn
C. the buttocks, knees, or feet are presented at the cervical opening
D. the shoulder is presented at the cervical opening
E. the top of the head, the brow, the face or the chin is presented at the cervical opening

8-140 Newborn congenital anomalies, often referred to as birth defects, have a variety of causes ranging from pregnancy or birth complications to genetic malformations to **conjoined twins** (two fetuses developed from the same ovum who are physically united at birth). In many cases, a congenital anomaly may have no known cause. Some examples of birth defects are **cleft palate**, a defect characterized by a cleft (division or fissure) in the midline of the palate, is often associated with **cleft lip**, one or more clefts in the upper lip; **esophageal atresia** (abnormal esophagus that is not continuous with the stomach); **gastroschisis** (incomplete closure of the abdominal wall); **respiratory distress syndrome** (acute lung disease occurring most often in premature babies); **spinal bifida** (developmental anomaly of the vertebra); and **fetal alcohol syndrome** (physical abnormalities that tend to appear in infants whose mothers consumed alcohol during pregnancy). The birth defects just described are also called _____ anomalies.

congenital

MATCH IT!

EXERCISE 39

_____ **1.** cleft palate
_____ **2.** esophageal atresia
_____ **3.** gastroscisis
_____ **4.** respiratory distress syndrome
_____ **5.** spina bifida

A. abnormal esophagus that is not continuous with the stomach
B. acute lung disease
C. developmental anomaly of the vertebra
D. fissure in the midline of the bony roof of the mouth
E. incomplete closure of the abdominal wall

> **BEYOND** THE BLUEPRINT Also called a nevus, a birthmark is a pigmented skin blemish that is usually benign. Any change in size, color, texture, or bleeding or itching should be called to the physician's attention.

SURGICAL AND THERAPEUTIC INTERVENTIONS

amnion

WORD ORIGIN

episiotomy *(G.)*
epision, pubic region;
-tomy, incision

episiotomy

laparorrhaphy

8-141 In a vaginal delivery, **amnio/tomy** is the deliberate rupture of the fetal membranes to induce labor. The literal translation of amniotomy is incision of the _____.

Oxytocin is a hormone that is produced by the pituitary gland and stimulates uterine contraction. Oxytocin (Pitocin) is also used as a drug to induce or augment uterine contractions. Other drugs, uterine relaxants, slow or stop labor by slowing or stopping uterine contractions.

An episiotomy facilitates delivery if the vaginal opening is too small. An **episio/tomy** is a surgical procedure in which an incision is made in the female perineum to enlarge the vaginal opening for delivery. The suffix -tomy will help you remember that an episiotomy involves an incision. Write this new term that means an incision that enlarges the vaginal opening to facilitate delivery: _____.

8-142 A cesarean section is performed when vaginal delivery would be hazardous to either the mother or baby. This type of delivery requires incision of the abdominal wall and uterus, and the baby is delivered trans/abdominally (see Fig. 8.40). Future births are not necessarily by C-section. Change the suffix of **laparotomy,** which means incision of the abdominal wall, to write a term that means suture of the abdominal wall: _____.

BUILD IT!

EXERCISE 40

Use the following word parts to build terms. (Some word parts will be used more than once.)
amni(o), cervic(o), lapar(o), -al, -rrhaphy, -rrhexis, -tomy

1. incision into the abdomen _____/_____
2. rupture of the inner membrane surrounding the fetus _____/_____
3. pertaining to the cervix _____/_____
4. suturing of the abdominal wall _____/_____

SEXUALLY TRANSMITTED DISEASES

TRANSMISSION

8-143 STDs or sexually transmitted infections (STIs) are usually caused by infectious organisms that have been passed from one person to another through anal, oral, or vaginal intercourse. STDs were formerly called **venereal diseases** (VDs), named for Venus, the Roman goddess of love. Abstinence is the only 100% reliable means of preventing infection with an STD by sexual activity. Latex condoms are the only other means that provide any protection.

KEY POINT Some organisms that cause STDs are transmitted only by sexual contact, some can be transmitted via body fluids (for example, AIDS via blood transfusion), and others can cause infections in other parts of the body. An example of the latter is an eye that has been infected by hands that are contaminated with organisms that cause gonorrhea. Some of the organisms that cause STDs can also be transmitted by other means that include the following:
- Blood transfusion or handling of contaminated products
- Needles or drug paraphernalia
- Intrauterine (within the uterus) transmission to the fetus
- Infection of the infant during childbirth

Most STDs start as lesions on the genital organs. A person who already has one STD can become infected with another STD. Different STDs are caused by specific types of viruses, bacteria, protozoa, fungi, and parasites. Without treatment, they can contribute to infertility, insanity, problem pregnancies, cancer, and death.

TYPES OF SEXUALLY TRANSMITTED DISEASES AND TREATMENTS

within

8-144 Gonorrhea (gon[o], genitals + -rrhea, discharge) is caused by the **gono/coccus** (GC), a gram-negative intracellular diplococcus. Intra/cellular means that the bacteria are located _____ the cells (in this case, white blood cells).

Gonorrhea causes a heavy urethral discharge in males, but females may be asymptomatic. See Fig. 8.51 for a common sign of gonorrhea and a stained urethral smear that is indicative of the disease. The disease can usually be treated with penicillin or with another antibiotic in penicillin-sensitive persons.

gonococcus

8-145 Many of the words in the medical dictionary that begin with gon(o) pertain to the GC, the type of bacteria that causes gonorrhea. Write the name of the microorganism that causes gonorrhea: _____.

The GC that causes gonorrhea, *Neisseria gonorrhoeae,* is a bacterium. When the presence of gram-negative intracellular diplococci is detected, a bacterial culture is generally performed to confirm that the organisms are gonococci. (Refer to Chapter 2, Frame 2-9, for a refresher about Gram stain.)

syphilis

8-146 Another STD, **syphilis,** is characterized by distinct stages over a period of years. Write the name of this STD, being careful of its spelling: _____.

The first stage of syphilis is characterized by swollen lymph nodes and the appearance of a painless sore called a **chancre** (Fig. 8.52, A). Do not confuse chancre with the word canker, which is an ulceration of the oral mucosa. The painless sore of syphilis that occurs usually on the genitals is called a _____.

chancre

Material from a chancre may be examined for the **spirochete** that causes syphilis (see Fig. 8.52, B). In addition, the fluorescent treponemal antibody absorption test (FTA-ABS) is a blood test for syphilis (see Fig. 8.52, C). The disease can spread to another person through sexual contact.

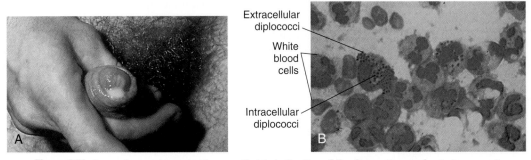

Figure 8.51 Gonorrhea and a stained smear that is indicative of the disease in a male. A, Gonococcal urethritis. Profuse, purulent drainage from the urethra. **B,** Gram-negative intracellular diplococci. The presence of gram-negative intracellular diplococci in a urethral smear is usually indicative of gonorrhea in males. The same finding in females is considered presumptive and is generally followed by culture to confirm the diagnosis. Note also the presence of many extracellular diplococci.

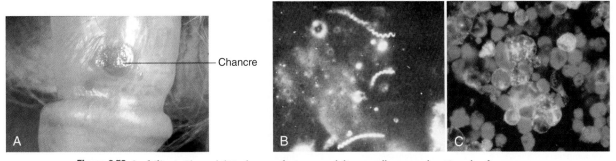

Figure 8.52 Syphilis. A, The syphilitic chancre of primary syphilis generally occurs about 2 weeks after exposure. **B,** Scrapings from the ulcer show spirochetes, the causative organism of syphilis, when examined microscopically using darkfield illumination. **C,** Fluorescent treponemal antibody absorption (FTA-ABS) test. If the patient's antibodies react with *Treponemal pallidum* on the slide, the result is fluorescence as shown in about 85% of primary syphilis cases and in 98% to 100% of secondary and late syphilis cases.

rash

8-147 If the disease is not treated with penicillin or another antibiotic, the second stage of syphilis occurs 2 weeks to 6 months after the chancre disappears. The results of blood tests for syphilis (VDRL or RPR tests) are generally positive at this time but should be confirmed by additional tests. The disease becomes systemic as organisms spread throughout the body, and a generalized rash appears. The disease can affect many organs. The outward sign that is characteristic of the second stage of syphilis is the _____. The second stage lasts 2 to 6 weeks and is followed by a fairly asymptomatic latent stage. Transmission of the disease can occur by blood transfer to another person during the latent stage.

Only about one third of untreated individuals progress to the third stage, which has irreversible complications, including changes in the cardiovascular and nervous system and soft rubbery tumors, called **gummas,** on any part of the body.

8-148 Before the problems of the third stage of syphilis were recognized, some "psychotic" patients in mental hospitals may have been suffering from **neuro/syphilis,** a complication of late syphilis.

> **BEYOND** THE BLUEPRINT The origin of syphilis is not clear, but the disease occurred throughout Europe shortly after the return of Christopher Columbus and his crew from the New World in 1493. Fever therapy (such as, intentional infection with malaria, which is a disease characterized by chills and fever) was used to treat mental illness in past times. Syphilitic patients who were infected with malaria developed high fever and improved. The organisms that cause syphilis, like many others, are adversely affected by high temperatures (sometimes a rise of as little as only 1° F or 2° F).

syphilis

8-149 **Congenital syphilis** is acquired by the fetus from the mother during pregnancy. The bacteria that cause syphilis can cross the placenta of an infected female and cause congenital _____. Infants who are born with congenital syphilis may have severe physical and mental defects and die within a few weeks after birth. An infant of an infected mother may be infected during childbirth. When the mother is known to be infected, a cesarean section is usually performed.

STDs and their causative organisms are shown in Table 8.3.

8-150 Chlamydial infection, **chlamyd/iosis,** is transmitted by intimate sexual contact and is treated with antibiotics.

Chancroid, another STD caused by a bacterium, produces painful ulcers.

Nonspecific genital infections are caused by a variety of microorganisms. **Non/gonococcal urethritis** is inflammation of the urethra by an organism other than the GC, the bacterium that causes _____.

gonorrhea

papillomavirus

8-151 AIDS, genital herpes, genital warts, and several types of hepatitis are caused by viruses. It is important to remember that genital warts, caused by the human _____ (HPV), is the only STD for which there is immunization.

Table 8.3   Sexually Transmitted Diseases and Their Causative Organisms

Disease	Causative Organism	Disease	Causative Organism
Bacterial		**Viral**	
Gonorrhea	*Neisseria gonorrhoeae*	Acquired immunodeficiency syndrome (AIDS)	Human immunodeficiency virus (HIV)
Syphilis	*Treponema pallidum,* a spirochete	Herpes genitalis (genital herpes)	Herpes simplex virus type 2 (HSV-2)
Chlamydial infection	*Chlamydia trachomatis*	Condyloma acuminatum (genital warts)	Human papillomavirus (HPV)
Chancroid (nonsyphilitic venereal ulcer)	*Haemophilus ducreyi*		
Nonspecific genital infection	Various organisms, not all of which are bacteria	Hepatitis B	Hepatitis B virus (HBV)
		Hepatitis C	Hepatitis C virus (HCV)
		Hepatitis D	Hepatitis D virus (HDV)
Protozoal			
Trichomoniasis	*Trichomonas vaginalis*	**Parasitic**	
		Pubic lice	*Phthirus pubis*
Fungal			
Candidiasis	*Candida albicans*		

MATCH IT!
EXERCISE 41

Match the terms in the left column with their descriptions.

_____ **1.** chancroid

_____ **2.** chlamydiosis

_____ **3.** gonorrhea

_____ **4.** syphilis

A. caused by a spirochete

B. caused by gram-negative intracellular diplococci

C. chlamydial infection

D. STD with a painful ulcer

WRITE IT!
EXERCISE 42

Case Study. *Answer the questions after reading the following report.*

Laboratory specimen of penile discharge for patient Hamad Basara, ID No. 013-0002, received 11/29/16. Gram stain shows the presence of both intracellular and extracellular negative diplococci. *Neisseria gonorrhoeae* grown in culture.

1. Name and describe the type of specimen received by the laboratory: _____

2. Describe intracellular vs. extracellular diplococci: _____

3. What is the name of the sexually transmitted disease that is implied? _____

4. What is the name of the organism that causes this disease? _____

5. How is this disease usually treated? _____

---

immunodeficiency

8-152 The abbreviation AIDS means **acquired _____ syndrome.** Immunodeficiency makes an individual susceptible to infection, cancer, and other diseases. As a result of the deficiency of antibodies, the immune response does not adequately protect the person from malignancies or opportunistic infections, which are infections that are caused by normally nonpathogenic organisms in someone whose resistance is decreased.

🔑 **KEY** POINT **AIDS is caused by HIV and is spread by sexual intercourse or exposure to contaminated blood, semen, breast milk, or other body fluids of infected persons.** The virus has a long incubation period (time between exposure and the onset of symptoms), and the disease we recognize as AIDS is the late, fatal stage of infection. Some persons with AIDS are susceptible to opportunistic infections and malignant neoplasms (tumors), especially **Kaposi sarcoma** (Fig. 8.53).

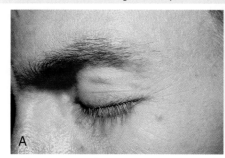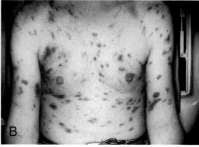

Figure 8.53 Kaposi sarcoma. A, An early lesion of Kaposi sarcoma. **B,** Advanced lesions of Kaposi sarcoma. Note widespread hemorrhagic plaques and nodules.

liver

8-153 Viral hepatitis is an inflammatory condition of the _____ caused by one of the hepatitis viruses, A, B, C, D, or E. Hepatitis A and E are not considered STDs, because transmission is generally through direct contact with contaminated food or water. Read about how Hepatitis B, C, and D are transmitted.

• Hepatitis B is transmitted by sexual contact, blood products, and contaminated needles. Hepatitis B vaccine is available, required by various educational institutions, and recommended for health care workers and others at greater than usual risk.

• Hepatitis C is primarily transmitted by blood products, shared needles, or shared straws for inhaling cocaine. It is transmitted less commonly by sexual intercourse. This type of hepatitis has a high likelihood of progressing to chronic hepatitis.

• Hepatitis D occurs only in patients who are infected with hepatitis B. It is transmitted by sexual contact and needle sharing.

Hepatitis B, C, and D are caused by hepatitis viruses B, C, and D, respectively. These viruses are abbreviated HBV, HCV, and HDV.

8-154 Herpes genitalis, a viral infection caused by the **herpes simplex virus** type 2 (HSV-2), is also known as _____ **herpes.**

genital

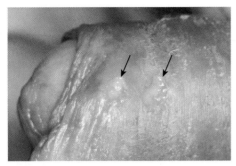

Figure 8.54 Genital herpes. These unruptured vesicles of (arrows) of herpes simplex virus type 2 (HSV-2) appear on the penis.

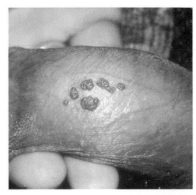

Figure 8.55 Genital warts. Multiple genital warts of the penis.

Painful genital blisters and ulcerations are characteristic of this disease (Fig. 8.54). The causative organism enters through the mucous membranes or breaks in the skin during contact with an infected person. Anti/viral agents may lessen the severity and duration of the symptoms. Active infection during pregnancy can lead to spontaneous abortion, stillbirth, or congenital birth defects. Delivery of the infant is often by cesarean section to prevent infection of the infant at the time of delivery.

warts

8-155 Condyloma acuminatum is commonly called **genital** _____, which also describes its major characteristic (Fig. 8.55). Persons who have had genital warts are at greater risk for genital malignancy, especially cervical cancer. The development of cervical cancer is very slow, and the pre/cancerous condition can be detected by a *Pap smear*. Pre/cancerous means likely to become cancerous.

Treatment to destroy the genital warts includes destruction with acid, laser, or cryo/therapy (cry[o], cold + -therapy, treatment). Cryo/therapy is destruction of the lesions using very

cold

_____ temperatures.

🔑 **KEY POINT Genital warts is the only STD, as well as the only cancer, for which a vaccine is available.** The vaccine prevents infection against the two types of HPV responsible for the majority of cervical cancer cases. To further reduce the risk of cervical cancer, it is recommended that women practice safe sex (using condoms) and limit their number of sexual partners, avoiding partners who participate in high-risk sexual activities. Cervical cancer is the third most common type of cancer in women worldwide.

Trochomonas

8-156 Trichomon/iasis is an infection caused by _____ *vaginalis*, a protozoon. Diagnosis is by microscopic examination of fresh urethral or vaginal secretions (Fig. 8.56). Symptoms of trichomoniasis include a frothy discharge with a bad odor in females; symptoms are minor or absent in males.

vulva

8-157 Candid/iasis, a fungal infection not limited to the genitals, can cause vulvo/vaginitis, which means inflammation of the _____ and the vagina. The infection is usually caused by *Candida albicans,* a yeast-type fungus (Fig. 8.57), and it

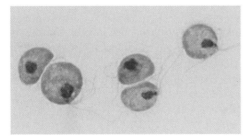

Figure 8.56 Microscopic *Trichomonas* in a stained smear.

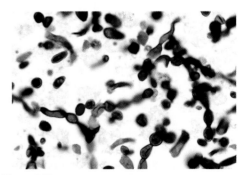

Figure 8.57 Microscopic appearance of *Candida albicans.*

mouth

sometimes occurs after administration of antibiotics for a bacterial infection or when immunity is suppressed.

It can be treated with oral and topical anti/fungal medications. Oral medications are taken by _____, and topical ones are applied directly to the affected area. *C. albicans* is also called **Monilia,** and the infection is sometimes called **moniliasis.**

8-158 Pubic lice are external parasites and are sometimes included with STDs, because they can be transmitted by sexual contact. They are also transmitted by close contact with contaminated objects, such as linens. They are commonly called *crab lice* and primarily infest the pubic region but are also found in armpits, beards, eyebrows, and eyelashes. The use of topical agents and particular attention to hygiene is used in treating lice.

8-159 The physician uses the patient's sexual history and symptoms to decide which diagnostic tests will be helpful in establishing the diagnosis of a STD. At times the patient has classic symptoms (such as, the blisters of genital herpes) and is treated without a positive diagnostic test. After the diagnosis of a STD, tests for syphilis, gonorrhea, and chlamydia are often recommended.

MATCH IT!
EXERCISE 43

Match the STDs in the left column with their characteristics in the right column.

_____ **1.** AIDS   **A.** fatal late stage of infection with HIV

_____ **2.** condyloma acuminatum   **B.** blisters and ulcerations of the genitals

_____ **3.** hepatitis B   **C.** caused by HBV

_____ **4.** hepatitis C   **D.** genital warts

_____ **5.** herpes genitalis   **E.** transmitted primarily by blood products, shared needles, etc.

PHARMACOLOGY

Drug Class: Effects and Uses

Alpha Blockers: Relax smooth muscle in the prostate to improve urinary flow
doxazosin (Cardura)   *tamsulosin (Flomax)*   *terazosin (Hytrin)*

Antiandrogens: Decrease specific androgen hormone levels to treat benign prostatic hyperplasia
dutasteride (Avodart)   *finasteride (Proscar)*

Antiretrovirals: Treat HIV infection (subtype of antivirals)
didanosine (Videx)   *lamivudine (Epivir)*   *ritonavir (Norvir)*
efavirenz (Sustiva)   *ribavirin (Virazole)*   *zidovudine (Retrovir)*

Aromatase Inhibitors: Block conversion of androgen hormones to estrogens to treat breast or ovarian cancer
anastrozole (Arimidex)   *exemestane (Aromasin)*   *letrozole (Femara)*

Contraceptives: Estrogen and progestin combination (or progestin alone) hormone therapy used to prevent pregnancy
Various routes of administration: *Oral, transdermal, intrauterine, vaginal, or by injection*
drospirenone/ethinyl estradiol (Yaz)   *norelgestromin/ethinyl estradiol (Ortho Evra)*   *norgestimate/ethinyl estradiol (Ortho*
medroxyprogesterone (Depo-Provera)   *norethindrone (Micronor)*   *Tri-Cyclen)*

Estrogens: Female hormones used for contraception or hormone replacement therapy, usually in combination with progestins
conjugated estrogens (Premarin)   *estradiol (Estrace, combination products)*   *estropipate (Ogen)*

Impotence Agents: Increase blood flow to penis to treat erectile dysfunction
alprostadil (Caverject)   *sildenafil (Viagra)*   *tadalafil (Cialis)*

Ovulation Stimulants: Fertility drugs used to promote ovulation
bromocriptine (Parlodel)   *clomiphene (Clomid)*
chorionic gonadotropin (Pregnyl)   *follitropin alfa (Follistim AQ)*

PHARMACOLOGY, cont'd

Oxytocics: Stimulate uterine contractions to promote labor or suppress postpartum uterine bleeding; also called uterotonics
methylergonovine (Methergine)   oxytocin (Pitocin)

Progestins: Progesterone hormones used for contraception or hormone replacement therapy, usually in combination with estrogens; or to treat menstrual disorders, endometriosis, or infertility
levonorgestrel (Mirena, combination products)   norgestimate (in combination, e.g., Ortho Tri-Cyclen)
medroxyprogesterone (Provera)

Tocolytics: Suppress uterine contractions to stop premature labor
indomethacin (Indocin)   magnesium sulfate (*no brand name)   terbutaline (Brethine)

WRITE IT! EXERCISE 44

Write a word in the blank to complete these sentences.

1. A class of pharmaceutics that decreases specific androgen hormone levels is _____.
2. Aromatase _____ are used to treat breast or ovarian cancer.
3. Fertility drugs used to promote ovulation are ovulation _____.
4. Oxytocics stimulate _____ contractions to promote labor.
5. A general term for subtypes of antivirals is _____.
6. The drug class used to suppress uterine contractions is called _____.

CHAPTER ABBREVIATIONS*

AIDS	acquired immunodeficiency syndrome	HSV-2	herpes simplex virus type 2 (genital herpes)
BBT	basal body temperature		
BPH	benign prostatic hyperplasia	IUD	intrauterine device
CPD	cephalopelvic disproportion	IVF	in vitro fertilization
CS or C-section	cesarean section	LH	luteinizing hormone
Cx	cervix	LMP	last menstrual period
D&C	dilation and curettage	OB	obstetrics
EDD	expected date of delivery	Pap	Papanicolaou
EFM	electronic fetal monitor	PID	pelvic inflammatory disease
FHR	fetal heart rate	PMS	premenstrual syndrome
FSH	follicle-stimulating hormone	PSA	prostate-specific antigen
FTA-ABS	fluorescent treponemal antibody absorption test	PVP	photoselective vaporization of the prostate; Green Light PVP
G	gravida (pregnant)	RPR	rapid plasma reagin test (for syphilis)
GC	gonococcus	STD	sexually transmitted disease
GPA	gravid/para/abortus	STI	sexually transmitted infection
GU	genitourinary	TPAL	term birth(s), premature birth(s), abortions, living children
GYN, Gyn, gyn	gynecology		
HBV	hepatitis B virus	TSS	toxic shock syndrome
hCG, HCG	human chorionic gonadotropin	TUMT	transurethral microwave thermotherapy
HCV	hepatitis C virus		
HDV	hepatitis D virus	TUNA	transurethral needle ablation
HIV	human immunodeficiency virus	TURP	transurethral resection of the prostate
HPV	human papillomavirus	VD	venereal disease
HRT	hormone replacement therapy	VDRL	Venereal Disease Research Laboratories

*Many of these abbreviations share their meanings with other terms.

Be Careful With These!

cervic(o)	*neck* or *uterine cervix*	orchi(o), orchid(o)	testicle
hyster(o)	uterus	vas(o)	*vessel* or *vas deferens*
metr(o)	*measurement* or *uterine tissue*	gravid vs. parity	*pregnancies* vs. *live births*

A Career as an IVF Embryologist

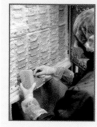

Yolanda Perez is an embryologist working in a private fertility institute in Arizona. She provides services to a broad range of male and female infertility and genetic cases. Using her biopsy skills, her work includes intra-cytoplasmic sperm injection and robotic micromanipulation. Here she is shown selecting one sample stored among thousands in the cryopreservation freezer. An embryologist requires a bachelor's degree in biological science and experience in clinical embryology. She is certified by the American College of Embryology; however, embryology certification is not required by all states. Yolanda supervises the work of embryology technicians who perform many laboratory tests, semen analysis and wash, processing cord blood samples, and cryopreservation of cells.

CHAPTER 8 SELF-TEST

Review the new word parts for this chapter. Work all of the following exercises to test your understanding of the material before checking your answers against those in Appendix IV.

BASIC UNDERSTANDING

Labeling

I. *Label the diagram with the following combining forms that correspond to numbered lines 1 through 5. (The first one is done as an example.):* cervic(o), colp(o), hyster(o), oophor(o), salping(o)

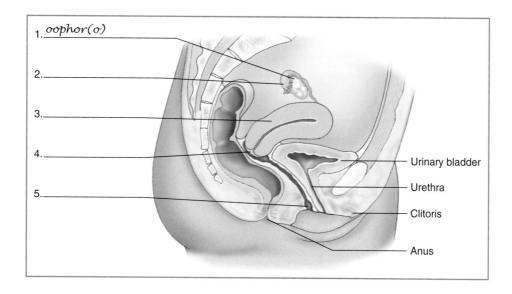

1. *oophor(o)*
2.
3.
4.
5.

Urinary bladder

Urethra

Clitoris

Anus

II.   *Label the diagram with the following combining forms that correspond to numbered lines 1 through 7. (The first one is done as an example.):* epididym(o), orchi(o), pen(o), prostat(o), scrot(o), urethr(o), vas(o)

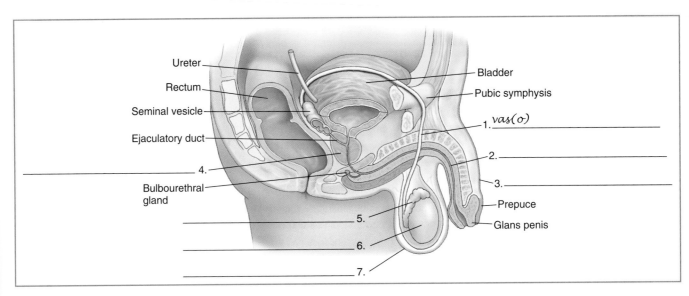

III.   *Label the following structures in the drawing:* amnion, amniotic fluid, chorion, placenta, umbilical cord, uterus

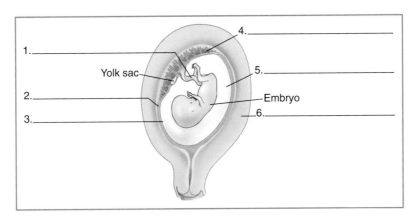

Matching

IV.   *Names of the three types of uterine tissue are in the left column. Match them with their locations in the uterus (A through C):*

_____ **1.** endometrium	**A.** innermost
_____ **2.** myometrium	**B.** middle
_____ **3.** perimetrium	**C.** outermost

V.   *Match terms in the left column with descriptions in the right column. (Selections A through F may be used more than once.)*

_____ **1.** ovary	**A.** gonad
_____ **2.** ovum	**B.** female sex cell
_____ **3.** sperm	**C.** male sex cell
_____ **4.** testis	**D.** normal site of implantation
_____ **5.** uterus	**E.** receives the sperm during intercourse
_____ **6.** uterine tube	**F.** usual site of fertilization
_____ **7.** vagina	

VI. Match terms in the left column with their descriptions in the right column.

_____ **1.** gamete	**A.**	afterbirth
_____ **2.** gonad	**B.**	important hormone of pregnancy
_____ **3.** placenta	**C.**	ovary or testis
_____ **4.** progesterone	**D.**	ovum or spermatozoon
_____ **5.** zygote	**E.**	product of fertilization

VII. Match the following pathologies of pregnancy with their descriptions.

_____ **1.** abruptio placentae	**A.**	abnormal implantation of the placenta in the uterus
_____ **2.** ectopic pregnancy	**B.**	onset of acute high blood pressure after the twenty-fourth week
_____ **3.** placenta previa	**C.**	false pregnancy
_____ **4.** preeclampsia	**D.**	implantation of a fertilized ovum outside the uterus
_____ **5.** pseudocyesis	**E.**	premature separation of the placenta from the uterine wall

Identifying Illustrations

VIII. Label these illustrations using one of the following: adhesiolysis, amniocentesis, azoospermia, cystocele, fetoscope, gastroschisis, primipara, sonogram, vasectomy, vulvectomy.

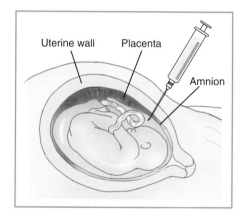

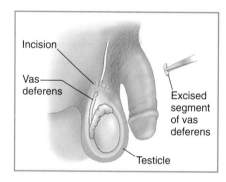

1. _____

2. _____

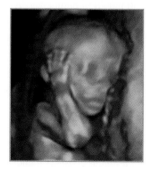

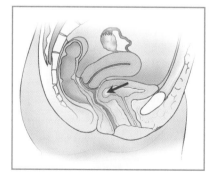

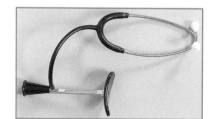

3. _____

4. _____

5. _____

IX. *The following diagrams represent displacements of the uterus. Label each as anteflexion, anteversion, retroflexion, or retroversion.*

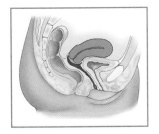 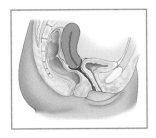 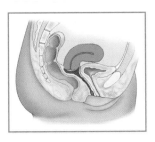 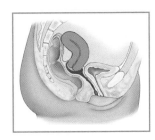

1. _____   2. _____   3. _____   4. _____

Deconstructing Words

X. *Divide the following words into their component parts, and write the meaning of each term.*

1. endometrium _____

2. erythroblastosis _____

3. hysteroscope _____

4. laparorrhaphy _____

5. neonatology _____

6. oophorectomy _____

7. proteinuria _____

8. salpingitis _____

9. spermatogenesis _____

10. vasovasostomy _____

Using Vocabulary

XI. *Circle one answer for each of the following questions.*

1. Belinda buys a pregnancy test at the local pharmacy, and the test is positive. Which hormone is tested for in a pregnancy test? (EIA, GPA, HCG, HDV)

2. A visit to Belinda's obstetrician confirms that she is pregnant, her history is taken, and a complete prenatal examination is performed. Vaginal palpation of specific bony landmarks that are used to estimate the size of the birth canal represents which clinical test? (amniocentesis, cephalopelvic disproportion, chorionic villus sampling, pelvimetry)

3. Cindy has a long and difficult labor. Which term describes this condition? (abortion, dystocia, eclampsia, stillbirth)

4. Gwen and Seth are new parents to a son with a genetic disorder of an extra chromosome. Which of the following is the likely name of the disorder? (Down syndrome, erythroblastosis fetalis, hemolytic anemia, pseudocyesis)

5. Becky developed high blood pressure, _____ hypertension in the eighth month of pregnancy. Which word completes the blank? (gestational, neonatal, ovulatory, postpartum)

6. During Becky's labor, the obstetrician finds that the fetus has entered the lesser pelvis, and the face is prominent at the cervical opening. Which type of fetal presentation is described? (breech, cephalic, shoulder, transverse)

7. When Pilar speaks to her gynecologist about birth control, she recommends a small intrauterine device that releases hormones on a regular schedule. Which type of contraceptive is described? (IUD, oral contraceptive, postcoital contraceptive, subdermal implant)

8. Cathy has had two pregnancies and two viable births. Which designation is described? (0-2-0-2, $G_1\,P_2$, 0-0-2-2, $G_2\,P_2$)

9. Tony is diagnosed with condyloma acuminatum. What is the common name of his sexually transmitted disease? (genital herpes, genital warts, moniliasis, venereal ulcer)

10. Phyllis has contracted a sexually transmitted disease caused by a fungus. Which of the following is a fungal disease? (candidiasis, chancroid, chlamydiosis, trichomoniasis)

11. Seventeen-year-old Indira has painful menstruation each month. Which condition does she suffer from? (amenorrhea, dysmenorrhea, metrorrhagia, menorrhea)

12. Which instrument does a gynecologist use in a routine gynecologic examination? (curet, hysterosalpingograph, hysteroscope, speculum)

13. Which examination of the abdominal cavity uses an instrument that is inserted through one or more small incisions in the abdominal wall? (dilation and curettage, hysteroscopy, laparoscopy, ultrasonography)

14. Halla complains of chronic pelvic pain. The gynecologist finds that her left ovary has numerous ovarian cysts with a great deal of inflammation. Which term means inflammation of an ovary? (cervicitis, oophoritis, salpingitis, vulvitis)

15. Which term means the first occurrence of menstruation? (amenorrhea, dysmenorrhea, menarche, mittelschmerz)

16. Which surgery is recommended to correct 60-year-old Salma's prolapsed uterus? (cervicectomy, hysterectomy, hysteropexy, leiomyomectomy)

17. Which term means a white, viscid discharge from the vagina and uterine cavity? (leukorrhea, occult blood, mittelschmerz, trichomoniasis)

18. Connie has debilitating abdominal pain during her menstrual periods. Laparoscopic surgery to remove ovarian cysts revealed an endometrial growth on the right ovary. Which term describes the endometrial growths on the ovary? (endometriosis, endometritis, hysteropathy, salpingopathy)

19. Which term means surgical repair of the vagina? (colpectomy, colpoplasty, colporrhaphy, oophorectomy)

20. Newborn Arturo has only one testicle. What is the name of this condition? (anorchidism, aspermia, oligospermia, orchidectomy)

21. Barry undergoes a bilateral vasectomy. Which of the following results is expected? (impotence, increased PSA, oligospermia, sterility)

22. Newborn Carlos undergoes circumcision. What tissue is removed in a circumcision? (glans penis, prepuce, prostate, testes)

23. Newborn Andrew has undescended testicles. What is the term for this condition? (cryptorchidism, orchidism, orchidorrhaphy, testalgia)

24. Billy suffers from twisting of the spermatic cord during wrestling practice. Which describes Billy's condition? (hydrocele, spermatocele, testicular torsion, varicocele)

25. Billy experienced a great deal of testicular pain. Which term describes this type of pain? (orchialgia, orchidism, orchiopathy, orchiotomy)

Filling in the Blanks

XII. Write a word in each blank to complete this paragraph.

The female reproductive cycle is composed of two cycles that occur simultaneously. The (1) _____ cycle reflects the changes that occur in the ovaries. The changes in the ovarian follicle are called follicle development, (2) _____, and the corpus luteal stage. Two important hormones secreted by the follicles are (3) _____ and progesterone. The (4) _____ cycle is also called the menstrual cycle. In this cycle, the endometrium thickens and prepares for a developing embryo. If fertilization does not occur, the endometrial lining is shed, a process that is called (5) _____.

Writing Terms

XIII. Write a term for each of the following phrases.

1. a newborn
2. a woman who has produced many viable offspring
3. an embryonic form of spermatozoa
4. attachment of a fertilized ovum to the endometrium
5. deliberate rupture of the fetal membranes to induce labor
6. excision of the prostate
7. excision of the uterus
8. heavy or long menstrual periods
9. herniation of a fallopian tube
10. incision made to enlarge the vaginal opening for delivery
11. incision of the vas deferens
12. inflammation of the cervix uteri
13. inflammation of the vulva and vagina
14. insufficient sperm in the semen
15. painless sore of syphilis
16. pertaining to the amnion and the chorion
17. pertaining to the fetus

18. release of an ovum from the ovary _____
19. surgical fixation of a fallopian tube _____
20. viewing the vagina and cervix with magnification _____

Making Connections

XIV. Describe the relationship of these terms.

1. ovaries and testes _____
_____

2. endometrium, myometrium, and perimetrium _____
_____

3. menarche and menstruation _____
_____

4. seminiferous tubules and spermatogenesis _____
_____

5. PSA and prostatic carcinoma _____
_____

6. amnion and chorion _____
_____

7. para 1 and primipara _____
_____

Finetuning Terms

XV. In addition to spelling, describe at least one difference in the following:

1. chancre and genital wart _____
_____

2. contraceptive patch and postcoital contraceptive _____
_____

3. ovarian cyst and ovarian cancer _____
_____

4. urethrovaginal fistula and vesicovaginal fistula _____
_____

5. vasectomy and vasovasostomy _____
_____

Opting for Opposites

XVI. Write a term that you learned that means the opposite of these words.

1. anteversion _____
2. spermatogenesis _____
3. antepartum _____
4. prenatal _____

GREATER COMPREHENSION

Using Pharmacologic Terms

XVII. Use all selections to match drug uses in the left column with the corresponding drug class.

_____ **1.** prevent pregnancy   **A.** antiandrogens
_____ **2.** treat BPH   **B.** antiretrovirals
_____ **3.** stimulate uterine contractions **C.** contraceptives
_____ **4.** suppress uterine contractions   **D.** oxytocics
_____ **5.** treat HIV infection   **E.** tocolytics

Health Care Reporting

XVIII. Read the following partial report of an emergency department record, and match each term in the left column with a description in the right column. (Not all selections with be used.)

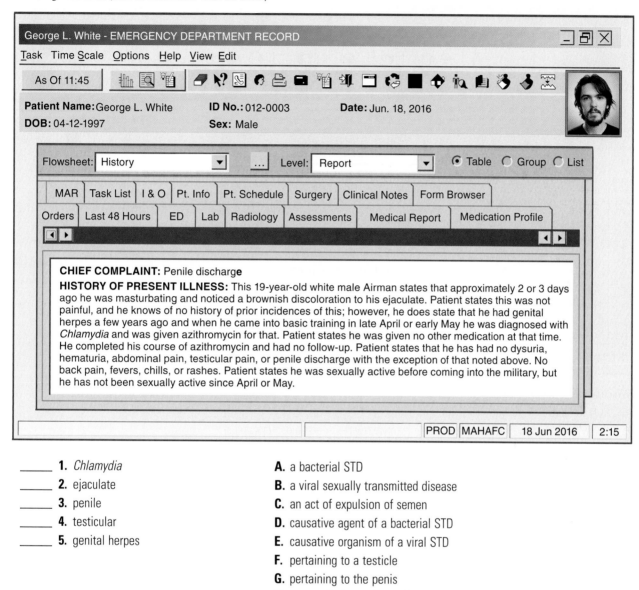

George L. White - EMERGENCY DEPARTMENT RECORD

Task Time Scale Options Help View Edit

As Of 11:45

Patient Name: George L. White   **ID No.:** 012-0003   **Date:** Jun. 18, 2016
DOB: 04-12-1997   **Sex:** Male

Flowsheet: History   Level: Report   ● Table ○ Group ○ List

MAR | Task List | I & O | Pt. Info | Pt. Schedule | Surgery | Clinical Notes | Form Browser

Orders | Last 48 Hours | ED | Lab | Radiology | Assessments | Medical Report | Medication Profile

CHIEF COMPLAINT: Penile discharge
HISTORY OF PRESENT ILLNESS: This 19-year-old white male Airman states that approximately 2 or 3 days ago he was masturbating and noticed a brownish discoloration to his ejaculate. Patient states this was not painful, and he knows of no history of prior incidences of this; however, he does state that he had genital herpes a few years ago and when he came into basic training in late April or early May he was diagnosed with *Chlamydia* and was given azithromycin for that. Patient states he was given no other medication at that time. He completed his course of azithromycin and had no follow-up. Patient states that he has had no dysuria, hematuria, abdominal pain, testicular pain, or penile discharge with the exception of that noted above. No back pain, fevers, chills, or rashes. Patient states he was sexually active before coming into the military, but he has not been sexually active since April or May.

PROD MAHAFC 18 Jun 2016 2:15

_____ **1.** *Chlamydia*
_____ **2.** ejaculate
_____ **3.** penile
_____ **4.** testicular
_____ **5.** genital herpes

A. a bacterial STD
B. a viral sexually transmitted disease
C. an act of expulsion of semen
D. causative agent of a bacterial STD
E. causative organism of a viral STD
F. pertaining to a testicle
G. pertaining to the penis
H. semen discharged in a single emission

Abbreviating

XIX. Write a letter in each blank that corresponds to the clue.

1. cephalopelvic disproportion ___ ___ ___
2. human chorionic gonadotropin ___ ___ ___
3. photoselective vaporization of the prostate ___ ___ ___
4. transurethral needle ablation ___ ___ ___ ___
5. virus that causes AIDS ___ ___ ___
6. virus that causes Hepatitis B ___ ___ ___

Health Care Reporting

XX. Read the following Office Visit Note, then circle one answer for each of the questions that follow the report.

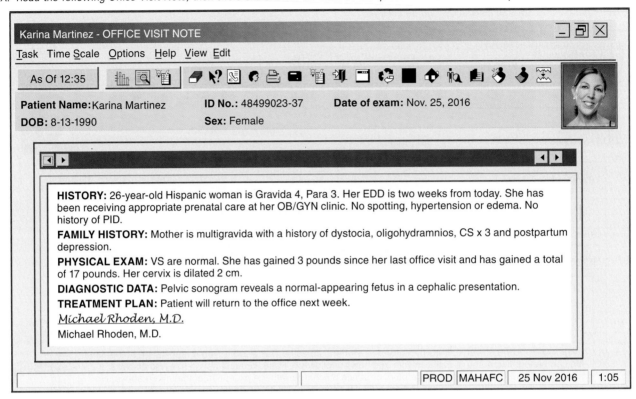

1. Which abbreviation refers to the branch of medicine dealing with childbirth?
   (CS, EDD, GYN, OB)
2. How many times has the patient been pregnant? (once, twice, three times, four times)
3. When did the patient's mother suffer depression? (after birth, before birth, during birth)
4. Which term in the report indicates difficult or painful labor?
   (cephalic, dystocia, oligohydramnios, para)
5. What is an alternate term for prenatal? (antenatal, antepartum, neonatal, postnatal)

Pronouncing Terms

XXI. Write the correct term for the following phonetic spellings.

1. an-**or**-ki-diz-um   _____
2. ā-zō-uh-**spur**-mē-uh   _____
3. kaw-tur-i-**zā**-shun   _____
4. ep-i-**did**-uh-mis   _____
5. **loo**-tē-in-ī-zing   _____
6. noor-ō-**sif**-i-lis   _____
7. ō-of-ur-**al**-juh   _____
8. pahr-tū-**ri**-shun   _____
9. spur-muh-tō-**zō**-uh   _____
10. ves-i-kō-**vaj**-i-nul   _____

Health Care Reporting

XXII. List and define/describe terms or phrases that relate to the reproductive system. Try to find as many as you can before seeing the answers. Challenge your classmates to see who recognizes the most terms.

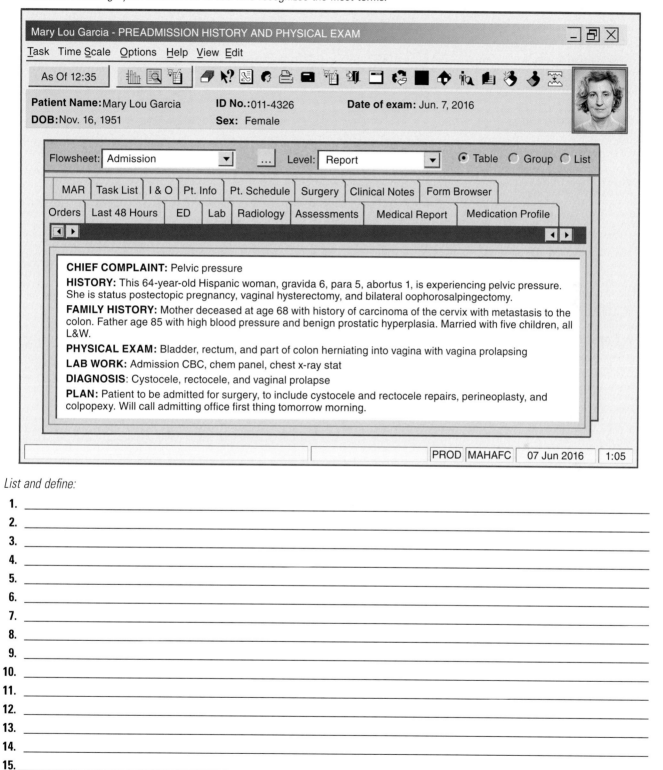

Mary Lou Garcia - PREADMISSION HISTORY AND PHYSICAL EXAM

Task   Time Scale   Options   Help   View   Edit

As Of 12:35

Patient Name: Mary Lou Garcia   **ID No.:** 011-4326   **Date of exam:** Jun. 7, 2016
DOB: Nov. 16, 1951   **Sex:** Female

Flowsheet: Admission   ...   Level: Report   ● Table   ○ Group   ○ List

MAR | Task List | I & O | Pt. Info | Pt. Schedule | Surgery | Clinical Notes | Form Browser

Orders | Last 48 Hours | ED | Lab | Radiology | Assessments | Medical Report | Medication Profile

CHIEF COMPLAINT: Pelvic pressure
HISTORY: This 64-year-old Hispanic woman, gravida 6, para 5, abortus 1, is experiencing pelvic pressure. She is status postectopic pregnancy, vaginal hysterectomy, and bilateral oophorosalpingectomy.
FAMILY HISTORY: Mother deceased at age 68 with history of carcinoma of the cervix with metastasis to the colon. Father age 85 with high blood pressure and benign prostatic hyperplasia. Married with five children, all L&W.
PHYSICAL EXAM: Bladder, rectum, and part of colon herniating into vagina with vagina prolapsing
LAB WORK: Admission CBC, chem panel, chest x-ray stat
DIAGNOSIS: Cystocele, rectocele, and vaginal prolapse
PLAN: Patient to be admitted for surgery, to include cystocele and rectocele repairs, perineoplasty, and colpopexy. Will call admitting office first thing tomorrow morning.

PROD | MAHAFC | 07 Jun 2016 | 1:05

List and define:

1. _____
2. _____
3. _____
4. _____
5. _____
6. _____
7. _____
8. _____
9. _____
10. _____
11. _____
12. _____
13. _____
14. _____
15. _____

Spelling

XXIII. Circle all misspelled terms, and write their correct spellings.

amniosentesis   contraseptive   extraembryonic   menarke   parturition   varicocele

Categorizing Terms and Practicing Pronunciation

XXIV. Classify the terms in the left column (1 through 15) by selecting A, B, C, D, or E from the right column.

_____ **1.** anorchidism
_____ **2.** antifungals
_____ **3.** antivirals
_____ **4.** balanitis
_____ **5.** cesarean section
_____ **6.** chorion
_____ **7.** colposcopy
_____ **8.** curettage
_____ **9.** episiotomy
_____ **10.** fetoscope use (office visit)
_____ **11.** hepatitis C
_____ **12.** hysterosalpingography
_____ **13.** laparorrhaphy
_____ **14.** preeclampsia
_____ **15.** trichomoniasis

A. anatomy
B. diagnostic test or procedure
C. pathology
D. surgery
E. nonsurgical therapy

(Be prepared to pronounce terms 1-15 in class after listening to Chapter 8 terms at *http://evolve.elsevier.com/Leonard/ building.* In addition, practice categorizing all boldface terms in this chapter.)

New Construction

XXV. Write the meaning of these terms. Even if you haven't seen the terms before, you may be able to divide the words into their component parts and determine their meanings.

1. balanoplasty _____
2. epididymoorchitis _____
3. fetoscopy _____
4. leiomyofibroma _____
5. oosperm _____
(Use Appendix IV to check your answers to the exercises.)

BMV LIST

Visit *http://evolve.elsevier.com/Leonard/ building* to listen to the boldface terms in Chapter 8. Look closely at the spelling of each term as it is pronounced.

abdominal hysterectomy (ab-**dom**-i-nul his-tur-**ek**-tuh-mē)
ablation (ab-**lā**-shun)
abortion (uh-**bor**-shun)
abruptio placentae (ab-**rup**-shē-ō pluh-**sen**-tē)
abstinence (**ab**-sti-nuns)
acquired immunodeficiency syndrome (uh-**kwīrd** im-ū-nō-duh-**fish**-un-sē **sin**-drōm)
adhesiolysis (ad-hē-sē-**ol**-i-sis)
alpha blockers (**al**-fuh **blok**-urz)
amenorrhea (uh-men-ō-**rē**-uh)
amniocentesis (am-nē-ō-sen-**tē**-sis)
amniochorial (am-nē-ō-**kor**-ē-ul)
amniochorionic (am-nē-ō-kor-ē-**on**-ik)
amnion (**am**-nē-on)
amnionic (am-nē-**on**-ik)
amniorrhexis (am-nē-ō-**rek**-sis)

amniotic (am-nē-**ot**-ik)
amniotomy (am-nē-**ot**-uh-mē)
anorchidism (an-**or**-ki-diz-um)
anorchism (an-**or**-kiz-um)
anovulation (an-ov-ū-**lā**-shun)
anteflexion (an-tē-**flek**-shun)
antenatal (an-tē-**nā**-tul)
antepartum (an-tē-**pahr**-tum)
anteversion (an-tē-**vur**-zhun)
antiandrogens (an-tē-**an**-druh-junz)
antiretrovirals (an-tē-ret-rō-**vī**-rulz)
aromatase inhibitors (uh-**rō**-muh-tās in-**hib**-i-turz)
aspermatogenesis (ā-spur-muh-tō-**jen**-uh-sis)
aspermia (uh-**spur**-mē-uh)
azoospermia (ā-zō-uh-**spur**-mē-uh)
balanitis (bal-uh-**nī**-tis)

Bartholin gland (**bahr**-tō-lin gland)

basal body temperature method (**bā**-sul bod-ē **tem**-per-uh-chur **meth**-ud)

benign prostatic hyperplasia (buh-**nīn** pros-**tat**-ik hī-pur-**plā**-zhuh)

breech presentation (brēch prē-zun-**tā**-shun)

bulbourethral gland (bul-bō-ū-**rē**-thrul gland)

calendar or rhythm method (**kal**-un-dur or **rith**-um **meth**-ud)

candidiasis (kan-di-**dī**-uh-sis)

cauterization (kaw-tur-i-**zā**-shun)

cauterize (**kaw**-tur-īz)

cephalic presentation (suh-**fal**-ik prē-zun-**tā**-shun)

cephalopelvic disproportion (sef-uh-lō-**pel**-vik dis-prō-**por**-shun)

cervical biopsy (**sur**-vi-kul **bī**-op-sē)

cervical cancer (**sur**-vi-kul **kan**-sur)

cervical cap (**sur**-vi-kul kap)

cervical dilation (**sur**-vi-kul dī-**lā**-shun)

cervical polyp (**sur**-vi-kul **pol**-ip)

cervicitis (sur-vi-**sī**-tis)

cervicocolpitis (sur-vi-kō-kol-**pī**-tis)

cervix (**sur**-viks)

cervix uteri (**sur**-viks **ū**-tur-ī)

cesarean section (suh-**zar**-ē-un **sek**-shun)

chancre (**shang**-kur)

chancroid (**shang**-kroid)

chlamydial infection (kluh-**mid**-ē-ul in-**fek**-shun)

chlamydiosis (kluh-mid-ē-**ō**-sis)

chorion (**kor**-ē-on)

chorionic (kor-ē-**on**-ik)

chorionic villi (kor-ē-**on**-ik **vil**-ī)

chorionic villus sampling (kor-ē-**on**-ik **vil**-us **sam**-pling)

circumcision (sur-kum-**sizh**-un)

cleft lip (kleft lip)

cleft palate (kleft **pal**-ut)

climacteric (klī-**mak**-tur-ik)

clitoris (**klit**-uh-ris)

coitus (**kō**-i-tus)

coitus interruptus (**kō**-i-tus in-tur-**rup**-tus)

colostrum (kuh-**los**-trum)

colpectomy (kol-**pek**-tuh-mē)

colpitis (kol-**pī**-tis)

colpocystitis (kōl-pō-sis-**tī**-tis)

colpodynia (kol-pō-**din**-ē-uh)

colpohysterectomy (kol-pō-his-tur-**ek**-tuh-mē)

colpoplasty (**kol**-pō-plas-tē)

colporrhagia (kol-pō-**rā**-juh)

colporrhaphy (kol-**por**-uh-fē)

colposcope (**kol**-pō-skōp)

colposcopy (kol-**pos**-kuh-pē)

conception (kun-**sep**-shun)

condyloma acuminatum (kon-duh-**lō**-muh uh-kū-mi-**nāt**-um)

congenital syphilis (kun-**jen**-i-tul **sif**-i-lis)

conjoined twins (kun-**joind** twinz)

contraception (kon-truh-**sep**-shun)

contraceptive patch (kon-truh-**sep**-tiv pach)

contraceptives (kon-truh-**sep**-tivz)

copulation (kop-ū-**lā**-shun)

corpus luteum (**kor**-pus **loo**-tē-um)

cryosurgery (krī-ō-**sur**-jur-ē)

cryotherapy (krī-ō-**ther**-uh-pē)

cryptorchidism (krip-**tor**-ki-diz-um)

curet (kū-**ret**)

cystocele (**sis**-tō-sēl)

cytology (sī-**tol**-uh-jē)

diaphragm with spermicide (**dī**-uh-fram with **sper**-mi-sīd)

dilatation (dil-uh-**tā**-shun)

dilation and curettage (dī-**lā**-shun and kū-ruh-**tahzh**)

Down syndrome (doun **sin**-drōm)

ductus deferens (**duk**-tus **def**-ur-enz)

dysmenorrhea (dis-men-uh-**rē**-uh)

dysplasia (dis-**plā**-zhuh)

dystocia (dis-**tō**-shuh)

eclampsia (uh-**klamp**-sē-uh)

ectopic pregnancy (ek-**top**-ik **preg**-nun-sē)

effacement (uh-**fās**-munt)

ejaculation (ē-jak-ū-**lā**-shun)

ejaculatory duct (ē-**jak**-yuh-luh-tor-ē dukt)

embryo (**em**-brē-ō)

endometrial ablation (en-dō-**mē**-trē-ul ab-**lā**-shun)

endometrial biopsy (en-dō-**mē**-trē-ul **bī**-op-sē)

endometriosis (en-dō-mē-trē-**ō**-sis)

endometritis (en-dō-mē-**trī**-tis)

endometrium (en-dō-**mē**-trē-um)

epididymis (ep-i-**did**-uh-mis)

epididymitis (ep-i-**did**-uh-**mī**-tis)

episiotomy (uh-piz-ē-**ot**-uh-mē)

erectile dysfunction (uh-**rek**-tīl dis-**funk**-shun)

erection (uh-**rek**-shun)

erythroblastosis fetalis (uh-rith-rō-blas-**tō**-sis fi-**ta**-lus)

esophageal atresia (uh-sof-uh-**jē**-ul uh-**trē**-zhuh)

estrogen (**es**-truh-jen)

expulsion (ek-**spul**-shun)

extraembryonic membrane (eks-truh-em-brē-**on**-ik **mem**-brān)

extrauterine pregnancy (eks-truh-**ū**-tur-in **preg**-nun-sē)

fallopian tube (fuh-**lō**-pe-un tōōb)

female condom (**fē**-māl **kon**-dum)

fetal (**fē**-tul)

fetal alcohol syndrome (**fē**-tul **al**-kuh-hol **sin**-drōm)

fetal presentation (**fē**-tul prē-zun-**tā**-shun)

fetoscope (**fē**-tō-skōp)

fetus (**fē**-tus)

fimbria (**fim**-brē-uh)

fistula (**fis**-tū-luh)

follicle-stimulating hormone (**fol**-i-kul **stim**-ū-lāt-ing **hor**-mōn)

fundus (**fun**-dus)

gamete (**gam**-ēt)

gastroschisis (gas-**tros**-ki-sis)

genital herpes (**jen**-i-tul **her**-pēz)

genital warts (**jen**-i-tul worts)

genitalia (jen-i-**tā**-lē-uh)

genitourinary (jen-i-tō-**ū**-ri-nar-ē)

gestation (jes-**tā**-shun)

glans penis (glanz **pē**-nis)

gonad (**gō**-nad)

gonadotropin (gō-nuh-dō-**trō**-pin)

gonococcus (gon-ō-**kok**-us)

gonorrhea (gon-ō-**rē**-uh)

graafian follicle (**grah**-fē-un **fol**-i-kul)

gravid (**grav**-id)

gravida (**grav**-i-duh)

gummas (**gum**-uz)

gynecologic (gī-nuh-kuh-**loj**-ik)

gynecology (gī-nuh-**kol**-uh-jē)

hemolytic disease of the newborn (hē-mō-**lit**-ik di-**zēz** ov the nōō-born)

hermaphroditism (hur-**maf**-ruh-di-tiz-um)

herpes genitalis (**hur**-pēz jen-i-**tal**-is)

herpes simplex virus (**hur**-pēz **sim**-pleks **vī**-rus)

human chorionic gonadotropin (**hū**-mun kor-ē-**on**-ik gō-nuh-dō-**trō**-pin)

hydrocele (**hī**-drō-sēl)

hydrocelectomy (hī-drō-sē-**lek**-tuh-mē)

hysterectomy (his-tur-**ek**-tuh-mē)

hysteropathy (his-tuh-**rop**-uh-thē)

hysteropexy (his-tur-ō-**pek**-sē)

hysteroptosis (his-tur-op-**tō**-sis)

hysterosalpingogram (his-tur-ō-sal-**ping**-gō-gram)

hysterosalpingography (his-tur-ō-sal-ping-**gog**-ruh-fē)

hysteroscope (**his**-tur-ō-skōp)

hysteroscopy (his-tur-**os**-kuh-pē)

implantation (im-plan-**tā**-shun)

impotence agents (**im**-puh-tuns **a**-junts)

infertility (in-fur-**til**-i-tē)

injectable contraceptive (in-**jek**-tuh-bul kon-truh-**sep**-tiv)

internal os (in-**tur**-nul os)

interstitial cells of Leydig (in-tur-**stish**-ul selz ov **lī**-dig)

intrauterine device (in-truh-**ū**-tur-in duh-**vīs**)

in vitro fertilization (in **vē**-trō fur-ti-li-**zā**-shun)

Kaposi sarcoma (**kah**-pō-shē sahr-**kō**-muh)

labia majora (**lā**-bē-uh muh-**jor**-uh)

labia minora (**lā**-bē-uh muh-**nor**-uh)

labor (**lā**-bur)

lactogenesis (lak-tō-**jen**-uh-sis)

laparohysterectomy (lap-uh-rō-his-tuh-**rek**-tuh-mē)

laparorrhaphy (lap-uh-**ror**-uh-fē)

laparoscope (**lap**-uh-rō-skōp)

laparoscopic oophorectomy (lap-uh-rō-**skop**-ik ō-of-uh-**rek**-tuh-mē)

laparoscopy (lap-uh-**ros**-kuh-pē)

laparotomy (lap-uh-**rot**-uh-mē)

leiomyoma (lī-ō-mī-**ō**-muh)

leukorrhea (lōō-kō-**rē**-uh)

luteinizing hormone (**lōō**-tē-in-ī-zing **hor**-mōn)

male condom (māl **kon**-dum)

menarche (muh-**nahr**-kē)

menopause (**men**-ō-pawz)

menorrhagia (men-uh-**rā**-juh)

menorrhea (men-uh-**rē**-uh)

menses (**men**-sēz)

menstrual cycle (**men**-strōō-ul **sī**-kul)

menstruation (men-strōō-**ā**-shun)

metritis (muh-**trī**-tis)

metrorrhagia (mē-trō-**rā**-juh)

mittelschmerz (**mit**-ul-shmertz)

Monilia (mō-**nil**-ē-uh)

moniliasis (mon-i-**lī**-uh-sis)

mons pubis (monz **pū**-bis)

multigravida (mul-tē-**grav**-i-duh)

multipara (mul-**tip**-uh-ruh)

myometritis (mī-ō-muh-**trī**-tis)

myometrium (mī-ō-**mē**-trē-um)

natural family planning methods (**nach**-uh-rul **fam**-i-lē **plan**-ing **meth**-udz)

neonatal (nē-ō-**nā**-tul)

neonate (**nē**-ō-nāt)

neonatologist (nē-ō-nā-**tol**-uh-jist)

neonatology (nē-ō-nā-**tol**-uh-jē)

neurosyphilis (noor-ō-**sif**-i-lis)

nongonococcal urethritis (non-gon-ō-**kok**-ul ū-ruh-**thrī**-tis)

nullipara (nuh-**lip**-uh-ruh)

obstetrician (ob-stuh-**tri**-shun)

obstetrics (ob-**stet**-riks)

oligospermia (ol-i-gō-**spur**-mē-uh)

ooblast (**ō**-ō-blast)

oogenesis (ō-ō-**jen**-uh-sis)

oophoralgia (ō-of-ur-**al**-juh)

oophorectomy (ō-of-uh-**rek**-tuh-mē)

oophoritis (ō-of-uh-**rī**-tis)

oophorohysterectomy (ō-of-uh-rō-his-tur-**ek**-tuh-mē)

oophoropathy (ō-of-uh-**rop**-uh-thē)

oophoropexy (ō-**of**-uh-rō-pek-sē)

oophorosalpingectomy (ō-of-uh-rō-sal-pin-**jek**-tuh-mē)

oophorosalpingitis (ō-of-uh-rō-sal-pin-**jī**-tis)

oral contraceptive (**or**-ul kon-truh-**sep**-tiv)

orchialgia (or-kē-**al**-juh)

orchidalgia (or-ki-**dal**-juh)

orchiditis (or-ki-**dī**-tis)

orchidopexy (**or**-ki-dō-pek-sē)

orchiectomy (or-kē-**ek**-tuh-mē)

orchiepididymitis (or-kē-ep-i-did-i-**mī**-tis)

orchiopathy (or-kē-**op**-uh-thē)

orchiopexy (**or**-kē-ō-pek-sē)

orchioplasty (**or**-kē-ō-plas-tē)

orchiorrhaphy (or-kē-**or**-uh-fē)

orchiotomy (or-kē-**ot**-uh-mē)

orchitis (or-**kī**-tis)

ova (**ō**-vuh)

ovarian (ō-**var**-ē-un)

ovarian cancer (ō-**var**-ē-un **kan**-sur)

ovarian cyst (ō-**var**-ē-un sist)

ovarian cystectomy (ō-**var**-ē-un sis-**tek**-tuh-mē)

ovary (**ō**-vuh-rē)

ovulation (ov-ū-**lā**-shun)

ovulation method (ov-ū-**lā**-shun **meth**-ud)

ovulation stimulants (ov-ū-**lā**-shun **stim**-ū-lunts)

ovum (**ō**-vum)

oxytocics (ok-sē-**tō**-siks)

oxytocin (ok-sē-**tō**-sin)
Pap smear (pap smēr)
Papanicolaou test (pap-uh-**nik**-ō-lā-o̅o̅ test)
paraurethral gland (par-uh-ū-**rē**-thrul gland)
parity (**par**-i-tē)
parous (**par**-us)
parturition (pahr-tū-**ri**-shun)
pelvic exenteration (**pel**-vik ek-sen-tur-**ā**-shun)
pelvic inflammatory disease (**pel**-vik in-**flam**-uh-tor-ē di-**zēz**)
pelvimetry (pel-**vim**-uh-trē)
penile (**pē**-nīl)
penile prosthesis (**pē**-nīl pros-**thē**-sis)
penis (**pē**-nis)
perimetrium (per-i-**mē**-trē-um)
perineal (per-i-**nē**-ul)
perineum (per-i-**nē**-um)
phimosis (fī-**mō**-sis)
placenta (pluh-**sen**-tuh)
placenta previa (pluh-**sen**-tuh **prē**-vē-uh)
placental stage (pluh-**sen**-tul stāj)
polycystic ovary syndrome (pol-ē-**sis**-tik **ō**-vuh-rē **sin**-drōm)
postcoital contraceptive (pōst-**koi**-tul kon-truh-**sep**-tiv)
postnatal (pōst-**nā**-tul)
postpartum (pōst-**pahr**-tum)
preeclampsia (prē-ē-**klamp**-sē-uh)
pregnancy (**preg**-nun-sē)
premenstrual syndrome (prē-**men**-stro̅o̅-ul **sin**-drōm)
prenatal (prē-**nā**-tul)
prepuce (**prē**-pūs)
preterm (prē-**term**)
primigravida (prī-mi-**grav**-i-duh)
primipara (prī-**mip**-uh-ruh)
progestins (prō-**jes**-tinz)
progesterone (prō-**jes**-tuh-rōn)
prostate (**pros**-tāt)
prostate-specific antigen (**pros**-tāt spuh-**sif**-ik **an**-ti-jun)
prostatectomy (pros-tuh-**tek**-tuh-mē)
prostatic (pros-**tat**-ik)
prostatic carcinoma (pros-**tat**-ik kahr-si-**nō**-muh)
prostatitis (pros-tuh-**tī**-tis)
proteinuria (prō-tē-**nū**-rē-uh)
pseudocyesis (so̅o̅-dō-sī-**ē**-sis)
pseudopregnancy (so̅o̅-dō-**preg**-nun-sē)
puberty (**pū**-bur-tē)
pubic lice (**pū**-bik līs)
puerpera (pū-**ur**-per-uh)
quadripara (kwod-**rip**-uh-ruh)
quickening (**kwik**-un-ing)
radical hysterectomy (**rad**-i-kul his-tur-**ek**-tuh-mē)
rapid plasma reagin test (**rap**-id **plaz**-muh **rē**-uh-jin test)
rectocele (**rek**-tō-sēl)
rectovaginal (rek-tō-**vaj**-i-nul)
respiratory distress syndrome (**res**-pur-uh-tor-ē dis-**tres** **sin**-drōm)
retroflexion (ret-rō-**flek**-shun)
retroversion (ret-rō-**vur**-zhun)
salpingectomy (sal-pin-**jek**-tuh-mē)

salpingitis (sal-pin-**jī**-tis)
salpingocele (sal-**ping**-gō-sēl)
salpingo-oophorectomy (sal-ping-gō-ō-of-uh-**rek**-tuh-mē)
salpingopexy (sal-**ping**-gō-pek-sē)
salpingorrhaphy (sal-ping-**gor**-uh-fē)
salpingostomy (sal-ping-**gos**-tuh-mē)
scrotal (**skrōt**-ul)
scrotum (**skrō**-tum)
secundipara (sē-kun-**dip**-uh-ruh)
semen (**sē**-mun)
seminal (**sem**-i-nul)
seminal vesicles (**sem**-i-nul **ves**-i-kulz)
seminiferous tubule (sem-i-**nif**-ur-us **to̅o̅**-būl)
shoulder presentation (**shōl**-dur prē-zun-**tā**-shun)
spermatic (spur-**mat**-ik)
spermatoblast (**spur**-muh-tō-blast)
spermatocele (**spur**-muh-tō-sēl)
spermatogenesis (spur-muh-tō-**jen**-uh-sis)
spermatozoa (spur-muh-tō-**zō**-uh)
spermatozoon (spur-muh-tō-**zō**-on)
spina bifida (**spī**-nuh **bif**-i-duh)
spirochete (**spī**-rō-kēt)
sponge (spunj)
stillbirth (**stil**-birth)
subdermal implant (sub-**dur**-mul **im**-plant)
symptothermal method (simp-tō-**thur**-mul **meth**-ud)
syphilis (**sif**-i-lis)
tertipara (tur-**tip**-uh-ruh)
testalgia (tes-**tal**-juh)
testicular (tes-**tik**-ū-lur)
testicular cancer (tes-**tik**-ū-lur **kan**-sur)
testicular torsion (tes-**tik**-ū-lur **tor**-shun)
testis (**tes**-tis)
testosterone (tes-**tos**-tuh-rōn)
tocolytics (tō-kō-**lit**-ics)
toxic shock syndrome (**tok**-sik shok **sin**-drōm)
transurethral microwave thermotherapy (trans-ū-**rē**-thrul **mī**-krō-wāv thur-mō-**ther**-uh-pē)
transurethral needle ablation (trans-ū-**rē**-thrul **nē**-dul ab-**lā**-shun)
transurethral resection prostatectomy (trans-ū-**rē**-thrul rē-**sek**-shun pros-tuh-**tek**-tuh-mē)
transverse presentation (trans-**vurs** prē-zun-**tā**-shun)
Trichomonas (trik-ō-**mō**-nus)
trichomoniasis (trik-ō-mō-**nī**-uh-sis)
trimester (trī-**mes**-tur)
tripara (**trip**-uh-ruh)
tubal ligation (**to̅o̅**-bul lī-**gā**-shun)
tubal ligation reversal (**to̅o̅**-bul lī-**gā**-shun rē-**vers**-ul)
urethra (ū-**rē**-thruh)
urethral discharge (ū-**rē**-thrul **dis**-chahrj)
urethrovaginal (ū-rē-thrō-**vaj**-i-nul)
urogenital (ū-rō-**jen**-i-tul)
uterine (**ū**-tur-in)
uterine cancer (**ū**-tur-in **kan**-sur)
uterine displacement (**ū**-tur-in dis-**plās**-munt)
uterine fibroid (**ū**-tur-in **fī**-broid)

uterine tube (**ū**-tur-in tōōb)
uterus (**ū**-tur-us)
vagina (vuh-**jī**-nuh)
vaginal (**vaj**-i-nul)
vaginal contraceptive ring (**vaj**-i-nul kon-truh-**sep**-tiv ring)
vaginal hysterectomy (**vaj**-i-nul his-tur-**ek**-tuh-mē)
vaginal speculum (**vaj**-i-nul **spek**-ū-lum)
vaginal spermicide (**vaj**-i-nul **spur**-mi-sīd)
vaginectomy (vaj-i-**nek**-tuh-mē)
vaginitis (vaj-i-**nī**-tis)
varicocele (**var**-i-kō-sēl)
vas deferens (vas **def**-ur-enz)
vasectomy (vuh-**sek**-tuh-mē)
vasostomy (vā-**zos**, vas-**os**-tuh-mē)
vasotomy (vā-**zot**-uh-mē)

vasovasostomy (vā-zō, vas-ō-vā-**zos**-tuh-mē)
venereal diseases (vuh-**nēr**-ē-ul di-**zēz**-uz)
vesicovaginal (ves-i-kō-**vaj**-i-nul)
vestibular glands (ves-**tib**-ū-lur glandz)
vestibule (**ves**-ti-būl)
viable offspring (**vī**-uh-bul **of**-spring)
viral hepatitis (**vī**-rul hep-uh-**tī**-tis)
visceral peritoneum (**vis**-ur-ul per-i-tō-**nē**-um)
vulva (**vul**-vuh)
vulval (**vul**-vul)
vulvar (**vul**-vur)
vulvectomy (vul-**vek**-tuh-mē)
vulvitis (vul-**vī**-tis)
vulvovaginitis (vul-vō-vaj-i-**nī**-tis)
zygote (**zī**-gōt)

Español ENHANCING SPANISH COMMUNICATION

English	Spanish (Pronunciation)
birth	nacimiento (nah-se-me-EN-to)
childbirth	parto (PAR-to)
circumcision	circuncisión (ser-koon-se-se-ON)
conception	concepción (kon-sep-se-ON)
condom	condón (kon-DON)
contraception	contracepción (kon-trah-sep-se-ON)
cream	crema (KRAY-mah)
diaphragm	diafragma (de-ah-FRAHG-mah)
erection	erección (ay-rek-se-ON)
feminine	femenina (fay-may-NEE-na)
fetus	feto (FAY-to)
foam	espuma (es-POO-mah)
hormone	hormona (or-MOH-nah)
impotency	impotencia (im-po-TEN-se-ah)
intercourse, sexual	cópula (KO-poo-lah)
masculine	masculino (mas-koo-LEE-no)
menopause	menopausia (may-no-PAH-oo-se-ah)
menstruation	menstruación (mens-troo-ah-se-ON)
newborn	recién nacida (ray-se-EN nah-SEE-dah)
ovarian	ovárico (o-VAH-re-ko)
ovary	ovario (o-VAH-re-o)
parturition	parto (PAR-to)
penis	pene (PAY-nay)
pregnancy	embarazo (em-bah-RAH-so)
pregnant	embarazada (em-bah-rah-SAH-dah)
prostate	próstata (PROS-tah-tah)
prostatic	prostático (pros-TAH-te-ko)
prostatitis	prostatitis (pros-ta-TEE-tis)
reproduction	reproducción (ray-pro-dook-se-ON)
rhythm method	método de ritmo (MAY-to-do day REET-mo)
sexual	sexual (sek-soo-AHL)
testicle	testículo (tes-TEE-koo-lo)
uterus	útero (OO-tay-ro)
vagina	vagina (vah-HEE-nah)

CHAPTER 9

Musculoskeletal System

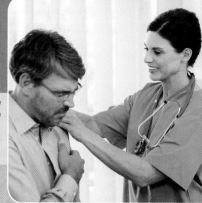

Orthopedics, a branch of surgery, specializes in the prevention and correction of deformities, disorders, or injury of the skeleton and associated structures, such as tendons and ligaments. Some orthopedists specialize in specific parts of the anatomy or certain diseases (back and spine, joint replacement, and sports medicine, for example).

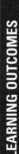

CONTENTS

LEARNING OUTCOMES

Basic Understanding

In this chapter, you will learn to do the following:

1. State the function of the musculoskeletal system, and analyze associated terms.
2. Write the meanings of the word parts associated with the musculoskeletal system, and use them to build and analyze terms.
3. Label the major bones of the body, and match them with their common names.
4. Name four major types of connective tissue of the musculoskeletal system.
5. List the three types of muscle tissue, and describe their functions.
6. Write the names of the diagnostic tests and procedures for assessment of the musculoskeletal system when given their descriptions, or match the procedures with their descriptions.
7. Write the names of musculoskeletal pathologies when given their descriptions, or match the pathologies with their descriptions.
8. Match surgical and therapeutic interventions with their descriptions, or write the names of the interventions when given their descriptions.
9. Build terms from word parts to label illustrations.

Greater Comprehension

10. Use word parts from this chapter to determine the meanings of terms in a health care report.
11. Spell the terms accurately.
12. Pronounce the terms correctly.
13. Write the meanings of the abbreviations.
14. Categorize terms as anatomy, diagnostic test or procedure, pathology, surgery, or nonsurgical therapy.
15. Recognize the meanings of general pharmacological terms from this chapter as well as the drug classes and their uses.

FUNCTION FIRST

The 206 named bones in the adult body are the body's skeleton, which changes through life with bone formation and bone destruction. The most widely known function of the skeletal system is that of support, providing form and shape for the body. Additional functions are protection of soft body parts, movement, blood cell formation, and storage. Bones provide a place for muscles and supporting structures to attach. Muscles function in the movement of body parts by contraction and relaxation of muscle fibers.

ANATOMY AND PHYSIOLOGY

muscles

9-1 Bones, as well as muscles, function in the movement of body parts, protected by a cushion of fat (Fig. 9.1). **Musculo/skeletal** means pertaining to the _____ and the skeleton. Because of the close association of the body's skeleton and muscles, the two systems are often referred to as one, such as in musculoskeletal disorders. Cells of the musculoskeletal system are derived from stem cells that mature and then begin to function as bone cells, muscle cells, and so on. This is not unlike cells of other body systems.

Characteristics of Bone

yellow

9-2 **Bone marrow** is the soft tissue that fills the cavities of the bones (Fig. 9.2). Red bone marrow functions in the formation of red blood cells, white blood cells, and platelets. In addition, bones store and release minerals, especially calcium, and are essential parts of mineral balance in the body. Fat is stored in the yellow bone marrow. The two types of bone marrow are red and _____ marrow.

9-3 The intercellular substance of bone contains an abundance of mineral salts, primarily calcium phosphate and calcium carbonate, which gives bone its unique hardness. Most of the calcium in our bodies is stored in the skeleton. The endocrine system controls the release of calcium from the bone when the level of _____ in the blood is decreased.

calcium

9-4 The chief characteristic of bone is its rigid nature, but it is important to remember that bone contains living cells and is richly supplied with blood vessels and nerves. Like other body tissues, bone requires oxygen and nutrients and produces wastes, the end products of metabolism.

🔑 **KEY** POINT **Bones may be classified as long, short, flat, or irregular.** Examples of long bones are those in the arm, leg, and thigh. Bones of the wrist are examples of short bones. Most of the bones of the skull are flat bones, and bones of the spine are classified as irregular bones. The general features of a long bone are shown in Fig. 9.3. The drawing shows that some parts of bone are hard and compact (compact bone), whereas other parts are spongy (spongy bone).

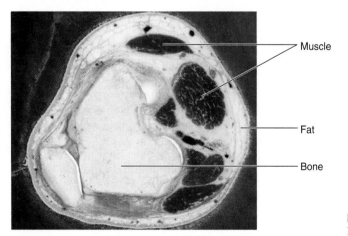

Figure 9.1 Digitized photograph of the upper arm in transverse section.
Bone, muscle, and fat identified.

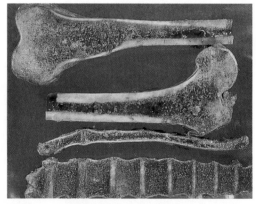

Figure 9.2 The interior appearance of bones, split to reveal marrow.
Note the red coloration of these bones, due to hemoglobin of red blood cells within the marrow. Note the width of the bones (from top to bottom), which are a lower leg bone, thigh bone, rib, and spinal bones.

compact

Does compact or spongy bony tissue serve as protection and support? _____

Os (plural, ossa) is used to write the formal names of bones. For example, os nasale refers to a bone of the nose. Be careful because os sometimes means an orifice (opening), an entrance, or outlet of a body cavity.

diaphysis

9-5 Answer these questions as you look at Fig. 9.3. The long shaft of the long bone is called the _____. This long shaft is thick, compact bone that surrounds yellow marrow in adults.

epiphysis

At each end of the diaphysis, there is an expanded portion called the _____.

The **epiphysis** is spongy bone that is covered by a thin layer of compact bone. The two ends are covered by articular cartilage to provide smooth surfaces for movement of the joints. Except in the areas where there is articular cartilage, the bone is covered with a tough membrane called **periosteum.** Analyzing the word parts of peri/ost/eum will help you remember its meaning. The

bone

prefix peri- means around, oste(o) means _____, and -ium means membrane. (In writing periosteum, an "i" is omitted to facilitate pronunciation.)

9-6 Locate the four types of bone tissue in Fig. 9.3.
- periosteum: Fibrous tissue that covers the bone
- compact bone: Lies just beneath the periosteum and has a system of small canals **(haversian canals)** that run parallel to the bone's long axis and contain blood vessels (see Fig. 9.3, B); canals are surrounded by concentric rings characteristic of mature bone
- spongy bone: Lighter than compact bone and contains large spongy meshworks called **trabeculae;** found largely in the epiphyses (plural form of epiphysis) and inner portions of long bones and is filled with red and yellow marrow
- yellow marrow: Found in the **medullary cavity**

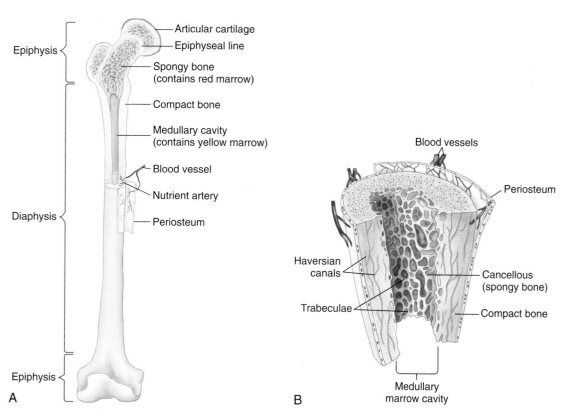

Figure 9.3 Typical long bone, partially sectioned. A, Major features of a long bone. The outer part is compact, dense bone. The inner part is spongy and contains large spaces filled with bone marrow. The epiphyseal line indicates a mature long bone. The line, once a cartilaginous epiphyseal plate, was responsible for increasing the length of the bone. However, around the end of puberty, cells stop duplicating. **B,** Cross-section of bone.

Learn the following word parts.

General Word Parts for Describing Bone

Word Part	Meaning
blast(o), -blast	embryonic form
myel(o)	bone marrow or spinal cord
osse(o)	bone or bony element
oste(o)	bone

Match combining forms with their meanings in the right column.

_____ **1.** blast(o)   **A.** bone

_____ **2.** myel(o)   **B.** bone marrow (sometimes the spinal cord)

_____ **3.** oste(o)   **C.** embryonic form

9-7 Calcium in bone is radiopaque; thus bones can obstruct x-rays so that they do not reach image receptors. Bones are represented by white areas in an x-ray image (Fig. 9.4). Unimpeded x-rays expose image receptors and cause a black or dark area in the image.

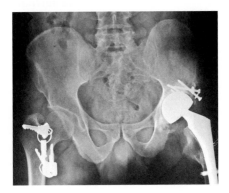

Figure 9.4 X-ray image of the pelvis. Keys were left in the pocket of a lightweight hospital robe during the examination, so radiography had to be repeated. Note also the metal fixation devices in the hip. Metal objects are radiopaque. Bones appear *white,* and soft tissue appears *gray.*

calcium

9-8 Calci/fication is the process by which organic tissue becomes hardened by deposit of what substance in tissue? _____

Normally calcium is deposited in bone in large amounts to give bone its hardness. Calcification in soft tissue is abnormal.

Draw a slash between the word parts in the following list of new terms. Then find the meanings of the word parts within the definitions. (Draw the slash, and then perform the remainder of the activity as a mental exercise.)

1. **myeloblast** embryonic bone marrow cell; myeloblasts mature into **myelocytes,** which mature into leukocytes normally found in blood

2. **osteoblast** an embryonic or early form of bone cell that develops into a mature bone cell

3. **osteocyte** mature bone cells that become embedded in the calcified intercellular substance of bone

4. **osteogenesis** or the formation of bone substance; same as **ossification.** Human embryos contain no bone but do contain cartilage, which is a more flexible tissue that is shaped like bone; ossification begins at the start of the fetal period (after the eighth week).

WRITE IT! EXERCISE 3

Write a word in each blank to complete these sentences.
1. The soft tissue that fills the cavities of the bones is bone _____.
2. The long shaft of a long bone is called the *diaphysis,* and the expanded portions at the ends are called the _____.
3. Most of the bone is covered with a tough membrane called _____.
4. An osteoblast is an embryonic form of a/an _____ cell.
5. A term that means pertaining to the muscles and the skeleton is _____.
6. Osteogenesis is also called _____.

Bones of the Skeleton

skeleton

WORD ORIGIN
skeletos (G.), skeleton
a dried body or a mummy

9-9 The human skeleton is the bony framework of the body. **Skeletal** means pertaining to the _____.

The skeletal system consists of the bones and the cartilages, ligaments, and tendons that are associated with the bones. Bones and muscles work together to enable us to bend our arms and legs, turn our heads, and perform other voluntary movements.

9-10 Although the adult human skeleton usually consists of 206 named bones, there are also a few others that vary in number from one individual to another, so they are not counted with the other 206 bones. The major bones are identified in Fig. 9.5. Study the names of the bones and their locations.

Note that the skeleton is divided into the axial skeleton and the appendicular skeleton. The division of the skeleton that forms the vertical axis of the body is the **axial skeleton.** The free appendages and their attachments are called the _____ **skeleton.**

appendicular

WRITE IT! EXERCISE 4

Write a word in each blank to complete these sentences.
1. The bony framework of the body is the _____.
2. A term that means pertaining to the skeleton is _____.
3. The division of the skeleton that forms the vertical axis of the body is the _____ skeleton.
4. Bones of the extremities and their attachments to the axial skeleton are called the _____ skeleton.

Axial Skeleton

axial

9-11 The skull, spinal column, sternum, and ribs make up the _____ skeleton.
It consists of 80 major bones. These bones form the vertical axis to which the appendicular skeleton attaches. Learn the word parts associated with bones of the axial skeleton.

Word Parts: Bones of the Axial Skeleton

Combining Form	Bone(s)	Common Name
cost(o)	costae	ribs
crani(o)	cranium	skull
rach(i), rachi(o), spin(o)	vertebral or spinal column	spine (backbone)
spondyl(o), vertebr(o)	vertebrae	bones of the spine
stern(o)	sternum	breastbone

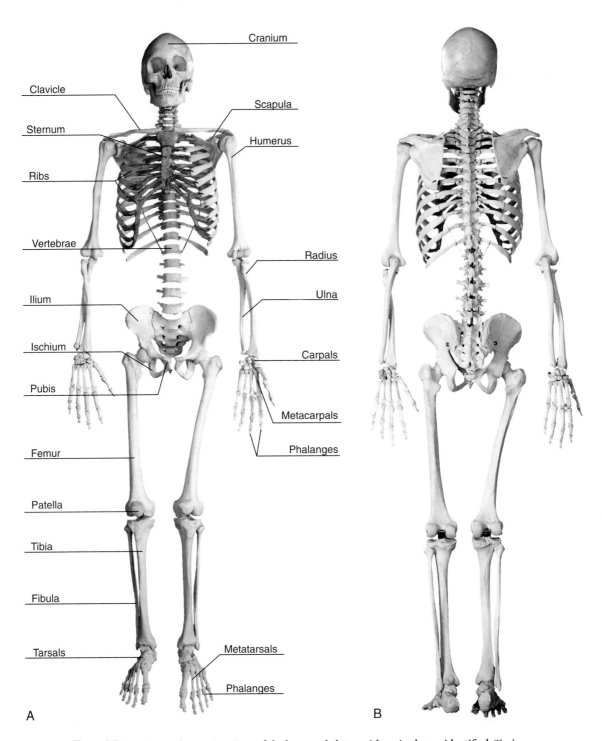

Cranium

Clavicle

Sternum

Ribs

Vertebrae

Ilium

Ischium

Pubis

Femur

Patella

Tibia

Fibula

Tarsals

Scapula

Humerus

Radius

Ulna

Carpals

Metacarpals

Phalanges

Metatarsals

Phalanges

A

B

Figure 9.5 Anterior and posterior views of the human skeleton with major bones identified. The bones are grouped in two divisions: The axial skeleton forms the vertical axis of the body and is shown here in *blue*. The appendicular skeleton includes the free appendages and their attachments and is shown as *bone colored*.

skull
WORD ORIGIN
facial *(L.)*
facialis, from; *facies,* face
ossicle *(L.)*
ossicle, little bone

9-12 The **cranium** serves as protection for the brain and forms the framework of the face. The common name for the cranium is the _____. It is composed of three types of bones: cranial bones; facial bones; and the six **auditory ossicles,** three tiny bones in each middle ear cavity (Fig. 9.6).

The bones that make up the skull are listed in Table 9.1. The opening at the base of the skull through which the spinal cord passes is called the **foramen magnum,** whose literal translation from Latin means large hole.

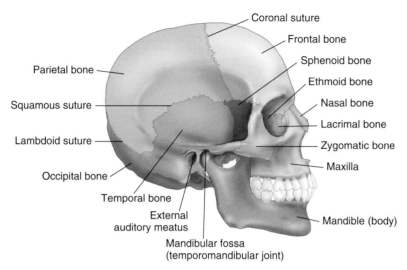

Figure 9.6 Major bones of the skull, lateral view. The cranium, that portion of the skull that encloses the brain, is composed of eight cranial bones (parietal, temporal, frontal, occipital, ethmoid, and sphenoid.) Sutures are immovable fibrous joints between many of the cranial bones. The 14 facial bones (not all are shown) form the basic framework and shape of the face. The auditory ossicles (not shown) are three tiny bones in each middle ear cavity. The external auditory meatus is the external opening of the ear.

Table 9.1   Named Bones of the Skull*

Cranial Bones		Facial Bones		Auditory Ossicles
Parietal (2)	Occipital (1)	Maxilla (2)	Palatine (2)	Malleus (2)
Temporal (2)	Ethmoid (1)	Zygomatic (2)	Inferior nasal concha (2)	Incus (2)
Frontal (1)	Sphenoid (1)	Mandible (1)	Lacrimal (2)	Stapes (2)
		Nasal (2)	Vomer (1)	

*Numbers represent the number of each bone.

You learned that crani(o) means cranium or skull. The cranium is the major portion of the skull, that which encloses and protects the brain. Write a word that means pertaining to the skull:

cranial

_____.

> **BEYOND** THE BLUEPRINT   The adult skull is made up of hard bones that serve as protection; however, newborns have "soft spots" called the *fontanels,* which are spaces covered by tough membranes between the soft bones of the skull (Fig. 9.7). These accommodate passage through the birth canal and allow for growth of the brain.

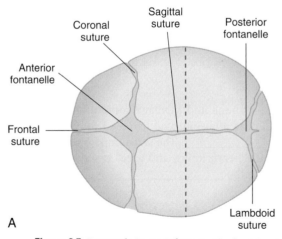

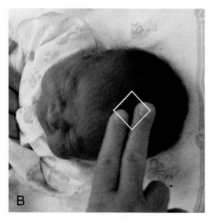

Figure 9.7 Fontanels in an infant. A, The frontal and posterior fontanels are located between soft cranial bones. Ossification of the sutures begins after completion of brain growth, at about 6 years of age, and is finished by adulthood at which time the sutures have become immovable joints. **B,** Demonstration of the anterior fontanelle of an infant.

WRITE IT! EXERCISE 5

Write a word in each blank to complete these sentences.

1. The axial skeleton is composed of the skull, the spinal column, the _____, and the ribs.

2. The combining form crani(o) means the _____ or the skull.

3. The combining form that means rib is _____.

4. The combining forms rach(i) and rachi(o) mean _____.

5. The combining form that means the breastbone is _____.

---

spine

9-13 The vertebral or spinal column is attached at the base of the skull. The **vertebral column** is commonly called the *backbone* or the _____, and it extends from the base of the skull to the pelvis. It encloses and protects the spinal cord, supports the head, and serves as a place of attachment for the ribs and muscles of the back.

spinal

The combining forms rach(i), rachi(o), and spin(o) mean spine. Combine spin(o) and -al to write a word that means pertaining to the spine: _____. Most medical terms pertaining to the spine use rach(i) and rachi(o), and the latter is more commonly used.

vertebrae

9-14 The vertebral column is composed of 26 **vertebrae**. Vertebrae is the plural form of **vertebra**. **Inter/vertebral** means between two adjoining _____. Cushions of cartilage between adjoining vertebrae are called **intervertebral disks**. These layers of cartilage absorb shock.

The vertebrae are named and numbered from the top downward (Fig. 9.8). Study the word parts for the types of vertebrae.

Types of Vertebrae (Uppermost to Lowermost)

Combining Form	Type of Vertebrae
cervic(o)	cervical vertebrae
thorac(o)	thoracic vertebrae
lumb(o)	lumbar vertebrae
sacr(o)	sacral vertebrae (fuse to form the **sacrum**)
coccyg(o)	coccygeal vertebrae (fuse to form the **coccyx**)

WRITE IT! EXERCISE 6

Write words to complete the blanks in the following sentences. Use Fig. 9.8, and count from above downward.

1. C1-C7 vertebrae in the area of the neck are _____ vertebrae.

2. T1-T12 vertebrae behind the chest cavity are _____ vertebrae.

3. L1-L5 vertebrae, which support the lower back, are _____ vertebrae.

4. S1-S5 vertebrae fused into the sacrum are _____ vertebrae.

5. The coccyx (tailbone) results from fusion of _____ vertebrae.

---

ribs

9-15 The combining form cost(o) means ribs. Another term for a rib is **costa,** and the plural is costae. **Inter/costal** is a term that means between the _____. Intercostal muscles lie between the ribs and draw adjacent ribs together to increase the volume of the thorax in breathing.

breastbone

9-16 Recall that the thorax is the cage of bone and cartilage containing the principal organs of respiration and circulation (Fig. 9.9). Locate the elongated flattened sternum. The common name of the **sternum** is the _____. The sternum is one of the bones that make up the thoracic cage, which protects the heart, lungs, and great vessels and also plays a role in breathing. **Thoracic** means pertaining to the _____.

thorax (chest)

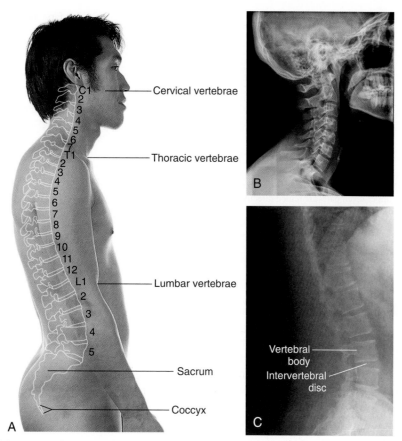

Figure 9.8 The vertebral column. A, The vertebrae are numbered from above downward. There are seven cervical vertebrae in the neck region, twelve thoracic vertebrae behind the chest cavity, five lumbar vertebrae supporting the lower back, five sacral vertebrae fused into one bone called the *sacrum*, and four coccygeal vertebrae fused into one bone called the *coccyx*. **B,** Lateral cervical spine x-ray. **C,** Thoraco-lumbar spine x-ray with vertebral body and intervertebral disk labeled.

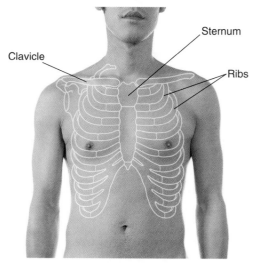

Figure 9.9 The thorax. The bones of the front part of the thorax are shown. The breastbone and ribs are part of the axial skeleton.

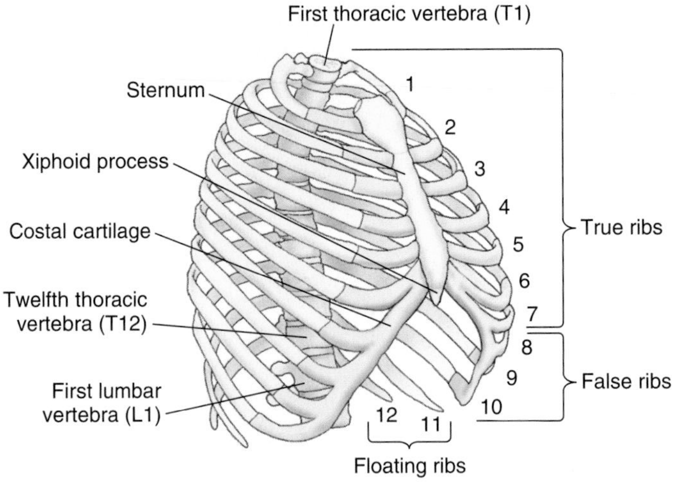

Figure 9.10 Anterolateral view of the thoracic cage. The ribs exist in pairs, twelve on each side of the chest, and are numbered from 1 to 12, beginning with the top rib. The upper seven pairs are joined directly with the sternum by a narrow strip of cartilage and are called *"true ribs."* The remaining five pairs are referred to as *"false ribs,"* because they do not attach directly to the sternum. The last two pairs of false ribs, the "floating ribs," are attached only on the posterior aspect.

9-17 Now view the sternum as part of the thoracic cage (Fig. 9.10). Attached to the sternum are the ribs that support the chest wall and protect the lungs and heart. The 12 pairs of ribs are numbered from the top rib, beginning with 1. The first seven ribs on each side join directly with the sternum by a strip of cartilage and are called _____ ribs.

true

Also note the **xiphoid process,** the smallest and lowermost part of the sternum, which is often used as a point of reference when examining the chest.

FIND IT!   **EXERCISE 7**

Draw a slash between the word parts in the following list of new terms. Then find the meanings of the word parts within the definitions. (Draw the slash, and then perform the remainder of the activity as a mental exercise.)

1. **costal** pertaining to the ribs
2. **infracostal** situated beneath a rib or all the ribs; same as **subcostal**
3. **infrasternal** beneath the sternum; **substernal**
4. **intrasternal** within the sternum
5. **retrosternal** situated or occurring behind the sternum
6. **sternal** pertaining to the sternum
7. **sternocostal** pertaining to the sternum and the ribs

8. **supracostal** situated above or upon a rib
9. **suprasternal** situated above the sternum
10. **thoracolumbar** pertaining to the thoracic and lumbar vertebrae
11. **vertebrocostal** pertaining to a vertebra and a rib; same as **costovertebral**
12. **vertebrosternal** pertaining to the vertebrae and the sternum; same as **sternovertebral**

BUILD IT!   **EXERCISE 8**

Use the following word parts to build terms. (Some word parts will be used more than once.)

infra-, inter-, supra-, cost(o), crani(o), lumb(o), stern(o), thorac(o), vertebr(o), -al, -ar

1. pertaining to the chest and the lower back   _____ / _____ / _____
2. pertaining to the skull   _____ / _____
3. pertaining to above a rib   _____ / _____ / _____
4. pertaining to beneath the breastbone   _____ / _____ / _____
5. between two adjoining spinal bones   _____ / _____ / _____

Appendicular Skeleton

appendicular

9-18 Bones of the extremities, the shoulder girdle, and the pelvic girdle comprise the appendicular skeleton. In other words, the appendicular skeleton includes the bones of the limbs and their attachments to the axial skeleton. The **shoulder girdle** includes the clavicle and the scapula, and the **pelvic girdle** includes the bones of the pelvis. The major division of the skeleton that attaches to the axial skeleton is called the _____ skeleton.

Learn the following word parts for the names of the bones of the appendicular skeleton.

Word Parts: Bones of the Appendicular Skeleton

Combining Form	Bone	Common Name	Combining Form	Bone	Common Name
clavicul(o)	clavicle	collarbone	**Bones of the Pelvic Girdle†**		
scapul(o)	scapula	shoulder blade	ili(o)	ilium	
Bones of the Lower Extremities			ischi(o)	ischium	
calcane(o)	calcaneus	heel bone	pub(o)	pubis	
femor(o)	femur	thigh bone	**Bones of the Upper Extremities**		
fibul(o)	fibula	calf bone	carp(o)	carpus	wrist
metatars(o)	metatarsals	bones of the feet	humer(o)	humerus	upper arm bone
patell(o)	patella	kneecap	metacarp(o)	metacarpals	bones of the hands
phalang(o)	phalanx*	toe	phalang(o)	phalanx*	finger
tars(o)	tarsus (sometimes edge of eyelid)	ankle	radi(o)	radius (or radiant energy)	bone of the forearm
tibi(o)	tibia	shin bone	uln(o)	ulna	bone of the forearm

*Plural, phalanges.
†These bones fuse to form the pelvic bone.

> **BEYOND** THE BLUEPRINT Note that the spelling of humerus is different from humorous, which means funny. A point near the lower end of the humerus is known as the *funny bone*, because if accidentally hit, a tingling sensation results.

WRITE IT! EXERCISE 9

Write a combining form for each of the following bones of the appendicular skeleton.

1. ankle _____
2. calf bone _____
3. collarbone _____
4. fingers or toes _____
5. heel bone _____
6. kneecap _____
7. shin bone _____
8. shoulder blade _____
9. thigh bone _____
10. upper arm bone _____
11. wrist _____

collarbone

9-19 The shoulder is the junction of the clavicle, scapula, and humerus (where the arm attaches to the trunk of the body). The **clavicle** is also known as the _____. The clavicles are long, curved horizontal bones that attach to the sternum and either the left or right scapula. The **scapula** is a large triangular bone that is commonly called the *shoulder blade*. Each scapula is joined to the **humerus,** the upper arm bone, by muscles and tendons. Locate these structures in Fig. 9.11.

> **BEYOND** THE BLUEPRINT The clavicle is the most frequently fractured bone in the body. Falling on the shoulder or an outstretched arm often transmits forces from the arm to the trunk and results in a fractured clavicle.

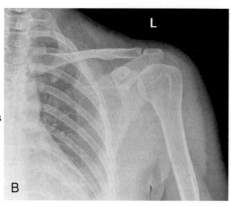

A   B

Figure 9.11 The shoulder. The posterior view of the shoulder shows the thin, flat, triangular scapula joining with the clavicle and humerus. **B,** Radiograph of shoulder. A complex of four muscles acts to provide stability while assisting with ROM.

FIND IT! **EXERCISE 10**

Draw a slash between the word parts in the following list of new terms. Then find the meanings of the word parts within the definitions. (Draw the slash, and then perform the remainder of the activity as a mental exercise.)

1. **costoclavicular** pertaining to or involving the ribs and the clavicle
2. **humeral** pertaining to the humerus
3. **humeroradial** pertaining to the humerus and the radius
4. **humeroscapular** pertaining to the humerus and the scapula
5. **humeroulnar** pertaining to the humerus and the ulna
6. **infraclavicular** below the clavicle

7. **infrascapular** below the scapula
8. **interscapular** between the two shoulder blades
9. **scapular** pertaining to the scapula
10. **scapuloclavicular** pertaining to the scapula and the clavicle
11. **sternoclavicular** pertaining to the sternum and the clavicle
12. **ulnoradial** pertaining to the ulna and the radius

---

forearm

carpus

carpals

next

carpal

fingers
phalanges

9-20 The **ulna** and the **radius** are bones of the _____.

The combining form carp(o) means the **carpus,** or wrist. Observe in Fig. 9.12 that the wrist consists of eight small bones, arranged in two transverse rows. **Carp/al** pertains to the _____. Bones of the wrist are called *carpals*. Therefore *carpals* is a word that means the same as carp/al bones. Bones of the hand also include **meta/carpals** and **phalanges**, which are bones of the fingers.

The wrist is composed of eight carpal bones, also called _____.

9-21 Many of the 126 bones that make up the appendicular skeleton are small and are found in the hands and feet, but several of the remaining bones in this part of the skeleton are the longest bones in the body. Bones of the appendicular skeleton are designed for movement.

The metacarpals connect the wrist bones (carpals) to the phalanges. You learned that meta- is a prefix that means a change or next, such as in a series. The meta/carpals lie _____ to the carpals. The five metacarpals constitute the palm. The proximal ends of the metacarpals join with the distal row of what type of bones?

_____

9-22 The distal ends of the metacarpals join with the phalanges. The combining form phalang(o) means phalanges. The phalanges are bones of the _____, as well as bones of the toes. **Carpo/phalang/eal** pertains to the carpus and the _____—in this case, the fingers.

See Fig. 9.12 to observe that there are three phalanges in each finger (a proximal, middle, and distal phalanx) except the thumb.

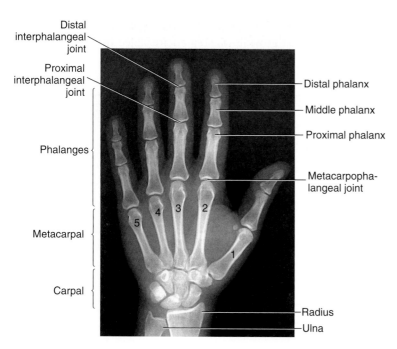

Figure 9.12 **Radiograph of the human hand, posteroanterior view.** The ulna and radius, as well as the bones of the hand, are identified. Eight small carpal bones make up the wrist. The palm of the hand contains five metacarpal bones, which are numbered 1 to 5 starting on the thumb side. There are three phalanges in each finger (a proximal, middle, and distal phalanx) except the thumb, which has two. The sesamoid bone is a small round bone embedded in the tendon that provides added strength for the thumb.

9-23 The pelvic girdle consists of two hipbones. Each of these bones consists of three separate bones in the newborn, but eventually the three fuse to form one bone. Names of the three bones are the ilium, the ischium, and the _____. Their combining forms are ili(o), ischi(o), and pub(o), respectively. The **ilium** is the largest of the three bones. The **ischium** is the posterior part of the pelvic girdle, and the **pubis** is the anterior part of the pelvic girdle. **Ili/ac, ischi/al,** and **pub/ic** mean pertaining to the ilium, the _____, and the pubis, respectively.

pubis

ischium

9-24 Locate these three bones that are fused to form each of the hipbones (Fig. 9.13). The hipbones join with the sacrum and coccyx to form the pelvis. Also compare the male pelvis with the female pelvis.

> **BEYOND** THE BLUEPRINT The size and shape of the female pelvis varies and is important in childbirth. It is generally less massive but wider and more circular than the male pelvis.

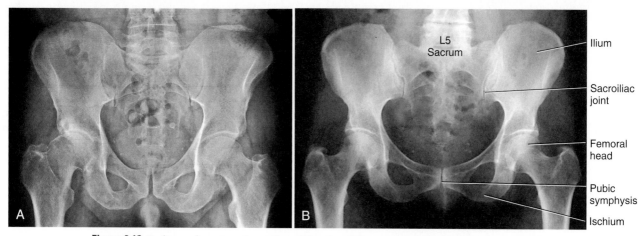

Figure 9.13 **Radiographs comparing male and female pelvis, anterior views. A,** Male pelvis. Bones of the male are generally larger and heavier. The pelvic outlet, the space surrounded by the lower pelvic bones, is heart shaped. **B,** Female pelvis. The pelvic outlet is larger and more oval than that of the male. L5 is the fifth lumbar vertebra. The pubic symphysis is the joint where the two pubic bones are joined.

The hairs growing over the pubic region are called **pubes.** This term is also used to denote the pubic region. The pubic region or the hairs that grow in this region are called the

pubes

_____.

The **pubic symphysis** is the **inter/pubic** joint where the two pubic bones meet.

FIND IT!   EXERCISE 11

Draw a slash between the word parts in the following list of new terms. Then find the meanings of the word parts within the definitions. (Draw the slash, and then perform the remainder of the activity as a mental exercise.)

1. **iliopubic** pertaining to the ilium and the pubis
2. **ischiococcygeal** pertaining to the ischium and the coccyx
3. **ischiopubic** pertaining to the ischium and the pubis
4. **subpubic** pertaining to a location beneath the pubis
5. **suprapubic** above the pubis

WRITE IT!   EXERCISE 12

1. List three bones that fuse to form the pelvic bone: _____; _____; _____
2. Write the names of the two bones of the forearm: _____; _____
3. Carpal means pertaining to the _____.
4. The shoulder girdle includes the clavicle and the _____.

ANALYZE IT!   EXERCISE 13

Break these words into their component parts by placing a slash between the word parts. Write the meaning of each term.

1. carpophalangeal _____
2. humeroscapular _____
3. interpubic _____
4. ulnoradial _____
5. metacarpal _____

9-25 The lower extremities, like the two upper extremities, are composed of 60 bones in the thigh, leg, foot, and the kneecap (or patella). The **femur,** or the thigh bone, is the longest and heaviest bone in the body (Fig. 9.14). The combining form femor(o) means femur. **Femor/al** pertains to

femur

the _____.

> **BEYOND** THE BLUEPRINT You've heard the expression of "breaking a hip." This expression refers to the femur, a weight-bearing bone; therefore, if it becomes weakened, as it sometimes does in older persons or those with osteoporosis, it cannot support the weight of the body, and the neck of the femur fractures. Many times it is more appropriate to say someone broke a hip and fell rather than fell and broke a hip.

9-26 The **patella,** or kneecap, is anterior to the knee joint. The lower leg is composed of two bones, the **tibia** and the **fibula.** The tibia, or shinbone, is the larger of the two bones. The combining form tibi(o) means tibia; the combining form fibul(o) means fibula.

fibula

Fibul/ar means pertaining to the _____.

9-27 The foot is composed of the ankle, instep, and toes. The ankle, or **tarsus,** consists of a group of seven short bones that resemble the bones of the wrist but are larger. The combining form tars(o) means the tarsus, or sometimes the edge of the eyelid.

Words used in the following frames refer to the ankle.

tarsus (or ankle)
tarsals

9-28 **Tars/al** means pertaining to the _____. The ankle is composed of seven tarsal bones called the _____. One of the tarsal bones is the **calcaneus,** or heel bone.

Bones of the feet are **metatarsals.** Like bones of the fingers, those of the toes are called *phalanges.*

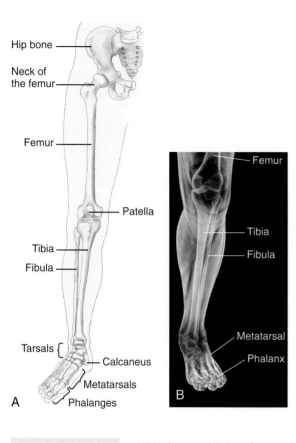

Figure 9.14 Lower extremity. A, Right lower extremity, anterior view. The lower extremity consists of the bones of the thigh, leg, foot, and patella. **B,** Colorized drawing of the left leg with joint areas in red.

calcaneus

9-29 The combining form calcane(o) refers to the calcaneus or heel bone. **Calcane/al** pertains to the calcaneus. **Calcaneo/plantar** pertains to the _____ and the sole. **Plantar** is a word that means concerning the sole.

distal

9-30 The bones between the tarsus and the toes are the metatarsals. Which end of the metatarsals joins with the toes? _____

phalang(o)

9-31 Bones of the toes are phalanges. Finger bones are also called _phalanges_. What is the combining form for phalanges? _____
There are two bones in the great toe and three in each of the lesser toes.

carpus (wrist)

Carpo/ped/al pertains to the _____ and the foot. A carpopedal spasm, for example, is involuntary contraction of the muscles of the hands and feet.

BUILD IT! EXERCISE 14

Use the following word parts to build terms. (Some word parts will be used more than once.)
carp(o), clavicul(o), femor(o), ili(o), ischi(o), phalang(o), pub(o), scapul(o), stern(o), -al, -ar, -eal, -ic
1. pertaining to the shoulder blade and the collarbone _____/_____/_____
2. pertaining to the wrist and fingers _____/_____/_____
3. pertaining to the ischium and the pubis _____/_____/_____
4. pertaining to the ilium and the thigh bone _____/_____/_____
5. pertaining to the sternum and the clavicle _____/_____/_____

FIND IT! EXERCISE 15

Draw a slash between the word parts in the following list of new terms. Then find the meanings of the word parts within the definitions. (Draw the slash, and then perform the remainder of the activity as a mental exercise.)
1. calcaneofibular pertaining to the calcaneus and the fibula
2. calcaneotibial pertaining to the calcaneus and tibia
3. iliofemoral pertaining to the ilium and the femur
4. infrapatellar below the patella
5. ischiofemoral pertaining to the ischium and the femur
6. patellofemoral pertaining to the patella and the femur
7. pubofemoral pertaining to the pubis and the femur

Joints, Tendons, and Ligaments

connective

9-32 Connective tissues, characterized by an abundance of intercellular material with relatively few cells, support and bind other body tissue and parts. Bone (the most rigid), cartilage, tendons, and ligaments are all connective tissues. Tissue that supports and binds other body tissue and parts is called _____ tissue.

🔑 **KEY** POINT A joint, or **articulation**, is a place of union between two or more bones. You are familiar with many joints—for example, the ankle, wrist, and knee. Joints are classified according to their structure and the amount of movement they allow. Types of joints and examples are immovable (sutures in the skull), slightly movable (joints that connect the ribs to the sternum), and freely movable (knee, shoulder, elbow).

Learn the following word parts for the joints, tendons, and ligaments.

Word Parts: Joints and Tendons

Combining Form	Meaning	Combining Form	Meaning
arthr(o), articul(o)	joint; articulation	synov(o), synovi(o)	synovial membrane
burs(o)	bursa	ten(o), tend(o), tendin(o)	tendon
chondr(o)	cartilage		

MATCH IT! EXERCISE 16

Match combining forms in the left column with descriptions in the right column.

_____ **1.** articul(o)   **A.** bursa

_____ **2.** burs(o)   **B.** cartilage

_____ **3.** chondr(o)   **C.** joint

_____ **4.** synovi(o)   **D.** synovial membrane

_____ **5.** ten(o)   **E.** tendon

joint

9-33 Articul/ar means pertaining to a _____. **Nonarticular** means not related to or involving the joints.

Most joints in the adult body are freely movable joints, which are also called **synovial joints.** The knee, the **tibio/femor/al** joint, is an example of a synovial joint. It is the body's largest joint. **Metatarsophalangeal joints** connect the toes with the metatarsals.

Articular cartilage covers the ends of the opposing bones in a synovial joint, and they are separated by a space called the *joint cavity* that is filled with synovial fluid for lubrication (Fig. 9.15). Synovial fluid is also called *synovia.*

🔑 **KEY** POINT Articular cartilage provides protection and support for the joints. Some joints also have pads and cushions that help stabilize the joint and act as shock absorbers. **Bursae** are fluid-filled sacs that help reduce friction. Note the location of the bursae in Fig. 9.15. Bursae are commonly located between the skin and underlying bone or between tendons and ligaments.

chondral

9-34 Embryos contain a great deal of translucent, elastic tissue that, for the most part, is transformed into bone as the embryo matures. This elastic tissue is **cartilage.** Not all cartilage becomes bone, as evidenced by cartilage found in several parts of the adult body, such as the nose and the ear. The combining form chondr(o) means cartilage. Use -al to write a term that means pertaining to cartilage: _____.

Chondr/oid means resembling cartilage. **Chondro/costal** means pertaining to the ribs and their associated cartilage. **Vertebro/chondral** means pertaining to a vertebra and the adjacent cartilage.

pertaining

9-35 Perichondrium is the membrane around the surface of cartilage. **Peri/chondrial** means _____ to or composed of perichondrium.

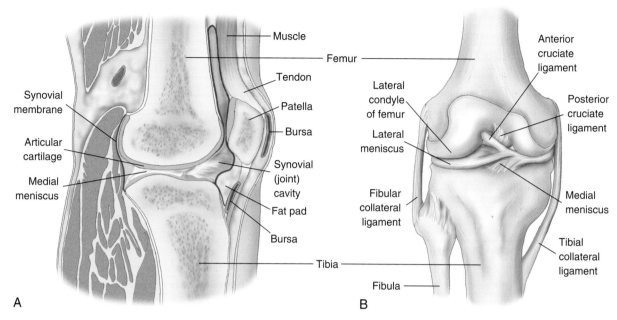

Figure 9.15 The knee joint. A, Lateral view, sagittal section. The hinged joint at the knee is a synovial joint. The ends of the opposing bones are covered by articular cartilage. The synovial membrane secretes synovial fluid into the joint cavity for lubrication. Menisci and bursae are special structures that act as protective cushions. **B,** Anterior view. Twelve ligaments, flexible bands of fibrous tissue, bind the structures of the knee to provide strength. Note how the anterior and posterior cruciate ligaments cross each other, a characteristic from which their name is derived (Latin: *crux*, cross; *ligare*, to bind).

9-36 The **temporomandibular joint** is one of a pair of joints connecting the mandible of the jaw to the temporal bone of the skull (Fig. 9.16). It is abbreviated TMJ.

9-37 Tendons are bands of strong, fibrous tissue that attach the muscles to the bones (Fig. 9.17). **Ligaments** connect bones or cartilage and serve to support and strengthen joints. What type of connective tissue attaches the muscles to the bones? _____

What type of connective tissue connects bones or cartilage? _____

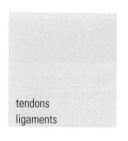

tendons
ligaments

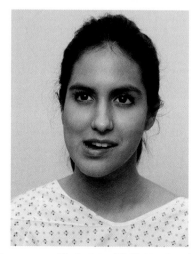

Figure 9.16 Temporomandibular joint (TMJ). TMJ lateral range of motion (ROM) is demonstrated.

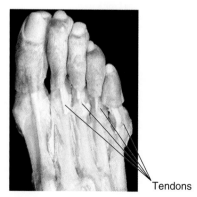

Figure 9.17 Tendons. Strong and flexible bands of dense fibrous connective tissue attach muscles to bones.

Write a word in each blank to complete these sentences.

1. Tissue that supports and binds other body tissue and parts is _____ tissue.

2. Another name for a joint is a/an _____.

3. Freely movable joints are filled with a fluid for lubrication and are called _____ joints.

4. Articular cartilage provides protection and support for the _____.

5. Fluid-filled sacs that help reduce friction in a joint are called _____.

6. Tissues that attach muscles to bones are _____.

7. Connective tissue that connects bones or cartilages and supports and strengthens joints is called a/an

   _____.

8. The membrane around the surface of cartilage is called the _____.

Muscles

embryonic

WORD ORIGIN
my(o) *(G.)*
myos, of muscle

9-38 A **myo/blast** is an _____ cell that develops into muscle fiber. Muscle is a type of tissue that is composed of fibers or cells that are able to contract, causing movement of body parts and organs. Before a skeletal muscle contracts, it receives an impulse from a nerve cell. The muscle exerts force on tendons, which in turn pull on bones, producing movement.

Hyper/tonicity of muscle is abnormally increased muscle tone or strength. **Hypo/tonicity** is diminished tone or tension in any body structure, such as in paralysis.

Word Parts: Muscle

Combining Form	Meaning	Combining Form	Meaning
fasci(o)	fascia	muscul(o), my(o)	muscle

muscle

9-39 Muscul/ar means pertaining to _____.

▶ **BEYOND** THE BLUEPRINT The muscular system is also closely associated with the nervous system, as indicated by the term *neuromuscular*, because a muscle fiber must first be stimulated by a nerve impulse before it can contract.

🔑 **KEY** POINT There are three types of muscle tissue in the body: skeletal, visceral, and cardiac. **Skeletal muscle,** with the primary function of movement of the body and its parts, is voluntarily controlled by the nervous system. **Visceral muscle,** which is located in the walls of organs and blood vessels, is involuntary and controlled by the autonomic nervous system as described in Chapter 10. **Cardiac muscle** is only located in the heart, is involuntary, and is also called **myocardium.** Characteristics of the three types of muscle tissues are shown in Fig. 9.18.

Nucleus of skeletal muscle cell —

Striations —

A   Skeletal muscle

Nucleus of smooth muscle cell —

B   Visceral muscle

Nucleus of cardiac muscle cell —

Striations —

C   Cardiac muscle

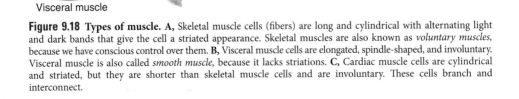

Figure 9.18 Types of muscle. A, Skeletal muscle cells (fibers) are long and cylindrical with alternating light and dark bands that give the cell a striated appearance. Skeletal muscles are also known as *voluntary muscles*, because we have conscious control over them. **B,** Visceral muscle cells are elongated, spindle-shaped, and involuntary. Visceral muscle is also called *smooth muscle*, because it lacks striations. **C,** Cardiac muscle cells are cylindrical and striated, but they are shorter than skeletal muscle cells and are involuntary. These cells branch and interconnect.

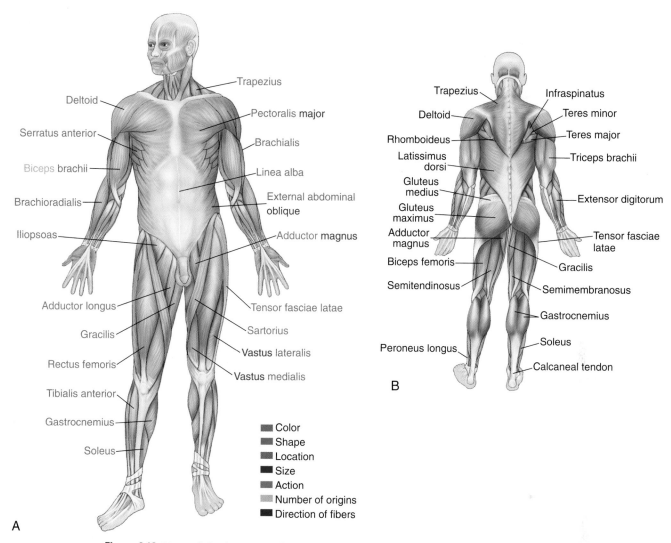

Figure 9.19 Major skeletal muscles of the body. A, Anterior view. Muscle features (such as, size, shape, direction of fibers, location, number of attachments, origin, and action) are often used in naming muscles (color-coding of the names on the anterior view). **B,** Posterior view.

9-40 More than 600 skeletal muscles are attached to and control movement of the skeletal bones. The major muscles are shown in Fig. 9.19.

Most skeletal muscles have names that describe some feature of the muscle—sometimes with several features combined in one name. Muscle features (such as, size, shape, direction of fibers, location and number of attachments, origin, and action) are often used in naming muscles. The name *pectoralis major* tells us it is a large muscle of the _____; *major* indicates the large size of the muscle. The names of the muscles in the anterior view have been color coded to indicate the origin of their names. For practice, color code as many muscles shown in the posterior view as you can, using terms you have learned together with a medical dictionary.

chest

9-41 A fibrous membrane called **fascia** covers, supports, and separates muscles. **Fascial** means pertaining to a _____.

Most skeletal muscles are attached to bones by tendons that span joints. When the muscle contracts, one bone moves relative to the other bone, and muscles sometimes work in groups to perform a particular movement. Muscles are arranged in antagonistic pairs. This means that when one muscle of the pair is contracted, the other is relaxed. For example, the biceps brachii muscle on the anterior arm bends the forearm at the elbow; the triceps brachii muscle on the posterior arm straightens the forearm at the elbow (see Fig. 3.8). When the former muscle contracts, the other is _____.

fascia

relaxed

WRITE IT! EXERCISE 18

List and describe the three types of muscles.

1. _____

2. _____

3. _____

extension

9-42 There are several commonly used terms to describe different types of movement brought about by muscular activity (Fig. 9.20). Use the information to write the answers in the following blanks.

The movement that straightens a limb is called _____ (Fig. 9.20, A).

The movement that is opposite and means to bend a limb is **flexion**. The muscles responsible for these movements are called **extensors** and **flexors**, respectively.

9-43 **Abduct/ion** is the drawing away from the midline of the body, and the responsible muscles are called **abductors**. The prefix ab- means away from. Abductors make movement possible away from the midline of the body. (Memory tool: In abduction, persons are often taken *away* against their own will.)

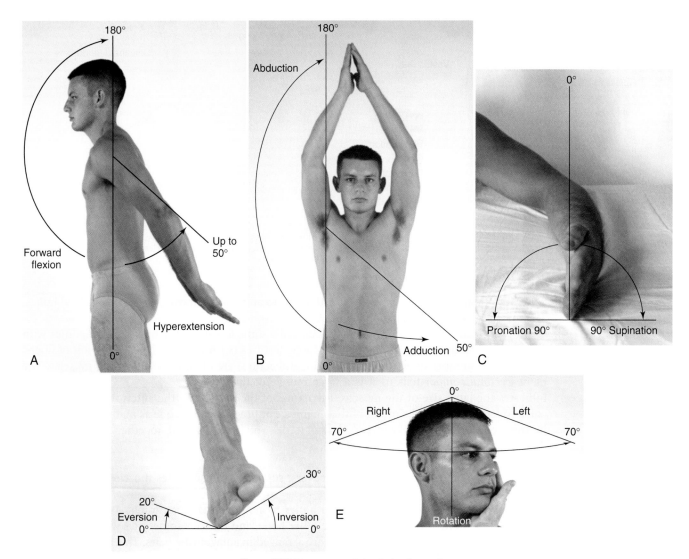

Figure 9.20 Movement of the skeletal muscles.

toward

The prefix ad- means toward. If ab/duction is the drawing away from the midline of the body, **ad/duction** is drawing _____ the midline (Fig. 9.20, B). The muscles responsible for adduction are called **adductors**. (Memory tool: Adhesives bring things together for bonding.)

A circular movement of a limb at the far end is **circumduction** (see Fig. 3.9, C). It is sometimes described as a combination of several movements (abduction, adduction, extension, and flexion).

supination

9-44 The rotation that allows the palm of the hand to turn up is called _____ (Fig. 9.20, C), whereas the rotation that turns the palm of the hand backward is **pronation**.

inversion

9-45 Eversion is a turning outward or inside out, such as a turning of the foot outward at the ankle. The opposite is turning inward, which is called _____ (Fig. 9.20, D).

➤ **BEYOND** THE BLUEPRINT Inversion has another meaning in genetics (a chromosome breaks off and reattaches in the reverse orientation), and it can also mean an abnormal condition in which an organ turns inside out, such as a uterine inversion.

9-46 Rotation is the movement of a bone around its own axis, and the muscle that is responsible for rotation is called a **rotator** (Fig. 9.20, E).

➤ **BEYOND** THE BLUEPRINT The rotator cuff is a group of muscles and their tendons in the shoulder that provides mobility and strength to the shoulder joint. Young people usually sustain a tear of the rotator cuff by substantial injury (throwing a ball or heavy lifting); however, older adults may experience tears related to aging or repetitive motions (Fig. 9.21).

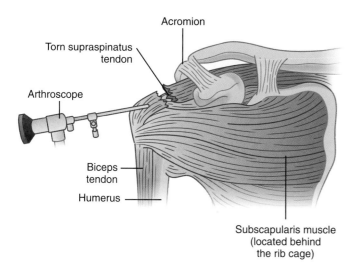

Figure 9.21 A torn rotator cuff. The acromion, an extension of the scapula, forms a joint with the clavicle. Manifestations of a tear in the rotator cuff include shoulder weakness and pain, as well as decreased ROM.

MATCH IT!

EXERCISE 19

Match the types of body movements in Numbers 1 through 5 with their meanings (A through I). Not all selections will be used.

_____ **1.** adduction

_____ **2.** circumduction

_____ **3.** eversion

_____ **4.** flexion

_____ **5.** supination

A. circular movement of a limb at the far end

B. drawing toward the midline of the body

C. movement of a bone around an axis

D. movement that allows turning the sole inward

E. movement that allows turning the sole outward

F. movement that bends a limb

G. movement that straightens a limb

H. rotation that turns the palm of the hand up

I. rotation that turns the palm of the hand down

DIAGNOSTIC TESTS AND PROCEDURES

9-47 Initial examination for musculoskeletal problems may include testing for range of motion (ROM), muscle strength, and reflexes. Muscle strength can be graded by asking the patient to apply resistance to the force exerted by the examiner (for example, the examiner tries to pull the bent arm down while the patient tries to raise it).

🔑 **KEY** POINT **ROM is measured as either active range of motion (AROM) or passive range of motion (PROM).** AROM is the range of movement through which a patient can actively, without assistance, move a joint by the adjacent muscles. PROM is the maximum range of movement through which the examiner can safely move a person's joint.

motion

ROM is the maximum amount of movement that a healthy joint is capable of, and it is measured in degrees of a circle (Fig. 9.22). ROM exercises are used to increase muscle strength and joint mobility. ROM means range of _____.

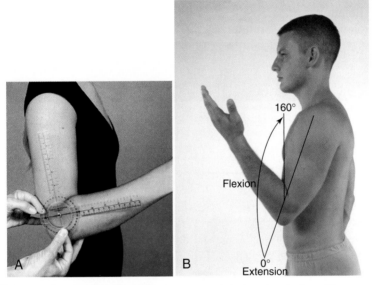

Figure 9.22 Range of motion (ROM) and its measurement. A, A goniometer is used to measure the angles of the ROM. **B,** Demonstration of the normal ROM of the elbow joint.

hammer

9-48 Reflex action is the immediate and involuntary functioning or movement of an organ or body part in response to a particular stimulus. The **reflex hammer** is a mallet with a rubber head that is used to tap tendons, nerves, or muscles to test reflex reactions (see Fig. 10.10, A and B). This instrument for testing reflex reactions is called a reflex _____.

electric

9-49 Electro/myo/graphy (EMG) is used to record the response of a muscle to _____ stimulation (Fig. 9.23). This is particularly useful in studying nerve damage and certain other disorders. The resulting record is called an **electromyogram.**

measures

9-50 Diagnostic studies of the bones and connective tissues include radiologic studies, bone scans, laboratory tests, and a few invasive procedures. Standard x-rays provide information about the joints and bone density or congenital deformities or fractures. Bone density testing, also called **bone densito/metry**, is any one of several methods of determining bone mass with a machine that _____ how well the rays penetrate the bone. This is helpful in diagnosing osteoporosis and determining the effectiveness of therapy.

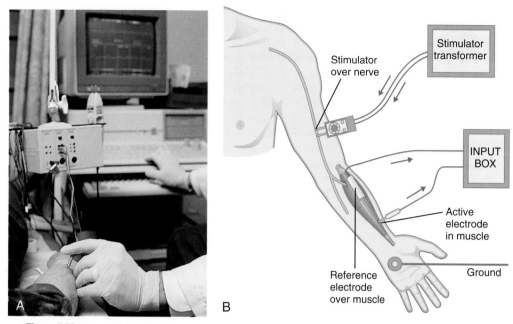

Figure 9.23 Electromyography (EMG). A, Patient and technician are shown with electromyographic equipment. Normal muscle at rest shows no electric activity. Needle electrodes are inserted into the muscle to record skeletal muscle activity when the muscle contracts. **B,** Schematic drawing of EMG, showing the stimulator transformer and the active electrode that has been placed in the muscle to detect skeletal muscle activity.

tomography

9-51 Bone tumors may be discovered during a routine radiologic examination. Computed tomography (CT), magnetic resonance imaging (MRI), bone scans, and biopsy are used to distinguish between benign and malignant tumors. Computed _____ produces an image of a cross-section of tissue. MRI is used to view soft tissue (for example, to visualize a cartilage tear). A **bone scan** is often useful in demonstrating malignant bone tumors, which appear as areas of increased uptake of radioactive material.

marrow

9-52 A bone marrow examination may include biopsy of the bone, as well as aspiration of bone marrow for microscopic study. These studies may be performed for other reasons, such as hemato/logic evaluation. Bone marrow studies are used to diagnose leukemia, identify tumors or other disorders of the bone marrow, and determine the extent of myelosuppression. **Myelo/suppression** is inhibition of the bone _____. (Read additional information about this in Frame 9-114).

The posterior iliac crest is generally the preferred site for **bone marrow aspiration** (Fig. 9.24). In adults the anterior iliac crest or the sternum may also be used.

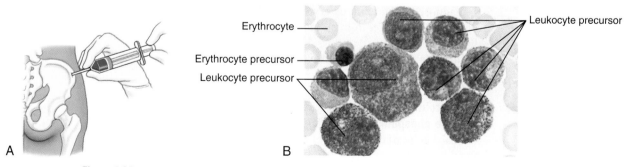

Figure 9.24 Bone marrow aspiration. A, Aspiration of bone marrow from the posterior iliac crest. **B,** Stained bone marrow. Numerous erythrocytes and leukocytes are normally present in bone marrow, and many are precursors (earlier forms) of cells that are seen in the circulating blood.

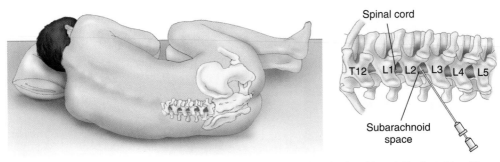

Figure 9.25 Lumbar puncture. The patient is generally positioned in the flexed lateral (fetal) position. The needle is inserted between the second and third or the third and fourth lumbar vertebrae. Cerebrospinal fluid can be removed or its pressure can be measured, and drugs can be introduced as done for spinal anesthesia.

vertebrae

joint

within

arthroscopy

puncture

9-53 A **lumbar puncture** (LP), commonly called a *spinal tap,* is performed for various therapeutic and diagnostic procedures. Diagnostic purposes include obtaining cerebrospinal fluid, measuring its pressure, or injecting substances for radiographic studies of the nervous system. Therapeutic indications include removing blood or pus, injecting drugs, and introducing an anesthetic for spinal anesthesia (Fig. 9.25).

The lumbar puncture is so named because the needle is inserted between two lumbar _____, usually L2-L3 or L3-L4.

9-54 Arthro/graphy is radiographic visualization of the inside of a _____. This is usually done by an intraarticular injection of a radiopaque substance. Both **intraarticular** and intra-articular mean _____ the joint.

The radiographic record produced after introduction of opaque contrast material into a joint is an **arthrogram.**

9-55 An **arthro/scope** is a fiberoptic instrument used for direct visualization of the interior of a joint. The process is called _____.

This procedure permits biopsy of cartilage or damaged synovial membrane, diagnosis of a torn cartilage, and, in some instances, removal of loose bodies in the joint space (Fig. 9.26).

9-56 Arthro/centesis is surgical _____ of a joint with a needle. This is performed to obtain samples of synovial fluid for diagnostic purposes, to remove excess fluid from joints to relieve pain, or to instill medications.

9-57 Several important laboratory tests are used to assess musculoskeletal disorders:

- **antinuclear antibody** (ANA) **test**: Serum is tested for antinuclear antibodies. Test is used primarily to diagnose systemic lupus erythematosus (described in the Arthritis and Connective Tissue Diseases section later in this chapter) although a positive result may indicate other autoimmune diseases.
- **erythrocyte sedimentation rate** (ESR): This is the rate at which erythrocytes settle out in a tube of blood that has been treated to prevent clotting. Elevated levels are found in many inflammatory processes.
- **rheumatoid factor** (RF): The RF test is positive in most patients with rheumatoid arthritis.
- **creatine phosphokinase** (CPK): Increased levels are found in skeletal muscle disorders and myocardial infarction (death of a portion of cardiac muscle, which is commonly called a *heart attack*).

In addition, serum calcium and serum phosphorus are decreased whenever there is excessive loss of calcium from the bone.

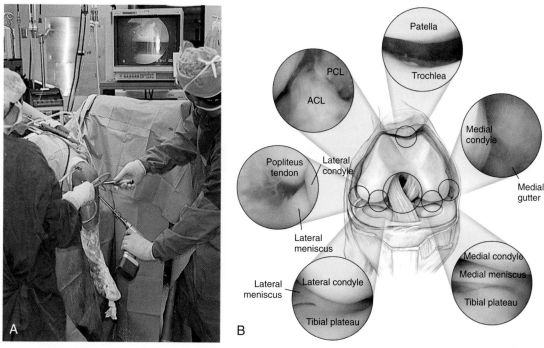

Figure 9.26 Arthroscopy of the knee. A, The examination of the interior of a joint is performed by inserting an arthroscope through a small incision, and then sterile fluid is pumped into the space to expand the joint and aid in its visualization. The arthroscope contains optical fibers and lenses that allow close visualization of the joint and is connected to a video camera. The doctor sees the appearance of the interior of the joint on a television monitor. **B,** Six points of the knee that can be seen. ACL and PCL are abbreviations for anterior and posterior cruciate ligament, respectively.

calcium	**9-58 Calci/uria** means _____ in the urine. Although calcium may be present in normal urine in minute amounts, it is not readily detectable. (Urinary excretion of calcium is affected by several things, including diet.) **Hyper/calciuria** is often seen in metastatic bone disease, in which there is rapid bone destruction.

WRITE IT! EXERCISE 20

Write a word in each blank to complete these sentences.
1. Bone density testing is also called bone _____.
2. EMG is the abbreviation for _____.
3. ROM means range of _____.
4. ESR means _____ sedimentation rate.
5. RF means _____ factor.
6. Arthrography is radiographic visualization of the inside of a/an _____.
7. A fiberoptic instrument that is used for direct visualization of the inside of a joint is a/an _____.
8. Surgical puncture of a joint is _____.

BUILD IT! EXERCISE 21

Use the following word parts to build terms.
intra-, articul(o), arthr(o), calc(i), electr(o), my(o), -ar, -gram, -graphy, -uria
1. radiographic visualization inside a joint _____/_____
2. calcium in the urine _____/_____
3. pertaining to within a joint _____/_____/_____
4. the record produced by electric stimulation of a muscle _____/_____/_____

PATHOLOGIES

9-59 Although injury is a primary cause of problems of the musculoskeletal system, the bones, muscles, and associated tissue are subject to various pathologies, including metabolic disturbances, infections, congenital disorders, and connective tissue diseases. You learned earlier that bone, cartilage, ligaments, and tendons are called _____ tissue, because they support and bind other tissues.

connective

Word Parts: Musculoskeletal Disorders

Combining Form	Meaning	Suffix	Meaning
ankyl(o)	stiff	-asthenia	weakness
scler(o)	hard	-sarcoma	malignant tumor from connective tissue
troph(o)	nutrition		

MATCH IT! **EXERCISE 22**

Match word parts in the left column with descriptions in the right column.

____ **1.** -asthenia   **A.** hard

____ **2.** -sarcoma   **B.** malignant tumor from connective tissue

____ **3.** ankyl(o)   **C.** nutrition

____ **4.** scler(o)   **D.** stiff

____ **5.** troph(o)   **E.** weakness

Stress and Trauma Injuries

pain

9-60 My/algia is muscular _____. Another word that means the same as myalgia is **myodynia**.

A muscle cramp is a painful, involuntary muscle spasm, often caused by inflammation of the muscle, but it can be a symptom of electrolyte imbalance. An example of the latter is **tetany**, a condition characterized by cramps, convulsions, twitching of the muscles, and sharp flexion of the wrists and ankle joints. It is caused by an imbalance in calcium metabolism.

9-61 Common musculoskeletal injuries include simple muscle strains, sprains, dislocations, and fractures:
- **strain:** Damage, usually muscular, results from excessive physical force
- **sprain:** A traumatic injury to the tendons, muscles, or ligaments around a joint, characterized by pain, swelling, and discoloration of the skin over the joint
- **dislocation:** Displacement of a bone from a joint; often evident on x-ray images of the affected bones (Fig. 9.27)
- **fracture** (fx): A break in a bone; usually evident on x-ray images of the affected bones
  If an x-ray image shows displacement of a bone from its joint, but no broken bone, the injury

dislocation

is a _____.

9-62 Fractures are described by the bone involved, the part of that bone, and the nature of the break, such as a compression fracture of the L4 vertebra. A **compression fracture** is a bone break caused by excessive vertical force. Pieces of the bone tend to move out in horizontal directions, and the affected bone collapses. The spinal cord is sometimes damaged in compression fractures of the vertebrae.

🔑 **KEY** POINT **Fractures are described as complete or incomplete and simple vs. compound.** They are classified as complete fractures with the break across the entire width of the bone, so it is divided into two sections, or incomplete fractures. They are also described by the extent of associated soft tissue damage as simple or compound. The bone protrudes through the skin in a **compound fracture**, which is also called an **open fracture.** If a bone is fractured but does not protrude through the skin, it is called a **simple** or **closed fracture** (Fig. 9.28).

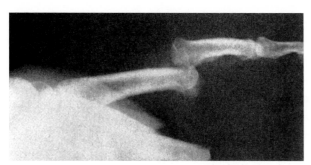

Figure 9.27 Radiograph demonstrating an interphalangeal dislocation of the finger.

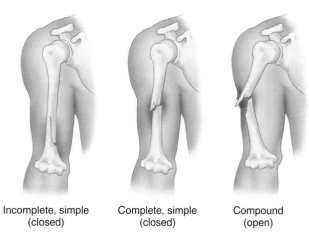

| Incomplete, simple (closed) | Complete, simple (closed) | Compound (open) |

Figure 9.28 **Classification and description of the severity of fractures.** Fractures are classified as either complete or incomplete and are described as either open or closed.

compound (or open)

Which type of fracture is a broken bone that causes an external wound?
_____

An incomplete fracture in which the bone is bent and fractured on one side only, as in Fig. 9.28, is called a **greenstick fracture** and is seen principally in children, whose bones are still pliant.

9-63 Fig. 9.29 illustrates four types of fractures:
- **impacted fracture:** One bone fragment is firmly driven into the fractured end of another fragment
- **comminuted fracture:** Bone is broken into many small fragments
- **spiral fracture:** Bone is twisted apart (also shows displacement)
- **transverse fracture:** The break in the bone is at right angles to the axis of the bone (also shows displacement)

transverse

Note that spiral and _____ fractures often result in open fractures.

9-64 Treatments for dislocations and fractures are included later in this chapter, but immobilization of fractures by use of a cast is common. Muscle shrinks when a limb is immobilized for a long period. The term **atrophy** means a decrease in the size of an organ or tissue. This type of atrophy

atrophy

is called disuse _____. Atrophy is noticeable in these cases, because the limb has decreased in size.

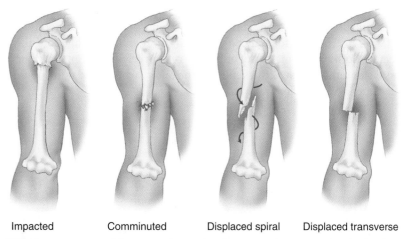

| Impacted | Comminuted | Displaced spiral | Displaced transverse |

Figure 9.29 **Common types of fractures.** The spiral and transverse fractures are also displaced. The ends of broken bones in displaced fractures often pierce the surrounding skin, resulting in open fractures; however, these two examples are closed fractures.

MATCH IT! **EXERCISE 23**

Match terms in the left column with those in the right column.

_____ **1.** atrophy

_____ **2.** comminuted fracture

_____ **3.** greenstick fracture

_____ **4.** impacted fracture

_____ **5.** myalgia

_____ **6.** spiral fracture

_____ **7.** transverse fracture

A. break in the bone is at right angles to the axis of the bone

B. bone is bent and fractured on one side only

C. bone is broken into small fragments

D. bone is twisted apart

E. decrease in size of an organ or tissue

F. one bone fragment is firmly driven into another

G. painful muscle

wrist

9-65 Carpal tunnel syndrome (CTS) is an example of trauma that results from prolonged, repetitive movements. CTS is a condition in which the median nerve in the wrist becomes compressed, causing pain and discomfort. Excessive hand exercise, a potential occupational hazard, can lead to a chronic condition of CTS. Carpal in its name will help you remember that CTS is a condition of the _____. Surgery to relieve the pressure on the nerve may be necessary.

➤ **BEYOND** THE BLUEPRINT Several studies have evaluated if there is association between extensive phone or computer use and carpal tunnel syndrome. Although these activities may cause a different form of hand pain, there is not enough evidence to support these as risk factors for carpal tunnel syndrome. Electrodiagnostic studies may be needed.

Tarsal tunnel syndrome is the ankle version of CTS. Treatment is similar to that for CTS.

WORD ORIGIN
temporomandibular *(L.)* *tempora*, the temples; *mandere*, to chew

temporomandibular

9-66 An abnormal condition characterized by facial pain and by mandibular dysfunction, apparently caused by a defective or dislocated temporomandibular joint (TMJ), is called *TMJ pain dysfunction syndrome* or is sometimes shortened to TMJ disorder. (The TMJ connects the temporal bone of the skull to the mandible of the jaw.)

Some indications of this disorder are clicking of the joint when the jaw moves, limitation of jaw movement, and temporomandibular dislocation. TMJ is an abbreviation for the _____ joint.

tarsus

hallux

9-67 Feet absorb considerable shock while running and walking, activities that can bring about a variety of disorders, particularly when structural weaknesses and other problems exist or improperly fitted shoes are worn.

Tarso/ptosis is prolapse of the _____. This is commonly called *flatfoot.*

Hallux means the great toe. **Hallux valgus** is a deformity of the foot, which is sometimes called a *bunion.* The great toe deviates laterally at the metatarsophalangeal (MTP) joint (Fig. 9.30, A). The medically correct name for bunion is _____ valgus.

A **hammertoe** is a toe that is permanently flexed at the midphalangeal joint, producing a clawlike appearance. This common abnormality often occurs simultaneously with hallux valgus (see Fig. 9.30, B). Hammertoe may be present in more than one digit, but the second toe is most often affected. **Corns** (hard masses of epithelial cells overlying a bony prominence) may develop on the dorsal side, and **calluses** (thickening of the outer layers of the skin at points of friction or pressure) may appear on the plantar surface.

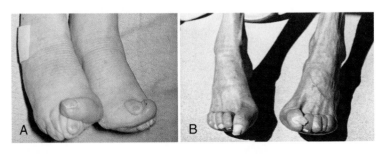

Figure 9.30 Deformities of the feet. A, Hallux valgus. The great toe rides over the second toe in this example. **B,** Hammertoe. The toes are permanently flexed. Hallux valgus and bunions are also present.

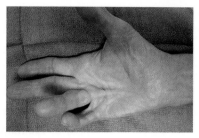

Figure 9.31 Dupuytren contracture. *This painless progressive shortening, thickening, and fibrosis of the subcutaneous tissue of the palm causes the fourth and fifth fingers to bend into the palm and resist extension.*

tumor

9-68 In **Morton neur/oma** a small, painful _____ grows in a digital nerve of the foot. Surgical removal of the neuroma is generally indicated if the pain persists and interferes with walking.

9-69 The cause is not known for some musculoskeletal disorders, such as **Dupuytren contracture,** a thickening and tightening of the palmar fascia, causing the fourth or fifth finger to bend into the palm and resist extension (Fig. 9.31).

9-70 Spinal stenosis, often a result of spinal degeneration, is narrowing of the spaces within the spine that can result in compression of the cauda equine in the lumbar spine. Symptoms include pain, paresthesias, and neurogenic cramplike pains in the lower extremities.

Low back pain that radiates down the buttock and below the knee, resulting from pressure on spinal nerve roots, is the most common symptom of a **herniated disk**, rupture of an intervertebral disk, the tough fibrous cushion between two vertebral bodies. This condition can result either from repeated stress or injury to the spine, or from natural degeneration with aging.

herniated

This is also called a *slipped disk,* but a more appropriate name is a _____ disk (Fig. 9.32).

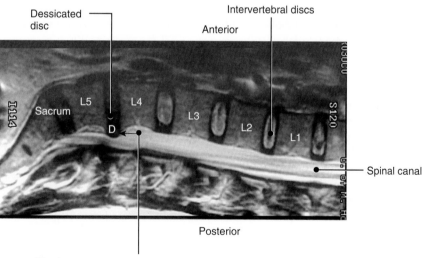

Figure 9.32 labels: Dessicated disc — Intervertebral discs — Anterior — L5 — L4 — L3 — L2 — L1 — Sacrum — D — Spinal canal — Posterior — Herniated disc of L4-L5 protruding into the spinal cord and compressing the nerve roots

Figure 9.32 A lumbar magnetic resonance imaging (MRI) scan of a herniated disk. The superior vertebrae are located to the right in the scan.

9-71 Common symptoms of persons with musculoskeletal disorders include pain, weakness, deformity, limitation of movement, stiffness, and **joint crepitus,** the crackling sound produced when a bone rubs against another bone or roughened cartilage.

Draw a slash between the word parts in the following list of new terms. Then find the meanings of the word parts within the definitions. (Draw the slash, and then perform the remainder of the activity as a mental exercise.)

1. **arthrochondritis** inflammation of the articular cartilage
2. **bursitis** inflammation of a bursa resulting from repetitive motion, trauma, infection or other disorders of the musculoskeletal system
3. **calcaneitis** inflammation of the heel bone
4. **calcaneodynia** painful heel
5. **chondralgia**, **chondrodynia** pain of the cartilage
6. **chondritis** inflammation of the cartilage. Inflammation of both bone and cartilage is **osteochondritis**.
7. **chondropathy** any disease of a cartilage
8. **ischialgia, ischiodynia** pain in the ischium
9. **rachialgia, rachiodynia** painful condition of the spine
10. **sacrodynia** pain in the sacrum
11. **spondylalgia** pain in a vertebra
12. **sternalgia** pain in the sternum
13. **synovitis** inflammation of a synovial joint
14. **tenalgia, tenodynia** pain in a tendon
15. **tendinitis** inflammation of a tendon. Sometimes occurs in conjunction with bursitis. Also spelled **tendonitis,** but tendinitis is the preferred spelling.
16. **tibialgia** pain in the tibia

Break these words into their component parts by placing a slash between the word parts. Write the meaning of each term.

1. tendinitis _____
2. spondylalgia _____
3. arthrochondritis _____
4. calcaneodynia _____
5. tarsoptosis _____

Metabolic Disturbances

9-72 Normal bone metabolism is affected by nutrition, hormones, and hereditary factors. Metabolic bone disorders include:

- **osteomalacia,** which is characterized by **decalcification**, a loss of calcium, and softening of the bone, accompanied by weakness, fracture, pain, anorexia, and weight loss.
- **osteoporosis,** which is a reduction in the amount of bone mass and increased porosity. The bones appear thin and fragile, and fractures are common (Fig. 9.33). Reduction in the amount of bone mass leads to subsequent fractures. It occurs most commonly in postmenopausal women, sedentary individuals, and patients receiving long-term steroid therapy. Bones appear thin and fragile. Loss of height and spinal deformities are common (Fig. 9.34). Dowager's hump is an abnormal curvature of the spine from front to back often seen in osteoporosis (caused by multiple fractures of the thoracic vertebrae).
- **Paget disease,** which is a skeletal disorder of unknown cause characterized by excessive bone destruction (**osteolysis**). The disease is named for Sir James Paget, an English surgeon; it is also called **osteitis deformans,** because it was originally thought to be an inflammatory process.

The metabolic bone disorder one associates more commonly with reduction in bone mass, which leads to loss of height and spinal deformity, is _____; the disorder more commonly associated with decalcification and softening of bone is _____; osteolysis is associated with _____ disease.

osteoporosis

osteomalacia; Paget

9-73 There is a delicate balance between bone destruction and bone formation. Excessive formation can lead to abnormal hardness and unusual heaviness of bone, called **osteo/sclerosis.**

Despite its density, osteosclerotic bone is brittle and subject to fracture. Literal interpretation of osteosclerotic is pertaining to bone that is _____.

hard

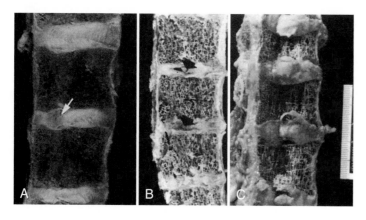

Figure 9.33 Normal versus osteoporotic vertebral bodies. The vertebral bodies are sectioned to show internal structure. **A,** Normal vertebral bodies. **B,** Vertebrae showing moderate osteoporosis. **C,** Vertebrae showing severe osteoporosis. **A** shows well-formed, normal vertebrae and disks. The *white arrow* points to a small focus of degeneration. In **B,** the overall shape of the vertebrae is preserved, but osteoporosis is already well developed. The disks show severe degeneration *(black arrows)*. Note in **C,** severe osteoporosis, how the vertebrae have been compressed by the bulging disks.

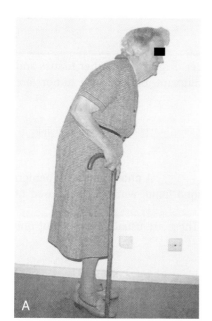

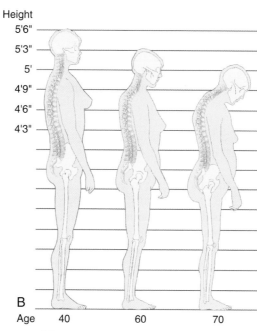

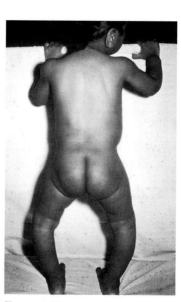

Figure 9.35 Rickets. This condition caused by deficiency of vitamin D results in abnormal bone formation, such as the bowed legs shown here (legs are bent outward at the knee).

Figure 9.34 Osteoporotic changes in the curvature of the spine. The spine appears normal at age 40 and shows osteoporotic changes at age 60 and 70. These changes bring about a loss of as much as 6 to 9 inches in height, and the so-called dowager's hump in the upper thoracic vertebrae.

calcium	

9-74 Vitamin D aids in the absorption of calcium from the intestinal tract. A deficiency of vitamin D results in insufficient calcium absorption and **calci/penia,** a deficiency of _____ in the body.

Osteomalacia is the adult equivalent of rickets in children.

Insufficient calcium for bone mineralization during the growing years causes **rickets.** Skeletal deformities of rickets (Fig. 9.35) are much more severe than those of osteomalacia in adults. In children, the disorder takes the form of _____.

rickets
osteomalacia

In adults, the disorder is called _____.

9-75 Osteo/penia is not a disease but a condition that is common to metabolic bone disease. **Osteopenia** is a reduced bone mass, which is usually the result of synthesis not compensating for the rate of destruction of bone. Write this term that means a reduced bone mass: _____.

osteopenia

Infections

bone

9-76 Oste/itis is inflammation of a _____. It may be caused by infection, degeneration, or trauma. Osteitis results in **oste/algia**, also called **osteo/dynia**, which means bone

pain

_____.

Osteo/mye/litis is an infection of the bone and bone marrow caused by infectious microorganisms that are introduced by trauma or surgery, by extension from a nearby infection, or via the bloodstream. Staphylococci are common causes of osteomyelitis.

9-77 Sometimes it is difficult to know if myel(o) in a word refers to bone marrow or the spinal cord, and in some words it can refer to either. For example, **myel/itis** means inflammation of either

marrow

the bone _____ or the spinal cord.

9-78 Cellul/itis is an acute, spreading, swollen, pus-forming inflammation of the deep subcutaneous tissues. It may be associated with abscess formation (see Fig. 13.29). If the muscle is also involved, it is called **myocellulitis**.

You learned earlier that cellul(o) means small cell, but that may not be helpful in remembering this term. Write the term that means an acute, pus-forming inflammation of the tissues and muscle:

myocellulitis

_____.

Tumors and Malignancies

9-79 The cause of bone tumors is largely unknown, unless cancer originates in other tissues and metastasizes to the bone. Bone tumors are either benign or malignant. Benign bone tumors are often asymptomatic.

🔑 **KEY POINT There are many types of benign bone tumors.** Benign tumors arise from several types of tissue. The major classifications include chondrogenic tumors, osteogenic tumors, and fibrogenic tumors.

cartilage

Chondro/genic tumors develop in the _____. A **chondr/oma** is a benign tumor or tumor-like growth of mature cartilage. An **osteo/chondr/oma,** which is composed of bone and cartilage, is the most common benign bone tumor.

bone

Osteo/genic tumors arise in the _____. These are usually benign, but one type, giant cell tumor of the bone, sometimes metastasizes.

Fibro/genic tumors are derived from fibrous tissue.

9-80 Metastatic bone cancer occurs far more frequently than primary bone cancer. Primary cancers of the breast, prostate, kidney, thyroid, and lung are sometimes called *bone-seeking cancers,* because they frequently metastasize to bone tissue, especially bone marrow.

🔑 **KEY POINT Terms using the word part -sarcoma name or describe malignant tumors.** There may be rare instances of misnomers. **Osteo/sarcoma** is the most common type of primary malignant bone tumor. In addition to osteosarcoma, other primary bone tumors include these cancers:

- **chondrosarcoma**
- **fibrosarcoma**
- **Ewing sarcoma**

malignant
cartilage

Words ending in sarcoma generally describe tumors that are _____.
A chondro/sarcoma is derived from _____, spreads to the bone, and destroys it.

fibrous

A fibro/sarcoma arises from _____ tissues. Ewing sarcoma is an aggressive bone tumor.

marrow

9-81 Multiple myel/oma is a malignant neoplasm of the bone _____ that disrupts and destroys bone marrow function. Both multiple myeloma and leukemia are white blood cell cancers with proliferation of certain types of cells and limited production of normal red blood cells, white blood cells, and platelets.

9-82 Leukemia is a broad term given to a group of malignant diseases that are characterized by replacement of bone marrow with proliferating immature leukocytes and abnormal numbers of immature leukocytes in the blood circulation.

🔑 **KEY** POINT **The classification of leukemia is complex, but the disease is classified according to the predominant type of proliferating leukocytes.** Acute leukemia has a sudden onset, whereas chronic leukemia develops slowly, and signs similar to those of acute leukemia may not appear for years. Diagnosis is made by blood tests and bone marrow biopsies.

lymphocytes

chronic

Lympho/cyt/ic or **lympho/blast/ic** and **myelo/cyt/ic** or **myelo/gen/ous** leukemias are broad classifications, and several subtypes exist. Lympho/blasts are immature cells that develop into _____. The immature cells in myelogenous leukemias are granulocytes.
ALL and CLL mean acute lymphocytic leukemia and chronic lymphocytic leukemia, respectively. Acute myelogenous leukemia is often abbreviated AML. CML means _____ myelogenous leukemia.

▶ **BEYOND** THE BLUEPRINT Environmental and genetic factors are believed to be involved in the development of leukemia, but the exact mechanism is generally unknown. Certain chemicals and drugs as well as ionizing radiation exposure (for example, the atomic bomb at Hiroshima or the Chernobyl nuclear accident) increase the risk for development of leukemia. The damage to genes that control cell growth changes cells from a normal to a malignant state.

BUILD IT! **EXERCISE 26**

Use the following word parts to build terms. (Some word parts will be used more than once.)
cellul(o), chondr(o), leuk(o), myel(o), my(o), oste(o), -emia, -itis, -sarcoma
1. inflammation of the bone   _____/_____
2. malignant tumor derived from cartilage   _____/_____
3. inflammation of the bone and bone marrow   _____/_____/_____
4. inflammation of muscle and deep subcutaneous tissues _____/_____/_____
5. blood condition with many immature white blood cells _____/_____

Congenital Defects

two

9-83 The skeletal system is affected by several developmental defects, including malformations of the spine. **Spina bifida** is a congenital abnormality characterized by defective closure of the bones of the spine. It can be so extensive that it allows herniation of the spinal cord (Fig. 9.36), or it might be evident only on radiologic examination. Remember that the prefix bi- in bi/fida means _____.

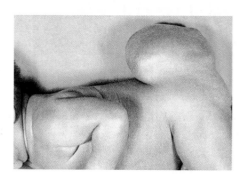

Figure 9.36 Spina bifida. This is a developmental defect in the lower spine. In cases where the separation is wide enough (as shown here), contents of the spinal canal protrude through the opening.

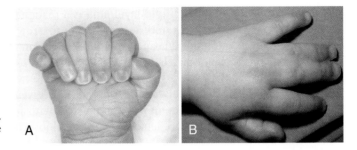

Figure 9.37 Comparison of the fingers in polydactyly and syndactyly.
A, Polydactyly. Note the presence of six fingers. **B,** Syndactyly. Note the webbing of the third and fourth phalanges.

9-84 The suffix -trophy means nutrition. **Dystrophy** is any abnormal condition caused by defective nutrition, often entailing a developmental change in muscles.

Muscular dystrophy is a group of inherited diseases that are characterized by weakness and atrophy of muscle without involvement of the nervous system. In all forms of muscular dystrophy, there is progressive disability and loss of strength. The name of this disease, the cause of which is

muscular | unknown but appears to be an inborn error of metabolism, is _____ dystrophy.

9-85 Each hand and foot normally has five digits. **Poly/dactyl/ism** or **poly/dactyly** is the presence

many | of _____ digits on the hands or feet. In either of these terms, it is understood that the number of digits is greater than the expected number of five (Fig. 9.37, A).

Syndactyly is a congenital anomaly of the hand or foot, marked by persistence of the webbing between adjacent digits, so they are more or less completely attached (Fig. 9.37, B). It can be so severe that there is complete union of the digits and fusion of the bones. Write this term that

syndactyly | means a congenital anomaly marked by webbing between adjacent digits: _____.

This is also called **syndactylism**. Compare polydactyly and syndactyly in Fig. 9.37.

Learn additional congenital disorders:

craniocele Hernial protrusion of the brain through a defect in the skull; **encephalocele**

kyphosis Abnormal convexity in the curvature of the thoracic spine as viewed from the side

lordosis Abnormal concavity of the lumbar spine as viewed from the side

rachischisis A **fissure** (split) of one or more vertebrae

sternoschisis Fissure of the sternum

scoliosis Lateral curvature of the spine, a fairly common abnormality of childhood, especially in females; sometimes it is caused by unequal leg lengths. Compare the three abnormal curvatures of the spine (Fig. 9.38).

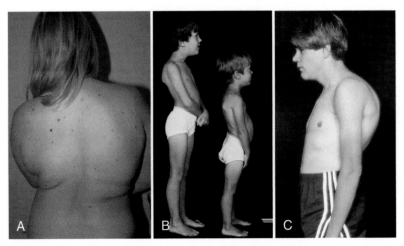

Figure 9.38 Three abnormal curvatures of the spine. A, Scoliosis, lateral curvature of the spine. **B,** Lordosis, abnormal anterior concavity of the lumbar spine. **C,** Severe kyphosis of the thoracic spine.

ANALYZE IT! **EXERCISE 27**	*Break these words into their component parts by placing a slash between the word parts. Write the meaning of each term.* **1.** craniocele _____ **2.** syndactylism _____ **3.** osteosclerosis _____ **4.** osteopenia _____ **5.** rachischisis _____

Arthritis and Connective Tissue Diseases

joints | **9-86 Arthr/itis** is any inflammatory condition of the _____, characterized by pain, heat, swelling, redness, and limitation of movement.

<table>
<tr><td rowspan="2">FIND IT! EXERCISE 28</td><td colspan="2">Draw a slash between the word parts in the following list of new terms. Then find the meanings of the word parts within the definitions. (Draw the slash, and then perform the remainder of the activity as a mental exercise.)</td></tr>
<tr><td>
1. ankylosing spondylitis inflammation and stiffening of the spine; the cause is unknown
2. ankylosis stiffening of a joint
3. arthralgia pain in a joint; arthrodynia
4. arthropathy any disease of the joints
5. arthrosclerosis hardening of the joints
6. dorsalgia pain in the back
7. osteoarthropathy a disease of the bones and joints
</td><td>
8. polyarthritis inflammation of more than one joint; the inflammation may migrate from one joint to the other, or several joints may be inflamed simultaneously
9. spondylarthritis spinal arthritis
10. spondyloarthropathy a general term that means any one of a group of inflammatory disorders that affect the joints and spine
</td></tr>
</table>

WORD ORIGIN
discoid *(G.)* *diskos,* flat plate *lupus, (L.)* wolf *erythros, (G.)* redness

diseases are characterized by altered function of the immune system and include the following diseases:

- **lupus erythematosus** (LE): Named for the characteristic butterfly rash that appears across the bridge of the nose in some cases (Fig. 9.39). Classified as **cutaneous** or **discoid lupus erythematosus** (DLE) and **systemic lupus erythematosus** (SLE).
- **systemic scleroderma:** Characterized by inflammation, fibrosis, and sclerosis of the skin and vital organs; also called **systemic sclerosis.** Cause is unknown, but autoimmunity is suspected.
- **Sjögren syndrome:** Characterized by deficient fluid production, which leads to dry eyes, dry mouth, and dryness of other mucous membranes, primarily affecting women older than 40 years.

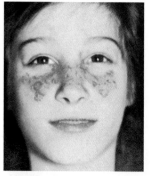

Figure 9.39 The characteristic "butterfly" rash of systemic lupus erythematosus (SLE). The rash is usually red, and thus the term *erythematous,* a Latin word meaning reddened, was added in naming this disease.

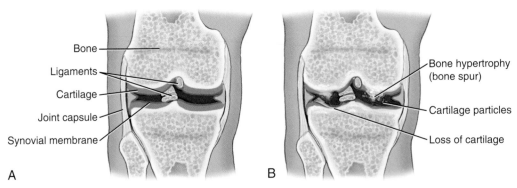

Figure 9.40 Joint changes that occur in degenerative joint disease (DJD) involving the knee. **A,** Normal knee joint. **B,** Bone hypertrophy and loss of cartilage in DJD of the knee.

9-88 Connective tissue diseases are a group of acquired disorders that cause immunologic and inflammatory changes in small blood vessels and connective tissue and include two important types of arthritis:

- **osteoarthritis:** A form of arthritis in which one or many joints undergo degenerative changes, particularly loss of articular cartilage (Fig. 9.40); it is also called *degenerative joint disease (DJD)*.
- **rheumatoid arthritis** (RA): The second most commonly occurring connective tissue disease. It is also the most destructive to joints, primarily affecting synovial joints. Joint deformity is common (Fig. 9.41).

rheumatoid

Osteoarthritis is the most common form of arthritis, but generally, _____ arthritis is more destructive to joints.

9-89 Some diseases are not primarily diseases of arthritis but are included because they affect the joints. **Gout** is a systemic disease associated with an inborn error of uric acid metabolism. Urate crystals deposit in the joints, myocardium, kidneys, and ears, causing inflammation. The disease can cause painful swelling of a joint, accompanied by chills and fever. Males are affected more often than females, and diet and medication are critical in the management of this disease called

gout

_____.

9-90 Lyme disease is an infection caused by the bite of an infected deer tick (Fig. 9.42, A). Symptoms in the early stages of the disease are a circular rash (Fig. 9.42, B), ill feeling, fever, headache, and muscle and joint aches. Prompt antibiotic treatment is effective. Without treatment, a small percentage of infected persons will develop arthritis as well as heart and neurologic problems. This disease,

Lyme

called _____ disease, is named for the place where it was originally described, Lyme, Connecticut.

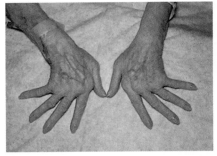

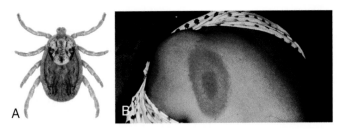

Figure 9.42 Lyme disease. **A,** The bite of this deer tick can cause Lyme disease. **B,** Note the target-like appearance of the bite of an infected tick.

Figure 9.41 **Hand deformities characteristic of chronic rheumatoid arthritis.** There is marked deformity of the metacarpophalangeal joints, causing deviation of the fingers to the ulnar side of the hand.

Muscular Disorders

many	**9-91 Polymyositis** is an inflammatory myo/pathy that involves _____ muscles, which leads to atrophy of the muscle. Weight loss, fatigue, and gradual weakness of the
myopathy	muscles are characteristic. A disease of the muscles is called a _____.
muscle	**9-92 Myo/fascial** pertains to a _____ and its fascia. Myofascial pain syndrome is pain in one region of the body, often diagnosed by palpation of a "trigger point" that causes pain and twitching of a muscle some distance away from the point of palpation. Myo/fascial means pertaining to a muscle and its fascia.
fatigue	**9-93 Chronic fatigue syndrome** is a disorder characterized by disabling fatigue accompanied by a variety of associated complaints, including muscle pain, joint pain, and headache. This disabling disorder that is named for its chief symptom is called chronic _____ syndrome.
muscles	**9-94 Poly/my/algia** means pain of many _____. **Polymyalgia rheumatica** is a chronic, inflammatory disease that primarily affects the arteries in muscles. The major symptoms are stiffness, weakness, and aching that occur most commonly in the shoulder or pelvic girdle.
joints	**9-95 Fibro/my/algia,** also called **fibromyalgia syndrome,** is characterized by widespread non-articular pain of the torso, extremities, and the face. It may be attributable to deep sleep deprivation. Non/articular means that the _____ are not involved in this chronic disorder.
softening	**9-96** Atrophy of muscle tissue occurs as one ages, but the rate is slowed by exercise. Therapeutic exercise that increases muscle strength and tone is helpful with balance in walking and provides support for the joints as one ages. **Myo/lysis** means disintegration or degeneration of muscle, and **myo/malacia** is abnormal _____ of muscular tissue.
myasthenia	**9-97 My/asthenia** is a term specifically applied to muscle weakness. The suffix -asthenia means weakness. Write this new word that means muscle weakness: _____. **Myasthenia gravis** is a disease of unknown cause, characterized by fatigue and muscle weakness resulting from a defect in the conduction of nerve impulses. It may either be restricted to one muscle group or become generalized. The disorder may affect any muscles of the body but especially those of the eyes, face, lips, tongue, neck, and throat.
muscle	**9-98** A **myo/cele** is herniation of a _____ through its ruptured sheath.
muscle	**9-99 Myo/fibr/osis** is a condition in which _____ tissue is replaced by fibrous tissue.

Case Study. *Write the meaning of terms 1-4.*

Prem Kamala, 70 years of age, fell while painting. Radiologic findings show a simple, complete fracture of the left fibula. He is able to move his left ankle and toes, suffers widespread arthralgia, and underwent right knee arthroscopy in 2016. Define these terms:

1. simple, complete fracture _____
2. fibula _____
3. arthralgia _____
4. arthroscopy _____

WRITE IT!
EXERCISE 30

Write a word in each blank space to complete these sentences.

1. A condition in which the median nerve in the wrist becomes compressed, causing pain, is _____ tunnel syndrome.
2. Inflammation of a bursa is _____.
3. Inflammation of an articular cartilage is _____.
4. TMJ disorder is a dysfunction of the _____ joint.
5. Another name for flatfoot is _____.
6. An osteosarcoma is a malignant bone _____.
7. A metabolic disorder that is characterized by decalcification, loss of calcium, and deterioration of bone tissue, is _____.
8. A congenital abnormality characterized by defective closure of the spine is called spina _____.
9. Degenerative joint disease is also called _____.
10. A disease of the nervous system that is characterized by fatigue and muscle weakness is called _____ gravis.

BUILD IT!
EXERCISE 31

Use the following word parts to build terms. (Some word parts will be used more than once.)
poly-, ankyl(o), arthr(o), dors(o), fibr(o), my(o), spondyl(o), -algia, -osis, -pathy

1. pain in the back _____/_____
2. condition of stiffening of a joint _____/_____
3. condition where muscle is replaced by fibrous tissue _____/_____/_____
4. pain in many muscles _____/_____/_____
5. disorder affecting the joints and spine _____/_____/_____

SURGICAL AND THERAPEUTIC INTERVENTIONS

reduction

9-100 **Orthopedics** is the branch of medicine that specializes in the prevention and correction of disorders of the musculoskeletal system. Orthopedic surgeons, also called **orthopedists,** restore fractures to their normal positions by **reduction,** pulling the broken fragments into alignment. Pulling a fracture into alignment is called _____.

A fracture is usually restored to its normal position by manipulation without surgery. This is called **closed reduction.**

🔑 **KEY** POINT **Management of a closed reduction usually involves immobilization with a splint, bandage, cast, or traction.** A **splint** immobilizes, restrains, or supports the injured part (for example, the finger) until healing occurs. A **cast** is a stiffer, more solid dressing form with plaster of Paris or other material. **Traction** is the use of a pulling force to a part of the body to produce alignment and rest, while decreasing muscle spasm and correcting or preventing deformity.

9-101 If a fracture must be exposed by surgery before the broken ends can be aligned, it is an **open reduction.** The fracture shown in Fig. 9.43 was corrected by surgery that included **internal fixation** to stabilize the alignment. Internal fixation uses pins, rods, plates, screws, and/or other materials to immobilize the fracture. After healing, the fixation devices may be either removed or left in place.

External fixation may be used in both open and closed reductions. This method uses metal pins attached to a compression device outside the skin surface (Fig. 9.44).

After a bone is broken, the body begins the healing process to repair the injury. Electric bone stimulation, bone grafting, and ultrasound treatment may be used when healing is slow or does not occur.

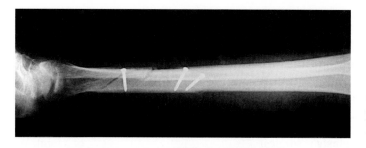

Figure 9.43 Internal fixation following a leg fracture. A lateral view of a lower leg break after reduction and internal fixation using screws.

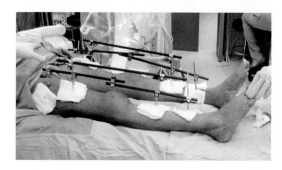

Figure 9.44 External fixation of a fracture. The fractured bone is held together by pins that are attached to a compression device. The pins are removed when the fracture is healed.

MATCH IT!
EXERCISE 32

Match the surgical terms in the left column with their meanings in the right column.

_____ **1.** closed reduction   **A.** exposing a broken bone by surgery and aligning it

_____ **2.** internal fixation   **B.** pulling a broken bone into alignment without surgery

_____ **3.** open reduction   **C.** surgery that uses pins or other materials to immobilize a broken bone

---

Word Parts: Orthopedics

Suffix	Meaning
-clasia	break
-desis	binding; fusion

---

binding or fusion

9-102 Analyze spondylo/syn/desis: spondyl(o) means vertebra; syn- means joined (or together); and -desis means _____.

   Spondylosyndesis is spinal fusion. It is fixation of an unstable segment of the spine, generally accomplished by surgical fusion with a bone graft or a synthetic device.

> **WORD ORIGIN**
> laminectomy *(L.)*
> *lamina*
> thin plate

laminectomy

9-103 Surgical removal of one or more bony arches of the vertebrae is a **lamin/ectomy,** and is largely performed to relieve the pain of herniated disks and compression fractures. This is surgical removal of the bony posterior arch of a vertebra to permit surgical access to the disk so that the herniated material can be removed. Write this term that means the surgical removal of the bony arch of a vertebra: _____.

   Complete excision of an intervertebral disk is a **disk/ectomy.**

vertebroplasty

9-104 Vertebral fractures can sometimes be repaired by **vertebro/plasty.** In this procedure, a plastic-like substance is injected on each side of the fractured vertebra to hold the fragments in position while the bone heals. The name of the procedure used to assist the healing of a fractured vertebra is called _____.

excision

9-105 A partial **fasciectomy** is generally performed to relieve Dupuytren contracture when function becomes impaired. A partial fasci/ectomy is _____ of fascia.

bunion

9-106 Numerous surgeries are performed to straighten the toes, remove bunions, and correct various deformities of the feet. A **bunion/ectomy** is excision of a _____. Surgical repair to straighten the great toe can be done at the same time. Surgery may be performed to correct the alignment in hammertoe also.

arthrotomy

9-107 Write a word that means incision of a joint, using arthr(o) and the suffix that means incision: _____. **Arthr/ectomy** is excision of a joint.

repair

9-108 **Arthro/plasty** is surgical _____ of a joint. When other measures are inadequate to provide pain control for degenerative joint disease, surgery may be indicated, often total joint replacement (TJR).

chondroplasty

9-109 Surgical repair of damaged cartilage is _____. This may be necessary if the cartilage becomes torn or displaced.
    Chondrectomy means surgical removal of cartilage.

> ➤ **BEYOND** THE BLUEPRINT Replacement of hips, knees, elbows, wrists, shoulders, and joints of the fingers and toes have become common. The knee follows hip replacement as the most common joint replacement. The patient has progressive exercise through physical therapy after knee surgery. The surgeon may prescribe a continuous passive motion (CPM) machine to keep the prosthetic knee in motion and prevent formation of scar tissue during the first few weeks of healing (Fig. 9.45).

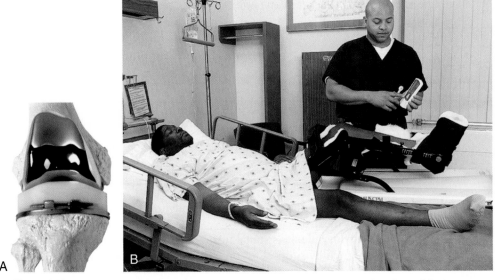

Figure 9.45 Knee replacement. A, With the patient under anesthesia, the diseased surfaces of the knee are removed, and a hinged prosthesis (such as the one shown) is inserted into the medullary cavities of the femur and tibia. **B,** After surgery, progressive exercise sometimes includes a continuous passive motion (CPM) machine.

arthrocentesis

9-110 Sometimes, excessive fluid accumulates in a synovial joint after injury and must be extracted with a needle. Write a word that means surgical puncture of a joint: _____.
    The suffix -desis means binding or fusion. Use this suffix with arthr(o) to form a word that literally means fusion of a joint: _____.

arthrodesis

    Arthrodesis is a surgical procedure that is used to immobilize a joint. It is artificial ankylosis. Fusing the bones together stabilizes painful joints that have become unable to bear weight. Thus a stiff but stable and painless joint results.

joint

9-111 **Arthro/clasia** is artificial breaking of an ankylosed _____ to provide movement. Arthroclasia is a surgical procedure that is used to break adhesions of an ankylosed joint. Another term that means operative loosening of adhesions in an ankylosed joint is formed by combining the word part for joint and the suffix that means dissolving or destruction. Use these word parts to write the new term: _____.

arthrolysis

FIND IT!

EXERCISE 33

Draw a slash between the word parts in the following list of new terms. Then find the meanings of the word parts within the definitions. (Draw the slash, and then perform the remainder of the activity as a mental exercise.)

1. **bursectomy** excision of a bursa
2. **carpectomy** excision of one or more of the bones of the wrist
3. **coccygectomy** excision of the coccyx
4. **costectomy** excision of a rib
5. **craniectomy** excision of a segment of the skull
6. **cranioplasty** surgical repair of the cranium
7. **craniotomy** incision into the cranium with a **craniotome.** Compare craniotomy and craniectomy (Fig. 9.46).
8. **myoplasty** surgical repair of a muscle
9. **myorrhaphy** suture of a torn or cut muscle
10. **osteectomy** excision of a bone or a portion of it; also called **ostectomy** (One "e" is often dropped.) An **osteotome** is an instrument used to cut bone.

11. **osteoplasty** surgical repair of a bone
12. **phalangectomy** excision of a bone of the finger or toe
13. **sternotomy** incision of the sternum, a common incision used in open-heart surgery
14. **tendoplasty** surgical repair of a tendon
15. **tenomyoplasty** surgical repair of a tendon and muscle
16. **tenorrhaphy** union of a divided tendon by suture
17. **tenotomy** incision of a tendon
18. **vertebrectomy** excision of a vertebra

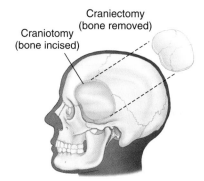

Craniotomy (bone incised)

Craniectomy (bone removed)

Figure 9.46 Craniotomy and craniectomy. Any surgical opening into the skull is a craniotomy. In this example, part of the skull is removed (a craniectomy) to remove a tumor. The bone may be replaced immediately after surgery or be temporarily left off to reduce pressure from swelling due to trauma caused by the surgery.

arthritis

9-112 Anti/arthritics are various forms of therapy that relieve the symptoms of _____, as well as antiarthritic agents, which reduce inflammation and pain.

Uricosurics are drugs that increase urinary excretion of uric acid in the treatment of gout.

9-113 Hematologists and oncologists treat persons with cancer or leukemia. The mode of treatment differs for different types of leukemia, but aggressive chemotherapy is common. A major side effect of chemotherapy is severe bone marrow suppression, so a combination of chemotherapy, antibiotics to prevent infection, and blood transfusions to replace red cells and platelets is often given. Write a word that is an adjective that means inhibiting bone marrow activity: _____.

myelosuppressive

9-114 Bone marrow transplantation (BMT) is used to stimulate the production of normal blood cells. The patient's bone marrow is first destroyed with radiation and chemotherapy. Healthy bone marrow cells (stem cells) are transfused into the patient's blood; they migrate to the spongy bone and multiply into cancer-free bone marrow cells. (Cord blood, collected immediately after birth, is rich in stem cells and may be an alternative to **bone marrow transplants.**) In **autologous transplants,** clients receive their own stem cells (which were collected before chemotherapy was begun).

bone

9-115 Bone cancers are treated with a combination of drugs and surgery. Excision of the tumor tissue is common in benign bone tumors. Oste/ectomy is excision of a _____.

The treatment of primary bone tumors is surgical, often combined with chemotherapy and radiation. Pain can be intense in malignant bone tumors, so controlling pain is an important part of a patient's care.

For more information, go the National Institute of Arthritis and Musculoskeletal and Skin Diseases (NIAMS) website: *www.niams.nih.gov.*

WRITE IT!

EXERCISE 34

Write terms for the following meanings.

1. breaking an ankylosed joint   _____
2. excision of a rib   _____
3. incision of a joint   _____
4. inhibiting bone marrow activity   _____
5. medications that reduce inflammation   _____
6. surgical removal of cartilage   _____
7. surgical repair of the skull   _____
8. suture of a torn or cut muscle   _____

ANALYZE IT!

EXERCISE 35

Break these words into their component parts by placing a slash between the word parts. Then write the meaning of each term.

1. craniotomy   _____
2. myorrhaphy   _____
3. tenomyoplasty   _____
4. spondylosyndesis   _____
5. fasciectomy   _____

PHARMACOLOGY

Many drugs are available to treat different forms of arthritis and other connective tissue diseases. In addition, numerous drugs are available to relieve pain and control the symptoms of musculoskeletal disorders.

Drug Class: Effect and Uses

Analgesics: Relieve pain
acetaminophen (Tylenol)   *celecoxib (Celebrex)*   *morphine (MS Contin)*
aspirin (Bayer)   *fentanyl (Duragesic)*   *oxycodone (OxyContin)*

Antigout Agents: *Treat gout*
colchicine (Colcrys)   *pegloticase (Krystexxa)*

Uricosurics: Increase urinary excretion of uric acid
probenecid (Benemid)

Xanthine Oxidase Inhibitors: Reduce production of uric acid
allopurinol (Zyloprim)

Antiinflammatories: Reduce inflammation
Corticosteroids and nonsteroidal antiinflammatory drugs (NSAIDs) act as antiinflammatories.
hydrocortisone (Cortef)   *ketorolac (Toradol)*   *prednisone (Rayos)*
ibuprofen (Motrin)   *methylprednisolone (Medrol)*   *triamcinolone (Kenalog)*

Antiosteoporotics: Used to treat osteoporosis
Some bisphosphonates and selective estrogen receptor modulatorsact as antiosteoporotics.
alendronate (Fosamax)   *raloxifene (Evista)*

Bisphosphonates: Affect bone formation to treat bone diseases such as osteoporosis
alendronate (Fosamax)   *ibandronate (Boniva)*

PHARMACOLOGY, cont'd

Disease-Modifying Antirheumatic Drugs (DMARDs): Slow progression of rheumatoid arthritis and other autoimmune diseases

auranofin (Ridaura)
etanercept (Enbrel)
infliximab (Remicade)
methotrexate (Trexall)
tocilizumab (Actemra)

Muscle Relaxants: Relax skeletal muscles to relieve pain due to muscle spasms

carisoprodol (Soma)
cyclobenzaprine (Flexeril)
metaxalone (Skelaxin)

Neuromuscular-Blocking Drugs: Induce muscle paralysis for surgery

cisatracurium (Nimbex)
pancuronium (Pavulon)
succinylcholine (Anectine)

WRITE IT! **EXERCISE 36**

Write a word in the blank to complete these sentences.

1. DMARDs means disease-modifying _____ drugs.
2. Drugs called _____ are used to treat osteoporosis.
3. Drugs that relieve inflammation are _____.
4. The class of pharmaceutical that relieves pain is _____.

CHAPTER ABBREVIATIONS*

ACL	anterior cruciate ligament	ACL	anterior cruciate ligament
ALL	acute lymphocytic leukemia	fx	fracture
AML	acute myelogenous leukemia	L1, L2, etc.	first, second, etc., lumbar vertebrae
ANA	antinuclear antibody	LE	lupus erythematosus
AROM	active range of motion	LP	lumbar puncture
BMT	bone marrow transplantation	MTP	metatarsophalangeal
C1, C2, etc.	first, second, etc., cervical vertebrae	NIAMS	National Institute of Arthritis and Musculoskeletal and Skin Diseases
CLL	chronic lymphocytic leukemia	NSAID	nonsteroidal antiinflammatory drug
CML	chronic myelogenous leukemia	PCL	posterior cruciate ligament
CPK	creatine phosphokinase	PROM	passive range of motion
CPM	continuous passive motion	RA	rheumatoid arthritis
CTS	carpal tunnel syndrome	RF	rheumatoid factor
DJD	degenerative joint disease	ROM	range of motion
DLE	discoid lupus erythematosus	SLE	systemic lupus erythematosus
DMARD	disease-modifying antirheumatic drug	T1, T2, etc.	first, second, etc., thoracic vertebrae
EMG	electromyography	TJR	total joint replacement
ESR	erythrocyte sedimentation rate	TMJ	temporomandibular joint

*Many of these abbreviations share their meanings with other terms.

A Career as an Athletic Trainer

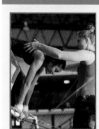

Tanya Palmer has been a certified athletic trainer for 5 years and never plans to stop. She is passionate about helping others achieve their goals. Her educational preparation took 4 years, but Tanya knew it would be worth the effort. Her father helped her start her own business, knowing that her success in gymnastics would draw many young athletes to her training facility. She helps individuals of all abilities and fitness levels. For more information, visit *www.nata.org*.

CHAPTER 9 SELF-TEST

Review the new word parts for this chapter. Work all of the following exercises to test your understanding of the material before checking your answers against those in Appendix IV.

BASIC UNDERSTANDING

Labeling

I. Label the diagram with the names of the bones and their combining forms. Number 1 is done as an example.

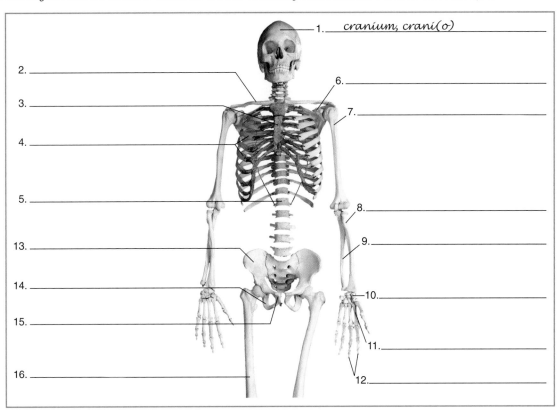

1. *cranium, crani(o)*
2. _____
3. _____
4. _____
5. _____
6. _____
7. _____
8. _____
9. _____
10. _____
11. _____
12. _____
13. _____
14. _____
15. _____
16. _____

Identifying Illustrations

II. Label the figures with the types of fractures: **A.** comminuted; **B.** impacted; **C.** spiral; **D.** transverse

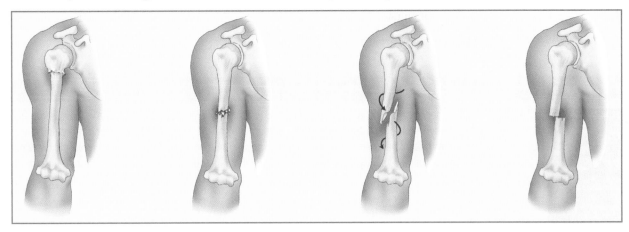

1. _____   2. _____   3. _____   4. _____

III. Label these illustrations using one of the following: adduction, arthroscopy, chondroplasty, electromyography, fasciectomy, myolysis.

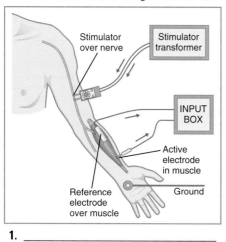

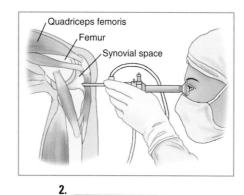

1. _____

2. _____

Matching

IV. Match the following anatomic structures with their descriptions.

_____ **1.** bone   **A.** connects bones or cartilages

_____ **2.** bursa   **B.** fluid-filled sac that helps reduce friction

_____ **3.** cartilage   **C.** fluid-secreting tissue lining the joint

_____ **4.** joint   **D.** place of union between two or more bones

_____ **5.** ligament   **E.** provides protection and support for a joint

_____ **6.** synovial membrane   **F.** strong, fibrous tissue that attaches muscles to bones

_____ **7.** tendon   **G.** the most rigid connective tissue

V. Match the types of body movements in 1 through 10 with their meanings (A through J).

_____ **1.** abduction   **A.** circular movement of a limb at the far end

_____ **2.** adduction   **B.** movement of a bone around an axis

_____ **3.** circumduction   **C.** movement of the sole of the foot inward

_____ **4.** eversion   **D.** movement of the sole of the foot outward

_____ **5.** extension   **E.** rotation that allows the palm of the hand to turn up

_____ **6.** flexion   **F.** rotation that turns the palm of the hand backward (down)

_____ **7.** inversion   **G.** to bend

_____ **8.** pronation   **H.** to bring together

_____ **9.** rotation   **I.** to straighten

_____ **10.** supination   **J.** to take away

VI. Match the bones in 1 through 10 with their common names (A through J).

_____ **1.** carpal   **A.** ankle bone

_____ **2.** clavicle   **B.** bones of the fingers and toes

_____ **3.** coccyx   **C.** breastbone

_____ **4.** femur   **D.** collarbone

_____ **5.** patella   **E.** hipbone

_____ **6.** pelvis   **F.** kneecap

_____ **7.** phalanges   **G.** shoulder blade

_____ **8.** scapula   **H.** tailbone

_____ **9.** sternum   **I.** thigh bone

_____ **10.** tarsal   **J.** wrist bone

Deconstructing Words

VII. Divide these words into their component parts, and then define each term.

1. carpophalangeal _____

2. chondrosarcoma _____

3. osteolysis _____

4. osteoarthropathy _____

5. scapuloclavicular _____

VIII. Label the types of vertebrae that are indicated in the illustration.

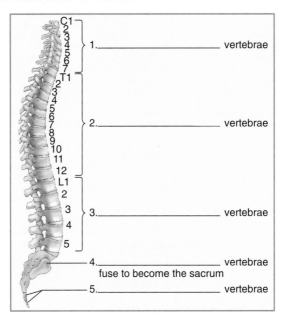

1. _____ vertebrae

2. _____ vertebrae

3. _____ vertebrae

4. _____ vertebrae
fuse to become the sacrum

5. _____ vertebrae

Listing

IX. List five functions of the skeletal system.

1. _____

2. _____

3. _____

4. _____

5. _____

X. List the three major types of muscle, and describe their functions.

1. _____

2. _____

3. _____

Using Vocabulary

XI. Circle the correct answers in the following multiple choice questions.

1. The neonatologist's report describes "a developmental defect in which the newborn's sternum is fissured as a result of incomplete fusion." What is a term for this defect? (costectomy, rachischisis, spondylosyndesis, sternoschisis)

2. Both bones of the forearm are fractured. Which term refers to both bones? (carpopedal, carpophalangeal, humeroulnar, ulnoradial)

3. Which of the following is a general term that means any disease of the joint, whether it is inflammatory, neurogenic, or another type of joint disease? (arthropathy, bursopathy, chrondropathy, osteopathy)

4. Susana is undergoing a test that records the electric activity associated with stimulation of skeletal muscle. What is the name of the record that is produced? (antinuclear antibodies, electromyogram, myograph, range of motion reading)

5. A physician on a medical mission trip to a remote region in Peru finds that some of the elderly villagers suffer from osteomalacia, which has resulted from loss of calcium from the bone. Which term means loss of calcium from bone?
(calcification, calciuria, decalcification, osteogenesis)

6. When Rita delivers a baby boy, the obstetrician counts six toes on the right foot and five toes on the left foot. What is the name of this condition? (carpopedal disease, Paget disease, phalangitis, polydactylism)

7. Lee has leukemia and has undergone chemotherapy and total body radiation to destroy leukemic cells from the soft material in the cavities of bones. What is the name of the soft tissue that fills the cavities of bones?
(bone marrow, diaphysis, epiphysis, periosteum)

8. The orthopedist examines radiographic images of Manuel's knee and explains a procedure in which a fiberoptic tube is inserted into the knee for direct visualization. What procedure is being explained? (arthrogram, arthrography, arthroscope, arthroscopy)

9. Kevin has had flat feet most of his life, and the orthopedist recommends orthotics to be worn in his shoes. What is the name of Kevin's condition? (Dupuytren contracture, hallux valgus, tarsal tunnel syndrome, tarsoptosis)

10. Some statistics estimate that one in two women older than 50 years will sustain a fracture during their lifetime that is related to this metabolic bone disease characterized by loss of bone density and deterioration of bone tissue. Which bone disease is described? (osteitis deformans, osteolysis, osteoporosis, Paget disease)

Writing Terms

XII. Write a term for each of the following meanings.

1. aligning a broken bone _____

2. between the ribs _____

3. degenerative joint disease _____

4. excision of the tailbone _____

5. herniation of a muscle _____

6. inflammation of a bone _____

7. lateral curvature of the spine _____

8. pertaining to muscle and fascia _____

9. pertaining to the joints _____

10. surgical puncture of a joint _____

Finetuning Terms

XIII. Describe the relationship of these terms.

1. myelocytes and myeloblasts _____

2. vertebrosternal and sternovertebral _____

Describing Differences

XIV. In addition to spelling, describe at least one difference in the following:

1. diaphysis and epiphysis _____

2. ligaments and tendons _____

Opting for Opposites

XV. Write a term that you learned that means the opposite of these words.

1. infrasternal _____

2. abductor _____

GREATER COMPREHENSION

Using Pharmacologic Terms

XVI. Use all selections to match terms in the left column with their descriptions in the right column.

_____ **1.** analgesics

_____ **2.** antiinflammatories

_____ **3.** bisphosphonates

_____ **4.** DMARDs

_____ **5.** myelosuppressives

_____ **6.** neuromuscular blocking drugs

_____ **7.** xanthine oxidase inhibitors

A. induce muscle paralysis

B. reduce uric acid production

C. relieve inflammation

D. relieve pain

E. slow progression of rheumatoid arthritis

F. suppression of bone marrow activity

G. treat osteoporosis

New Construction

XVII. Break the following words apart, and then write the meaning of each term.

1. bursopathy _____

2. musculotendinous _____

3. osteochondral _____

4. suprapatellar _____

5. tenosynovitis _____

Health Care Reporting

XVIII.   Read the following report; then select one-word answers to complete the sentences.

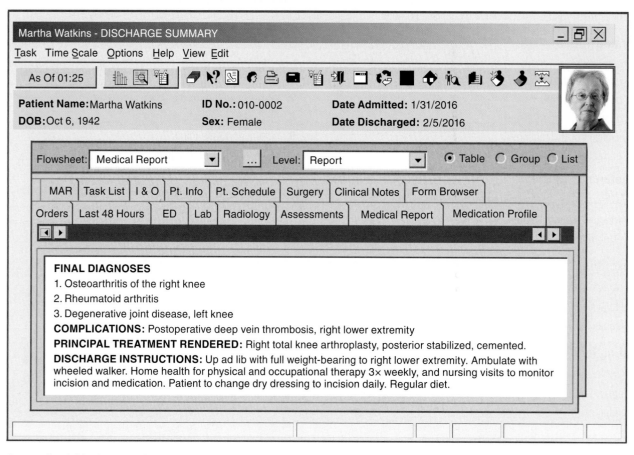

Martha Watkins - DISCHARGE SUMMARY

Task Time Scale Options Help View Edit

As Of 01:25

Patient Name: Martha Watkins   **ID No.:** 010-0002   **Date Admitted:** 1/31/2016
DOB: Oct 6, 1942   **Sex:** Female   **Date Discharged:** 2/5/2016

Flowsheet: Medical Report   ...   Level: Report   ● Table ○ Group ○ List

MAR | Task List | I & O | Pt. Info | Pt. Schedule | Surgery | Clinical Notes | Form Browser

Orders | Last 48 Hours | ED | Lab | Radiology | Assessments | Medical Report | Medication Profile

FINAL DIAGNOSES
1. Osteoarthritis of the right knee
2. Rheumatoid arthritis
3. Degenerative joint disease, left knee
COMPLICATIONS: Postoperative deep vein thrombosis, right lower extremity
PRINCIPAL TREATMENT RENDERED: Right total knee arthroplasty, posterior stabilized, cemented.
DISCHARGE INSTRUCTIONS: Up ad lib with full weight-bearing to right lower extremity. Ambulate with wheeled walker. Home health for physical and occupational therapy 3× weekly, and nursing visits to monitor incision and medication. Patient to change dry dressing to incision daily. Regular diet.

1. A type of arthritis that sometimes has an autoimmune component is _____ arthritis.

2. An operation to restore the integrity and function of a joint is _____.

3. Another term for degenerative arthritis is _____.

4. The right leg and foot is the right _____.

5. The term that means to walk is _____.

Abbreviating

XIX. Write a letter for an abbreviation in each blank that corresponds to the clue.

1. acute leukemia with many lymphoblasts __ __ __

2. creatine phosphokinase __ __ __

3. joint movement with maximum of 360° __ __ __

4. metatarsophalangeal __ __ __

5. resulting record is an electromyogram __ __ __

6. osteoarthritis __ __ __

Spelling

XX. Circle all misspelled terms and write their correct spelling.

adductor   anomaly   femoral   fissure   ileofemoral

Health Care Reporting

XXI. Read the following ED Visit Note and select the correct answers.

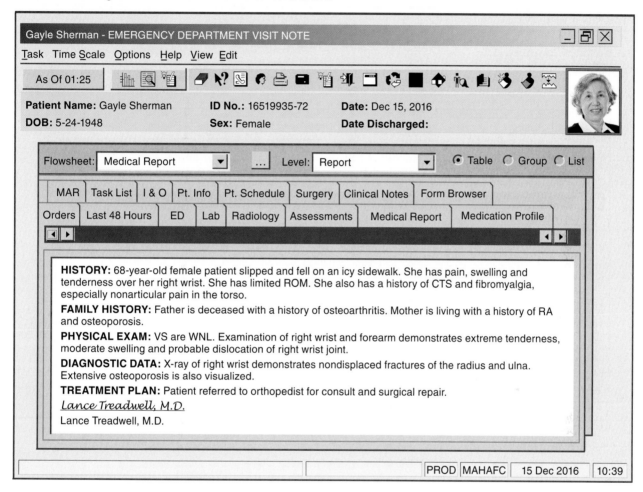

Gayle Sherman - EMERGENCY DEPARTMENT VISIT NOTE			

Task   Time Scale   Options   Help   View   Edit

As Of 01:25

Patient Name: Gayle Sherman   **ID No.:** 16519935-72   **Date:** Dec 15, 2016
DOB: 5-24-1948   **Sex:** Female   **Date Discharged:**

Flowsheet: Medical Report   ...   Level: Report   ⦿ Table   ○ Group   ○ List

| MAR | Task List | I & O | Pt. Info | Pt. Schedule | Surgery | Clinical Notes | Form Browser |
| Orders | Last 48 Hours | ED | Lab | Radiology | Assessments | Medical Report | Medication Profile |

HISTORY: 68-year-old female patient slipped and fell on an icy sidewalk. She has pain, swelling and tenderness over her right wrist. She has limited ROM. She also has a history of CTS and fibromyalgia, especially nonarticular pain in the torso.

FAMILY HISTORY: Father is deceased with a history of osteoarthritis. Mother is living with a history of RA and osteoporosis.

PHYSICAL EXAM: VS are WNL. Examination of right wrist and forearm demonstrates extreme tenderness, moderate swelling and probable dislocation of right wrist joint.

DIAGNOSTIC DATA: X-ray of right wrist demonstrates nondisplaced fractures of the radius and ulna. Extensive osteoporosis is also visualized.

TREATMENT PLAN: Patient referred to orthopedist for consult and surgical repair.

Lance Treadwell, M.D.

Lance Treadwell, M.D.

| | | PROD | MAHAFC | 15 Dec 2016 | 10:39 |

1. The abbreviation that indicates a connective tissue disease that primarily affects synovial joints is (CTS, DJD, RA, ROM)
2. Osteoarthritis refers to inflammation of a bone and a (intervertebral disk, ligament, joint, tendon).
3. Mrs. Sherman's history indicates widespread nonarticular pain in the torso. This description means that what part of the body is NOT involved? (extremities, joints, muscles, torso)
4. There is a reduction in the amount of (bone, calcaneal, medullary, muscle) mass with increased porosity in osteoporosis.
5. CTS refers to a disorder involving the (pelvis, skull, spine, wrist).

Pronouncing Terms

XXII. Use the BMV List at the end of this chapter. Write the term that corresponds to each pronunciation.

1. ahr-thrō-**klā**-zhuh   _____
2. bis-**fos**-fuh-nāts   _____
3. kon-drō-sahr-**kō**-muh   _____
4. mī-us-**thē**-nē-uh   _____
5. rā-**kis**-ki-sis   _____
6. stur-nō-**kos**-tul   _____

Health Care Reporting

XXIII. List and define/describe terms or phrases that relate to the musculoskeletal system. Try to find as many as you can before seeing the answers, using the glossary or a medical dictionary, if necessary. Challenge your classmates to see who is first to correctly identify the terms.

Prem Kamala - PREOPERATIVE HISTORY AND PHYSICAL

Task Time Scale Options Help View Edit

As Of 2:15

Patient Name: Prem Kamala   **ID No.:** 010-0001   **Date of exam:** Feb 11, 2014
DOB: 09-27-1943   **Sex:** Male   **Attending Physician:** John T. Riley, M.D.   **Date of Surgery:** Feb 12, 2014

Flowsheet: History   ...   Level: Report   ● Table ○ Group ○ List

MAR | Task List | I & O | Pt. Info | Pt. Schedule | Surgery | Clinical Notes | Form Browser

Orders | Last 48 Hours | ED | Lab | Radiology | Assessments | Medical Report | Medication Profile

HPI: 70-year-old man who fell yesterday, injuring left leg. Radiologic findings show comminuted proximal left femur fracture. Admitted for surgical repair of fracture.

ROS: A 12-point ROS is negative except for edema, left thigh. Sensation intact in left foot. Able to move left ankle and toes.

MEDICATIONS: insulin, Neurontin, Effexor, Paxil

ALLERGIES: penicillin, which causes hives and swelling of the tongue

PAST MEDICAL HISTORY: Insulin-dependent diabetes mellitus, neuropathy, herniated disk, arthralgias, depression

PAST SURGICAL HISTORY: Spinal laminectomy; right knee arthroscopy in the past

FAMILY HISTORY: Diabetes mellitus in his father; osteoporosis in his mother

1. _____
2. _____
3. _____
4. _____
5. _____
6. _____

Categorizing Terms and Practicing Pronunciation

XXIV. Categorize the terms in the left columns (1 through 10) by selecting A, B, C, D, or E.

_____	**1.** antiarthritics	_____	**6.** fibromyalgia	**A.** anatomy
_____	**2.** atrophy	_____	**7.** infrapatellar	**B.** diagnostic test or procedure
_____	**3.** bone densitometry	_____	**8.** reflex hammer	**C.** pathology
_____	**4.** calcaneofibular	_____	**9.** vertebroplasty	**D.** surgery
_____	**5.** epiphysis	_____	**10.** xiphoid process	**E.** nonsurgical therapy

(Be prepared to pronounce terms 1-10 in class after listening to the Chapter 9 terms at *http://evolve.elsevier.com/Leonard/building/*. In addition, practice categorizing all boldface terms in this chapter.) (Use Appendix IV to check your answers to the exercises.)

BMV LIST

Visit *http://evolve.elsevier.com/Leonard/building/* to listen to the boldface terms in Chapter 9. Look closely at the spelling of each term as it is pronounced.

abduction (ab-**duk**-shun)
abductor (ab-**duk**-tor)
adduction (uh-**duk**-shun)
adductor (uh-**duk**-tur)
analgesics (an-ul-**jē**-ziks)
ankylosing spondylitis (ang-kuh-**lō**-sing spon-duh-**lī**-tis)
ankylosis (ang-kuh-**lō**-sis)
antiarthritic (an-tē-ahr-**thrit**-ik)
antigout (an-tē-**gout**)
antiinflammatory (an-tē-in-**flam**-uh-tor-ē)
antinuclear antibody test (an-tē-**nōō**-klē-ur **an**-ti-bod-ē test)
anti-osteoporotics (an-tē-os-tē-ō-puh-**rot**-iks)
appendicular skeleton (ap-en-**dik**-ū-lur **skel**-uh-tun)
arthralgia (ahr-**thral**-juh)
arthrectomy (ahr-**threk**-tuh-mē)
arthritis (ahr-**thrī**-tis)
arthrocentesis (ahr-thrō-sen-**tē**-sis)
arthrochondritis (ahr-thrō-kon-**drī**-tis)
arthroclasia (ahr-thrō-**klā**-zhuh)
arthrodesis (ahr-thrō-**dē**-sis)
arthrodynia (ahr-thrō-**din**-ē-uh)
arthrogram (**ahr**-thrō-gram)
arthrography (ahr-**throg**-ruh-fē)
arthrolysis (ahr-**throl**-i-sis)
arthropathy (ahr-**throp**-uh-thē)
arthroplasty (**ahr**-thrō-plas-tē)
arthrosclerosis (ahr-thrō-skluh-**rō**-sis)
arthroscope (**ahr**-thrō-skōp)
arthroscopy (ahr-**thros**-kuh-pē)
arthrotomy (ahr-**throt**-uh-mē)
articular (ahr-**tik**-ū-lur)
articulation (ahr-tik-ū-**lā**-shun)
atrophy (**at**-ruh-fē)
auditory ossicle (**aw**-di-tor-ē **os**-i-kul)
autoimmune disease (aw-tō-i-**mūn** di-**zēz**)
autologous transplant (aw-**tol**-uh-gus **trans**-plant)
axial skeleton (**ak**-sē-ul **skel**-uh-tun)
bisphosphonates (bis-**fos**-fuh-nāts)
bone densitometry (bōn den-si-**tom**-uh-trē)
bone marrow (bōn **mar**-ō)
bone marrow aspiration (bōn **mar**-ō as-pi-**rā**-shun)
bone marrow transplant (bōn **mar**-ō **trans**-plant)
bone scan (bōn skan)
bunionectomy (bun-yun-**ek**-tuh-mē)
bursae (**bur**-sē)
bursectomy (bur-**sek**-tuh-mē)
bursitis (bur-**sī**-tis)
calcaneal (kal-**kā**-nē-ul)
calcaneitis (kal-kā-nē-**ī**-tis)
calcaneodynia (kal-kā-nē-ō-**din**-ē-uh)
calcaneofibular (kal-kā-nē-ō-**fib**-ū-lur)
calcaneoplantar (kal-kā-nē-ō-**plan**-tur)

calcaneotibial (kal-kā-nē-ō-**tib**-ē-ul)
calcaneus (kal-**kā**-nē-us)
calcification (kal-si-fi-**kā**-shun)
calcipenia (kal-si-**pē**-nē-uh)
calciuria (kal-sē-**ū**-rē-uh)
callus (**kal**-us)
cardiac muscle (**kahr**-dē-ak **mus**-ul)
carpal (**kahr**-pul)
carpal tunnel syndrome (**kahr**-pul **tun**-ul **sin**-drōm)
carpals (**kahr**-pulz)
carpectomy (kahr-**pek**-tuh-mē)
carpopedal (kahr-pō-**ped**-ul)
carpophalangeal (kahr-pō-fuh-**lan**-jē-ul)
carpus (**kahr**-pus)
cartilage (**kahr**-ti-luj)
cast (kast)
cellulitis (sel-ū-**lī**-tis)
chondral (**kon**-drul)
chondralgia (kon-**dral**-juh)
chondrectomy (kon-**drek**-tuh-mē)
chondritis (kon-**drī**-tis)
chondrocostal (kon-drō-**kos**-tul)
chondrodynia (kon-drō-**din**-ē-uh)
chondrogenic (kon-drō-**jen**-ik)
chondroid (**kon**-droid)
chondroma (kon-**drō**-muh)
chondropathy (kon-**drop**-uh-thē)
chondroplasty (**kon**-drō-plas-te)
chondrosarcoma (kon-drō-sahr-**kō**-muh)
chronic fatigue syndrome (**kron**-ik fuh-**tēg sin**-drōm)
circumduction (sur-kum-**duk**-shun)
clavicle (**klav**-i-kul)
closed fracture (klōzd **frak**-chur)
closed reduction (klōzd rē-**duk**-shun)
coccygectomy (kok-si-**jek**-tuh-mē)
coccyx (**kok**-siks)
comminuted fracture (kom-i-**nōōt**-ud **frak**-chur)
compound fracture (**kom**-pound **frak**-chur)
compression fracture (kom-**presh**-un **frak**-chur)
connective tissue (kuh-**nek**-tiv **tish**-ōō)
connective tissue disease (kuh-**nek**-tiv **tish**-ōō di-**zēz**)
corns (kornz)
costa (**kos**-tuh)
costal (**kos**-tul)
costectomy (kos-**tek**-tuh-mē)
costoclavicular (kos-tō-kluh-**vik**-ū-lur)
costovertebral (kos-tō-**vur**-tuh-brul)
cranial (**krā**-nē-ul)
craniectomy (krā-nē-**ek**-tuh-mē)
craniocele (**krā**-nē-ō-sēl)
cranioplasty (**krā**-nē-ō-plas-tē)
craniotome (**krā**-nē-ō-tōm)

craniotomy (krā-nē-**ot**-uh-mē)
cranium (**krā**-nē-um)
creatine phosphokinase (**krē**-uh-tin fos-fō-**kī**-nās)
cutaneous lupus erythematosus (kū-**tā**-nē-us l̄oo-pus
    er-uh-them-uh-**tō**-sis)
decalcification (dē-kal-si-fi-**kā**-shun)
diaphysis (dī-**af**-uh-sis)
discoid lupus erythematosus (**dis**-koid l̄oo-pus
    er-uh-them-uh-**tō**-sis)
disease-modifying antirheumatic drugs (di-**zēz** **mod**-i-fī-ing
    an-tē-r̄oo-**mat**-ik drugz)
diskectomy (dis-**kek**-tuh-mē)
dislocation (dis-lō-**kā**-shun)
dorsalgia (dor-**sal**-juh)
Dupuytren contracture (dū-pwē-**trah** kun-**trak**-chur)
dystrophy (**dis**-truh-fē)
electromyogram (ē-lek-trō-**mī**-ō-gram)
electromyography (ē-lek-trō-mī-**og**-ruh-fē)
encephalocele (en-**sef**-uh-lō-sēl)
epiphysis (uh-**pif**-uh-sis)
erythrocyte sedimentation rate (uh-**rith**-rō-sīt sed-i-mun-**tā**-
    shun rāt)
eversion (ē-**vur**-zhun)
Ewing sarcoma (**ū**-ing sahr-**kō**-muh)
extension (ek-**sten**-shun)
extensor (ek-**sten**-sor)
external fixation (ek-**stur**-nul fik-**sā**-shun)
fascia (**fash**-ē-uh)
fascial (**fash**-ē-ul)
fasciectomy (fas-ē-**ek**-tuh-mē)
femoral (**fem**-uh-rul)
femur (**fē**-mur)
fibrogenic (fī-brō-**jen**-ik)
fibromyalgia (fī-brō-mī-**al**-juh)
fibromyalgia syndrome (fī-brō-mī-**al**-juh **sin**-drōm)
fibrosarcoma (fī-brō-sahr-**kō**-muh)
fibula (**fib**-ū-luh)
fibular (**fib**-ū-lur)
fissure (**fish**-ur)
flexion (**flek**-shun)
flexor (**flek**-sor)
foramen magnum (fō-**rā**-mun **mag**-num)
fracture (**frak**-chur)
gout (gout)
greenstick fracture (**grēn**-stik **frak**-chur)
hallux valgus (**hal**-uks **val**-gus)
hammertoe (**ham**-ur-tō)
haversian canals (huh-**ver**-zhun kuh-**nalz**)
herniated disk (**hur**-nē-āt-ud disk)
humeral (**hū**-mur-ul)
humeroradial (hū-mur-ō-**rā**-dē-ul)
humeroscapular (hū-mur-ō-**skap**-ū-lur)
humeroulnar (hū-mur-ō-**ul**-nur)
humerus (**hū**-mur-us)
hypercalciuria (hī-pur-kal-sē-**ū**-rē-uh)
hypertonicity (hī-pur-tō-**nis**-i-tē)
hypotonicity (hī-pō-tō-**nis**-i-tē)

iliac (**il**-ē-ak)
iliofemoral (il-ē-ō-**fem**-uh-rul)
iliopubic (il-ē-ō-**pū**-bik)
ilium (**il**-ē-um)
impacted fracture (im-**pak**-tud **frak**-chur)
infraclavicular (in-fruh-kluh-**vik**-ū-lur)
infracostal (in-fruh-**kos**-tul)
infrapatellar (in-fruh-puh-**tel**-ur)
infrascapular (in-fruh-**skap**-ū-lur)
infrasternal (in-fruh-**stur**-nul)
intercostal (in-tur-**kos**-tul)
internal fixation (in-**tur**-nul fik-**sā**-shun)
interpubic (in-tur-**pū**-bik)
interscapular (in-tur-**skap**-ū-lur)
intervertebral (in-tur-**vur**-tuh-brul)
intervertebral disk (in-tur-**vur**-tuh-brul disk)
intraarticular (in-truh-ahr-**tik**-ū-lur)
intrasternal (in-truh-**stur**-nul)
inversion (in-**vur**-zhun)
ischial (**is**-kē-ul)
ischialgia (is-kē-**al**-juh)
ischiococcygeal (is-kē-ō-kok-**sij**-ē-ul)
ischiodynia (is-kē-ō-**din**-ē-uh)
ischiofemoral (is-kē-ō-**fem**-uh-rul)
ischiopubic (is-kē-ō-**pu**-bik)
ischium (**is**-kē-um)
joint crepitus (joint **krep**-i-tus)
kyphosis (kī-**fō**-sis)
laminectomy (lam-i-**nek**-tuh-mē)
leukemia (l̄oo-**kē**-mē-uh)
ligament (**lig**-uh-munt)
lordosis (lor-**dō**-sis)
lumbar puncture (**lum**-bur **punk**-chur)
lupus erythematosus (l̄oo-pus er-uh-them-uh-**tō**-sis)
Lyme disease (līm di-**zēz**)
lymphoblastic leukemia (lim-fō-**blas**-tik l̄oo-**kē**-mē-uh)
lymphocytic leukemia (lim-fō-**sit**-ik l̄oo-**kē**-mē-uh)
medullary cavity (**med**-uh-lar-ē **kav**-i-tē)
metacarpals (met-uh-**kahr**-pulz)
metatarsals (met-uh-**tahr**-sulz)
metatarsophalangeal joint (met-uh-tahr-sō-fuh-**lan**-jē-ul joint)
Morton neuroma (**mor**-tun noo-**rō**-muh)
multiple myeloma (**mul**-ti-pul mī-uh-**lō**-muh)
muscle relaxants (**mus**-ul rē-**lak**-sunts)
muscular (**mus**-kū-lur)
muscular dystrophy (**mus**-kū-lur **dis**-truh-fē)
musculoskeletal (mus-kū-lō-**skel**-uh-tul)
myalgia (mī-**al**-juh)
myasthenia (mī-us-**thē**-nē-uh)
myasthenia gravis (mī-us-**thē**-nē-uh **grav**-is)
myelitis (mī-uh-**lī**-tis)
myeloblast (**mī**-uh-lō-blast)
myelocyte (**mī**-uh-lō-sīt)
myelocytic leukemia (mī-uh-lō-**sit**-ik l̄oo-**kē**-mē-uh)
myelogenous leukemia (mī-uh-**loj**-uh-nus l̄oo-**kē**-mē-uh)
myelosuppression (mī-uh-lō-suh-**presh**-un)
myelosuppressive (mī-uh-lō-suh-**pres**-iv)

myoblast (**mī**-ō-blast)
myocardium (mī-ō-**kahr**-dē-um)
myocele (**mī**-ō-sēl)
myocellulitis (mī-ō-sel-ū-**lī**-tis)
myodynia (mī-ō-**din**-ē-uh)
myofascial (mī-ō-**fash**-ē-ul)
myofibrosis (mī-ō-fī-**brō**-sis)
myolysis (mī-**ol**-i-sis)
myomalacia (mī-ō-muh-**lā**-shuh)
myopathy (mī-**op**-uh-thē)
myoplasty (**mī**-ō-plas-tē)
myorrhaphy (mī-**or**-uh-fē)
neuromuscular blocking drugs (noor-ō-**mus**-kū-lur **blok**-ing drugz)
nonarticular (non-ahr-**tik**-ū-lur)
open fracture (**ō**-pun **frak**-chur)
open reduction (**ō**-pun rē-**duk**-shun)
orthopedics (or-thō-**pē**-diks)
orthopedist (or-thō-**pē**-dist)
ossification (os-i-fi-**kā**-shun)
ostealgia (os-tē-**al**-juh)
ostectomy (os-**tek**-tuh-mē)
osteectomy (os-tē-**ek**-tuh-mē)
osteitis (os-tē-**ī**-tis)
osteitis deformans (os-tē-**ī**-tis di-**for**-mans)
osteoarthritis (os-tē-ō-ahr-**thrī**-tis)
osteoarthropathy (os-tē-ō-ahr-**throp**-uh-thē)
osteoblast (**os**-tē-ō-blast)
osteochondritis (os-tē-ō-kon-**drī**-tis)
osteochondroma (os-tē-ō-kon-**drō**-muh)
osteocyte (**os**-tē-ō-sīt)
osteodynia (os-tē-ō-**din**-ē-uh)
osteogenesis (os-tē-ō-**jen**-uh-sis)
osteogenic (os-tē-ō-**jen**-ik)
osteolysis (os-tē-**ol**-uh-sis)
osteomalacia (os-tē-ō-muh-**lā**-shuh)
osteomyelitis (os-tē-ō-mī-uh-**lī**-tis)
osteopenia (os-tē-ō-**pē**-nē-uh)
osteoplasty (**os**-tē-ō-plas-tē)
osteoporosis (os-tē-ō-puh-**rō**-sis)
osteosarcoma (os-tē-ō-sahr-**kō**-muh)
osteosclerosis (os-tē-ō-skluh-**rō**-sis)
osteotome (**os**-tē-ō-tōm)
Paget disease (**paj**-et di-**zēz**)
patella (puh-**tel**-uh)
patellofemoral (puh-tel-ō-**fem**-uh-rul)
pelvic girdle (**pel**-vik **gir**-dul)
perichondrial (per-i-**kon**-drē-ul)
perichondrium (per-i-**kon**-drē-um)
periosteum (per-ē-**os**-tē-um)
phalangectomy (fal-un-**jek**-tuh-mē)
phalanges (fuh-**lan**-jēz)
plantar (**plan**-tur)
polyarthritis (pol-ē-ahr-**thrī**-tis)
polydactylism (pol-ē-**dak**-tul-iz-um)
polydactyly (pol-ē-**dak**-tuh-lē)
polymyalgia (pol-ē-mī-**al**-juh)

polymyalgia rheumatica (pol-ē-mī-**al**-juh rōō-**mat**-ik-uh)
polymyositis (pol-ē-mī-ō-**sī**-tis)
pronation (prō-**nā**-shun)
pubes (**pū**-bēz)
pubic (**pū**-bik)
pubic symphysis (**pū**-bik **sim**-fi-sis)
pubis (**pū**-bis)
pubofemoral (pū-bō-**fem**-uh-rul)
rachialgia (rā-kē-**al**-juh)
rachiodynia (rā-kē-ō-**din**-ē-uh)
rachischisis (rā-**kis**-ki-sis)
radius (**rā**-dē-us)
reduction (rē-**duk**-shun)
reflex hammer (**rē**-fleks **ham**-ur)
retrosternal (ret-rō-**stur**-nul)
rheumatoid arthritis (**rōō**-muh-toid ahr-**thrī**-tis)
rheumatoid factor (**rōō**-muh-toid **fak**-tur)
rickets (**rik**-uts)
rotation (rō-**tā**-shun)
rotator (**rō**-tā-tur)
sacrodynia (sā-krō-**din**-ē-uh)
sacrum (**sā**-krum)
scapula (**skap**-ū-luh)
scapular (**skap**-ū-lur)
scapuloclavicular (skap-ū-lō-kluh-**vik**-ū-lur)
scoliosis (skō-lē-**ō**-sis)
shoulder girdle (**shōl**-dur **gir**-dul)
simple fracture (**sim**-pul **frak**-chur)
Sjögren syndrome (**shō**-grun **sin**-drōm)
skeletal (**skel**-uh-tul)
skeletal muscle (**skel**-uh-tul **mus**-ul)
spina bifida (**spī**-nuh **bif**-i-duh)
spinal (**spī**-nul)
spiral fracture (**spī**-rul **frak**-chur)
splint (splint)
spondylalgia (spon-di-**lal**-juh)
spondylarthritis (spon-dul-ahr-**thrī**-tis)
spondylarthropathy (spon-duh-lō-ahr-**throp**-uh-thē)
spondylosyndesis (spon-duh-lō-sin-**dē**-sis)
sprain (sprān)
sternal (**stur**-nul)
sternalgia (stur-**nal**-juh)
sternoclavicular (stur-nō-kluh-**vik**-ū-lur)
sternocostal (stur-nō-**kos**-tul)
sternoschisis (stur-**nos**-ki-sis)
sternotomy (stur-**not**-uh-mē)
sternovertebral (stur-nō-**vur**-tuh-brul)
sternum (**stur**-num)
strain (strān)
subcostal (sub-**kos**-tul)
subpubic (sub-**pū**-bik)
substernal (sub-**stur**-nul)
supination (sōō-pi-**nā**-shun)
supracostal (sōō-pruh-**kos**-tul)
suprapubic (sōō-pruh-**pū**-bik)
suprasternal (sōō-pruh-**stur**-nul)
syndactylism (sin-**dak**-tuh-liz-um)

syndactyly (sin-**dak**-tuh-lē)
synovial joint (si-**nō**-vē-ul joint)
synovitis (si-nō-**vī**-tis)
systemic lupus erythematosus (sis-**tem**-ik l̄oo-pus
    er-uh-them-uh-**tō**-sis)
systemic scleroderma (sis-**tem**-ik sklēr-ō-**dur**-muh)
systemic sclerosis (sis-**tem**-ik skluh-**rō**-sis)
tarsal (**tahr**-sul)
tarsal tunnel syndrome (**tahr**-sul **tun**-ul **sin**-drōm)
tarsals (**tahr**-sulz)
tarsoptosis (tahr-sop-**tō**-sis)
tarsus (**tahr**-sus)
temporomandibular joint (tem-puh-rō-man-**dib**-ū-lur joint)
tenalgia (tē-**nal**-juh)
tendinitis (ten-di-**nī**-tis)
tendon (**ten**-dun)
tendonitis (ten-duh-**nī**-tis)
tendoplasty (**ten**-dō-plas-tē)
tenodynia (ten-ō-**din**-ē-uh)
tenomyoplasty (ten-ō-**mī**-ō-plas-tē)
tenorrhaphy (tuh-**nor**-uh-fē)
tenotomy (tuh-**not**-uh-mē)

tetany (**tet**-uh-nē)
thoracic (thuh-**ras**-ik)
thoracolumbar (thor-uh-kō-**lum**-bur)
tibia (**tib**-ē-uh)
tibialgia (tib-ē-**al**-juh)
tibiofemoral (tib-ē-ō-**fem**-or-ul)
trabeculae (truh-**bek**-ū-lē)
traction (**trak**-shun)
transverse fracture (trans-**vers frak**-chur)
ulna (**ul**-nuh)
ulnoradial (ul-nō-**rā**-dē-ul)
uricosurics (ū-ri-kō-**sū**-riks)
vertebra (**vur**-tuh-bruh)
vertebrae (**vur**-tuh-brē)
vertebral column (**vur**-tuh-brul **kol**-um)
vertebrectomy (vur-tuh-**brek**-tuh-mē)
vertebrochondral (vur-tuh-brō-**kon**-drul)
vertebrocostal (vur-tuh-brō-**kos**-tul)
vertebroplasty (**vur**-tuh-brō-plas-tē)
vertebrosternal (vur-tuh-brō-**stur**-nul)
visceral muscle (**vis**-ur-ul **mus**-ul)
xiphoid process (**zif**-oid, **zī**-foid **pros**-us)

Español ENHANCING SPANISH COMMUNICATION

English	Spanish (Pronunciation)
ankle	tobillo (to-BEEL-lyo)
back	espalda (es-PAHL-dah)
bones	huesos (oo-AY-sos)
calcium	calcio (KAHL-se-o)
cartilage	cartílago (kar-TEE-lah-go)
cheek	mejilla (may-HEEL-lyah)
chew, to	masticar (mas-te-KAR)
collarbone	clavícula (klah-VEE-koo-lah)
cranium	cráneo (KRAH-nay-o)
elbow	codo (KO-do)
extremity	extremidad (ex-tray-me-DAHD)
forearm	antebrazo (an-tay-BRAH-so)
fracture	fractura (frak-TOO-rah)
heel	talón (tah-LON)
jaw	mandíbula (man-DEE-boo-lah)
joint	articulacíon (ar-te-koo-lah-se-ON), coyuntura (ko-yoon-TOO-rah)
knee	rodilla (ro-DEEL-lyah)
kneecap	rótula (RO-too-lah)
ligament	ligamento (le-gah-MEN-to)
movement	movimiento (mo-ve-me-EN-to)
neck	cuello (koo-EL-lyo)
phalanges	falanges (fah-LAHN-hays)

English	Spanish (Pronunciation)
phosphorus	fósforo (FOS-fo-ro)
reduction	reducción (ray-dook-se-ON)
sacrum	hueso sacro (oo-AY-so SAH-kro)
shoulder	hombro (OM-bro)
shoulder blade	espaldilla (es-pal-DEEL-lyah)
skeleton	esqueleto (es-kay-LAY-to)
spinal column	columna vertebral (ko-LOOM-nah ver-tay-BRAHL)
spine	espinazo (es-pe-NAH-so)
spiral	espiral (es-pe-RAHL)
sprain, to	torcer (tor-SERR)
sternum	esternón (es-ter-NON)
stiff	tieso (te-AY-so)
support	sustento (sus-TEN-to)
tear	lágrima de los ojos (LAH-gre-mah day los O-hos)
temple	sien (se-AYN)
tendon	tendón (ten-DON)
thumb	pulgar (pool-GAR)
toe	dedo del pie (DAY-do del pe-AY)
vertebral column	columna vertebral (ko-LOOM-nah ver-tay-BRAHL)
weakness	debilidad (day-be-le-DAHD)

Nervous System

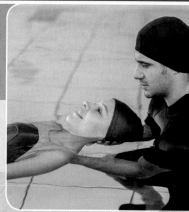

Aquatic physical therapy or pool therapy uses the benefits of heat and the buoyancy of water to reduce the stress on joints and assist in healing and strengthening of muscles in stroke survivors, or of persons with osteoarthritis, and those recovering from shoulder, hip, or knee replacement.

LEARNING OUTCOMES

Basic Understanding

In this chapter, you will learn to do the following:

1. State the function of the nervous system, and analyze associated terms.
2. Write the meaning of word parts associated with the nervous system, and use them to build and analyze terms.
3. Distinguish between the structures of the central nervous system and those of the peripheral nervous system, and define the terms associated with these structures.
4. Write the names of the diagnostic tests and procedures for assessment of the nervous system when given their descriptions, or match the procedures with the descriptions.
5. Write the names of nervous system pathologies when given their descriptions, or match the pathologies with their descriptions.
6. Write the names of psychologic disorders when given their descriptions, or match the disorders with their descriptions.
7. Write the terms for surgical and therapeutic interventions for nervous system pathologies and psychologic disorders when given their descriptions, or match the interventions with their descriptions.
8. Build terms from word parts to label illustrations.

Greater Comprehension

9. Use word parts from this chapter to determine the meaning of terms in a health care report.
10. Spell the terms accurately.
11. Pronounce the terms correctly.
12. Write the meaning of the abbreviations.
13. Categorize terms as anatomy, diagnostic test or procedure, pathology, surgery, or nonsurgical therapy.
14. Recognize the meanings of general pharmacological terms from this chapter as well as the drug classes and their uses.

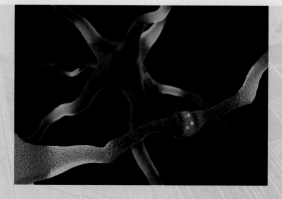

FUNCTION FIRST

The nervous system is the body's control center and communications network. It performs these functions:

- stimulates movement
- senses changes both within and outside the body
- provides us with thought, learning, and memory
- maintains homeostasis (a dynamic equilibrium of the internal environment of the body) along with the help of the hormonal system.

The nervous system keeps the other body systems coordinated, and its activities can be grouped as sensory functions (receptors detect changes inside and outside the body), integrative functions (create sensations, produce thoughts and memory, and make decisions), and motor functions (enable us to respond to a stimulus).

ANATOMY AND PHYSIOLOGY

nerve

10-1 The nervous system is the network of structures that activates, coordinates, and controls all functions of the body. The terms **nervous** and **neur/al** mean pertaining to a _____ or the nerves, but the nervous system includes the brain and spinal cord as well as the nerves.

10-2 The nervous system is the body's most organized and complex system. It affects both psychologic and physiologic functions. In addition to being the center of thinking and judgment, the nervous system influences other body systems. For example, damage to the spinal nerves that supply nerve impulses to the diaphragm may result in respiratory arrest.

Organization of the Nervous System

10-3 There are two principal divisions of the nervous system (Fig. 10.1):

- **central nervous system** (CNS): Brain and spinal cord
- **peripheral nervous system** (PNS): Various nerves and nerve masses that connect the brain and spinal cord with receptors, muscles, and glands

central

CNS is an abbreviation for _____ nervous system.

peripheral

PNS is an abbreviation for _____ nervous system.

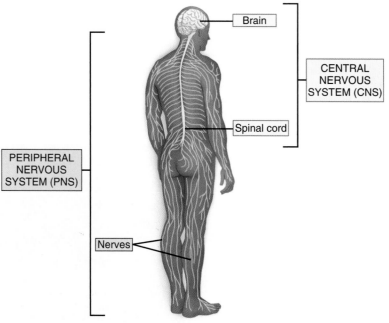

Figure 10.1 A simplified view of the nervous system.

> ➤ **BEYOND** THE BLUEPRINT The brain has an anatomic feature, the blood–brain barrier, which prevents or slows the passage of chemical compounds, toxins, pathogens, microorganisms, and some drugs. For example, penicillin can be used to treat infections in other parts of the body but cannot cross the blood–brain barrier.

WRITE IT!   EXERCISE 1

Write words in the blanks to complete the following.

1. List four functions of the nervous system: _____

_____

2. The various activities of the nervous system can be grouped as detecting changes, producing thoughts and making decisions, and causing an effect in muscles or glands. What are the names of these three activities?

_____, _____, and _____ functions

3. Name the two principal divisions of the nervous system: _____

and _____.

---

efferent

afferent

nerve

WORD ORIGIN
glia *(G.)*
glia, glue

10-4 Observe the two divisions of the CNS in Fig. 10.2, the brain and spinal cord. You also see that the PNS is divided into two systems: the sensory or **afferent system** and the motor or **efferent system.** Which of these two systems, afferent or efferent, conveys information from the CNS to muscles and glands? _____

Which system, afferent or efferent, conveys information from the receptors to the CNS? _____.

10-5 The nervous system is composed of two types of cells: neurons and neuroglia. Both types of cells that comprise nervous tissue are named using neur(o), which means _____.

Neurons conduct impulses either to or from the CNS. **Neuroglia,** or **glia cells,** provide special support and protection. If a neuron is destroyed, it cannot replace itself. However, neuroglia are far more numerous and, because they can reproduce, are the only source of primary malignant brain tumors, those originating in the brain.

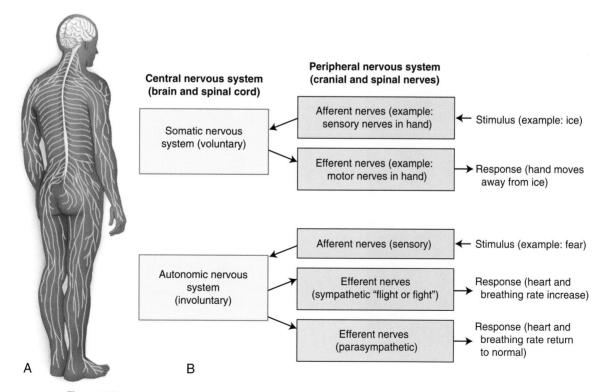

Figure 10.2 Divisions of the nervous system. A, The central nervous system (CNS) *(yellow)* includes the brain and spinal cord. The peripheral nervous system (PNS) *(blue)* is made up of nerves that take impulses away from and toward the CNS to receptors, muscles, and glands. **B,** Schematic drawing of the interrelationship of the CNS and PNS.

Learn the following word parts.

Word Parts: Cells of the Nervous System

Combining Form	Meaning
dendr(o)	tree
gli(o)	neuroglia or a sticky substance
nerv(o), neur(o)	nerve

Write the combining form(s) for these meanings.

1. nerve   _____

2. neuroglia   _____

3. tree   _____

10-6 The neuron, or nerve cell, is the basic unit of the nervous system. Neurons carry out the function of the nervous system by conducting nerve impulses. Each neuron has a cell body, a single **axon,** and one or more **dendrites** (Fig. 10.3).

axon

The axon and dendrites are cytoplasmic projections, or processes, that extend from the cell body. They are sometimes called *nerve fibers.* An axon carries impulses away from the cell body. Dendrites transmit impulses to the cell body. Which type of cytoplasmic projection carries a nervous impulse away from the cell body? _____

dendrite

The combining form dendr(o) means tree. Which type of cytoplasmic projection has numerous branches? _____

10-7 Many axons are surrounded by a white lipid covering called a **myelin sheath.** The myelinated axons appear whitish and are called *white matter.* Those that are not myelinated appear grayish

gray

and are called _____ matter.

In a myelinated fiber, the nerve impulse "jumps" from one **node of Ranvier** (see Fig. 10.3, B) to the next and results in a faster rate of conduction than in an unmyelinated nerve fiber. If the myelin sheath becomes damaged, as it does in certain diseases (such as multiple sclerosis [MS]), conduction of the impulse is impaired.

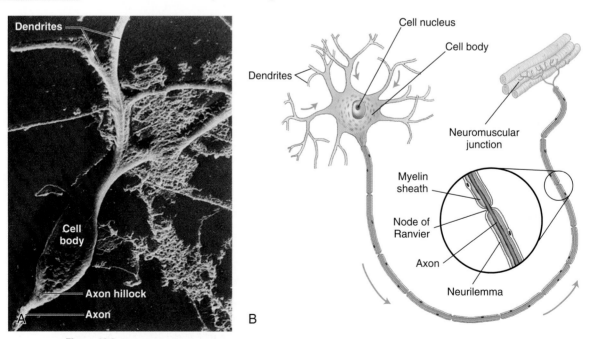

Figure 10.3 Structure of a typical neuron. A, Micrograph of a neuron with labeled nerve processes: dendrites and an axon. The axon hillock is its point of attachment to the nerve cell. **B,** The basic parts of a neuron are the cell body, a single axon, and several dendrites. Arrows indicate the direction that an impulse travels to or from the cell body. Some axons are surrounded by a segmented myelin sheath. The myelinated regions provide much faster conduction of the nerve impulse than parts of the axon that are not myelinated.

🔑 **KEY** POINT The region of communication between one neuron and another is called the **synapse**. An axon terminates in several short branches that together form a **synaptic bulb.** The synaptic bulb releases a chemical neurotransmitter that either inhibits or enhances a nervous impulse.

Some of the best known neurotransmitters are **acetylcholine** (ACh), **epinephrine, dopamine, serotonin,** and **endorphins.** To prevent prolonged reactions, a neurotransmitter is quickly inactivated by an enzyme.

nerves

10-8 Neuro/muscul/ar means concerning both _____ and muscles.

🔑 **KEY** POINT A neuro/muscular junction is the area of contact between a neuron and adjoining skeletal muscle. When a nerve impulse reaches the neuromuscular junction, ACh is released, which leads to contraction of the muscle. ACh acts rapidly on muscle tissue, and most of it is then promptly inactivated by an enzyme, **acetylcholinester/ase.** Certain drugs can block transmission of impulses to the skeletal muscle. The transmission is blocked at the neuromuscular junction.

10-9 Conduction of nervous impulses is often described as a **reflex arc.** A reflex is an automatic, involuntary response to some change, which is either inside or outside the body. Reflexes help maintain homeostasis by making constant adjustments to our blood pressure, breathing rate, and pulse. A common reflex is that of quickly removing your hand from a hot object.

A **deep tendon reflex** (DTR) is one way of assessing the reflex arc. For example, a sharp tap on the tendon just below the kneecap normally causes extension of the leg at the knee. This is called the **patellar response** or knee jerk response. A normal response indicates an intact reflex arc between the nervous system and the muscles that are involved in the response. Other areas are also assessed for reflex activities. An automatic, involuntary response to some change, either inside

reflex

or outside the body, is called a _____.

10-10 The reflex arc involves two types of neurons: a sensory neuron and a motor neuron. **Sensory neurons** transmit nerve impulses toward the spinal cord and the brain. **Motor neurons** transmit nerve impulses from the brain and the spinal cord (Fig. 10.4).

motor

Note that the _____ neuron causes the muscle to contract.

WRITE IT! **EXERCISE 3**

Write words in the blanks to complete these sentences.
1. The PNS is divided into the afferent or _____ system and the motor system.
2. The CNS is divided into the _____ and spinal cord.
3. Name the two types of cells of the nervous system: _____ and _____, or glial cells.
4. Name the two types of cytoplasmic projections of a basic nerve cell: _____ and _____.
5. Acetylcholinesterase is an enzyme that inactivates _____.
6. DTR is the abbreviation for deep tendon _____.
7. Motor _____ transmit nerve impulses from the brain to the spinal cord.

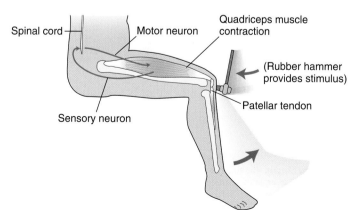

Spinal cord
Motor neuron
Quadriceps muscle contraction
(Rubber hammer provides stimulus)
Patellar tendon
Sensory neuron

Figure 10.4 Conceptual drawing of the reflex arc. A receptor detects the stimulus, the tap on the patellar tendon with the reflex hammer. The sensory neuron transmits the nerve impulse to the spinal cord. The motor neuron conducts a nervous impulse that causes the quadriceps muscle to contract. Extension of the leg at the knee, also called *knee jerk,* is the normal patellar response.

Central Nervous System

10-11 The brain is that part of the CNS contained within the skull. This soft mass of tissue weighs approximately 1360 grams (3 pounds) in the average adult, receives thousands of bits of information, and integrates all the data to determine the appropriate response. The brain is surrounded by the **cranium** (skull), and the spinal cord is protected by the vertebrae. In addition to the skull and vertebrae, the brain and spinal cord are protected by three membranes called **meninges** and circulating **cerebrospinal fluid** (CSF). The singular form of meninges is meninx.

Learn the following word parts.

Word Parts: Central Nervous System

Combining Form	Meaning
arachn(o)	spider or arachnoid (a meningeal membrane)
cerebell(o)	cerebellum
cerebr(o), encephal(o)	brain (cerebr[o] sometimes means cerebrum)
myel(o)	spinal cord (sometimes means bone marrow)
mening(i), mening(o)	meninges

WRITE IT!
EXERCISE 4

Write the meanings of the following.

1. arachn(o) _____
2. cerebell(o) _____
3. cerebr(o) _____

4. mening(o) _____
5. myel(o) _____

10-12 The meninges enclose the brain and the spinal cord (Fig. 10.5). **Meningeal** means pertaining to the meninges.

🔑 **KEY POINT Remember the three meningeal layers.** The tough outer layer, the **dura mater,** lies just inside the cranial bones and lines the vertebral canal. The middle layer is the **arachnoid,** a thin layer with numerous threadlike strands that attach it to the innermost layer. The combining form arachn(o) means either the arachnoid membrane or spider. The innermost layer, the **pia mater,** is thin and delicate and is tightly attached to the surface of the brain and spinal cord. (dura mater *[L.] durus,* hard; *mater,* mother. pia *[L.] pia,* tender)

dura
pia

The outer layer is the _____ mater. The middle layer is the arachnoid, and the innermost layer is the _____ mater.

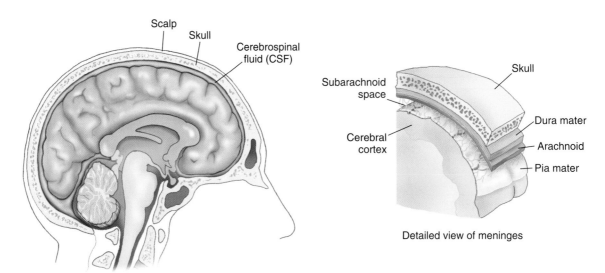

Scalp
Skull
Cerebrospinal fluid (CSF)
Subarachnoid space
Cerebral cortex
Skull
Dura mater
Arachnoid
Pia mater

Detailed view of meninges

Figure 10.5 The brain and its protective coverings, the meninges. The tough outer membrane, the dura mater, lies just inside the skull. The threadlike strands of the middle layer, the arachnoid, resemble a cobweb. The pia mater is the innermost meningeal layer and is so tightly bound to the brain that it cannot be removed without damaging the surface.

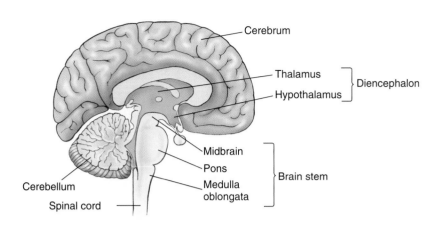

Figure 10.6 **Midsagittal view of the principal structures of the brain.** The brain stem consists of the midbrain, the pons, and the medulla. Its lower end is a continuation of the spinal cord. The diencephalon is above the brain stem and consists of the thalamus and the hypothalamus. The cerebrum is about seven eighths of the total weight of the brain and spreads over the diencephalon. The cerebellum is inferior to the cerebrum.

below (or beneath)

10-13 Sub/dural means _____ the dura mater, so it refers to the area between the dura mater and the arachnoid. The potential space between these two membranes is the **subdural space.**

10-14 The brain consists of several parts: the cerebrum, diencephalon, brain stem, and cerebellum (Fig. 10.6). The **cerebellum** lies just under the cerebrum, the largest portion of the brain. The **thalamus** and **hypothalamus** are parts of the _____.

diencephalon

stem

> WORD ORIGIN
> foramen *(L.)*
> *foramina,* hole

The **midbrain, pons,** and **medulla** are parts of the **brain** _____. The medulla is continuous with the spinal cord at an opening in the skull called the **foramen magnum.**

10-15 The **cerebrum** is the largest and uppermost portion of the brain, and the combining form cerebr(o) means either the cerebrum or the brain in general. The cerebrum is concerned with interpretation of impulses and all voluntary muscle activities. It is the center of higher mental faculties.

cerebrum

cranium (skull)

Cerebr/al means pertaining to the _____.
Craniocerebral means pertaining to the _____ and the cerebrum.

10-16 A longitudinal fissure almost completely divides the cerebrum into two **cerebral hemispheres** (hemi-means half). The surface of each hemisphere (right and left) is covered with a convoluted layer of gray matter called the **cerebral cortex.** Division of the cortex into lobes provides useful reference points (Fig. 10.7).

frontal

The lobe that is located near the front of the cerebrum is the _____ **lobe.**

temporal

The regions of the head in front of the ears are known as the *temples.* The parts of the cerebrum that are located in the areas of the temples are called the _____ **lobes.**

occipital

parietal

Occipital is an adjective that means concerning the back part of the head. The lobe that is located at the back of the head, just behind the temporal lobe, is the _____ **lobe.**
Another lobe, just above the occipital lobe, is the _____ **lobe.** The lobe deep within the brain is the **insula.**

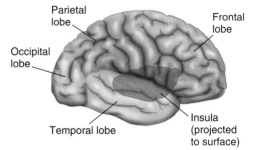

Figure 10.7 **Lateral view of the cerebrum.** The surface of the cerebrum is marked by convolutions. The pia mater closely follows the convolutions and goes deep into the grooves (sulci). Each cerebral hemisphere is divided into five lobes: the frontal lobe, the parietal lobe, the occipital lobe, the temporal lobe, and an insula that is covered by parts of the other lobes.

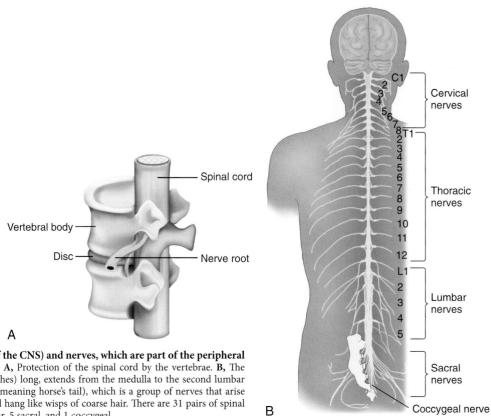

Figure 10.8 **The spinal cord (part of the CNS) and nerves, which are part of the peripheral nervous system, emerging from it. A,** Protection of the spinal cord by the vertebrae. **B,** The spinal cord, about 44 cm (16 to 18 inches) long, extends from the medulla to the second lumbar vertebra. It ends as the cauda equina (meaning horse's tail), which is a group of nerves that arise from the lower portion of the cord and hang like wisps of coarse hair. There are 31 pairs of spinal nerves: 8 cervical, 12 thoracic, 5 lumbar, 5 sacral, and 1 coccygeal.

> **BEYOND** THE BLUEPRINT Note that different lobes are associated with different functions. The frontal lobes are associated with personality, behavior, emotion, and intellectual functions. The temporal lobes are associated with hearing and smell, the occipital lobes are associated with vision, and the parietal lobes are associated with language and the general function of sensation.

10-17 The **spinal cord** is a cylindric structure located in the canal of the vertebral column Fig. 10.8, A. Thirty-one pairs of spinal nerves arise from the spinal cord and are named and numbered according to the region and level of the spinal cord from which they emerge (Fig. 10.8, B).

within

10-18 Intra/thecal means _____ a sheath (such as, the spinal canal). An intrathecal injection is an injection into the subarachnoid space (between the arachnoid and pia mater membranes) for diffusion of a contrast material throughout the spinal fluid (see lumbar puncture, Fig. 9.25).

WORD ORIGIN
intrathecal *(L.)*
intra, within;
theca, sheath

brain

10-19 In addition to the protection offered by the meninges, CSF surrounds and cushions the spinal cord and brain. **Cerebro/spinal** means pertaining to the _____ and the spinal cord.
    CSF is formed in the ventricles, which are four cavities in the brain. The fluid circulates through the ventricles, the subarachnoid space, and the central canal of the spinal cord. Cavities in the brain that produce CSF are called **cerebral** _____.

ventricles

cerebellum

10-20 Cerebell/ar pertains to the _____.

ANALYZE IT! EXERCISE 5	*Break these words into their component parts by placing a slash between the word parts. Write the meaning of each term.* **1.** cerebrospinal _____ **2.** craniocerebral _____ **3.** meningeal _____ **4.** neuromuscular _____ **5.** subdural _____

Peripheral Nervous System

10-21 The PNS is that portion of the nervous system that is outside the CNS. **Peripheral** means located away from the center. The PNS is located away from the nervous system control center.

🔑 **KEY POINT** **The PNS forms the communication network between the CNS and the rest of the body.** The PNS consists of the nerves that branch out from the brain and spinal cord, which communicate with the rest of the receptors, muscles, and glands. It is further divided into the **sensory** (afferent) and **motor** (efferent) **systems.** Special sense organs (for example, the eyes, ears and nose) have receptors that detect sensations, and then sensory neurons transmit the information to the CNS. Motor neurons carry impulses that initiate muscle contraction.

sciatic

The **sciatic nerve** is actually two nerves bound together by a common sheath of connective tissue but is collectively called the *sciatic nerve*. It is often considered to be the largest nerve in the body, arising from spinal nerves on either side, and is called the _____ nerve. It supplies the entire musculature of the leg and foot. Irritation or injury to this nerve causes pain, often from the thigh down its branches into the toes. Neuralgia along the course of the sciatic nerve is called *sciatica*.

sensory

10-22 Receptors are sensory nerve endings that respond to various kinds of stimulation. The awareness that results from the stimulation is what we know as sensation. The major senses are sight, hearing, smell, taste, and touch. Receptors are _____ nerve endings. (See Chapter 11 for more information.)

The PNS consists of nerves that connect with **somatic** tissues (skin and muscles that are involved in conscious activities) and also nerves that link the CNS to **autonomic** tissues (the visceral organs, such as the stomach and heart, which function without conscious effort). These further divisions of the PNS are illustrated in Fig. 10.9.

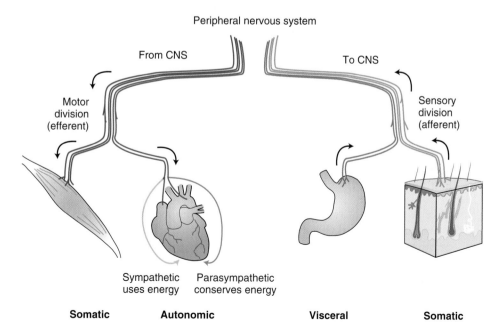

Figure 10.9 Schematic drawing of the divisions of the peripheral nervous system (PNS). The motor (efferent) division is subdivided into the somatic and autonomic systems. The sensory (afferent) division is subdivided into the visceral and somatic systems.

The autonomic system regulates and coordinates visceral activities without our conscious effort. This helps maintain a stable internal environment. The autonomic system has two divisions, the sympathetic and parasympathetic nervous systems.

autonomic

10-23 **Sympathetic** and **parasympathetic** systems are divisions of the _____ nervous system. In general, impulses transmitted by the nerve fibers of one division stimulate an organ, whereas impulses from the other division either decrease or halt organ activity.

Activation of the sympathetic division causes a series of physiologic responses called the *fight-or-flight response*. These responses increase the heart and breathing rates and prepare the body for fighting off danger. When danger is past, which system would counteract these responses?

parasympathetic

_____ system

10-24 Sympathetic and parasympathetic nerve fibers, like other axons of the nervous system, release neurotransmitters and are classified on the basis of the substance produced. **Cholinergic** fibers release acetylcholine. **Adrenergic** fibers release epinephrine. (Epinephrine is also called **adrenaline;** hence the term adren/ergic.)

acetylcholine
epinephrine

Cholinergic fibers release _____.
Adrenergic fibers release _____.

WRITE IT! **EXERCISE 6**

Write words in the blanks to complete the following.

1. The _____ nervous system forms the communication between the CNS and the rest of the body.
2. The PNS connects with both _____ and autonomic tissues.
3. Sensory nerve endings that respond to stimuli are called _____.
4. Cholinergic fibers release _____.
5. Adrenergic fibers release _____.

 ## DIAGNOSTIC TESTS AND PROCEDURES

10-25 Consciousness is responsiveness of the mind to the impressions made by the senses. A change in the level of consciousness may be the first indication of a decline in CNS function. Memory, another means of assessing neurologic function, is classified as long-term, recent, and immediate memory. Loss of memory is often an early sign of neurologic problems.

The **Glasgow Coma Scale** is a standardized system for assessing the degree of conscious impairment in the critically ill (especially those with head injuries) and for predicting the duration and ultimate outcome of coma. The system involves determination of the degree of eye opening, verbal response, and motor response.

KEY POINT **Levels of consciousness are a cognitive function involving arousal mechanisms of the brain.** The levels of consciousness include alert wakefulness (normal); response to stimuli, although it may be slow; drowsiness; **stupor** (patient is vaguely aware of the environment); and **coma** (patient does not appear to be aware of the environment).

consciousness

The various stages of response of the mind to stimuli are called the levels of _____.

10-26 A number of radiographic examinations are available to assess the nervous system. Plain x-ray studies of the skull and spine are often helpful in diagnosing fractures, abnormal curvatures, or other bony abnormalities.

Computed tomography (CT) and magnetic resonance imaging (MRI) are used to assess structural changes of the brain and spinal cord. CT is particularly helpful in detecting intracranial bleeding, lesions, and cerebral edema (see Fig. 2.38).

brain

Encephalo/graphy is radiography of the _____. It is accomplished by withdrawal and replacement of the CSF by a gas. Because of the risks involved, it is generally used only when results of CT and MRI are not definitive.

Sleep studies are not invasive and are used to diagnose sleep disorders such as **sleep apnea,** which is a sleep disorder characterized by short periods in which respiration is absent. These tests are performed in a sleep laboratory where the patient is monitored electronically (including electroencephalography [EEG] as well as recording heart and respiration rates) while sleeping. The patient must be very quiet or asleep during EEG (see Fig. 10.12).

10-27 Positron emission tomography (PET) is a computerized nuclear medicine technique that uses radioactive substances to assess the function of various body structures, particularly the brain.

> 🔑 **KEY** POINT **The PET equipment constructs color-coded images that indicate the intensity of metabolic activity.** The patient either inhales or is injected with radioactive material. The positrons of the injected material are absorbed by body cells and the equipment constructs color-coded images of the gamma rays that result. The radioactivity used in PET is short lived, so patients are exposed to only small amounts of radiation.

function

An important advantage of PET is that it assesses _____, whereas most radiographic imaging studies of the brain assess structure.

10-28 Deep tendon reflex (DTR) and superficial reflex are used to assess neurologic and muscular damage. A DTR, a brisk contraction of a muscle in response to a sharp tap by a finger or rubber hammer on a tendon, is often helpful in diagnosing a stroke (Fig. 10.10). A **superficial reflex** is evaluated by stimulation of the skin, such as stroking the sole of the foot to evaluate the response.

tendon

The two types of reflex that are easily tested are the deep _____ reflex and the superficial reflex.

10-29 In a lumbar puncture (see Fig. 9.25), the pressure of the CSF can be measured and a sample of fluid may be withdrawn for analysis (measurement of protein, glucose, and other chemicals, RBCs, WBCs, or detection of microorganisms, as well as tumor cells). In addition, intrathecal

cerebrospinal

medicines can be administered. CSF means the _____ fluid.

10-30 Brain scans include CT, MRI, and PET scans. Using contrast materials, both CT and MRI provide images of the brain and spinal cord. PET scans are especially helpful in detecting malignancies and evaluating brain abnormalities. CT, MRI, and PET scans all represent brain

scans

_____.

Doppler ultrasound studies are helpful in studying blood flow in the intracranial arteries, as well as the carotids (that supply blood to the head and neck).

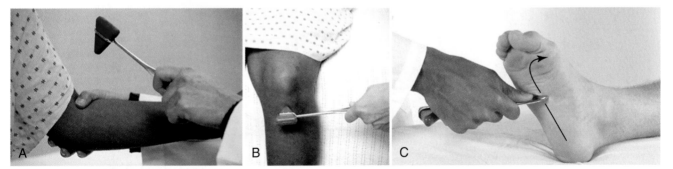

Figure 10.10 Deep tendon reflex (A and B) versus superficial reflex (C). A, Biceps reflex. The examiner elicits the biceps reflex by placing the thumb over the biceps tendon and striking the thumb with a hammer. **B,** Patellar reflex. This reflex is elicited by striking the patellar tendon just below the kneecap. The normal response is extension of the leg. **C,** Superficial plantar reflex is tested by stroking the lateral side of the foot from the heel to the ball and then curve across the ball of the foot to the medial side. Plantar flexion of all toes, as shown here, should occur.

Read about additional diagnostic procedures.

cerebral angiography A radiographic procedure used to visualize the vascular system of the brain after injection of a radiopaque contrast medium; not used as often as less invasive CT but can be used to diagnose abnormalities such as an **aneurysm,** which is a ballooning out of the wall of a vessel (Fig. 10.11).

echoencephalography The use of ultrasound to study intracranial structures. The record produced is an **echoencephalogram.**

electroencephalography The process of recording the electrical activity of the brain using an **electroencephalograph** (Fig. 10.12, A). The record produced is an **electroencephalogram** (Fig. 10.12, B) and is sometimes required for the diagnosis of brain death, generally defined as loss of brain function.

myelography Radiography of the spinal cord after injection of a contrast medium; record produced is a **myelogram;** can be useful in studying spinal lesions, spinal injuries, or disk disease.

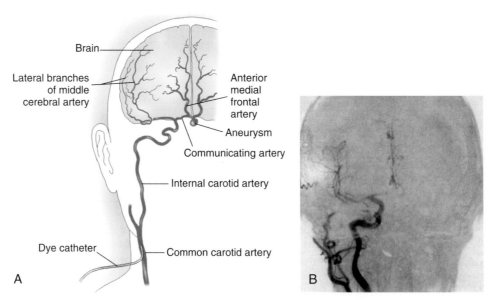

Figure 10.11 Cerebral aneurysm. A, Diagram of an aneurysm and the major cerebral arteries visible in cerebral angiography. **B,** A cerebral angiogram. Cerebral angiography is used to study intracranial circulation and is especially helpful in visualizing aneurysms and vascular occlusions. A contrast medium is used that outlines the vessels of the brain.

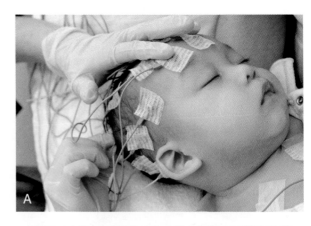

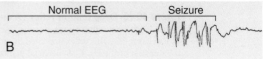

Figure 10.12 Electroencephalography (EEG). A, Baby undergoing EEG. This procedure is painless, but the patient must be quiet during the procedure. **B,** An electroencephalogram showing the comparison of the normal part on an EEG, followed by seizure activity.

Match diagnostic procedures in the left columns with their descriptions in the right column.

_____ **1.** brain scan	**A.** brisk muscular contraction in response to stimuli
_____ **2.** cerebral angiography	**B.** imaging of the brain using radioisotopes
_____ **3.** deep tendon reflex	**C.** radiography of the spinal cord
_____ **4.** echoencephalography	**D.** use of ultrasound to study brain structure
_____ **5.** myelography	**E.** visualization of blood vessels of the brain

PATHOLOGIES

10-31 Pain, which is caused by stimulation of the sensory nerve endings, is the most common symptom for which patients seek medical advice. Disturbances of the CNS vary from acute to chronic, short term to long term, and minor to life-threatening. Pathologies include trauma, congenital disorders, infections, tumors, degenerative disorders, diseases of the sense organs, and psychologic disturbances.

KEY POINT **The nervous system is a complicated body system, and many of its functions are not well understood, particularly in the realm of psychologic disorders.** Some disorders of the nervous system do not fit into the categories presented here. For example, the learning disorder **dyslexia** is an impairment of the ability to read, spell, and write words; it results from a variety of pathologic conditions, some of which are associated with the nervous system. Dyslexic persons often reverse letters and words, cannot adequately distinguish the letter sequences in written words, and have difficulty determining right from left. The exact cause of dyslexia is not known, but it is unrelated to intelligence (dyslexia *[G.] dys-,* bad, difficult; *lexis,* word).

Learn the meanings of the following word parts.

Additional Word Parts: Nervous System Pathologies

Combining Form	Meaning	Suffix	Meaning
pseud(o)	false	-algesia, -esthesia	sensitivity to pain
		-asthenia	weakness
		-lexia	words, phrases
		-orexia	hunger

10-32 **Sciatica** is inflammation of the sciatic nerve, usually marked by pain and tenderness along the course of the nerve through the thigh and leg. This may arise from problems in the lower back as a result of a herniated intervertebral disk (see Fig. 9.32) or arthritis and is accompanied by lower back pain (LBP). Write this term that means inflammation of the sciatic nerve: _____.

sciatica

Draw a slash between the word parts in the following list of new terms. Then find the meanings of the word parts within the definitions. (Draw the slash, and then perform the remainder of the activity as a mental exercise.)

1. **algesia** refers to sensitivity to pain and is also used as a suffix. **Hyperalgesia** is increased sensitivity to pain. **Hypalgesia** or **hypoalgesia** means a decrease in sensation in response to stimulation of the sensory nerves.

2. **dyskinesia** impairment of the ability to execute voluntary movements.

3. **neuralgia** pain of a nerve. **Polyneuralgia** is a type of neuralgia that affects many nerves simultaneously.

4. **paresthesia** subjective sensation, experienced as numbness, tingling, or "pins and needles" feeling, often in the absence of an external stimulus

5. **polyneuropathy** a condition in which many peripheral nerves are affected. An example is **polyneuritis,** which is inflammation of many nerves simultaneously.

6. **pseudesthesia** imaginary or false sensation; a sensation occurring in the absence of the appropriate stimulus, which can occur in a lost arm or leg after amputation; also known as **pseudoesthesia**

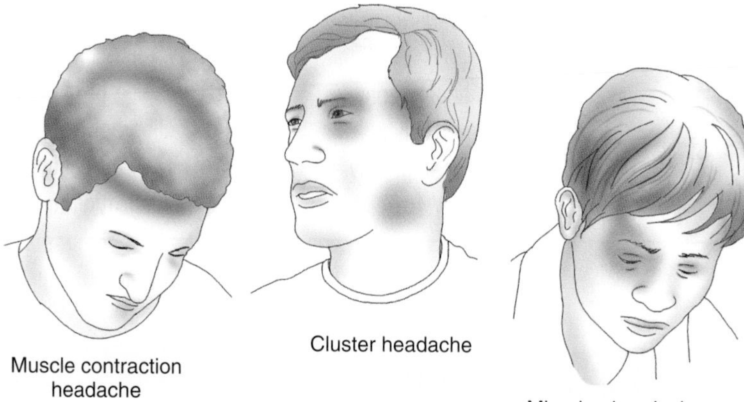

Figure 10.13 Three types of headaches. Shaded areas show regions of most intense pain.

Muscle contraction headache

Cluster headache

Migraine headache

Headaches

headache

10-33 A headache, which is pain in the head from any cause, is a symptom. Most headaches do not indicate serious disease. **Cephal/algia**, often shortened to **ceph/algia**, is a synonym for

_____.

The most common types of headaches are pain related to the eyes, ears, teeth, and paranasal structures (for example, a sinus headache). Other kinds of headaches include tension headaches (muscle contraction headaches), cluster headaches, and migraine headaches (Fig. 10.13):

- **muscle contraction headaches (tension headaches):** Result from the long-sustained contraction of skeletal muscles around the scalp, face, neck, and upper back
- **cluster headaches:** Characterized by intense unilateral pain; very painful, occurring in clusters, and do not last long
- **migraine headaches:** Characterized by recurrent throbbing headaches, often accompanied by loss of appetite, photophobia [phot(o), light + -phobia, fear; abnormal sensitivity to light], and nausea with or without vomiting; a vascular disorder

> **BEYOND** THE BLUEPRINT Migraine headaches occur more often in females than in males and sometimes begin in childhood. The classic migraine begins with depression, irritability, restlessness, and perhaps loss of appetite. There may also be transient neurologic disturbances, including visual problems (flashes of light, distorted or double vision, seeing spots), dizziness, and nausea. The headache increases in severity until it becomes intense and may last a few hours or up to several days if not treated.

BUILD IT! **EXERCISE 9**

Use the following word parts to build terms.

dys-, hyper-, poly-, cephal(o), neur(o), phot(o), -algia, -algesia, -itis, -lexia, -phobia

1. headache _____/_____
2. sensitivity to or fear of light _____/_____
3. inflammation of many nerves _____/_____
4. increased sensitivity to pain _____/_____
5. condition of difficulty with reading _____/_____

Trauma

10-34 Craniocerebral trauma is commonly called _head trauma_ or _head injury_. It is a traumatic insult to the brain caused by an external physical force that may produce a diminished or altered state of consciousness. It may result in impairment of cognitive abilities (perception, reasoning, judgment, and memory) or physical functions and may be temporary or permanent. Head trauma is either open or closed:

- Skull fractures or gunshot wounds that disrupt the integrity of the skin are examples of open head traumas.
- Blunt trauma as seen in motor vehicle accidents or athletic injuries can lead to **concussions, contusions** (bruises), or tearing of the brain.

concussion

10-35 A **cerebral concussion** usually causes loss of consciousness. A concussion is an injury to the brain resulting from violent jarring or shaking, such as a blow or an explosion. A blow to the head can cause a cerebral _____.

> **BEYOND** THE BLUEPRINT Repeated concussions may contribute to the development of symptoms that mimic Lou Gehrig disease (discussed later in the Degenerative Disorders section), which is a devastating degenerative disease named after the baseball great who was its famous victim.

A person who is responsive to signals received by the senses is said to be conscious. A person who is **semi/conscious** is only partially aware of his or her surroundings.

A **coma** is a profound unconsciousness from which the patient cannot be aroused. Using semiconscious as a model, write a word that means a partial or mild coma from which the patient can be aroused: _____.

semicoma

brain

10-36 Head injuries can also result in a spinal cord injury (SCI). An **encephalo/myelo/pathy** is any disease involving the _____ and the spinal cord.

Forceful injuries to the vertebral column can damage the spinal cord and lead to neurologic problems. Injuries to the vertebral column that can result in damage to the spinal cord include excessive rotation, hyperextension, hyperflexion, and vertical compression (Fig. 10.14).

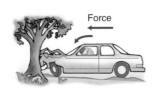

Force

Hyperflexion injury of the cervical spine

A

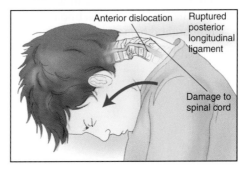

Anterior dislocation Ruptured posterior longitudinal ligament

Damage to spinal cord

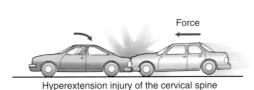

Force

Hyperextension injury of the cervical spine

B

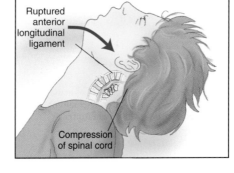

Ruptured anterior longitudinal ligament

Compression of spinal cord

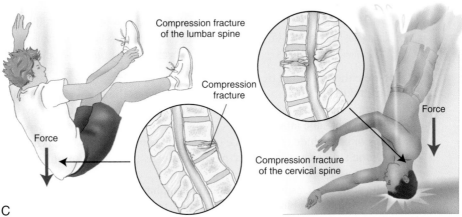

Compression fracture of the lumbar spine

Compression fracture

Force

Force

Compression fracture of the cervical spine

C

Figure 10.14 Closed spinal cord injuries. Fractures and dislocations to the vertebral column can result in injury to the spinal cord. These types of vertebral injuries occur most often at points where a relatively mobile portion of the spine meets a relatively fixed segment. **A,** Hyperflexion of the cervical vertebrae. **B,** Hyperextension of the cervical vertebrae. **C,** Vertical compression of the cervical spine and the lumbar spine.

disease

carpoptosis

speech

WORD ORIGIN
dysarthria *(G.)*
dys, bad or difficult;
arthroun, to articulate

blood

10-37 The peripheral nerves are subject to many types of trauma. A **peripheral neuropathy** is any _____ of the peripheral nerves. Those of the extremities are commonly affected. An example is wristdrop, in which nerve damage results in the hand remaining in a flexed position at the wrist, and it cannot be extended. Write the term that means wristdrop by combining carp(o) and -ptosis: _____.

10-38 An abnormal condition in which language function is absent or disordered because of an injury to certain areas of the cerebral cortex can result in **a/phasia** or **dys/phasia.** Literal translation of a/phasia is absence of _____.

Difficult, poorly articulated speech, usually caused by damage to a central or peripheral motor nerve, is called **dys/arthria.**

10-39 You learned earlier that a hematoma is a collection of _____ in the tissues of the skin or in an organ. Three types of **hematomas** are associated with head injuries (Fig. 10.15):
- **epidural hematoma:** Accumulation of blood in the epidural space. Epi/dural means situated on or outside the dura mater. The hematoma compresses the dura mater and thus compresses the brain.
- **subdural hematoma:** Accumulation of blood between the dura mater and the arachnoid; it is often the result of an arachnoid tear associated with a head injury.
- **intracerebral hematoma:** Bleeding within the brain itself, associated with a cerebral tear; it has a high mortality rate, but fortunately, this type is less common than the other two types.

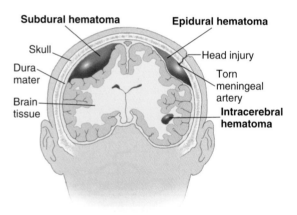

Figure 10.15 Three types of hematomas associated with head injuries: subdural hematoma, epidural hematoma, and intracerebral hematoma.

10-40 **Cerebro/vascular accident** (CVA) is also called *stroke* or *stroke syndrome.*

🔑 **KEY** POINT **Normal blood supply to the brain has been disrupted in CVA.** CVA results in insufficient oxygen to brain tissue, caused by hemorrhage, occlusion (closing), vasospasm, or constriction of the blood vessels that normally supply oxygen to the brain. Go to the National Institute of Neurological Disorders and Stroke (NINDS) website, *www.ninds.nih.gov,* for more information.

Strokes are either ischemic or hemorrhagic (Fig. 10.16):
1. **Ischemic strokes** result from inadequate blood flow to the brain caused by partial or complete occlusion of a cerebral artery. Ischemic strokes are generally preceded by warning signs, such as a **transient ischemic attack** (TIA), caused by a brief interruption in cerebral blood flow. TIA symptoms often include disturbance of normal vision, dizziness, weakness, and numbness.
   - **thrombotic strokes** are caused by plaque deposits that build up on the interior of a cerebral artery.
   - **embolic strokes** are caused by a **cerebral embolus,** which is a plug of matter (usually a blood clot) brought by the blood to the cerebral artery.
2. **Hemorrhagic strokes** are caused by the rupture of a cerebral artery. This may be preceded by a **cerebral aneurysm,** which is an abnormal, localized dilation of a cerebral artery that ruptures and produces a **cerebral hemorrhage.**

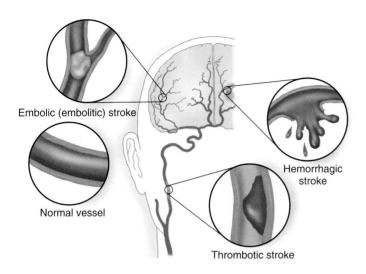

Embolic (embolitic) stroke

Normal vessel

Hemorrhagic stroke

Thrombotic stroke

Figure 10.16 Types of stroke. A cerebrovascular accident (CVA), commonly referred to as a *stroke,* is a disruption in the normal blood supply to the brain. Most strokes are either embolic or thrombotic strokes in which a cerebral artery is partially or completely occluded. A hemorrhagic stroke is caused by the rupture of a cerebral artery.

MATCH IT! **EXERCISE 10**

Match items in the left column with those in the right column.

_____ **1.** cerebral concussion

_____ **2.** cerebrovascular accident

_____ **3.** coma

_____ **4.** dysarthria

A. damage to the brain caused by jarring or shaking

B. poorly articulated speech

C. profound unconsciousness

D. results from inadequate oxygen to brain tissue

Paralysis

paralysis

10-41 Paralysis is the loss of muscle function, loss of sensation, or both and is a sign of an underlying problem. Paralysis may be caused by trauma, disease, or poisoning. Injury to different areas of the spinal cord results in different types of paralysis.

In **para/plegia,** the upper limbs are not affected. Para/plegia is _____ of the lower portion of the body and both legs. The prefix para- means near, beside, or abnormal. Some interpretation is needed in the term *paraplegia.* Compare three types of paralysis (Fig. 10.17).

facial

10-42 Facial paralysis, or **Bell palsy,** is a neuropathy that drastically affects the body image (Fig. 10.18). The cause is unknown; the onset is acute and is characterized by a drawing sensation with paralysis of all facial muscles on the affected side. Bell palsy is acute paralysis of a cranial nerve affecting one side of the face, also called _____ paralysis.

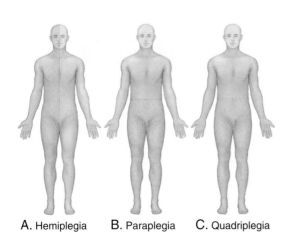

A. Hemiplegia   B. Paraplegia   C. Quadriplegia

Figure 10.17 Comparison of affected areas in three types of paralysis. A, Hemiplegia. **B,** Paraplegia. **C,** Quadriplegia.

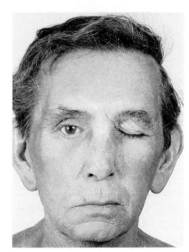

Figure 10.18 Bell palsy. Unilateral paralysis of the facial nerve, often resulting in inability to close the eye on the affected side.

Draw a slash between the word parts in the following list of new terms. Then find the meanings of the word parts within the definitions. (Draw the slash, and then perform the remainder of the activity as a mental exercise.)

1. **diplegia** paralysis of similar parts on both sides of the body
2. **hemiplegia** paralysis of one side of the body
3. **monoplegia** paralysis of one limb
4. **quadriplegia** paralysis of all four extremities

Congenital and Genetic Disorders

meninges

meninges

palsy

WORD ORIGIN
chorea *(G.)*
choreia, dance

Huntington

10-43 Congenital defects of the nervous system may be obvious at birth and may vary from minor to severe. An abnormal protrusion near the spine may be a meningocele or meningo/myelo/cele. A **meningo/cele** is hernial protrusion of _____ through a defect in the skull or vertebral column (Fig. 10.19).

A **meningo/myelo/cele** is hernial protrusion of parts of the _____ and spinal cord through a defect in the vertebral column. Both these congenital defects are generally repaired by surgery, but either defect may result in residual motor and sensory deficits.

10-44 Cerebral palsy is a motor function disorder caused by a permanent, nonprogressive brain defect present at birth or occurring shortly thereafter (Fig. 10.20). It may result in spastic paralysis in various forms, seizures, and varying degrees of impaired speech, vision, and hearing. It is often associated with asphyxia during birth. This congenital defect is called cerebral _____.

10-45 Huntington disease, also called **Huntington chorea,** is a hereditary disorder that affects both genders equally. Symptoms begin between 30 and 50 years of age. The two main signs and symptoms are progressive mental status changes leading to dementia and rapid, jerky movements in the trunk, facial muscles, and extremities. Neurotransmitters have been implicated in the symptoms of this inherited disorder called _____ disease.

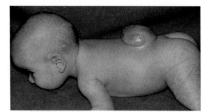

Figure 10.19 Meningocele. The spinal meninges have formed a hernial cyst that is filled with cerebrospinal fluid (CSF) and is protruding through a defect in the vertebral column.

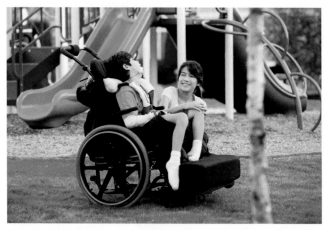

Figure 10.20 Cerebral palsy. Sister sits next to disabled brother in wheelchair. Early identification facilitates highly individualized treatment.

Infections

Infections of the CNS include the following diseases:

botulism An often fatal form of food poisoning, most often from improperly canned food, caused by the toxin of a bacterium, *Clostridium botulinum,* which is toxic to nervous tissue and causes paralysis of both voluntary and involuntary motor activity. Symptoms usually appear 12 to 36 hours after eating contaminated food.

cerebellitis Inflammation that is confined to the cerebellum

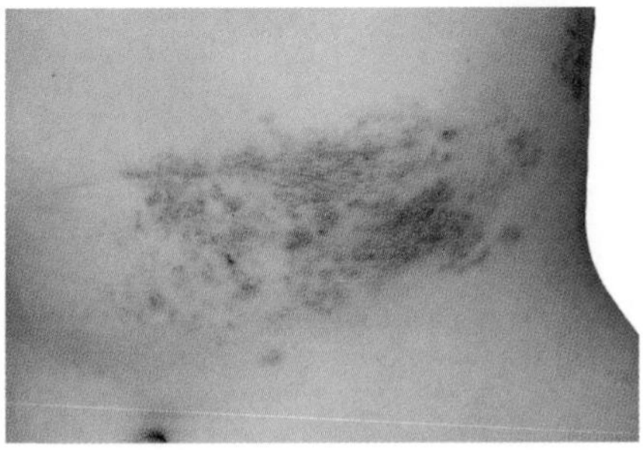

Figure 10.21 Shingles. These painful skin eruptions follow the underlying route of cranial or spinal nerves that are inflamed by the virus.

encephalitis Inflammation of the brain tissue, often caused by a virus, usually having gained access to the bloodstream from a viral infection elsewhere in the body

encephalomeningitis Inflammation of the brain and its coverings

encephalomyelitis Inflammation of the brain and spinal cord

meningitis Inflammation of the meninges of the brain and spinal cord, usually caused by bacterial or viral organisms

poliomyelitis An acute viral disease that attacks the gray matter of the spinal cord and parts of the brain; can be asymptomatic, mild, or paralytic; can be prevented by immunization; informally called *polio* (G. *polios*, gray)

rabies An acute, often fatal, disease of the CNS transmitted to humans by infected animals. Without medical interven-tion and possibly the use of vaccine, coma and death are likely; obsolete name is **hydrophobia,** the name given after observation that rabid animals avoid water (because paralysis prevents them from being able to swallow).

shingles an acute infection caused by reactivation of the latent chickenpox virus. This infection mainly affects adults. The cause of reactivation is not known, but it is linked to aging, immune impairment, and stress; herpes zoster (Fig. 10.21).

tetanus An acute, potentially fatal infection of the CNS caused by the toxin of an anaerobic bacillus, *Clostridium tetani,* which attacks the nervous system and results in muscle rigidity and spasms; also known as *lockjaw,* taking its name from the resulting rigidity of the jaw; easily preventable through immunization.

ventriculitis Inflammation of a ventricle of the brain

ANALYZE IT! | **EXERCISE 12**

Break these words into their component parts by placing a slash between the word parts. Write the meaning of each term.

1. cerebellitis _____
2. encephalomeningitis _____
3. hemiplegia _____
4. meningomyelocele _____
5. ventriculitis _____

Tumors

10-46 Primary brain tumors arise within the brain structures and rarely spread outside the brain. Glia cells are the only source of primary malignant brain tumors. The tumors are called *gliomas.* A **gli/oma,** a primary tumor of the brain, is composed of which type of nerve cell?

neuroglia

_____

10-47 A **meningi/oma** is a tumor of the meninges that grows slowly and may invade the skull. Tumors within the skull can invade and compress brain tissue, which generally leads to increased intracranial pressure (ICP), headaches, and many neurologic problems, such as a **neuro/genic bladder,** a dysfunction of the urinary bladder caused by a lesion (a tumor) of the nervous system. Normal control of urination and emptying of the bladder is usually absent.

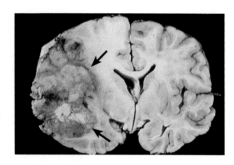

Figure 10.22 **A primary brain tumor.** This autopsy specimen of the brain shows a large tumor *(arrows)*. This patient had multiple distant metastases in the lung and spine. Compare the size of the two cerebral hemispheres.

within

10-48 You know that crani(o) means the cranium, or skull, therefore **intra/cranial** means _____ the skull. Brain tumors can become quite large, occupying considerable intracranial space, as shown in Fig. 10.22.

Apraxia means an impairment in the ability to perform purposeful acts or to manipulate objects without a loss of strength, coordination, or sensation. Motor apraxia is an inability to handle small objects (although aware of their proper use) or carry out planned movement. This condition results from a lesion in the frontal cortex. Apraxia of speech interferes with speech although understanding of speech remains intact.

water; head

10-49 Disorders, such as brain tumors, that interfere with the flow of CSF cause fluid accumulation in the skull, which is called *hydrocephalus*. Translated literally, hydro/cephalus means _____ in the _____. **Hydrocephalus** is a pathologic condition characterized by an abnormal accumulation of CSF within the skull and is usually accompanied by increased ICP. When this happens in an infant, before the cranial bones fuse, the cranium enlarges (see Fig. 3.37). In an older child or adult, the pressure damages the soft brain tissue.

tumor

10-50 A **neur/oma** is a benign _____ composed chiefly of neurons and nerve fibers. Although neuromas are benign, they can be painful (for example, a Morton neuroma that occurs in the foot) or can compress brain tissue (for example, an acoustic neuroma).

Seizure Disorders

seizure

10-51 A **seizure** is an abnormal, sudden, excessive discharge of electric activity within the brain. Seizures are also known as **convulsions.** This abnormal activity is assessed in EEG. A seizure may be recurrent, such as in a seizure disorder, or transient and acute, such as after a concussion. A concussion is damage to the brain caused by a violent jarring or shaking.

Remember that the suffix -lepsy means _____. **Epilepsy** is a group of chronic neurologic disorders characterized by recurrent episodes of convulsive seizures, sensory disturbances, loss of consciousness, or all of these.

narcolepsy

10-52 Narcolepsy is uncontrollable, brief episodes of sleep and uses the combining form narc(o), which means stupor. In narcolepsy the person cannot prevent a sudden attack of sleep while performing daytime activities. Its cause is unknown, and no pathologic lesions are found in the brain. The person may experience momentary loss of muscle tone. Visual or auditory hallucinations often occur at the onset of sleep. Stimulant drugs are often prescribed to prevent the sudden attacks of sleep at inappropriate times. The name of this disorder is _____.

Case Study. *Select terms from the report to match the descriptions.*

In the 1900s, George Goodwin was referred to neurologist Dr. Thomas Smith for severe cephalgia of 2 months' duration. Test results were negative and there was no indication of dyskinesia, dysphasia, or dyslexia. Family history indicated a father who suffered frequent narcolepsy. George was admitted to the hospital. Hydrocodon-APAP 5-325 four times a day was effective in treating the pain and he was sent home after three days with a Rx for this medication. The son notified us four months later that Mr. Goodwin had died. Autopsy showed an inoperable brain tumor.

1. headache _____

2. impairment of voluntary movement _____

3. inability to read, spell, and write words _____

4. recurrent, uncontrollable brief episodes of sleep _____

Degenerative Disorders

10-53 Degenerative disorders are those in which there is deterioration of structure or function of tissue. Included in this section are neurologic disorders that affect motor ability or nerve transmission (Parkinson disease, MS, amyotrophic lateral sclerosis (ALS), myasthenia gravis) and involve mental deterioration (dementia, Alzheimer disease).

Parkinson disease is a slowly progressing, debilitating, neurologic disease that affects motor ability. It is characterized by muscle rigidity, bradykinesia, and tremor. The suffix -kinesia means

slow   movement. **Brady/kinesia** means _____ movement, or slowness of all voluntary movement or speech. **Tremor** is rhythmic, purposeless, quivering involuntary movement. A characteristic posture and masklike facial expression are often seen (Fig. 10.23).

(A tremor is common in benign essential tremors, such as an involuntary shaking of the hand, head or face; however no other sign of Parkinson disease is present.)

> **BEYOND** THE BLUEPRINT Film and TV star Michael J. Fox, whose roles include *Back to the Future, Family Ties,* and *Spin City,* and *The Michael J. Fox Show* was diagnosed with Parkinson disease in 1991. He first noticed his finger twitching while filming *Doc Hollywood.* Parkinson disease occurs most often in people older than 50 years and results from widespread degeneration of a part of the brain that produces dopamine. Michael's diagnosis at a younger age has not stopped him from being an enthusiastic spokesperson for the Michael J. Fox Foundation, which is dedicated to finding a cure for Parkinson disease.

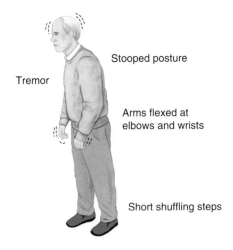

Tremor

Stooped posture

Arms flexed at elbows and wrists

Short shuffling steps

Figure 10.23 Latter stage of Parkinson disease. Characteristics of this degenerative neurologic disorder include resting tremor, pill rolling of the fingers, muscle rigidity and weakness, a shuffling gait, a masklike and immobile facial expression, and forward flexion of the trunk. Some of the latter signs are evident in this patient.

10-54 Amyotrophic lateral sclerosis (ALS) is also called *Lou Gehrig disease.* It is characterized by atrophy (wasting) of the hands, forearms, and legs. The disease results in paralysis and death. The cause of the disease is unknown. Analyzing the parts of a/myo/trophic, a- means without, my(o)

muscle   means _____, and -trophic means nutrition.

This rare degenerative disease of the motor neurons, characterized by weakness and atrophy of

amyotrophic   the muscles, is ALS, which means _____ lateral sclerosis.

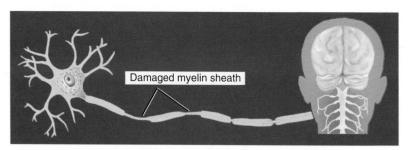

Figure 10.24 Nerve damage to the spinal cord and brain in multiple sclerosis (MS). This results in multiple areas of scar tissue. Depending on where the damage occurs, symptoms may include problems with muscular control, balance, speech, or vision.

> ➤ **BEYOND** THE BLUEPRINT It is said that his accomplishments in baseball made Lou Gehrig an authentic American hero and his tragic death, dying of ALS at age 37, made him a legend. For years, his endurance and strength earned him the nickname "Iron Horse." Playing for the New York Yankees with other greats, Babe Ruth and Joe DiMaggio, they outhomered most teams in baseball. Gehrig was diagnosed with ALS in 1937, quickly became disabled, and never played baseball again. The cause of most cases of ALS is not known, and only 5% of the cases are genetic. Statistics show that military veterans have a 60% more likely chance of having ALS (implying the possibility of chemical exposure); also one who has experienced repeated concussions may develop a traumatic encephalopathy that mimics ALS.

sclerosis

10-55 Multiple sclerosis (MS) is a progressive degenerative disease that affects the myelin sheath and conduction pathways of the CNS. This disease that is named for the multiple areas of sclerotic tissue that replace the myelin sheath is multiple _____.

🔑 **KEY** POINT In MS, the myelin sheath deteriorates and is replaced by scar tissue that interferes with normal transmission of the nerve impulse (Fig. 10.24). One of the earliest signs is paresthesia, which is abnormal sensations in the extremities or on one side of the face. The disease is characterized by periods of remission and exacerbation (flare). Disability increases as the disease progresses, and the periods of exacerbation become more frequent.

muscle

myasthenia

10-56 My/asthenia gravis, meaning grave muscle weakness, is a chronic neuromuscular disease characterized by muscular weakness and fatigue. The suffix -asthenia means weakness, so my/asthenia means weakness of the _____.

This degenerative condition results from a defect in the conduction of nerve impulses at the neuromuscular junction. Characterized by chronic fatigue and muscle weakness, it is called _____ gravis.

10-57 Dementia is a progressive mental disorder of the brain. **Agnosia,** also called agnosis, is a total or partial loss of the ability to recognize familiar objects or persons through sensory stimuli as a result of dementia or organic brain damage.

🔑 **KEY** POINT Because there are many causes of dementia, conditions that cause the decline may be treatable or partially reversible. Dementia is characterized by confusion, disorientation, deterioration of memory and intellectual abilities, and personality disintegration. Dementia occurs most often in older adults. Dementia caused by drug intoxication, insulin shock, hydrocephalus, or certain other causes may be reversed by treating the underlying cause. Organic forms of dementia, such as Alzheimer disease, are generally considered incurable.

Alzheimer

Alzheimer disease is chronic, progressive mental deterioration that is sometimes called *dementia, Alzheimer type.* This accounts for more than half of the persons with dementia who are older than 65 years of age. It is less common in people in their 40s and 50s. Although the exact cause is not known, both chemical and structural changes occur in the brain (Fig. 10.25). The disease is characterized by confusion, memory failure, disorientation, inability to carry out purposeful activities, and speech and gait disturbances. It involves irreversible loss of memory. The patient becomes increasingly mentally impaired, severe physical deterioration takes place, and death occurs. This type of dementia is called _____ disease.

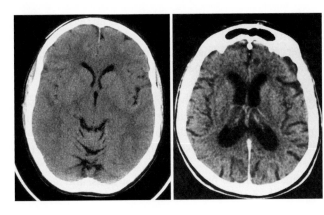

Figure 10.25 Normal computed tomography (CT) scan versus CT scan of Alzheimer disease. The CT scan on the *left* shows a normal brain. In the CT scan on the *right*, however, note the dark patches in the cerebral cortex (damage typical of Alzheimer disease).

BUILD IT!
EXERCISE 14

Use the following word parts to build terms.

a-, brady-, intra-, crani(o), gli(o), my(o), narc(o), troph(o), -al, -ic, -kinesia, -lepsy, -oma

1. slow movement _____/_____
2. uncontrollable brief episodes of sleep (or stupor) _____/_____
3. pertaining to the area within the skull _____/_____/_____
4. tumor of glial cells _____/_____
5. pertaining to a lack of muscle nutrition _____/_____/_____/_____

Psychologic Disorders

10-58 Psychologic disorders are unlike most diseases or disorders that confront health professionals, because there often is no change in the body structure and sometimes not even detectable changes in chemistry, thus making the abnormalities difficult to demonstrate and treat in the usual sense. A psychologist is one who is trained in methods of psychologic analysis, therapy, and research. You learned in Chapter 1 that the medical specialty that deals with the diagnosis, treatment, and prevention of mental illness is _____.

psychiatry

A mental health disorder is a disturbance of emotional equilibrium with impaired functioning, caused by genetic, physical, chemical, biological, psychological, or social and cultural factors. This is also called a mental illness, emotional illness, or psychiatric disorder.

Learn the meanings of the following combining forms related to psychology.

Additional Word Parts: Psychology

Combining Form	Meaning
ment(o), psych(o)	mind
phren(o)	mind or diaphragm
pyr(o)	fire
schist(o), schiz(o)	split

MATCH IT!
EXERCISE 15

Match items in the left column with those in the right column. Items A through C may be used more than once.

_____ 1. phren(o)   **A.** fire
_____ 2. psych(o)   **B.** mind
_____ 3. pyr(o)   **C.** split
_____ 4. schiz(o)

10-59 Several disorders are discussed in this section, including mental deterioration, anxiety disorders, phobias, obsessions and compulsions, schizophrenia, and mood disorders.

Only a few psychologic disorders have observable pathologic conditions of the brain. Examples of observable pathologic conditions are dementia and Alzheimer disease. (These disorders were discussed earlier in this chapter.)

Neurodevelopmental disorders are impairments of the growth and development of the brain or CNS (sometimes it refers to disorders of brain function that affect emotion, learning ability, and memory that unfold as the individual grows). These include intellectual disabilities, communication disorders, attention deficit/hyperactivity disorders, autism spectrum disorders, and certain motor disorders.

Communication disorders include stuttering, inability to produce certain sounds, and language disorder (a disruption or inability to understand and/or produce the conventional symbols or words of one's native language).

WORD ORIGIN
autism *(G.)*
autos, self

autism

10-60 Signs of psychologic disorders can appear in a very young child. Such is the case with autism and attention deficit disorder. Conduct disorder is a behavioral pattern occurring primarily in children and adolescents that is characterized by aggression and violations of the rights of others. **Autism** is characterized by withdrawal and impaired development in social interaction and communication. Write the name of this disorder that may be characterized by extreme withdrawal: _____.

Attention deficit disorder and **attention deficit hyperactivity disorder** are abbreviated ADD and ADHD, respectively. These are characterized by several patterns of behavior, such as short attention span and poor concentration in multiple settings, and, in ADHD, hyperactivity. Hyperactivity is also called **hyper/kinesia.** Translated literally, hyper/kinesia or **hyper/kinesis** is above normal

movement

_____.

Intellectual disability, autism spectrum disorder, and Tourette syndrome are other disorders that are usually diagnosed in childhood.

10-61 Anxiety disorders are characterized by anticipation of impending danger and dread, the source of which is largely unknown or unrecognized (Fig. 10.26). An anxiety attack is an acute, psychobiologic reaction that usually includes several of the following: restlessness, tension, tachycardia, and breathing difficulty. A **psycho/biological response** involves both the _____

mind

and the physical body.

WORD ORIGIN
obsession *(L.)*
obsidere, to haunt

11-62 An **obsessive-compulsive disorder** (OCD) is an anxiety disorder characterized by recurrent and persistent thoughts, ideas, and feelings of obsessions or compulsions sufficiently severe to cause distress, consume considerable time, or interfere with the person's occupational, social, or interpersonal functioning. An **obsession** is a persistent thought or idea that occupies the mind and cannot be erased by logic or reasoning. A **compulsion** is an irresistible, repetitive impulse to act contrary to one's ordinary standards. An OCD is a pattern of persistent behaviors that involve

obsession

compulsion to act on an _____.

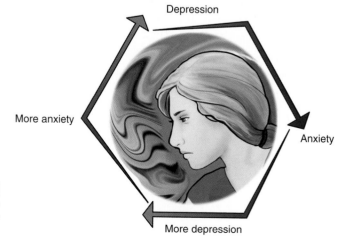

Figure 10.26 Schematic of the anxiety cycle. A permanent state of nervousness, worry, and apprehension can lead to depression. An anxiety disorder can be a build-up, over time, of everyday stress from problems.

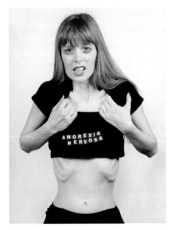

Figure 10.27 Anorexia nervosa in a young female. The prominent ribs and gaunt face are consistent with prolonged refusal to eat.

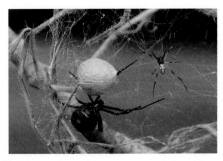

Figure 10.28 Black widow spiders. The larger female, shown with the egg case, has a powerful neurotoxin that causes pain and sometimes death.

WORD ORIGIN
bulimia *(G.)*
bous, ox;
limos, hunger

10-63 Both anorexia nervosa and bulimia are eating disorders that have psychological components. **Bulimia** is characterized by insatiable craving for food, often resulting in episodes of continuous eating, and followed by depression and purging. **Anorexia nervosa** is characterized by a prolonged refusal to eat, resulting in emaciation, amenorrhea, emotional disturbance concerning body image, and fear of becoming obese, and it is usually associated with anxiety, irritation, fear, and anger. The condition is seen primarily in adolescents and predominantly in girls (Fig. 10.27).

appetite

Both bulimia and anorexia nervosa have psychological components. Literal translation of anorexia indicates a lack of _____, but anorexia nervosa is representative of an emotional disturbance that affects at least two body systems.

fear

10-64 Phobias are obsessive, irrational, and intense fears of an object, an activity, or a physical situation. The suffix -phobia means abnormal _____. Phobias range from abnormal fear of public places, which is known as **agoraphobia,** to abnormal fear of animals, which is known as **zoophobia,** and they even include an abnormal fear of acquiring a phobia, which is known as **phobophobia. Arachnophobia** is a morbid fear of spiders.

WORD ORIGIN
agoraphobia *(G.)*
agora, marketplace;
phobos, fear

> **BEYOND** THE BLUEPRINT The bite of some spiders is dangerous to humans, including the black widow (Fig. 10.28), the brown recluse, and species of jumping spiders and tarantulas. Spider venom may contain enzymatic proteins that are capable of affecting neuromuscular transmission or cardiovascular function.

acrophobia

fear

Write a word that means an irrational fear of heights by using the combining form for extremity and -phobia: _____.

Claustro/phobia is a morbid _____ of closed places. A claustrum (L., *claustrum,* a closing) is a barrier.

> **BEYOND** THE BLUEPRINT Claustrophobic individuals generally tolerate open MRI, because they are not enclosed within the magnetic resonance unit, but the scan generally takes longer to complete than a regular MRI.

An abnormal fear of fire is **pyro/phobia.**

after

10-65 Posttraumatic stress disorder is characterized by an acute emotional response _____ a traumatic event or situation involving severe environmental stress, such as a physical assault or military combat.

10-66 A panic disorder or **panic attack** is an episode of acute anxiety that occurs unpredictably with feelings of intense apprehension or terror, accompanied by dyspnea (difficult breathing), dizziness, sweating, trembling, and chest pain.

panic

When these signs and symptoms occur unpredictably with feelings of extreme apprehension, the disorder is called a _____ attack.

10-67 Emotional conflicts are so repressed in a **dissociative disorder** that a separation or split in the personality occurs, resulting in an altered state of consciousness or a confusion in identity. Existence within a person of two or more separate identities is an example of a _____ disorder. Symptoms may include amnesia, and in this case the loss of memory is generally caused by severe emotional trauma.

dissociative

10-68 A **mood disorder** is a variety of conditions characterized by a disturbance in mood as the main feature. In severe cases, they may be a sign of depressive disorder or may be symptomatic of a bipolar disorder. Conditions characterized by a disturbance in mood are called _____ disorders.

mood

10-69 Most persons experience occasional feelings of sadness or discouragement resulting from personal loss or tragedy; however, **clinical depression** is an abnormal emotional state characterized by exaggerated feelings of sadness, despair, discouragement, emptiness, and hopelessness. It is important to remember that the feelings of sadness and hopelessness are _____ in clinical depression.

exaggerated

10-70 A **mania** is an unstable emotional state that includes excessive excitement, elation, ideas, and psychomotor activities. In an extreme manic episode, a delusion of grandeur may occur. The suffix -mania is used to write terms pertaining to excessive preoccupation. **Megalo/mania** is an abnormal mental state in which one believes oneself to be a person of great importance, power, fame, or wealth. You learned earlier that -mania means excessive preoccupation; therefore the literal translation of megalo/mania is excessive _____ with greatness.

preoccupation

A **bipolar disorder** is a major mental disorder characterized by the occurrence of manic episodes, major depressive episodes, or mixed moods. The term *bipolar* in the name indicates that the disorder has two distinct aspects. Megalomania may occur in an extreme manic episode of bipolar disorder.

10-71 The combining form pyr(o) means fire. **Pyro/mania** is excessive preoccupation with _____. A **pyro/maniac** has an obsessive preoccupation with fires. Pyro/mania is a compulsion to set fires or watch fires.

fire

Klepto/mania is characterized by an abnormal, uncontrollable, and recurrent urge to steal.

WORD ORIGIN
kleptomania *(G.)*
kleptein, to steal;
mania, madness

> **BEYOND** THE BLUEPRINT Kleptomania (shoplifting for the thrill, rather than for need), often coexists with other mental disorders, such as OCD or bulimia. Some studies suggest that 0.6% of the general population may have kleptomania and that it is more common in females. The high-profile celebrities reported for shoplifting support that statistic.

10-72 **Sexual disorders** are those caused at least in part by psychologic factors. Such a disorder, characterized by a decrease or disturbance in sexual desire that is not the result of a general medical condition, is called a *sexual dysfunction*. Sexual perversion or deviation, in which the sexual instinct is expressed in ways that are biologically undesirable, socially prohibited, or socially unacceptable, is termed **para/phil/ia.** Sexual dysfunctions and paraphilia are classified as _____ disorders.

sexual

10-73 **Somatoform disorders** are any of a group of disorders characterized by symptoms suggesting physical illness or disease, for which there are no demonstrable organic causes or physiologic dysfunctions. Somato/form is derived from somat(o), meaning _____ and -form, which is a suffix for shape.

body

What was formerly called **hypochondriasis** or **hypochondria** has been replaced by two diagnoses: somatic symptom disorder and illness anxiety disorder (IAD). To meet the criteria for somatic symptom disorder, patients must have one or more chronic somatic symptoms about which they are excessively preoccupied or fearful. Patients with IAD may or may not have a medical condition, but have heightened bodily sensations, are anxious about the possibility of an undiagnosed illness, and devote excessive time and energy to health concerns.

weakness

10-74 The suffix -asthenia means weakness. **Neur/asthenia** is a nervous disorder characterized by _____ and sometimes nervous exhaustion. It is often associated with a depressed state and is believed by some to be **psychosomatic** (having body symptoms of emotional origin).

Pseudo/mania is a false or pretended mental disorder. **Pseudo/plegia** is hysterical paralysis. There is loss of muscle power without real paralysis.

10-75 A psychotic disorder, or **psychosis,** is any major mental disorder characterized by a gross impairment in reality testing. Normal reality is an ego function that enables one to differentiate between external reality and any inner imaginative world and to behave in a manner that exhibits an awareness of accepted norms. Impairment of reality testing is indicative of a disturbance that may lead to psychosis.

🔑 **KEY** POINT **Schizo/phrenia is any of a large group of psychotic disorders.** Schizophrenia is characterized by gross distortion of reality, hallucinations, disturbances of language and communication, and disorganized or catatonic behavior (psychologically induced immobility with muscular rigidity that is interrupted by agitation).

split

The combining form schiz(o) means _____. Translated literally, schizophrenia means split mind and relates to the splitting off of a part of the psyche, which may dominate the psychic life of the patient even though it may express behavior contrary to the original personality. The concept of multiple personalities, two or more distinct subpersonalities, is not necessarily a characteristic of schizophrenia.

10-76 A number of personality disorders exist with which you may already be familiar. These include antisocial personality disorder, paranoid personality disorder and others. **Anti/social** behavior is acting _____ the rights of others.

against

Paranoid personality disorder (commonly shortened to paranoia) is characterized by persistent delusions of persecution, mistrust, and combativeness.

A number of general symptomatic terms associated with mental disorders are amnesia (loss of memory), catatonia (psychologically induced immobility at times interrupted by agitation), defense mechanism, delirium (frenzied excitement), delusion (persistent belief or perception), dementia (persistent organic mental disintegration), hallucination (sensory perception that does not result from an external stimulus in the waking state), illusion (false interpretation of an external sensory stimulus) libido (psychic energy associated with sexual desire or pleasure), and somnambulism (complex motor activity during sleep that usually culminates in sleepwalking). Somn/ambulism may be easier to remember, since you know that ambulate means to walk.

WORD ORIGIN
catatonia, G.
kata, down
tonos, tension
illusion
L. illuder
to mock
somnambulism
L. somnus, sleep
ambulare, to walk

10-77 Substance abuse is the overindulgence in and dependence on a stimulant, depressant, or other chemical substance, leading to the detriment of the individual's physical or mental health, or the welfare of others. Several terms related to substance abuse are intoxication, dependence, delirium tremens (DTs), tolerance, harmful use, and withdrawal symptoms (unpleasant, sometimes life-threatening physiological changes that occur when some drugs are withdrawn after prolonged, regular use). Delirium tremens is an acute and sometimes fatal psychotic reaction caused by abrupt cessation of excessive intake of alcoholic beverages.

Additional information about psychologic disorders can be found in the *Diagnostic and Statistical Manual of Mental Disorders* (DSM), which is published by the American Psychiatric Association (*www.dsm5.org/Pages/Default.aspx*).

It is based on the International Classification of Disease and uses diagnostic codes, which are fundamental to medical record keeping, greatly facilitating data record keeping and retrieval. DSM

Diagnostic

means _____ *and Statistical Manual of Mental Disorders.*

BUILD IT!
EXERCISE 16

Use the following word parts to build terms.

hyper-, neur(o), pseudo-, psych(o), pyr(o), -asthenia, -kinesia, -mania, -osis, -phobia

1. false or pretended mental disorder _____/_____

2. major mental disorder _____/_____

3. nervous disorder characterized by muscular weakness _____/_____

4. abnormal fear of fire _____/_____

5. excessive movement _____/_____

SURGICAL AND THERAPEUTIC INTERVENTIONS

skull (cranium)

10-78 Cranial surgery may be needed for brain tumors, trauma, brain abscesses, or vascular abnormalities. The individual's need determines the particular type of surgery. Selected cranial surgical procedures are presented in Table 10.1.

In reading Table 10.1, you see that a **burr hole** is a hole drilled into the _____. It is particularly used to drain or irrigate an abscess.

Table 10.1	Types of Cranial Surgery
Type	**Description**
Burr hole	Opening into the cranium with a drill; used to remove localized fluid and blood beneath the dura
Craniotomy	Opening into the cranium with removal of a bone flap, and opening of the dura to remove a lesion, repair a damaged area, drain blood, or relieve increased intracranial pressure (ICP)
Craniectomy	Excision into the cranium to cut away a bone flap
Cranioplasty	Repair of a cranial defect resulting from trauma, malformation, or previous surgical procedure; artificial material used to replace damaged or lost bone
Shunt procedures	Alternate pathway to redirect cerebrospinal fluid (CSF) from one area to another using a tube or implanted device; for example, a ventriculoperitoneal shunt
Stereotaxis	Precision localization of a specific area of the brain using a frame or a frameless system based on three-dimensional coordinates; procedure is used for biopsy, radiosurgery, or dissection

Modified from Lewis SM, Heitemper MM, Dirksen SR: *Medical-surgical nursing,* St Louis, 2004, Mosby.

10-79 Any surgical opening into the skull is a **craniotomy** (See Fig. 9.46).

🔑 **KEY** POINT **Craniotomies are performed to gain access to the brain, relieve ICP, or control bleeding inside the skull.** Surgical removal of a portion of the skull in order to perform surgery on the brain is a **craniectomy.** This type of surgery may be necessary to repair the brain or its vessels, remove a brain tumor, or repair an aneurysm.

excision
repair
cerebrotomy

An **aneurysm/ectomy** is _____ of an aneurysm.
Cranio/plasty is surgical _____ of the skull after surgery or injury to the skull.
Use cerebr(o) to write a word that means incision of the brain: _____.

ventricle

10-80 **Shunts** are used to redirect CSF from one area to another using a tube or an implanted device. A **ventriculo/peritone/al shunt** creates a passageway between a cerebral _____ and the peritoneum for the draining of CSF from the brain in hydrocephalus (Fig. 10.29).

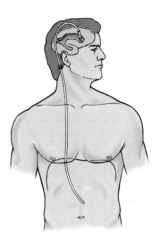

Figure 10.29 Ventriculoperitoneal shunt. This type of shunt consists of plastic tubing between a cerebral ventricle and the peritoneum for the draining of excess cerebrospinal fluid (CSF) from the brain in hydrocephalus.

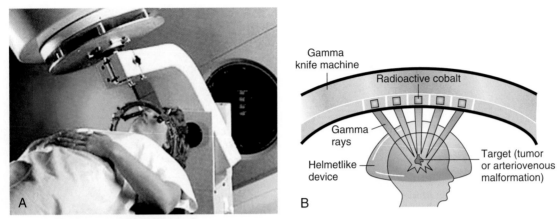

Figure 10.30 **Gamma knife treatment assisted by stereotaxis. A,** The stereotactic frame holds the head in a fixed position. **B,** In a gamma knife treatment, beams are intense only at the targeted area.

10-81 Stereotaxis uses a system of three-dimensional coordinates to locate a site to be operated on or irradiated. In **stereotactic surgery** the surgeon is assisted by a computer-guided apparatus that is used to target a specific area of the brain.

Stereotactic radiosurgery involves closed-skull destruction of a target (for example, a tumor) using ionizing radiation. The patient's head is held in a stereotactic frame (Fig. 10.30, A). In a **gamma knife procedure,** a high dose of radiation is delivered to precisely targeted tumor tissue. In naming this procedure, "knife" was used because controlled destructive radiation replaces the surgical knife (see Fig. 10.30, B). The Cyberknife® system uses unique robotic mobility and continuous image guidance, which follows the target through the treatment (eliminating the need for restrictive head frame).

In combination with stereotactic procedures, surgical lasers are also used to destroy tumors.

destruction

10-82 Neuro/lysis is _____ of nerves. Neurolysis has several meanings, but all of them have to do with nervous tissue. The word is used to mean release of a nerve sheath by cutting it longitudinally, loosening of adhesions surrounding a nerve, or disintegration of nerve tissue.

neuroplasty

Write a word that means surgical repair of a nerve: _____.
Neuro/rrhaphy specifically means suture of a nerve. **Neuro/tripsy** is surgical crushing of a nerve. **Neurectomy** is excision of a nerve.

WRITE IT!
EXERCISE 17

Write a term for each of the following.
1. device used to redirect body fluid to another area _____
2. excision of an aneurysm _____
3. surgical removal of a portion of the skull _____
4. suture of a nerve _____
5. surgical crushing of a nerve _____

---

nerve

10-83 Pain management may be for a short time (for example, after surgery) or longer (chronic pain) and may include both drug therapy and nondrug treatments. Nerve blocks are used to reduce pain by temporarily or permanently blocking transmission of _____ impulses. **Nerve block anesthesia** is produced by injecting an anesthetic along the course of a nerve to inhibit the conduction of impulses to and from the area supplied by the nerve.

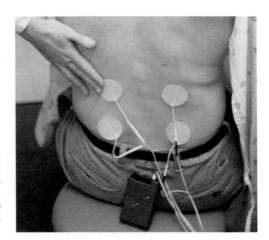

Figure 10.31 Transcutaneous electrical nerve stimulation (TENS). The TENS unit is being used in this example to control low back pain. Electrodes are placed on the skin and attached to a stimulator by flexible wires. The electric impulses block transmission of pain signals to the brain. TENS is not addictive and has no known side effects, but it is contraindicated in patients with artificial cardiac pacemakers.

Sympathectomy is a surgical procedure in which one or more sympathetic nerves are severed. This surgery has special uses, including alleviation of pain.

10-84 Epidural anesthesia is injection of an anesthetic into the epidural space, which contains spinal fluid and spinal nerves. Epidurals, most commonly performed in the lumbar area, can be tailored to numb an area of the body from the lower extremities to the upper abdomen. They are often used in labor and childbirth. Epidural injections, containing various combinations of cortisone and anesthetics, are used by pain specialists to alleviate chronic pain of the lower back.

10-85 Trans/cutane/ous electrical nerve stimulation (TENS) is a method of pain control by the application of electric impulses to the nerve endings (Fig. 10.31). Pain signals to the brain are blocked by electric impulses generated by a stimulator that is attached to electrodes placed on the skin. Literal translation of transcutaneous is across or performed through the _____.

skin

10-86 Many drugs, including hypnotics and antipyretics, act on the CNS.
Hypnotics are drugs often used as sedatives to produce a calming effect. Functional activity, irritability, and excitement are decreased by sedatives.
Anti/pyretics act _____ fever.

WORD ORIGIN
hypnotics *(G.)*
hypnos, sleep

against

10-87 If a cerebral embolus is caused by a blood clot, a thrombo/lytic may be used. **Thrombolytics** _____ blood clots.

dissolve

10-88 A **vago/tomy** is severing of various branches of the vagus nerve and is done to reduce the amount of acid secreted in the stomach. This is done to prevent the recurrence of an ulcer. Write this term that means severing of the vagus nerve: _____.

vagotomy

10-89 Psycho/analysis is a method of diagnosing and treating disorders of the _____. This is accomplished by ascertaining and studying the facts of the patient's mental condition.
Psycho/therapy is treatment of disorders of the mind by psychologic means rather than by physical means.

mind

ANALYZE IT!
EXERCISE 18

Break these words into their component parts by placing a slash between the word parts. Write the meaning of each term.
1. neurolysis _____
2. psychotherapy _____
3. vagotomy _____
4. transcutaneous _____

Match terms in the left columns with descriptions in the right column.

_____ **1.** epidural   **A.** application of electric impulses to the nerve endings

_____ **2.** thrombolytics   **B.** injection of anesthesia to produce numbness in the lower part of the body

_____ **3.** TENS   **C.** agents used to dissolve blood clots

PHARMACOLOGY

The nervous system innervates many other body systems and thus indirectly influences their functions. The following drug classes relate more specifically to the central nervous system and psychological and emotional disorders.

🔑 **KEY** POINT **Psycho/pharmacology is the study of the action of drugs on functions of the mind. Anti/anxiety drugs** are used to relieve feelings of anxiety. **Tranquilizers** are prescribed to calm anxious or agitated persons, ideally without decreasing their consciousness. **Narcotic drugs** produce stupor or sleep.

Drug Class: Effect and Uses

Analgesics: Relieve pain

Narcotic analgesics (also called **Opioid** *analgesics): Potential for addiction or abuse; used for severe pain; may alter one's perception; produce tolerance or dependency*

codeine (Tylenol with codeine #3, with acetaminophen)	meperidine (Demerol)	oxycodone (OxyContin)
	methadone (Dolophine)	tramadol (Ultram)
fentanyl (Duragesic)	morphine (MS Contin)	

Nonnarcotic analgesics: No potential for addiction or abuse

acetaminophen (Tylenol)   NSAIDs (see below for examples)

Nonsteroidal antiinflammatory drugs (NSAIDs): Mild to moderate pain relief

aspirin (Bayer)   ibuprofen (Motrin)

celecoxib (Celebrex)   naproxen (Aleve)

Antialcoholics: Discourage use of alcohol

disulfiram (Antabuse)

Anticonvulsants: Treat epilepsy and other seizure disorders

carbamazepine (Tegretol)	gabapentin (Neurontin)	phenytoin (Dilantin)
divalproex (Depakote)	lacosamide (Vimpat)	topiramate (Topamax)
ethosuximide (Zarontin)	lamotrigine (Lamictal)	

Antidepressants: Treat depression and other mental disorders by affecting the balance of neurotransmitters in the brain.
Types of antidepressants include tricyclic, tetracyclic, monoamine oxidase inhibitors, serotonin modulators, selective serotonin reuptake inhibitors (SSRIs), selective serotonin and norepinephrine reuptake inhibitors (SSNRIs), and atypical.

amitriptyline (Elavil)	fluoxetine (Prozac)	venlafaxine (Effexor)
bupropion (Wellbutrin)	mirtazapine (Remeron)	vilazodone (Viibryd)
citalopram (Celexa)	phenelzine (Nardil)	
duloxetine (Cymbalta)	trazodone (Oleptro)	

Antimigraine drugs: Treat migraine headaches

ergotamine (Cafergot, with caffeine)   sumatriptan (Imitrex)

rizatriptan (Maxalt)   zolmitriptan (Zomig)

Antiparkinsonian agents: Relieve symptoms of Parkinson disease and parkinsonian syndromes
Types include catechol O-methyltransferase (COMT) inhibitors, dopamine agonists, and certain anticholinergics

amantadine (Symmetrel)	levodopa/carbidopa (Sinemet)	selegiline (Eldepryl)
benztropine (Cogentin)	pramipexole (Mirapex)	tolcapone (Tasmar)

PHARMACOLOGY, cont'd

Antipsychotics/neuroleptics: Manage the symptoms of psychoses, such as hallucinations, delusions, or mania

aripiprazole (Abilify)	*haloperidol (Haldol)*	*risperidone (Risperdal)*
asenapine (Saphris)	*lurasidone (Latuda)*	*thioridazine (Mellaril)*
chlorpromazine (Thorazine)	*olanzapine (Zyprexa)*	
clozapine (Clozaril)	*quetiapine (Seroquel)*	

Anxiolytics (also called antianxiety drugs): Induce relaxation to relieve anxiety
Many drugs in this class may also be considered hypnotics (promote sleep) or sedatives (depress central nervous system)
Some antidepressants and the beta-blocker propranolol are also used to treat anxiety

buspirone (BuSpar)	*hydroxyzine (Vistaril)*
doxepin (Silenor)	*meprobamate (Equanil)*

Benzodiazepines: Sedatives used to treat anxiety

alprazolam (Xanax)	*diazepam (Valium)*	*temazepam (Restoril)*
chlordiazepoxide (Librium)	*lorazepam (Ativan)*	
clonazepam (Klonopin)	*midazolam (Versed)*	

Cholinesterase inhibitors: Increase levels of acetylcholine to treat cognitive failures associated with dementia

donepezil (Aricept)	*galantamine (Razadyne)*	*rivastigmine (Elexon)*

Mood stabilizers: Balance neurotransmitters in the brain to prevent severe mood swings (mania and depression) and to treat bipolar disorder
lithium (Lithobid)

Stimulants: Increase synaptic activity in the brain to treat attention-deficit disorder, narcolepsy, fatigue, or to suppress the appetite

dextroamphetamine (Dexedrine)	*methylphenidate (Ritalin)*	*phentermine (Adipex-P)*

WRITE IT! **EXERCISE 20**

Write words in the blanks to complete these sentences.

1. Antipsychotics, also called _____, manage the symptoms of psychoses.
2. The drug class _____ is used to treat epilepsy and other seizure disorders.
3. Opioid _____ are used for severe pain.
4. The drug class, _____, is used to induce relaxation to relieve anxiety.
5. The drug class, _____ inhibitors, treat cognitive failures associated with dementia.

CHAPTER ABBREVIATIONS*

ACh	acetylcholine		**EEG**	electroencephalography
ADD	attention deficit disorder		**IAD**	illness anxiety disorder
ADHD	attention deficit hyperactivity disorder		**ICP**	intracranial pressure
ALS	amyotrophic lateral sclerosis		**LBP**	lower back pain
CNS	central nervous system		**MS**	multiple sclerosis
CSF	cerebrospinal fluid		**OCD**	obsessive-compulsive disorder
CVA	cerebrovascular accident, costovertebral angle		**PNS**	peripheral nervous system
DSM	*Diagnostic and Statistical Manual of Mental Disorders*		**SCI**	spinal cord injury
			TENS	transcutaneous electrical nerve stimulation
DTs	delirium tremens		**TIA**	transient ischemic attack
DTR	deep tendon reflex			

*Many of these abbreviations share their meanings with other terms.

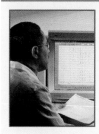

A Career as an Electroencephalography Technologist

Joyce is an EEG and polysomnography technologist. She enjoys her work at a center that studies sleep disorders. She knows that the test results help physicians determine treatment and that improving patients' sleep is one of the best aids to better health. Joyce studied electroneurodiagnostic technology (most programs are about 1 to 2 years), earned her associate's degree, and passed the national board examination. There are also programs that specifically focus on polysomnographic technology. For more information, visit *www.aset.org.*

CHAPTER 10 SELF-TEST

Review the new word parts for this chapter. Work all of the following exercises to test your understanding of the material before checking your answers against those in Appendix IV.

BASIC UNDERSTANDING

Labeling

I.   *Label the drawing of the meninges with arachnoid, dura mater, and pia mater.*

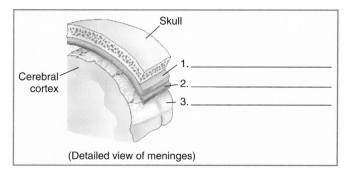

(Detailed view of meninges)

II.   *Label the following structures in the drawing: brain stem, cerebellum, cerebrum, diencephalon, and spinal cord.*

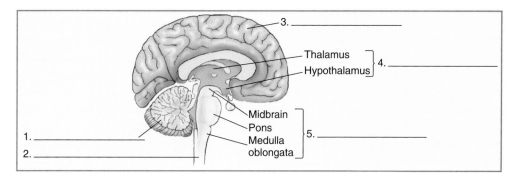

Deconstructing Terms

III.   *Break these words apart, and write the meaning of each term.*

1. polyneuralgia   _____

2. aneurysmectomy   _____

3. neurogenic   _____

4. craniotomy   _____

5. subdural   _____

Identifying Illustrations

IV. *Label these illustrations using one of the following: cholinesterase, hemiplegia, hypochondriasis, meningocele, paraplegia,*
     ventriculoperitoneal, shingles

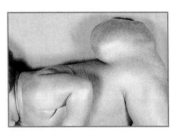

1. _____

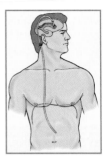

2. _____ shunt

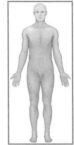

3. _____

Matching

V. *Assign structures in the left column to the correct division of the nervous system by choosing either A or B.*

_____ **1.** brain   **A.** central nervous system

_____ **2.** sense organs   **B.** peripheral nervous system

_____ **3.** spinal cord

Using Vocabulary

VI. *Circle the correct answer for each of the following:*

1. Danielle is riding on the back of a motorcycle when it is hit by an automobile. The ER physician's findings include evidence of a
   fracture at the base of the skull, accompanied by facial paralysis and a soft bruise behind the left ear, indicating a tear of the
   outermost of the three meningeal membranes. What is the name of the outermost membrane?
   (arachnoid, cochlea, dura mater, pia mater)

2. Harry B., 75-years-old and living at home with his wife, shows signs of a type of dementia that involves irreversible loss of memory,
   disorientation, and speech and gait disturbances. Which disorder has been described?
   (Alzheimer disease, Lou Gehrig disease, Meniere syndrome, multiple sclerosis)

3. A vehicle in which Scott was riding while serving in Iraq was hit by an IED. He sustained a spinal cord injury (SCI) and has paralysis
   of both legs and the lower body. Which type of paralysis does he have? (diplegia, hemiplegia, paraplegia, quadriplegia)

4. Khalida, age 75, sees her internist and complains of symptoms that he recognizes as transient ischemic attacks (TIAs).
   After extensive testing, which is normal except for hypertension, he prescribes antihypertensives and warns her of the
   characteristics of a stroke. Which of the following is another name for stroke?
   (cerebrovascular accident, craniocerebral trauma, monoplegia, polyneuropathy)

5. Xavier undergoes radiography that includes injection of contrast medium to detect lesions of the spinal cord. Which of the following
   terms is a record of his test? (encephalogram, encephalography, myelogram, myelography)

6. Cameron has suffered a morbid fear of becoming trapped in a closed place as long as she can remember. Which of the following is
   her condition? (acrophobia, agoraphobia, claustrophobia, zoophobia)

7. A newborn will undergo surgery for a saclike protrusion of the meninges through a defect in the vertebral column. Which term
   describes the newborn's pathology? (meningitis, meningocele, myelocyte, myelomalacia)

8. Which reaction is the nurse practitioner testing when she strikes the patient's patellar tendon, just below the kneecap?
   (biceps reflex, deep tendon reflex, kneecap reflex incontinence, superficial reflex)

9. Fifteen-year-old Brittany is experiencing insatiable episodes of continuous eating and afterward experiencing depression and
   purging. Which disorder is described? (anorexia nervosa, bulimia, cerebral concussion, hypochondriasis)

10. Tests indicate that Yash suffers from paralysis and loss of sensation in his right leg. Which term correctly describes his loss of
    sensitivity to pain? (algesia, hypalgesia, hyperalgesia, parakinesis)

Filling in the Blanks

VII. Write the appropriate word in each blank.

Three membranes collectively known as (1) _____ cover the brain and spinal cord.
The largest and uppermost portion of the brain is the (2) _____. A fluid called
(3) _____ fluid surrounds and cushions the brain and spinal cord. The nervous system is composed of two types
of cells. The basic unit of the nervous system is called a (4) _____. The other type of cell that serves as support
is a (5) _____ cell.

A cytoplasmic projection that carries impulses away from the cell body of the neuron is called an (6) _____.
Another type of cytoplasmic process that carries an impulse to the cell body is a (7) _____.

Writing Terms

VIII. Write one term for each of the following meanings.

1. a record produced by the electrical impulses of the brain   _____

2. agent used to treat the symptoms of depression   _____

3. false or pretended mental disorder   _____

4. inflammation of the brain and spinal cord   _____

5. irrational fear of public places where escape is difficult   _____

6. partially aware of one's surroundings   _____

7. radiography of the spinal cord   _____

8. recording the electric activity of the brain   _____

9. surgical breaking up of adhesions around a nerve   _____

10. uncontrollable, brief episodes of sleep   _____

Making Connections

IX. Describe the relationship of these terms.

1. neurons and neuroglia   _____

_____

2. axon and dendrite   _____

_____

3. dura mater and pia mater   _____

_____

Finetuning Terms

X. In addition to spelling, describe at least one difference in the following:

1. central nervous system and peripheral nervous system   _____

_____

2. somatic nervous system and autonomic nervous system   _____

_____

GREATER COMPREHENSION

Abbreviating

XI. Write a letter in each blank for the abbreviation that corresponds to the clue.

1. Acute psychotic reaction resulting from abrupt cessation of excessive alcohol intake is __ __ __.

2. Cerebrospinal fluid is __ __ __.

3. Lou Gehrig disease is __ __ __.

4. The abbreviation for acetylcholine is __ __ __.

5. The disorder that was formerly called hypochondriasis is __ __ __.

Health Care Reporting

XII. Read the following Death Summary, and match terms with their descriptions. (Not all selections will be used.)

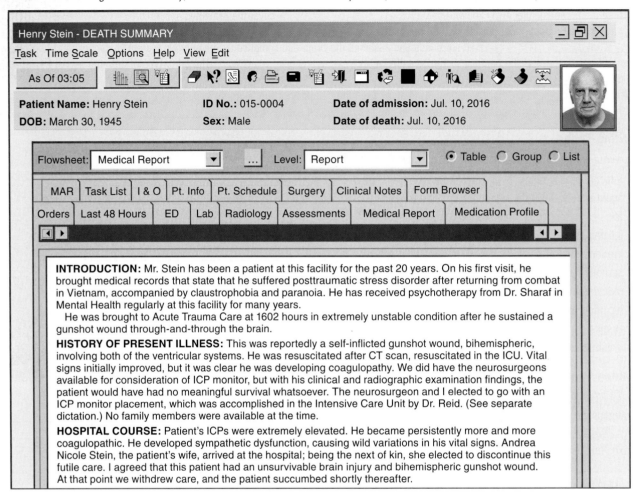

Henry Stein - DEATH SUMMARY

Task Time Scale Options Help View Edit

As Of 03:05

Patient Name: Henry Stein   **ID No.:** 015-0004   **Date of admission:** Jul. 10, 2016
DOB: March 30, 1945   **Sex:** Male   **Date of death:** Jul. 10, 2016

Flowsheet: Medical Report   ...   Level: Report   ● Table ○ Group ○ List

MAR | Task List | I & O | Pt. Info | Pt. Schedule | Surgery | Clinical Notes | Form Browser
Orders | Last 48 Hours | ED | Lab | Radiology | Assessments | Medical Report | Medication Profile

INTRODUCTION: Mr. Stein has been a patient at this facility for the past 20 years. On his first visit, he brought medical records that state that he suffered posttraumatic stress disorder after returning from combat in Vietnam, accompanied by claustrophobia and paranoia. He has received psychotherapy from Dr. Sharaf in Mental Health regularly at this facility for many years.

He was brought to Acute Trauma Care at 1602 hours in extremely unstable condition after he sustained a gunshot wound through-and-through the brain.

HISTORY OF PRESENT ILLNESS: This was reportedly a self-inflicted gunshot wound, bihemispheric, involving both of the ventricular systems. He was resuscitated after CT scan, resuscitated in the ICU. Vital signs initially improved, but it was clear he was developing coagulopathy. We did have the neurosurgeons available for consideration of ICP monitor, but with his clinical and radiographic examination findings, the patient would have had no meaningful survival whatsoever. The neurosurgeon and I elected to go with an ICP monitor placement, which was accomplished in the Intensive Care Unit by Dr. Reid. (See separate dictation.) No family members were available at the time.

HOSPITAL COURSE: Patient's ICPs were extremely elevated. He became persistently more and more coagulopathic. He developed sympathetic dysfunction, causing wild variations in his vital signs. Andrea Nicole Stein, the patient's wife, arrived at the hospital; being the next of kin, she elected to discontinue this futile care. I agreed that this patient had an unsurvivable brain injury and bihemispheric gunshot wound. At that point we withdrew care, and the patient succumbed shortly thereafter.

_____ **1.** bihemispheric	**A.** behavior associated with delusions of persecution
_____ **2.** claustrophobia	**B.** characterized by acute emotional response to a traumatic event
_____ **3.** ICP monitor	**C.** device to monitor a patient's intracranial pressure
_____ **4.** paranoia	**D.** dysfunction of the autonomic nervous system
_____ **5.** posttraumatic stress disorder	**E.** measuring of the acetycholine level
_____ **6.** psychotherapy	**F.** morbid fear of closed spaces
_____ **7.** sympathethic dysfunction	**G.** pertaining to both sides of the cerebrum
	H. pertaining to the cerebellum
	I. psychologically induced immobility
	J. therapy by psychologic means

Spelling

XIII. Circle all misspelled terms, and write their correct spelling.

acetylcoline   Alzheimer   cerebrul   neurektomy   ocipital

Health Care Reporting

XIV. Read the health care report, then write terms from the report that match the descriptions.

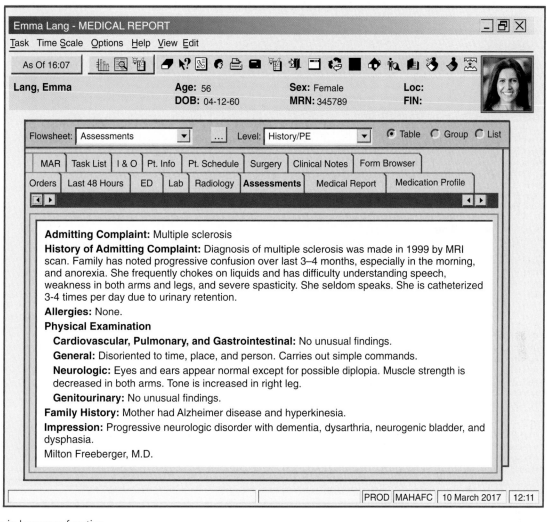

Emma Lang - MEDICAL REPORT

Task Time Scale Options Help View Edit

As Of 16:07

Lang, Emma **Age:** 56 **Sex:** Female **Loc:**
DOB: 04-12-60 **MRN:** 345789 **FIN:**

Flowsheet: Assessments ... Level: History/PE ⦿ Table ○ Group ○ List

MAR | Task List | I & O | Pt. Info | Pt. Schedule | Surgery | Clinical Notes | Form Browser

Orders | Last 48 Hours | ED | Lab | Radiology | Assessments | Medical Report | Medication Profile

Admitting Complaint: Multiple sclerosis

History of Admitting Complaint: Diagnosis of multiple sclerosis was made in 1999 by MRI scan. Family has noted progressive confusion over last 3–4 months, especially in the morning, and anorexia. She frequently chokes on liquids and has difficulty understanding speech, weakness in both arms and legs, and severe spasticity. She seldom speaks. She is catheterized 3-4 times per day due to urinary retention.

Allergies: None.

Physical Examination

　Cardiovascular, Pulmonary, and Gastrointestinal: No unusual findings.

　General: Disoriented to time, place, and person. Carries out simple commands.

　Neurologic: Eyes and ears appear normal except for possible diplopia. Muscle strength is decreased in both arms. Tone is increased in right leg.

　Genitourinary: No unusual findings.

Family History: Mother had Alzheimer disease and hyperkinesia.

Impression: Progressive neurologic disorder with dementia, dysarthria, neurogenic bladder, and dysphasia.

Milton Freeberger, M.D.

PROD | MAHAFC | 10 March 2017 | 12:11

1. difficulty in language function _____

2. abnormally increased motor function _____

3. progressive, degenerative disease of the brain _____

4. loss of appetite _____

5. chronic disease characterized by progressive destruction of the myelin sheaths of neurons _____

Pronouncing Terms

XV. Write the correct term for the following phonetic spellings.

1. al-**jē**-zē-uh _____

2. an-ū-riz-**mek**-tuh-mē _____

3. **ef**-ur-unt _____

4. kō-lin-**es**-tur-āse _____

5. ser-uh-**brot**-uh-mē _____

6. sī-kō-**ther**-uh-pē _____

Health Care Reporting

XVI. Read the following report and select one answer for Questions 1-6.

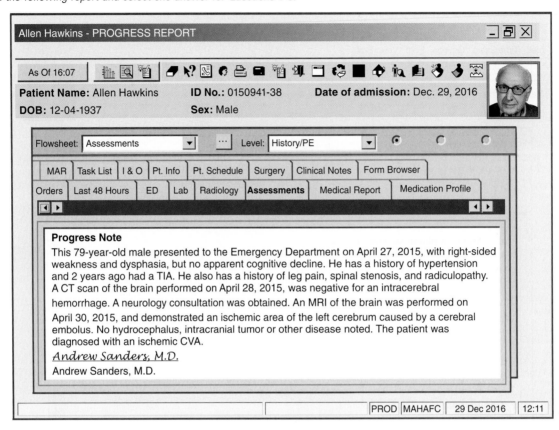

Allen Hawkins - PROGRESS REPORT

Patient Name: Allen Hawkins   **ID No.:** 0150941-38   **Date of admission:** Dec. 29, 2016
DOB: 12-04-1937   **Sex:** Male

Flowsheet: Assessments   Level: History/PE

MAR | Task List | I & O | Pt. Info | Pt. Schedule | Surgery | Clinical Notes | Form Browser
Orders | Last 48 Hours | ED | Lab | Radiology | **Assessments** | Medical Report | Medication Profile

Progress Note
This 79-year-old male presented to the Emergency Department on April 27, 2015, with right-sided weakness and dysphasia, but no apparent cognitive decline. He has a history of hypertension and 2 years ago had a TIA. He also has a history of leg pain, spinal stenosis, and radiculopathy. A CT scan of the brain performed on April 28, 2015, was negative for an intracerebral hemorrhage. A neurology consultation was obtained. An MRI of the brain was performed on April 30, 2015, and demonstrated an ischemic area of the left cerebrum caused by a cerebral embolus. No hydrocephalus, intracranial tumor or other disease noted. The patient was diagnosed with an ischemic CVA.
Andrew Sanders, M.D.
Andrew Sanders, M.D.

PROD | MAHAFC | 29 Dec 2016 | 12:11

1. The term in the report which refers to inadequate blood flow is (embolus, hydrocephalus, ischemic, stenosis)
2. The "T" in the abbreviation "TIA" stands for (temporal, transient, transcutaneous, tumor)
3. Dysphasia is a condition which refers to a patient's (attention span, cognition, movement, speech)
4. The abbreviation which indicates a stroke is (CVA, CT, MRI, TIA)
5. The prefix in the term "intracerebral" means (brain, disease, nerve, within)
6. The term for a mass of undissolved matter present in a blood vessel is (dysphasia, embolus, hemorrhage, stenosis)

Using Pharmacologic Terms

XVII. Use all selections to match terms in the left column with their descriptions in the right column.

_____ **1.** anticonvulsants   **A.** treat ADD, narcolepsy, fatigue or suppress the appetite
_____ **2.** analgesics   **B.** treat epilepsy and other seizure disorders
_____ **3.** neuroleptics   **C.** relieve pain
_____ **4.** anxiolytics   **D.** antipsychotics
_____ **5.** cholinesterase inhibitors   **E.** relieve anxiety
_____ **6.** mood stabilizers   **F.** increase levels of acetycholine
_____ **7.** stimulants   **G.** balance neurotransmitters to prevent severe mood swings

Categorizing Terms and Practicing Pronunciation

XVIII. Classify the terms in the left column by selecting A, B, C, D, or E.

_____	**1.** antipsychotics	**A.** anatomy
_____	**2.** botulism	**B.** diagnostic test or procedure
_____	**3.** burr hole	**C.** pathology
_____	**4.** carpoptosis	**D.** surgery
_____	**5.** cerebral angiography	**E.** nonsurgical therapy
_____	**6.** insula	
_____	**7.** myelogram	
_____	**8.** opioid analgesics	
_____	**9.** sciatica	
_____	**10.** sympathectomy	

(Be prepared to pronounce terms 1-10 in class after listening to Chapter 11 terms at *http://evolve.elsevier.com/Leonard/building/*. In addition, practice categorizing all boldface terms in this chapter.)

New Construction

XIX. Divide these words into their component parts, and write the meaning of each term.

1. arachnitis _____

2. cardiophobia _____

3. cerebrocerebellar _____

4. encephalomalacia _____

5. meningoencephalomyelitis _____

(Use Appendix IV to check your answers to the exercises.)

BMV LIST

Visit *http://evolve.elsevier.com/Leonard/building/* to listen to the boldface terms in Chapter 10. Look closely at the spelling of each term as it is pronounced.

acetylcholine (as-uh-tul-, as-uh-tēl-**kō**-lēn)
acetylcholinesterase (as-uh-tul-, as-uh-tēl-kō-li-**nes**-tuh-rās)
acrophobia (ak-rō-**fō**-bē-uh)
adrenaline (uh-**dren**-uh-lin)
adrenergic (ad-ren-**ur**-jik)
afferent system (**af**-ur-unt **sis**-tum)
agnosia (ag-**nō**-zhuh)
agoraphobia (ag-uh-ruh-**fō**-bē-uh)
algesia (al-**jē**-zē-uh)
Alzheimer disease (**awltz**-hī-mur di-**zēz**)
amyotrophic lateral sclerosis (ā-mī-ō-**trō**-fik **lat**-ur-ul skluh-**rō**-sis)
analgesic (an-ul-**jē**-zik)
aneurysm (**an**-ū-riz-um)
aneurysmectomy (an-ū-riz-**mek**-tuh-mē)
anorexia nervosa (an-ō-**rek**-sē-uh nur-**vō**-suh)
antialcoholics (an-tē-al-kō-**hol**-iks)
antianxiety drugs (an-tē-ang-**zī**-uh-tē drugz)
anticonvulsant (an-tē-kun-**vul**-sunt)
antidepressant (an-tē-dē-**pres**-unt)
antimigraine drugs (an-tē-**mī**-grān drugz)
antiparkinsonian agents (an-tē-pahr-kin-**sō**-nē-un **ā**-junts)
antipsychotic (an-tē-sī-**kot**-ik)
antipyretic (an-tē-pī-**ret**-ik)

antisocial (an-tē-**sō**-shul)
anxiety disorders (ang-**zī**-uh-tē dis-**or**-durz)
anxiolytics (ang-zē-ō-**lit**-iks)
aphasia (uh-**fā**-zhuh)
apraxia (uh-**prak**-sē-uh)
arachnoid (uh-**rak**-noid)
arachnophobia (uh-rak-nō-**fō**-bē-uh)
attention deficit disorder (uh-**ten**-shun **def**-i-sit dis-**or**-dur)
attention deficit hyperactivity disorder (uh-**ten**-shun **def**-i-sit hī-pur-ak-**tiv**-i-tē dis-**or**-dur)
autism (**aw**-tiz-um)
autonomic (aw-tuh-**nom**-ik)
axon (**ak**-son)
Bell palsy (bel **pawl**-zē)
bipolar disorder (bī-**pō**-lur dis-**or**-dur)
botulism (**boch**-uh-liz-um)
bradykinesia (brad-ē-ki-**nē**-zhuh)
brain scan (brān skan)
brain stem (brān stem)
bulimia (boo-**lē**-mē-uh)
burr hole (bur hōl)
carpoptosis (kahr-pop-**tō**-sis)
central nervous system (**sen**-trul **nur**-vus **sis**-tum)
cephalalgia (sef-uh-**lal**-juh)

cephalgia (suh-**fal**-juh)
cerebellar (ser-uh-**bel**-ur)
cerebellitis (ser-uh-bel-**ī**-tis)
cerebellum (ser-uh-**bel**-um)
cerebral (suh-**rē**-brul, **ser**-uh-brul)
cerebral aneurysm (suh-**rē**-brul, **ser**-uh-brul **an**-ū-riz-um)
cerebral angiography (suh-**rē**-brul, **ser**-uh-brul an-jē-**og**-ruh-fē)
cerebral concussion (suh-**rē**-brul, **ser**-uh-brul kun-**kush**-un)
cerebral cortex (suh-**rē**-brul, **ser**-uh-brul **cor**-teks)
cerebral embolus (suh-**rē**-brul, **ser**-uh-brul **em**-bō-lus)
cerebral hemisphere (suh-**rē**-brul, **ser**-uh-brul **hem**-i-sfēr)
cerebral hemorrhage (suh-**rē**-brul, **ser**-uh-brul **hem**-uh-ruj)
cerebral palsy (suh-**rē**-brul, **ser**-uh-brul **pawl**-zē)
cerebral ventricle (suh-**rē**-brul, **ser**-uh-brul **ven**-tri-kul)
cerebrospinal (ser-uh-brō-**spī**-nul)
cerebrospinal fluid (ser-uh-brō-**spī**-nul **floo**-id)
cerebrotomy (ser-uh-**brot**-uh-mē)
cerebrovascular accident (ser-uh-brō-**vas**-kū-lur **ak**-si-dunt)
cerebrum (**ser**-uh-brum, suh-**rē**-brum)
cholinergic (kō-lin-**ur**-jik)
cholinesterase inhibitors (kō-lin-**es**-tur-ās in-**hib**-i-turz)
claustrophobia (klaws-trō-**fō**-bē-uh)
clinical depression (**klin**-i-kul di-**presh**-un)
cluster headache (**klus**-tur **hed**-āk)
coma (**kō**-muh)
compulsion (kom-**pul**-shun)
concussion (kun-**kush**-un)
contusion (kun-**too**-zhun)
convulsion (kun-**vul**-shun)
craniectomy (krā-nē-**ek**-tuh-mē)
craniocerebral (krā-nē-ō-**ser**-uh-brul)
cranioplasty (**krā**-nē-ō-plas-tē)
craniotomy (krā-nē-**ot**-uh-mē)
cranium (**krā**-nē-um)
deep tendon reflex (dēp **ten**-dun **rē**-fleks)
dementia (duh-**men**-shuh)
dendrite (**den**-drīt)
diencephalon (dī-un-**sef**-uh-lon)
diplegia (dī-**plē**-jē-uh)
dissociative disorders (di-**sō**-shē-āt-iv dis-**or**-durz)
dopamine (**dō**-puh-mēn)
dura mater (**doo**-ruh **mā**-tur)
dysarthria (dis-**ahr**-thrē-uh)
dyskinesia (dis-ki-**nē**-zhuh)
dyslexia (dis-**lek**-sē-uh)
dysphasia (dis-**fā**-zhuh)
echoencephalogram (ek-ō-en-**sef**-uh-luh-gram)
echoencephalography (ek-ō-en-sef-uh-**log**-ruh-fē)
efferent system (**ef**-ur-unt **sis**-tum)
electroencephalogram (ē-lek-trō-en-**sef**-uh-luh-gram)
electroencephalograph (ē-lek-trō-en-**sef**-uh-luh-graf)
electroencephalography (ē-lek-trō-en-sef-uh-**log**-ruh-fē)
embolic stroke (em-**bol**-ik strōk)
encephalitis (en-sef-uh-**lī**-tis)
encephalography (en-sef-uh-**log**-ruh-fē)
encephalomeningitis (en-sef-uh-lō-men-in-**jī**-tis)
encephalomyelitis (en-sef-uh-lō-mī-uh-**lī**-tis)

encephalomyelopathy (en-sef-uh-lō-mī-uh-**lop**-uh-thē)
endorphin (en-**dor**-fin)
epidural anesthesia (ep-i-**doo**-rul an-es-**thē**-zhuh)
epidural hematoma (ep-i-**doo**-rul hē-muh-**tō**-muh)
epilepsy (**ep**-i-lep-sē)
epinephrine (ep-i-**nef**-rin)
foramen magnum (fō-**rā**-mun **mag**-num)
frontal lobe (**frun**-tul **lōb**)
gamma knife procedure (**gam**-uh nīf prō-**sē**-jur)
Glasgow Coma Scale (**glas**-gō **kō**-muh skāl)
glia cell (**glī**-uh sel)
glioma (glī-**ō**-muh)
hematoma (hē-muh-**tō**-muh)
hemiplegia (hem-ē-**plē**-juh)
hemorrhagic stroke (hem-uh-**raj**-ik strōk)
Huntington chorea (**hun**-ting-tun kuh-**rē**-uh)
hydrocephalus (hī-drō-**sef**-uh-lus)
hydrophobia (hī-drō-**fō**-bē-uh)
hypalgesia (hī-pal-**jē**-zē-uh)
hyperalgesia (hī-pur-al-**jē**-zē-uh)
hyperkinesia (hī-pur-ki-**nē**-zhuh)
hyperkinesis (hī-pur-ki-**nē**-sis)
hypnotic (hip-**not**-ik)
hypoalgesia (hī-pō-al-**jē**-zē-uh)
hypochondria (hī-pō-**kon**-drē-uh)
hypochondriasis (hī-pō-kon-**drī**-uh-sis)
hypothalamus (hī-pō-**thal**-uh-mus)
insula (**in**-suh-luh)
intracerebral hematoma (in-truh-**ser**-uh-brul hē-muh-**tō**-muh)
intracranial (in-truh-**krā**-nē-ul)
intrathecal (in-truh-**thē**-kul)
ischemic stroke (is-**kē**-mik strōk)
kleptomania (klep-tō-**mā**-nē-uh)
mania (**mā**-nē-uh)
medulla (muh-**dul**-uh)
megalomania (meg-uh-lō-**mā**-nē-uh)
meningeal (muh-**nin**-jē-ul)
meninges (muh-**nin**-jēz)
meningioma (muh-nin-jē-**ō**-muh)
meningitis (men-in-**jī**-tis)
meningocele (muh-**ning**-gō-sēl)
meningomyelocele (muh-ning-gō-**mī**-uh-lō-sēl)
midbrain (**mid**-brān)
migraine headache (**mī**-grān **hed**-āk)
monoplegia (mon-ō-**plē**-juh)
mood disorders (**mood** dis-**or**-durz)
mood stabilizers (**mood** **stā**-bi-lī-zerz)
motor neuron (**mō**-tur **noor**-on)
motor system (**mō**-tur **sis**-tum)
multiple sclerosis (**mul**-ti-pul skluh-**rō**-sis)
muscle contraction headache (**mus**-ul kun-**trak**-shun **hed**-āk)
myasthenia gravis (mī-us-**thē**-nē-uh **grav**-is)
myelin sheath (**mī**-uh-lin shēth)
myelogram (**mī**-uh-lō-gram)
myelography (mī-uh-**log**-ruh-fē)
narcolepsy (**nahr**-kō-lep-sē)
narcotic drugs (nahr-**kot**-ik drugz)

nerve block anesthesia (nurv blok an-es-**thē**-zhuh)

nervous (**nur**-vus)

neural (**noor**-ul)

neuralgia (noo-**ral**-juh)

neurasthenia (noor-us-**thē**-nē-uh)

neurectomy (noo-**rek**-tuh-mē)

neurodevelopmental disorders (noor-ō-dē-vel-op-**men**-tul dis-**or**-durz)

neurogenic bladder (noor-ō-**jen**-ik **blad**-ur)

neuroglia (noo-**rog**-lē-uh)

neuroleptics (noor-ō-**lep**-tiks)

neurolysis (noo-**rol**-i-sis)

neuroma (noo-**rō**-muh)

neuromuscular (noor-ō-**mus**-kū-lur)

neuron (**noor**-on)

neuroplasty (**noor**-ō-plas-tē)

neurorrhaphy (noo-**ror**-uh-fē)

neurotripsy (noor-ō-**trip**-sē)

node of Ranvier (nōd ov rahn-**vyā**)

obsession (ob-**sesh**-un)

obsessive-compulsive disorder (ub-**ses**-iv-kum-**pul**-siv dis-**or**-dur)

occipital lobe (ok-**sip**-i-tul **lōb**)

opioid analgesics (**ō**-pē-oid an-ul-**jē**-ziks)

panic attack (**pan**-ik uh-**tak**)

paralysis (puh-**ral**-i-sis)

paranoid personality disorder (**par**-uh-noid pur-suh-**nal**-i-tē dis-**or**-dur)

paraphilia (par-uh-**fil**-ē-uh)

paraplegia (par-uh-**plē**-juh)

parasympathetic (par-uh-sim-puh-**thet**-ik)

paresthesia (par-es-**thē**-zhuh)

parietal lobe (puh-**rī**-uh-tul lōb)

Parkinson disease (**pahr**-kin-sun di-**zēz**)

patellar response (puh-**tel**-ur rē-**spons**)

peripheral (puh-**rif**-ur-ul)

peripheral nervous system (puh-**rif**-ur-ul **nur**-vus **sis**-tum)

peripheral neuropathy (puh-**rif**-ur-ul noo-**rop**-uh-thē)

phobia (**fō**-bē-uh)

phobophobia (fō-bō-**fō**-bē-uh)

pia mater (**pī**-uh, **pē**-uh **mā**-tur)

poliomyelitis (pō-lē-ō-mī-uh-**lī**-tis)

polyneuralgia (pol-ē-noo-**ral**-juh)

polyneuritis (pol-ē-noo-**rī**-tis)

polyneuropathy (pol-ē-noo-**rop**-uh-thē)

pons (ponz)

positron emission tomography (**poz**-i-tron ē-**mish**-un tō-**mog**-ruh-fē)

posttraumatic stress disorder (pōst-traw-**mat**-ik stres dis-**or**-dur)

pseudesthesia (sōōd-es-**thē**-zhuh)

pseudoesthesia (sōō-dō-es-**thē**-zhuh)

pseudomania (sōō-dō-**mā**-nē-uh)

pseudoplegia (sōō-dō-**plē**-juh)

psychoanalysis (sī-kō-uh-**nal**-i-sis)

psychobiological response (sī-kō-bī-ō-**loj**-i-kul rē-**spons**)

psychopharmacology (sī-kō-fahr-muh-**kol**-uh-jē)

psychosis (sī-**kō**-sis)

psychosomatic (sī-kō-sō-**mat**-ik)

psychotherapy (sī-kō-**ther**-uh-pē)

pyromania (pī-rō-**mā**-nē-uh)

pyromaniac (pī-rō-**mā**-nē-ak)

pyrophobia (pī-rō-**fō**-bē-uh)

quadriplegia (kwod-ri-**plē**-juh)

rabies (**rā**-bēz, **rā**-bē-ēz)

receptor (rē-**sep**-tur)

reflex arc (**rē**-fleks ark)

schizophrenia (skit-sō-**frē**-nē-uh)

sciatic nerve (sī-**at**-ik nurv)

sciatica (sī-**at**-i-kuh)

seizure (**sē**-zhur)

semicoma (sem-ē-**kō**-muh)

semiconscious (sem-ē-**kon**-shus)

sensory neuron (**sen**-suh-rē **noor**-on)

sensory system (**sen**-suh-rē **sis**-tum)

serotonin (ser-ō-**tō**-nin)

sexual disorders (**sek**-shōō-ul dis-**or**-durz)

shingles (**shing**-gulz)

shunt (shunt)

sleep apnea (slēp **ap**-nē-uh)

somatic (sō-**mat**-ik)

somatoform disorders (sō-**mat**-ō-form dis-**or**-durz)

spinal cord (**spī**-nul kord)

stereotactic radiosurgery (ster-ē-ō-**tak**-tik rā-dē-ō-**sur**-jur-ē)

stereotactic surgery (ster-ē-ō-**tak**-tik **sur**-jur-ē)

stereotaxis (ster-ē-ō-**tak**-sis)

stimulants (**stim**-ū-lunts)

stupor (**stōō**-pur)

subdural (sub-**doo**-rul)

subdural hematoma (sub-**doo**-rul hē-muh-**tō**-muh)

subdural space (sub-**doo**-rul spās)

superficial reflex (sōō-pur-**fish**-ul **rē**-fleks)

sympathectomy (sim-puh-**thek**-tuh-mē)

sympathetic (sim-puh-**thet**-ik)

synapse (**sin**-aps)

synaptic bulb (si-**nap**-tik bulb)

temporal lobe (**tem**-puh-rul lōb)

tension headache (**ten**-shun **hed**-āk)

tetanus (**tet**-uh-nus)

thalamus (**thal**-uh-mus)

thrombolytic (throm-bō-**lit**-ik)

thrombotic stroke (throm-**bot**-ik strōk)

tranquilizers (**trang**-kwi-līz-urz)

transcutaneous electrical nerve stimulation (trans-kū-**tā**-nē-us ē-**lek**-tri-kul nurv stim-ū-**lā**-shun)

transient ischemic attack (**tran**-shent, **tran**-sē-unt is-**kē**-mik uh-**tak**)

tremor (**trem**-ur)

vagotomy (vā-**got**-uh-mē)

ventriculitis (ven-trik-ū-**lī**-tis)

ventriculoperitoneal shunt (ven-trik-ū-lō-per-i-tō-**nē**-ul shunt)

zoophobia (zō-ō-**fō**-be-uh)

Español | ENHANCING SPANISH COMMUNICATION

English	Spanish (pronunciation)
adrenaline	adrenalina (ah-dray-nah-LEE-nah)
analgesic	analgésico (ah-nal-HAY-se-ko)
antidepressant	antidepresivo (an-te-day-pra-SI-vo)
anxiety	ansiedad (an-se-ay-DAHD)
aphasia	afasia (ah-FAY-see-ah)
arachnoid	arachnoides (ah-rak-NO-e-des)
botulism	botulismo (bo-too-LEES-mo)
cephalgia	cefalalgia (say-fah-lahl-HE-ah)
cerebrum	cerebro (say-RAY-bro)
coma	coma (KO-mah), letargo (lay-TAR-go)
concussion	concusión (kon-koo-se-ON)
conscious	consciente (kons-se-EN-tay)
consciousness	conciencia (kon-se-EN-se-ah)
contusion	contusión (kon-too-se-ON)
convulsion	convulsión (kon-vool-se-ON)
cranium	cráneo (KRAH-nay-o)
dementia	demencia (day-MEN-se-ah)
depression	depresión (day-pre-se-ON)
epilepsy	epilepsia (ay-pe-LEP-se-ah)
fatigue	fatiga (fah-TEE-gah)
gray	gris (grees)
headache	dolor de cabeza (do-LOR day kah-BAY-sa)
hemiplegia	hemiplejia (am-me-PLAY-he-ah)
hypnotic	hipnótico (ip-NO-te-ko)
kleptomania	cleptomanía (klep-to-mah-NEE-ah)

English	Spanish (pronunciation)
lobe	lóbulo (LO-boo-lo)
mood	disposición (dis-po-se-se-ON)
neck	cuello (koo-EL-lyo)
nervous	nervioso (ner-ve-O-so)
neuron	neurona (nay-oo-RO-nah)
obsession	obsesión (ob-say-se-ON)
painful	doloroso (do-lo-RO-so)
panic	pánico (PAH-ne-ko)
paralysis	parálisis (pah-RAH-le-sis)
paraplegia	paraplejia (pah-rah-PLAY-he-ah)
psychosis	psicosis (se-KO-sis)
psychosomatic	psicosomático (se-co-so-MAH-te-ko)
psychotherapy	psicoterapia (se-ko-tay-RAH-pe-ah)
rabies	rabia (RAH-be-ah)
schizophrenia	esquizofrenia (es-ke-so-FRAY-ne-ah)
seizure	ataque (ah-TAH-kay)
sensation	sensación (sen-sah-se-ON)
sleep	sueño (soo-AY-nyo)
spinal column	columna vertebral (ko-LOOM-nah ver-tay-BRAHL)
stroke	ataque de apoplejía (ah-TAH-kay day ah-po-play-HEE-ah)
stupor	estupor (es-too-POR)
tetanus	tétano (TAY-tah-no)
tranquilizer	calmante (kal-MAHN-tay)
tremor	temblor (tem-BLOR)

Peripheral Nervous System
Special Sense Organs

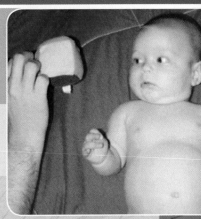

Pregnant women report that fetuses kick after sudden loud noises. At birth, an infant may turn toward a parent who is whispering. Here an audiologist demonstrates how a 3-month-old infant responds to interesting sounds by looking in the direction of the sound.

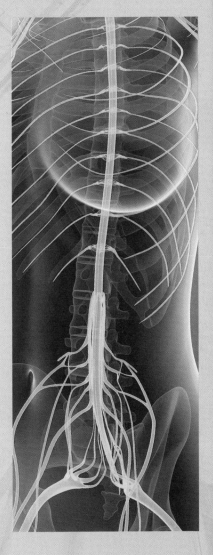

LEARNING OUTCOMES

Basic Understanding

In this chapter, you will learn to do the following:

1. Recognize or write the function of the peripheral nervous system.
2. Recognize or write the meaning of receptors in the peripheral nervous system.
3. List or recognize the names of the special sense organs.
4. Recognize or write the meanings of Chapter 11 word parts, and use them to build or analyze terms.
5. Write terms for selected structures of the special sense organs or match terms with their descriptions.
6. Write the names of the diagnostic terms and procedures studied in this chapter when given descriptions, or match the procedures with their descriptions.
7. Match the names of pathologies related to the special sense organs with their descriptions, or write the names of the pathologies when given their descriptions.
8. Match surgical and therapeutic interventions in Chapter 11 with their descriptions, or write the names of the interventions when given their descriptions.
9. Build terms from word parts to label illustrations.

Greater Comprehension

10. Use word parts from this chapter to determine the meanings of terms in a health care report.
11. Spell the terms accurately.
12. Pronounce the terms correctly.
13. Write the meaning of the abbreviations.
14. Categorize terms as anatomy, diagnostic test or procedure, pathology, surgery, or nonsurgical therapy.
15. Recognize the meanings of general pharmacological terms from this chapter as well as the drug classes and their uses.

FUNCTION FIRST

The peripheral nervous system (PNS) forms the communication network between the central nervous system (CNS) and the rest of the body. The PNS consists of the nerves that branch out from the brain and spinal cord, which communicate with the rest of the receptors, muscles, and glands (see Chapter 10).

Receptors are sensory nerve endings that respond to various kinds of stimulation. The awareness that results is what we know as sensation. Special **sense organs**—the eyes, ears, skin, mouth, and nose—have receptors that detect sensations. Then sensory neurons transmit the signals to the CNS where they are interpreted as sight, hearing, touch, taste, or smell.

SPECIAL SENSE ORGANS

11-1 Senses are how stimuli are perceived. Conditions outside and within the body are distinguished and evaluated. The major sense organs will be studied here, but keep in mind that the body has other senses that include thirst, hunger, fullness, and visceral sensations. Five special sense organs—the eyes, ears, skin, mouth, and nose—are emphasized in this chapter.

Sense organs (like the eye, for example) contain receptors that are activated by specific stimuli. This activation initiates nerve impulses that lead to the brain (the optic nerve in this example). The brain interprets the signal. A simple example shows how light is transmitted to the brain:

Light → Receptors cells in the eye → Optic nerve → Brain translates
(Stimulus)   (Sense Organ)   stimuli into visual images

EYES

ANATOMY AND PHYSIOLOGY

11-2 The eyes are paired organs of sight (right eye, OD; left eye OS; each eye OU). Several accessory structures (muscles, eyelids, and eyebrows, for example) are associated with the eyes.

Label the structures in Fig. 11.1 as you read the next paragraphs.

11-3 Light rays enter the **pupil** (1), the small dark circular structure located in the center of the eye that is surrounded by the colored portion of the eye that we regularly see, the **iris** (2). Muscles of the iris constrict the pupil in bright light and dilate the pupil in dim light, thereby regulating the amount of light entering the eye. The tough outer layer of the eye is composed of the **sclera** (3), the white opaque membrane covering most of the eyeball. Light first enters the eye through the _____.

pupil

🔑 **KEY** POINT **Remember that scler(o) means the sclera of the eye as well as hard.** Scler/itis means inflammation of the sclera; however, sclerose means to harden or to cause hardening.

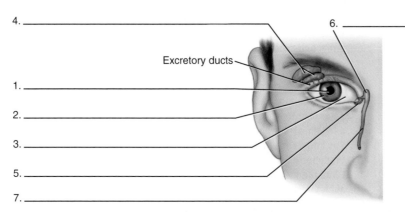

4. _____   6. _____

Excretory ducts

1. _____

2. _____

3. _____

5. _____

7. _____

Figure 11.1 Major structures of the eye, anterior view.

11-4 Associated with the eye are certain accessory organs: muscle, fascia, eyebrow, eyelid, conjunctiva, and the lacrimal glands. The **conjunctiva** is the mucous membrane lining the inner surface of the eyelid and acts as a protective covering for the exposed surface of the eye. You'll learn in this chapter that lacrim(o) means tear, tearing, or crying. The **lacrimal glands** (4) produce and store tears **(lacrimal fluid)** that keep the eyeballs moist.

Tears produced by the lacrimal gland wash over the eyeball and are drained through small openings in the inner corner of the eye. Tears pass through these openings into small **lacrimal ducts** (5) that drain into the **nasolacrimal sac** (6). From here the tears pass into the large **nasolacrimal duct** (7) that ends in the nasal cavity. If more tears are produced than can be removed, we say the person is crying. This is also called **tearing**. Tears are _____ fluid.

lacrimal

> 🌟 **TOOL TIP!**
>
> *Be sure to note the difference in the ways that "tear" is used. It can refer to "a tear" as in lacrimal fluid; "to tear" as for an eye to water or to cry; or "to tear" as to rip or pull apart by force. Of course, the last "tear" is pronounced differently than the first word.*

11-5 Observe and label Fig. 11.2, A, as indicated in the following discussion. The eyeball is composed of three layers:

- **sclera:** The tough outer layer that covers most of the eye, which you labeled in Fig. 11.1. Locate it in Fig. 11.2.
- **cornea** (8): The transparent structure at the front of the eyeball that bends or refracts light rays so that they are focused properly on the sensitive receptor cells in the posterior of the eye.
- **choroid** (9): A dark brown membrane inside the sclera; it is continuous with the iris and the **ciliary body** (10) on the anterior surface of the eye. The choroid is a vascular layer of tissue that supplies blood to the outer retina.

The ciliary body surrounds the outside of the **lens** (11) in a circular fashion, allowing change in shape and thickness of the lens. These changes cause **refraction** of light rays, in the posterior region of the eye, causing flattening of the lens (for distant vision) or thickening and rounding of the lens (for close vision). This refractory adjustment for close vision is called **accommodation.**

The ciliary body also secretes a fluid called *aqueous humor,* which is found in the **anterior chamber** (12). Another cavity of the eye is the **vitreous chamber** (13), which is filled with a soft, jelly-like material, the **vitreous humor.** Escape of this fluid due to trauma may result in significant damage to the eye.

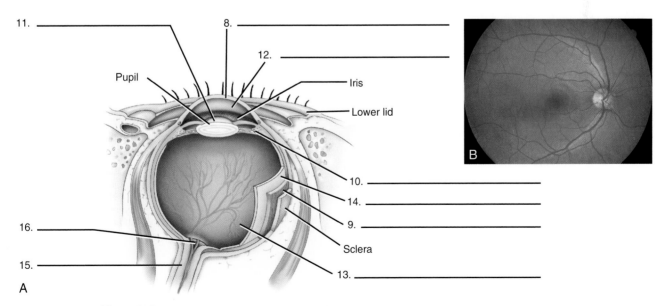

Figure 11.2 Structures of the eyeball, sectioned, superior view. A, Numbered structures in transverse section. **B,** Ophthalmoscopic view of the interior of the eye. A normal retina and optic nerve are shown. The normal retina and blood vessel walls are mainly transparent. Note that the branching points of the blood vessels "point" toward the optic nerve.

The **retina** (14) is the delicate nervous tissue membrane of the eye, which is continuous with the **optic nerve** (15) and enables vision. The **optic disc** (16), the region of the eye where the optic nerve meets the retina, has no light receptors; therefore it is known as the blind spot of the eye. The blind spot is clearly visible in the **ophthalmo/scopic** view (see Fig. 11.2, B).

Perhaps this simple schematic will help you remember the most important structures involved in vision:

pupil → lens → retina → optic nerve → brain

In addition to names of the structures, remember that the changes in the shape and thickness of the lens bring about _____ of light rays, and refractory adjustment for close vision is _____.

Two slightly different images to the brain produce depth of vision.

Intra/ocular and **extra/ocular** mean inside and outside the eye, respectively. Eyelids open and close the eye and keep foreign objects from entering most of the time. Each of our eyes is encased in a protective, bony socket. Our binocular vision sends two slightly different images to the brain, which the brain uses to determine depth of vision. Eye dominance is an unconscious preference to use one eye rather than the other for certain purposes, such as looking through a telescope or a monocular microscope. This unconscious preference to use one eye rather than the other for certain purposes, such as looking through a mononuclear microscope is called eye _____.

11-6 Light waves travel through the eye so that they are focused on photo/receptor cells of the retina called the **rods and cones** (Fig. 11.3). Photo/receptor means that rods and cones are receptive to _____. Rods are responsible for peripheral vision, night vision, and detection of motion. Three types of cones function in bright light and are responsible for color and central vision.

11-7 Most cases of color blindness affect either the green or red receptor cones so that the two colors cannot be distinguished from each other. This is called **daltonism;** and in most cases, it is not a blindness, but a weakness in perceiving colors distinctly. It is an inherited, sex-linked disorder. This sex-linked disorder in which there is a weakness in perceiving colors distinctly is _____.

Total color blindness, or **achromatic vision,** is characterized by an inability to see any color at all. It may be the result of a defect or absence of the cones. Normal color vision sees various shades of color in a color blindness chart (Fig. 11.4).

See Table 11.1 for a summary of eye structures and their functions.

refraction
accommodation

dominance

light

daltonism

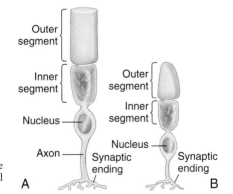

Figure 11.3 Drawings of rod and cone photoreceptor cells of the eye. Note the difference in the shape of rods and cones. There are about 100 million rods and 3 million cones in the retina. **A,** Retinal rod. **B,** Retinal cone.

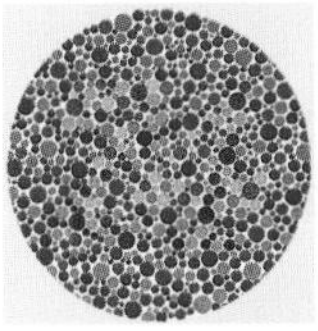

Figure 11.4 Color blindness chart. A person with normal color vision sees different shades of green (representing the number 74) red, and orange. A person with daltonism sees different shades, but does not see different colors distinctly.

Table 11.1	Functions of the Major Components of the Eye
Structure	**Function**
Cornea	Refraction of light
Choroid	Blood supply
Ciliary body	Secretion of vitreous fluid; helps change the shape of lens
External ocular muscles	Movement of the globe
Eyelid	Protection for the eye
Iris	Contracts or relaxes to control the amount of light entering the eye through the pupil
Lacrimal glands	Secretion of tears
Lens	Light refraction
Optic nerve	Transmission of visual information to the brain
Retina	Transforms optic signals into nerve impulses
Rods	Distinguish light from dark; perceive shape and movement
Cones	Color vision
Sclera	External protection

WRITE IT!

EXERCISE 1

Write a word in each blank to complete these sentences.

1. Communication between the central nervous system and the rest of the body is accomplished by

   the _____ nervous system.

2. Sensory nerve endings that respond to various stimuli are called _____.

3. List the names of the five special sense organs: _____

   _____

MATCH IT!

EXERCISE 2

Match the anatomical terms in the left column with correct responses in the right column.

_____ **1.** ciliary body

_____ **2.** conjunctiva

_____ **3.** cornea

_____ **4.** iris

_____ **5.** lacrimal gland

_____ **6.** nasolacrimal duct

_____ **7.** optic disc

_____ **8.** pupil

_____ **9.** retina

_____ **10.** sclera

A. also known as the blind spot

B. channel that carries tears from the nasolacrimal sac to the nose

C. colored portion of the eye

D. delicate, nervous tissue of the eye

E. lines the inner surface of the eyelid

F. produces and stores tears

G. small, round dark circular structure located in the center of the eye

H. surrounds the outside of the lens and causing flattening or thickening of it

I. transparent structure at the front of the eye that refracts light rays

J. white, opaque membrane covering most of the eyeball

Use Appendix IV to check your answers to all the exercises in Chapter 11.

Learn these word parts:

Word Parts: Eye

Combining Form	Meaning	Combining Form	Meaning
choroid(o)	choroid	ocul(o), ophthalm(o)	eye
chrom(o)	color	opt(o), optic(o)	vision
conjunctiv(o)	conjunctiva	presby(o)	old or old age
corne(o), kerat(o)*	cornea	pupill(o)**	pupil
dacry(o), lacrim(o)	tear	retin(o)	retina
ir(o), irid(o)	iris	ton(o)	tone or tension

*Kerat(o) sometimes means hard or horny.
**Note that pupill(o) has two l's.

WRITE IT!   EXERCISE 3

Write the meanings of these combining forms.

1. conjunctiv(o) _____
2. dacry(o) _____
3. corne(o) _____
4. irid(o) _____

5. kerat(o) _____
6. lacrim(o) _____
7. ocul(o) _____
8. retin(o) _____

FIND IT!   EXERCISE 4

Write the combing forms and their meanings for these new terms.

1. **choroidal**
   pertaining to the choroid
   choroid(o), choroid _____
2. **conjunctival**
   pertaining to the conjunctiva
   _____
3. **corneal**
   pertaining to the cornea
   _____
4. **iridic**
   pertaining to the iris
   _____
5. **lacrimal**
   pertaining to the tears
   _____
6. **ocular, optic** (also **ophthalmic**)
   of, pertaining to, or affecting the eye
   _____
7. **pupillary**
   pertaining to the pupil
   _____
8. **retinal**
   pertaining to the retina
   _____

DIAGNOSTIC TESTS AND PROCEDURES

🔑 **KEY POINT Optometrists** and their assistants test the eyes and prescribe corrective glasses or contact lens as well as topical medications. **Ophthalmologists** are medical doctors who specialize in the anatomy and physiology, diagnosis and treatment of disorders of the eyes.

ophthalmoscopy

11-8 You studied in an earlier chapter that an **ophthalmoscope** is an instrument used in _____, visual examination of the eyes (see Fig. 2.32, A).

11-9 Visual acuity is a measure of the ability to distinguish letters and numbers at a given distance. A **Snellen chart** (Fig. 11.5) is one of several charts that test visual acuity. An individual who can read at 20 feet what the average person can read at this distance has 20/20 vision, whereas an individual who can read at 20 feet what the average person can read at 30 feet has 20/30 vision. Visual acuity can be tested using a _____ chart.

Snellen

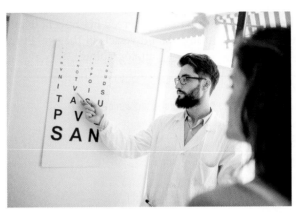

Figure 11.5 Snellen chart. Charts test visual acuity by distinguishing letters and numbers ordinarily seen at different distances.

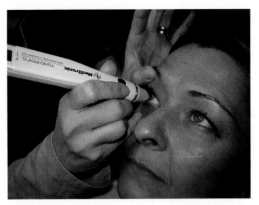

Figure 11.6 Tono-Pen tonometry. Several types of tonometers are used. The Tono-Pen method measures and records the resistance of the eyeball to indentation after exerting a tiny pressure.

➤ **BEYOND** THE BLUEPRINT Legal blindness is defined in most states as best corrected visual acuity less than 20/200 in the better eye or marked constriction of the visual fields.

The Tumbling E chart, as well as other nonalphabet charts, are available for young children or those who are unable to use the Snellen chart.

Accommodation reflex is an adjustment of the eyes for near vision. Specially designed charts are used to test near vision.

measure

11-10 A **keratometer** is an instrument used to _____ the cornea, and is sometimes called an **ophthalmometer**.

11-11 **Tonometry** is measuring of intraocular pressure (IOP) using a **tonometer** (Fig. 11.6) usually after numbing the eye with an anesthetic. Everyone who has gone for an eye exam has probably experienced tonometry, which is measurement of _____ pressure.

intraocular

11-12 **Assessment of visual fields** determines the physical space visible to an individual in a fixed position (Fig. 11.7). VF means visual field. Ophthalmologists also commonly perform a **slit-lamp examination** (Fig. 11.8), which examines the various layers of the eye with a bright light, usually after the pupils have been dilated using a **mydriatic** (agent that dilates the pupil), often an anesthetic, and sometimes a dye. Write this term that means an agent that dilates the pupil:

mydriatic

_____.

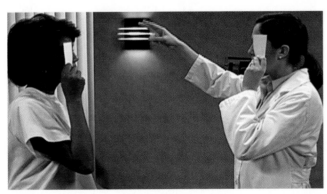

Figure 11.7 Assessment of visual fields. A normal test is 65 degrees upward, 75 degrees downward, 60 degrees inward, and 90 degrees outward. Defects in the vision that remain constant are usually caused by damage to the retina or visual pathways.

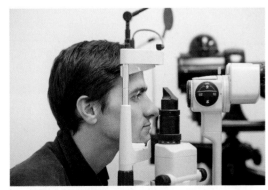

Figure 11.8 Slit-lamp examination. A high intensity beam of light is projected through a narrow slit and a cross section of the illuminated part of the eye is examined through a magnifying lens.

fluorescein

11-13 The **fluorescein angiography** procedure uses fluorescein (a bright green fluorescent dye) and rapid serial photography to study movement of blood through blood vessels in the eye. Practice writing the name of this procedure: _____ angiography.

Match the terms on the left with their meanings in the right column.

_____ **1.** accommodation reflex

_____ **2.** keratometer

_____ **3.** mydriatic

_____ **4.** tonometry

_____ **5.** visual acuity

_____ **6.** visual fields

A. ability to distinguish letters or numbers at a given distance

B. adjustment of the eyes for near vision

C. agent that dilates the pupil

D. instrument used to measure the cornea

E. measurement of intraocular pressure

F. physical space visible when head is held still

PATHOLOGIES

WORD ORIGIN
presbyopia *(G.)*
presby, old man;
-opia, vision

presbyopia

11-14 Diseases of the eye are common, and minor visual problems are not even considered to be true diseases. For example, eyeglasses and eye drops can be bought without a prescription. Optometrists treat eye problems such as nearsightedness or farsightedness; ophthalmologists are medical doctors who treat other pathologies of the eye.

People often notice a change in their vision as they become older. **Presby/opia** is hyperopia and impairment of vision due to advancing years or old age. Write this term that means impairment of vision in older persons: _____.

11-15 Three additional common irregularities in vision are refractive disorders, because the light rays are not focused appropriately to the retina.

- **hyperopia:** Farsightedness, or inability of the eyes to focus on nearby objects; rays of light entering the eye are brought to focus behind the retina.
- **myopia:** Nearsightedness; parallel rays entering the eye are focused in front of the retina.
- **astigmatism:** Uneven focusing of the image, resulting from distortion of the curvature of the lens or cornea. (Compare these three irregularities illustrated in Fig. 11.9.)

hyperopia
astigmatism

Which disorder means farsightedness? _____

Which disorder results in uneven focusing of the image? _____

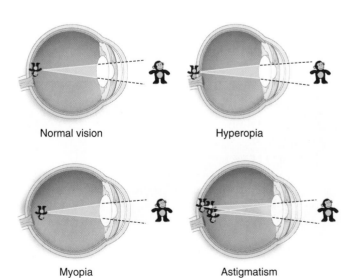

Normal vision   Hyperopia

Myopia   Astigmatism

Figure 11.9 Refraction of the eye. Normal vs. three common irregularities.

MATCH IT!
EXERCISE 6

Match the terms on the left with their meanings in the right column.

_____ **1.** astigmatism

_____ **2.** hyperopia

_____ **3.** myopia

_____ **4.** presbyopia

A. a distortion of the curvature of the lens

B. farsightedness

C. impairment of vision due to advancing age

D. nearsightedness

Abnormal conditions of the eye or vision are included in the following list:

amblyopia Reduced vision in one eye, not correctable by glasses but by wearing eye patch; also called **strabismus** (Fig. 11.10)

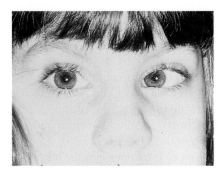

Figure 11.10 Amblyopia. Lazy eye

cataract An abnormal progressive condition of the lens, characterized by loss of transparency (Fig. 11.11). Cataract comes from the Latin word, *cataracta*, meaning waterfall. Congenital cataracts are usually hereditary; senile cataracts are the result of old age.

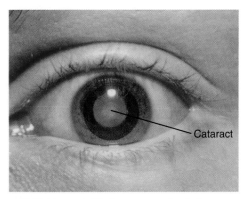

Figure 11.11 Cataract. The lens appears cloudy due to cataract.

color vision deficiencies
    achromatic vision (see Frame 11-7)
    achromatopsia Profound inability to see color
    daltonism (see Frame 11-7)
conjunctivitis Inflammation of the conjunctiva; also called *red eye* or *pink eye*

glaucoma An abnormal condition of increased pressure within the eye. Prolonged pressure can damage the retina and optic nerve.

macular degeneration (MD) A progressive deterioration of the retina associated with new vessel formation that can progress to blindness (Fig. 11.12)

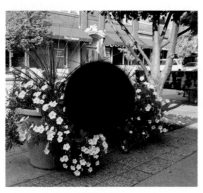

Figure 11.12 Macular degeneration. The blind spot in the center shows the loss of central vision.

nyctalopia Poor vision at night or in dim light
photophobia Excessive sensitivity of the eyes to light
retinal detachment Separation of the retina (tear) from the choroid, usually resulting from a hole or tear in the retina (Fig. 11.13). If detachment is not halted, total blindness of the eye ultimately results.

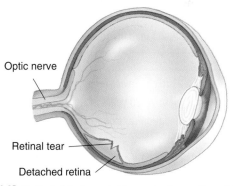

Optic nerve

Retinal tear

Detached retina

Figure 11.13 Retinal detachment. The onset of separation of the retina from the back of the eye is usually sudden and painless. The person may experience bright flashes of light or floating dark spots in the affected eye. Sometimes there is loss of visual field, as though a curtain is being pulled over part of the visual field.

retinopathy Any disease of the retina. Diabetic retinopathy is an abnormality of the retina caused by diabetes mellitus (Fig. 11.14).

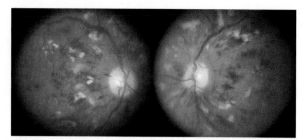

Figure 11.14 Ophthalmoscopic view in diabetic retinopathy. Note several retinal hemorrhages and abnormal pigmentations.

xerophthalmia Dry corneas and conjunctival areas [xer(o), dry]

Disorders of the eyelid and nearby structures

Several irregularities of accessory structures of the eye follow:
blepharedema Swelling of the eyelid

blepharitis Inflammation of the eyelid (Fig. 11.15)

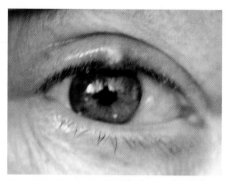

Figure 11.15 Blepharitis caused by a sty. This infection of a gland of the eye shows a great deal of redness and swelling.

dacryocystitis Infection of the lacrimal sac caused by obstruction of the lacrimal ducts
ectropion Turning outward (eversion) of the eyelid
entropion Turning inward of the eyelid
hordeolum Sty or stye, resulting from an infected sebaceous gland of an eyelash (see Fig. 11.15)
ptosis Drooping of the upper eyelids; **blepharoptosis**

WRITE IT! EXERCISE 7

Write terms for the following meanings.

1. any disease of the retina _____
2. drooping of the upper eyelids _____
3. poor vision at night or in dim light _____
4. red eye or pink eye _____
5. condition of increased pressure within the eye _____
6. inflammation of the eyelid _____
7. also called strabismus _____
8. excessive sensitivity of the eyes _____
9. sty _____
10. profound inability to see color _____

WRITE IT! EXERCISE 8

Case Study. Select terms from the report to match the descriptions.

Rachel Harlow, 80 years of age, was examined by Dr. Chein in the Ophthalmology Clinic for blurry vision and nyctalopia. Accommodation reflex and visual field are normal. Tono-Pen tonometry showed increased pressure in the right eye, likely glaucoma.

1. ability of the eye to adjust to variations in distance _____
2. increased pressure within the eye _____
3. measuring of intraocular pressure _____
4. physical space visible to an individual in a fixed position _____
5. poor vision at night or in dim light _____

SURGICAL AND THERAPEUTIC INTERVENTIONS

iris

11-16 Covering an eye in childhood is one example of a therapeutic intervention. Glaucoma is often treated with eyedrops and a laser; in extreme cases, **iridectomy** (surgical removal of part of the _____) is performed to restore proper drainage.

eyelid

11-17 Blepharoplasty is surgical repair of the _____ to repair ptosis.

corneal

11-18 A **corneal transplant** is transplantation of _____ tissue from a donor or the patient's own cornea.

cold

11-19 Ophthalmic cryosurgery is a general term for the use of extreme _____ to remove a cataract or to cause the edges of a detached retina to heal. **Cryo/extraction** is removal of a cataract using an extremely cold probe.

cornea

11-20 As a therapeutic measure, **corneal abrasion** means scraping away of the outer layers of the _____, perhaps to smooth one that is abnormally buckled.

lens

11-21 Extraction of the lens means removal of the lens to treat a cataract. **Intraocular lens transplant** is replacing the _____ with an artificial lens. This surgery may also be used for patients with extreme myopia, diplopia, and certain other abnormalities. IOL means intraocular lens.

> **BEYOND** THE BLUEPRINT Corneas are easily transplanted for people with scarred or opaque corneas. Transplants are generally successful, because antibodies responsible for rejection of foreign tissue usually do not reach the avascular, transplanted cornea.

retina

11-22 Laser retinal photocoagulation uses a laser to make pinpoint scars to stabilize a detached _____.

myopia

11-23 Laser-assisted in-situ keratomileusis **(LASIK)** is corneal surgery in which the excimer laser and a microkeratome (instrument used to create a thin hinged flap on the surface of the cornea) are combined to correct nearsightedness, also called _____.

within

11-24 Treatment of macular degeneration includes intraocular injections, laser, and vitamins. **Intra/ocular** means _____ the eyeball.

MATCH IT! EXERCISE 9

Match the terms in the left column with their meanings in the right column.

_____ **1.** blepharoplasty
_____ **2.** cryoextraction
_____ **3.** intraocular lens transplant
_____ **4.** laser retinal photocoagulation
_____ **5.** LASIK

A. corneal surgery using a laser and a microtome
B. removal of a cataract
C. replacing the lens with an artificial lens
D. stabilizing a detached retina with the use of laser
E. surgical repair of the eyelids
F. use of extreme cold to remove cataracts or reattach a detached retina

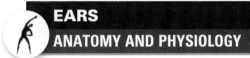

EARS

ANATOMY AND PHYSIOLOGY

hear

11-25 The ears have receptors that detect touch, pain, heat and cold, but we usually think of the ears as enabling us to _____. We depend on our ears not only for hearing but also for the sense of equilibrium (commonly called *balance*). Important abbreviations to remember are AD (right ear), AS (left ear), and AU (each ear).

WORD ORIGIN
cerumen *(L.)*
cera, wax

cerumen

11-26 Several glands secrete a yellowish, brown, waxy substance called **cerumen**, which lubricates and protects the ear. Write this term that means the yellowish, brown, waxy substance normally found in the ear: _____.

11-27 Refer to Fig. 11.16. Anatomically, the ear is divided into the external ear, middle ear, and inner ear:
- external ear: The visible part of the ear; ends at the **tympanic membrane** (eardrum)
- middle ear: Air-filled cavity containing three tiny bones
- inner ear **labyrinth:** Contains the cochlea and semicircular canals

tympanic

cochlea

The external ear ends at the _____ membrane; the middle ear contains three tiny bones, and the inner ear contains the _____ and the semicircular canals.

11-28 The external ear functions in collecting sound waves and directing them into the ear canal, where they strike the tympanic membrane. As the eardrum vibrates, it moves three small bones (**ossicles**) in the middle ear (**malleus, incus,** and the **stapes**) that conduct the sound waves through the middle ear. The malleus, incus, and stapes are three small bones in the middle ear called the

ossicles

_____. Locate these bones in Fig. 11.16.

A simplified schematic of the pathway of sound is as follows:

Sound → auditory canal → eardrum → ossicles → cochlea → auditory nerve fibers → auditory region of the brain

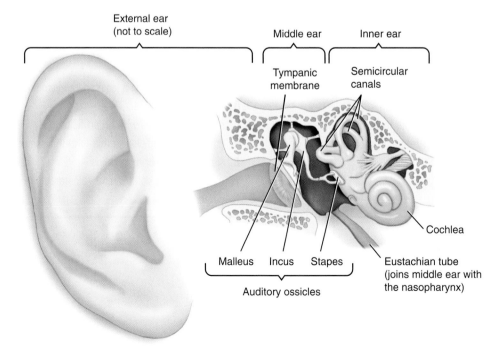

Figure 11.16 Structures of the ear.

canals

11-29 As the stapes moves, it touches a membrane called the **oval window,** which separates the middle ear from the inner ear. The inner ear is a complex inner structure that contains receptors for hearing (cochlea) and the sense of balance (semicircular canals). The **cochlea** is a spiral tunnel, resembling a snail shell and containing the sense of hearing.

The **semicircular canals** are fluid-filled _____ that open into the cochlea and are important in our sense of balance.

The **auditory** or **eustachian tube** leads from the middle ear to the pharynx (throat). This tube can prevent damage to the eardrum by equalizing pressure in the middle ear to the atmospheric pressure.

> **BEYOND** THE BLUEPRINT Normally the pressure of air in the middle ear is equal to that of the environment; however if you ascend to high altitudes (flying or climbing a high mountain), the atmospheric pressure in the middle ear is greater than that in the outer ear, causing the eardrum to bulge outward. Swallowing opens the eustachian tube so that air can leave the middle ear until the pressures are balanced. The eardrum relaxes and avoids the danger of bursting.

Learn the following word parts.

Word Parts

Combining Form	Meaning	Suffixes	Meaning
acoust(o), audi(o)	hearing	-ory	pertaining to
aur(o), auricul(o), ot(o)	ear		
cerumin(o)	ear wax		
cochle(o)	cochlea		
myring(o), tympan(o)	eardrum		
salping(o)*	eustachian tube		

*Be careful! salping(o) also means uterine tube.

FIND IT! **EXERCISE 10**

Find the combining form in these new terms, and write its meaning. A short definition is provided for each term.

Term	Combining Form	Meaning of Combining Form
1. acoustic	_____	_____
pertaining to sound or hearing		
2. audible	_____	_____
capable of being heard		
3. auditory	_____	_____
pertaining to the sense of hearing and the organs involved		
4. aural, auricular, otic	_____	_____
pertaining to the ear		
5. cochlear	_____	_____
pertaining to the cochlea		

DIAGNOSTIC TESTS AND PROCEDURES

otoscopy

11-30 An **otoscopic examination**, also called **otoscopy,** is examination of the ear using an **otoscope** (see Fig. 2.31). An otoscopic exam is the same as _____.

11-31 Audiology is a field of research and clinical practice devoted to the study of hearing disorders, measuring hearing, and other aspects of preserving and improving hearing.

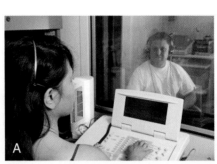
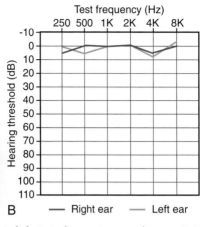
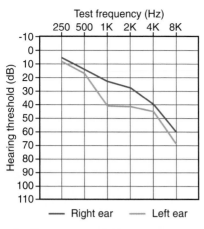

Test frequency (Hz)

Figure 11.17 Audiometry. A, Audiologist is shown using an audiometer. **B,** Normal audiogram pattern (left) vs. audiogram showing hearing loss (right).

 KEY POINT   An **audiologist** is a health professional who detects and evaluates hearing loss and determines how a patient can best make use of remaining hearing. An **audio/meter** is an electronic device for measuring hearing. The record produced in **audiometry** is an **audiogram** (Fig. 11.17).

audiologist

Write the name of the health professional who detects and evaluates hearing: _____.

Hearing is tested by using tones from very low to very high frequencies at various decibels (dBs) of intensity. The lowest intensity at which a young, normal ear can detect sound (about 51% of the time) is nearly 0 dB. Conversational speech is around 60 dBs, and sounds at that decibel intensity are not harmful. Exposure to loud noises, even for a short time, can damage the cochlear hair cells and result in hearing loss. Looking at Table 11.2, note that 3 minutes is considered a safe exposure time if you are sitting in the front row at a rock concert. **Deafness** is inability to hear. Having some degree of hearing impairment is "hearing impaired."

Table 11.2   Decibel Intensity and Safe Exposure Time for Common Sounds

Sound	Decibel (dB) Intensity	Safe Exposure Time*	Sound	Decibel (dB) Intensity	Safe Exposure Time*
Threshold of hearing	0		Chain saw	100	2 hours
Whispering	20		Rock concert, front row	120	3 minutes
Average residence or office	40		Jet engine	140	Immediate danger
Conversational speech	60				
Car traffic	70	>8 hours	Rocket launching pad	180	Immediate danger
Motorcycle	90	8 hours			

From Ignatavicius DD, Workman ML: *Medical-surgical nursing: critical thinking for collaborative care,* ed 5, St Louis, 2006, Saunders.
*For every 5-dB increase in intensity, the safe exposure time is cut in half.

auditory

11-32 Various **tuning fork tests** screen for both function of the auditory nerve and ability of ear structures to conduct sound waves to the inner ear. Weber's tuning using a fork is shown in Fig. 11.18. Tuning fork tests screen for function of the _____ nerve and ear structures to conduct sound waves.

PATHOLOGIES

ears

11-33 Anotia is a congenital absence of one or both _____. Ear trauma can occur from a blow by a blunt object. The eardrum can be damaged by extended exposure to loud noises, penetrating injury, rupture, or perforation by shock waves from an explosion, deep sea diving, trauma, or acute middle ear infections. A perforated eardrum can be seen during an otoscopic examination, which is an examination of the _____ using an otoscope (Fig. 11.19).

ear

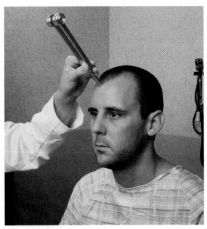

Figure 11.18 Weber's tuning fork test. By placing the stem of a vibrating tuning fork in the center of the forehead or the top of the head as shown, the loudness of the sound should be equal in both ears if hearing is normal or if there is symmetric hearing loss.

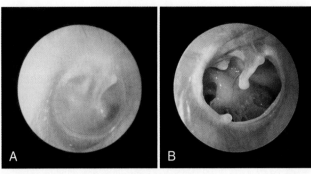

Figure 11.19 Comparison of the appearance of a normal eardrum and a perforated eardrum. A, Otoscopic view of a normal intact eardrum. **B,** Otoscopic view of a perforated eardrum.

ear

WORD ORIGIN
media *(L.)*
medius, middle

WORD ORIGIN
myringitis *(L.)*
myringa, eardrum

11-34 Otitis means inflammation of the _____. Otitis may produce **ot/algia,** pain in the ear, which is also called an *earache.*

    Otitis media is inflammation of the middle ear. The middle ear is separated from the external ear by the eardrum. **Myringitis** means inflammation of the tympanic membrane. **Mastoiditis** is an infection of one of the mastoid bones of the skull, which is usually an extension of a middle ear infection. It is difficult to treat and can result in hearing loss. Antibiotic therapy is aimed at treating middle ear infections before they progress to mastoiditis.

    Otitis externa means an external ear infection, often caused by fungus, also called **otomycosis** (commonly called *swimmer's ear*). **Otitis interna** is an inner ear infection, which is inflammation of the inner ear, and can affect both hearing and equilibrium. A discharge from the ear, **otorrhea,** may accompany otitis. Otorrhea may contain blood, pus, or even spinal fluid. Ear infections are just one cause of otorrhea.

otosclerosis

11-35 Otosclerosis is hardening of the ear. This condition is caused by formation of spongy bone around structures of the middle and inner ear, and it leads to hearing impairment. Write this term that means hardening of the ear: _____.

cholesteatoma

11-36 A **cholesteatoma** (*[G.] chole,* bile; *stear,* fat) is a cystic mass composed of epithelial cells and cholesterol that is found in the middle ear, which may occlude the middle ear or destroy the adjacent bones. Write the name of this new term: _____.

Meniere

11-37 Tinnitus, ear noise, is one of the most common complaints of persons with ear or hearing disorders. The noise includes ringing, buzzing, roaring or clicking. It may be a sign of something as simple as accumulation of earwax or cerumen, or as serious as **Meniere disease**. The latter is a chronic disease of the inner ear with recurring episodes of hearing loss, tinnitus, and vertigo. **Vertigo** is also called *dizziness.* Write the eponym that is a chronic disease of the inner ear with recurring episodes of hearing loss, ear noise, and dizziness: _____ disease.

MATCH IT! EXERCISE 11

Match the terms in the left column with their descriptions in the right column.

_____ **1.** cerumen	**A.** abnormal hardening of the bones in the middle ear
_____ **2.** otalgia	**B.** ear wax
_____ **3.** otorrhea	**C.** discharge or draining from the ear
_____ **4.** otosclerosis	**D.** dizziness
_____ **5.** tinnitus	**E.** earache
_____ **6.** vertigo	**F.** ringing or other noise in one or both ears

SURGICAL AND THERAPEUTIC INTERVENTIONS

cochlea

11-38 An assistive listening device (ALD) or hearing aid is an electronic device that amplifies sound. In complete hearing loss, a **cochlear implant** assists hearing by electrically stimulating the cochlea (Fig. 11.20). A cochlear implant is implanted surgically into the _____ of a deaf individual's ear.

repair

11-39 Otoplasty is surgical _____ or reconstruction of the external ear.

> **BEYOND** THE BLUEPRINT Otoplasty is a common procedure in which, for cosmetic reasons, some of the cartilage of the external ear is removed to bring the ears closer to the head.

eardrum

11-40 Tympanostomy is surgical creation of an opening through the _____ to promote drainage and/or allow the introduction of artificial tubes (pressure-equalizing tubes) to maintain the opening (Fig. 11.21).

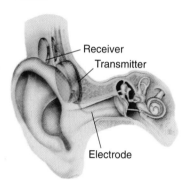

Receiver
Transmitter
Electrode

Figure 11.20 Cochlear implant. An electronic device that is surgically implanted into the cochlea of a deaf person.

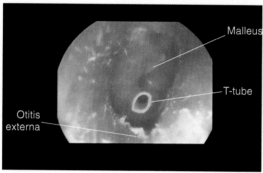

Malleus
T-tube
Otitis externa

Figure 11.21 Pressure-equalizing tube in place in the eardrum. An incision is made in the eardrum, and a temporary tube is positioned to relieve pressure and release pus or fluid from the middle ear. The tube is left in place for a time to allow the ear to drain.

WRITE IT! EXERCISE 12

Write a word in each blank to complete these sentences.
1. A term for surgical creation of an opening through the eardrum is _____.
2. Surgical repair or reconstruction of the ear is _____.
3. A _____ implant assists hearing by electrically stimulating the _____.

SKIN
SENSORY NERVE ENDINGS

11-41 The skin is equipped with several sensory nerve endings that respond to various kinds of stimulation. In addition, modified skin structures continue into various parts of the body, such as mucous membrane in the lining of the nose, the mouth, nose, and the eyes.

Learn these word parts.

Word Parts: Types of Receptors

Combining Form	Meaning	Combining Form	Meaning
chem(o)	chemical	phot(o)	light
mechan(o)	mechanical	therm(o)	heat
noc(i)	cause harm, injury, or pain		

touch

light

temperature

nociceptors

touch

pain

nerves

11-42 Mechano/receptors that are sensitive to mechanical changes in touch or pressure are widely distributed in the skin. Mechanoreceptors for hearing are located within the ear. Mechanoreceptors sense mechanical changes in _____ or pressure.

11-43 The eyes contain **photoreceptors** that detect _____.

11-44 Thermoreceptors are located immediately under the skin and are widely distributed in the body. By their name, you know that thermo/receptors detect changes in _____, sensing both cool and heat, as the name implies.

11-45 The sense of pain is initiated by special receptors called **nociceptors** that are widely distributed throughout the skin and internal organs. Write the name of the receptors that initiate the sensation of pain: _____.

11-46 It is fairly easy for health professionals to recognize those who are hearing or sight impaired. Patients will generally complain if they do not taste food.

Pain and light touch are commonly assessed sensory functions. Assessment of the sensory nerve endings is very important in patients with conditions affecting the spinal cord or spinal nerves, such as trauma, tumors, infections, or stenosis. For testing the ability to feel touch, the patient closes his or her eyes and the health care provider touches him or her (on the arm, for example) and asks the patient to point to the area touched. This is a simple test for the ability to feel _____.

11-47 Pain sensation is assessed with an object perceived as being sharp or dull; for example, a paper clip or a cotton-tipped applicator has a dull end and a sharp end. After demonstrating what will be done while the patient has their eyes open, the patient closes his or her eyes and indicates whether the object is sharp or dull, thereby providing an easy test for the sensation of _____. A sensation reported as dull when the stimulus was sharp indicates the need for more specialized testing.

11-48 Neuropathies, or disease or degeneration of the peripheral _____, such as those of diabetes mellitus and vascular problems, may have a PNS cause and may affect the entire extremity or both extremities. Sensory deficits from spinal cord injuries vary with the location of the injury.

WRITE IT! EXERCISE 13

Write a word in each blank to complete these sentences.

1. Nerve endings that detect light are called _____.
2. Nerve endings that detect changes in temperature are called _____.
3. Nerve endings that detect pain are called _____.
4. Receptors that are sensitive to mechanical changes in touch or pressure are called _____.

MOUTH AND NOSE

chemoreceptors

11-49 Chemoreceptors are nerve endings in the nose, mouth, and tongue that are adapted for excitation by chemicals that enable taste. With openings on the surface of the tongue and mouth, **taste buds** are taste organs that have chemoreceptors for sweet, sour, bitter, and salty tastes (Fig. 11.22). It is important to remember that the nerve endings in the nose and mouth that enable taste are _____.

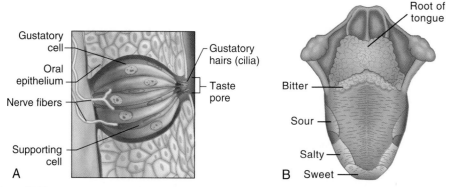

Figure 11.22 Taste buds and the regions of the tongue. A, Drawing of an individual taste bud. Each taste bud rests in a pocket. Many taste buds are distributed over the tongue and the roof of the mouth. **B,** Taste regions of the tongue. In addition to the four basic taste sensations (sweet, sour, bitter, and salty), there are combined perceptions plus the input from olfactory receptors.

Learn this word part.

Word Parts

Suffix	Meaning
-osmia	sense of smell

smell

absence

11-50 The nose is also responsible for the sense of smell, and this sense is intricately linked with chemoreceptors that enable us to experience different tastes of food and other substances. The term **olfaction** means the sense of smell, and **olfactory** means pertaining to the sense of _____.

11-51 Olfactory receptors are sensitive to smell, and they are also easily fatigued, explaining why odors that are very noticeable at first are no longer sensed after a short time.

Hyper/osmia is an abnormally increased sensitivity to odors. **An/osmia** is impairment or _____ of the sense of smell, and it can occur either as a temporary condition when one has a respiratory infection, or as a permanent anosmia when the olfactory nerve is destroyed.

Advancing age may bring about reduced function of the sense of smell. Temporary loss of sensitivity to smells often results from colds and other nasal infections. Also, because of the damaging effects of the pollutants in tobacco smoke, reduction of the sense of smell is often seen in smokers.

MATCH IT!
EXERCISE 14

Match the terms in the left column with their descriptions in the right column.

_____ **1.** anosmia   **A.** increased sensitivity to odors

_____ **2.** chemoreceptors   **B.** loss or impairment of the sense of smell

_____ **3.** hyperosmia   **C.** nerve endings that are adapted for detecting chemicals

_____ **4.** olfactory   **D.** pertaining to the sense of smell

PHARMACOLOGY

Numerous ophthalmic creams, ointments, or liquid drops are prescribed to relieve pressure within the eye, to provide moisture, or as anesthetic or antibiotic preparations for the eye. Antibiotics are used to treat bacterial ear and skin infections.

Drug Class: Effect and Uses

Antiglaucoma Drugs: Decrease the intraocular pressure in the eye to treat glaucoma
Types include carbonic anhydrase inhibitors, alpha agonists, beta-blockers, cholinergics, and prostaglandin analogs

acetazolamide (Diamox)	*dorzolamide (Trusopt)*	*pilocarpine (Isopto Carpine)*
bimatoprost (Lumigan)	*latanoprost (Xalatan)*	*timolol (Timoptic)*
brimonidine (Alphagan)		

Ceruminolytics: Soften and break down earwax
carbamide peroxide (Debrox)

Cycloplegics (*[G.] kylos,* round or recurring; *plege,* stroke): Paralyze accommodation of the eye. All cycloplegics also act as mydriatics.
atropine (Atropisol)   *cyclopentolate (Cyclogyl)*   *homatropine (Isopto Homatropine)*

Miotics: (*[G.] mio-,* less + -tic, pertaining to): Constrict the pupil of the eye
echothiophate (Phospholine Iodide)

Mydriatics: Dilate the pupil of the eye. Many mydriatics also act as cycloplegics.
atropine (Atropisol)   *phenylephrine (Cyclomydril)*
cyclopentolate (Cyclogyl)   *tropicamide (Mydriacyl)*

WRITE IT! **EXERCISE 15**

Write a term in each blank to complete the sentences.
1. Agents used to break down earwax are called _____.
2. Agents used to constrict the _____ of the eye are miotics.
3. Agents used to dilate the pupils are _____.
4. Agents used to treat glaucoma are _____ drugs.
5. Agents which paralyze accommodation of the eye are _____, which also act as mydriatics.

CHAPTER ABBREVIATIONS

AD	right ear	LASIK	laser-assisted in-situ keratomileusis
ALD	assistive listening device	MD*	macular degeneration
AS	left ear	OD	right eye (L. *oculus dexter*)
AU	each ear	OS	left eye (L. *oculus sinister*)
dB	decibel	OU	each eye (L. *oculus uterque*)
IOL	intraocular lens	VF	visual fields

*Also, medical doctor.

Be Careful With These!

accommodation vs. refraction	daltonism vs. achromatic vision
anosmia vs. hyperosmia	myopia vs. hyperopia
cornea vs. choroid	retinal rods vs. cones

A Career as a Doctor of Optometry

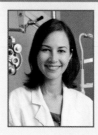

Danielle Mueller is a Doctor of Optometry (OD) and enjoys the patient contact in her career and knowing that she is helping patients maintain the amazing sense of sight. After taking as many courses as possible in anatomy and biochemistry, she completed her degree in biology, and then obtained a four-year doctoral-level degree, concentrating primarily on structure, function, and disorders of the eye. For additional information, go to the website for ASCO, the Association of Schools and Colleges of Optometry: *www.opted.org.*

CHAPTER 11 SELF-TEST

Review the new word parts for this chapter. Work all of the following exercises to test your understanding of the material before checking your answers against those in Appendix IV.

Matching

I.   Match the terms on the left with the descriptions on the right.

_____ **1.** chemoreceptor   **A.** a vascular layer inside the sclera

_____ **2.** cornea   **B.** filled with a soft, jelly-like material

_____ **3.** choroid   **C.** produces and stores tears

_____ **4.** lacrimal gland   **D.** sensory nerve ending that responds to various stimuli

_____ **5.** pupil   **E.** small, dark circular structure located in the center of the eye

_____ **6.** vitreous chamber   **F.** transparent structure that bends or refracts light rays

Filling in the Blanks

II.   Write a word to complete each sentence.

1. The sense organs that are continuous with the optic nerve and enable vision are the _____.

2. Total color blindness is the same as _____.

3. Use of a tonometer to measure intraocular pressure is called _____.

4. The ear structure that contains receptors for hearing is the _____.

5. The auditory or _____ tube leads from the middle ear to the pharynx.

6. An _____ is one who is trained to detect and evaluate hearing.

7. Otitis _____ means inflammation of the middle ear.

8. The organ or modifications of it that is associated with mechanoreceptors, photoreceptors, nociceptors, and mechanoreceptors is the _____.

9. The nose and _____ have chemoreceptors that enable one to smell and taste food.

10. Three major bones of the middle ear are the malleus, incus, and _____.

Making Connections

III.   Describe the relationship of these terms.

1. amblyopia and strabismus   _____

_____

2. vision accommodation and refraction   _____

_____

Identifying Illustrations

IV. *Label these illustrations using one of the following: cholesteatoma, cochlear, ectropion, entropion, hyperopia, myopia, mydriatic.*

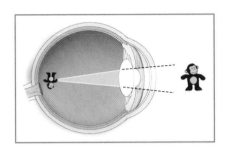

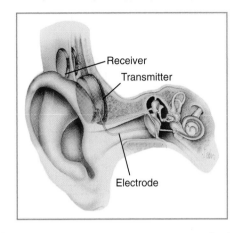

1. _____

2. _____ implant

Using Vocabulary

V. *Circle the correct answer for each of the following.*

1. Kallie is a 72-year-old female who tells the optometrist that her eyes do not adjust as quickly when she goes into a dark theater as they used to. Muscles of which eye structure regulate the amount of light entering the eye? (conjunctiva, choroid, cornea, iris)

2. Dr. Jindal explains to Seth that he has total color blindness. Which of the following is Seth's condition? (achromatic vision, day vision, double vision, night vision)

3. What is tested when Dr. Johnson uses a Tono-Pen tonometer during an ophthalmic examination? (assessment of visual field, intraocular pressure, refractory adjustment, sensory nerve response)

4. Hashim is told he needs blepharoplasty to correct droopy eyelids. What problem does blepharoplasty correct? (amblyopia, ptosis, nyctalopia, retinopathy)

5. The flight attendant told Carrie to swallow when she experienced painful pressure in the middle ear while flying, and the pressure was relieved. How did swallowing help equalize the pressure in her ears? (opening of the eustachian tube, response of the oval window, vibration of the bones in the middle ear, vibration of the eardrum)

6. Which part of the ear is responsible for the sense of balance? (cochlea, semicircular canals, stapes, tympanic membrane)

7. Tina is 65 years old, and her vision is deteriorating. What is the name of vision impairment due to advancing years? (abrasion, astigmatism, photophobia, presbyopia)

8. What is the term for the agent that the optical assistant drops in Tina's eyes to dilate the pupils? (mydriatic, nyctalopia, photocoagulation, tinnitus)

Writing Terms

VI. *Write one word for each of the following clues.*

1. earwax _____

2. farsightedness _____

3. loss or impairment of the sense of smell _____

4. pertaining to the sense of smell _____

5. receptor that detects pain _____

6. receptor that is sensitive to mechanical change _____

7. removal of a cataract using an extremely cold probe _____

8. swelling of the eyelid _____

9. synonym for ptosis _____

10. the congenital absence of one or both ears _____

Labeling

VII. Label numbers 1 to 5 with the following structures of the eye: lacrimal duct, iris, nasolacrimal duct, pupil, sclera.

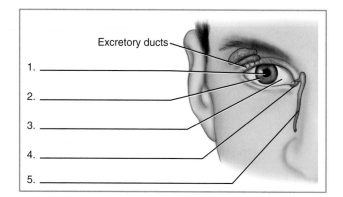

Excretory ducts

1. _____
2. _____
3. _____
4. _____
5. _____

Finetuning Terms

VIII. In addition to spelling, describe at least one difference in the following:

1. anosmia vs. hyperosmia _____

_____

2. daltonism vs. achromatic vision _____

_____

GREATER COMPREHENSION

Spelling

IX. Circle all incorrectly spelled terms, and write the correct spellings.

aricular   floroscein angiography   glaucoma   pupillary   vitrus humor

Pronouncing Terms

X. Write the correct term for the following phonetic spellings.

1. ek-**trō**-pē-on   _____

2. **lā**-sik   _____

3. mid-rē-**at**-ik   _____

4. ō-**tal**-juh   _____

5. suh-rōō-mi-nō-**lit**-iks   _____

6. ū-**stā**-kē-un   _____

Categorizing Terms and Practicing Pronunciation

XI. Classify the terms in the left column by selecting A, B, C, D, or E.

_____ **1.** astigmatism	**A.** anatomy
_____ **2.** audiometry	**B.** diagnostic test or procedure
_____ **3.** ceruminolytics	**C.** pathology
_____ **4.** hordeolum	**D.** surgery
_____ **5.** iridectomy	**E.** nonsurgical therapeutic intervention
_____ **6.** macular degeneration	
_____ **7.** otitis interna	
_____ **8.** photoreceptors	
_____ **9.** vertigo	
_____ **10.** vitreous chamber	

(Be prepared to pronounce terms 1 to 10 in class after listening to the Chapter 11 terms at *http://evolve.elsevier.com/Leonard/building/*. In addition, practice categorizing all boldface terms in this chapter.)

Health Care Reporting

XII. Read the health report and circle the correct answer in #1-5.

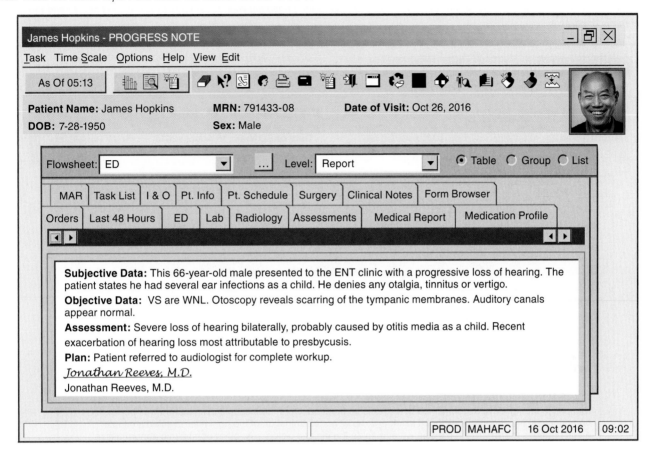

1. The term "otalgia" means (earwax, ear infection, ear pain, hearing loss)
2. The term "auditory" refers to (ear, hearing, noise, sound)
3. The tympanic membrane is also referred to as the (cochlea, eardrum, Eustachian tube, stapes)
4. The patient's inflammatory condition is located in the (auditory ossicles, external ear, inner ear, middle ear)
5. Vertigo is characterized by (buzzing, clicking, dizziness, ringing)

Abbreviating

XIII. Write a letter in each blank for the abbreviation that corresponds to the clue.

1. assistive listening device __ __ ___
2. L. *oculus uterque* __ __
3. intraocular lens __ __ ___

4. left ear __ __
5. left eye __ __
6. right ear __ __

Using Pharmacologic Terms

XIV. Use all selections to match terms in the left column with their descriptions in the right column.

___ **1.** antiglaucoma drugs
___ **2.** ceruminolytics
___ **3.** cycloplegics
___ **4.** miotics

A. constrict the pupil of the eye
B. decrease intraocular pressure
C. paralyze accommodation of the eye
D. soften and break down earwax

Health Care Reporting

XV. *List and define/describe ten terms or phrases that relate to the special sense organs. Try to find as many as you can before seeing the answers, using the Glossary or a medical dictionary, if necessary. Challenge your classmates to see who is first to find the ten terms or phrases.*

Carl M. White - CONSULTATION ⎽ 🗗 ☒

Task Time Scale Options Help View Edit

| As Of 05:13 |

Patient Name: Carl M. White   **ID No.:** 015-0423   **Date of ED Visit:** 15 August 2014
DOB: 01-01-86   **Sex:** Male

Flowsheet: ES   ...   Level: Report   ⦿ Table ○ Group ○ List

| MAR | Task List | I & O | Pt. Info | Pt. Schedule | Surgery | Clinical Notes | Form Browser |
| Orders | Last 48 Hours | ED | Lab | Radiology | Assessments | Medical Report | Medication Profile |

Chief Complaint: Pain in right eye

History of Present Illness: This 28-year-old male was breaking up concrete on the back patio of his home when he began to experience severe pain in his right eye. He replied "No" when asked if he had been wearing protective goggles.

Allergies: None

Family History: 55-year-old mother: diabetes, diabetic retinopathy, nyctalopia; 62-year-old father: Meniere disease, tinnitus

Physical Examination: This 28-year-old body builder appears in remarkable physical condition, except for redness in the right eye accompanied by extreme lacrimation. Ophthalmoscopic examination was performed on both eyes: No abnormalities found in left eye; however, examination of the right eye revealed a minute piece of debris (concrete?) in the sclera just outside the iris at 3 o'clock. No other ophthalmic abnormalities were noted.

Treatment: The minute piece of debris in right eye was easily removed with forceps. Eye was flushed with normal saline, followed by two drops of Cortisporin Ophthalmic Drops. Patient instructed to stay away from dusty environments for a week to allow healing; then use goggles when doing jobs such as breaking up concrete.

Diagnosis/Plan: Trauma to right eye caused by minute piece of debris, which was easily removed. Patient to make appointment with an ophthalmologist for follow-up and continue with Cortisporin Ophthalmic Suspension Drops, 1 drop every 3-4 hours in the right eye until his appointment or for one week.

Charlene R. Noradello, M.D.

| PROD | MAHAFC | 15 Aug 2014 | 09:02 |

---

1. _____
2. _____
3. _____
4. _____
5. _____
6. _____
7. _____
8. _____
9. _____
10. _____

New Construction

XVI. Divide these words into their component parts, and write the meaning of each term.

1. dacryolithiasis _____

2. extraocular _____

3. iritis _____

4. keratitis _____

5. pupilloplegia _____

BMV LIST

Visit http://evolve.elsevier.com/Leonard/building/ to listen to the boldface terms in Chapter 11. Look closely at the spelling of each term as it is pronounced.

accommodation (uh-kom-uh-**dā**-shun)
accommodation reflex (uh-kom-uh-**dā**-shun **rē**-fleks)
achromatic vision (ak-rō-**mat**-ik **vizh**-un)
achromatopsia (uh-krō-muh-**top**-sē-uh)
acoustic (uh-**kōōs**-tik)
amblyopia (am-blē-**ō**-pē-uh)
anosmia (an-**oz**-mē-uh)
anotia (an-**ō**-shuh)
anterior chamber (an-**tēr**-ē-ur **chām**-bur)
antiglaucoma drugs (an-tē-glaw-**kō**-muh drugz)
assessment of visual fields (uh-**ses**-munt uv **vizh**-ōō-ul fēldz)
astigmatism (uh-**stig**-muh-tiz-um)
audible (**aw**-duh-bul)
audiogram (**aw**-dē-ō-gram)
audiologist (aw-dē-**ol**-uh-jist)
audiology (aw-dē-**ol**-uh-jē)
audiometer (aw-dē-**om**-uh-tur)
audiometry (aw-dē-**om**-uh-trē)
auditory (**aw**-di-tor-ē)
auditory tube (**aw**-di-tor-ē tōōb)
aural (**aw**-rul)
auricular (aw-**rik**-ū-lur)
blepharedema (blef-ur-i-**dē**-muh)
blepharitis (blef-uh-**rī**-tis)
blepharoplasty (**blef**-uh-rō-plas-tē)
blepharoptosis (blef-uh-rop-**tō**-sis)
cataract (**kat**-uh-rakt)
cerumen (suh-**rōō**-mun)
ceruminolytics (suh-rōō-mi-nō-**lit**-iks)
chemoreceptors (kē-mō-rē-**sep**-turz)
cholesteatoma (kō-luh-stē-uh-**tō**-muh)
choroid (**kor**-oid)
choroidal (kor-**oid**-ul)
ciliary body (**sil**-ē-ar-ē **bod**-ē)
cochlea (**kok**-lē-uh)
cochlear (**kok**-lē-ur)
cochlear implant (**kok**-lē-ur **im**-plant)
color vision deficiencies (**kul**-ur **vizh**-un dē-**fish**-un-sēz)
conjunctiva (kun-**junk**-ti-vuh)
conjunctival (kun-**junk**-ti-vul)
conjunctivitis (kun-junk-ti-**vī**-tis)
cornea (**kor**-nē-uh)

corneal (**kor**-nē-ul)
corneal abrasion (**kor**-nē-ul uh-**brā**-zhun)
corneal transplant (**kor**-nē-ul **trans**-plant)
cryoextraction (krī-ō-ek-**strak**-shun)
cycloplegics (sī-klō-**plē**-jiks)
dacryocystitis (dak-rē-ō-sis-**tī**-tis)
daltonism (**dawl**-tun-iz-um)
deafness (**def**-nis)
ectropion (ek-**trō**-pē-on)
entropion (en-**trō**-pē-on)
eustachian tube (ū-**stā**-kē-un tōōb)
extraction of the lens (ek-**strak**-shun uv thuh lenz)
extraocular (eks-truh-**ok**-ū-lur)
fluorescein angiography (flōō-**res**-ēn an-jē-**og**-ruh-fē)
glaucoma (glaw-, glou-**kō**-muh)
hordeolum (hor-**dē**-ō-lum)
hyperopia (hī-pur-**ō**-pē-uh)
hyperosmia (hī-pur-**oz**-mē-uh)
incus (**ing**-kus)
intraocular (in-truh-**ok**-ū-lur)
intraocular lens transplant (in-truh-**ok**-ū-lur lenz **trans**-plant)
iridectomy (ir-i-**dek**-tuh-mē)
iridic (ī-**rid**-ik)
iris (**ī**-ris)
keratometer (ker-uh-**tom**-uh-tur)
labyrinth (**lab**-uh-rinth)
lacrimal (**lak**-ri-mul)
lacrimal ducts (**lak**-ri-mul dukts)
lacrimal fluid (**lak**-ri-mul **flōō**-id)
lacrimal glands (**lak**-ri-mul glandz)
laser retinal photocoagulation (**lā**-zur **ret**-i-nul fō-tō-kō-ag-ū-**lā**-shun)
LASIK (**lā**-sik)
lens (lenz)
macular degeneration (**mak**-ū-lur dē-jen-ur-**ā**-shun)
malleus (**mal**-ē-us)
mastoiditis (mas-toid-**ī**-tis)
mechanoreceptors (mek-uh-nō-rē-**sep**-turz)
Meniere disease (me-**nyār** di-**zēz**)
miotics (mī-**ot**-iks)
mydriatic (mid-rē-**at**-ik)
myopia (mī-**ō**-pē-uh)

myringitis (mir-in-**jī**-tis)
nasolacrimal duct (na-zō-**lak**-ri-mul dukt)
nasolacrimal sac (na-zō-**lak**-ri-mul sak)
neuropathies (noo-**rop**-uh-thēz)
nociceptors (nō-si-**sep**-turz)
nyctalopia (nik-tuh-**lō**-pē-uh)
ocular (**ok**-ū-lur)
olfaction (ol-**fak**-shun)
olfactory (ol-**fak**-tuh-rē)
ophthalmic (of-**thal**-mik)
ophthalmic cryosurgery (of-**thal**-mik kri-ō-**sur**-jur-ē)
ophthalmologist (of-thul-**mol**-uh-jist)
ophthalmometer (of-thul-**mom**-uh-tur)
ophthalmoscope (of-**thal**-mō-skōp)
ophthalmoscopic (of-thal-muh-**skop**-ik)
ophthalmoscopy (of-thul-**mos**-kuh-pē)
optic (**op**-tik)
optic disc (**op**-tik disk)
optic nerve (**op**-tik nurv)
optometrist (op-**tom**-uh-trist)
ossicles (**os**-i-kulz)
otalgia (ō-**tal**-juh)
otic (**ō**-tik)
otitis (ō-**tī**-tis)
otitis externa (ō-**tī**-tis eks-**tur**-nuh)
otitis interna (ō-**tī**-tis in-**tur**-nuh)
otitis media (ō-**tī**-tis **mē**-dē-uh)
otomycosis (ō-tō-mī-**kō**-sis)
otoplasty (**ō**-tō-plas-tē)
otorrhea (ō-tō-**rē**-uh)
otosclerosis (ō-tō-skluh-**rō**-sis)
otoscope (**ō**-tō-skōp)
otoscopic examination (ō-tō-**skōp**-ik eg-zam-i-**nā**-shun)
otoscopy (ō-**tos**-kuh-pē)
oval window (**ō**-vul **win**-dō)

photophobia (fō-tō-**fō**-bē-uh)
photoreceptors (fō-tō-rē-**sep**-turz)
presbyopia (pres-bē-**ō**-pē-uh)
ptosis (**tō**-sis)
pupil (**pū**-pil)
pupillary (**pūp**-i-lar-ē)
receptors (rē-**sep**-turz)
refraction (rē-**frak**-shun)
retina (**ret**-i-nuh)
retinal (**ret**-i-nul)
retinal detachment (**ret**-i-nul dē-**tach**-munt)
retinopathy (ret-i-**nop**-uh-thē)
rods and cones (rodz and kōnz)
sclera (**sklēr**-uh)
semicircular canals (sem-ē-**sur**-kyuh-lur kuh-**nalz**)
sense organs (sens **or**-gunz)
slit-lamp examination (slit lamp eg-zam-i-**nā**-shun)
Snellen chart (**snel**-un chahrt)
stapes (**stā**-pēz)
strabismus (struh-**biz**-mus)
taste buds (tāst budz)
tearing (**tēr**-ing)
thermoreceptors (thur-mō-rē-**sep**-turz)
tinnitus (**tin**-i-tus, ti-**nī**-tus)
tonometer (tō-**nom**-uh-tur)
tonometry (tō-**nom**-uh-trē)
tuning fork tests (**tōōn**-ing fork tests)
tympanic membrane (tim-**pan**-ik **mem**-brān)
tympanostomy (tim-puh-**nos**-tuh-mē)
vertigo (**vur**-ti-gō)
visual acuity (**vizh**-ōō-ul uh-**kū**-i-tē)
vitreous chamber (**vit**-rē-us **chām**-bur)
vitreous humor (**vit**-rē-us **hū**-mur)
xerophthalmia (zēr-of-**thal**-mē-uh)

Español ENHANCING SPANISH COMMUNICATION

English	Spanish (Pronunciation)
buzzing	zumbido (soom-BEE-do)
cornea	cornea (KOR-ne-ah)
cry	lloro (YO-ro)
earwax	cerilla (say-REEL-yah)
eyeball	globo del ojo (GLO-bo del O-ho)
hear (to)	oír (o-EER)
optic	óptico (OP-te-ko)
nose	nariz (nah-REES)
retina	retina (ray-TEE-nah)
smell (to)	oler (o-LEER)
taste	sabor (sah-BOR)

Endocrine System

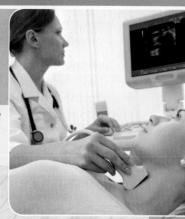

A sonographer scans the patient's thyroid using the ultrasound probe, and images are captured and projected on the screen. Permanent records are made for study to determine if a mass is present, and cysts are differentiated from solid masses/tumors.

Basic Understanding

In this chapter, you will learn to do the following:

1. State the function of the endocrine system, and analyze associated terms.
2. Write the meaning of the word parts associated with the endocrine system, and use them to build and analyze terms.
3. Define homeostasis, and describe two ways in which the pituitary gland cooperates with the nervous system to maintain it.
4. Write the names of the other glands of the endocrine system, describe their functions, and define the terms associated with these structures.
5. Recognize the hormones associated with the major endocrine organs and their target organs or functions.
6. Write the names of the diagnostic tests and procedures used for assessment of the endocrine system when given descriptions of the procedures, or match the procedures with their descriptions.
7. Write the names of endocrine system pathologies when given their descriptions, or match the pathologies with their descriptions.
8. Match the terms for endocrine system surgical and therapeutic interventions with their descriptions, or write the names of the interventions when given their descriptions.
9. Build terms with word parts to label illustrations.

LEARNING OUTCOMES

Greater Comprehension

10. Use word parts from this chapter to determine the meanings or answer questions about the terms in a health care report.
11. Spell the terms accurately.
12. Pronounce the terms correctly.
13. Write the meanings of the abbreviations.
14. Categorize terms as anatomy, diagnostic test or procedure, pathology, surgery, or nonsurgical therapy.
15. Recognize the meanings of general pharmacological terms from this chapter as well as the drug classes and their uses.

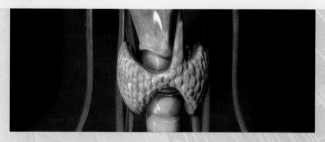

FUNCTION FIRST

The **endocrine system** cooperates with the nervous system to maintain homeostasis by regulating body activities. This is accomplished by endocrine hormones that affect various processes throughout the body, such as growth, metabolism, and secretions from other organs. Homeostasis (home[o], sameness or constant + -stasis, stopping or controlling) is a relative constancy in the internal environment of the body.

The nervous system communicates with the endocrine system through nerve impulses. The endocrine system acts through chemical messengers called *hormones.*

ANATOMY AND PHYSIOLOGY

secrete

12-1 You have learned that the combining form crin(o) means to _____. The endocrine (endo-, inside + -crine, to secrete) system is composed of the ductless glands and other structures that secrete hormones into the bloodstream. The ductless glands are **endocrine glands,** which secrete **hormones,** special chemical substances, into the blood that are carried to another part of the body, where they exert specific physiologic effects. Write the name of the chemical secretions of endocrine glands: _____.

hormones

12-2 A **gland** is an organ that has specialized cells that secrete or excrete substances that are not related to the gland's ordinary metabolism. There are many glands in the body.

🔑 **KEY** POINT **Glands are classified as either exocrine or endocrine glands.** The prefix exo- means outside, and **exo/crine glands** have ducts that enable them to empty secretions onto an external or an internal body surface. A sweat gland is an example of an exocrine gland. Endocrine glands (for example, the thyroid and pituitary glands) are ductless, so they secrete their hormones into the bloodstream. Compare endocrine and exocrine glands (Fig. 12.1).

ducts

Unlike exocrine glands, endocrine glands have no _____, so they secrete their hormones into the bloodstream.

12-3 Dysfunctions in hormone production fall into two categories: either a deficiency or an excess in secretion. A deficiency is called **hypo/secretion.** Excess secretion is called _____.

hypersecretion

The organ or structure toward which the effects of a hormone are primarily directed is called the **target organ.** If a hormone has a specific effect on the thyroid gland, then the thyroid is the target organ. If a hormone has a specific effect on the ovaries, then the ovary is the _____ organ. The target cell concept explains how only certain cells of specific organs are affected by a specific hormone (Fig. 12.2).

target

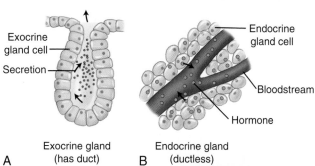

Figure 12.1 Comparison of the structure of an exocrine gland vs. an endocrine gland. A, Exocrine glands, such as sweat glands, are simple glands that have a duct that enable them to empty secretions onto a body surface. **B,** Endocrine glands are ductless and produce and secrete hormones into the blood or lymph nodes.

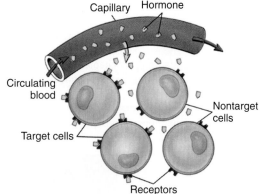

Figure 12.2 The target cell concept. The hormone recognizes the target tissue through receptors (the site that interacts with the hormone), so the hormones act only on cells that have receptors specific for that hormone. The shape of the receptor determines which hormone can react with it.

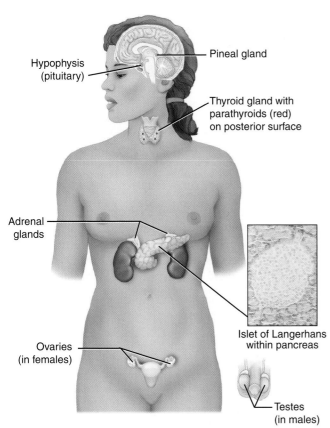

Figure 12.3 **Location of major glands of the endocrine system.**

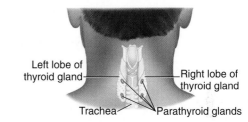

Figure 12.4 **Parathyroid glands.** Each parathyroid gland, embedded in the posterior surface of the thyroid, is about the size of a grain of rice.

12-4 Hormones are either proteins or steroids. Most hormones in the human body are proteins, with the exception of the sex hormones and those from the adrenal cortex, which are **steroids** (a special group of lipids). Proteins are quickly inactivated in the digestive tract, so if there is a deficiency, these hormones are administered by injection. Sex hormones and other steroids can be taken orally.

12-5 Locations of the major glands of the endocrine system are shown in Fig. 12.3. Read descriptions of the major endocrine glands:

- **pituitary gland:** A small, round structure about 1 cm (or ½ inch) in diameter that is attached by a stalk at the base of the brain; also called the **hypophysis**
- **adrenal glands:** One lies above each of the two kidneys; also called the **supra/renal** glands
- **gonads**—ovaries and testes: Glands that provide ova and sperm, respectively
- **pineal gland:** Shaped like a pine cone and is attached to the posterior part of the brain; also called the *pineal body*
- **thyroid:** Consists of bilateral lobes that are connected by a narrow strip of thyroid tissue and located at the front of the neck; also called the *thyroid gland*
- **parathyroid glands:** Embedded in the posterior surface of the thyroid; the name implies that they are located "near or beside" the thyroid (Fig. 12.4)
- **pancreas:** An elongated structure that has digestive functions as well as endocrine functions; the **islets of Langerhans** are microscopic clusters of cells responsible for the endocrine work of the pancreas.

WORD ORIGIN
pineal *(L.)*
pineus, pine cone

WRITE IT!   EXERCISE 1

1. Write the names of seven major glands of the endocrine system: _____

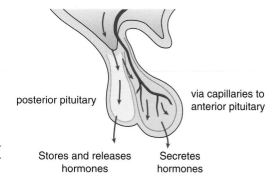

posterior pituitary

via capillaries to anterior pituitary

Stores and releases hormones

Secretes hormones

Figure 12.5 The pituitary, the master gland. The anterior pituitary is composed of glandular tissue, and the posterior pituitary is composed of nervous tissue.

12-6 Some hormones of the endocrine glands are released in response to the nervous system (for example, the adrenal gland releases adrenaline in response to the sympathetic nervous system in stressful situations). In addition, the pituitary gland supplies hormones that act directly on cells or stimulate other glands that govern numerous vital processes (Fig. 12.5). Because many endocrine glands respond to hormones produced by the pituitary gland, it is nicknamed "the **master gland.**"

🔑 **KEY** POINT   **The pituitary gland has many names.** The pituitary gland is also called the *pituitary*, the *hypophysis cerebri*, or simply the *hypophysis*. The suffix -physis means growth. The pituitary is nicknamed "the master gland."

under (beneath)

The hypo/physis was so named because it grows _____ the cerebrum.

WRITE IT!   **EXERCISE 2**

Fill in the blanks in these sentences.
1. The endocrine system and the _____ system cooperate to maintain homeostasis.
2. The name of the master gland is the _____.
3. An organ that has specialized cells that secrete or excrete substances that are not related to its ordinary metabolism is called a/an _____.
4. Chemical substances that are produced in one part of organ and initiate or regulate the activity of an organ in another part are called _____.

Learn the meanings of the following terms.

Word Parts: Endocrine Anatomy and Physiology

Combining Form	Meaning	Combining Form	Meaning
Associated With Anatomy		**Associated With Function**	
aden(o)	gland	andr(o)	male or masculine
adren(o), adrenal(o)	adrenal gland	calc(i)	calcium
cortic(o)	cortex	dwarf/o	dwarf
gonad(o)	gonad	gigant(o)	large
mamm(o), mast(o)	breast	gluc(o)	glucose
pancreat(o)	pancreas	glyc(o), glycos(o)	sugar
parathyroid(o)	parathyroid glands	insulin(o)	insulin
pituitar(o), hypophys(o)	pituitary gland	iod(o)	iodine
thyr(o), thyroid(o)	thyroid gland	ket(o), keton(o)	ketone
		lact(o)	milk
		trop(o)	to stimulate
		Suffix	
		-crine	secrete
		-dipsia	thirst
		-physis	growth
		-tropic	stimulating
		-tropin	that which stimulates

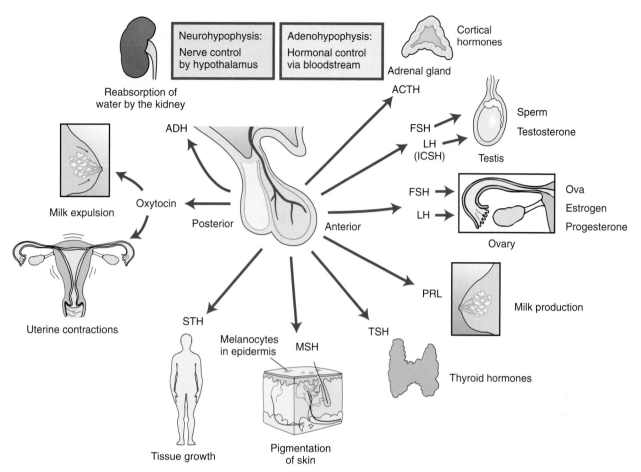

Figure 12.6 The pituitary, the master gland. The posterior pituitary lobe *(shown on the left)* is controlled by nervous stimulation by the hypothalamus and releases two hormones. In contrast, the anterior pituitary lobe is controlled by hypothalamic hormones brought by the bloodstream and secretes many hormones.

12-7 Examine the diagram of the pituitary and its target organs in Fig. 12.6. The pituitary is divided structurally and functionally into an anterior lobe and a posterior lobe.

The posterior lobe of the pituitary is called the **neurohypophysis.** The combining form neur(o) means _____. This lobe contains ends of neurons, the cell bodies of which are located in the **hypothalamus,** a portion of the lower part of the brain. The hormones of the neurohypophysis are stored in the axon endings and are released when a nerve impulse travels down the axon.

The anterior lobe of the pituitary is called the **adenohypophysis.** The word part aden(o) refers to a _____. This lobe is the glandular part of the hypophysis. The release of hormones from the adenohypophysis is controlled by regulating hormones produced by the hypothalamus.

12-8 Look again at Fig. 12.6. Abbreviations such as ADH, STH, and MSH stand for pituitary hormones; their meanings are antidiuretic hormone, somatotropic hormone and melanocyte-stimulating hormone, respectively. The two hormones produced by the posterior lobe of the pituitary act directly on specific cells of the kidneys, the breasts, and the uterus.

nerve

gland

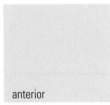

anterior

The anterior lobe of the pituitary produces many hormones, several of which act on other endocrine glands, causing them also to secrete hormones. The green arrows in Fig. 12.6 represent anterior pituitary hormones. Note that luteinizing hormone (LH) in males is also called interstitial cell–stimulating hormone (ICSH). (Interstitial in the name refers to certain cells of the testes.) Which lobe of the pituitary releases the greater number of hormones? _____ lobe

---

MATCH IT! **EXERCISE 3**

Match the word parts in the left columns with their description in the right. (Choices may be used more than once.)

_____ **1.** aden(o)	_____ **8.** hypophys(o)
_____ **2.** andr(o)	_____ **9.** lact(o)
_____ **3.** -crine	_____ **10.** mamm(o)
_____ **4.** -dipsia	_____ **11.** mast(o)
_____ **5.** gigant(o)	_____ **12.** -physis
_____ **6.** glyc(o)	_____ **13.** -tropin
_____ **7.** glycos(o)	_____ **14.** trop(o)

A. breast
B. gland
C. growth
D. large
E. male or masculine
F. milk
G. pituitary
H. secrete
I. sugar
J. that which stimulates
K. thirst
L. to stimulate

WRITE IT! **EXERCISE 4**

Fill in the blanks.

1. List the names or abbreviations of the two hormones that are stored in the neurohypophysis and released into the bloodstream after nervous stimulation by the hypothalamus: _____ and

_____.

2. List the abbreviations of the seven hormones of the adenohypophysis:

_____   _____

_____   _____

_____   _____

_____

ANALYZE IT! **EXERCISE 5**

Break these words into their component parts by placing a slash between the word parts. Write the meaning of each term.

1. adenohypophysis _____

2. neurohypophysis _____

3. hypothalamus _____

4. exocrine _____

5. homeostasis _____

Hormones of the Neurohypophysis

Antidiuretic Hormone and Oxytocin

posterior

12-9 The hypothalamus controls the neurohypophysis, the _____ lobe, by direct nervous stimulation.

🔑 **KEY** POINT **The hypothalamus synthesizes two hormones that are stored in the neurohypophysis.** Antidiuretic hormone and oxytocin are synthesized in the hypothalamus and transported to the neurohypophysis for storage. On stimulation by the hypothalamus, the neurohypophysis releases them into the bloodstream.

against

> WORD ORIGIN
> diuresis (G.)
> *dia,* through;
> *ouron,* urine

12-10 Antidiuretic hormone (ADH) affects the volume of urine excreted. The prefix anti- means _____. **Diuretic** means increasing urine excretion or the amount of urine. It also means an agent that promotes urine excretion. Anti/diuretic hormone acts against a diuretic. It acts in the kidneys to reabsorb water from the urine, producing concentrated urine. Absence of this hormone produces **diuresis,** passage of large amounts of dilute urine.

increase

12-11 Some common caffeinated drinks (tea, coffee, soda) and even water can act as diuretics. Physicians also prescribe diuretic drugs to rid the body of excess fluid in patients with edema. Diuretics (increase or decrease?) _____ urination. Anti/diuretic hormone causes a decrease in the amount of water lost in urination. A simple diagram may help:

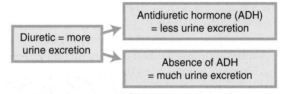

oxytocin

12-12 The second hormone, **oxytocin,** is released in large quantities just before a female gives birth. It causes uterine contractions, thus inducing childbirth. It also acts on the mammary glands to stimulate the release of milk. Write the name of the pituitary hormone that causes contraction of the uterus and acts on the mammary glands: _____. Here's a quick summary:

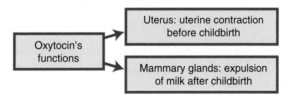

Hormones of the Adenohypophysis

TSH, FSH, LH, STH, MSH

12-13 The hypothalamus regulates the adenohypophysis, the anterior lobe, by producing regulatory and inhibitory hormones.

🔑 **KEY** POINT **Regulatory and inhibitory hormones stimulate or inhibit the adenohypophysis.** Hypothalamic regulatory and inhibitory hormones act on the adenohypophysis to either stimulate or inhibit the secretion of its hormones. When the adenohypophysis secretes its hormones, they travel through the bloodstream and bring about changes in other organs, often another endocrine gland. Note that the control from the hypothalamus to the adenohypophysis is hormonal, whereas the control of the neurohypophysis—as mentioned earlier—is through nervous stimulation.

The adenohypophysis releases several hormones that regulate a large range of body activities. Look again at the target organs of these hormones (see Fig. 12.6). Most of these pituitary secretions stimulate other glands, and many of their names contain trop(o), which means to stimulate or turn. **Tropic** is an adjective that means to _____.

stimulate

thyroid

12-14 Looking at Fig. 12.6, you see that the pituitary secretes TSH, which causes the glandular cells of the _____ to produce thyroid hormones. TSH means **thyroid-stimulating hormone** and is also called **thyrotropin.**

thyroid

12-15 The gland located at the front of the neck that is stimulated by TSH is the _____. **Eu/thyroid** means a normally functioning thyroid, because eu- means good or normal.

> **KEY** POINT The major functions of the thyroid gland are regulation of body metabolism, normal growth and development, and the storage of calcium in bone tissue. It accomplishes these functions by secretion of three hormones: thyroxine, triiodothyronine, and thyrocalcitonin.

iodine

12-16 The majority of the hormones secreted by the thyroid gland is **thyroxine,** abbreviated T_4, which is **tetra/iodo/thyro/nine,** because the molecule contains four atoms of _____ in its chemical structure.

iodine

Another hormone produced by the thyroid gland, but in far lower quantities, is **tri/iodo/thyronine,** which is abbreviated T_3. Both of these hormones are synthesized by the thyroid using iodine. If there is a deficiency of _____ in the diet, the thyroid will not be able to produce sufficient T_3 and T_4 for metabolism.

thyroid

A third hormone produced by the thyroid gland is **thyro/calcitonin** (TCT, also called **calcitonin**). This hormone is involved in the homeostasis of the blood calcium level. TCT is a hormone produced by the _____. The combining form calc(i) means calcium. To recap:

Thyroid gland → T3 / T4 / Thyrocalcitonin

12-17 The combining form gonad(o) means gonads (ovaries or testes).

> **KEY** POINT Two important pituitary hormones have the gonads as target organs. **Gonado/tropic hormones** stimulate the ovaries of the female and the testes of the male. **Follicle-stimulating hormone** (FSH) and **luteinizing hormone** (LH) are produced by the adenohypophysis.

gonadotropin

Write a word that means a hormone that stimulates the gonads: _____.
FSH and LH are gonadotropins.

gonads

12-18 Gonad/al means pertaining to the _____. **Gonadotropic** is an adjective that means stimulating the gonads. The first gonadotropic hormone, FSH, stimulates the ovaries to secrete estrogen and acts on the follicle (as its name implies). FSH stimulates production of sperm in the testes of males.

LH stimulates ovulation and production of progesterone in the female ovary. LH often is called **interstitial cell–stimulating hormone** (ICSH) in male individuals, because it promotes the growth of the interstitial cells of the testes and the secretion of testosterone. Here's a summary:

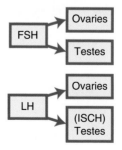

FSH → Ovaries / Testes

LH → Ovaries / (ISCH) Testes

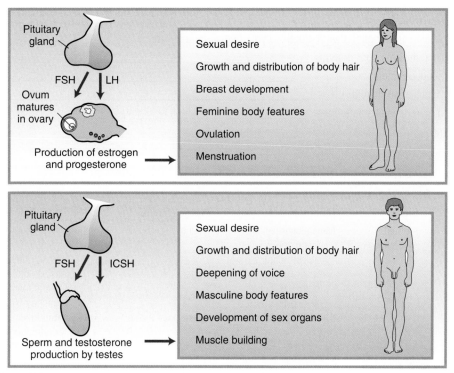

Figure 12.7 Secondary female and male sexual characteristics. The changes that occur at puberty are brought about by the hypothalamus and the anterior pituitary. Changes in the secretions of FSH and LH bring about changes in the ovaries and testes and the hormones they produce.

testosterone

12-19 The period of life at which reproduction becomes possible is **puberty.** It is recognized by maturation of the genitals and appearance of secondary sex characteristics. The onset of puberty is triggered by the hypothalamus and the anterior pituitary. FSH and LH act on the testes and ovaries (Fig. 12.7). Male sex hormones are collectively called **androgens,** and **testosterone** is the most abundant.

Fig. 12.7 reinforces the concept that the main hormones secreted by the ovaries and testes are estrogen and _____, respectively. **Progesterone** is another important female hormone produced mainly by the ovaries (and by the placenta during pregnancy) and in minute amounts by the adrenal cortex.

🔑 **KEY POINT** Ovaries produce estrogen (largely responsible for female sexual characteristics) and progesterone (also produced by the placenta), which maintains pregnancy.

male

masculine

12-20 The combining form andr(o) means _____ or masculine. Testosterone is the most potent androgen and is produced in large quantities by the testes, making that produced by the adrenal glands insignificant in most cases. **Andro/genic** means producing _____ characteristics or masculinization. In women, the masculinization effect of androgen secretion may become evident after menopause.

🔑 **KEY POINT** Testes produce testosterone, which is responsible for male sexual characteristics.

stimulates

somatotropin

12-21 Growth hormone (GH) is also called **somato/tropic hormone** (STH), or **somatotropin.** The suffix -tropin refers to that which stimulates. Somato/tropin is the hormone that _____ body growth.

This hormone increases the rate of growth and maintains size once growth is attained. It is called GH or _____.

black

12-22 Melanocyte-stimulating hormone (MSH) from the pituitary stimulates melanocytes distributed throughout the epidermis. MSH promotes pigmentation and controls the amount of melanin produced by melanocytes. The name melanin implies the color _____. **Melanin** is a black or dark brown pigment that occurs naturally in the hair, skin, and parts of the eye.

Use the following word parts to build terms.

eu-, andr(o), melan(o), somat(o), thyr(o), trop(o), -cyte, -genic, -ic, -oid, -tropin

1. that which stimulates body growth _____/_____

2. cell that produces melanin _____/_____

3. normally functioning thyroid _____/_____/_____

4. producing masculine characteristics _____/_____

5. stimulating _____/_____

Table 12.1	Hormones Secreted by the Adrenal Gland		
Gland	**Hormone**	**Target Tissue**	**Principal Action**
Adrenal cortex	Mineralocorticoids (main one is aldosterone)	Kidney	Increases water retention by changing sodium and potassium reabsorption in the kidney tubules
	Glucocorticoids (main ones are cortisol and cortisone)	Most body tissue	Increases blood glucose levels; inhibits inflammation and the immune response
	Androgens, estrogens	Most body tissue	Secreted in such small amounts that the effect is generally masked by ovarian and testicular hormones
Adrenal medulla	Epinephrine, norepinephrine	Heart and blood vessels, liver, skeletal muscles	Increases heart rate and blood pressure, increases blood flow and blood glucose level, helps the body cope with stress

ACTH and Prolactin

12-23 Each adrenal gland has two parts, a cortex and a medulla, and each part has its own functions. The outer **cortex** makes up the bulk of the gland, and the inner portion is called the **medulla.** Table 12.1 lists the important hormones produced by the adrenal glands.

🔑 **KEY POINT** **The cortex and medulla of the adrenal gland are stimulated by different means, and they secrete different hormones.** The hypothalamus influences both portions, but the medulla receives direct nervous stimulation. The cortex is stimulated by **adrenocorticotropin,** also called **adrenocorticotropic hormone** (ACTH), which is brought by the circulating blood.

cortex

glucose

12-24 Use Table 12.1 to write answers for Frames 12-24 and 12-25. Mineralocorticoids, gluco-corticoids, androgens, and estrogens are secreted by the adrenal _____. **Mineralo/corticoids** help maintain water balance in the body. As the name implies, **gluco/corticoids** increase blood _____, but they also inhibit inflammation. **Cortisone** is used to relieve pain and inflammation in topical preparations and is also injected in the joints. Androgens have masculinizing effects, and **estrogens** have feminizing effects.

norepinephrine

12-25 The adrenal medulla secretes two hormones: **epinephrine,** which stimulates the heart, and _____, which causes constriction of blood vessels.

Epinephrine is also called **adrenaline,** which you have probably heard before, so this may help you remember that these two hormones are sometimes called the *fight-or-flight hormones,* because they prepare the body for strenuous activity.

milk

12-26 **Prolactin** (PRL) is also the **lactogenic hormone,** because it causes production of _____ by the mammary glands. PRL has no known function in males.

mammary

12-27 The **mammary glands** are the two glands of the female breasts that secrete milk. The female breasts are accessory organs of the reproductive system. The breasts are located anterior to the chest muscles, and each breast contains 15 to 20 lobes of glandular tissue that radiate around the nipple. The milk-producing glands of the female are called the _____ glands.

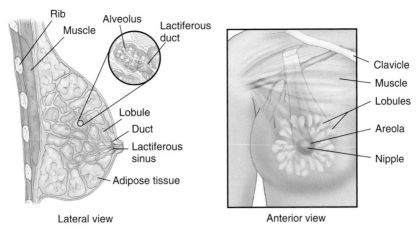

Figure 12.8 Structure of the adult female breast, lateral and anterior views. The breasts are mammary glands and function as part of both the endocrine and reproductive systems.

Structural aspects of the breast are shown in Fig. 12.8. The circular pigmented area of skin surrounding the nipple is the **areola. Lobule** means small lobe. The lobes are separated by connective and adipose (fatty) tissue. The amount of adipose tissue determines the size of the breasts but not the amount of milk that can be produced.

12-28 **Lacto/genic** means inducing the secretion of milk (lact[o] means milk).

KEY POINT **Changes in the mammary glands prepare the breasts of a pregnant female for lacto/genesis, the production of milk.** The most important hormone that stimulates milk production is PRL. The mammary glands secrete a cloudy fluid called **colostrum** during the first few days after a female gives birth. Because of both high antibody and protein content, colostrum serves adequately as food for the infant until milk production begins 2 to 3 days after birth.

12-29 Each breast lobule is drained by its own **lactiferous** duct, which has a dilated portion called a *sinus* that serves as a reservoir for milk. The nipple, located near the center of the breast, contains the openings of the milk ducts.

Lactation is the secretion or ejecting of milk. Milk ejection is a normal reflex in a lactating woman and is elicited by tactile stimulation of the nipple (such as, nursing by the infant). Impulses from the nipple to the hypothalamus stimulate the release of _____ by the pituitary gland, which brings about contractions that eject the milk from the breast (Fig. 12.9). If a lactating mother stops nursing, milk production usually ceases within a few days.

oxytocin

12-30 Several adjectives are used when describing locations near the breasts. Remembering that inter- means between, **inter/mammary** means situated _____ the breasts. **Retro/mammary** means behind the breast.

between

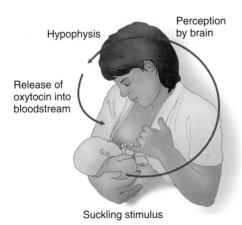

Figure 12.9 Interrelationships of hypothalamus, neurohypophysis, and breast. Suckling by the infant stimulates nerve endings at the nipple. Impulses are carried to the hypothalamus, which causes the neurohypophysis to secrete oxytocin into the bloodstream. The oxytocin is carried to the breast, where it causes milk to be expressed into the ducts. Milk begins to flow within 30 seconds to 1 minute after a baby begins to suckle.

Table 12.2 summarizes the major hormones of the pituitary, the target organs, and resulting actions or secretions.

Table 12.2 Major Hormones and Target Organs of the Master Gland

Hormone	Target Organ or Gland (Hormone Secreted)/Actions
Neurohypophysis*	
Antidiuretic hormone (ADH)	Kidney cells/conserve water
Oxytocin	Uterus during pregnancy/uterine contractions; mammary glands of lactating female/release of milk
Adenohypophysis	
Adrenocorticotropin (ACTH)	Adrenal cortex (mineralocorticoids, glucocorticoids, androgens, and estrogens); see Table 12.1
Follicle-stimulating hormone (FSH)	Ovarian follicles (estrogen)/ova; testes/sperm
Luteinizing hormone (LH)[†]	Ovaries (progesterone); testes (testosterone)
Melanocyte-stimulating hormone (MSH)	Melanocytes in epidermis; pigmentation
Prolactin (PRL)	Mammary glands; production of milk
Somatotropin (growth hormone [GH])	Body cells; growth or maintenance of size
Thyrotropin (TSH)	Thyroid gland (triiodothyronine [T_3], thyroxine [T_4], and thyrocalcitonin [TCT]); body metabolism and growth

*Action of the neurohypophysis on the adrenal medulla to secrete epinephrine and norepinephrine is nervous stimulation/nonhormonal.
[†]In males, LH is often called *interstitial cell–stimulating hormone (ICSH)*.

ANALYZE IT! EXERCISE 7

Break these words into their component parts by placing a slash between the word parts. Write the meaning of each term.

1. lactogenic _____
2. adrenal _____
3. retromammary _____
4. lactation _____
5. adrenocorticotropic _____

Other Endocrine Tissues

12-31 In addition to the endocrine glands that have been studied in previous sections, the pineal gland, the pancreas, and the parathyroids are considered here with a few other organs that have hormonal activity.

The exact functions of the pineal gland have not been established, but there is evidence that it secretes the hormone **melatonin**—so-named because its release is stimulated by darkness. The pineal gland usually begins to diminish around the age of 7 years. If degeneration does not occur, the production of melatonin remains high, and puberty may be delayed in girls. This indicates that melatonin may inhibit the activities of the ovaries.

Melatonin is secreted by the _____ gland. In addition to a regulatory function in sexual development, effects of melatonin may influence the sleepiness–wakefulness cycle and mood and may cause a decrease in skin pigmentation.

12-32 Strict regulation of hormonal secretion is important to maintain homeostasis.

> WORD ORIGIN
> melatonin *(G.)*
> *melas,* black

pineal

KEY POINT The body uses three different methods to regulate hormones: direct nervous stimulation, secretion of hormones in response to other hormones, and a negative feedback mechanism.

The adrenal medulla is an example of direct nervous stimulation. The adrenal medulla secretes epinephrine and norepinephrine in response to stimulation by sympathetic nerves.

Tropic hormones cause secretion of other hormones. For example, thyrotropin (TSH) from the anterior pituitary gland causes the thyroid gland to secrete the _____ hormones.

The interaction between two important pancreatic hormones and the concentration of glucose in the blood is an example of a negative feedback system. In negative feedback a gland is sensitive to the concentration of a substance that it regulates. Continue reading to see how this works.

12-33 The pancreas has an exocrine portion that secretes digestive enzymes that are carried through a duct to the small intestine and an endocrine portion that secretes hormones into the blood. The endocrine portion consists of many small cell groups called *islets of Langerhans*. These cells secrete two hormones that have a role in regulating blood glucose levels.

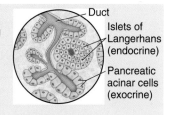

🔑 KEY POINT The islets of Langerhans secrete two important hormones, **glucagon** and **insulin**, which regulate each other through negative feedback (a decreased function in response to a stimulus). Here's how it works: The action of glucagon is to increase blood sugar levels, thus preventing **hypoglycemia** from occurring between meals. As glucose levels rise, they "turn off" or negatively affect the secretion of glucagon. In response to the high concentration of glucose in the blood, insulin is secreted, which promotes the uptake and utilization of glucose for energy. As glucose levels decrease, insulin levels decrease and the process begins again with the secretion of glucagon in response to hypoglycemia (Fig. 12.10).

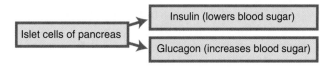

12-34 Food contains carbohydrates, which are broken down into glucose for energy. Glucose is the type of sugar found in blood. After eating a meal that contains carbohydrates, hyperglycemia results. Then which hormone is secreted, glucagon or insulin, that promotes the uptake and utilization of glucose? _____. As the level of glucose drops, glucagon is secreted to prevent blood sugar from dropping too low between meals, and the cycle begins again. The action of insulin and glucagon are opposite or antagonistic to each other, one causing the blood glucose to increase, the other causing it to decrease.

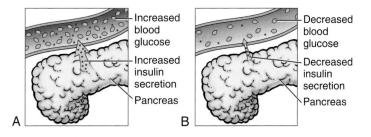

Figure 12.10 Feedback mechanism between blood glucose and insulin. A, Elevated blood glucose levels stimulate the secretion of insulin from the pancreas. **B,** As blood glucose levels decrease, the stimulus for insulin secretion also decreases. **C,** A schematic representation of the actions of glucagon and insulin in response to the levels of blood glucose.

Insufficient insulin activity results in **diabetes mellitus** (DM) and the resulting hyperglycemia. DM is caused by a deficiency or a complete lack of insulin secretion or resistance to insulin by target cells. For additional information, go to *www.diabetes.org.* Although heredity plays an important role in DM, it is believed that excess weight and physical inactivity contribute to insulin resistance. Learn more at *http://diabetes.niddk.nih.gov/dm/pubs/insulinresistance/index.aspx#resistance* and *http://www.nhlbi.nih.gov/health/health-topics/topics/ms/atrisk.html.*

12-35 The parathyroid gland (any of four small structures attached to the dorsal surface of the thyroid) is an endocrine gland that is not directly controlled by the pituitary but is closely linked with the thyroid gland.

🔑 **KEY** POINT **The thyroid gland regulates the parathyroid glands by negative feedback.** Parathyroid glands secrete **parathyroid hormone** (PTH) or **parathormone** (para- is used here to mean near or beside). PTH increases the blood calcium level, and its production and release is regulated by a negative feedback mechanism.

calcium

Negative feedback of PTH means that it is secreted in response to low levels of _____ in the blood.

thyroid

PTH has the opposite effect, or is antagonistic, to calcitonin secreted by the _____ gland. To recap:

Parathyroid glands ⟶ Parathyroid hormone (PTH) ⟶ ↑blood calcium

12-36 In addition to the endocrine glands that you have studied, other organs that have some hormonal activity include the stomach, small intestines, thymus, heart, and placenta.

The lining of the stomach produces **gastrin,** which stimulates the production of hydrochloric acid, and the enzyme **pepsin,** each being a substance that is used in the digestion of food. The hormone gastrin (gastr[o] means stomach) is secreted in response to food in the stomach. Hormones secreted by the lining of the small intestine stimulate the pancreas and the gallbladder to produce substances that aid in digestion.

The **thymus** is located near the middle of the chest cavity behind the breastbone. It produces **thymosin,** which assists in the development of lymphocytes, blood cells that function in immunity. The thymus, usually largest at puberty, diminishes in size as an individual reaches adulthood. The hormone produced by the thymus is called _____.

thymosin

Special cells in the atria, the upper chambers of the heart, produce a hormone, **atriopeptin,** which increases the loss of sodium and water in urine.

The placenta of a pregnant female produces **human chorionic gonadotropin** (HCG), estrogen, and progesterone, which function to maintain the uterine lining during pregnancy.

WORD ORIGIN
prostaglandin *(G.)*
prostates, standing before;
glans (L.), acorn

12-37 The cells of most tissues throughout the body can produce prostaglandins when stimulated, particularly by injury. **Prostaglandins,** potent chemical regulators, are hormonelike substances that have a localized, immediate, and short-term effect on or near the cells where they are produced.

Prostaglandins have many effects, and the same substance sometimes has opposite effects on different tissues. Some of the effects include smooth muscle contraction, involvement in blood clotting, and many aspects of fever and pain. They are believed to be implicated in the symptoms of severe menstrual cramps, premenstrual syndrome, and premature labor. Write the name of these hormonelike substances: _____.

prostaglandins

The major endocrine glands and their secretions are summarized in Table 12.3. For more information, go to *http://endocrine.niddk.nih.gov/.*

Table 12.3 Major Endocrine Glands and Their Secretions

Gland	Primary Secretions
Pituitary gland, anterior lobe	Adrenocorticotropic hormone (ACTH), follicle-stimulating hormone (FSH), growth hormone (GH), interstitial cell–stimulating hormone (ICSH), luteinizing hormone (LH), prolactin (PRL), melanocyte-stimulating hormone (MSH), thyrotropin (TSH)
Pituitary gland, posterior lobe	Antidiuretic hormone (ADH) and oxytocin
Adrenal glands, cortex	Aldosterone, cortisol, and androgens
Adrenal glands, medulla	Epinephrine and norepinephrine
Gonads, ovaries	Estrogen, progesterone, and human chorionic gonadotropin (HCG)
Gonads, testes	Testosterone
Pancreas (islets of Langerhans)	Insulin and glucagon
Parathyroid glands	Parathormone (PTH)
Thyroid gland	Thyroxine (T_4), triiodothyronine (T_3), and calcitonin
Pineal gland	Melatonin and serotonin
Thymus	Thymosin

MATCH IT! EXERCISE 8

Match the hormones in the left columns with the glands on the right that secrete them.

_____ **1.** adrenocorticotropic hormone   _____ **7.** luteinizing hormone   **A.** adrenals

_____ **2.** antidiuretic hormone   _____ **8.** melanocyte-stimulating hormone   **B.** gonads

_____ **3.** epinephrine   _____ **9.** oxytocin   **C.** pancreas

_____ **4.** follicle-stimulating hormone   _____ **10.** testosterone   **D.** pituitary

_____ **5.** growth hormone   _____ **11.** thyrocalcitonin   **E.** thyroid

_____ **6.** insulin   _____ **12.** thyrotropin

WRITE IT! EXERCISE 9

Name the target organ for each of the following hormones.

1. adrenocorticotropic hormone _____   **4.** luteinizing hormone _____

2. antidiuretic hormone _____   **5.** prolactin _____

3. follicle-stimulating hormone _____   **6.** thyrotropin _____

DIAGNOSTIC TESTS AND PROCEDURES

12-38 Most endocrine glands are not accessible for examination in a routine physical examination; however, the thyroid gland and the male gonads are exceptions. The patient's neck can be observed for any unusual bulging over the thyroid area, and the gland can be palpated (Fig. 12.11, A). Both enlargement and masses are abnormal findings and indicate additional testing is necessary.

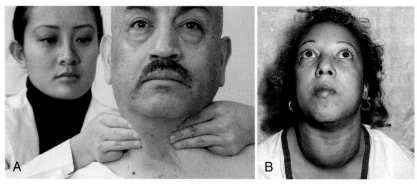

Figure 12.11 Physical examination of the thyroid gland. A, Using the hands to feel for thyroid enlargement or masses. **B,** Observing the patient for thyroid enlargement and exophthalmos (or exophthalmia), which is protrusion of the eyeballs. This patient shows both exophthalmos and a goiter, which is an enlarged thyroid gland evidenced by the swelling in the neck.

palpation

Likewise, the testicles are examined visually for a difference in size and are palpated for masses. The method of using the hands or fingers to examine an organ is called _____.

Physical indications of endocrine dysfunctions include unusually tall or short stature, coarsening of facial features, edema (accumulation of fluid in the interstitial tissues), hair loss, or excessive facial hair in females.

increased

12-39 Hyper/thyroid/ism is abnormally _____ activity of the thyroid. A classic finding associated with hyper/thyroid/ism is **ex/ophthal/mos**—that is, protrusion (bulging outward) of the eyeballs. Hyperthyroidism is not always the cause of exophthalmos, and further tests are required. The patient in Fig. 12.11, B, has exophthalmos and a **goiter,** which is an enlarged thyroid gland that is usually evident as a pronounced swelling in the neck. The metabolic processes of the body are accelerated as a result of the hypersecretion of thyroid hormones. Signs and symptoms include nervousness, fatigue, constant hunger, weight loss, heat intolerance, and palpitations (pounding or racing of the heart).

12-40 Laboratory testing includes blood tests and urine tests, depending on the symptoms. Pituitary studies include blood tests for levels of GH, gonadotropins, and other hormones secreted by the

luteinizing

pituitary gland. The gonadotropins are FSH and _____ hormone.

MRI is useful in identifying tumors involving the pituitary or the hypothalamus. Ultrasound is used to examine the thyroid, as well as the testes. Radioimmunoassay (RIA) studies are nuclear medicine tests, which use radioactive chemicals and antibodies to detect minute concentrations of a substance in the blood.

12-41 There are a number of blood tests and radiologic tests to determine thyroid function. Blood studies include testing for TSH, T_4, and T_3. (T_3 and T_4 are sometimes collectively called thyroid hormone.)

Because the thyroid gland absorbs iodine from the blood to synthesize T_3 and T_4, radioactive iodine can be used to study the gland. Radioactive iodine, ^{131}I, like all radionuclides (radioisotopes), gives off radiation. The **radioactive iodine uptake** (RAIU) **test** measures the ability of the thyroid gland to trap and retain the ^{131}I after oral ingestion. A radiation counter determines the amount of ^{131}I uptake by the thyroid gland. If a less than normal quantity of radioactive iodine is absorbed by the thyroid gland, which condition is expected, hypothyroidism or hyperthyroidism?

hypothyroidism

_____

Thyroid scans consist of administration of a radiopharmaceutical, followed by passage of a scanner over the thyroid, and creation of an image of the spatial distribution of the radionuclide.

parathyroid

12-42 Measurement of the levels of PTH, calcium, and phosphate in the blood helps to determine the functioning of the _____ gland.

Several hormones secreted by the adrenal glands can be measured in the blood and urine, as can the level of ACTH in the blood. Computed tomography, sometimes using contrast agents, can be used to detect tumors of the adrenal gland.

12-43 Blood tests to study pancreatic function include fasting blood sugar (FBS), **glycosylated hemoglobin** (HbA₁c), and oral **glucose tolerance tests** (GTTs). The FBS measures the glucose level in circulating blood. **Hyper/glyc/emia** is a greater than normal amount of glucose in the blood, and **hypo/glyc/emia** is a _____ than normal amount of blood glucose.

less

A GTT is a test of the body's ability to use carbohydrates by giving a standard dose of glucose to the patient and measuring the blood and urine for glucose levels at regular intervals.

KEY POINT The HbA₁c level provides a more accurate reflection of uncontrolled diabetes than a FBS level. Rather than only measuring the concentration of FBS on the particular day of testing, results of the HbA₁c represent the average blood glucose levels over the previous 3 or 4 months. In controlled DM, the HbA₁c concentration is within the normal range, but in uncontrolled cases, the levels may be three or four times the normal.

12-44 Urine studies to evaluate pancreatic function include testing for glucose and ketones. Neither glucose nor ketone levels are detectable in normal urine specimens. Use glycos(o) and -uria to write a word that means the presence of sugar, especially glucose, in the urine: _____.

glycosuria

Ketones are products of abnormal use of fat in the body (as in diabetes). Excessive production of ketones leads to their excretion in the urine. Combine keton(o) and -uria to write a word that means the presence of ketones in the urine: _____.

ketonuria

Radiologic testing to identify pancreatic tumors or cysts usually includes computed tomography, with or without a contrast medium. Ultrasound is also used in diagnosis of pancreatic disorders.

12-45 The breasts are part of several body systems, including the endocrine system. Self-examination of the breasts should be done periodically. A breast self-examination includes observing and palpating the breasts for changes that could indicate disease. Early diagnosis of breast cancer greatly improves the chance of survival.

▶ **BEYOND** THE BLUEPRINT Breast cancer may look like a rash of the nipple. A woman often may assume that a rash is a skin infection or allergy. Note the uneven superficial red appearance of more than half of the nipple in this surgical specimen of breast cancer, which had invaded the underlying breast tissue.

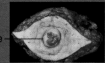

Nipple

Mammo/graphy is a diagnostic procedure that uses x-rays to study the soft tissues of the breast (Fig. 12.12, A). It is used as a screening test to detect various benign conditions and malignant tumors of the breast. The radiographic image produced in mammography is called a

mammogram

_____.

Fig. 12.12, C is a mammogram showing carcinoma of the breast. Sonography is also used in the diagnosis of breast disorders; it can distinguish cystic from solid growths.

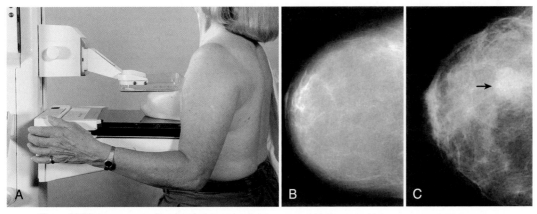

Figure 12.12 Mammography. A, Clinical setting for mammography. **B,** Normal Mammogram. **C,** Mammogram of cancer of the breast. The *arrow* indicates carcinoma.

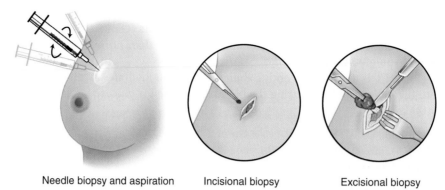

Needle biopsy and aspiration   Incisional biopsy   Excisional biopsy

Figure 12.13 Breast biopsy techniques. Needle biopsy and aspiration is used if fluid is present. The needle is rotated, moved back and forth, and moved slightly in or out to aspirate a specimen that is representative of several areas. If no fluid is aspirated, tissue is removed by incisional biopsy or excisional biopsy, the latter performed to remove all of the mass itself.

Digital breast tomosynthesis (DBT), using multiple images of the entire breast, is an advanced type of 3-dimensional mammogram that can offer earlier and more accurate cancer detection. The machine looks similar, the breast is compressed in the same way as for a mammogram, but the x-ray tube moves in a circular arc around the breast, and the image is sent to a computer, which produces a focused 3-D image.

12-46 Breast masses are one of the most common disorders of the breast; and fortunately, most masses are benign.

🔑 **KEY** POINT **Several diagnostic tools are available to evaluate a breast mass.** In addition to mammography, any of several diagnostic tools may be indicated, such as needle biopsy and aspiration, incisional biopsy, or excisional biopsy (Fig. 12.13). Needle aspiration is the removal of fluid and tissue from the breast mass through a large-bore needle. An **incisional biopsy** is the surgical removal of tissue from the breast mass, and **excisional biopsy** removes the mass itself. The fluid and tissue removed in these procedures is examined histologically.

When fluid or tissue is removed through a large-bore needle, this is called needle biopsy and
aspiration
_____.

MATCH IT! EXERCISE 10	Match the descriptions in the left column with the test or abbreviation on the right.	
	_____ **1.** blood test of fasting glucose level	**A.** goiter
	_____ **2.** examination with the hands or fingers	**B.** RAIU
	_____ **3.** test of thyroid's ability to trap and retain iodine	**C.** palpation
	_____ **4.** test of hemoglobin attached to a glucose molecule	**D.** FBS
	_____ **5.** enlarged thyroid gland	**E.** HbA$_{1c}$

BUILD IT! **EXERCISE 11**

Use the following word parts to build terms. (Some word parts will be used more than once.)
hyper-, hypo-, glyc(o), glycos(o), keton(o), mamm(o), thyroid(o), -emia, -graphy, -ism, -uria

1. increased activity of the thyroid gland _____/_____/_____

2. less than normal amount of glucose in the blood _____/_____/_____

3. presence of ketones in the urine _____/_____

4. presence of sugar in the urine _____/_____

5. radiographic examination of the breast _____/_____

PATHOLOGIES

adenopathy

12-47 Too little or too much of a specific hormone leads to a dysfunction of the endocrine system. Write a term that has a literal translation of any disease of a gland: _____.
This term means any disease of a gland, but remember that the term is sometimes used to mean any disease of the lymph nodes.

> **BEYOND** THE BLUEPRINT Body builders sometimes take steroid hormones to achieve muscular definition, which can lead to endocrine disorders. Physicians can order tests of steroids when they see overdevelopment of muscles in a patient and suspect abuse.

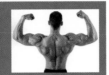

An **aden/oma** is a benign tumor in which the cells are clearly derived from glandular tissue. In contrast, **adeno/carcinoma** means any of a large group of malignant tumors of the glands.

FIND IT! EXERCISE 12

Draw a slash between the word parts in the following list. Then find the meanings of the word parts within the definitions. (Draw the slash, and then perform the remainder of the activity as a mental exercise.)

1. **hyperpituitarism** increased activity of the pituitary gland; a common cause is the presence of a benign tumor, especially a pituitary adenoma; overproduction or underproduction of GH during childhood leads to **gigantism,** characterized by excessive stature or **dwarfism,** extreme shortness and often other defects

(Fig. 12.14). Compare a pituitary-deficient child with a normal 3-year-old (Fig. 12.15).

2. **hypopituitarism** decreased activity of the pituitary gland; deficiency of one or more anterior pituitary hormones

3. **polydipsia** excessive thirst

4. **polyuria** excessive urination

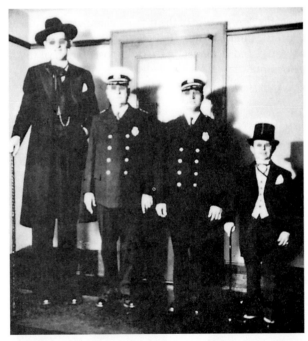

Figure 12.14 Gigantism and dwarfism, resulting from abnormal secretions of growth hormone (GH). Hypersecretion of GH during the early years results in gigantism *(person on far left).* The person usually has normal body proportions and normal sexual development. Hyposecretion of GH during the early years produces a dwarf *(person on far right)* unless the child is treated with injections of GH.

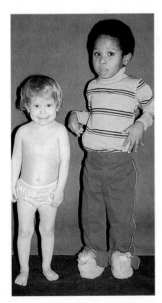

Figure 12.15 Childhood deficiency of growth hormone (GH). Compare the normal 3-year-old boy with the short 3-year-old girl who exhibits the characteristic small stature and "Kewpie doll" appearance, suggesting a deficiency of GH.

Pituitary, Thyroid, and Parathyroid Disorders

12-48 Pituitary dysfunction can result in hypo/secretion or hyper/secretion of the pituitary hormones. Disorders of the posterior lobe of the pituitary are usually related to a deficiency or excess of ADH, which is the _____ hormone.

antidiuretic

Disorders of the posterior lobe of the pituitary include the following:

- **diabetes insipidus:** A disorder associated with a deficiency of ADH or inability of the kidneys to respond to ADH, polyuria, and polydipsia; do not confuse with DM, the well-known type of diabetes that is associated with insufficient or improper use of insulin by the body.
- **syndrome of inappropriate ADH secretion:** Excessive release of ADH that usually develops in association with other diseases; abbreviation is SIADH

12-49 The effects and hormones of anterior pituitary disorders are excessive or deficient growth (somatotropin), metabolism (PRL, STH, ACTH, and MSH), or sexual development (FSH and LH). Untreated endocrine dysfunctions during childhood generally have longer lasting and greater effects than those that occur after puberty. Because of better knowledge and improved testing, many endocrine dysfunctions in children are treated, and long-lasting effects are avoided.

Disorders of the anterior lobe of the pituitary include the following:

acromegaly Oversecretion of GH in adults, characterized by thickening of the bones of the feet, hands, cheeks, and jaws (Fig. 12.16); may also involve other pituitary hormones

goiter A descriptive term that means an enlarged thyroid gland, evident as a pronounced swelling in the neck (see Fig. 12.11, B)

hyperthyroidism Excessive secretion of two hormones of the thyroid gland, resulting in increased metabolic rate; the patient becomes excitable and nervous, exhibiting moist skin, rapid pulse, increased metabolic activity, weight loss, and exophthalmos, marked protrusion of the eyeballs (see Fig. 12.11, B); the most common form of hyperthyroidism is **Graves disease**, which is believed to be an autoimmune disease. A life-threatening form of Graves disease is thyroid storm, also called **thyrotoxicosis.**

hypothyroidism Decreased activity of the thyroid gland; in childhood, results in **cretinism,** characterized by arrested physical and mental development (Fig. 12.17)

myxedema Severe form of adult hypothyroidism (deficiency of T_4 and T_3) with severe swelling, especially facial puffiness

pituitary cachexia A state of ill health, malnutrition, and wasting, caused by hyposecretion of the pituitary gland in adults

thyropathy Any disease of the thyroid gland; thyroid diseases include inflammation (**thyroiditis**) or enlargement of the thyroid and hypersecretion or hyposecretion of thyroid hormones

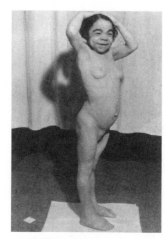

Figure 12.17 Cretinism. This 33-year-old untreated adult cretin exhibits characteristic features. She is only 44 inches tall, and has underdeveloped breasts, protruding abdomen, umbilical hernia, widened facial features, and scant axillary and pubic hair.

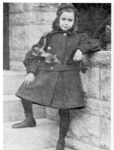 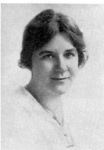 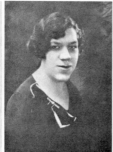 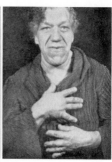

Figure 12.16 Progression of acromegaly. The patient is shown at age 9, age 16, age 33 with well-established acromegaly, and age 52 in the late stages of acromegaly.

Draw a slash between the word parts in the following list. Then find the meanings of the word parts within the definitions. (Draw the slash, and then perform the remainder of the activity as a mental exercise.)

1. **hyperparathyroidism** increased secretion of the parathyroids, which causes **hypercalcemia,** greater than normal concentration of calcium in the blood

2. **hypoparathyroidism** insufficient secretion of the parathyroids, which causes **hypocalcemia,** less than normal concentration of calcium in the blood

3. **pituitary hypogonadism** decreased secretion of FSH or LH by the pituitary gland

4. **hypogonadism** decreased functional activity of the gonads; results in a deficiency of the hormones produced by the affected organs (ovaries or testes)

Break these words into their component parts by placing a slash between the word parts. Write the meaning of each term.

1. adenocarcinoma _____

2. polydipsia _____

3. hypopituitarism _____

Adrenal, Pancreas, and Breast Disorders

enlargement
adrenopathy

12-50 Adreno/megaly is _____ of one or both adrenal glands. Using adren(o), write a word that means any disease of the adrenals: _____.

adrenals

12-51 Hyper/adrenal/ism is increased secretory activity of the _____. Hypersecretion of the adrenal cortex causes **Cushing syndrome** (Fig. 12.18), which is characterized by increased blood glucose levels, edema resulting from imbalance of water in the body, and masculinization in female individuals.

Tumors that result in hypersecretion of androgens or estrogens before puberty usually have dramatic effects. This is called the **adrenogenital syndrome** or **adrenal virilism.** There is a rapid onset of puberty and sex drive in males. In females, the masculine distribution of body hair develops, and the clitoris enlarges to look more like a penis.

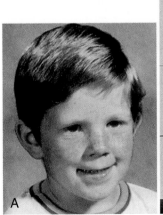
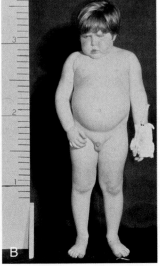

Figure 12.18 Cushing syndrome. These photographs show the dramatic changes associated with Cushing syndrome. **A,** Patient before the onset of Cushing syndrome. **B,** Patient 4 months later, now drastically affected by hypersecretion of the adrenal cortex.

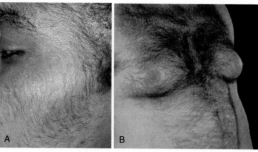

Figure 12.19 Examples of estrogen and androgen imbalances. A, Hirsutism, excessive body hair in a masculine distribution pattern, can result from several causes, including heredity, hormonal dysfunction, and/or medication. **B,** Gynecomastia, a noninflammatory enlargement of both breasts in males, can be temporary and benign. The most common cause is a disturbance of the normal ratio of androgen to estrogen and may occur as a side effect of drug therapy.

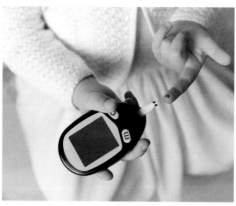

Figure 12.20 Glucometer. This is a battery-operated unit used by persons with diabetes to determine their blood glucose from as little as one drop of blood.

hair

12-52 Several dysfunctions of the gonadal hormones are discussed in Chapter 9. Hirsutism and gynecomastia are other disorders resulting from imbalances in estrogens and androgens.

Excessive growth and male distribution of body hair in the female is **hirsutism** (Fig. 12.19, A). It has several causes, including heredity, hormonal dysfunction, and medication. Decreased estrogen levels or other hormonal dysfunction can result from abnormalities of the ovaries or adrenals. Hirsutism, however, means excessive growth of _____.

andropathy

Occasionally an adrenal tumor secretes excess estrogens. When this occurs, the male patient experiences development of gyneco/mast/ia, which translated literally means a female breast condition (see Fig. 12.19, B). **Gynecomastia** means excessive growth of the male mammary glands.

Andro/pathy means any disease peculiar to the male gender, such as gynecomastia. Write this word that means a disease seen only in males: _____.

decreased

cortex

12-53 Hypo/adrenal/ism is _____ adrenal activity. The loss of medullary activity does not cause as drastic an effect as the loss of adrenocortical activity. **Adreno/cortical** pertains to the adrenal _____.

Hyposecretion of epinephrine produces no significant effect. Hypersecretion, usually from a tumor, puts the body in a prolonged or continual fight-or-flight mode.

hyposecretion

12-54 Hyposecretion of the adrenal cortex in which all three classes of adrenal corticosteroids are reduced leads to **Addison disease.** This life-threatening condition is characterized by dehydration, low blood glucose levels, bronzing of the skin, and general ill health. Partial or complete failure of the adrenal glands can result from auto/immune processes, infection, tumors, or hemorrhage within the gland. Addison disease results from _____ of the adrenal cortex.

pancreatitis

insulin

12-55 The pancreas is subject to inflammation and cancer, and both conditions can lead to insufficient secretion of insulin. Write a term that means inflammation of the pancreas: _____. This disorder, as well as pancreatic cancer, can result in a deficiency of insulin secretion by the pancreas. **Hypo/insulin/ism** is a deficient secretion of _____ by the pancreas.

greater

12-56 Diabetes mellitus (DM) is primarily a result of resistance to insulin or a deficiency or complete lack of insulin secretion by the insulin-producing cells of the pancreas. Without insulin, glucose builds up in the blood and hyperglycemia results. Hyper/glycem/ia means a _____ than normal level of glucose in the blood. Diabetics are urged to control blood glucose levels to significantly reduce complications of uncontrolled diabetes. A blood glucose monitor called a glucometer (Fig. 12.20) can be used by diabetics to monitor their blood glucose levels.

excessive

Hyperglycemia causes serious fluid and electrolyte imbalances, ultimately resulting in the classic symptoms of diabetes: polyphagia, polyuria, and polydipsia. See Table 12.4 to compare characteristics of diabetes insipidus and diabetes mellitus. **Polyphagia** (poly-, many + -phagia, eating) means excessive hunger and uncontrolled eating. Polyuria (-uria, urination) means _____ urination, and polydipsia (-dipsia, thirst) means excessive thirst.

Table 12.4   Comparison of Diabetes Insipidus With Diabetes Mellitus

Characteristic	Diabetes Insipidus	Diabetes Mellitus
ADH deficiency	Yes	No
Polyuria	Yes	Yes
Polydipsia	Yes	Yes
Insufficient or improper use of insulin	No	Yes*
Two types, I and II	No	Yes
Hyperglycemia	No	Yes
Glycosuria	No	Yes

*Diabetes mellitus is classified as type 1 or type 2.

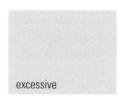

WORD ORIGIN
diabetes *(G.)*
diabainein, to pass
through

mellitus

12-57 When used alone, the term *diabetes* generally refers to diabetes mellitus, but one should be aware that the term *diabetes* means excessive excretion of urine, and diabetes insipidus, for example, is so named because of its classic symptoms, not because of its relationship to DM.

Broad classifications of DM are type 1, type 2, gestational, and other types. **Type 1 diabetes mellitus** is genetically determined and results in absolute insulin deficiency. Individuals with this particular gene produce little or no insulin and are classified as having type 1 diabetes _____. This disease was previously called *insulin-dependent diabetes mellitus (IDDM).*

🔑 **KEY** POINT **Chronic complications of DM include vascular diseases and neuro/pathy.** Vascular diseases include diseases of the heart and major vessels, as well as smaller vessels (e.g., **diabetic nephro/pathy,** which is damage to the small vessels of the kidneys and is the leading cause of end-stage renal disease in the United States). **Diabetic retino/pathy,** another complication, is a disorder of the retinal blood vessels of the eye that can eventually lead to blindness. **Diabetic neuropathy** is nerve damage associated with DM. Foot complications are a common problem for the patient with diabetes (Fig. 12.21), particularly the development of **peripheral vascular disease** (PVD), which can lead to amputation.

insulin

12-58 The specific genetic link and development of **type 2 diabetes mellitus** is unclear. Contributing causes may be genetic and environmental factors, as well as the aging process and obesity. It is characterized by insulin resistance, rather than insufficient _____ secretion. Type 2 DM was formerly called *non–insulin-dependent diabetes mellitus (NIDDM),* but this term was misleading because some individuals with type 2 diabetes require insulin.

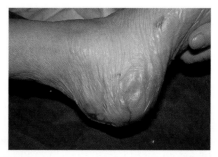

Figure 12.21 Early pressure damage to the heel in diabetic neuropathy.
Diabetes is associated with a wide range of neuropathies, especially noninflammatory disease processes of the heel and toes.

gestational

12-59 Gestational diabetes mellitus (GDM), first recognized during pregnancy, is carbohydrate intolerance, usually caused by a deficiency of insulin. It disappears after delivery of the infant but in a significant number of cases, returns years later. This type of diabetes is called _____ diabetes mellitus.

There are some other less common types of DM in addition to type 1, type 2, and gestational DM. An example is the type of DM associated with hyperthyroidism.

decreased

12-60 Hyper/insulin/ism is excessive insulin in the body. Hyperinsulinism results in hypo/glyc/emia, which is a _____ amount of glucose in the blood.

Hypo/glycemia is a less than normal amount of glucose in the blood. It is caused by administration of too much insulin, excessive secretion of insulin by the pancreas, or dietary deficiency. An individual with hypoglycemia usually experiences weakness, headache, hunger, visual disturbances, and anxiety. If untreated, hypoglycemia can lead to coma and death. Write the term that means less than normal levels of glucose in the blood: _____.

hypoglycemia

12-61 The mammary glands are lactiferous glands in the female breasts that are the target organs of oxytocin and PRL. Many problems associated with the breast are not a result of hormones. However, hormones may be related to breast disorders, for example, inappropriate lactation (nipple discharge).

breast

12-62 Mast/itis is an inflammatory condition of the _____ that occurs most frequently in lactating women. It is usually caused by bacterial infection. If mastitis is untreated, abscesses may form. **Mamm/algia, masto/dynia,** and **mast/algia** mean breast

pain

_____.

12-63 Frequently encountered breast disorders include fibrocystic disease, breast cancer, and benign tumors. **Fibro/cystic breast disease** is a disorder characterized by single or multiple benign cysts of the breast. The cysts must be considered potentially malignant until diagnostic tests indicate otherwise; thereafter, the breasts should be observed carefully for change. The cysts often occur as a result of cyclic breast changes that accompany the menstrual cycle. This disorder characterized by benign cysts of the breast is called _____ breast disease.

fibrocystic

12-64 A number of breast tumors (for example, fibroadenoma, which is a nontender encapsulated tumor [Fig. 12.22]) are benign and can be differentiated from cancerous tumors by mammography and biopsy. Excluding skin cancer, breast cancer has been the most common malignancy among women in the United States for years. The cause of breast cancer is still unknown, but early detection and improved treatment have contributed to a decrease in mortality rates. Breast cancer in females is still a major cause of cancer death. Breast cancer in males is rare.

Breast cancer often begins as a small, painless lump; dimpled skin; or nipple retraction. As the cancer progresses, there may be nipple discharge, pain, and ulceration.

cancer

Masto/carcinoma is a term that means breast _____. Ductal carcinoma in situ (DCIS) is any of a large group of carcinomas confined to the lactiferous duct where it is formed.

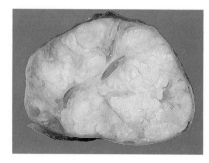

Figure 12.22 Fibroadenoma. This benign (2.5 cm) tumor is nontender, encapsulated, round, movable, and firm, usually located in the upper outer quadrant of the breast and occurs most frequently in women younger than 30 years of age.

WRITE IT!

EXERCISE 15

Case Study. Select terms from the report to match the descriptions.

Humberto Cordova suddenly began experiencing polyuria, polydipsia, and polyphagia. Laboratory findings showed a normal level of antidiuretic hormone, but hyperglycemia, glycosuria, and ketonuria. Further testing indicated diabetes mellitus.

1. a greater than normal amount of glucose in the blood _____

2. excessive, uncontrolled eating _____

3. increased urination _____

4. pertaining to the suppression of urine excretion _____

5. presence of sugar, especially glucose, in the urine _____

BUILD IT!

EXERCISE 16

Use the following word parts to build terms. (Some word parts will be used more than once.)

hyper-, adrenal(o), carcin(o), insulin(o), mast(o), pancreat(o), -dynia, -ism, -itis, -oma

1. inflammation of the pancreas _____/_____

2. pain in the breast _____/_____

3. cancer of the breast _____/_____/_____

4. increased secretory activity of the adrenals _____/_____/_____

5. excessive insulin in the body _____/_____/_____

MATCH IT!

EXERCISE 17

Match the pathologies in the left column with their characteristics in the right column.

_____ **1.** acromegaly

_____ **2.** Addison disease

_____ **3.** Cushing syndrome

_____ **4.** cretinism

_____ **5.** diabetes mellitus

_____ **6.** exophthalmos

_____ **7.** gigantism

_____ **8.** goiter

_____ **9.** hypogonadism

_____ **10.** myxedema

A. decreased functional activity of the ovaries or testes

B. enlarged thyroid gland

C. hypersecretion of the adrenal cortex

D. hypersecretion of GH in adults

E. hypersecretion of somatotropin during childhood

F. hyposecretion of the adrenal cortex

G. hyposecretion of T_4 and T_3 during adulthood

H. hypothyroidism in childhood

I. insufficient secretion or resistance to insulin

J. outward protrusion of the eyeballs

SURGICAL AND THERAPEUTIC INTERVENTIONS

12-65 The goal of treatment of diabetes mellitus is to maintain a balance of the body's insulin and glucose. Type 1 diabetes is controlled by administration of insulin, proper diet, and exercise. Insulin is administered by injection on a regular basis, either sub/cutaneous injection or via an insulin pump. An **insulin pump** is a portable battery-operated instrument that delivers a measured amount of insulin through the abdominal wall. It can be programmed to deliver doses of insulin according to the body's needs (Fig. 12.23). The individual with type 1 diabetes requires an outside source of _____ to sustain life.

insulin

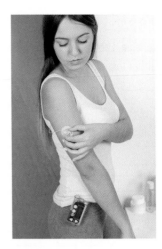

Figure 12.23 External insulin pump. This insulin pump is about the size of a small cell phone and is worn externally. It delivers precise doses of rapid-acting insulin to closely match your body's needs. Additional insulin can be delivered "on demand" before an unusually large meal or to correct a high blood sugar.

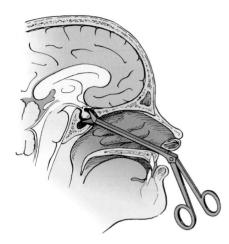

Figure 12.24 Hypophysectomy. Surgical removal of the pituitary gland may be performed to excise a pituitary tumor or to slow the growth and spread of endocrine-dependent malignant tumors. It is done only if other treatment fails to destroy all pituitary tissue.

Insulin is a **glucose-lowering agent.** Type 2 diabetes is controlled by diet, exercise, oral agents, and sometimes insulin. Oral agents are another means of lowering blood glucose.

Proper nutrition is important in gestational diabetes. Insulin is given if nutritional therapy is insufficient.

12-66 Treatment of hypoglycemia may consist of a glucose paste placed inside the cheek, administration of glucose (dextrose), such as that found in orange juice, or intravenously if the person is unconscious. Strict attention to diet is important for patients with hypoglycemia caused by

excessive

_____ secretion of insulin.

12-67 Because the most common cause of hypopituitarism is a pituitary tumor, treatment consists of surgery or radiation to remove the tumor, followed by administration of the deficient hormones.

Certain types of pituitary tumors can cause overproduction of GH, and the treatment of choice is surgery to remove the tumor. Irradiation of the tumor and drugs may also be indicated. **Hypophysectomy** is surgical removal or destruction of the hypophysis (Fig. 12.24). Hypophys/ectomy is

hypophysis (pituitary)

removal or destruction of the _____. Increased production of a single tropic hormone (such as TSH) usually causes oversecretion by the target organ (e.g., overproduction of T_4 and T_3). Drug therapy may be useful in suppressing the hormone production.

12-68 The treatment of hyperthyroidism is destruction of large amounts of the thyroid tissue by either surgery or radioactive materials or the use of **anti/thyroid drugs** to block the production of

excision

thyroid hormones. **Thyroid/ectomy** is _____ of the thyroid.

12-69 It may be necessary to surgically remove adrenal tumors that cause the adrenals to produce excess corticoids. Using adrenal(o), write a word that means excision of an adrenal gland:

adrenalectomy

_____.

12-70 Removal of one or more parathyroids is **parathyroidectomy**.

Build a word that means removal of the pancreas:

pancreatectomy

_____.

A surgical procedure that is used to treat pancreatic cancer is **pancreatoduodenostomy**, removal of the pancreas and duodenum. A radical procedure that removes the duodenum, the head of the pancreas, and part of the stomach and the common bile duct is called a Whipple procedure.

mastopexy

12-71 Masto/ptosis is sagging or prolapsed breasts. Write a word using mast(o) that means surgical fixation of the breasts: _____.

Mastopexy is performed to correct a pendulous breast. (This is also called a *breast lift*.)

12-72 The extent and location of metastases determines the therapeutic strategy in breast cancer. For breast cancer with distant metastases, nonsurgical treatment (chemotherapy, hormone therapy, and sometimes radiation) may be prescribed. For women with breast cancer at a stage for which surgery is recommended, follow-up after the surgery with chemotherapy, radiation, hormone therapy, or targeted therapy may be prescribed.

Excision of the lump with removal of varying amounts of tissue is often the treatment of choice in breast cancer. The amount of extra tissue removed ranges from a small amount of surrounding healthy tissue to the entire breast. A **lumpectomy** is surgical excision of a tumor that is known to

breast

be or suspected of being cancer. **Mast/ectomy** is removal of the _____.
Only breast tissue is removed in a simple mastectomy, whereas axillary lymph nodes and muscles of the chest are removed in a radical mastectomy (Fig. 12.25).

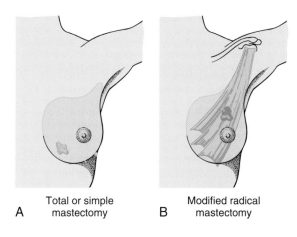

A   Total or simple
mastectomy

B   Modified radical
mastectomy

Figure 12.25 Simple vs. radical mastectomy. These are most commonly performed to remove a malignant tumor. **A,** In a simple mastectomy, only breast tissue is removed. **B,** In a radical mastectomy, axillary lymph nodes and some of the muscles of the chest are removed with the breast.

breast

12-73 Breast reconstruction may begin during the original mastectomy or soon after surgical removal of the breast, using saline or silicone breast implants. **Mammo/plasty** is plastic surgery of the _____.

reduce

Mammoplasty, surgical reshaping of the breasts, can be done to reduce or lift large or sagging breasts and sometimes to enlarge small breasts. **Augmentation mammoplasty** is plastic surgery to increase the size of the female breast. **Reduction mammoplasty** is plastic surgery to _____ the size of the breast.

WRITE IT!
EXERCISE 18

Write a term for each of the following meanings.

1. excision of a lump in the breast   _____

2. excision of the thyroid   _____

3. plastic surgery of the breast   _____

4. removal of the adrenal gland   _____

5. surgical fixation of the breasts   _____

6. surgical removal of a breast   _____

! Be Careful With These!

diabetes insipidus vs.   *diabetic nephropathy* vs.   *diuresis* vs. *diuretic*   *type 1 diabetes mellitus* vs.
   diabetes mellitus   *diabetic neuropathy*   *type 2 diabetes mellitus*

Watch out for all the abbreviations in this chapter!

PHARMACOLOGY

Drug Class: Effect and Uses

Antidiabetics/Antihyperglycemic Agents: Control blood glucose levels to treat diabetes mellitus
Types include alpha-glucosidase inhibitors, biguanides, glucagon-like peptide-1 (GLP-1) receptor agonists, insulins, meglitinides, sulfonylureas, and thiazolidinediones

acarbose (Precose)	*insulin glargine (Lantus)*	*pioglitazone (Actos)*
glipizide (Glucotrol)	*liraglutide (Victoza)*	*repaglinide (Prandin)*
glyburide (DiaBeta)	*metformin (Glucophage)*	*rosiglitazone (Avandia)*
insulin recombinant human (Humulin R)	*miglitol (Glyset)*	

Antithyroid Drugs: Reduce production of thyroid hormones to treat hyperthyroidism or goiter
methimazole (Tapazole) *propylthiouracil (PTU)*

Corticosteroids: Replacement therapy to treat under functioning adrenal glands
dexamethasone (Decadron) *prednisone (Rayos)*
methylprednisolone (Medrol) *triamcinolone (Kenalog)*

Growth Hormone: Treat growth failure
somatropin (Nutropin)

Posterior Pituitary Hormones: Replacement antidiuretic hormone to manage symptoms of diabetes insipidus
vasopressin (Pitressin)

Thyroid Drugs: Replacement thyroid hormones to treat hypothyroidism
levothyroxine (Synthroid) *liotrix (Thyrolar)*

WRITE IT! **EXERCISE 19**

1. Agents used to treat hyperthyroidism are called _____ drugs.
2. Antidiabetic drugs are also called _____ agents.
3. Replacement therapy for hypofunctioning adrenals are _____.
4. A pharmacological agent used to treat growth failure is growth _____.
5. Thyroid drugs are replacement thyroid hormones to treat _____.

CHAPTER ABBREVIATIONS*

ACTH	adrenocorticotropic hormone	**LH**	luteinizing hormone
ADH	antidiuretic hormone	**MSH**	melanocyte-stimulating hormone
DCIS	ductal carcinoma in situ	**NIDDM**	non–insulin-dependent diabetes mellitus
DM	diabetes mellitus	**PRL**	prolactin
FBS	fasting blood sugar	**PTH**	parathyroid hormone; parathormone
FSH	follicle-stimulating hormone	**PVD**	peripheral vascular disease
GDM	gestational diabetes mellitus	**RIA**	radioimmunoassay
GH	growth hormone	**RAIU**	radioactive iodine uptake
GTT	glucose tolerance test	**SIADH**	syndrome of inappropriate ADH secretion
HbA$_{1c}$	glycosylated hemoglobin	**STH**	somatotropic hormone
hCG or HCG	human chorionic gonadotropin	**T$_3$**	triiodothyronine
^{131}I	radioactive iodine	**T$_4$**	thyroxine
ICSH	interstitial cell–stimulating hormone	**TCT**	thyrocalcitonin
IDDM	insulin-dependent diabetes mellitus	**TSH**	thyroid-stimulating hormone

*Many of these abbreviations share their meanings with other terms.

A Career as a Physical Therapist

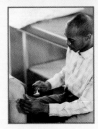

Aaron Toma graduated with a Doctor of Physical Therapy (DPT) degree only last year and works in a facility associated with a large group of medical specialists. His favorite part of the job is helping patients regain strength and improve mobility. Physical therapists treat individuals of all ages who have medical problems or health-related conditions that limit their abilities to move and perform functional daily activities. They help improve mobility and relieve pain, many times reducing the need for surgery and prescription drugs. Physical therapists pass a state-administered national exam after completing either a 3+3 program with specific pre-professional (undergraduate/pre-PT) or a bachelor's degree plus three years in a DPT program. For more information, go *www.apta.org*.

CHAPTER 12 SELF-TEST

Review the new word parts for this chapter. Work all of the following exercises to test your understanding of the material before checking your answers against those in Appendix IV.

BASIC UNDERSTANDING

Listing

I.   Write the names of the seven major endocrine glands: _____
_____

II. Describe two ways in which the pituitary cooperates with the nervous system to maintain homeostasis.

1. _____

2. _____

Matching

III. Match each hormone with its target gland. (Some selections will be used more than once.)

_____ **1.** antidiuretic hormone   **A.** breasts

_____ **2.** follicle-stimulating hormone **B.** gonads

_____ **3.** luteinizing hormone   **C.** kidneys

_____ **4.** oxytocin   **D.** thyroid gland

_____ **5.** thyrotropin

IV. Match each hormone with the gland(s) that secrete them.

_____ **1.** adrenocorticotropin   _____ **8.** melanocyte-stimulating hormone   **A.** adrenals

_____ **2.** antidiuretic hormone   _____ **9.** oxytocin   **B.** gonads

_____ **3.** epinephrine   _____ **10.** testosterone   **C.** pancreas

_____ **4.** follicle-stimulating hormone _____ **11.** thyrocalcitonin   **D.** pituitary

_____ **5.** growth hormone   _____ **12.** thyrotropin   **E.** thyroid

_____ **6.** insulin   _____ **13.** thyroxine

_____ **7.** luteinizing hormone

V.   Match these hormones with their principal action.

_____ **1.** calcitonin   _____ **5.** melanocyte-stimulating hormone   **A.** have antidiuretic effect

_____ **2.** epinephrine   _____ **6.** mineralocorticoids   **B.** decreases blood calcium level

_____ **3.** insulin   _____ **7.** parathormone   **C.** decreases blood glucose level

_____ **4.** glucocorticoids   **D.** increases blood calcium level

                                                                                      E. increases blood glucose level

                                                                                      F. increases heart rate and blood pressure

                                                                                      G. promotes pigmentation of skin and hair

Analyzing Terms

VI.   Break these words into their component parts, and define each term.

1. adrenocortical   _____

2. endocrine   _____

3. hypercalcemia   _____

4. mastectomy   _____

5. somatotropin   _____

Identifying Illustrations

VII.   Label these illustrations using one of the following: adrenocorticotropin, hypophysectomy, mammogram, mastalgia, mastectomy, thyroidectomy

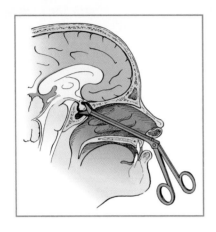

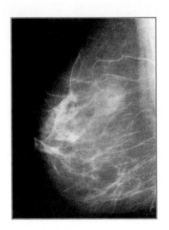

1. _____   **2.** _____

Using Vocabulary

VIII. Circle the correct answer for each of the following questions.

1. The anatomy class is studying glands. Which of the following is an exocrine gland? (adrenal gland, pituitary, sweat gland, thyroid)

2. Anthony is undergoing puberty. Which of the following hormones produce masculine sex characteristics? (androgens, estrogens, prolactins, triiodothyronine)

3. Andria is having a diagnostic procedure that uses radiation to study the soft tissues of the breast. What is the name of the diagnostic procedure? (mammogram, mammography, radioactive iodine uptake test, reduction mammoplasty)

4. Darius suffers from hypersecretion of the adrenal gland. Which pathology is more likely? (Addison disease, Cushing syndrome, gigantism, thyrotoxicosis)

5. Sixty-year-old Christina is found to have increased secretion of growth hormone. Which condition is associated with this finding? (acromegaly, cretinism, gigantism, gonadopathy)

6. Justin has a deficiency of ADH. Which disorder is associated with this deficiency? (cretinism, diabetes insipidus, hyperaldosteronism, pituitary dwarfism)

7. Forty-eight-year old Abdul is found to have a deficiency of T_4 and T_3. Which disorder is likely? (cretinism, Graves disease, hypogonadism, myxedema)

8. The physician explains to Cody that the islets of Langerhans secrete insulin. The islets of Langerhans are found in which structure? (adrenal gland, kidney, pancreas, thyroid)

9. Luis is diabetic. Which test is more accurate for determining the degree of blood glucose control? (fasting blood sugar, glycosylated hemoglobin, radioactive iodine uptake, urinary ketones)

10. Palpation of Brianna's thyroid gland indicates enlargement. Which term describes an enlarged thyroid gland? (goiter, hyperadrenalism, hyperthyroidism, hypothyroidism)

Opting for Opposites

IX.   Write a term that you learned that means the opposite of these words.

1. diuretic _____

2. hyperpituitarism _____

Writing Terms

X. Write a term for each of the following.

1. adrenaline _____

2. decreased thyroid activity _____

3. excessive growth of hair _____

4. gland that produces either ova or sperm _____

5. increased level of blood glucose _____

6. lactogenic hormone _____

7. master gland _____

8. producing masculine characteristics _____

9. stability in the normal body state _____

10. sugar in the urine _____

Making Connections

XI. Describe the relationship of these terms.

1. adrenal gland and suprarenal gland _____
_____

2. pituitary and thyroid gland _____

3. insulin and glucose-lowering agent _____
_____

Finetuning Terms

XII. In addition to spelling, describe at least one difference in the following:

1. endocrine gland and exocrine gland _____
_____

2. follicle-stimulating hormone and estrogen _____

3. type 1 diabetes mellitus and type 2 diabetes mellitus _____
_____

GREATER COMPREHENSION

Pronouncing Terms

XIII. Write the correct term for the following phonetic spellings.

1. ā-trē-ō-**pep**-tin _____

4. kuh-**kek**-sē-uh _____

2. fī-brō-**sis**-tik _____

5. mik-suh-**dē**-muh _____

3. glī-**kō**-suh-lāt-ud _____

6. thī-**rot**-ruh-pin _____

Spelling

XIV. Circle each misspelled term in the following list, and write its correct spelling.

adrenohypophysis   calcitonin   homostasis   neurohypophysis   tyrotropin

Abbreviating

XV. Write a letter in each blank for the abbreviation that corresponds to the clue.

1. a hormone that decreases urine production   __ __ __

4. somatotropic hormone   __ __ __

2. follicle-stimulating hormone   __ __ __

5. thyrocalcitonin   __ __ __

3. parathormone   __ __ __

Health Care Reporting

XVI. Read the Report, and answer the questions.

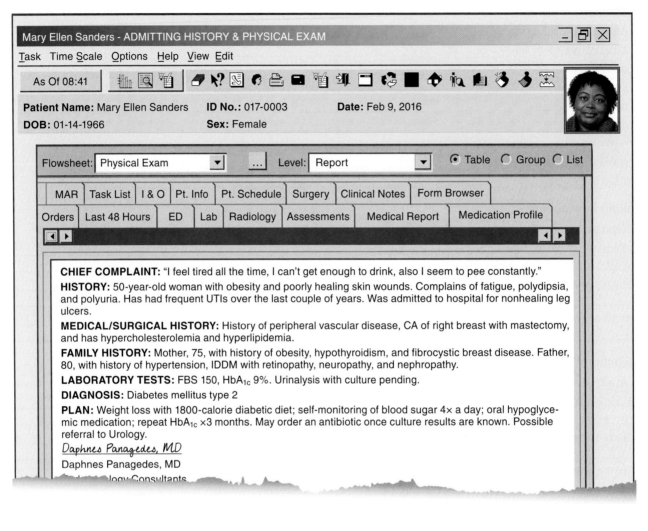

Mary Ellen Sanders - ADMITTING HISTORY & PHYSICAL EXAM

Task   Time Scale   Options   Help   View   Edit

As Of 08:41

Patient Name: Mary Ellen Sanders   **ID No.:** 017-0003   **Date:** Feb 9, 2016
DOB: 01-14-1966   **Sex:** Female

Flowsheet: Physical Exam   ...   Level: Report   ○ Table   ○ Group   ○ List

| MAR | Task List | I & O | Pt. Info | Pt. Schedule | Surgery | Clinical Notes | Form Browser |

| Orders | Last 48 Hours | ED | Lab | Radiology | Assessments | Medical Report | Medication Profile |

CHIEF COMPLAINT: "I feel tired all the time, I can't get enough to drink, also I seem to pee constantly."

HISTORY: 50-year-old woman with obesity and poorly healing skin wounds. Complains of fatigue, polydipsia, and polyuria. Has had frequent UTIs over the last couple of years. Was admitted to hospital for nonhealing leg ulcers.

MEDICAL/SURGICAL HISTORY: History of peripheral vascular disease, CA of right breast with mastectomy, and has hypercholesterolemia and hyperlipidemia.

FAMILY HISTORY: Mother, 75, with history of obesity, hypothyroidism, and fibrocystic breast disease. Father, 80, with history of hypertension, IDDM with retinopathy, neuropathy, and nephropathy.

LABORATORY TESTS: FBS 150, HbA$_{1c}$ 9%. Urinalysis with culture pending.

DIAGNOSIS: Diabetes mellitus type 2

PLAN: Weight loss with 1800-calorie diabetic diet; self-monitoring of blood sugar 4× a day; oral hypoglycemic medication; repeat HbA$_{1c}$ ×3 months. May order an antibiotic once culture results are known. Possible referral to Urology.

Daphnes Panagedes, MD

Daphnes Panagedes, MD
...logy Consultants

1. Explain the complaints that the patient has had with her urinary tract. _____

2. Which term indicates that she had a cancerous breast removed? _____

3. Indicate the terms related to her levels of cholesterol and lipids, and explain their meanings. _____

4. Explain two things that the H&P tells us about her skin. _____

5. Define *retinopathy, neuropathy,* and *nephropathy.* _____

6. What part of the H&P reports the glycosylated hemoglobin? Explain its meaning. _____

Using Pharmacologic Terms

XVII. Use all selections to match terms in the left column with descriptions in the right column.

_____ **1.** antithyroid drugs   **A.** treat diabetes
_____ **2.** antihyperglycemic agents   **B.** treat hyperthyroidism
_____ **3.** corticosteroids   **C.** treat hypofunctioning adrenals
_____ **4.** thyroid drugs   **D.** treat hypothyroidism

Health Care Reporting

XVIII. Read the surgical report, and define the terms that follow it.

Humberto Cardova - SURGICAL REPORT   ▢ ▣ ☒

Task   Time Scale   Options   Help   View   Edit

As Of 09:53

Patient Name: Humberto Cardova   **ID No.:** 017-0004   **Date of Surgery:** Jun 13, 2016
DOB: 03-02-1996   **Sex:** Male

Flowsheet: [Post-operative ▼]   [...]   Level: [Report ▼]   ⦿ Table ○ Group ○ List

| MAR | Task List | I & O | Pt. Info | Pt. Schedule | Surgery | Clinical Notes | Form Browser |

| Orders | Last 48 Hours | ED | Lab | Radiology | Assessments | Medical Report | Medication Profile |

PREOPERATIVE DIAGNOSIS: Bilateral gynecomastia

POSTOPERATIVE DIAGNOSIS: Bilateral gynecomastia

SURGEON: Frank J. Wright, MD   **ASSISTANT:** Jane Stewart, MD

ANESTHETIST: Ron DeVittori, MD   **ANESTHESIA:** General endotracheal via intubation and Marcaine infiltration

SPONGE COUNT VERIFIED: Correct at end of case

MATERIAL FORWARDED TO THE LABORATORY FOR EXAMINATION

1. Right breast tissue   2. Left breast tissue

OPERATION PERFORMED: Bilateral subcutaneous mastectomies

COMPLICATIONS: None

INDICATIONS: This 20-year-old Hispanic male patient, referred by Dr. Panagedes, has gynecomastia, which has been persistent for more than 1½ years and is affecting his social development and behavior. Desires surgical correction.

DESCRIPTION OF OPERATION

After discussion of risks, benefits, and alternatives, and after answering all questions, the patient signed informed consent and was taken to the operating room, sleep induced, intubated, and fully anesthetized. He was positioned squarely and symmetrically on the board with both arms out without hyperextension of the arms and with a pillow under the knees. Sterile prep with Betadine scrub and paint, sterile towels and drapes, was performed on the bilateral chest, shoulders, arms, and upper abdomen, and the patient was draped out. An incision was made in a semicircle under each breast with a 5-mm extension to the right and left of the nipples. The incision was at the edge of the areola. Leaving an adequate depth of tissue behind the nipples to avoid nipple necrosis, the breasts were divided under the nipples; then the breast and fat pads surrounding the breasts were excised using electrocautery dissection on the right and left sides. Care was taken to avoid making the flap too thin. Good hemostasis was achieved. The pectoralis fascia was left intact; the axillary fat pad was left undisturbed.

Both wounds were irrigated with warm sterile saline solution. Good hemostasis was achieved. With the patient symmetric and midline marked, the breast tissue was examined with the skin flaps reapproximated.

| PROD | MAHAFC | 13 Jun 2016 | 1:41 |

Define:

1. gynecomastia _____

2. bilateral mastectomies _____

3. areola _____

4. hemostasis _____

5. axillary fat pad _____

6. reapproximated _____

XIX. Read the Office Note, then circle one answer for each multiple-choice question.

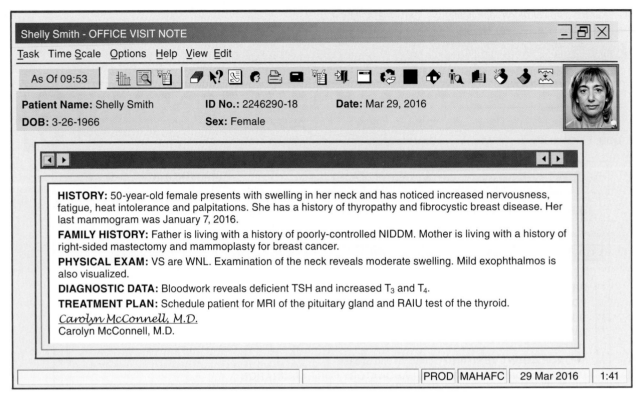

1. The term in the report that refers to protruding eyes is (exophthalmos, goiter, palpitations, thyropathy)
2. The "I" in the abbreviation "RAIU" stands for (infection, inflammation, insulin, iodine)
3. The patient's mother had a history of mammoplasty, which involves (surgical incision, surgical puncture, surgical removal, surgical repair) of the breast.
4. NIDDM is also known as (gestational diabetes mellitus, type 1 diabetes mellitus, type 2 diabetes mellitus, diabetes insipidus)
5. The "H" in the abbreviation "TSH" refers to a special chemical substance termed a (gonad, gland, hormone, steroid)

Categorizing Terms and Practicing Pronunciation

XX. Classify the terms in the left columns by selecting A, B, C, D, or E.

_____	**1.** acromegaly	_____	**6.** lobule	**A.** anatomy
_____	**2.** dwarfism	_____	**7.** mammogram	**B.** diagnostic test or procedure
_____	**3.** glucose-lowering agent	_____	**8.** mastectomy	**C.** pathology
_____	**4.** hirsutism	_____	**9.** radioactive iodine uptake	**D.** surgery
_____	**5.** hypogonadism	_____	**10.** thyroiditis	**E.** nonsurgical therapy

(Be prepared to pronounce terms 1-10 in class after listening to the Chapter 12 terms at *http://evolve.elsevier.com/Leonard/building/.* In addition, practice categorizing all boldface terms in this chapter.)

New Construction

XXI. Divide each of these terms into its component parts. Then write the meaning of each term.

1. parathyrotropic   _____

2. endocrinopathy   _____

3. lactosuria   _____

4. pituitarism   _____

5. thyrogenic   _____

(Use Appendix IV to check your answers to the exercises.)

BMV LIST

Visit *http://evolve.elsevier.com/Leonard/building/* to listen to the boldface terms in Chapter 12. Check spellings carefully.

acromegaly (ak-rō-**meg**-uh-lē)
Addison disease (**ad**-i-sun di-**zēz**)
adenocarcinoma (ad-uh-nō-kar-si-**nō**-muh)
adenohypophysis (ad-uh-nō-hī-**pof**-uh-sis)
adenoma (ad-uh-**nō**-muh)
adenopathy (ad-uh-**nop**-uh-thē)
adrenal gland (uh-**drē**-nul gland)
adrenal virilism (uh-**drē**-nul **vir**-i-liz-um)
adrenalectomy (uh-drē-nul-**ek**-tuh-mē)
adrenaline (uh-**dren**-uh-lin)
adrenocortical (uh-drē-nō-**kor**-ti-kul)
adrenocorticotropic hormone (uh-drē-nō-kor-ti-kō-**trō**-pik
    hor-mōn)
adrenocorticotropin (uh-drē-nō-kor-ti-kō-**trō**-pin)
adrenogenital syndrome (uh-drē-nō-**jen**-i-tul **sin**-drōm)
adrenomegaly (uh-drē-nō-**meg**-uh-lē)
adrenopathy (ad-run-**op**-uh-the)
androgen (**an**-drō-jun)
androgenic (an-drō-**jen**-ik)
andropathy (an-**drop**-uh-thē)
antidiabetics (an-tē-dī-uh-**bet**-iks)
antidiuretic hormone (an-tē-dī-ū-**ret**-ik **hor**-mōn)
antihyperglycemic agents (an-tē-hī-pur-glī-**sē**-mik **ā**-junts)
antithyroid drugs (an-tē-**thī**-roid drugz)
areola (uh-**rē**-ō-luh)
atriopeptin (ā-trē-ō-**pep**-tin)
augmentation mammoplasty (awg-men-**tā**-shun **mam**-ō-plas-tē)
calcitonin (kal-si-**tō**-nin)
colostrum (kuh-**los**-trum)
cortex (**kor**-teks)
corticosteroids (kor-ti-kō-**ster**-oidz)
cortisone (**kor**-ti-sōn)
cretinism (**krē**-tin-iz-um)
Cushing syndrome (**koosh**-ing **sin**-drōm)
diabetes insipidus (dī-uh-**bē**-tēz in-**sip**-i-dus)
diabetes mellitus (dī-uh-**bē**-tēz **mel**-luh-tus, muh-**lī**-tis)
diabetic nephropathy (dī-uh-**bet**-ik nuh-**frop**-uh-thē)
diabetic neuropathy (dī-uh-**bet**-ik noo-**rop**-uh-thē)
diabetic retinopathy (dī-uh-**bet**-ik ret-i-**nop**-uh-thē)
diuresis (dī-ū-**rē**-sis)
diuretic (dī-ū-**ret**-ik)
dwarfism (**dworf**-iz-um)
endocrine glands (**en**-dō-krin glandz)
endocrine system (**en**-dō-krin **sis**-tum)
epinephrine (ep-i-**nef**-rin)
estrogen (**es**-truh-jun)
euthyroid (ū-**thī**-roid)
excisional biopsy (ek-**sizh**-un-ul **bī**-op-sē)
exocrine glands (**ek**-sō-krin glandz)
exophthalmos (ek-sof-**thal**-mos)
fibrocystic breast disease (fī-brō-**sis**-tik brest di-**zēz**)
follicle-stimulating hormone (**fol**-i-kul **stim**-ū-lāt-ing **hor**-mōn)
gastrin (**gas**-trin)

gestational diabetes mellitus (jes-**tā**-shun-ul dī-uh-**bē**-tēz
    mel-luh-tus, muh-**lī**-tis)
gigantism (jī-**gan**-tiz-um)
gland (gland)
glucagon (**glōō**-kuh-gon)
glucocorticoid (glōō-kō-**kor**-ti-koid)
glucose-lowering agent (**glōō**-kōs **lō**-wur-ing **ā**-junt)
glucose tolerance tests (**glōō**-kōs **tol**-ur-uns tests)
glycosuria (glī-kō-**sū**-rē-uh)
glycosylated hemoglobin (glī-**kō**-suh-lāt-ud **hē**-mō-glō-bin)
goiter (**goi**-tur)
gonad (**gō**-nad)
gonadal (gō-**nad**-ul)
gonadotropic (gō-nuh-dō-**trō**-pik)
gonadotropic hormones (gō-nuh-dō-**trō**-pik **hor**-mōnz)
gonadotropin (gō-nuh-dō-**trō**-pin)
Graves disease (grāvz di-**zēz**)
growth hormone (grōth **hor**-mōn)
gynecomastia (gī-nuh-kō-**mas**-tē-uh)
hirsutism (**hur**-sōōt-iz-um)
hormone (**hor**-mōn)
human chorionic gonadotropin (**hū**-mun kor-ē-**on**-ik
    gō-nuh-dō-**trō**-pin)
hyperadrenalism (hī-pur-uh-**drē**-nul-iz-um)
hypercalcemia (hī-pur-kal-**sē**-mē-uh)
hyperglycemia (hī-pur-glī-**sē**-mē-uh)
hyperinsulinism (hī-pur-**in**-suh-lin-iz-um)
hyperparathyroidism (hī-pur-par-uh-**thī**-roid-iz-um)
hyperpituitarism (hī-pur-pi-**tōō**-i-tuh-riz-um)
hypersecretion (hī-pur-sē-**krē**-shun)
hyperthyroidism (hī-pur-**thī**-roid-iz-um)
hypoadrenalism (hī-pō-uh-**drē**-nul-iz-um)
hypocalcemia (hī-pō-kal-**sē**-mē-uh)
hypoglycemia (hī-pō-glī-**sē**-mē-uh)
hypogonadism (hī-pō-**gō**-nad-iz-um)
hypoinsulinism (hī-pō-**in**-su-lin-iz-um)
hypoparathyroidism (hī-pō-par-uh-**thī**-roid-iz-um)
hypophysectomy (hī-pof-uh-**sek**-tuh-mē)
hypophysis (hī-**pof**-uh-sis)
hypopituitarism (hī-pō-pi-**tōō**-i-tuh-riz-um)
hyposecretion (hī-pō-suh-**krē**-shun)
hypothalamus (hī-pō-**thal**-uh-mus)
hypothyroidism (hī-pō-**thī**-roid-iz-um)
incisional biopsy (in-**sizh**-un-ul **bī**-op-sē)
insulin (**in**-suh-lin)
insulin pump (**in**-suh-lin pump)
intermammary (in-tur-**mam**-uh-rē)
interstitial cell–stimulating hormone (in-tur-**stish**-ul
    sel-**stim**-ū-lāt-ing **hor**-mōn)
islets of Langerhans (**ī**-lets ov **lahng**-uhr-hahnz)
ketone (**kē**-tōn)
ketonuria (kē-tō-**nū**-rē-uh)
lactation (lak-**tā**-shun)

lactiferous (lak-**tif**-ur-us)
lactogenesis (lak-tō-**jen**-uh-sis)
lactogenic (lak-tō-**jen**-ik)
lactogenic hormone (lak-tō-**jen**-ik **hor**-mōn)
lobule (**lob**-ūl)
lumpectomy (lum-**pek**-tuh-mē)
luteinizing hormone (**lōō**-tē-in-ī-zing **hor**-mōn)
mammalgia (muh-**mal**-juh)
mammary gland (**mam**-uh-rē gland)
mammogram (**mam**-uh-gram)
mammography (muh-**mog**-ruh-fē)
mammoplasty (**mam**-ō-plas-tē)
mastalgia (mas-**tal**-juh)
mastectomy (mas-**tek**-tuh-mē)
master gland (**mas**-tur gland)
mastitis (mas-**tī**-tis)
mastocarcinoma (mas-tuh-kahr-si-**nō**-muh)
mastodynia (mas-tō-**din**-ē-uh)
mastopexy (**mas**-tō-pek-sē)
mastoptosis (mas-top-**tō**-sis)
medulla (muh-**dul**-uh)
melanin (**mel**-uh-nin)
melanocyte-stimulating hormone (**mel**-uh-nō-sīt, muh-**lan**-ō-
  sīt-**stim**-ū-lāt-ing **hor**-mōn)
melatonin (mel-uh-**tō**-nin)
mineralocorticoid (min-ur-al-ō-**kor**-ti-koid)
myxedema (mik-suh-**dē**-muh)
neurohypophysis (noor-ō-hī-**pof**-uh-sis)
norepinephrine (nor-ep-i-**nef**-rin)
oxytocin (ok-sē-**tō**-sin)
pancreas (**pan**-krē-us)
pancreatectomy (pan-krē-uh-**tek**-tuh-mē)
pancreatitis (pan-krē-uh-**tī**-tis)
pancreatoduodenostomy (pan-krē-uh-tō-dōō-ō-duh-**nos**-tuh-mē)
parathormone (par-uh-**thor**-mōn)
parathyroid glands (par-uh-**thī**-roid glandz)
parathyroid hormone (par-uh-**thī**-roid **hor**-mōn)
parathyoidectomy (par-uh-thī-roid-**ek**-tuh-mē)
pepsin (**pep**-sin)
peripheral vascular disease (puh-**rif**-ur-ul **vas**-kū-lur di-**zēz**)
pineal gland (**pin**-ē-ul gland)
pituitary cachexia (pi-**tōō**-i-tar-ē kuh-**kek**-sē-uh)

pituitary gland (pi-**tōō**-i-tar-ē gland)
pituitary hypogonadism (pi-**tōō**-i-tar-ē hī-pō-**gō**-nad-iz-um)
polydipsia (pol-ē-**dip**-sē-uh)
polyphagia (pol-ē-**fā**-juh)
polyuria (pol-ē-**ū**-rē-uh)
posterior pituitary hormones (pos-**tēr**-ē-ur pi-**tōō**-i-tar-ē
  hor-mōnz)
progesterone (prō-**jes**-tuh-rōn)
prolactin (prō-**lak**-tin)
prostaglandin (pros-tuh-**glan**-din)
puberty (**pū**-bur-tē)
radioactive iodine uptake test (rā-dē-ō-**ak**-tiv ī-ō-dīn **up**-tāk
  test)
reduction mammoplasty (rē-**duk**-shun **mam**-ō-plas-tē)
retromammary (ret-rō-**mam**-ur-ē)
somatotropic hormone (sō-muh-tō-**trō**-pik **hor**-mōn)
somatotropin (**sō**-muh-tō-trō-pin)
steroid (**ster**-oid)
suprarenal (sōō-pruh-**rē**-nul)
syndrome of inappropriate ADH secretion (**sin**-drōm ov
  i-nuh-**prō**-prē-ut ADH sē-**krē**-shun)
target organ (**tahr**-gut **or**-gun)
testosterone (tes-**tos**-tuh-rōn)
tetraiodothyronine (tet-ruh-ī-ō-dō-**thī**-rō-nēn)
thymosin (thī-**mō**-sin)
thymus (**thī**-mus)
thyrocalcitonin (thī-rō-kal-si-**tō**-nin)
thyroid (**thī**-roid)
thyroid drugs (**thī**-roid drugz)
thyroid-stimulating hormone (**thī**-roid-**stim**-ū-lāt-ing **hor**-mōn)
thyroidectomy (thī-roid-**ek**-tuh-mē)
thyroiditis (thī-roid-**ī**-tis)
thyropathy (thī-**rop**-uh-thē)
thyrotoxicosis (thī-rō-tok-si-**kō**-sis)
thyrotropin (thī-**rot**-ruh-pin)
thyroxine (thī-**rok**-sin)
triiodothyronine (trī-ī-ō-dō-**thī**-rō-nēn)
tropic (**trō**-pik)
type 1 diabetes mellitus (tīp 1 dī-uh-**bē**-tēz **mel**-luh-tus,
  muh-**lī**-tis)
type 2 diabetes mellitus (tīp 2 dī-uh-**bē**-tēz **mel**-luh-tus,
  muh-**lī**-tis)

Español   ENHANCING SPANISH COMMUNICATION

English	Spanish (Pronunciation)	English	Spanish (Pronunciation)
adrenal	suprarenal (soo-prah-ray-NAHL)	hormone	hormona (or-MOH-nah)
adrenaline	adrenalina (ah-dray-nah-LEE-nah)	insulin	insulina (in-soo-LEE-nah)
augmentation	aumento (ah-oo-MEN-to)	iodine	yodo (YO-do)
diabetes	diabetes (de-ah-BAY-tes)	masculine	masculino (mas-koo-LEE-no)
dwarf	enano (ay-NAH-no)	nipple	pezón (pay-SON)
giant	gigante (he-GAHN-tay)	pancreas	páncreas (PAHN-kray-as)
glucose	glucosa (gloo-KO-sah)	pituitary	pituitario (pe-too-e-TAH-re-o)
goiter	papera (pah-PAY-rah)	synthesis	síntesis (SEEN-tay-sis)
growth	crecimiento (kray-se-me-EN-to)	thyroid	tiroides (te-RO-e-des)

Integumentary System

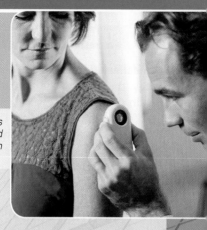

Dermatology is the study of the skin, including its pathologic characteristics and the diagnosis and treatment of skin disorders. A dermatologist is shown examining the patient for skin cancer.

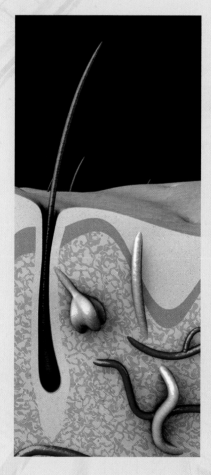

LEARNING OUTCOMES

Basic Understanding

In this chapter, you will learn to do the following:

1. State the function of the integumentary system, and analyze associated terms.
2. Write the meaning of the word parts associated with the integumentary system, and use them to build and analyze terms.
3. Match the epidermis, dermis, and adipose tissue with their characteristics.
4. List the four accessory skin structures, and describe their functions.
5. Write the names of the diagnostic tests and procedures for integumentary system assessment when given descriptions of the procedures, or match the procedures with their descriptions.
6. Match the names of integumentary system pathologies with their descriptions, or write the names of the pathologies when given their descriptions.
7. Match the different types of skin lesions with their descriptions.
8. Match the integumentary system terms for surgical and therapeutic interventions with their descriptions, or write the names of the interventions when given their descriptions.
9. Build terms with word parts to label illustrations.

Greater Comprehension

10. Use word parts from this chapter to determine the meanings of terms in a health care report.
11. Spell the terms accurately.
12. Pronounce the terms correctly.
13. Recognize or use abbreviations presented in this chapter.
14. Categorize terms as anatomy, diagnostic test or procedure, pathology, surgery or nonsurgical therapy.
15. Recognize the meanings of general pharmacological terms from this chapter as well as the drug classes and their uses.

FUNCTION FIRST

A **dermato/logist** is a physician who specializes in **dermatology,** the study of the skin and diagnosis and treatment of skin disorders.

The skin (integument) is the external covering of the body and is the largest organ of the body. It has many important functions and the mnemonic, DERMA, will help you remember them:

- **D** vitamin synthesis
- **E**limination of wastes through perspiration
- **R**egulation of body temperature through perspiration
- **M**akes information about the environment available to the brain
- **A**cts as barrier to pathogens

ANATOMY AND PHYSIOLOGY

The Skin

integumentary

13-1 The term **integument** means a covering or skin. The **integumentary** system is the skin and its glands, hair, nails, and other structures that are derived from it. Because it is on the outside of our bodies, we are more familiar with the skin than with any other organ. Write the name of this body system that includes the skin and other structures derived from it: _____ system.

Modified skin continues into various parts of the body, for example, the mucous membrane that lines the mouth, the nose, the intestines, and other cavities or canals that open to the outside. The skin that is studied in this chapter is the body covering, the integument.

Learn the following word parts and their meanings.

Word Parts: Anatomy and Physiology of the Skin

Word Part	Meaning	Combining Form	Meaning
Skin Layers		**Accessory Skin Structures and Substances**	
adip(o), lip(o)	fat	hidr(o)	sweat
cutane(o), derm(a), derm(o), dermat(o)	skin	onych(o), ungu(o)	nail
		pil(o), trich(o)	hair
kerat(o)	horny or cornea	seb(o)	sebum
-derm	skin or germ layer		

WRITE IT! **EXERCISE 1**

Use the mnemonic, DERMA, to help you remember the functions of the skin.

1. D _____
2. E _____
3. R _____
4. M _____
5. A _____

MATCH IT! **EXERCISE 2**

Match the word parts in the left column with their description in the right column. (Choices may be used more than once.)

_____ **1.** adip(o)	**A.** fat	
_____ **2.** cutane(o)	**B.** horny or cornea	
_____ **3.** hidr(o)	**C.** hair	
_____ **4.** kerat(o)	**D.** nail	
_____ **5.** lip(o)	**E.** sebum	
_____ **6.** onych(o)	**F.** skin	
_____ **7.** pil(o)	**G.** sweat	
_____ **8.** seb(o)		
_____ **9.** trich(o)		
_____ **10.** ungu(o)		

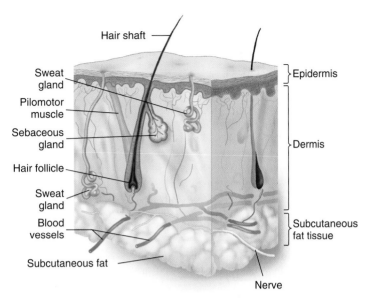

Figure 13.1 The skin. The epidermis, the thin outer layer, is composed of four to five layers. Underneath the epidermis is the thicker dermis, composed of connective tissue containing lymphatics, nerves, blood vessels, hair follicles, sebaceous glands, and sweat glands. Beneath the dermis is a layer of subcutaneous adipose tissue.

above

13-2 The skin consists of two main parts: the epidermis and the dermis. Remembering that epi- means above or on, where is the epi/dermis located? _____ the dermis

13-3 Locate the dermis and the epidermis in the drawing of the skin (Fig. 13.1). The **epidermis** consists of four or five layers. **Epidermal** means pertaining to or resembling epidermis.

🔑 **KEY** POINT **The palms and soles have the greatest number of epidermal layers.** The outermost layer of epidermis consists of cells that are nonliving and are constantly being shed and replaced. These cells contain **keratin,** a waterproofing protein that hardens over several days. Keratin is a **sclero/protein,** a type of protein that is insoluble and has a fibrous structure, which helps to describe the scaly, or horny, nature of keratin.

horny

The combining form kerat(o) means either horny or the cornea—the convex, transparent structure at the front of the eye. When kerat(o) is used in discussions regarding the skin, it means hard or horny.

Kerato/genesis is the formation of keratin, a _____ material.

dermis

13-4 The **dermis,** also called the **corium,** is the thicker layer of the skin. It is a noncellular connective tissue that is composed of collagen and elastic fibers that provide strength and flexibility. The dermis contains numerous blood vessels, nerves, and glands. Hair follicles also are embedded in this layer. Which layer of the skin is thicker, the epidermis or the dermis? _____

▶ **BEYOND** THE BLUEPRINT The upper region of the dermis has many fingerlike projections. The ridges marking the outermost layer of the skin are caused by the size and arrangement of these projections. The ridge patterns on the fingertips and thumbs (fingerprints) are different for each person.

below

13-5 Locate the subcutaneous adipose tissue in Fig. 13.1. Dermal and cutaneous mean pertaining to the skin. Sub/cutaneous means pertaining to _____ the skin.

The **subcutaneous adipose tissue** lies just under the dermis. It serves as a cushion against shock and insulates the body. The combining form adip(o) means fat. **Adipose** means pertaining to

fat

_____.

▶ **BEYOND** THE BLUEPRINT As the skin ages, the number of elastic fibers decreases and much of the adipose tissue is lost. This causes the skin to wrinkle and sag. Loss of collagen fibers makes the skin more fragile, and reduced sebaceous gland activity causes dry, itchy skin.

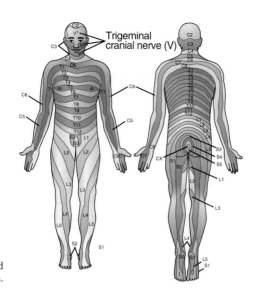

Figure 13.2 Dermatome distribution of spinal nerves. The dermatomes are named *C, T, L,* and *S* (cervical, thoracic, lumbar, and sacral), which correspond to the spinal nerves that innervate them.

13-6 The skin is derived from a tissue layer called **ectoderm** that forms during embryonic development. Sense receptors of the skin, as well as other parts of the nervous system, are also derived from ectoderm.

🔑 **KEY POINT   Three germ layers form during early stages of embryonic development.** Soon after fertilization, the fertilized egg undergoes cell division, producing a ball of cells that eventually differentiates into three distinct layers: **endoderm, mesoderm,** and ectoderm. The suffix -derm means either skin or a germ layer. Here it is used to refer to a germ layer, which is a primary layer of cells of the developing embryo from which various organ systems develop.

ectoderm

Endo/derm, meso/derm, and ectoderm are the innermost, middle, and outermost germ layers, respectively. Skin is derived from which germ layer? _____

13-7 The term **dermatome** has three different meanings:
- In embryology, dermatome refers to a layer of tissue in early human development.
- In surgery, a dermatome is an instrument used to cut thin slices of skin for grafting.
- In anatomy and physiology, a dermatome refers to the skin surface area innervated (supplied) by a spinal nerve. A dermatome is named according to the nerve's source from the spinal cord. Dermatomes C, T, L, and S designate cervical, thoracic, lumbar, and sacral accordingly (Fig. 13.2).

ANALYZE IT!   EXERCISE 3

Break these words into their component parts by placing a slash between the word parts. Then write the meaning of each term.

1. keratogenesis   _____

2. subcutaneous   _____

3. ectoderm   _____

4. dermatologist   _____

5. endoderm   _____

Accessory Skin Structures

13-8 The **accessory skin structures** include hair, nails, sebaceous glands, and sweat glands. They are embedded in the dermis.

Hair protects the scalp from injury, eyebrows and eyelashes protect the eyes, and hair in the nostrils and external ear canals protects these structures from dust and insects. The differing distribution of hair in male and female individuals is controlled by hormones. At puberty, hair develops in the armpit (**axillary** region) and pubic regions and, in the male, on the face and other parts of the body.

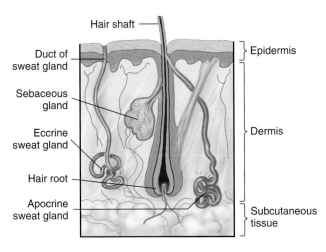

Figure 13.3 The structure of hair and associated glands. The hair shaft extends beyond the surface of the epidermis, and the root is the portion of the hair that is below the surface of the skin. Hair contains no nerves. Two types of glands (sebaceous glands and apocrine sweat glands) have ducts that open into hair follicles, and their secretions are transported to the skin surface. Stimulation of the eccrine sweat glands causes perspiration through ducts that open onto the surface of the skin. This is the single most important factor in the regulation of body temperature.

Observe the structure of a hair in Fig. 13.3. The hair root is embedded in the dermis and is the portion of the hair below the surface. The shaft protrudes above the surface of the skin.

The **arrector pili muscles** (also known as pilomotor muscles; see Fig. 13.1) contract under stresses of cold or fright, straighten the hair follicles, and raise the hairs, producing goose bumps or gooseflesh.

Observing Fig. 13.3, the names of the two glands that are directly connected with the hair follicle are the **apocrine sweat gland** and the _____ gland.

> sebaceous

Most **sebaceous glands** are structurally associated with hair follicles, but those of the eyelids, nipples, and genitalia are freestanding. Sebaceous glands are found in all areas of the body that have hair. **Sebum,** the oily material secreted by the sebaceous gland, keeps hair and skin soft and pliable and also inhibits growth of bacteria on the skin.

The **sudoriferous gland,** or sweat gland, is another type of gland found in the skin.

13-9 Sweat glands are found in most parts of the skin and are the most numerous in the palms and soles. Look again at Fig. 13.3, and study the two types of sweat glands. Those that are associated with the hair follicles interact with bacteria on the skin to produce a characteristic body odor. Sweat glands that are not associated with hair follicles open to the surface of the skin through pores. When stimulated by temperature increases or emotional stress, these glands produce perspiration that evaporates on the skin surface and has a cooling effect.

WORD ORIGIN
sweat (L.)
sudor, sweat

> **KEY POINT Perspiration, or sweat, is the substance produced by the sweat glands.** Sweat is a mixture of water, salt, and other waste products. Although elimination of waste is a function of the sweat glands, their principal function is to help regulate body temperature. As sweat evaporates on the skin surface, the skin is cooled and the body temperature is decreased.

Use hidr(o) to write terms pertaining to sweat. Do not confuse hidr(o) and hydr(o). The combining form hydr(o) means _____, whereas hidr(o) means sweat or perspiration.

> water

Fingernails and toenails, modifications of the horny epidermal cells, are composed of keratin. (See the fingernail components in Fig. 13.4. The cuticle, which is the thin edge of hardened epithelial cells at the base of the nail, is not shown in the illustration.)

WORD ORIGIN
cuticle (L.)
cuticula, little skin

WORD ORIGIN
lunula (L.)
luna, moon

Nails are thin plates of dead epidermis that contain a very hard type of keratin, which protects the fingers and toes and helps us pick up small objects. The nail matrix is responsible for growth of the nail and appears as a whitish, crescent-shaped area called the **lunula.**

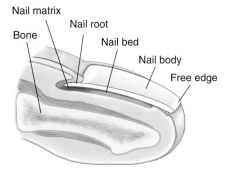

Figure 13.4 Structures of the nail. Each nail has a free edge, a nail body (the visible part), and a nail root, which is covered with skin. The nail bed is thickened to form the nail matrix, which is responsible for growth of the nail. The matrix is under the part of the nail body that appears as a whitish, crescent-shaped area called the *lunula.* Nails appear pinkish because of the rich supply of blood vessels in the underlying dermis.

nails

Onycho/phagia is the habit of nail biting. An **onycho/phag/ist** habitually bites the _____.

nail

13-10 Another combining form, ungu(o), also means nail. It is used to write an adjective, **ungual,** which means pertaining to the _____.

WRITE IT! EXERCISE 4

Write a word in each blank.
1. Name the two layers of the skin: _____ and _____.
2. Name the germ layer from which the skin is derived: _____.
3. Write the name of the oily material secreted by sebaceous glands: _____.
4. Write another term for a sweat gland: _____.
5. Write an adjective that means pertaining to the nail: _____.

DIAGNOSTIC TESTS AND PROCEDURES

13-11 Diagnostic tests are generally performed when inspection of the skin is not sufficient to diagnose a suspected condition. A biopsy (Bx, bx) is performed to remove samples of lesions if malignancy is suspected. Laboratory cultures are performed to identify the cause of an infection, and skin tests are used to determine the existence of allergies.

biopsy

Of the diagnostic tests just described, which term means the removal of a small piece of living tissue? _____

13-12 A skin biopsy may involve removal of part of a lesion, either a punch biopsy or a shaved specimen. In a **punch biopsy** an instrument called a _punch_ is used to remove a small amount of material (at least to the level of the dermis) for microscopic study (Fig. 13.5). A **shaved specimen** is performed on superficial lesions, using a razor blade to obtain the specimen. Material may also be obtained by **curettage,** the scraping of material from a lesion using an instrument called a **curet** (Fig. 13.6).

curettage

Write the name of the procedure that uses a curet to scrape material from a lesion for testing: _____.

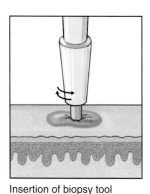

Insertion of biopsy tool

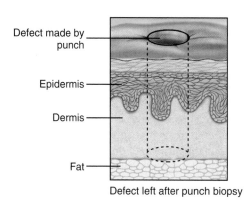

Defect made by punch

Epidermis

Dermis

Fat

Defect left after punch biopsy

Figure 13.5 Punch biopsy. With the use of a punch, living tissue is removed for microscopic examination.

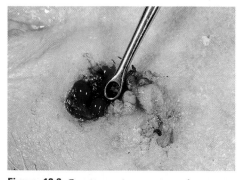

Figure 13.6 Curettage. A curet is used to scrape material from the surface of a wound. Curettage is performed to obtain tissue for either microscopic examination or culture or to clear unwanted material from areas of chronic infection.

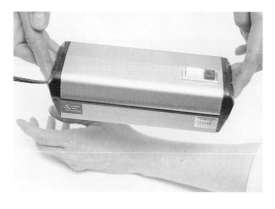

Figure 13.7 Wood lamp. This type of lamp is used to help diagnose certain bacterial and fungal infections. The light causes hairs infected with particular microorganisms to become fluorescent.

fungi

13-13 Tissue or fluids (obtained by needle aspiration) can be examined microscopically, and bacterial and fungal cultures may be done in an effort to grow the causative organisms in an artificial culture medium to establish the cause of an infection. Special microscopic studies can demonstrate the presence of fungal or bacterial infections and the presence of certain parasites, such as lice. Fungal or bacterial infections are those caused by _____ or bacteria.

Some fungi are fluorescent when viewed with a Wood lamp, which is an ultraviolet (UV) light that is also called a *black lamp* (Fig. 13.7).

allergy

13-14 A skin test is one that is performed to determine the reaction of the body to a substance by observing the results of either injecting the substance or applying it to the skin. When it is done to determine whether an allergy to a particular substance exists, it is called an *allergy test.*

A skin test called an _____ test is performed to detect allergic reactions.

sweat

13-15 A sweat test is specifically performed to diagnose **cystic fibrosis,** a congenital disorder that causes abnormally thick secretions of mucus, particularly in the lungs. Increased levels of sodium and chloride are present in the sweat of individuals who have cystic fibrosis, and _____ tests are used to diagnose the disorder.

WRITE IT! EXERCISE 5

Write an answer in each blank in the following sentences.

1. The test in which a sample of living tissue is removed for diagnostic purposes is called a/an _____.
2. Fluids can be removed from a wound by _____ aspiration.
3. A/An _____ test is one that is done to determine the reaction to a substance by observing the results of either injecting the substance or applying it to the skin.
4. A/An _____ test demonstrates increased levels of sodium and chloride in cystic fibrosis.

PATHOLOGIES

away

13-16 An important characteristic of skin is its ability to communicate information to the trained observer. Normal skin has an even tone that is free of lesions, bruises, or signs of inflammation (pain, heat, redness, or swelling).

You learned that ex- means out, without, or away from. **Ex/foliation** is a falling _____ of tissue in scales or layers. **Induration** is hardening of a tissue, especially the skin, and is usually caused by edema and inflammation.

13-17 Different appearances of the skin can indicate different conditions. For example, it can be excessively red in high blood pressure, or appear very pale in anemia.

Learn the following word parts and their meanings.

Word Parts: Skin Pathologies and Treatments

Combining Form	Meaning	Combining Form	Meaning
cry(o)	cold	rhytid(o)	wrinkle
erythemat(o)	erythema or redness	seps(o), sept(o)*	infection
follicul(o)	follicle	xer(o)	dry
heli(o)	sun	**Suffix**	
ichthy(o)	fish	-phoresis	transmission
necr(o)	dead or death		

*Sometimes sept(o) means septum.

MATCH IT!
EXERCISE 6

Match the words in the left column with the word parts in the right column.

_____ **1.** cold   **A.** cry(o)

_____ **2.** dead or death   **B.** erythemat(o)

_____ **3.** dry   **C.** heli(o)

_____ **4.** fish   **D.** ichthy(o)

_____ **5.** infection   **E.** necr(o)

_____ **6.** redness or erythema   **F.** rhytid(o)

_____ **7.** sun   **G.** seps(o) or sept(o)

_____ **8.** wrinkle   **H.** xer(o)

Read about additional conditions that affect the skin's appearance.

albinism A partial or total absence of pigment in the skin, hair and eyes. It is present at birth and is due to a defect in melanin precursors (see Fig. 2.22). An **albino** is a person affected with albinism.

cyanosis A bluish discoloration of the skin and mucous membranes (see Fig. 2.23).

discoid lupus erythematosus (DLE) A chronic systemic disease characterized by lesions that are covered with scales; named because of the reddish facial rash that appears in some patients (see Fig. 9.41); believed to be an autoimmune disease.

erythema Redness or inflammation of the skin (for example, sunburn) or mucous membranes that is the result of dilation of the superficial capillaries.

ichthyosis Any of several skin conditions in which the skin is dry and scaly, resembling fish skin. Some forms are hereditary, and the skin is described as **ichthyoid**, resembling fish skin (Fig. 13.8).

jaundice A yellow discoloration of the skin, mucous membranes, and whites of the eyes (see Fig. 2.24).

pediculosis Infestation by human lice, *Pediculus*, of the scalp, skin, or pubic hair region.

scleroderma A general term for hardening and thickening of the skin, which is a finding in various diseases. Systemic scleroderma is an autoimmune disease.

xeroderma A mild nonhereditary form of ichthyosis, which is characterized by roughness and dryness of the skin.

xerosis Excessive dryness of the skin, causing it to be vulnerable to scaling, thinning, and injury; the term also means abnormal dryness of the eye, skin, or mouth.

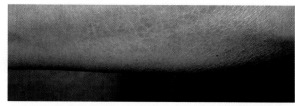

Figure 13.8 **Ichthyosis.** The type shown here is hereditary and is characterized by large dry, dark scales.

BUILD IT! **EXERCISE 7**

Use the following word parts to build terms. (Some word parts will be used more than once.)

albin(o), cyan(o), ichthy(o), scler(o), xer(o), -derma, -ism, -osis

1. lack of pigment in the skin, hair, and eyes _____/_____

2. bluish discoloration _____/_____

3. skin condition resembling a fish _____/_____

4. hardening and thickening of the skin _____/_____

5. condition of dryness _____/_____

Skin Lesions

13-18 A skin **lesion** is any visible, local abnormality of the tissues of the skin, such as a sore, a rash, or a tumor. Most skin lesions are benign, but one type, a melanoma, is among the most malignant of all kinds of cancer.

Trauma, such as cuts, punctures, or burns, exposes the underlying tissue to infection. Climate, hygiene, and general health also play a part. An **abscess** is any pus-containing cavity that is surrounded by inflamed tissue and is characteristically caused by infection with staphylo/cocci. Healing usually occurs when the abscess drains or is incised. Staphylococci, often abbreviated staph, are pyo/genic bacteria, which means they produce _____.

pus

13-19 A **cyst** is a closed sac in or under the skin that contains fluid or semisolid material. A **sebaceous cyst** contains a collection of yellow, cheesy sebum, and is sometimes open to the surface (Fig. 13.9, A). A **pilonidal cyst** often develops in the sacral region of the skin, and is sometimes considered a poorly drained anaerobic abscess, rather than a true cyst (Fig. 13.9, B).

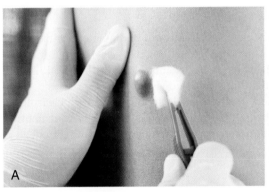 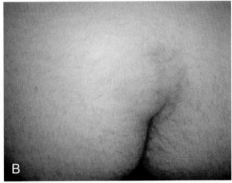

Figure 13.9 Two types of cysts. A, Sebaceous cyst. The physician examines a sebaceous cyst that is draining sebum. **B,** Pilonidal cyst, a cyst that often develops in the sacral region of the skin and contains hairs. Sometimes these open to the surface and drain.

A **nodule** is a solid elevated lesion 1 cm or more in diameter, for example, an enlarged lymph node. Observe the two types of lesions shown in Fig. 13.10. Both a cyst and a nodule cause a raised area of the overlying skin, but the cyst is filled with fluid or a semisolid material, whereas the _____ is solid, more than 1 cm wide, and can be detected by touch.

nodule

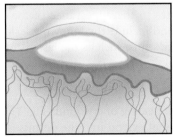 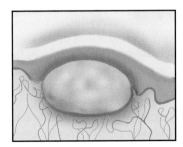

Figure 13.10 Schematic drawing of a cyst and a nodule. Palpation by a physician will usually distinguish between a fluid-filled cyst and a solid nodule.

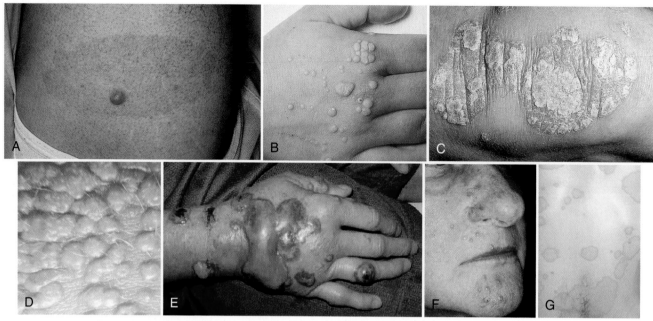

Figure 13.11 Primary lesions of the skin. These initial reactions to an underlying problem alter one of the structural components of the skin. **A,** Macules; **B,** papules; **C,** plaques; **D,** vesicles; **E,** bullae resulting from a burn; **F,** pustules; **G,** wheals.

13-20 Examine the appearance of other types of lesions presented in Fig. 13.11. The lesions are **primary lesions,** because they are initial reactions to an underlying problem:

- **macule:** A nonraised, small dark spot on the skin; for example, freckles or some rashes (Fig. 13.11, A)
- **papule:** A solid raised lesion that is less than 1 cm in diameter; for example, a mole (Fig. 13.11, B)
- **plaque:** A flat, dry, often raised patch; for example, dandruff (Fig. 13.11, C)
- **vesicles:** Small blisters containing clear fluid (Fig. 13.11, D)
- **bullae:** Singular *bulla;* blisters greater than 1 cm and filled with clear fluid (Fig. 13.11, E)
- **pustules:** Small circumscribed elevation of the skin containing purulent fluid (Fig. 13.11, F)
- **wheals:** Transient, elevated, and irregularly-shaped lesions resulting from an allergic skin eruption called **urticaria** (Fig. 13.11, G). Treatment includes antihistamines and removal of the stimulus or allergen.

MATCH IT!
EXERCISE 8

Match the skin lesions in the left columns with their characteristics in the right column.

_____ **1.** bulla   **A.** blister, larger than 1 cm

_____ **2.** cyst   **B.** lesions resulting from allergic skin reaction

_____ **3.** wheals   **C.** discolored spot, not elevated

_____ **4.** macule   **D.** fluid-filled sac containing pus

_____ **5.** papule   **E.** sac filled with clear fluid

_____ **6.** pustule   **F.** solid elevation, less than 1.0 cm in diameter

13-21 **Secondary lesions** are changes in the appearance of the primary lesion that occur with normal progression of the disease and include the following lesions:

- **fissures:** Linear cracks in the epidermis, such as the lesions of athlete's foot or other cracklike lesions of the skin (Fig. 13.12, A)
- **scales:** Dried fragments of sloughed epidermis; frequently seen in **psoriasis,** which is a common chronic skin disease (Fig. 13.12, B)
- **scar:** A mark remaining after the healing of a wound (Fig. 13.12, C)
- **ulcers:** Deep, irregular erosions that extend into the dermis (Fig. 13.12, D)
- **atrophy:** Thinning of the skin with loss of skin markings (Fig. 13.12, E)
- **excoriation:** A scratch; an injury to the surface of the body caused by trauma (Fig. 13.12, F)

WORD ORIGIN
excoriation *(L.)*
excoriare, to flay

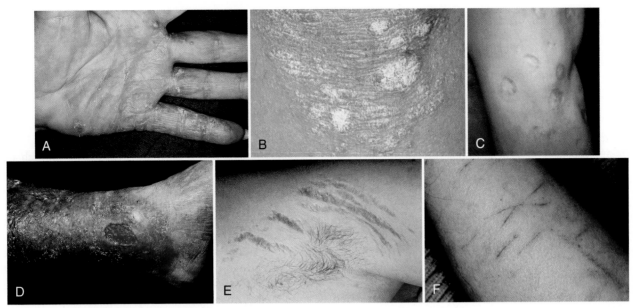

Figure 13.12 Secondary lesions of the skin. The linear lines of atrophy, ulcerations, and fissures result from changes in the initial skin lesion. **A,** Fissures; **B,** scales; **C,** scars; **D,** ulcer; **E,** atrophy; **F,** excoriation.

Dermatitis and Skin Infections

skin

13-22 Dermat/itis is an inflammatory condition of the _____.

It may be acute or chronic and is a very general term that applies to any type of inflammation of the skin, including skin infections. Sunburn is a type of dermatitis that results from overexposure to the sun. **Contact dermatitis** results from exposure to an irritant that initiates an allergic response, such as poison ivy or a reaction to a chemical (Fig. 13.13).

13-23 Skin infections are caused by specific types of bacteria, viruses, and fungi. A **verruca** is a benign warty skin lesion (wart) with a rough surface caused by a common contagious virus (Fig.

verruca

13.14). The term for a wart is a _____.

Herpes simplex virus (HSV) infection is the most common viral infection of adult skin. Herpes simplex virus type 1 (HSV-1) causes the classic fever blisters (see Fig. 13.15). Another type of herpes virus, herpes zoster, causes shingles and occurs with reactivation of the herpes virus in individuals who have previously had chickenpox. The cause of fever blisters is an infection with

herpes

the type 1 _____ simplex virus. HSV-1 is not to be confused with herpes simplex virus type 2 (HSV-2), which causes genital herpes infections that are generally limited to the genital region.

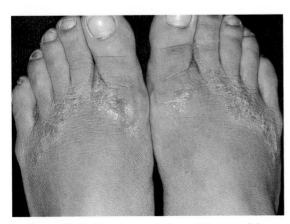

Figure 13.13 Allergic contact dermatitis to sandals.

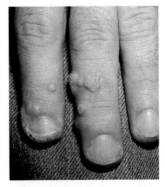

Figure 13.14 A wart is a skin infection. A verruca, commonly called a *wart,* has a rough surface and is caused by a virus.

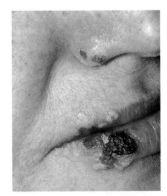

Figure 13.15 Fever blisters. This infection is caused by a virus and has an affinity for mucous membranes of the mouth and nose.

13-24 Many bacterial infections produce pus. A **furuncle,** commonly called a *boil,* is a localized **suppurative** infection that begins with infection of a hair follicle or sebaceous gland by pathogenic staphylococci.

Three words that mean the production of pus are **suppuration, purulence,** and **pyogenesis.** Remember the meanings of suppuration and purulence, although they do not contain word parts that you necessarily recognize. Like _____, suppuration and purulence mean production of pus.

pyogenesis

Read about other types of dermatitis and skin infections.

dermatomycosis A superficial fungal infection; called also **myco/dermat/itis. Ringworm,** or **tinea,** is a group of dermatomycoses that affect various parts of the body (Fig. 13.16).

eczema A superficial dermatitis of unknown cause and confined to the surface of the skin.

herpes zoster An acute infection caused by reactivation of the dormant chickenpox virus, characterized by the development of painful blisterlike eruptions that follow the underlying route of cranial or spinal nerves (Fig. 10.21); commonly called *shingles.* Vaccination to prevent herpes zoster is available.

photodermatitis Inflammation of the skin resulting from an abnormal skin reaction to light; this is a common symptom of DLE.

scabies A contagious dermatitis caused by the itch mite and transmitted by close contact (Fig. 13.17).

seborrhea Excessive production of sebum, the oily secretion of the sebaceous glands. Increased activity of these glands at puberty may block the hair follicle and cause blackheads or pus-filled pimples, which lead to acne, also called **acne vulgaris,** which is characterized by blackheads, whiteheads, pimples, nodules, and cysts (Fig. 13.18). Blackheads are partially-blocked sebum plugs, whereas whiteheads are closed. Pimples are small pustules.

seborrheic dermatitis A chronic inflammatory condition of the skin that is characterized by greasy scales and yellowish crusts. Dandruff is an example.

skin infection Invasion of the skin by pathogenic microorganisms (Table 13.1).

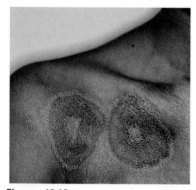

Figure 13.16 Ringworm, a superficial fungal infection of the nonhairy skin of the body. The disease is named for the characteristic circular lesions.

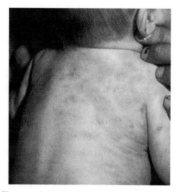

Figure 13.17 Scabies rash in an infant.

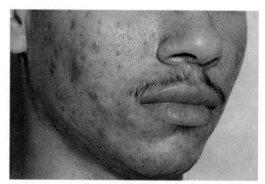

Figure 13.18 Acne vulgaris on the lower face. Acne is common where sebaceous glands are numerous (face, upper back, and chest).

Table 13.1   Skin Eruptions Caused by Infectious Microorganisms

Bacterial	Fungal	Viral
Erysipelas*	Candidiasis	Herpes simplex virus type 1 fever blisters
Furuncles (boils) and carbuncles	Onychomycosis	Herpes zoster (shingles)
Impetigo	Tinea capitis (ringworm of scalp)	Rubella (German measles)
Leprosy	Tinea corporis (generalized)	Rubeola (measles)
Lyme disease	Tinea pedis (athlete's foot)	Varicella (chickenpox)
Meningococcemia		Verrucae (warts)
Paronychia (infection of marginal structures around nail)		
Scarlet fever		
Syphilis		

*Consult a medical dictionary for explanations of the terms.

MATCH IT!
EXERCISE 9

Match the skin conditions in the left column with their characteristics in the right column.

_____ **1.** dermatitis   **A.** any inflammatory condition of the skin
_____ **2.** dermatomycosis   **B.** characterized by greasy scales and yellowish crusts
_____ **3.** furuncle   **C.** commonly called a boil
_____ **4.** pyogenesis   **D.** fungal skin infection
_____ **5.** seborrheic dermatitis **E.** production of pus
_____ **6.** verruca   **F.** warty skin infection

Other Skin Abnormalities

WORD ORIGIN
petechiae *(l.)*
petecchie, flea bite

petechiae

ecchymosis

nevus

tumor

13-25 Dried serum, sebum, blood, or pus on the skin surface produces a **crust.** Crusts frequently result from broken vesicles, bullae, or pustules.

Petechiae are tiny purple or red spots appearing on the skin as a result of tiny hemorrhages within the dermal or submucosal layers (see Fig. 13.19, A). They are flush with the skin and range in size from pinpoint to pinhead size. Write the term for the spots that result from tiny hemorrhages in the skin: _____.

An **ecchymosis** is a hemorrhagic spot, larger than a petechia. It forms a nonelevated blue or purplish patch (see Fig. 13.19, B). Write the term for this large hemorrhagic spot: _____.

13-26 A new growth of tissue characterized by a disordered growth of cells is a tumor, also called a *neoplasm.* Several benign tumors have already been mentioned, for example, warts and moles. Another term for a mole is a **nevus**; the plural is nevi. Write the term that means a mole: _____.

13-27 The combining form lip(o) means fats. A **lip/oma** is a common, benign _____ consisting of mature fat cells, usually removed by surgical excision.

A **kerat/oma,** also called a *callus,* is a flat, poorly-defined mass, usually at locations of external pressure. A **corn** is also caused by pressure or friction but, unlike a callus, is round or conical and usually painful.

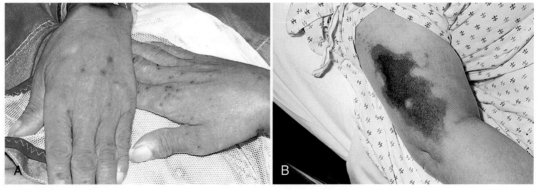

Figure 13.19 Petechiae and ecchymosis. A, Petechiae appear on the skin as a result of tiny hemorrhages beneath the surface. **B,** An ecchymosis is an escape of blood into the subcutaneous tissues.

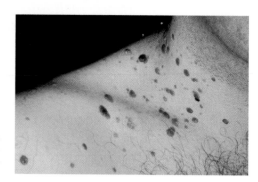

Figure 13.20 Seborrheic keratoses. Numerous seborrheic keratoses are present; some of which are deeply pigmented with melanin. The large lesions show the characteristic stuck-on appearance. Seborrheic keratoses are benign tumors that can be removed by curettage, cryotherapy, and application of caustic agents.

13-28 Kerat/osis is a condition of the skin characterized by the formation of horny growths or excessive development of the epithelium. One type of keratosis, **sebo/rrhe/ic keratosis,** is a consequence of aging. This common benign lesion may occur anywhere on the body of an older person but is more commonly found on the face, neck, upper trunk, and arms (Fig. 13.20). An abnormal appearance of the skin such as this, with well-defined edges and definite boundaries, is described as a circumscribed lesion, because one could easily draw a circle around it.

Actinic keratosis is a premalignant lesion that is common in people with chronically sun-damaged skin. Write the name of the type of keratosis that is considered a premalignant lesion: _____ keratosis. These premalignant lesions may progress to skin cancer if the lesions are not removed. They are usually removed, because this type of keratosis can progress to **squamous cell carcinoma.**

13-29 Basal cell and squamous cell cancers are common types of skin cancer that are rarely invasive. In other words, they rarely spread to other organs. **Basal cell carcinoma** is a malignant epithelial cell tumor that begins as a papule and continues to enlarge. One type of skin cancer that is included in cancer statistics is malignant melanoma. Because about half of malignant melanomas arise from moles, nevi with irregular edges or variegated colors are usually surgically removed and examined microscopically to determine their cell type. Literal interpretation of melan/oma is a black _____.

A **malignant melanoma,** often shortened to melanoma, is a pigmented neoplasm that originates in the skin and is composed of **melano/cytes.** It is highly metastatic, one of the most aggressive of all skin cancers, and causes a high mortality rate in affected individuals. Fig. 13.21 shows a melanoma with two other common types of skin cancer. Squamous cell carcinoma, basal cell carcinoma, and malignant melanoma are all types of skin _____.

13-30 Kaposi sarcoma is the most common malignancy associated with acquired immunodeficiency syndrome (AIDS). The lesions are small, purplish-brown papules that spread throughout the skin, the lymph nodes, and the internal organs. Other disorders associated with this lesion include diabetes and malignant lymphoma. The name of the lesion is _____ sarcoma (see Fig. 8.53).

WORD ORIGIN
actinic *(G.)*
aktis, ray

actinic

tumor

cancer (or carcinoma)

Kaposi

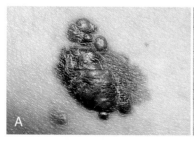
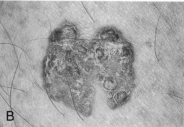
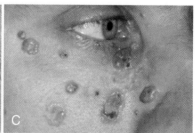

Figure 13.21 **Three common types of skin cancer. A,** Malignant melanoma. **B,** Squamous cell carcinoma. **C,** Basal cell carcinoma.

WRITE IT! EXERCISE 10

Write a word in each blank to complete the sentences.

1. Tiny purple or red spots that result from tiny hemorrhages within the dermal or submucosal layers are called

   _____.

2. Another name for a mole is a/an _____.

3. A condition of the skin characterized by the formation of horny growths or excessive development of the horny growth

   is called a/an _____.

4. A common, benign tumor consisting of mature fat cells is called a/an _____.

5. The most common malignancy associated with AIDS is _____ sarcoma.

Injuries to the Skin

13-31 A **wound** is a physical injury involving a break in the skin, usually caused by an act or accident other than a disease.

🔑 **KEY** POINT **Unintentional wounds often take longer to heal, and the risk for infection is greater than for intentional wounds, which are the result of planned invasive therapy or treatment, as in surgery.** Intentional wound edges are clean, bleeding is controlled, the wound is usually made under sterile conditions, and the risk of infection is low. Unintentional wounds occur from unexpected trauma or forcible injury, such as in scrapes, burns, or stabbing. This type of wound usually occurs in an unsterile environment, the edges are jagged, and bleeding may be uncontrolled.

intentional

A surgical incision can be classified as which type of wound, intentional or unintentional?

_____

13-32 The skin is subject to many injuries because of its exposure to the external environment. Trauma to the skin and underlying tissues requires healing to repair the defect, whether the wound was created by a surgical incision or an accident. A surgical wound generally heals quickly because of its aseptic (free of infection) nature. **A/septic** means free of pathogenic organisms or

infected

_____ material.

🔑 **KEY** POINT **Infection is just one of several things that slow the healing process.** Factors that slow the process of healing include the following:

- Infection, presence of foreign material, or necrotic tissue
- Movement (lack of immobilization) of the wound
- Poor blood circulation in the area of an abscess or in the individual in general

- Decreased number of white blood cells in the blood
- Deficiency of antibodies in the blood
- Malnutrition in the individual

13-33 A pressure ulcer is a special type of injury to the skin that occurs almost exclusively in people with limited mobility. Also called *bedsores* or **decubitus ulcers,** these sores occur in the skin over a bony prominence as a result of mechanical trauma and lack of adequate blood circulation to the affected area (Fig. 13.22). Once formed, they are slow to heal. Ulcerations that occur almost

pressure or decubitus

exclusively in persons with limited mobility are called _____ ulcers.

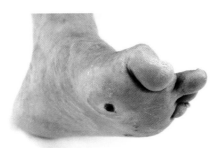

Figure 13.22 A decubitus ulcer. This type of injury is also known as a pressure sore or bed sore.

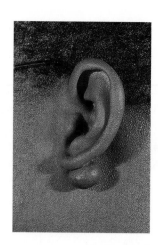

Figure 13.23 Keloid. This is an overgrowth of scar tissue.

keloid

A mark that is left by healing of a lesion where excess collagen was produced to replace the injured tissue is called a *scar.* Excessive overgrowth of unsightly scar tissue, called a **keloid,** occurs in some individuals, especially African Americans (Fig. 13.23). Write the word that means overgrowth of scar tissue: _____.

13-34 A **laceration** is a torn, jagged wound (Fig. 13.24, A). A **puncture** is a wound made by piercing. Skin is scraped or rubbed away by friction in an **abrasion.** One type of injury, a **contusion,** is caused by a blow to the body that causes subcutaneous bleeding and does not disrupt the integrity of the skin. A contusion is called a *bruise* and is characterized by swelling, discoloration, and pain (see Fig. 13.24, B).

laceration

A torn, jagged wound is called a _____, whereas a wound that is made by piercing is called a *puncture.*

abrasion

When skin is scraped away by friction, it is called an _____.

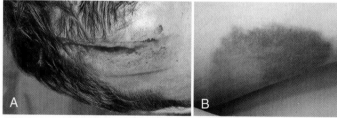

Figure 13.24 Two types of wounds. A, A laceration is a torn, jagged wound. **B,** A contusion is a bruise.

Case Study. *Match terms from the report with descriptions 1-5.*

Dermatologist Amy Sadighi examined three patients and made the following diagnoses: Follow-up visit with Adam Burns, keloid resulting from laceration requiring stitches one month ago; 17-year-old Noah Dearing, acne vulgaris with several cysts, abscesses, and scarring; 45-year-old Ardith Castillo has developed severe urticaria with various-sized wheals post-antibiotic.

1. sacs under the skin filled with fluid or semi-solid material _____

2. elevated and irregularly shaped lesions _____

3. excessive overgrowth of unsightly scar tissue _____

4. skin eruption that is also known as hives _____

5. torn, jagged wound _____

13-35 Burns are tissue injuries resulting from excessive exposure to heat, electricity, chemicals, radiation, or gases, in which the extent of the injury is determined by the amount of exposure and the nature of the agent that causes the burn. The magnitude of the injury is based on the depth and extent of the total body surface area (TBSA) that is burned.

Burns are sometimes classified as first-, second-, third-, and fourth-degree injuries. The American Burn Association (ABA) advocates categorizing the burn injury according to the depth of tissue destruction as a **superficial** or **deep partial-thickness burn** or as a **full-thickness burn** (third or fourth degree). Study Fig. 13.25, and read the descriptions of skin layer destruction and appearances of the burns.

In comparing superficial partial-thickness burns and full-thickness burns, _____-thickness burns destroy deeper layers of tissue.

The superficial burn does not extend beyond which layer of skin? _____

In a deep partial-thickness burn, damage does not extend beyond which layer of skin? _____

Muscle and bone are exposed in a _____ full-thickness burn.

Which type of burn is characterized by blisters? deep _____ thickness burn

13-36 Burned tissue usually represents various levels of damage. In addition to the burn depth, burn severity takes into consideration factors, such as the size and location of the burn, mechanism of injury, duration and intensity of the burn, and the age and health of the individual. The very young as well as older persons are at greatest risk. The magnitude of the burn is determined by how much of the TBSA is affected. TBSA means total body _____ area.

Margin answers:
full
epidermis

dermis
deep
partial

surface

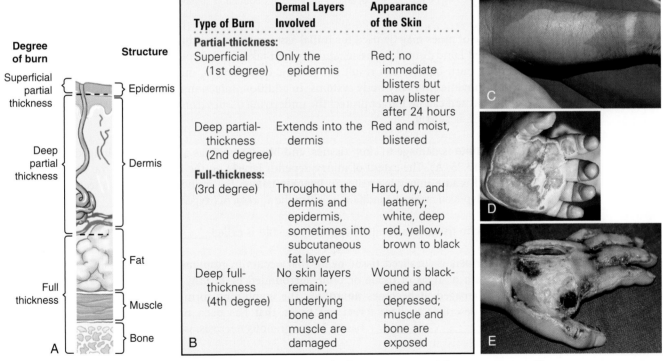

Figure 13.25 Degree of burn and structures involved. A, Cross-section of skin. **B,** Description of burns. **C,** partial-thickness burn. **D,** Deep partial-thickness burn. **E,** Full-thickness burn.

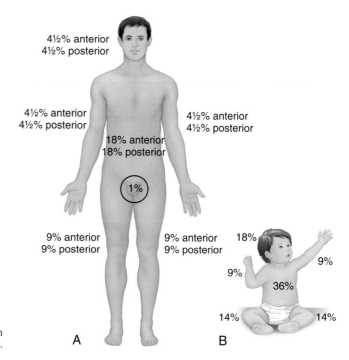

Figure 13.26 **The rule of nines for estimating burn percentage. A,** In an adult. **B,** Modified in infant because of the proportionally larger head size.

🔑 **KEY POINT** **The "rule of nines" calculates the size of a burn injury.** The **rule of nines** is a formula for estimating the percentage of adult body surface covered by burns (Fig. 13.26) and is modified in infants and children because of the proportionately larger head size.

The rule of nines may be used for initial assessment of an adult burn patient; however, a more complicated Lund-Browder classification system takes into account the patient's age.

Serious burn injuries can result in systemic disturbances, including fluid and protein losses, and abnormalities in many body systems. In addition, infection is a serious threat when the skin is destroyed and can no longer protect the underlying tissues from microorganisms. Another term for infection is **sepsis.**

13-37 **Frostbite** is damage to skin, tissues, and blood vessels as a result of prolonged exposure to cold (Fig. 13.25, A). The extent of injury depends largely on the intensity and the duration of the exposure. Because injury is greater in **hypoxic tissue,** the individual's health affects the severity

below ⟶ of injury. Hyp/oxia means a condition in which the amount of oxygen is _____ normal.

frostbite ⟶ Damage to tissue as a result of exposure to cold is called _____.

13-38 **Necr/osis** is localized tissue death that occurs in response to disease or injury—in other words, death of areas of tissue or bone surrounded by healthy parts (Fig. 13.27). When tissue is badly damaged, it becomes **necro/tic.** The combining form necr(o) means dead or death. Necro/tic describes a characteristic of tissue that has been broken down. Necrotic tissue is

dead ⟶ _____ tissue. In gangrenous necrosis, ischemia combined with bacterial action causes tissue decay.

WRITE IT! **EXERCISE 12**

Write a word in each blank to complete these sentences.
1. In a deep partial-thickness burn, damage does not extend beyond the layer of skin called the _____.
2. A physical injury involving a break in the skin is a _____.
3. An injury that causes subcutaneous bleeding but does not result in a break in the skin is a _____.
4. Skin damage that results from exposure to cold is _____.

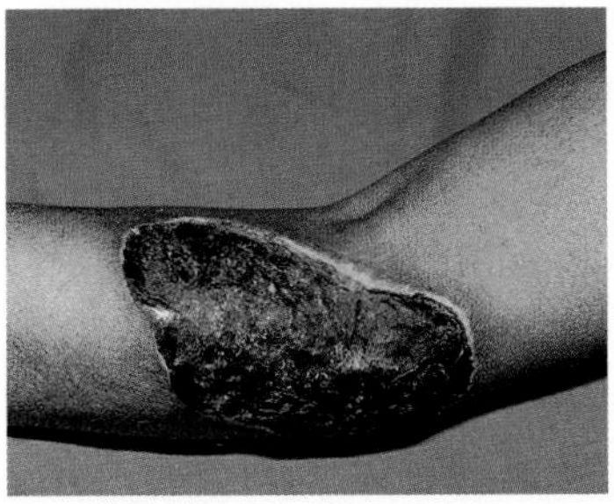

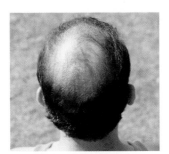

Figure 13.27 Skin necrosis. This skin eruption began as red, painful plaques that became necrotic.

Figure 13.28 Alopecia prematura. This man is in his early 30s and is experiencing premature baldness.

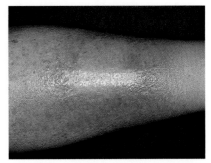

Figure 13.29 Cellulitis. Bacteria invade the deep subcutaneous tissue.

Disorders of Accessory Skin Structures

alopecia

13-39 Pathologies also occur with the hair, nails, sebaceous glands, and sweat glands. Baldness is **alopecia.** Write this new word for baldness: _____.
Alopecia prematura is baldness that occurs early in life (Fig. 13.28).

FIND IT!

EXERCISE 13

Draw a slash between the word parts in the following list of new terms. Then find the meanings of the word parts within the definitions. (Draw the slash, and then perform the remainder of the activity as a mental exercise.)

1. **folliculitis** a superficial bacterial infection involving the hair follicles. Without treatment, folliculitis can progress to **cellulitis** a localized bacterial invasion of subcutaneous tissue (Fig. 13.29).
2. **hidradenitis** inflammation of a sweat gland. A chronic form is caused by closure of the pores with secondary bacterial infection of apocrine glands, chiefly in the axillary and anogenital areas, forming an abscess or a cyst.
3. **leukoderma** localized loss of skin pigment. One form is **vitiligo**, irregular depigmentation of patches of the skin (Fig. 13.30).

4. **onycholysis** separation of a nail from its nail bed, beginning at the free margin, associated with dermatitis, fungal infection, or psoriasis (Fig. 13.31).
5. **onychomalacia** abnormal softening of the nails
6. **onychopathy** any disease of the nails
7. **onychosis** atrophy or other unhealthy condition of the nails
8. **onychomycosis** a fungal condition of the nails (Fig. 13.32).
9. **trichopathy** any disease of the hair
10. **trichosis** an abnormal growth or development of hair

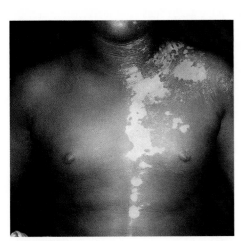

Figure 13.30 Vilitigo. The cause of this acquired skin disorder is unknown. The cause of these hypopigmented areas is unknown.

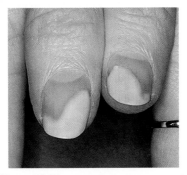

Figure 13.31 Onycholysis. Separation of a nail from its bed.

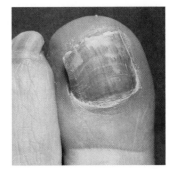

Figure 13.32 Onychomycosis. This is a fungal condition of the nails. Note the discoloration of the nail and the redness around the nail, indicating inflammation.

transmission

13-40 Dia/phoresis means excessive sweating. The suffix -phoresis means transmission. Translated literally, dia/phoresis means _____ through, so you will need to remember that diaphoresis means excessive sweating (or perspiration).

Perspiration is only one means of ridding the body of excess heat. The level of heat produced within the body and lost from the body surface is regulated and controlled by the brain.

below

13-41 Prolonged exposure to cold temperatures can lead to **hypo/therm/ia,** a condition in which the body temperature is _____ normal. Literal translation of hypothermia is a condition of less than normal heat.

13-42 Hyperthermia is a state in which an individual's body temperature is elevated above his or her normal range. In a healthy person, internal body temperature is maintained within a narrow range by the brain, resulting in a balance between generation and conservation of heat.

KEY POINT Understand the difference between pyrexia and hyperthermia. Pyrexia, or fever, is an increased body temperature that is mediated by an increase in the heat regulatory set point. In contrast, hyperthermia overrides or bypasses normal heat regulation. Heatstroke and sunstroke are examples of hyperthermia. These conditions are caused by prolonged exposure to excessive heat or the sun and may be life-threatening. **Thermo/plegia** is another name for heatstroke or sunstroke.

paralysis

Translated literally, thermoplegia means heat _____, but you know it means heatstroke or sunstroke.

SURGICAL AND THERAPEUTIC INTERVENTIONS

against

13-43 Most surgical procedures involving the skin are for the purposes of repairing or treating damaged skin, removing lesions, or penetrating the skin to perform diagnostic or surgical procedures.

Wound irrigation is the flushing of an open wound using a medicated solution, water, sterile saline (a salt solution, usually an isotonic solution of sodium chloride), or an antimicrobial liquid preparation. **Anti/microbial** means pertaining to a substance that acts _____ microorganisms, either killing or inhibiting their growth.

This type of irrigation is done to cleanse and remove debris or excessive drainage. The wound is irrigated and the rinsing solution is aspirated and discarded until the returning solution is clear. After irrigation is completed, the area is dried and some type of dressing is applied.

13-44 Wound management depends on the type and characteristics of the wound. Some types of wounds are left uncovered; others require coverings ranging from medicated transparent sprays to sterile dressings.

KEY POINT Superficial wounds often heal without suturing. Deep wounds with gaping edges or wounds located over joints where movement opens the cut edges are generally stapled or sutured to stop the bleeding, hold the tissues together, and enhance the healing process. Adhesive sprays are used for closing certain wounds, but deep wounds generally require suturing.

Negative-pressure wound therapy (vacuum-assisted closure [VAC]) uses suction and controlled negative pressure (vacuum) to remove drainage and speed wound healing. The VAC system pulls infectious materials and other fluids from the wound via tubing. Wounds suitable for this type of therapy include acute or traumatic wounds, chronic ulcerated wounds, or surgical wounds that have dehisced. You probably remember from an earlier chapter that **dehiscence** is the rupture of a wound closure or the separation of a surgical incision, typically an abdominal incision.

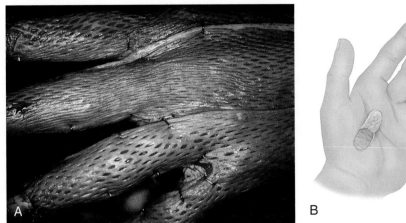
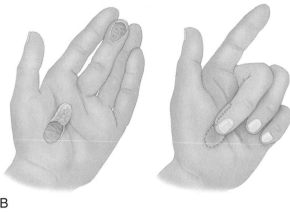

Figure 13.33 Skin graft. A, This skin graft, covering a severe burn to the hand, has multiple slits allowing the grafted piece of skin to stretch over a larger area. **B,** Flap graft. A near graft from the palm to the finger. The surgeon may apply a plaster splint to keep the graft immobilized while healing, usually 2 to 3 weeks, which is then removed and the graft is released.

13-45 Severe burns of the arms or legs can require **amputation,** the surgical removal of a limb or part of the body. All depths of burns except superficial partial-thickness burns may involve skin grafting.

🔑 **KEY** POINT A skin graft is transplantation of skin to cover areas where skin has been lost through a burn or other trauma or to replace diseased skin that has been removed (Fig. 13.33, A). A **derma/tome** is used to cut thin slices of skin for grafting.

self

If the graft is from the patient's own body, it is called an **autograft,** for which the literal translation is _____ graft. (A product in research harvests a patient's stem cells from a small area of unwounded skin [usually one square inch], cultures them, then sprays them onto the wound, where new skin begins to grow at the cellular level.)

A **skin flap** (Fig. 13.33, B) is a special type of skin graft that involves moving a section of skin to a nearby area without cutting off the end of the transplanted tissue. This is done to leave some of the blood circulation intact.

tissue

13-46 An **allograft** is a graft of tissue between two genetically different individuals of the same species. **Histo/compatibility** is necessary for a successful transplant of any organ or tissue. Histo-compatibility means that the transplanted _____ is capable of surviving without ill effects. If the tissue is not compatible, this is called **in/compatibility.**

Learn the following terms for various surgical procedures:

cryosurgery Destruction of small growths, such as warts, by application of extreme cold; **cryotherapy**

débridement The removal of foreign material and dead or damaged tissue, especially from a wound. To **débride** is to remove by dissection.

electrodessication Destruction of superficial skin growths by burning with an electric spark

escharotomy Surgical incision of constricting necrotic tissue resulting from a severe burn, done to relieve pressure from severe swelling and restore blood flow

incision and drainage (I&D) Opening of an infected wound and withdrawal of its fluids and discharges

onychectomy Excision of a nail; declawing of an animal

MATCH IT!
EXERCISE 14

Match the terms in the surgical list in the left column with their descriptions on the right.

_____ **1.** allograft
_____ **2.** autograft
_____ **3.** débridement
_____ **4.** escharotomy

A. cutting away of dead or damaged tissue in a wound
B. surgical incision to relieve pressure after a severe burn
C. tissue graft between two genetically different individuals
D. tissue graft whereby one's tissue is transplanted to another site of one's body

13-47 Plastic surgery is the replacement or restoration of parts of the body and is performed to correct a structural or cosmetic defect. Although females are more likely to seek plastic surgery, males increasingly use plastic surgery (for example, hair transplantation or removal of tattoos).

In hair transplantation, grafts or plugs of skin containing hair follicles are transplanted from some other part of the body to the head. An oral medication is effective in restoring hair in certain types of hair loss but must be taken the remainder of one's life to prevent hair loss.

Increased expenditures on cosmetics, surgery, and other treatments to improve our appearance attest to how we value our physical appearance.

Types of plastic surgery include the following:

collagen injections A reconstructive technique to enhance the lips or "plump" sagging facial skin. This is sometimes used with injections of botulinum toxin (Botox) also called *botulinum toxin type A*, a potent bacterial toxin that relaxes facial wrinkles (Fig. 13.34, A). Botox is also used to relax the muscles involved in spasm of the eyelid or spastic ailments.

dermabrasion Physical "sanding of the skin" to remove superficial scars or tattoos on the skin. Alternatives to dermabrasion are chemical peels or laser destruction of the outermost epidermal layers.

electrolysis Destruction of a tissue, such as a hair follicle, by passing electric current through it

laser treatments Destruction of skin imperfections, dark spots or hair follicles (see Fig. 13.34, B)

liposuction, suction **lipectomy** Excision of subcutaneous fat from the neck, legs, arms, belly, and elsewhere by placing a narrow tube under the skin and applying a vacuum (see Fig. 13.34, C). Injection **lipolysis,** the breakdown or destruction of fat by injection, or laser treatments are alternatives for liposuction.

rhytidoplasty Surgical repair for wrinkles; facelift. Skin of the face is tightened, and the skin is made to appear firm and smooth.

tattoo removal Multiple treatments, either dermabrasion or laser removal (see Fig. 13.34, D). The age, density, type and color of ink, and depth of pigment insertion determine the number of treatments.

Medications applied to the skin:

aerosol A liquid that is vaporized and propelled into the air by gas under pressure within a chamber

antibiotics Antimicrobial agents derived from cultures of microorganisms or produced synthetically

antipruritics Agents that relieve or prevent itching

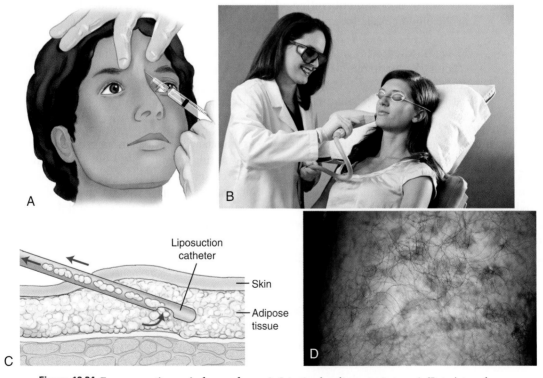

Figure 13.34 Four cosmetic surgical procedures. A, Injecting botulinum toxin type A (Botox) to reduce frown lines. **B,** Removal of hair and destruction of the hair follicle with laser. **C,** Liposuction, also called *suction lipectomy,* removes adipose tissue with a suction pump device. **D,** Laser destruction of a tattoo.

antiseptics Substances that inhibit the growth of microorganisms without necessarily killing them

ointment (ung) A medicated, fatty, soft substance for external application

retinoids Compounds that increase the sloughing of epithelial cells; often used to treat acne, they are structurally related to substances that exhibit vitamin A activity.

topical medications Drugs placed directly on the skin. Topical antimicrobial agents and dressings are applied to injured or burned tissue to prevent infection. Topical anesthetics are applied to the skin to prevent feeling. **Antibacterials, antifungals,** and **antivirals** treat bacterial, fungal, and viral infections, respectively.

transdermal drug delivery A method of applying a drug to the skin (often called a *skin patch*), which is absorbed through the skin and enters the circulatory system (see Fig. 3.10); used particularly for estrogen, nicotine, and scopolamine (for prevention of motion sickness).

13-48 Several physical treatments are available for various skin conditions. UV light therapy is a common physical treatment in psoriasis and other skin conditions. UV radiation, one of the types of energy that is included in sunlight, is more readily accessible and easier to control than exposure to the sun.

treatment

Helio/therapy is _____ of disease by exposing the body to sunlight. The combining form heli(o) means the sun.

water

Certain wounds require **heat hydro/therapy.** By its name, you know that heat hydrotherapy makes use of warm _____.

13-49 The remaining types of physical therapy have to do with treatments for muscle pain, reduction of tissue swelling, or increasing circulation. The skin is involved in many cases, however, because the treatment is delivered through the skin.

sound

Ultrasound is used therapeutically as a penetrating deep-heating agent for soft tissue. Ultrasound uses high-frequency _____ waves.

heat

Another method of generating heat in soft tissue is **diathermy.** Both diathermy and ultrasound are used to increase circulation to an inflamed area. Dia/therm/y means passing high-frequency current through tissue to generate _____ in a particular part of the body.

13-50 Various types of stimulation to the skin and subcutaneous tissue offer pain relief. **Trans/cutaneous electric nerve stimulation** (TENS) is one of these methods (see Fig. 10.31). Trans/cutaneous means that the electrical current is delivered across (or through) the

skin

_____.

Electrodes are placed over the painful sites, and small amounts of electric current are delivered to painful areas.

For more information, go to *www.nlm.nih.gov/medlineplus/skinconditions.html.*

MATCH IT! EXERCISE 15

Match the types of therapy in the left column with their characteristics on the right.

_____ **1.** diathermy

_____ **2.** heat hydrotherapy

_____ **3.** heliotherapy

_____ **4.** TENS

A. delivers electric current through the skin to painful areas

B. exposes the body to the sun

C. uses high-frequency current to generate heat for healing

D. uses warm water

PHARMACOLOGY

Topical medications are drugs placed directly on the skin. Topical antimicrobial agents and dressings are applied to injured or burned tissue to prevent infection.

Drug Class: Effect and Uses

Anesthetics, Topical: Relieve pain at the site of contact
benzocaine (Orajel)   *lidocaine (Xylocaine)*

Antihistamines, Topical: Relieve surface allergy symptoms
diphenhydramine (Benadryl)

Antiinfectives, Topical: Inhibit the growth of or kill microorganisms on the skin

Antibacterials: Treat bacterial infections
clindamycin (Cleocin)   *neomycin, polymyxin B sulfate (Neosporin)*
mupirocin (Bactroban)   *silver sulfadiazine (Silvadene)*

Antifungals: Treat fungal infections
butenafine (Mentax)   *ciclopirox (Loprox)*   *clotrimazole (Lotrimin AF)*

Antivirals: Treat viral infections
acyclovir (Zovirax)   *penciclovir (Denavir)*

Antiinflammatories, Topical: Reduce inflammation

Corticosteroids: Treat various skin disorders
amcinonide (Cyclocort)   *hydrocortisone (Cortizone)*

Immunosuppressants: Treat atopic dermatitis or eczema
pimecrolimus (Elidel)   *tacrolimus (Protopic)*

Antipruritics: Topical antiinflammatories, anesthetics, antihistamines, or counterirritants that may be used to relieve itching
See relevant drug classes in this section

Antipsoriatics: Treat psoriasis
anthralin (Drithocreme)   *calcipotriene (Dovonex)*   *tazarotene (Tazorac)*

Antiseborrheic Drugs: Reduce amount of sebum produced to treat dandruff
selenium sulfide (Selsun Blue)   *zinc pyrithinone (Dandrop, with ketoconazole)*

Astringents: Dry and contract skin tissue
calamine lotion (Calamine Plain)   *witch hazel*

Counterirritants/Rubefacients: Create inflammation topically to relieve local pain and swelling
camphor (Vicks VapoRub)   *menthol (Halls)*

Keratolytics: Shed top layer of skin to treat acne or remove warts, corns, or other lesions
azelaic acid (Azelex)   *benzoyl peroxide (Benzac AC)*   *salicylic acid (Compound W)*

Retinoids: Regulate epithelial cell growth to treat acne, psoriasis, and other skin problems
adapalene (Differin)   *tazarotene (Tazorac)*   *tretinoin (Retin-A)*

Scabicides/Pediculicides: Kill scabies, lice, or mites
lindane (Scabene)   *permethrin (Nix)*

PHARMACOLOGY, cont'd

WRITE IT!
EXERCISE 16

Choose from these terms to complete the sentences:

anesthetics, antipruritics, antiseborrheic, astringents, keratolytics, pediculicides, rubefacients, transdermal

1. Another name for counterirritants is _____.
2. Another name for scabicides is _____.
3. Applying a drug to the skin where it is absorbed and enters the circulatory system is called _____ drug delivery.
4. Medications called _____ are used to dry and contract skin tissue.
5. Medications called _____ shed the top layer of skin to treat acne or remove warts.
6. Topical medications called _____ relieve itching.
7. Medications to treat dandruff that reduce the amount of sebum are _____ drugs.
8. Topical medications called _____ relieve pain at the site of contact.

CHAPTER ABBREVIATIONS*

ABA	American Burn Association	**I&D**	incision and drainage
AIDS	acquired immunodeficiency syndrome	**STAPH**	staphylococci
Bx, bx	biopsy	**TBSA**	total body surface area
DLE	discoid lupus erythematosus	**TENS**	transcutaneous electric nerve stimulation
HSV	herpes simplex virus	**ung**	ointment
HSV-1	herpes simplex virus type 1	**VAC**	vacuum-assisted closure
HSV-2	herpes simplex virus type 2		

*Many of these abbreviations share their meanings with other terms.

A Career as a Nurse Practitioner

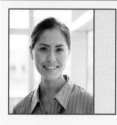

Shannon Chen is a nurse practitioner (NP) providing care to patients from newborns to the elderly in a busy dermatology practice. She worked several years as a registered nurse while getting her master's degree and acquired the competence, expert knowledge base, and complex decision-making skills needed for her job. She examines patients, orders diagnostic procedures, prescribes medications, takes biopsies, and makes referrals in a busy dermatology clinic. Nurse practitioners are in high demand as health care services dramatically increase. For additional information, go to *aanp.org*.

! Be Careful With These!

allograft vs. *autograft*	*ectoderm* vs. *endoderm* vs.	*keratolytic* vs. *onycholytic*	*vesicles* vs. *bullae*
cyst vs. *nodule*	*mesoderm*	*scleroderma* vs. *xeroderma*	

CHAPTER 13 SELF-TEST

Review the new word parts for this chapter. Work all of the following exercises to test your understanding of the material before checking your answers against those in Appendix IV.

BASIC UNDERSTANDING

Labeling

I.   Label the degree of burn (1 to 3) and the structures (4 to 6) in the following illustration of the skin and underlying structures.

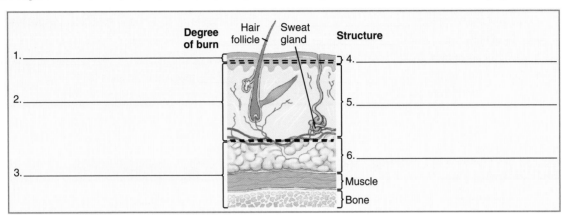

Listing

II.   List five functions of the skin.

1. _____
2. _____
3. _____
4. _____
5. _____

III.   List the accessory skin structures, and describe their functions.

1. _____
2. _____
3. _____
4. _____

Matching

IV.   Match skin lesions in the left column with their characteristics in the right column.

_____ **1.** bulla

_____ **2.** cyst

_____ **3.** fissure

_____ **4.** macule

_____ **5.** papule

_____ **6.** pustule

_____ **7.** keloid

_____ **8.** vesicle

A. blister, larger than 1 cm

B. blister, smaller than 1 cm

C. cracklike lesion of the skin

D. discolored spot, not elevated

E. excess collagen production after injury

F. fluid-filled sac containing pus

G. sac filled with clear fluid

H. solid elevation, less than 1 cm in diameter

Identifying Illustrations

V. Identify the following illustrations using one of these terms: atrophy, excoriation, fissure, keratosis, papules, petechiae, scleroderma.

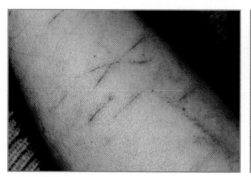 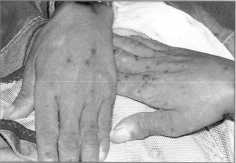 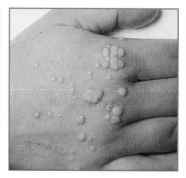

1. _____

2. _____

3. _____

Analyzing Terms

VI. Divide these words into their component parts, and write the meaning of each term.

1. electrolysis _____

2. ichthyosis _____

3. keratogenesis _____

4. melanocyte _____

5. scleroderma _____

Using Vocabulary

VII. Circle the correct answer for each multiple choice question.

1. Eight-year-old Rosaura is undergoing skin tests in which small quantities of allergens are injected intracutaneously. What is the name of this test? (needle aspiration, punch biopsy, skin culture, allergy testing)

2. Tom, age 82, has numerous skin tags and warts that the doctor removes by using destructive subfreezing temperatures. Which treatment is described? (cryosurgery, electrodessication, heliotherapy, ultrasound)

3. Dr. Pratt is examining a high school athlete for an injury sustained while sliding into home plate. Radiography reports are negative, and the wound needs to be cleaned before it is bandaged. Which of the following means cleaning of debris and damaged tissue from the wound? (débridement, necrosis, pyemia, rhytidectomy)

4. The doctor is examining a swelling of Katherine's right armpit, which he believes to be a swelling of the lymph node, but orders appropriate tests to rule out a tumor. What region is the physician examining? (adipose, alopecia, apocrine, axillary)

5. Nalini, age 72, complains to the visiting nurse about her continued scalp problems of yellowish crusts and scales. Which skin disease is described? (acne vulgaris, basal cell carcinoma, seborrheic dermatitis, verruca)

6. The pediatrician examines an infant who may have cystic fibrosis. Which diagnostic test is she likely to request? (shaved specimen, skin biopsy, sebum analysis, sweat test)

7. Sixty-year-old Anna complains of hardened areas in her face and fingers. The internist suspects a systemic disease and orders the appropriate tests. Which disease/disorder is more likely? (ecchymosis, Kaposi sarcoma, keratosis, scleroderma)

8. Ray has been confined to bed for the past several months and has developed a bedsore on the skin of the lumbar area. What is another name for the lesion? (decubitus ulcer, keratoma, mole, wart)

9. A child touches her hand to a hot burner and is brought to the emergency department with a burn that extends throughout the epidermis and into the dermis. Which type of burn does she have? (deep partial-thickness, deep full-thickness, full-thickness, superficial partial-thickness)

10. While swimming near Crystal Beach, a jellyfish brushes Julie's leg, resulting in "bands" of destroyed skin that came in contact with the jellyfish. Which term pertains to the skin destruction? (actinic, cyanotic, necrotic, purulent)

Filling in the Blanks

VIII. Complete the sentences by writing a term in each blank space.

1. Cells of the epidermis contain _____, which is a scleroprotein.

2. The corium is another name for the layer of skin called the _____.

3. An oily material secreted by the sebaceous glands is called _____.

4. Sweat glands, also called _____ glands, produce perspiration.

5. Diaphoresis means excessive _____.

Writing Terms

IX.   Write words for each of the following clues.

1. a boil   _____

2. a contagious dermatitis caused by the itch mite   _____

3. a torn, jagged wound   _____

4. absence of pigment in the skin, hair, and nails   _____

5. another name for a bruise   _____

6. any disease of the nails   _____

7. baldness   _____

8. condition in which the skin is dry and scaly   _____

9. heatstroke or sunstroke   _____

10. superficial infection involving hair follicles   _____

Making Connections

X.   Describe the relationship of these terms.

1. dermis and epidermis   _____

_____

2. curet and curettage   _____

_____

Finetuning Terms

XI.   In addition to spelling, describe at least one difference in the following:

1. cyst and nodule   _____

_____

2. topical drug and transdermal drug   _____

_____

GREATER COMPREHENSION

Spelling

XII.   Circle each misspelled term in this list, and write the correct spelling.

abrasion   aerosol   ektoderm   hydradenitis   onykectomy

Abbreviating

XIII. Write a letter in each blank for the abbreviation that corresponds to the clue.

1. acquired immunodeficiency syndrome   __ __ __ __

2. biopsy   __ __

3. virus that causes fever blisters   __ __ __

4. ointment   __ __ __

5. used to calculate the magnitude of a burn   __ __ __ __

Health Care Reporting

XIV. Read the following operative report, and using your critical thinking skills, answer the questions that follow the report.

Ames M. Weaver - OPERATION REPORT

Task Time Scale Options Help View Edit

As Of 06:27

Patient Name: Ames M. Weaver   **ID No.:** 016-0003   **Date of surgery:** Jul 11, 2016
DOB: 06-04-1992   **Sex:** Male   **Surgeon:** Mark Bonneville, MD   **Anesthesia:** General endotracheal by Dr. Reid

Flowsheet: Post-operative   ▼   ...   Level: Report   ▼   ⦿ Table ○ Group ○ List

| MAR | Task List | I & O | Pt. Info | Pt. Schedule | Surgery | Clinical Notes | Form Browser |

| Orders | Last 48 Hours | ED | Lab | Radiology | Assessments | Medical Report | Medication Profile |

PREOPERATIVE DIAGNOSIS: Improvised explosive device (IED) soft-tissue wounds, right lower extremity
POSTOPERATIVE DIAGNOSIS: Improvised explosive device (IED) soft-tissue wounds, right lower extremity
MATERIAL FORWARDED TO THE LABORATORY: Cultures were taken from his small proximal wound for microbiology
OPERATIONS PERFORMED
1. Irrigation and débridement   2. Wound VAC, right thigh wounds
Estimated blood loss: Minimal
Preop antibiotics: Ancef 2 grams
Complications: None
Tourniquet time: None
PREOPERATIVE HISTORY: Patient is a 24-year-old active duty airman assigned to Air Force Special Forces in Iraq. On 3 July, he sustained wounds from an IED and was initially treated with tourniquet, then had débridements in Iraq, then in Landstuhl. He was brought to PCL Clinic 9 July where he underwent irrigation and débridement by the General Surgery team. He was immediately transferred to my service when Dr. Janskin had to go out of the country.
Past Medical History: Negative. **Past Surgical History:** Childhood tonsillectomy. **Allergies:** None.
Medications: Just what he has been given at PCL.

I discussed all the risks of repeat surgery and our recommendations with the patient. He is a Senior Airman in the Air Force. I also discussed with him the need to consider stopping tobacco use. He indicated his understanding of all the many risks of surgery. He also understood the recommendations for repeated irrigation and débridement. Patient gave informed consent.
DESCRIPTION OF OPERATION: The patient was identified in the preoperative area, and his operative site was signed. He was brought to the operating room where a final time-out was called. He then underwent satisfactory endotracheal anesthesia. He was placed in the left lateral decubitus position. His large lateral thigh wound required minimal débridement. His other, smaller wounds also required minimal débridement. Copious irrigation was carried out.
The wound VAC was placed in his large lateral thigh wound with vessel loops. In addition, his distal thigh wound, which was the largest of the three smaller wounds, had a wound VAC placed. A bridge was placed on top of plastic, not on top of skin. His other two wounds were temporarily closed with plans to reopen and repeat I&D of them. Cultures were taken from his small proximal wound.
The patient was extubated and taken to recovery room in good condition.

| PROD | MAHAFC | 11 Jul 2016 | 10:14 |

---

1. What is meant by débridement? _____

_____

2. What is meant by irrigation as described in the operation? _____

_____

3. Explain wound VAC. _____

_____

4. What does the abbreviation I&D mean? _____

_____

XV. After reading the following consultation, match the descriptions (1 to 7) to the terms or phrases (A to G).

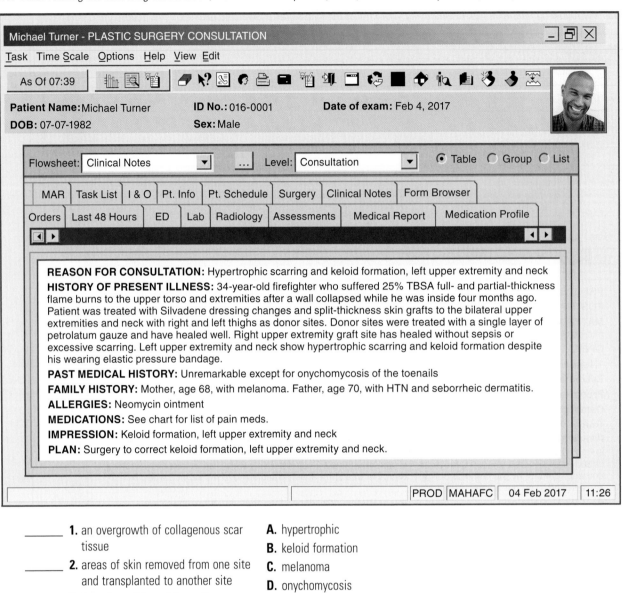

Michael Turner - PLASTIC SURGERY CONSULTATION

Task Time Scale Options Help View Edit

As Of 07:39

Patient Name: Michael Turner   **ID No.:** 016-0001   **Date of exam:** Feb 4, 2017
DOB: 07-07-1982   **Sex:** Male

Flowsheet: Clinical Notes   ...   Level: Consultation   ⦿ Table ○ Group ○ List

| MAR | Task List | I & O | Pt. Info | Pt. Schedule | Surgery | Clinical Notes | Form Browser |

| Orders | Last 48 Hours | ED | Lab | Radiology | Assessments | Medical Report | Medication Profile |

REASON FOR CONSULTATION: Hypertrophic scarring and keloid formation, left upper extremity and neck
HISTORY OF PRESENT ILLNESS: 34-year-old firefighter who suffered 25% TBSA full- and partial-thickness flame burns to the upper torso and extremities after a wall collapsed while he was inside four months ago. Patient was treated with Silvadene dressing changes and split-thickness skin grafts to the bilateral upper extremities and neck with right and left thighs as donor sites. Donor sites were treated with a single layer of petrolatum gauze and have healed well. Right upper extremity graft site has healed without sepsis or excessive scarring. Left upper extremity and neck show hypertrophic scarring and keloid formation despite his wearing elastic pressure bandage.
PAST MEDICAL HISTORY: Unremarkable except for onychomycosis of the toenails
FAMILY HISTORY: Mother, age 68, with melanoma. Father, age 70, with HTN and seborrheic dermatitis.
ALLERGIES: Neomycin ointment
MEDICATIONS: See chart for list of pain meds.
IMPRESSION: Keloid formation, left upper extremity and neck
PLAN: Surgery to correct keloid formation, left upper extremity and neck.

PROD MAHAFC   04 Feb 2017   11:26

_____ **1.** an overgrowth of collagenous scar tissue

_____ **2.** areas of skin removed from one site and transplanted to another site

_____ **3.** fungal condition of the nails

_____ **4.** infection

_____ **5.** malignant skin cancer

_____ **6.** pertaining to an increase in size

_____ **7.** the classification of the type of burn

A. hypertrophic

B. keloid formation

C. melanoma

D. onychomycosis

E. sepsis

F. split-thickness skin grafts

G. 25% total body surface area (TBSA) full- and partial-thickness

Pronouncing Terms

XVI. Write the correct term for the following phonetic spellings.

1. **bul**-uh   _____

2. dē-**his**-uns   _____

3. ē-lek-trō-des-i-**kā**-shun   _____

4. **fū**-rung-kul   _____

5. **rit**-i-dō-plas-tē   _____

6. **sup**-ū-rā-tiv   _____

Health Care Reporting

XVII. Read the medical report and select one answer in the multiple-choice questions.

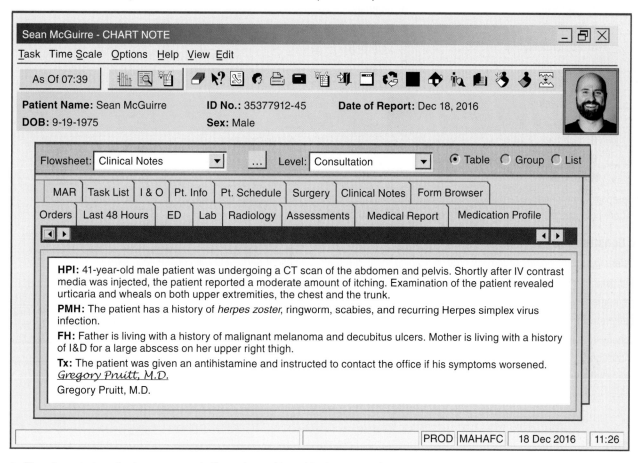

Sean McGuirre - CHART NOTE

Task Time Scale Options Help View Edit

As Of 07:39

Patient Name: Sean McGuirre   **ID No.:** 35377912-45   **Date of Report:** Dec 18, 2016
DOB: 9-19-1975   **Sex:** Male

Flowsheet: Clinical Notes   Level: Consultation   ⦿ Table ○ Group ○ List

MAR | Task List | I & O | Pt. Info | Pt. Schedule | Surgery | Clinical Notes | Form Browser

Orders | Last 48 Hours | ED | Lab | Radiology | Assessments | Medical Report | Medication Profile

HPI: 41-year-old male patient was undergoing a CT scan of the abdomen and pelvis. Shortly after IV contrast media was injected, the patient reported a moderate amount of itching. Examination of the patient revealed urticaria and wheals on both upper extremities, the chest and the trunk.

PMH: The patient has a history of *herpes zoster*, ringworm, scabies, and recurring Herpes simplex virus infection.

FH: Father is living with a history of malignant melanoma and decubitus ulcers. Mother is living with a history of I&D for a large abscess on her upper right thigh.

Tx: The patient was given an antihistamine and instructed to contact the office if his symptoms worsened.
Gregory Pruitt, M.D.
Gregory Pruitt, M.D.

PROD | MAHAFC | 18 Dec 2016 | 11:26

1. The alternate term for herpes zoster is (furuncle, scabies, shingles, verruca).
2. Which term in the report means irregularly-shaped lesions? (decubitus, scabies, urticaria, wheals)
3. Herpes simplex virus is the cause of (acne vulgaris, fever blisters, eczema, seborrheic keratosis).
4. Ringworm is a disorder caused by a (bacteria, fungus, protozoa, virus)
5. The term in the report which refers to an allergic skin eruption is (abscess, decubitus, ulcers, urticaria)

Using Pharmacologic Terms

XVIII. Use all selections to match terms in the left column with descriptions in the right column.

___ **1.** antipruritics	**A.** kill scabies, lice, or mites
___ **2.** antiseborrheic	**B.** reduce sebum
___ **3.** keratolytics	**C.** relieve itching
___ **4.** pediculicides	**D.** used as counterirritants
___ **5.** rubefacients	**E.** used to remove warts or corns

Categorizing Terms and Practicing Pronunciations

XIX. Classify the terms in the left column by selecting A, B, C, D, or E.

____ **1.** diathermy	**A.** anatomy
____ **2.** eczema	**B.** diagnostic test or procedure
____ **3.** escharotomy	**C.** pathology
____ **4.** liposuction	**D.** surgery
____ **5.** pediculosis	**E.** nonsurgical therapy
____ **6.** rhytidectomy	
____ **7.** shaved specimen	
____ **8.** skin flap	
____ **9.** ungual	
____ **10.** xerosis	

(Be prepared to pronounce terms 1-10 in class after listening to Chapter 13 terms at *http://evolve.elsevier.com/Leonard/building/*. In addition, practice categorizing all boldface terms in this chapter.)

New Construction

XX. Determine the meanings of these words by dividing them into their component parts, and then define each term.

1. anhidrosis _____

2. dermatographia _____

3. hyperkeratosis _____

4. onychodystrophy _____

5. trichophagia _____

(Use Appendix IV to check your answers to the exercises.)

BMV LIST

Visit *http://evolve.elsevier.com/Leonard/building/* to listen to the boldface terms in Chapter 13. Look closely at the spelling of each term as it is pronounced.

abrasion (uh-**brā**-zhun)
abscess (**ab**-ses)
accessory skin structures (ak-**ses**-uh-rē skin **struk**-churz)
acne vulgaris (**ak**-nē vul-**gar**-is)
actinic keratosis (ak-**tin**-ik ker-uh-**tō**-sis)
adipose (**ad**-i-pōs)
aerosol (**ār**-ō-sol)
albinism (**al**-bi-niz-um)
albino (al-**bī**-nō)
allograft (**al**-ō-graft)
alopecia (al-ō-**pē**-shuh)
amputation (am-pū-**tā**-shun)
anesthetics (an-us-**thet**-iks)

antibacterials (an-tē-bak-**tēr**-ē-ulz)
antibiotic (an-tē-bī-**ot**-ik)
antifungals (an-tē-**fung**-gulz)
antihistamines (an-tē-**his**-tuh-mēnz)
antiinfectives (an-tē-in-**fek**-tivz)
antiinflammatories (an-tē-in-**flam**-uh-tor-ēz)
antimicrobial (an-tē-mī-**krō**-bē-ul)
antipruritic (an-tē-prōō-**rit**-ik)
antipruritics (an-tē-prōō-**rit**-iks)
antipsoriatics (an-tē-sor-ē-**at**-iks)
antiseborrheic drugs (an-tē-seb-ō-**rē**-ik drugz)
antiseptic (an-ti-**sep**-tik)
antivirals (an-tē-**vī**-rulz)

apocrine sweat gland (**ap**-ō-krin swet gland)
arrector pili muscle (uh-**rek**-tor **pī**-lī **mus**-ul)
aseptic (ā-**sep**-tik)
astringents (uh-**strin**-junts)
atrophy (**at**-ruh-fē)
autograft (**aw**-tō-graft)
axillary (**ak**-si-lar-ē)
basal cell carcinoma (**bā**-sul sel kahr-si-**nō**-muh)
bulla (**bul**-uh)
burn (burn)
cellulitis (sel-ū-**lī**-tis)
collagen injection (**kol**-uh-jun in-**jek**-shun)
contact dermatitis (**kon**-takt dur-muh-**tī**-tis)
contusion (kun-**tōō**-zhun)
corium (**kor**-ē-um)
corn (korn)
counterirritants (coun-tur-**ir**-i-tunts)
crust (krust)
cryosurgery (krī-ō-**sur**-jur-ē)
cryotherapy (krī-ō-**ther**-uh-pē)
curet (kū-**ret**)
curettage (kū-ruh-**tahzh**)
cyanosis (sī-uh-**nō**-sis)
cyst (sist)
cystic fibrosis (**sis**-tik fī-**brō**-sis)
débride (dā-**brēd**)
débridement (dā-brēd-**maw**)
decubitus ulcer (dē-**kū**-bi-tus **ul**-sur)
deep partial-thickness burn (dēp **par**-shul **thik**-nus burn)
dehiscence (dē-**his**-uns)
dermabrasion (dur-muh-**brā**-zhun)
dermatitis (dur-muh-**tī**-tis)
dermatologist (dur-muh-**tol**-uh-jist)
dermatology (dur-muh-**tol**-uh-jē)
dermatome (**dur**-muh-tōm)
dermatomycosis (dur-muh-tō-mī-**kō**-sis)
dermis (**dur**-mis)
diaphoresis (dī-uh-fuh-**rē**-sis)
diathermy (**dī**-uh-thur-mē)
discoid lupus erythematosus (**dis**-koid **lōō**-pus
   er-uh-them-uh-**tō**-sis)
ecchymosis (ek-i-**mō**-sis)
ectoderm (**ek**-tō-durm)
eczema (**ek**-zuh-muh)
electrodessication (ē-lek-trō-des-i-**kā**-shun)
electrolysis (ē-lek-**trol**-uh-sis)
endoderm (**en**-dō-durm)
epidermal (ep-i-**dur**-mul)
epidermis (ep-i-**dur**-mis)
erythema (er-uh-**thē**-muh)
escharotomy (es-kuh-**rot**-uh-mē)
excoriation (eks-kō-rē-**ā**-shun)
exfoliation (eks-fō-lē-**ā**-shun)
fissure (**fish**-ur)
folliculitis (fuh-lik-ū-**lī**-tis)
frostbite (**frost**-bīt)
full-thickness burn (fool **thik**-nus burn)

furuncle (**fū**-rung-kul)
heat hydrotherapy (hēt hī-drō-**ther**-uh-pē)
heliotherapy (hē-lē-ō-**ther**-uh-pē)
herpes simplex virus (**hur**-pēz **sim**-pleks **vī**-rus)
herpes zoster (**hur**-pēz **zos**-tur)
hidradenitis (hī-drad-uh-**nī**-tis)
histocompatibility (his-tō-kum-pat-i-**bil**-i-tē)
hyperthermia (hī-pur-**thur**-mē-uh)
hypothermia (hī-pō-**thur**-mē-uh)
hypoxic tissue (hī-**pok**-sik **tish**-ōō)
ichthyoid (**ik**-thē-oid)
ichthyosis (ik-thē-ō-**sis**)
incision and drainage (in-**sizh**-un and **drān**-uj)
incompatibility (in-kum-pat-i-**bil**-i-tē)
induration (in-dū-**rā**-shun)
integument (in-**teg**-ū-munt)
integumentary (in-teg-ū-**men**-tar-ē)
jaundice (**jawn**-dis)
Kaposi sarcoma (**kah**-pō-shē sahr-**kō**-muh)
keloid (**kē**-loid)
keratin (**ker**-uh-tin)
keratogenesis (ker-uh-tō-**jen**-uh-sis)
keratolytics (ker-uh-tō-**lit**-iks)
keratoma (ker-uh-**tō**-muh)
keratosis (ker-uh-**tō**-sis)
laceration (las-ur-**ā**-shun)
laser treatments (**lā**-zur **trēt**-munts)
lesion (**lē**-zhun)
leukoderma (lōō-kō-**der**-muh)
lipectomy (li-**pek**-tuh-mē)
lipolysis (li-**pol**-uh-sis)
lipoma (lip-**ō**-muh)
liposuction (lip-ō-**suk**-shun)
lunula (**lōō**-nū-luh)
macule (**mak**-ūl)
malignant melanoma (muh-**lig**-nunt mel-uh-**nō**-muh)
melanocyte (**mel**-uh-nō-sīt, muh-**lan**-ō-sīt)
mesoderm (**mez**-ō-durm)
mycodermatitis (mī-kō-dur-muh-**tī**-tis)
necrosis (nuh-**krō**-sis)
necrotic (nuh-**krot**-ik)
nevus (**nē**-vus)
nodule (**nod**-ūl)
ointment (**oint**-munt)
onychectomy (on-i-**kek**-tuh-mē)
onycholysis (on-i-**kol**-i-sis)
onychomalacia (on-i-kō-muh-**lā**-shuh)
onychomycosis (on-i-kō-mī-**kō**-sis)
onychopathy (on-i-**kop**-uh-thē)
onychophagia (on-i-kō-**fā**-juh)
onychophagist (on-i-**kof**-uh-jist)
onychosis (on-i-**kō**-sis)
papule (**pap**-ūl)
pediculicides (puh-**dik**-ū-li-sīdz)
pediculosis (puh-dik-ū-**lō**-sis)
perspiration (pur-spi-**rā**-shun)
petechia (puh-**tē**-kē-uh)

photodermatitis (fō-tō-dur-muh-**tī**-tis)
pilonidal cyst (pī-lō-**nī**-dul sist)
plaque (plak)
primary lesions (**prī**-mar-ē **lē**-zhunz)
psoriasis (suh-**rī**-uh-sis)
punch biopsy (punch **bī**-op-sē)
puncture (**punk**-chur)
purulence (**pū**-rōō-luns)
pustule (**pus**-tūl)
pyogenesis (pī-ō-**jen**-uh-sis)
pyrexia (pī-**rek**-sē-uh)
retinoid (**ret**-i-noid)
rhytidoplasty (**rit**-i-dō-plas-tē)
ringworm (**ring**-wurm)
rubefacients (rōō-buh-**fā**-shunts)
rule of nines (rōōl ov nīnz)
scabicides (**skā**-bi-sīdz)
scabies (**skā**-bēz)
scales (skālz)
scar (skahr)
scleroderma (sklēr-ō-**dur**-muh)
scleroprotein (sklēr-ō-**prō**-tēn)
sebaceous cyst (suh-**bā**-shus sist)
sebaceous gland (suh-**bā**-shus gland)
seborrhea (seb-ō-**rē**-uh)
seborrheic dermatitis (seb-ō-**rē**-ik dur-muh-**tī**-tis)
seborrheic keratosis (seb-ō-**rē**-ik ker-uh-**tō**-sis)
sebum (**sē**-bum)
secondary lesions (**sek**-un-dar-ē **lē**-zhunz)
sepsis (**sep**-sis)
shaved specimen (shāvd **spes**-i-mun)

skin flap (skin flap)
skin infection (skin in-**fek**-shun)
squamous cell carcinoma (**skwā**-mus sel kahr-si-**nō**-muh)
subcutaneous adipose tissue (sub-kū-**tā**-nē-us **ad**-i-pōs **tish**-ōō)
sudoriferous gland (sōō-dō-**rif**-ur-us gland)
superficial partial-thickness burn (sōō-pur-**fish**-ul **par**-shul **thik**-nus burn)
suppuration (sup-ū-**rā**-shun)
suppurative (**sup**-ū-rā-tiv)
suturing (**sōō**-chur-ing)
tattoo removal (ta-**tōō** ri-**mōō**-vul)
thermoplegia (thur-mō-**plē**-juh)
tinea (**tin**-ē-uh)
topical medication (**top**-i-kul med-i-**kā**-shun)
transcutaneous electrical nerve stimulation (trans-kū-**tā**-nē-us ē-**lek**-tri-kul nurv stim-ū-**lā**-shun)
transdermal drug delivery (trans-**dur**-mul drug dē-**liv**-ur-ē)
trichopathy (tri-**kop**-uh-thē)
trichosis (tri-**kō**-sis)
ulcer (**ul**-sur)
ungual (**ung**-gwul)
urticaria (ur-ti-**kar**-ē-uh)
verruca (vuh-**rōō**-kuh)
vesicle (**ves**-i-kul)
vitiligo (vit-i-**lī**-gō)
wheal (hwēl, wēl)
wound (wōōnd)
wound irrigation (wōōnd ir-i-**gā**-shun)
xeroderma (zēr-ō-**dur**-muh)
xerosis (zēr-**ō**-sis)

Español ENHANCING SPANISH COMMUNICATION

English	Spanish (Pronunciation)	English	Spanish (Pronunciation)
allergy	alergia (ah-LEHR-he-ah)	hives	roncha (RON-chah)
burn	quemadura (kay-mah-DOO-rah)	injury	daño (DAH-nyo)
dermatology	dermatología (der-mah-to-lo-HEE-ah)	nails	uñas (OO-nyahs)
eyebrow	ceja (SAY-hah)	perspiration	sudor (soo-DOR)
eyelash	pestaña (pes-TAH-nyah)	skin	piel (pe-EL)
gland	glándula (GLAN-doo-lah)	ulcer	ulcera (OOL-say-rah)
hair	pelo (PAY-lo)	wound	lesión (lay-se-ON)

CHAPTER 14

Oncology
Cancer Can Occur in Any Body System

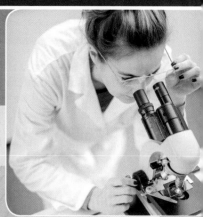

Anatomical pathologists study tissue from biopsy, surgery, or autopsy. To see the tissue under a microscope, the sections are processed, and histological sections are placed on glass slides and stained before they are examined by the pathologist.

LEARNING OUTCOMES

Basic Understanding

1. Distinguish between benign and malignant tumors.
2. Distinguish between primary and metastatic tumors.
3. Recognize that cancer is the second leading cause of death in the United States.
4. Name or recognize the four modes of cancer metastasis.
5. Recognize the difference in tumor grading and tumor staging.

6. Write the names of the diagnostic tests and procedures used for assessment of tumors when given their descriptions, or match them with their descriptions.
7. Write the names of cancer pathologies when given their descriptions, or match them with their descriptions.
8. Match the terms for surgical and therapeutic interventions for cancer with their descriptions, or write the interventions when given their descriptions.

Greater Comprehension

9. Spell the terms accurately.
10. Pronounce the terms correctly.
11. Recognize or use abbreviations presented in this chapter.
12. Categorize terms as anatomy, diagnostic test or procedure, pathology, surgery, or nonsurgical therapy.

13. Recognize the meanings of general pharmacological terms from this chapter as well as the drug classes and their uses.
14. Use terms from this chapter to read and understand health care reports.

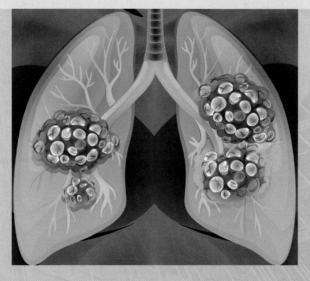

FUNCTION FIRST

Cancer (or carcinoma) is defined in 2 ways:
- a neoplasm characterized by the uncontrolled growth of cells that tend to invade surrounding tissue and metastasize to distant body sites
- any of a large group of malignant neoplastic diseases characterized by the presence of malignant cells.

Oncology is the branch of medicine that specializes in the study and treatment of neoplastic diseases, particularly cancer, a significant public health problem in the United States and throughout the world. A physician who specializes in the study and treatment of neoplastic diseases is an oncologist.

CARCINOGENESIS

cancer

14-1 You learned in Chapter 2 that cancer(o) and carcin(o) mean cancer. **Carcino/genesis** is the process by which normal cells undergo malignant transformation to become _____ cells and may take years to complete. This can result from exposure to chemicals or radiation, viral infections, and factors such as smoking and diet as well as unknown factors.

🔑 **KEY** POINT **Differentiation is a developmental process in which unspecified cells or tissues are modified to become different types of tissues (such as bone or muscle).** All human beings start as a single cell that begins to divide, then the cells begin to differentiate into different types of cells and produce different types of tissue that have different functions. This is called cellular differentiation. Cancer cells originate as a particular type of tissue, but then lose the ability to differentiate and revert back to immature, **undifferentiated cells.**

new

14-2 A **neo/plasm** is considered abnormal and is translated literally as a _____ growth, but not all neoplasms are cancerous.

Cancer arises when defects in the genes (DNA sequences on chromosomes) that regulate cellular production and repair are not corrected, and most often is caused by mutations that occur over the course of a lifetime. Cancer is uncontrolled growth of cells that tend to invade surrounding tissue.

▶ **BEYOND** THE BLUEPRINT The discovery of an abnormal chromosome in chronic myelogenous leukemia by Peter Nowell who worked in Philadelphia provided evidence in 1960 for a genetic link to cancer. The abnormal chromosome was thus named the Philadelphia chromosome.

14-3 A neoplasm that is at the original site where it first arose is called a **primary tumor** (example, lung cancer that has originated in the lung). That cancer can metastasize and spread to other tissues (**metastatic cancer**). An example of metastatic cancer is advanced lung cancer that has spread to nearby organs, such as the liver.

DEATH AND CANCER STATISTICS

carcinogens

14-4 The cause of most human cancer is not known, but many potential **carcinogens,** substances or agents that cause or increase the incidence of cancer, have been identified (Table 14.1). Cancer may be caused not only by environmental factors, but also by heredity (for example, certain inherited types of colon, breast, or kidney cancer). Substances or agents that cause or increase the incidence of cancer are called _____.

heart

14-5 Five major causes of U.S. deaths (in the order in which they occur) are heart disease, cancer (slightly less than heart disease), chronic lower respiratory diseases, stroke, and accidents; however the general profile of leading causes varies by the age at death. Accidents, homicide, and suicide are the leading causes of death in those aged 1 to 24 years. Overall, the leading cause of death in the United States is _____ disease, and the second leading cause of death is cancer.

cancer

14-6 You have already learned that neoplasms are also called tumors. Benign tumors do not invade surrounding tissue or spread to distant sites. However, a malignant neoplasm is the same as _____.

Table 14.1   Selected Known Human Carcinogens

Alcoholic beverage consumption
Arsenic
Asbestos
Benzene
Cadmium
Coal tar
Coke oven emissions
Environmental tobacco smoke
Estrogen postmenopausal therapy
Formaldehyde
Infection with Epstein-Barr virus, HBV, HCV, and HPV
Smokeless tobacco
Solar radiation and exposure to sunlamps and sunbeds
Soot
Tobacco smoking
Vinyl chloride

Selections from Report on known and probable human carcinogens, American Cancer Society, www.cancer.org.

Table 14.2   Leading Sites of New Cancer Cases and Deaths: 2016 Estimates

Men	Women
Estimated New Cases for the Three Major Causes	
Prostate (21%)	Breast (29%)
Lung and bronchus (14%)	Lung and bronchus (13%)
Colon and rectum (8%)	Colon and rectum (8%)
Estimated Deaths for the Three Major Causes	
Lung and bronchus (27%)	Lung and bronchus (26%)
Prostate (8%)	Breast (14%)
Colon and rectum (8%)	Colon and rectum (8%)

Data from Cancer Statistics, 2016, American Cancer Society, www.cancer.org. Excludes basal and squamous cell skin cancers and *in situ* carcinomas.

14-7 Cancer can occur in persons of all ages and can occur anywhere in the body. Many potential causes of cancer are recognized, but the majority of cancers are attributed to cigarette smoking, exposure to carcinogenic chemicals, radiation, and ultraviolet rays. Carcino/genic refers to the

cause   ability to _____ cancer.

14-8 Each year the American Cancer Society (ACS) estimates the number of new cancer cases and deaths expected in the United States.

The incidence of cancer and cancer death varies by type in men and women. Look at estimated incidences and deaths for men and women in Table 14.2. Look first at the estimated new cases in American men. The site of the greatest number of estimated new cancer cases in men is the

prostate   _____. In women, what is the site of the greatest number of estimated
breast   new cancer cases? _____.
lung   Notice that cancer of the _____ and bronchus ranks number one in estimated deaths from cancer for all adults.

14-9 Lung cancer remains a highly lethal disease, although significant improvements in treatment have occurred.

🔑 **KEY** POINT **The most important cause of lung cancer is tobacco smoking.** Besides cigarettes, exposure to airborne asbestos, uranium, radon, and high doses of ionizing radiation have been linked to increased incidence of lung cancer, according to the ACS. Cigarette smoking increases the risk of lung cancer more than the risk of cancer at any other site, but cigarette smoking—as well as pipe smoking—also multiplies the risk of cancers of the lip, mouth, tongue, and throat.

tobacco   The greatest cause of lung cancer is smoking _____.

➤ **BEYOND** THE BLUEPRINT Most skin cancers and most *in situ* cancers are not included in cancer predictions and statistics about cancer deaths. *In situ* is Latin and means localized and not invading the surrounding tissue. In other words, it means not metastasized or spread.

14-10 Table 14.2 gives only the major causes of estimated new cancer cases and deaths in the United States, and cervical cancer is not listed. But worldwide, cervical cancer is the third most common type of cancer in women. Cervical cancer starts in the cervix, the lower part of the uterus that opens at the top of the vagina. Almost all cervical cancers are caused by human papillomavirus,
cervix   for which a vaccine was developed in 2006. Cervical cancer is cancer of the _____.

WRITE IT!

EXERCISE 1

Write a word in each blank to complete theses sentences.

1. Cancer cells lose their ability to differentiate and revert back to _____ cells.

2. The process by which cancer cells undergo transformation to become cancer cells is called _____.

3. A term for a new growth is _____.

4. Substances or agents that cause or increase the incidence of cancer are _____.

5. The number one cause of death in the United States is _____ disease.

6. The number two cause of death in the United States is _____.

7. Vaccines that prevent hepatitis B and most types of _____ cancer are available.

BENIGN VS. MALIGNANT TUMORS

malignant

14-11 As stated, although all cancers are neoplasms (new growths), not all neoplasms are cancerous. Some neoplasms are benign neoplasms; in other words, benign neoplasms are not _____ and do not invade surrounding tissue. **Malignant tumors** invade surrounding tissue and metastasize to distant sites.

Table 14.3 lists some benign skin growths and malignant neoplasms that have been presented in earlier chapters of this book.

malignant

14-12 Review the differences in benign and malignant tumors in Fig. 14.1. Note that malignant tumors invade other tissues; malignant cells move through the membrane and gain access to nearby tissue, blood and lymph vessels. **Metastasis** is the process in which tumor cells move from their primary location to remote colonies. You see that benign tumors are well-differentiated and nonmetastatic, while _____ tumors are anaplastic/undifferentiated and metastatic. **Anaplasia**, characteristic of malignancy, is a change in the structure and orientation of cells, characterized by a loss of differentiation and reversion to a more primitive form.

A. Benign Tumor
Slow growing
Encapsulated/not invasive
Well-differentiated
Not metastatic

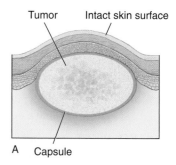

Tumor   Intact skin surface

A   Capsule

B. Malignant Tumor
Rapid growing
Invasive
Anaplastic/undifferentiated
Metastatic

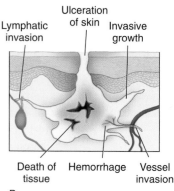

Lymphatic invasion   Ulceration of skin   Invasive growth

Death of tissue   Hemorrhage   Vessel invasion

B

Figure 14.1 Comparison of benign and malignant tumors.

Table 14.3 Examples of Benign Skin Growths vs. Malignant Neoplasms	
Benign	**Malignant**
angioma	basal cell carcinoma
nevus (mole)	cancer of almost every organ
lipoma	Kaposi sarcoma
sebaceous keratosis	malignant melanoma
blisters, wheals	squamous cell carcinoma

14-13 Not all malignant cells are capable of metastasis. In metastasis (meta-, next + -stasis, stop), cells move from their primary location. Common sites to which cells metastasize are lymph nodes, bone, lung, brain, and liver. There are four ways in which cancer cells **metastasize,** or form new cancers in other places (Fig. 14.2).

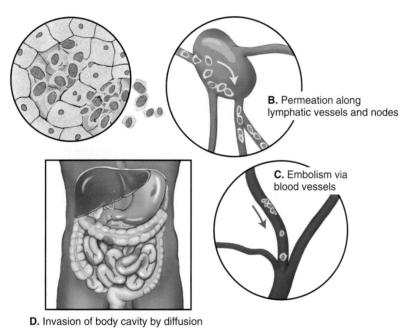

A. Direct extension into neighboring tissue

B. Permeation along lymphatic vessels and nodes

C. Embolism via blood vessels

D. Invasion of body cavity by diffusion

Figure 14.2 **Modes of metastasis of cancer. A,** Extension into neighboring tissue. **B,** Invasion of the lymphatic system. **C,** Picked up and spread to other parts by the blood. **D,** Invasion of a body cavity.

MATCH IT! **EXERCISE 2**

Match descriptions in the left column with either A or B.

___ **1.** anaplastic   **A.** benign tumor
___ **2.** metastatic   **B.** malignant tumor
___ **3.** not invasive
___ **4.** rapid growing
___ **5.** well-differentiated

WRITE IT **EXERCISE 3**

Using Fig. 14.2, describe four ways in which cancer metastasizes.

1. _____
2. _____
3. _____
4. _____

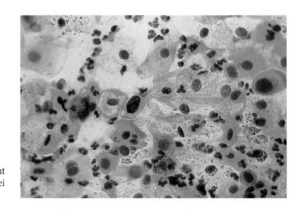

Figure 14.3 Malignant cells in a vaginal Papanicoloau smear. The nuclei of malignant cells have enlarged nuclei and have absorbed the pink stain, in contrast to the small nuclei of normal cells.

14-14 Pathologists distinguish between cells from benign tumors and cells of malignant tumors. One major difference is in the nuclei and cytoplasm. Whereas the nucleus of a benign cell is a small part of the total cell volume, many of the nuclei of malignant cells are greatly enlarged, and both the cytoplasm and nuclei vary in size and shape (Fig. 14.3).

Naming Tumors

benign

14-15 Tumors are named according to the cell type they resemble most. Benign tumors are generally named by adding -oma to the name for the cell type. For example, adenoma, chondroma, fibroma, and lipoma represent _____ tumors.

The names of malignant tumors generally are **sarcomas, carcinomas,** and **adenocarcinomas.** There are exceptions to these general rules, and some major exceptions are lymphomas and gliomas, both types of malignant tumors. Any name accompanied by terms such as metastatic or metastases is clearly malignant. Occasionally a tumor will have the name of the physician who first described it, such as Hodgkin's disease, Kaposi's sarcoma, or Ewing's sarcoma.

malignant

In general, the suffix -oma is used to name benign tumors, and sarcomas, carcinomas, and adenocarcinomas represent _____ tumors.

Staging and Grading Tumors

14-16 **Anatomical pathology** is the study of body structures. Anatomical pathologists assess the overall appearance of tissue samples and surgical specimens sent to the anatomy laboratory before selecting samples for further study. Histology technicians prepare and stain sections of body tissue on glass slides so that pathologists and histologic technologists can study the cellular makeup of the stained tissue. Special staining techniques aid in the study of cellular components. **Cytopathology** studies free cells or tissue fragments after staining.

Pathologists study the microscopic appearance of tumor cells and use a **malignancy grading system** that is based on the cells' maturity or differentiation. The **tumor's grade** indicates how much the cells appear different from their original form. Grade 1 cells are well differentiated, closely resembling the normal parent cell (sometimes called low-grade tumors). Grades 2 and 3 are moderately to poorly differentiated. Grade 4 tumors are so undifferentiated that their origin may be difficult to determine.

differentiated

Of the four grades for malignant tumors, Grade 1 cells are well _____ and closely resemble the normal parent cell.

14-17 After clinical assessment of the tumor (physical examination, diagnostic procedures, sometimes surgical exploration, and histological examination), tumors are classified on the basis of microscopic appearance, tissue of origin, and extent of spread. **Cancer staging** describes the exact location, size, and extent that a malignant tumor has spread, and is used to plan treatment and predict prognosis.

Some systems also use I to IV or alphabetically A to D; however, the American Joint Committee for Cancer Staging and End Results developed the TNM staging system. Reporting uses the following initials for cancer staging:
- T (**t**umor size)
- N (regional lymph **n**ode involvement)
- M (distant **m**etastases)

staging

size

Subscripts in each category indicate the degree of dissemination. According to this system $T_1N_0M_0$ designates a small **localized tumor** (not spreading), whereas $T_4N_3M_3$ is a very large lesion involving regional nodes and distant sites. Cancer _____ describes the location, size, and extent of the tumor spread.

In the TNM staging system, T stands for _____ of the tumor, N represents the regional lymph node involvement, and M stands for distant metastases.

WRITE IT! EXERCISE 4

Write a word in each blank to complete the following sentences

1. Adenomas, chondromas, and fibromas represent _____ tumors.

2. Sarcomas and carcinomas are types of _____ tumors.

3. The tumor's _____ indicates how much the cells appear unlike their original form.

4. Cancer _____ describes the location, size, and extent that the tumor has spread.

DIAGNOSTIC TESTS AND PROCEDURES

14-18 The American Cancer Society (ACS; www.cancer.org) has listed some general signs and symptoms of cancer of which you should be aware. But remember, having any of these does not mean you have cancer. (For example, an unexplained weight loss of 8 or 10 pounds may or may not be the first sign of cancer.) Looking at the list, hyper/pigmentation is a darkening of the skin.

Individuals who have a high risk of lung cancer sometimes have low-dose computed tomography (LDCT) scanning of the chest to detect early lesions.

KEY POINT ACS general cancer signs and symptoms include unexplained weight loss, persistent fever, fatigue that doesn't get better with rest, pain that does not go away with treatment, and skin changes such as hyperpigmentation, jaundice, erythema, pruritis, and excessive hair growth.

core

14-19 Biopsy of a suspicious lesion is often necessary. This includes **endoscopic biopsy,** for example samples removed from suspicious polyps that may be removed during a colonoscopy.

Instead of excising tissue, sometimes a **core needle biopsy** is performed, one in which a needle is used to extract a small amount of tissue from a tumor for study. A biopsy that uses a core needle to extract the tissue is called a _____ needle biopsy.

spread

14-20 A **sentinel lymph node biopsy** (SNB) is performed to determine if cancer, especially breast cancer, has spread to the nearby lymph nodes, whereby it may metastasize to other organs. This test to identify the sentinel node is performed by injecting dye or radioisotope, a radioactive form of an element, into the tumor site, then tracking the dye's path in the underarm (axillary) lymph nodes to identify the sentinel (first) node(s), the first in the axillary chain and most likely to contain metastases of breast cancer. The node is removed and biopsied; the tumor has not metastasized or _____ if the sentinel node is negative for tumor cells (Fig. 14.4).

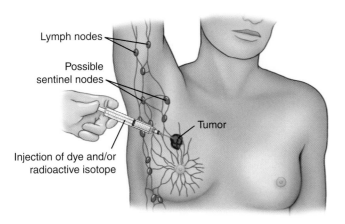

Lymph nodes

Possible sentinel nodes

Tumor

Injection of dye and/or radioactive isotope

Figure 14.4 Sentinel lymph node biopsy. Dye or radioisotope is injected into the tumor site and tracked to the axillary nodes to identify the sentinel (first) lymph node. The breast cancer has not spread if the sentinel node is negative for tumor cells.

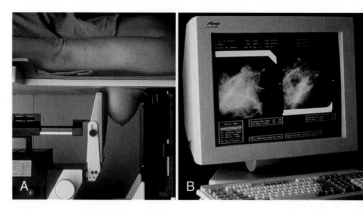

Figure 14.5 **Stereotactic breast biopsy.** This technique combines mammography and computer-assisted biopsy. **A,** Prone positioning of the patient. **B,** Digital mammogram. The exact location of the lesion is shown on the digital mammogram and is used for placement of the biopsy needle to obtain the specimen.

stereotactic

14-21 Radiography may reveal suspicious areas that look different than the surrounding tissue, since tumor tissue is usually more dense than surrounding healthy tissue. Mammography is especially useful in early detection of breast cancer. **Stereotactic mammography** uses 3-D breast imaging to perform a needle breast biopsy and differentiate a benign from a malignant lesion, assisting in locating the lesion and placement of the needle (Fig. 14.5). This special type of mammography is called _____ mammography.

cytology

14-22 A Pap smear to detect cancer of the uterine cervix or vagina is an example of **exfoliative cytology,** where cells are scraped from a region and examined. Exfoliative pertains to the peeling or sloughing off of tissue cells. Exfoliative _____ is the microscopic examination of sloughed off cells for diagnostic purposes.

marrow

14-23 A **bone marrow biopsy,** aspiration of bone marrow fluid using a needle, followed by a microscopic tissue examination is used to diagnose a number of conditions, including leukemia, lymphoma, leukemia, and multiple myeloma. In a bone marrow biopsy, the fluid studied is bone _____.

marker

14-24 **Tumor marker tests,** also called **biomarkers,** measure the levels of biochemical substances in the body (in the blood, urine, or body tissues) that may be associated with the presence of a certain types of cancer. The tumor markers are the tumor substances in the body that may be associated with cancer. These tests, tumor _____ tests are used in combination with other cancer tests. Examples include PSA (prostate specific antigen) in which increased levels may be due to prostate cancer or BPH (benign prostatic hypertrophy), so other tests are indicated for diagnosis (Fig. 14.6).

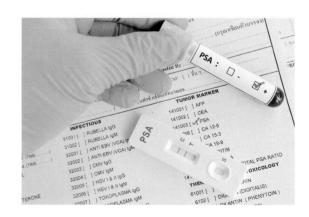

Figure 14.6 PSA test for prostate cancer screening and diagnosis.

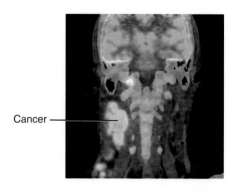

Cancer

Figure 14.7 **High resolution PET scan.** Providing information about the metabolism of an internal structure, this PET scan shows neck cancer (arrow).

14-25 CT, MRI, as well as nuclear medicine scans provide information about a tumor's size, shape, and location. **Nuclear medicine imaging,** using injected, ingested, or inhaled radioactive material and a scanning device is also called **radionuclide organ imaging.** These tests are particularly helpful in locating and staging cancer of the bone and the thyroid.

A PET scan provides information about the metabolism, size, and shape of an internal structure (Fig. 14.7). SPECT (single-photon emission computed tomography), a variation of CT, uses a rotating camera and radioactive substances to create 3-D images, and is especially useful in identifying bone metastases (Fig. 14.8). This special type of computed tomography is abbreviated _____.

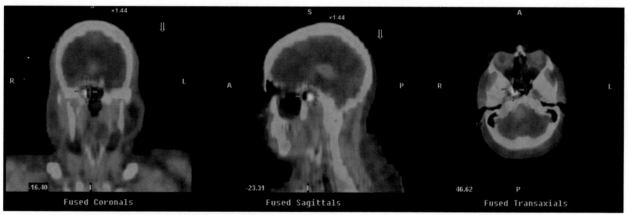

Fused Coronals   Fused Sagittals   Fused Transaxials

Figure 14.8 **SPECT imaging of the brain.** The radioactivity measures the blood flow that indirectly indicates metabolic activity, with higher metabolic activity indicated by the yellow-orange color. This computer generated image is not as sharp as a regular photograph.

14-26 Radioimmunoassay (RIA) is an in vitro test that is used to determine the concentration of proteins in a patient's blood. It involves the injection of radioactively labeled substance that reacts with a particular protein.

A **radioisotope scan** shows the concentration of a radioisotope in a body site, such as the thyroid gland, brain or kidney. Radioisotopes may be administered intravenously or orally. In a thyroid scan, an iodine **radionuclide** (isotope that undergoes radioactive decay, thus emitting energy that

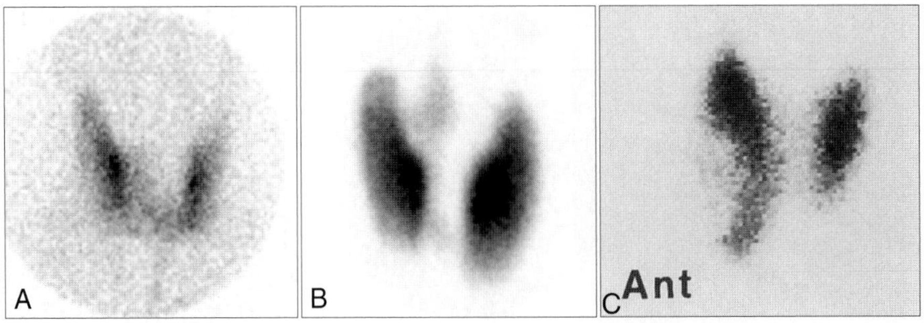

Figure 14.9 **Comparison of thyroid scans. A,** A normal thyroid scan. **B,** A "hot nodule" which shows increased uptake of iodine, indicating an active nodule, probably benign. **C,** A "cold nodule" indicates decreased uptake, a common occurrence when malignancy is present.

iodine

is measurable with a detector) is administered orally or intravenously, the thyroid absorbs the radionuclide and the scan reveals the size and position of the thyroid gland (Fig. 14.9). The radionuclide used in a thyroid scan is _____ radionuclide.

In contrast, a **radioactive iodine uptake** (RAIU) test assesses the function of the thyroid by giving the patient radioactive iodine (which is absorbed by the thyroid gland more readily than other tissues) and a sensor is placed over the thyroid. The thyroid function test which uses a sensor to detect radioactive iodine in the thyroid gland is called a radioactive iodine

uptake

_____ test.

WRITE IT!   **EXERCISE 5**

Write a word in each blank space to complete these sentences.

1. A Pap smear to detect cancer of the uterine cervix or vagina is an example of _____ cytology.

2. A radioactive iodine uptake test assesses the function of the _____.

3. An isotope that undergoes radioactive decay, emitting measurable energy is a/an _____.

4. Bone marrow _____, aspiration of bone marrow and microscopic tissue examination, is helpful in diagnosing leukemia and other bone marrow diseases.

5. Determining the concentration of proteins in the blood using an in vitro test is _____.

6. Nuclear medicine _____ uses injected, ingested, or inhaled radioactive material and a scanning device.

7. Single-photon _____ computed tomography uses a rotating camera and radioactive substances.

8. Stereotactic _____ uses 3-D breast images to perform a needle breast biopsy.

9. Tumor _____ are the tumor substances in the body that may be associated with cancer.

10. Using a core needle to extract a small amount of tissue from a tumor is called a core needle _____.

PATHOLOGIES

14-27 Cancer is a group of hundreds of diseases, and each cancer is distinguished by the site, nature, or cause of the lesion. Incidence of different kinds of cancer varies greatly with gender, age, geographic location, and ethnic group. Early signs of cancer may include anorexia (lack of appetite), fatigue, bruising, and wasting.

Table 14.4 Selected Examples of Cancer

Circulatory System (Chapter 4)
Cardiovascular (cardi[o], heart; vascul[o], vessel)
  blood-forming tissue: leukemias (leuk[o], white; -emia, blood)
  bone marrow: multiple myeloma (myel[o], bone marrow; -oma, tumor)
  blood vessel tissue: angiosarcoma (angi[o], vessel)
  lymphatics/immune: Hodgkin lymphoma, non-Hodgkin lymphoma
  thymus: malignant thymoma
Respiratory System (Chapter 5)
  epithelial tissue of respiratory tract, lung, bronchus: adenocarcinoma of the lung, small cell carcinoma,
    mesothelioma, bronchogenic carcinoma (aden[o], gland; carcin[o], cancer; bronch[o]), bronchus; -genic,
    produced in)
Gastrointestinal (Chapter 6) (gastr[o], stomach)
  adenocarcinoma of the esophagus, stomach, colon, pancreas, and/or rectum
Urinary (Chapter 7) (urin[o], urine)
  kidney: nephroma/renal cell carcinoma, Wilms tumor/nephroblastoma (nephr[o], ren[o], kidney; blast[o],
    immature)
  bladder: bladder cancer
Reproductive System (Female, Chapter 8)
  ovaries: ovarian carcinoma
  uterus: endometrial carcinoma (endo-, inside; metr[o], uterine tissue)
  uterine cervix: squamous cell carcinoma of the cervix
Reproductive System (Male, Chapter 8)
  prostate: prostatic cancer
  testis: adenocarcinoma of the testes, seminoma, teratoma (semin[o], semen)
Musculoskeletal (Chapter 9) (muscul[o], muscle)
  bone: Ewing sarcoma, osteosarcoma (oste[o], bone)
  cartilage: chondrosarcoma (chondr[o], cartilage; sarcoma, malignant tumor)
  muscle: leiomyosarcoma (my[o], muscle)
Nervous System (Chapter 10)
  CNS: glioblastoma multiforme (gli[o], neuroglia; blast[o], embryonic form; multi-, many)
Special Sense Organs (Chapter 11)
  eyes: retinoblastoma (retin[o], retina)
Endocrine (Chapter 12)
  thyroid: thyroid carcinoma
Integumentary, skin (Chapter 13)
  basal cell carcinoma, squamous cell carcinoma, malignant melanoma, Kaposi sarcoma

Some warning signs of cancer are sores that don't heal or unusual bleeding, changes in a wart or mole, changes in bowel or bladder function, a lump under the tissue, persistent hoarseness or cough, chronic indigestion, or what is perceived as bone pain located on only one side. During the physical examination of the body systems, the physician examines areas in which lymph nodes are accessible (side of the neck, for example). The patient may be aware of "lumps," which can be extremely important as signs of infection or possible malignancy. It is important to know that not all enlarged lymph nodes are pathological (for example, a small cervical or submandibular node may be normal or result from a respiratory infection).

Premalignant (precancerous) skin lesions are not yet cancerous, but may become cancerous over time and continued exposure to sunlight or irritation. Watch for skin cancer by being particularly careful about changes in a wart or _____.

mole

Review Table 14.4 for examples of cancer associated with body systems presented in this book.

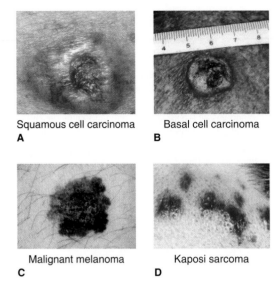

Squamous cell carcinoma
A

Basal cell carcinoma
B

Malignant melanoma
C

Kaposi sarcoma
D

Figure 14.10 Examples of skin cancer lesions. A, Squamous cell carcinoma. **B,** Basal cell carcinoma. **C,** Malignant melanoma. **D,** Kaposi sarcoma of AIDS.

14-28 Table 14.4 includes basal and squamous cell carcinomas, but metastases of these two types of skin cancer are rare. However, local invasion destroys underlying and adjacent tissue, and occurs most frequently in sun-exposed areas of the body, such as the face, scalp, and ears; so removal is recommended. An annual skin examination is recommended, and have suspicious growths examined by a dermatologist. The two types of skin cancer in which metastasis is rare are basal and _____ cell carcinoma.

squamous

🔑 **KEY** POINT **Basal cell carcinoma** is a malignant epithelial cell tumor that begins as a papule and enlarges peripherally, but metastasis is rare. **Squamous cell carcinoma** is a slow-growing malignant tumor of squamous epithelium (flattened scalelike tissue cells). Local invasion of either type of tumor destroys underlying and adjacent tissue.

14-29 Malignant melanoma is a tumor originating from melanocytes and is related to sun or ultraviolet light exposure. It may metastasize and is among the most malignant of all skin cancers. Melanoma is rare in blacks, and races with little skin pigment are most susceptible. About one-third to one half of all malignant melanomas originate in preexisting lesions (for example, freckles and preexisting moles). Learn the ABCDE rule for self-detection of skin cancer:

- A   asymmetry (growths that look lopsided)
- B   border (that are irregular)
- C   color (changes in the color of a mole or appearance of multiple colors)
- D   diameter (larger than a pencil eraser, $\frac{1}{4}$ inch in diameter)
- E   elevation (raised above the skin and has an uneven appearance) or evolution (change in the look or feel of the lesion over time)

one-fourth

In other words, examine skin growths for asymmetry, irregular borders, changes in the color, growths larger than _____ inch, and look different over time. Have all new growths examined by a dermatologist. How many of the ABCDE's can you see? (Fig. 14.10)

🔑 **KEY** POINT Remember these three types of skin cancers: basal cell carcinoma, squamous cell carcinoma, and melanoma. Metastasis of the first two types of skin cancer listed is rare.

MATCH IT!

EXERCISE 6

Match these types of cancer with the correct body system.

_____	**1.** adenocarcinoma of the stomach	_____	**10.** osteosarcoma	**A.** circulatory
_____	**2.** basal cell carcinoma	_____	**11.** ovarian carcinoma	**B.** endocrine
_____	**3.** bladder cancer	_____	**12.** prostatic cancer	**C.** gastrointestinal
_____	**4.** endometrial carcinoma	_____	**13.** retinoblastoma	**D.** integumentary
_____	**5.** gliobastoma multiforme	_____	**14.** seminoma	**E.** musculoskeletal
_____	**6.** leukemia	_____	**15.** small cell lung cancer	**F.** nervous system
_____	**7.** melanoma	_____	**16.** thymoma	**G.** reproductive
_____	**8.** mesothelioma	_____	**17.** thyroid cancer	**H.** respiratory
_____	**9.** nephroma			**I.** special sense organs
				J. urinary

WRITE IT!

EXERCISE 7

Write the ABCDE term that corresponds to the following descriptions:

1. A: for _____, growths that look lopsided

2. B: for _____, growths that are irregular

3. C: for changes in the _____ of a mole or appearance of multiple hues

4. D: for _____, should be no larger than a pencil eraser, $\frac{1}{4}$ inch in diameter

5. E: _____, looks or feels different over time

SURGICAL AND THERAPEUTIC INTERVENTIONS

remission

14-30 Remission, whether spontaneous or the result of therapy, is the disappearance of the characteristics of a malignant tissue. The disappearance of the characteristics of malignant tissue is called _____.

14-31 Three major methods of treating cancer are:
- surgical excision
- radiation therapy
- systemic or biological therapy (chemotherapy, bone marrow transplant and immunotherapy)

excision

Surgical excision is the primary treatment for cancer; however, cancer removal requires the cancer to be small and present in only one organ that can be removed (in other words, the cancer has not spread). **Surgical biopsy** of the following may be successful at stopping cancer if it has not spread: skin, stomach, colon, lung, breast, and uterus. Therefore, when possible, the primary way to remove cancer is surgical _____.

Resection is excision of a significant part of an organ plus surrounding tissue that contains lymph nodes, whereas **exenteration** is extensive surgical removal of the tumor, its origin, and all surrounding tissue; evisceration. Exenteration is more extensive than resection.

debulking

14-32 Debulking is sometimes used to remove as much of a tumor's primary mass as possible, followed by radiation and/or chemotherapy to prevent further spread. Write this term that means excision of part of a bulky tumor to reduce its size when it's not possible to remove all of it: _____.

breast

14-33 A **simple mast/ectomy** is removal of a cancerous _____, whereas a **radical mastectomy** is the removal of a cancerous breast, along with the lymph nodes, and the underlying muscle. A **lump/ectomy** is removal of the tumor only.

burning

14-34 Cauterization is burning tissue to destroy it, using a chemical, dry ice, or laser. Cauterization is _____ tissue to destroy it. The use of subfreezing temperatures to destroy tissue is **cryosurgery.**

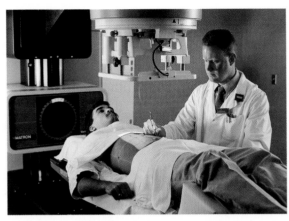

Figure 14.11 **Male patient being prepared to receive radiation therapy.** The external beam of radiation is generated by the equipment.

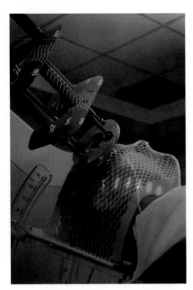

Figure 14.12 **Patient receiving radiotherapy treatments for brain cancer.**

14-35 Radiotherapy, also called radiation therapy, is the treatment of neoplastic disease by using x-rays or gamma rays to destroy malignant cells (Figs. 14.11 and 14.12). Some cancers are treated solely with radiation, but radiation is sometimes done before surgical removal to shrink the tumor or after excision of the tumor.

The goal of radiotherapy is to deliver a maximum dose of radiation to the tumor tissue and a minimal dose to the surrounding normal tissue. Cancerous tumors that are destroyed by radiation are said to be **radiosensitive,** whereas those that are not affected are **radioresistant.** Radiotherapy is another term for _____ therapy.

radiation

14-36 When **fractionation** is used in radiology, radiation is administered in smaller units over time to minimize tissue damage compared to a single large dose. Write this term that is used when radiation is administered several times in smaller units: _____

fractionation

14-37 A **linear accelerator** (LINAC) is an apparatus used in radiology that accelerates charged subatomic particles to deliver supervoltage x-rays for radiotherapy (Fig. 14.13). Write this new term that is abbreviated LINAC: linear _____.

accelerator

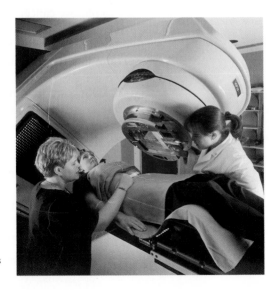

Figure 14.13 Linear accelerator. Also called photon therapy, since it uses photon beams produced by a linear accelerator.

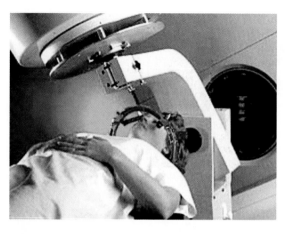

Figure 14.14 **Stereotactic radiosurgery.** The stereotactic frame holds the head in a fixed position.

brachytherapy

14-38 Brachy/therapy, internal radiotherapy, is implantation of radiation seeds or beads of radioactive material directly into the tumor or a cavity of the tumor, and these may be temporary or permanent. Write the name of this type of cancer therapy that uses radioactive beds or seeds: _____.

stereotactic

14-39 Stereotactic radiosurgery (gamma knife stereotactic surgery) delivers a large dose of radiation from several different angles to treat small intracranial tumors or to destroy a vascular abnormality (arteriovenous malformation in the brain) (Fig. 14.14). Write this term for gamma knife surgery: _____ radiosurgery.

chemicals

14-40 Chemotherapy is the use of _____ to treat cancer and is included in the next section of this book, *Pharmacology.* Chemotherapy may be used alone or in combination with radiation and/or surgery (Fig. 14.15). Many agents used in chemotherapy can be injected intravenously; in addition, various types of catheters may be used.

WORD ORIGIN
apheresis
aphaeresis (Gk.),
removal

apheresis

14-41 Apheresis (sometimes called **hemapheresis**) is a procedure in which blood is temporarily withdrawn, one or more components are selectively removed, and the rest of the blood is returned (reinfused) to the patient. This process is used in treating various diseases, such as leukemia, and also for procuring blood elements from donors. Write this term that means the procedure where blood is temporarily withdrawn, certain components are removed, and the rest of the blood is returned to the patient or donor: _____.

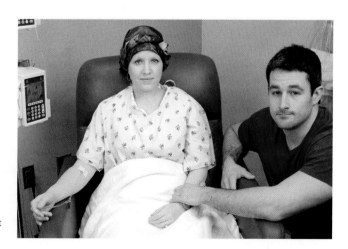

Figure 14.15 **Chemotherapy.** Patient receives chemotherapy to treat breast cancer.

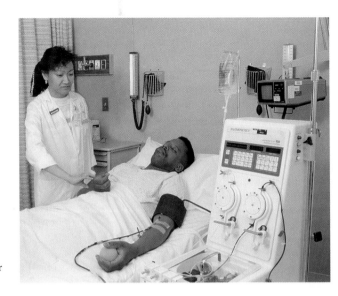

Figure 14.16 Patient on a blood pheresis machine. He is being treated for leukemia and excess leukocytes are being removed.

14-42 The apheresis department in a hospital commonly processes platelets, leukocytes, and plasma. Apheresis often shortened to pheresis, involving these blood components are **platelet/pheresis, leuk/apheresis,** and **plasma/pheresis,** respectively. (Note that the *a* is omitted when forming some terms with apheresis.) An excess of a patient's leukocytes can be removed. For example, leuka/pheresis is a process in which blood is withdrawn, _____

white

blood cells (leukocytes) are removed, and the remaining blood is reinfused into the donor (Fig. 14.16).

Plateletpheresis involves collection of platelets from a donor using apheresis. The platelets are then infused into a patient who has thrombocyto/penia, which you remember is a deficiency of blood _____.

platelets

Plasmapheresis is removal of plasma from the blood; however, in this procedure, the blood is withdrawn from the donor and it then receives special treatment to replace the plasma with saline (an isotonic solution). This treatment concentrates and separates out the red blood cells, which can be given to a patient who needs red blood cells but not whole blood.

14-43 Biological therapy includes bone marrow transplant and immunotherapy, both using the body's own defenses to fight cancer. A **bone marrow transplant** (BMT) may use bone marrow from a matching donor to stimulate normal blood cell growth in specific types of leukemia. Bone marrow is ideally harvested from the donor on the day it is infused into the patient. BMT means bone marrow _____.

transplant

14-44 Immunotherapy is the use of immunostimulants and immunosuppressants to prevent and treat disease. This includes the transfer of immunocompetent cells from one person to another. **Stem cell transplantation** is collection of stem cells from a compatible donor and administration to a recipient. Patients with certain malignancies are candidates for this procedure. Both patient and recipient undergo conditioning processes before donation or receiving the stem cells. In autologous stem cell transplantion, the patient's own stem cells are collected, then reinfused after chemotherapy.

Collection of stem cells, then administration to a recipient, is called stem cell

transplantation

_____.

> **BEYOND** THE BLUEPRINT Historically, the major players in cancer therapy has been radiotherapy, chemotherapy and surgery – but immunotherapy is becoming an important part of cancer treatment. There are times when immunotherapy will be used alone, and sometimes it will be used in conjunction with other therapies. The Food and Drug Administration recently approved an immunotherapy drug that stimulates the body's immune system for the treatment of metastatic non–small-cell lung cancer. In other words, the drug could be the first treatment that a patient receives for the disease, instead of chemotherapy.

WRITE IT! EXERCISE 8

Write words in the blanks to complete these sentences.
1. The disappearance of the characteristics of malignant tissue is _____.
2. The primary method of treating a small tumor that has not spread is _____.
3. Excision of a significant part of an organ plus surrounding tissue and less extensive than exenteration is _____.
4. Removing as much of a tumor's primary mass when unable to remove all of the tumor is _____.
5. Removal of a cancerous breast is _____.
6. Removal of only the tumor in breast cancer is _____.
7. Burning tissue to destroy it is _____.
8. Describing a cancerous tumor that is destroyed by radiation is _____.
9. Administering smaller units of radiation to minimize tissue damage is _____.
10. Internal radiation by implanting radioactive material is _____.
11. Hemapheresis is often shortened to _____.
12. The use of immunostimulants and immunosuppressants to prevent and treat disease is _____.

WRITE IT! EXERCISE 9

List three traditional methods of treating cancer.
1. _____
2. _____
3. _____

PHARMACEUTICS

Chemotherapy is the use of drugs to treat cancer. Ideally, the cytotoxic drug selectively kills large numbers of tumor cells without harming healthy cells. These chemotherapeutic agents are often used in combination with other cancer treatments, such as radiation therapy.

Certain vaccinations can reduce the risk of developing cancer associated with specific chronic infections: hepatitis B vaccine and human papilloma virus (HPV) vaccine.

Antineoplastic/Cytotoxic/Chemotherapeutic Agents: Destroy or inhibit growth of cancerous cells. Subclasses include alkylating agents, anthracyclines, antimetabolites, terpenoids, plant alkaloids, topoisomerase inhibitors, and monoclonal antibodies

cisplatin (Platinol)	melphalan (Alkeran)	tamoxifen (Soltamox)
cyclophosphamide (Cytoxan)	methotrexate (Trexall)	vincristine (Oncovin)
doxorubicin (Doxil)	paclitaxel (Taxol)	
fluorouracil (Efudex)	rituximab (Rituxan)	

Immunosuppressants: Inhibit immune system

azathioprine (Imuran)	everolimus (Zortress)	mycophenolate (CellCept)
cyclosporine (Neoral)	glatiramer (Copaxone)	tacrolimus (Prograf)

Radiopharmaceuticals: Assess various internal functions (diagnostic) or treat certain cancers or tissue hyperfunction (therapeutic)

iodine-131 sodium iodide (Hicon)	technetium-99m MDP (Technescan MDP)	thallium-201 thallous chloride
samarium-153 lexidronam (Quadramet)	technetium-99m tetrofosmin (Myoview)	

WRITE IT! EXERCISE 10

Write words in the blanks to complete these sentences.
1. The use of drugs to treat cancer is _____.
2. Vaccines are currently available to prevent cancer from human _____ virus and hepatitis B.
3. Drugs that inhibit the immune system are called _____.
4. Radioactive substances used to assess or treat cancers or tissue hyperfunction are called _____.

CHAPTER ABBREVIATIONS

ACS	American Cancer Society	PSA	prostate-specific antigen
BPH	benign prostatic hypertrophy	RAIU	radioactive iodine uptake test
DNA	deoxyribonucleic acid	RIA	radioimmunoassay
HPV	human papilloma virus	SNB	sentinel node biopsy
LDCT	low dose computed tomography	SPECT	single photon emission computed tomography
LINAC	linear accelerator	TNM	staging system for cancer

A Career in Apheresis Nursing

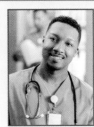

Charles is a nurse in the apheresis department of a large metropolitan hospital. His comprehensive nursing background and an extensive training program in the apheresis lab helped prepare him to assess patient and donor needs, monitor vital signs, and interpret them to recognize the early signs of adverse reactions. He transfuses blood and blood products and manages fluid volume in plasma exchange. One of the aspects of his job that he enjoys most is the daily communication with patients, donors, and other health care professionals.

Be Careful With These!

benign vs. *malignant neoplasms*   *cancer grading system* vs. *cancer staging system*   *carcinogen* vs. *carcinogenesis*   *primary cancer* vs. *metastatic cancer*

CHAPTER 14 SELF TEST

Work all of the following exercises to test your understanding of the material before checking your answers against those in Appendix IV.

BASIC UNDERSTANDING

Matching

I.   *Match tumor characteristics with either benign tumor (A) or malignant tumor (B).*

_____ **1.** cell nucleus is greatly enlarged   _____ **5.** name generally ends in -oma   **A.** benign tumor

_____ **2.** adenomas and fibromas   _____ **6.** adenocarcinomas and sarcomas   **B.** malignant tumor

_____ **3.** encapsulated   _____ **7.** slow growing

_____ **4.** invasive   _____ **8.** undifferentiated

II. *Match these tumors and the body system with which they are usually associated.*

_____ **1.** leukemia   _____ **9.** prostatic cancer   **A.** circulatory

_____ **2.** multiple myeloma   _____ **10.** seminoma   **B.** endocrine

_____ **3.** angiosarcoma   _____ **11.** teratoma   **C.** gastrointestinal

_____ **4.** mesothelioma   _____ **12.** glioblastoma multiforme   **D.** integumentary

_____ **5.** bronchogenic carcinoma   _____ **13.** retinoblastoma   **E.** musculoskeletal

_____ **6.** renal cell carcinoma   _____ **14.** thyroid carcinoma   **F.** nervous

_____ **7.** nephroblastoma   _____ **15.** basal cell carcinoma   **G.** respiratory

_____ **8.** endometrial carcinoma   _____ **16.** Kaposi sarcoma   **H.** reproductive

I. special sense organs

J. urinary

Listing

III. Write the ABCDE terms associated with skin cancer self-detection that correspond to the following descriptions of skin growths.

1. A for _____.

2. B for _____.

3. C for _____.

4. D for _____.

5. E for _____ or _____.

IV. Name four modes of metastasis of cancer.

1. _____

2. _____

3. _____

4. _____

V. Name three traditional methods of treating cancer.

1. _____

2. _____

3. _____

Using Vocabulary

VI. Circle the correct answer for each multiple choice question.

1. What is the developmental process whereby cells become different types of tissues? (carcinogenesis, cytopathology, differentiation, metastasis)

2. Which of the following measures the levels of biochemical substances in the body that may be associated with cancer? (tumor marker tests, exfoliative cytology, tumor metastasis, tumor grading)

3. Which of the following describes the location, size, and extent that the tumor has spread? (cancer anaplasia, cancer metastasis, cancer oncology, cancer staging)

4. Which of the following does a pathologist use to indicate how much the cells in a tissue appear different than their original form? (cytopathology, plasmapheresis, sentinel biopsy, tumor grading system)

5. Which of the following in vitro tests is used to determine the concentration of proteins in the blood? (radioimmunoassay, thyroid scan, tumor grading, radionuclide organ imaging)

6. Which of the following is a noninvasive surgery that uses gamma radiation to destroy a brain tumor? (gamma knife radiation, excision, exenteration, lumpectomy)

7. Which of the following is a variation of computed tomography? (needle biopsy, SNB, SPECT, stereotactic mammography)

8. Which of the following is considered the most malignant of all skin cancers? (basal cell carcinoma, chondrosarcoma, malignant melanoma, squamous cell carcinoma)

9. Which of the following procedures uses 3-D breast imaging? (PSA test, stereotactic mammography, tumor grading, tumor marker tests)

10. Which of the following represents examination of the first lymph node that receives drainage from a primary tumor? (core exfoliative cytology, needle biopsy, endoscopic biopsy, sentinel lymph node biopsy)

11. Which of the following substances is associated with prostate cancer? (ACS, HPV, PSA, TNM)

12. Which of the letters in the TNM system represent the regional lymph node involvement? (T, N, M, none of the letters)

13. Which ranking does cancer have among causes of death in the United States (first, second, third, fourth)

14. Which term means a change in the structure and orientation of cells and reversion to a more primitive form? (anaplasia, invasion, metastasis, permeation)

15. Which term means selective removal of blood components and reinfusing the rest of the patient's blood? (apheresis, differentiation, fractionation, resection)

Writing Terms

VII. Write words for each of the following clues.

1. administraton of smaller doses of radiaton over time _____
2. capable of being changed by reacting to radioactive emissions _____
3. disappearance of malignant tissue characteristics _____
4. excision of a significant part of an organ _____
5. internal radiation by implanting radioactive material _____
6. process by which cells become cancer cells _____
7. removal of a cancerous breast _____
8. removal of only the primary mass of a tumor _____
9. the use of chemicals to treat cancer _____
10. unchanged or not affected by radioactive emissions _____

GREATER UNDERSTANDING

Health Care Reporting

VIII. Select terms from the report to complete the blanks that follow the report.

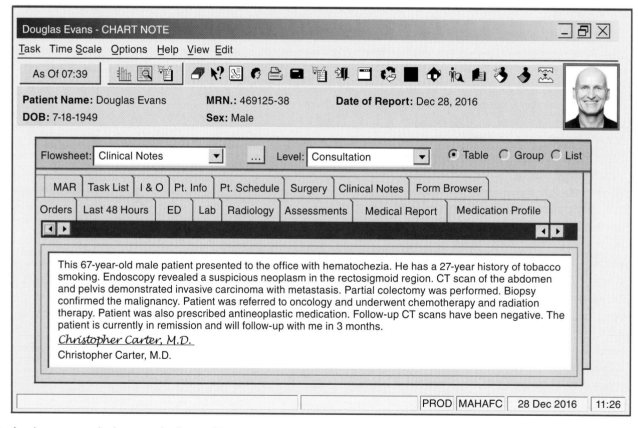

1. An alternate term in the report for "cancer" is _____ .
2. Two terms in the report that refer to the spread of a cancer to other areas of the body are *invasive* and _____ .
3. The term from the report that indicates that the patient is currently free of cancer-related symptoms is _____ .
4. Which term is a cancer treatment using chemicals? _____ .
5. Which term from the report means a new growth? _____ .

IX. Read the sentences that follow the report and write "T" for True or "F" for False.

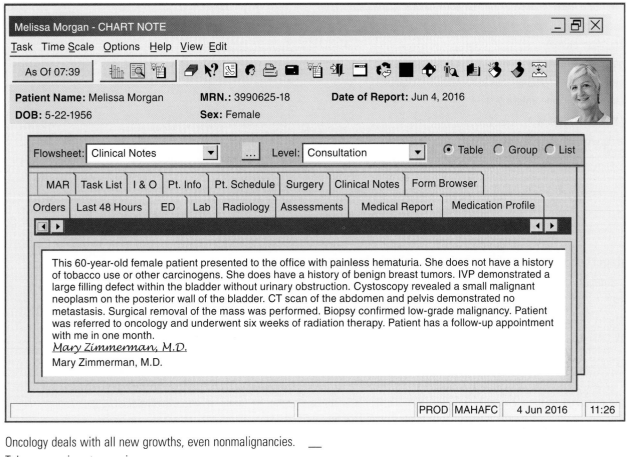

| Melissa Morgan - CHART NOTE | ▬ ⬜ ✕ |

Task Time Scale Options Help View Edit

As Of 07:39

Patient Name: Melissa Morgan   **MRN.:** 3990625-18   **Date of Report:** Jun 4, 2016
DOB: 5-22-1956   **Sex:** Female

Flowsheet: Clinical Notes ▼   …   Level: Consultation ▼   ⦿ Table ○ Group ○ List

| MAR | Task List | I & O | Pt. Info | Pt. Schedule | Surgery | Clinical Notes | Form Browser |

| Orders | Last 48 Hours | ED | Lab | Radiology | Assessments | Medical Report | Medication Profile |

This 60-year-old female patient presented to the office with painless hematuria. She does not have a history of tobacco use or other carcinogens. She does have a history of benign breast tumors. IVP demonstrated a large filling defect within the bladder without urinary obstruction. Cystoscopy revealed a small malignant neoplasm on the posterior wall of the bladder. CT scan of the abdomen and pelvis demonstrated no metastasis. Surgical removal of the mass was performed. Biopsy confirmed low-grade malignancy. Patient was referred to oncology and underwent six weeks of radiation therapy. Patient has a follow-up appointment with me in one month.
Mary Zimmerman, M.D.
Mary Zimmerman, M.D.

| | | PROD | MAHAFC | 4 Jun 2016 | 11:26 |

1. Oncology deals with all new growths, even nonmalignancies. __

2. Tobacco use is not a carcinogen. __

3. Malignant cancers can also be termed benign. __

4. Radiotherapy is an alternate term for radiation therapy. __

5. Radiology is the study of tumors. __

Pronouncing Terms

X. Write the correct term for the following phonetic spellings.

1. an-uh-**plā**-zhuh _____

2. kaw-tur-i-**zā**-shun _____

3. muh-**tas**-tuh-sīz _____

4. ong-**kol**-uh-jē _____

5. rā-dē-ō-fahr-muh-**sōo**-ti-kul _____

6. ster-ē-ō-**tak**-tik _____

Spelling

XI. Circle all incorrectly spelled terms and write the correct spelling.

anaplasia   exfoliative   radioimunoassay   remision   sitopathology

Abbreviating

XII. Write a letter in each blank that corresponds to the clue.

1. deoxyribonucleic acid __ __ __

2. linear accelerator __ __ __ __ __

3. nonmalignant, noninflammatory prostate enlargement __ __ __

4. prostatic protein (sometimes associated with cancer) __ __ __

5. radioactive iodine uptake test __ __ __ __

6. radioimmunoassay __ __ __

Using Pharmacologic Terms

XIII. Select descriptions from the right column that define terms in the left column.

_____ **1.** antineoplastics	**A.**	drugs that inhibit new growth of cells
_____ **2.** chemotherapy	**B.**	drugs that inhibit the immune system
_____ **3.** immunosuppressants	**C.**	using drugs to treat cancer

Categorizing Terms and Practicing Pronunciation

XIV. Categorize the terms by selecting A, B, C, D, or E.

_____ **1.** cauterization	_____ **6.** mastectomy	**A.**	anatomy
_____ **2.** bone marrow biopsy	_____ **7.** sentinel node	**B.**	diagnostic test or procedure
_____ **3.** fractionation	_____ **8.** radioimmunoassay	**C.**	pathology
_____ **4.** immunosuppressant	_____ **9.** radioisotope scan	**D.**	surgery
_____ **5.** leukapheresis	_____ **10.** sarcoma	**E.**	nonsurgical therapy

(Be prepared to pronounce terms 1-10 in class after listening to Chapter 14 terms at *http://evolve.elsevier.com/Leonard/building/*. In addition, practice categorizing all boldface terms in this chapter.)

BMV LIST

Visit *http://evolve.elsevier.com/Leonard/building/* to listen to the boldface terms in Chapter 14. Look closely at the spelling of each term as it is pronounced.

adenocarcinoma (ad-uh-nō-kahr-si-**nō**-muh)
anaplasia (an-uh-**plā**-zhuh)
anatomical pathology (an-uh-**tom**-i-kul puh-**thol**-uh-jē)
antineoplastic (an-tē-nē-ō-**plas**-tik)
apheresis (af-uh-**rē**-sis)
basal cell carcinoma (**bā**-sul sel kahr-si-**nō**-muh)
biomarkers (**bī**-ō-mahr-kurz)
bone marrow biopsy (bōn **mar**-ō **bī**-op-sē)
bone marrow transplant (bōn **mar**-ō **trans**-plant)
brachytherapy (brak-ē-**ther**-uh-pē)
cancer staging (**kan**-sur **stā**-jing)
carcinogen (kahr-**sin**-uh-jen)
carcinogenesis (kahr-si-nō-**jen**-uh-sis)
carcinoma (kahr-si-**nō**-muh)
cauterization (kaw-tur-i-**zā**-shun)
chemotherapeutic (kē-mō-ther-uh-**pū**-tik)
chemotherapy (kē-mō-**ther**-uh-pē)
core needle biopsy (kor **nē**-dul **bī**-op-sē)
cryosurgery (crī-ō-**sur**-jur-ē)
cytopathology (sī-tō-puh-**thol**-uh-jē)
cytotoxic (sī-tō-**tok**-sik)
debulking (dē-**bulk**-ing)
differentiation (dif-ur-en-shē-**ā**-shun)

endoscopic biopsy (en-dō-**skop**-ik **bī**-op-sē)
exenteration (ek-sen-tur-**ā**-shun)
exfoliative cytology (eks-**fō**-lē-uh-tiv sī-**tol**-uh-jē)
fractionation (frak-shun-**ā**-shun)
hemapheresis (hē-muh-fuh-**rē**-sis)
immunosuppressant (im-ū-nō-suh-**pres**-unt)
immunotherapy (im-ū-nō-**ther**-uh-pē)
leukapheresis (loo-kuh-fuh-**rē**-sis)
linear accelerator (**lin**-ē-ur ak-**sel**-ur-ā-tur)
localized tumor (**lō**-kul-īzd **too**-mur)
lumpectomy (lum-**pek**-tuh-mē)
malignancy grading system (muh-**lig**-nun-sē **grād**-ing **sis**-tum)
malignant melanoma (muh-**lig**-nunt mel-uh-**nō**-muh)
malignant tumor (muh-**lig**-nunt **too**-mur)
metastasis (muh-**tas**-tuh-sis)
metastasize (muh-**tas**-tuh-sīz)
metastatic cancer (met-uh-**stat**-ik **kan**-sur)
neoplasm (**nē**-ō-plaz-um)
nuclear medicine imaging (**noo**-klē-ur **med**-i-sin **im**-uh-jing)
oncology (ong-**kol**-uh-jē)
plasmapheresis (plaz-muh-fuh-**rē**-sis)
plateletpheresis (plāt-lut-fuh-**rē**-sis)

primary carcinoma (**prī**-mar-ē kahr-si-**nō**-muh)
primary tumor (**prī**-mar-ē **too**-mur)
radical mastectomy (**rad**-i-kul mas-**tek**-tuh-mē)
radioactive iodine uptake test (rā-dē-ō-**ak**-tiv **ī**-ō-dīn **up**-tāk test)
radioimmunoassay (rā-dē-ō-im-ū-nō-**as**-ā)
radioisotope scan (rā-dē-ō-**ī**-suh-tōp skan)
radionuclide (rā-dē-ō-**noo**-klīd)
radionuclide organ imaging (rā-dē-ō-**noo**-klīd **or**-gun **im**-uh-jing)
radiopharmaceutical (rā-dē-ō-fahr-muh-**soo**-ti-kul)
radioresistant (rā-dē-ō-rē-**zis**-tunt)
radiosensitive (rā-dē-ō-**sen**-si-tiv)
radiotherapy (rā-dē-ō-**ther**-uh-pē)

remission (rē-**mish**-un)
resection (rē-**sek**-shun)
sarcoma (sahr-**kō**-muh)
sentinel lymph node biopsy (**sen**-ti-nul limf nōd **bī**-op-sē)
simple mastectomy (**sim**-pul mas-**tek**-tuh-mē)
squamous cell carcinoma (**skwā**-mus sel kahr-si-**nō**-muh)
stem cell transplantation (stem sel trans-plan-**tā**-shun)
stereotactic mammography (ster-ē-ō-**tak**-tik muh-**mog**-ruh-fē)
stereotactic radiosurgery (ster-ē-ō-**tak**-tik rā-dē-ō-**sur**-jur-ē)
surgical biopsy (**sur**-ji-kul **bī**-op-sē)
surgical excision (**sur**-ji-kul ek-**sizh**-un)
tumor marker tests (**too**-mur **mahrk**-ur tests)
tumor's grade (**too**-murz grād)
undifferentiated cells (un-dif-ur-**en**-she-āt-ud selz)

Español ENHANCING SPANISH COMMUNICATION

English	Spanish (Pronunciation)
benign	benigno (bay-NEEG-no)
biopsy	biopsia (be-OP-see-ah)
breast	seno (SAY-no)
chemotherapy	quimioterapia (kee-mee-oh-the-rah-PEE-ah)
freckles	pecas (PAY-kah)
imaging	imagen (e-MAH-hen)
immunity	inmunidad (in-moo-ne-DAHD)
malignant	maligno (mah-LEEG-no)
microscope	microscopio (me-kros-KO-pe-o)
mole	lunar (loo-NAR)
nuclear medicine	medicina nuclear (meh-dee-SEE-nah noo-kleh-AHR)
radiation	radiacion (rah-de-ah-se-ON)
therapy	therapia (ther-ah-PEE-ah); tratamiento (trah-tah-me-EN-to)
ultrasound	ultrasonido (ool-trah-soh-NEE-do)
x-rays	radiografia (rah-de-o-grah-FEE-ah); rayos-x (rah-yohs A-kiss)

Self Test: Mini-Review of Book

Basic Understanding

After completing Chapters 1 through 14, you will be able to do the following:

1. Match terms pertaining to anatomy, diagnostic tests or procedures, pathology, surgery, or therapy with their meanings or descriptions.

The review is a sample of chapter material but does not include every term. Before taking the test that your instructor prepares, refer to your study sheet several times and study the list of terms at the end of each chapter, being sure you remember the meaning of each term.

Circle the correct answer for each of the following questions.

CHAPTER 1

1. Cynthia is pregnant. Which type of specialist should she see to care for her during her pregnancy, labor, and delivery? (gerontologist, obstetrician, orthopedist, otologist)
2. Which of the following physicians specializes in the diagnosis and treatment of newborns through the age of 28 days? (geriatrician, gynecologist, neonatologist, urologist)
3. Luja injures her arm while ice skating. The emergency room physician orders an x-ray examination. Which type of physician is a specialist in interpreting x-ray films? (gynecologist, ophthalmologist, plastic surgeon, radiologist)
4. What does the word neuron mean? (medical specialty that deals with the nervous system, nerve cell, neurosurgery, specialist in diseases of the nervous system)
5. Which physician is certified in the laboratory study of disease? (clinical pathologist, gastroenterologist, internist, surgical pathologist)

CHAPTER 2

6. Rita tells the doctor that she has a sore throat. Which term describes the sore throat? (diagnosis, prognosis, sign, symptom)
7. Mr. Chader has plastic surgery on his hand. What is the name of this procedure? (carpectomy, chiroplasty, ophthalmoplasty, otoplasty)
8. Which term means a record of the electric impulses of the heart? (electrocardiogram, electrocardiograph, electrocardiography, telecardiography)
9. Which of the following describes an unfavorable response to medical treatment? (autoimmune, contagious, iatrogenic, functional)
10. Which term means a medication that relieves pain? (analgesic, approximate, ptosis, radiopharmaceutical)

CHAPTER 3

11. Which term describes a structure that can be seen with the naked eye?
(macroscopic, microscopic, ophthalmoscopic, ophthalmoscopy)

12. In which type of injection is the needle placed in the muscular layer?   (intradermal, intramuscular, intravenous, subcutaneous)

13. Which term means a set of symptoms that occur together and characterize a particular disease or condition?
(dysphoria, symptomatic, syndrome, tachyphasia)

14. Interstitial fluid fills the spaces   (around, between, inside, outside) most of the cells of the body.

15. A decrease in the number of blood platelets is called   (hemophilia, leukemia, leukocytosis, thrombopenia).

CHAPTER 4

16. Charlie, a 60-year-old man, has just been diagnosed as having a coronary occlusion. He is most at risk for which of the following?
(atrioventricular block, congenital heart disease, myocardial infarction, rheumatic fever)

17. Charlie is told that he has a form of arteriosclerosis in which yellowish plaque has accumulated on the walls of the arteries. What is the name of this form of arteriosclerosis?   (aortostenosis, atherosclerosis, cardiomyopathy, coarctation)

18. Agustin developed a blood clot in a coronary artery. What is Jim's condition called?
(hypotension, coronary artery bypass, coronary thrombosis, fibrillation)

19. Baby Harish is born with cyanosis and a heart murmur. Which congenital heart disease does the neonatologist think is most likely?
(atrial septal defect, atrioventricular block, megalocardia, pericarditis)

20. Ten-year-old Aafiya had a sore throat for several days before he developed painful joints and a fever. Which disease does the physician suspect that can cause damage to the heart valves?   (defibrillator, pericardium, lymphoma, rheumatic fever)

CHAPTER 5

21. Mrs. Estafan's doctor tells her that she has pneumonia. What is another name for her diagnosis?
(congestive heart disease, pneumonitis, pulmonary edema, pulmonary insufficiency)

22. Which term means coughing up and spitting out sputum?   (expectorate, expiration, exhalation, extrapleural)

23. What is the serous membrane that lines the walls of the thoracic cavity?   (parietal pleura, rhinorrhea, silicosis, visceral pleura)

24. Which of the following expand the air passages?   (antitussives, antihistamines, antineoplastics, bronchodilators)

25. Mrs. Chadar has difficulty breathing except when sitting in an upright position. What is the term for her condition?
(anoxia, hypocapnia, inspiration, orthopnea)

CHAPTER 6

26. Jean Jones' physician orders CT of the pancreas. What is the name of this diagnostic test?
(barium enema, barium meal, pancreatography, esophagogastroscopy)

27. Tests show that Cal has a gallstone in the common bile duct. Which of the following is a noninvasive conservative procedure to alleviate Cal's problem?   (cholecystostomy, choledochostomy, choledochojejunostomy, extracorporeal shock wave lithotripsy)

28. Linda M., a 16-year-old girl, is diagnosed as having self-induced starvation. Which of the following is the name of the disorder associated with Linda's problem?   (anorexia nervosa, aphagia, malaise, polyphagia)

29. Unless there is intervention for Linda's self-induced starvation, which condition will result?   (adipsia, atresia, emaciation, volvulus)

30. A 70-year-old man is diagnosed with cancer of the colon. Which term indicates a surgical intervention for this condition?
(colectomy, colonoscope, colonic irrigation, colonic stasis)

CHAPTER 7

31. Which of the following terms means making radiographic images of the urinary system after the urine has been rendered opaque by a contrast medium?   (cystoscopy, cystoureteroscopy, intravenous urography, nephrotomography)

32. Which of the following conditions is indicated if the blood urea nitrogen is elevated?   (pyelostomy, pyuria, renal clearance, renal failure)

33. Which term means pertaining to the urinary bladder and a ureter?   (cystourethral, extracystic, urethrovaginal, vesicoureteral)

34. Which term means excretion of an abnormally large quantity of urine?   (anuria, dysuria, oliguria, polyuria)

35. Which of the following is not a type of urinary tract catheterization?
(endoscopy tube, nephrostomy tube, suprapubic tube, urethral tube)

CHAPTER 8

36. Which term means difficult or painful menstruation?   (amenorrhea, dysmenorrhea, metrorrhagia, menorrhea)

37. Which term means a condition in which tissue that contains typical endometrial elements is present outside the uterus?
(endometriosis, endometritis, hysteropathy, salpingopathy)

38. Which term means absence of a testis?   (anorchidism, aspermia, oligospermia, orchidectomy)

39. Which term means abnormal or difficult labor?   (abortion, dystocia, eclampsia, stillbirth)

40. Which of the following is the common name for condyloma acuminatum?   (genital herpes, genital warts, moniliasis, venereal ulcer)

CHAPTER 9

41. Which term means congenital fissure of the breastbone?   (costectomy, rachischisis, spondylosyndesis, sternoschisis)

42. Which term means pertaining to two bones of the forearm?   (carpopedal, carpophalangeal, humeroulnar, ulnoradial)

43. Which term means any disease of the joints?   (arthropathy, bursopathy, chondropathy, osteopathy)

44. Which of the following is the record produced in a procedure that records the response of a muscle to electric stimulation?
(arthrocentesis, electromyogram, myograph, range-of-motion reading)

45. What is the term for the presence of extra fingers or toes?   (carpopedal disease, Paget disease, phalangitis, polydactylism)

CHAPTER 10

46. Which part of the nervous system contains the brain and spinal cord?
(peripheral nervous system, autonomic nervous system, central nervous system, thalamus)

47. Which term means paralysis of the lower portion of the body and both legs?   (diplegia, hemiplegia, paraplegia, quadriplegia)

48. Which of the following means hernial protrusion of the meninges through a defect in the vertebral column?
(meningitis, meningocele, myelocele, myelomalacia)

49. Which term means the use of ultrasound to study intracranial structures?
(brain scan, myelogram, echoencephalography, cerebral angiography)

50. Which of the following is chronic, progressive mental deterioration that involves irreversible loss of memory, disorientation, and speech and gait disturbances?   (Alzheimer disease, Lou Gehrig disease, Meniere syndrome, multiple sclerosis)

CHAPTER 11

51. Carmelite is a 72-year-old female who tells the optometrist that her eyes do not adjust as quickly when she goes into a dark theater as they used to. Muscles of which eye structure regulate the amount of light entering the eye?   (conjunctiva, choroid, cornea, iris)

52. The ophthalmologist explains to Seth that he has total color blindness. Which of the following is Seth's condition?
(achromatic vision, day vision, double vision, night vision)

53. Albert is told he needs blepharoplasty to correct droopy eyelids. What problem does blepharoplasty correct?
(ambylopia, ptosis, nyctalopia, retinopathy)

54. Which part of the ear is responsible for the sense of balance?   (cochlea, semicircular canals, stapes, tympanic membrane)
55. What is the term for the agent that the optical assistant drops in Tina's eyes to dilate the pupils?
    (mydriatic, nyctolopia, photocoagulation, tinnitus)

CHAPTER 12

56. The islets of Langerhans are structures in which of the following?   (adrenal, kidney, pancreas, thyroid)
57. Which of the following terms means an enlarged thyroid gland?   (goiter, hyperadenism, hyperthyroidism, hypothyroidism)
58. What is the name of the diagnostic procedure that uses x-rays to study the breast?
    (mammogram, mammography, radioactive iodine uptake test, reduction mammoplasty)
59. Which of the following disorders is associated with a deficiency of ADH?
    (cretinism, diabetes insipidus, hyperaldosteronism, pituitary dwarfism)
60. Which of the following pathologies is associated with hypersecretion of the glucocorticoids?
    (Addison disease, Cushing syndrome, gigantism, thyrotoxicosis)

CHAPTER 13

61. Which of the following means removal of foreign material and dead or contaminated tissue from an infected or traumatic lesion
    until surrounding healthy tissue is exposed?   (débridement, necrosis, pyemia, rhytidectomy)
62. Which of the following is an inflammatory skin disease that begins on the scalp but may involve other areas, particularly the
    eyebrows?   (acne vulgaris, basal cell carcinoma, seborrheic dermatitis, verruca)
63. Which term means a disease characterized by chronic hardening and thickening of the skin?
    (ecchymosis, Kaposi sarcoma, keratosis, scleroderma)
64. In describing a burn by "thickness," which type of burn is characterized by blisters immediately after the injury?
    (deep partial-thickness, deep full-thickness, full-thickness, superficial partial-thickness)
65. Which term means the death of areas of tissue or bone surrounded by healthy parts?   (atrophy, erosion, fissure, necrosis)

CHAPTER 14

66. What is the developmental process whereby cells become different types of tissues?
    (carcinogenesis, cytopathology, differentiation, metastasis)
67. Which of the following in vitro tests is used to determine the concentration of proteins in the blood?
    (radioimmunoassay, thyroid scan, tumor grading, radionuclide organ imaging)
68. Which of the following is a variation of computed tomography?   (needle biopsy, SNB, SPECT, stereotactic mammography)
69. Which ranking does cancer have among causes of death in the United States?   (first, second, third, fourth)
70. Which of the following represents examination of the first lymph node that receives drainage from a primary tumor?
    (exfoliative cytology, needle biopsy, endoscopic biopsy, sentinel lymph node biopsy)

Appendix I: Medical Abbreviations

Abbreviations are presented in this book because many are still commonly used, but particular caution must be taken in both using and reading abbreviations. Note that many of these abbreviations share their meanings with other terms. If a common abbreviation is missing, you may wish to check to see if its use is discouraged by the Institute for Safe Medication Practices (**www.ismp.org**).

A&O	alert and oriented	BPH	benign prostatic hypertrophy
a.c.	before meals (*ante cibum*)	BUN	blood urea nitrogen
ABA	American Burn Association	Bx, bx	biopsy
ABG	arterial blood gas	C	Celsius
ACA	Affordable Care Act	C&S	culture and sensitivity
ACh	acetylcholine	C1, C2, etc.	first, second, etc., cervical vertebrae
ACL	anterior cruciate ligament	CABG	coronary artery bypass graft
ACS	American Cancer Society, acute coronary syndrome	CAD	coronary artery disease
		CAL	chronic airflow limitation
ACTH	adrenocorticotropic hormone	CBC, cbc	complete blood cell
AD	right ear	CC	chief complaint
ADD	attention deficit disorder	CDC	Centers for Disease Control and Prevention
ADH	antidiuretic hormone	CHF	congestive heart failure
ADHD	attention deficit hyperactivity disorder	CK (CPK)	creatine kinase (formerly called creatine phosphokinase)
ADL	activity of daily living		
ad lib.	freely as needed, at pleasure (*ad libitum*)	CLL	chronic lymphocytic leukemia
AFib	atrial fibrillation	cm	centimeter
AHF	antihemophilic factor	CML	chronic myelogenous leukemia
AI	aortic insufficiency (and several others)	CMV	cytomegalovirus
AIDS	acquired immunodeficiency syndrome	CNS	central nervous system
ALD	assistive listening device	CO_2	carbon dioxide
ALL	acute lymphocytic leukemia	COLD	chronic obstructive lung disease
ALS	amyotrophic lateral sclerosis	COPD	chronic obstructive pulmonary disease
ALT	alanine aminotransferase	CPAP	continuous positive airway pressure (for sleep apnea)
AMA	American Medical Association		
AML	acute myelogenous leukemia	CPD	cephalopelvic disproportion
ANA	antinuclear antibody	CPK	creatine phosphokinase
AP	anteroposterior (also others)	CPM	continuous passive motion
aq.	water (*aqua*)	CPR	cardiopulmonary resuscitation
ARDS	acute (or adult) respiratory distress syndrome	CPT	Current Procedural Terminology
		CRF	chronic renal failure
ARF	acute renal failure	CS, C-section	cesarean section
AROM	active range of motion	CSF	cerebrospinal fluid
AS	left ear	CSR	Cheyne-Stokes respiration
ASHD	arteriosclerotic heart disease	CT, CAT	computed tomography, computed axial tomography
AST	aspartate aminotransferase		
AU	each ear	CTS	carpal tunnel syndrome
AV, A-V	atrioventricular	CVA	cerebrovascular accident (also costovertebral angle)
AVB	atrioventricular block		
baso	basophil	Cx	cervix
BBT	basal body temperature	D&C	dilation and curettage
b.i.d.	twice a day (*bis in die*)	dB	decibel
BMI	body mass index	DCIS	ductal carcinoma in situ
BMT	bone marrow transplant	DIC	disseminated intravascular coagulation
BP	blood pressure	DJD	degenerative joint disease
BPH	benign prostatic hyperplasia	dL	deciliter

DLE	discoid lupus erythematosus	HbA$_{1c}$	glycosylated hemoglobin
DM	diabetes mellitus	HBV	hepatitis B virus
DMARD	disease-modifying antirheumatic drug	hCG, HCG	human chorionic gonadotropin
DNA	deoxyribonucleic acid	HCPCS	Healthcare Common Procedure Coding
DOB	date of birth		System
DRG	diagnosis-related group	HCT, Hct	hematocrit
DRI	dietary reference intake	HCV	hepatitis C virus
DSA	digital subtraction angiography	HDL	high-density lipoprotein
DSM	*Diagnostic and Statistical Manual of Mental*	HDN	hemolytic disease of the newborn
	Disorders	HDV	hepatitis D virus
DTs	delirium tremens	HEENT	head, eye, ear, nose, throat
DTR	deep tendon reflex	HEV	hepatitis E virus
Dx	diagnosis	HHx	health history
EBV	Epstein-Barr virus	HIPAA	Health Insurance Portability and
ECCE	extracapular cataract extraction		Accountability Act
ECG, EKG	electrocardiogram	HIV	human immunodeficiency virus
ECMO	extracorporeal membrane oxygenator	HPF	high-power field
ED	emergency department	HPI	history of present illness
EDD	expected date of delivery	HPV	human papillomavirus
EEG	electroencephalogram;	HRT	hormone replacement therapy
	electroencephalography	HSV	herpes simplex virus
EFM	electronic fetal monitor	HSV-1	herpes simplex virus type 1
EGD	esophagogastroduodenoscopy	HSV-2	herpes simplex virus type 2
EMG	electromyography	HTN	hypertension
EMS	emergency medical service	Hx	history
ENT	ear, nose, and throat	^{131}I	radioactive iodine
eos	eosinophil	I&D	incision and drainage
ESR	erythrocyte sedimentation rate	I&O	intake and output
ESWL	extracorporeal shock wave lithotripsy	IAD	illness anxiety disorder
F	Fahrenheit	IBD	inflammatory bowel disease
FBS	fasting blood sugar	IBS	irritable bowel syndrome
FDA	Food and Drug Administration	ICD-9	International Classification of Diseases, 9th
FEMA	Federal Emergency Management Agency		revision
FH	family history	ICD-10	International Classification of Diseases, 10th
FHR	fetal heart rate		revision
FSH	follicle-stimulating hormone	ICP	intracranial pressure
FTA-ABS	fluorescent treponemal antibody absorption	ICSH	interstitial cell–stimulating hormone
	test	IDDM	insulin-dependent diabetes mellitus
fx	fracture	IED	improvised explosive device
g	gram	INR	International Normalized Ratio
G	gravida (pregnant)	IOL	intraocular device
GC	gonococcus	IP	inpatient
GDM	gestational diabetes mellitus	IUD	intrauterine device
GERD	gastroesophageal reflux disease	IV	intravenous
GFR	glomerular filtration rate	IVF	in vitro fertilization
GH	growth hormone	IVP	intravenous pyelography
GI	gastrointestinal	IVU	intravenous urography
GP	general practitioner	kg	kilogram
GPA	gravid/para/abortus	KUB	kidneys, ureters, and bladder
GTT	glucose tolerance test	L	liter
GU	genitourinary	L&W	living and well
GYN, Gyn, gyn	gynecology	L1, L2, etc.	first, second, etc., lumbar vertebrae
h	hour (*hora*)	LA	left atrium
H&P	history and physical	lab	laboratory
H2RA	histamine 2 receptor antagonist	LASIK	laser-assisted in-situ keratomileusis
HAV	hepatitis A virus	LBP	lower back pain
Hb, Hgb	hemoglobin	LDCT	low-dose computed tomography

LDH	lactate dehydrogenase (enzyme elevated after MI)	PCL	posterior cruciate ligament
LDL	low-density lipoprotein	PDA	patent ductus arteriosus (also posterior descending [coronary] artery)
LE	lupus erythematosus	PE	physical examination, pulmonary embolism
LFT	liver function test	PET	positron emission tomography
LH	luteinizing hormone	PFT	pulmonary function test
LINAC	linear accelerator	pH	potential hydrogen; hydrogen ion concentration
LLQ	left lower quadrant		
LMP	last menstrual period	PID	pelvic inflammatory disease
LP	lumbar puncture	PMH	past medical history
LPF	low-power field	PMS	premenstrual syndrome
LTRA	leukotriene receptor antagonist	PNS	peripheral nervous system
LUQ	left upper quadrant	p.o.	orally (per os)
LV	left ventricle	PPI	proton pump inhibitor
lymph	lymphocyte	PRL	prolactin
mcg	microgram	p.r.n.	as the occasion arises, as needed (pro re nata)
MD	doctor of medicine; macular degeneration		
mg	milligram	PROM	passive range of motion
MI	myocardial infarction	PSA	prostate-specific antigen
MIDCAB	minimally invasive direct coronary artery bypass	Pt	patient
		PT	prothrombin time (also physical therapy)
min	minutes		
MIS	minimally invasive surgery	PTCA	percutaneous transluminal coronary angioplasty
mL	milliliter		
mm Hg	millimeters of mercury	PTH	parathyroid hormone; parathormone
mono	monocyte	PTT	partial thromboplastin time
MRI	magnetic resonance imaging	PVC	premature ventricular contraction
MRSA	methicillin-resistant *Staphylococcus aureus*	PVD	peripheral vascular disease
MS	multiple sclerosis	PVP	photoselective vaporization of the prostate; Green Light PVP
MSH	melanocyte-stimulating hormone		
MTP	metatarsophalangeal	q.	every (quaque)
MVP	mitral valve prolapse	q.i.d.	four times a day (quater in die)
N&V	nausea and vomiting	R	respirations
neut	neutrophil	RA	right atrium; rheumatoid arthritis
NG	nasogastric	RAIU	radioactive iodine uptake
NIAMS	National Institute of Arthritis and Musculoskeletal and Skin Diseases	RBC	red blood cell, red blood cell count
		RDS	respiratory distress syndrome
NIDDM	non–insulin-dependent diabetes mellitus	RF	rheumatoid factor
NIH	National Institutes of Health	Rh	rhesus (a blood group)
NPO	nothing by mouth (nil per os)	RIA	radioimmunoassay
NSAID	nonsteroidal antiinflammatory drug	RLQ	right lower quadrant
O₂	oxygen	ROM	range of motion
OB	obstetrics	ROS	review of systems
OCD	obsessive-compulsive disorder	RPFT	registered pulmonary function therapist
OD	overdose; right eye (oculus dexter)	RPR	rapid plasma reagin test (for syphilis)
OP	outpatient	RUQ	right upper quadrant
OPCAB	off-pump coronary artery bypass	RV	right ventricle
Ophth	opthalmology	Rx	prescription
OR	operating room	SA	sinoatrial
OTC	over-the-counter (drug that can be obtained without a prescription)	SARS	severe acute respiratory syndrome
		SCI	spinal cord injury
P	pulse	SGOT	serum glutamate-oxaloacetic transaminase (enzyme test of heart and liver function, now called AST)
PA	posteroanterior (also others)		
PACU	postanesthesia care unit		
Pap	Papanicolaou	SGPT	serum glutamate-pyruvate transaminase (enzyme test of liver function, now called ALT)
PAT	paroxysmal atrial tachycardia		
PCI	percutaneous coronary intervention		

SIADH	syndrome of inappropriate ADH secretion	TPAL	term birth(s), premature birth(s), abortions, living children
SIDS	sudden infant death syndrome	TPN	total parenteral nutrition
SLE	systemic lupus erythematosus	TSH	thyroid-stimulating hormone
SNB	sentinel node biopsy	TSS	toxic shock syndrome
SOB	shortness of breath	TTO	transtracheal oxygen
SPECT	single-photon emission computed tomography	TUMT	transurethral microwave thermotherapy
		TUNA	transurethral needle ablation
SSN	social security number	TUR	transurethral resection
staph	staphylococci	TURP	transurethral resection of the prostate
stat.	immediately *(statim)*	Tx	treatment
STD	sexually transmitted disease	UA, U/A	urinalysis
STH	somatotropic hormone	UGI	upper gastrointestinal (or upper GI)
STI	sexually transmitted infection	ung	ointment
strep	streptococci	URI	upper respiratory infection
T	temperature	US	ultrasound
T1, T2, etc.	first, second, etc., thoracic vertebrae	UTI	urinary tract infection
T_3	triiodothyronine	UV	ultraviolet
T_4	thyroxine	VAC	vacuum-assisted closure
TB	tuberculosis	VC	vital capacity
TBSA	total body surface area	VCUG	voiding cystourethrogram
TCT	thyrocalcitonin	VD	venereal disease
TEE	transesophageal echocardiogram	VDRL	Venereal Disease Research Laboratories
TENS	transcutaneous electric nerve stimulation	VF	visual fields
TIA	transient ischemic attack	VS	vital signs
t.i.d.	three times a day *(ter in die)*	WBC	white blood cell, white blood cell count
TJC	The Joint Commission	WD, WN	well developed, well nourished
TJR	total joint replacement	WHO	World Health Organization
TMJ	temporomandibular joint	WMD	weapons of mass destruction
TNM	staging system for cancer	WNL	within normal limits

Appendix II: Enhancing Spanish Communication

English	Spanish (pronunciation)	English	Spanish (pronunciation)
abdomen	abdomen (ab-DOH-men), vientre (ve-EN-tray)	anesthetic	anestésico (ah-nes-TAY-se-ko)
		aneurism	aneurisma (ah-neh-REES-mah)
abscess	absceso (ab-SAY-so), apostema (ah-pos-TAY-ma)	angina	angina (ahn-HEE-nah)
		ankle	tobillo (to-BEEL-lyo)
acidity	acidez (ah-se-DES)	antibiotic	antibiótico (an-te-be-O-te-ko)
acute	agudo (ah-GOO-do)	anticoagulant	anticoagulante (an-te-ko-ah-goo-LAHN-tay)
adrenal	suprarenal (soo-prah-ray-NAHL)		
adrenaline	adrenalina (ah-dray-nah-LEE-nah)	antidepressant	antidepresivo (an-te-day-pra-SI-vo)
aged	envejecido (en-vay-hay-SEE-do)	antigen	antígeno (an-TEE-hay-no)
albumin	albúmina (al-BOO-me-nah)	antihistamine	antihistamina (an-te-es-tay-ME-nah)
allergy	alergia (ah-LEHR-he-ah)	anxiety	ansiedad (an-se-ay-DAHD)
analgesic	analgésico (ah-nal-HAY-se-ko)	aphasia	afasia (ah-FAY-see-ah)
anatomy	anatomía (ah-nah-to-MEE-ah)	appendix	apéndice (ah-PEN-de-say)
anemia	anemia (ah-NAY-me-ah)	appetite	apetito (ah-pay-TEE-to)
anesthesia	anestesia (ah-nes-TAY-se-ah)	arachnoid	arachnoides (ah-rak-NO-e-des)
anesthesiology	anestesiología (an-es-te-se-o-lo-HE-ah)	arm	brazo (BRAH-so)
		artery	arteria (ar-TAY-re-ah)

English	Spanish (pronunciation)
asphyxia	asfixia (as-FEEK-se-ah)
aspirate	aspirar (as-pe-RAR)
asthma	asma (AHS-mah)
augmentation	aumento (ah-oo-MEN-to)
bacilli	bacilos (bah-SE-los)
back	espalda (es-PAHL-dah)
belch	eructo (ay-ROOK-to)
belly	barriga (bar-REE-gah)
benign	benign (bay-NEEG-no)
biopsy	biopsia (be-OP-see-ah)
birth	nacimiento (nah-se-me-EN-to)
black	negro (NAY-gro)
blood	sangre (SAHN-gray)
blood pressure	presión sanguínea (pray-se-ON san-GEE-nay-ah)
blood sample	muestra de sangre (moo-AYS-trah day SAHN-gray)
blood transfusion	transfusión de sangre (trans-foo-se-ON day SAHN-gray)
blood vessel	vaso sanguine (VAH-so san-GEE-nay)
blue	azul (ah-SOOL)
body	cuerpo (koo-ERR-po)
bone	hueso (oo-AY-so)
bones	huesos (oo-AY-sos)
botulism	botulismo (bo-too-LEES-mo)
brain	cerebro (say-RAY-bro)
breast	seno (SAY-no)
breathe	alentar (ah-len-TAR), respirar (res-pe-RAR)
breathing	respiración (res-pe-rah-se-ON)
burn	quemadura (kay-mah-DOO-rah)
buzzing	zumbido (soom-BEE-do)
calcium	calcio (KAHL-se-o)
calculus	cálculo (KAHL-coo-lo)
cancer	cáncer (KAHN-ser)
capillary	capilar (kah-pe-LAR)
cartilage	cartílago (kar-TEE-lah-go)
catheter	catéter (kah-TAY-ter)
cells	célula (SAY-LU-AH)
cephalgia	cefalalgia (say-fah-lahl-HE-ah)
cerebrum	cerebro (say-RAY-bro)
cheek	mejilla (may-HEEL-lyah)
chemotherapy	quimioterapia (kee-mee-oh-the-rah-PEE-ah)
chest	pecho (PAY-cho)
chest pain	dolor en el pecho (do-LOR en el PAY-cho)
chew, to	masticar (mas-te-KAR)
child	niña (NEE-nya), niño (NEE-nyo)
childbirth	parto (PAR-to)
cholesterol	colesterol (ko-les-tay-ROL)
chronic	crónico (KRO-ne-ko)
circumcision	circuncisión (ser-koon-se-se-ON)
clinical	clinico (KLE-ne-ko)
clot	coágulo (ko-AH-goo-lo)
coagulant	coagulante (ko-ah-goo-LAHN-tay)
coagulation	coagulación (ko-ag-oo-lah-se-ON), coágulo (ko-AH-goo-lo)
cold	frio (FRE-o)
collarbone	clavícula (klah-VEE-koo-lah)

English	Spanish (pronunciation)
coma	coma (KO-mah), letargo (lay-TAR-go)
conception	concepción (kon-sep-se-ON)
concussion	concusión (kon-loo-se-ON)
condom	condón (kon-DON)
congenital	congénito (kon-HE-ne-to)
conscious	consciente (kons-se-EN-tay)
consciousness	conciencia (kon-se-EN-se-ah)
constipation	estreñimiento (es-tray-nye-me-EN-to)
contagious	contagioso (kon-tay-HEYO-so)
contraception	contracepción (kon-trah-sep-se-ON)
contusion	contusión (kon-too-se-ON)
convulsion	convulsión (kon-vool-se-ON)
cornea	cornea (KOR-ne-ah)
cough	tos (tos)
cranium	cráneo (KRAH-nay-o)
cream	crema (KRAY-mah)
cry	lloro (YO-ro)
cystitis	cystitis (sis-TEE-tis)
defecate	evacuar (ay-vah-koo-AR)
dehydration	deshidración (des-e-dra-se-ON)
dementia	demencia (day-MEN-se-ah)
dentist	dentista (den-TEES-tah)
depression	depresión (day-pre-se-ON)
dermatology	dermatología (der-mah-to-lo-HEE-ah)
destruction	destrucción (des-trook-se-ON)
diabetes	diabetes (de-ah-BAY-tes)
diagnosis	el diagnóstico (al de-ag-NOS-te-ko)
diagnostic	diagnóstico (de-ag-NOS-te-ko)
dialysis	diálisis (de-AH-le-sis)
diaphragm	diafragma (de-ah-FRAHG-mah)
diarrhea	diarrea (de-ar-RAY-ah)
digestion	digestión (de-hes-te-ON)
dilatation	dilatación (de-lah-tah-se-ON)
disease	enfermedad (en-fer-may-DAHD)
disseminate	diseminar (de-say-me-NAR)
dizziness	vértigo (VERR-te-go)
dwarf	enano (ay-NAH-no)
dyspnea	disnea (dis-NAY-ah)
ear	oreja (o-RAY-hah)
earwax	cerilla (say-REEL-yah)
edema	hidropesía (e-dro-pay-SEE-ah)
elbow	codo (KO-do)
electricity	electricidad (ay-lec-tre-se-DAHD)
electrocardiogram	electrocardiograma (a-lek-tro-kahr-de-o-GRAH-ma)
embolus	émbolo (EM-bo-lo)
emergency	emergencia (a-mar-han-SE-ah), urgencia (ur-han-SE-ah)
endocrine	endocrino (and-o-KRE-no)
endoscopy	endoscopía (an-do-sko-PEE-ah)
enlargement	aumento (ah-oo-MEN-to)
enzyme	enzima (en-SEE-mah)
epidemic	epidemia (ep-ah-day-ME-ah)
epilepsy	epilepsia (ay-pe-LEP-se-ah)
erect, straight	derecho (day-RAY-cho)
erection	erección (ay-rek-se-ON)
erythrocyte	erithrocito (a-rith-ro-SEE-to)
esophagus	esófago (ay-SO-fah-go)

English	Spanish (pronunciation)
excretion	excreción (ex-kray-se-ON)
extremity	extremidad (ex-tray-me-DAHD)
eye	ojo (O-ho)
eyeball	globo del ojo (GLO-bo del O-ho)
eyebrow	ceja (SAY-hah)
eyelash	pestaña (pes-TAH-nyah)
eyelid	párpado (PAR-pah-do)
face	cara (KAH-rah)
fainting	languidez (lan-gee-DES), desmayo (des-MAH-yo)
fatigue	fatiga (fah-TEE-gah)
fear	miedo (me-AY-do)
feces	excremento (ex-kray-MEN-to)
female	mujer (mu-HAR)
feminine	femenina (fay-may-NEE-na)
fetus	feto (FAY-to)
fever	fiebre (fe-AY-bray)
fiber	fibra (FEE-brah)
fibrin	fibrina (fe-BREE-nah)
finger	dedo (DAY-do)
fingerprint	impresión digital (im-pray-se-ON de-he-TAHL)
fire	fuego (foo-AY-go)
fluid	fluido (floo-EE-do)
foam	espuma (es-POO-mah)
foot (pl., feet)	pie (PE-ay), pies (PE-ays)
forearm	antebrazo (an-tay-BRAH-so)
forensic	forense (fo-RAN-sa)
fracture	fractura (frak-TOO-rah)
freckles	pecas (PAY-kah)
fungus	hongo (ONG-go)
gallbladder	vesícula biliar (vay-SEE-koo-la be-le-AR)
gallstone	cálculo biliar (KAHL-koo-lo be-le-AR)
gastric	gástrico (GAS-tre-ko)
genetic	genetic (he-NE-te-kah)
geriatrics	geriatriá (gay-re-ah-TRE-ah)
giant	gigante (he-GAHN-tay)
gland	glándula (GLAN-doo-lah)
glucose	glucosa (gloo-KO-sah)
goiter	papera (pah-PAY-rah)
gray	gris (grees)
green	verde (VERR-day)
growth	crecimiento (kray-se-me-EN-to)
gum, gingiva	encía (en-SEE-ah)
gynecology	ginecología (he-nay-ko-lo-HEE-ah)
hair	pelo (PAY-lo)
hand	mano (MAH-no)
head	cabeza (kah-BAY-sah)
headache	dolor de cabeza (do-LOR day kah-BAY-sa)
hear (to)	oír (o-EER)
heart	corazón (ko-rah-SON)
heat	calor (kah-LOR)
heel	talón (tah-LON)
hemiplegia	hemiplejia (am-me-PLAY-he-ah)
hemophilia	hemophilia (ay-mo-FEE-le-ah)
hemorrhage	hemorragia (ay-mor-RAH-he-ah)
hernia	hernia (AYR-ne-ah), quebradura (kay-brah-DOO-rah)

English	Spanish (pronunciation)
high blood pressure	hipertensión, presión alta (e-per-ten-se-ON, pray-se-ON AHL-tah)
hip	cadera (kah-DAY-rah)
hives	roncha (RON-chah)
hormone	hormona (or-MOH-nah)
hunger	hambre (AHM-bray)
hydrocephalus	hidrocéfalo (e-dro-SAY-fah-lo)
hypnotic	hipnótico (ip-NO-te-ko)
hypodermic	hipodérmico (e-po-DER-me-co)
imaging	imagen (e-MAH-hen)
immunity	inmunidad (in-moo-ne-DAHD)
immunology	inmunologia (en-mu-no-lo-HE-ah)
imperfect	imperfecto (im-per-FEK-to)
impotency	impotencia (im-po-TEN-se-ah)
incontinence	incontinencia (in-kon-te-NEN-se-ah)
infection	infección (en-fek-SYON)
infectious	infeccioso (en-fek-SYO-so)
inflammation	inflamación (in-flah-mah-se-ON)
influenza	gripe (GREE-pay)
injury	daño (DAH-nyo)
instrument	instrumento (ins-troo-MEN-to)
insulin	insulina (in-soo-LEE-nah)
intercourse, sexual	cópula (KO-poo-lah)
internal medicine	medicina interna (may-de-SE-na in-TER-nah)
intestine	intestino (in-tes-TEE-no)
iodine	yodo (YO-do)
jaw	mandíbula (man-DEE-boo-lah)
joint	articulacíon (ar-te-koo-lah-se-ON), coyuntura (ko-yoon-TOO-rah)
kidney	riñon (ree-NYOHN)
kleptomania	cleptomanía (klep-to-mah-NEE-ah)
knee	rodilla (ro-DEEL-lyah)
kneecap	rótula (RO-too-lah)
larynx	laringe (lah-REN-gay)
laxative	purgante (poor-GAHN-tay)
leg	pierna (pe-ERR-nah)
leukemia	leucemia (lay-oo-SAY-me-ah)
life	vida (VEE-dah)
ligament	ligamento (le-gah-MEN-to)
lips	labios (LAH-be-os)
lithotripsy	litotricia (le-to-TREE-see-ah)
lithotripter	lithotritor (le-to-tre-TOR)
liver	hígado (EE-ga-do)
lobe	lóbulo (LO-boo-lo)
lung	pulmón (pool-MON)
lymph	linfa (LEEN-fa)
lymphatic	linfático (lin-FAH-te-ko)
malignant	maligno (mah-LEEG-no)
masculine	masculino (mas-koo-LEE-no)
membrane	membrana (mem-BRAH-nah)
menopause	menopausia (may-no-PAH-oo-se-ah)
menstruation	menstruación (mens-troo-ah-se-ON)
microscope	microscopio (me-kros-KO-pe-o)
milk	leche (LAY-chay)
mind	mente (MEN-te)
mole	lunar (loo-NAR)
mood	disposición (dis-po-se-se-ON)
mouth	boca (BO-kah)

English	Spanish (pronunciation)	English	Spanish (pronunciation)
movement	movimiento (mo-ve-me-EN-to)	procedure	procedimiento (pro-se-de-MYEN-to)
mucous	mucoso (moo-KO-so)	prolapse	prolapso (pro-LAHP-so)
mucus	moco (MO-ko)	prostate	próstata (PROS-ta-tah)
murmur	murmullo (moor-MOOL-lyo)	prostatic	prostático (pros-TAH-te-ko)
muscle	músculo (MOOS-koo-lo)	prostatitis	prostatitis (pros-ta-TEE-tis)
nails	uñas (OO-nyahs)	protection	proteccion (pro-tek-se-ON)
narcotic	narcótico (nar-KO-te-ko)	psychiatry	psiquiatría (se-ke-ah-TREE-ah)
narrow	estrecho (es-TRAY-cho)	psychology	psicología (se-ko-lo-HEE-ah)
navel	ombligo (om-BLEE-go)	psychosis	psicosis (se-KO-sis)
neck	cuello (koo-EL-lyo)	psychosomatic	psicosomático (se-co-so-MAH-te-ko)
nephrectomy	nefrectomia (nay-fra-to-MEE-ah)	psychotherapy	psicoterapia (se-ko-tay-RAH-pe-ah)
nephritis	nefritis (nay-FREE-tis)	pulmonary	pulmonary (pool-mo-NAR)
nephrotomy	nefrotomia (nay-fro-to-MEE-ah)	pulmonary	thrombosis pulmonary (throm-BO-
nerve	nervio (NERR-ve-o)	thrombosis	ses pool-mo-NAR)
nervous	nervioso (ner-ve-O-so)	pulse	pulso (POOL-so)
neurology	neurología (nay-oo-ro-lo-HEE-ah)	puncture	perferación (per-fo-ra-SYON)
neuron	neurona (nay-oo-RO-nah)	purulent	purulento (poo-roo-LEN-to)
newborn	recién nacido (boy), nacida (girl) (ray-se-EN nah-SEE-do, nah-SEE-dah)	rabies	rabia (RAH-be-ah)
		radiation	radiación (rah-de-ah-se-ON)
nipple	pezón (pay-SON)	rectum	recto (REK-to)
nose	nariz (nah-REES)	red	rojo (RO-ho)
nostril	orificio de la nariz (or-e-FEE-se-o day lah nah-REES)	redness	rojo (RO-ho)
		reduction	reducción (ray-dook-se-ON)
nuclear medicine	medicina nuclear (meh-dee-SEE-nah noo-kleh-AHR)	renal artery	arteria renal (ar-TAY-re-ah ray-NAHL)
nutrition	nutrición (noo-tre-se-ON)	renal calculus	cálculo renal (KAHL-koo-lo ray-NAHL)
obsession	obsesión (ob-say-se-ON)	repair (to)	reparar (ray-puh-rahr)
obstruction	obstrucción (obs-trook-se-ON)	reproduction	reproducción (ray-pro-dook-se-ON)
optic	óptico (OP-te-ko)	resistance	resistencia (ray-sis-TEN-tay)
orthodontist	ortodóntico (or-to-DON-te-ko)	respiration	respiración (res-pe-rah-se-ON)
ovarian	ovárico (o-VAH-re-ko)	retina	retina (ray-TEE-nah)
ovary	ovario (o-VAH-re-o)	rheumatic fever	fiebre reumatica (fe-AY-bray ray-oo-MAT-e-kah)
oxygen	oxígeno (ok-SEE-hay-no)	rheumatism	reumatismo (ru-may-TEZ-mo)
pain	dolor (do-LOR)	rhythm	ritmo (REET-mo)
painful	doloroso (do-lo-RO-so)	rhythm method	método de ritmo (MAY-to-do day REET-mo)
pallor	palidez (pah-le-DAS)		
palm	palma (PAHL-mah)	rib	costilla (kos-TEEL-lyah)
pancreas	páncreas (PAHN-kray-as)	ringing	zumbido (zoom-BEE-do)
panic	pánico (PAH-ne-ko)	rupture	ruptura (roop-TOO-rah)
paralysis	parálisis (pah-RAH-le-sis)	sacrum	hueso sacro (oo-AY-so SAH-kro)
paraplegia	paraplejia (pah-rah-PLAY-he-ah)	saliva	saliva (sah-LEE-vah)
parasite	parásito (pah-RAH-se-to)	sangionous	sanguine (san-GEE-no)
parturition	parto (PAR-to)	schizophrenia	esquizofrenia (es-ke-so-FRAY-ne-ah)
pathology	patología (pah-to-lo-HEE-ah)		
penis	pene (PAY-nay)	secrete	secretar (say-kra-TAR)
perineum	perineo (pay-re-NAY-o)	secretion	secreción (say-kray-se-ON)
perspiration	sudor (soo-DOR)	seizure	ataque (ah-TAH-kay)
perspire	sudar (soo-DAR)	sensation	sensación (sen-sah-se-ON)
pertussis	tos ferina (TOS fay-REE-nah)	serum	suero (soo-AY-ro)
phagocyte	fagocito (fah-go-SEE-to)	sexual	sexual (sex-soo-AHL)
phalanges	falanges (fah-LAHN-hays)	shoulder	hombro (OM-bro)
phosphorus	fósforo (FOS-fo-ro)	shoulder blade	espaldilla (es-pal-DEEL-lyah)
physical examination	examen físico (ek-SAH-men FEE-se-co)	signs	signos (SAYG-nos)
		skeleton	esqueleto (es-kay-LAY-to)
pituitary	pituitario (pe-too-e-TAH-re-o)	skin	piel (pe-EL)
pneumonia	neumonía (nay-oo-mo-NEE-ah), pulmonía (pool-mo-NEE-ah)	skull	cráneo (KRAH-nay-o)
		sleep	sueño (soo-AY-nyo)
pregnancy	embarazo (em-bah-RAH-so)	smell (to)	oler (o-LEER)
pregnant	embarazada (em-bah-rah-SAH-dah)		
prescription	receta (ray-SAY-tah)		

English	Spanish (pronunciation)	English	Spanish (pronunciation)
sole	planta (PLAHN-tah)	thrombus	coagulo (ko-AG-goo-loh)
sound	sonido (so-NE-do)	thumb	pulgar (pool-GAR)
spasm	espasmo (es-PAHS-mo)	thyroid	tiroides (te-RO-e-des)
specimen	muestra (moo-AYS-trah)	tissue	tejido (TAY-he-do)
speech	habla (AH-blah), lenguaje (len-goo-AH-hay)	toe	dedo del pie (DAY-do del pe-AY)
		tongue	lingua (LEN-goo-ah)
spinal column	columna vertebral (ko-LOOM-nah ver-tay-BRAHL)	tonsil	tonsila (ton-SEE-lah), amígdala (ah-MEEG-dah-lah)
spine	espinazo (es-pe-NAH-so)	toxin	toxina (tox-SEE-nah)
spiral	espiral (es-pe-RAHL)	trachea	tráquea (TRAH-kay-ah)
spleen	bazo (BAH-so)	tranquilizer	calmante (kal-MAHN-tay)
sprain, to	torcer (tor-SERR)	transfusion	transfusión (trans-foo-se-ON)
sputum	esputo (es-POO-to)	trauma	daño (DAH-nyo), herida (ay-REE-dah)
starch	almidón (al-me-DON)		
sternum	esternón (es-ter-NON)	treatment	tratamiento (trah-tah-MYEN-to)
stiff	tieso (te-AY-so)	tremor	temblor (tem-BLOR)
stomach	estómago (es-TOH-mah-go)	twisted	torcido (tor-SE-do)
stone	cálculo (KAHL-koo-lo)	ulcer	ulcera (OOL-say-rah)
stroke	ataque de apoplejía (ah-TAH-kay day ah-po-play-HEE-ah)	ultrasonic	ultrasonic (ul-trah-SO-ne-ko)
		ultrasound	ultrasonido (ul-trah-so-NEE-do)
stupor	estupor (es-too-POR)	urea	urea (oo-RAY-ah)
sugar	azúcar (ah-SOO-kar)	urinalysis	urinálisis (oo-re-NAH-le-sis)
support	sustento (sus-TEN-to)	urinary	urinario (oo-re-NAH-re-o)
surgeon	cirujano(a) (se-roo-HAH-no) (na)	urinary bladder	vejiga (vah-HEE-gah)
surgery	cirugía (se-roo-HEE-ah)	urinary system	sistema urinario (sis-TAY-mah oo-re-NAH-re-o)
susceptibility	susceptibilidad (soos-sep-te-be-le-DAHD)		
		urinate	orinar (o-re-NAR)
suture	sutura (soo-TOO-rah)	urination	urinación (oo-re-nah-se-ON)
swallow	tragar (trah-GAR)	urine	orina (o-REE-nah)
sweat	sudor (soo-DOR)	urology	urología (oo-ro-lo-HEE-ah)
swelling	hinchar (in-CHAR); prominencia (pro-me-NEN-se-ah)	uterus	útero (OO-tay-ro)
		vaccination	vacunación (vah-koo-nah-se-ON)
symptom	síntoma (SEEN-to-mah)	vagina	vagina (vah-HEE-nah)
syncope	síncope (SEEN-ko-pay)	varicose veins	venas varicosas (VAH-nahs vah-re-KO-sas)
synthesis	síntesis (SEEN-tay-sis)		
taste	sabor (sah-BOR)	vein	vena (VAY-nah)
tear	lágrima de los ojos (LAH-gre-mah day los O-hos)	vertebral column	columna vertebral (ko-LOOM-nah ver-tay-BRAHL)
tears	lágrimas de los ojos (LAH-gre-mahs day los O-hos)	vessel	vaso (VAH-so)
		voice	voz (vos)
teeth	dientes (de-AYN-tays)	voided specimen	orinado (o-re-NAH-do)
temperature	temperatura (tem-pay-rah-TOO-rah)	voiding	urinar (oo-re-NAR)
temple	sien (se-AYN)	vomiting	vómito (VO-me-to)
tendon	tendón (ten-DON)	water	agua (AH-goo-ah)
testicle	testículo (tes-TEE-koo-lo)	weakness	debilidad (day-be-le-DAHD)
tests	pruebas (proo-AY-bahs)	whisper	voz baja (voz BAH-hah)
tetanus	tétano (TAY-tah-no)	white	blanco (BLAHN-ko)
therapy	therapia (ther-ah-PEE-ah), tratamiento (trah-tah-me-EN-to)	wound	lesión (lay-se-ON)
		wrist	muñeca (moo-NYAY-kah)
thigh	muslo (MOOS-lo)	x-ray	radiografía (rah-de-o-grah-FEE-ah)
thirst	sed (sayd)	x-rays	rayos-x (rah-yohs A-kiss)
throat	garganta (gar-GAHN-tah)	yellow	amarillo (ah-mah-REEL-lyo)

Appendix III: Word Parts

This appendix has two parts.
A. Alphabetized Word Parts and Meanings
B. English Words and Corresponding Word Parts

A. Alphabetized Word Parts and Meanings

Word Part	Meaning
a-	no, not, without
ab-	away from
abdomin(o)	abdomen
-able	capable of, able to
-ac	pertaining to
acid(o)	acid
acoust(o)	hearing
acr(o)	extremities (arms and legs)
ad-	toward
aden(o)	gland
adenoid(o)	adenoids
adip(o)	fat
adren(o), adrenal(o)	adrenal gland
-al	pertaining to
alb(o), albin(o)	white
albumin(o)	albumin
algesi(o), -algesia	sensitivity to pain
-algia	pain
alkal(o)	alkaline, basic
alveol(o)	alveoli, air sac
amni(o)	amnion
amyl(o)	starch
an-	no, not, without
-an	belonging or pertaining to
ana-	upward, excessive, again
an(o)	anus
andr(o)	male or masculine
aneurysm(o)	aneurysm
angi(o)	vessel
ankyl(o)	stiff
-ant	that which causes
ante-	before in time or in place
anter(o)	anterior or front
anthrac(o)	coal
anti-	against
aort(o)	aorta
apic(o)	apex
append(o), appendic(o)	appendix
-ar	pertaining to
arachn(o)	spider or arachnoid membrane
arter(o), arteri(o)	artery
arteriol(o)	arteriole
arthr(o), articul(o)	joint; articulation
-ary	pertaining to
-ase	enzyme
-asthenia	weakness

Word Part	Meaning
-ate	to cause an action or the result of an action
atel(o)	imperfect or incomplete
ather(o)	yellowish, fatty plaque
-ation	process
atri(o)	atrium
audi(o)	hearing
aur(o), auricul(o)	ear
aut(o)	self
axill(o)	axilla (armpit)
bacter(i), bacteri(o)	bacteria
balan(o)	glans penis
bi-	two
bi(o)	life or living
bil(i)	bile or gall
blast(o), -blast	immature, embryonic form
blephar(o)	eyelid
brady-	slow
bronch(o), bronchi(o)	bronchi
bronchiol(o)	bronchioles
bucc(o)	cheek
burs(o)	bursa
calc(i)	calcium
calcane(o)	calcaneus (heel bone)
cancer(o)	cancer
-capnia	carbon dioxide
carcin(o)	cancer
cardi(o)	heart
carp(o)	carpus (wrist)
caud(o)	tail or toward the tail
cec(o)	cecum
-cele	hernia
cellul(o)	little cell or compartment
-centesis	surgical puncture to aspirate or remove fluid
centi-	one hundred or one hundredth
cephal(o)	head
cerebell(o)	cerebellum
cerebr(o)	brain, cerebrum
cerumin(o)	ear wax
cervic(o)	neck; cervix uteri
cheil(o)	lip
chem(o)	chemical
chir(o)	hand
chlor(o)	green
chol(e)	bile

Word Part	Meaning
cholecyst(o)	gallbladder
choledoch(o)	common bile duct
chondr(o)	cartilage
chori(o)	chorion
choroid(o)	choroid
chrom(o)	color
-cidal	killing
circum-	around
-clasia	break
clavicul(o)	clavicle (collarbone)
coagul(o)	coagulation
coccyg(o)	coccyx (tail bone)
cochle(o)	cochlea
col(o), colon(o)	colon or large intestine
colp(o)	vagina
coni(o)	dust
conjunctiv(o)	conjunctiva
contra-	against
corne(o)	cornea
coron(o)	crown
cortic(o)	cortex
cost(o)	costae (ribs)
crani(o)	cranium (skull)
crin(o)	to secrete
-crine	secrete
cry(o)	cold
crypt(o)	hidden
cutane(o)	skin
cyan(o)	blue
-cyesis	pregnancy
cyst(o)	bladder, cyst, fluid-filled sac
cyt(o), -cyte	cell
dacry(o)	tear
dactyl(o)	finger or toe (digit)
de-	down, from, or reversing
deci-	one tenth (1/10)
dendr(o)	tree
dent(i), dent(o)	tooth
derm(a), derm(o), dermat(o)	skin
-derm	skin or germ layer
-desis	binding, fusion
di-	two
dia-	through
dipl(o), diplo-	double
-dipsia	thirst
dist(o)	distant, far
diverticul(o)	diverticula
dors(o)	dorsal, back
duoden(o)	duodenum
dwarf(o)	dwarf
-dynia	pain
dys-	bad, difficult
-eal	pertaining to
ech(o)	sound
-ectasia, ectasis	dilatation (dilation, enlargement) or stretching of a structure or part
ecto-	out, without, away from
-ectomy	excision (surgical removal or cutting out)
-edema	swelling

Word Part	Meaning
electr(o)	electricity
embol(o)	embolus
-emesis	vomiting
-emia	blood condition
en-, end-, endo-	inside
encephal(o)	brain
endocardi(o)	endocardium
enter(o)	small intestine; intestines
epi-	above, on
epididym(o)	epididymis
epiglott(o)	epiglottis
-er	one who
erythemat(o)	erythema or redness
erythr(o)	red
esophag(o)	esophagus
esthesi(o)	feeling or sensation
-esthesia	sensitivity to pain
eu-	good, normal
-eum	membrane
ex-, exo-, extra-	out, without, away from
fasci(o)	fascia
femor(o)	femur
fet(o)	fetus
fibr(o)	fiber or fibrous
fibrin(o)	fibrin
fibul(o)	fibula
fluor(o)	emitting or reflecting light
follicul(o)	follicle
fung(i)	fungus
gastr(o)	stomach
gen(o)	beginning, origin
-gen	that which generates
-genesis	producing or forming
-genic	produced by or in
genit(o)	organs of reproduction
ger(a), ger(o), geront(o)	elderly
gigant(o)	large
gingiv(o)	gums
gli(o)	neuroglia or a sticky substance
glomerul(o)	glomerulus
gloss(o)	tongue
gluc(o)	glucose
glyc(o), glycos(o)	sugar
gon(o)	genitals or reproduction
gonad(o)	gonad
-gram	a record
-graph	instrument for recording
-graphy	process of recording
-gravida	pregnant female
gynec(o)	female
heli(o)	sun
hem(a), hem(o), hemat(o)	blood
hemi-	half, partly
hemoglobin(o)	hemoglobin
hepat(o)	liver
herni(o)	hernia
hidr(o)	perspiration, sweat
hist(o)	tissue
home(o)	sameness, constant

Word Part	Meaning
humer(o)	humerus (upper arm bone)
hydr(o)	water
hyper-	excessive, more than normal
hypo-	beneath or below normal
hypophys(o)	pituitary gland (hypophysis)
hyster(o)	uterus
-ia	condition or theory
-iac	one who suffers
-iasis	condition
iatr(o)	physician or treatment
-iatrician	practitioner
-iatrics, -iatry	medical profession or treatment
-ible	able to, capable of
-ic, -ical	pertaining to
ichthy(o)	fish
idi(o)	individual
-ile	belonging to or pertaining to
ile(o)	ileum
ili(o)	ilium
immun(o)	immune, immunity
in-	not or inside (in)
infer(o)	lowermost or below
infra-	beneath, under
insulin(o)	insulin
inter-	between
intestin(o)	intestines
intra-	within
iod(o)	iodine
ipsi-	same
ir(o), irid(o)	iris
is(o)	equal
ischi(o)	ischium
-ism	condition or theory
-ist	one who
-itis	inflammation
-ium	membrane
-ive	pertaining to
jejun(o)	jejunum
kal(i)	potassium
kary(o)	nucleus
kerat(o)	cornea; hard, horny
ket(o), keton(o)	ketone bodies
kinesi(o)	movement
-kinesia, -kinesis	movement, motion
lacrim(o)	tear
lact(o)	milk
lapar(o)	abdominal wall
laryng(o)	larynx
later(o)	side
leps(o), -lepsy	seizure
leuk(o); occasionally leuc(o)	white
-lexia	words, phrases
lingu(o)	tongue
lip(o)	fat, lipid
lith(o), -lith	stone; calculus
lob(o)	lobe
log(o)	knowledge, words
-logic, -logical	pertaining to the science or study of
-logist	one who studies; specialist

Word Part	Meaning
-logy	study or science of
lumb(o)	lower back
lymph(o)	lymph, lymphatics
lymphaden(o)	lymph node
lymphangi(o)	lymph vessel
lymphat(o)	lymphatics
lys(o)	destruction, dissolving
-lysin	that which destroys
-lysis	process of loosening, freeing, or destroying
-lytic	capable of destroying
macro-	large or great
mal-	bad
-malacia	soft; abnormal softening
mamm(o)	breast
mandibul(o)	mandible
-mania	excessive preoccupation
-maniac	one who shows excessive preoccupation
mast(o)	breast
maxill(o)	maxilla
mechan(o)	mechanical
medi(o), medio-	middle
mediastin(o)	mediastinum
mega-, megal(o), megalo-	large, enlarged, or great
-megaly	enlargement
melan(o)	black
men(o)	month
mening(i), mening(o)	meninges
ment(o)	mind
meso-	middle
meta-	change; next, as in a series
metacarp(o)	metacarpals (hand bones)
metatars(o)	metatarsals (foot bones)
metr(o)	measure; uterine tissue
-meter	instrument used to measure
-metry	process of measuring
micro-	small
mid-	middle
milli-	one thousandth
mono-	one
morph(o)	shape; form
muc(o)	mucus
multi-	many
muscul(o)	muscle
myc(o)	fungus
myel(o)	bone marrow or spinal cord
my(o)	muscle
myocardi(o)	myocardium
myring(o)	eardrum
narc(o)	stupor
nas(o)	nose
nat(o)	birth
natr(o)	sodium
ne(o)	new
necr(o)	dead or death
nephr(o)	kidney
nerv(o), neur(o)	nerve
noc(i)	cause harm, injury, or pain

Word Part	Meaning
noct(i)	night
norm(o)	normal
nos(o)	disease
nucle(o)	nucleus
nulli-	none
nyct(o)	night
o(o)	egg (ovum)
obstetr(o)	midwife
ocul(o)	eye
odont(o)	teeth
-oid	resembling
-ole	small
olig(o)	few, scanty
-oma	tumor
omphal(o)	umbilicus (navel)
onc(o)	tumor
onych(o)	nail
oophor(o)	ovary
ophthalm(o)	eye
-opia, opt(o), optic(o)	vision
or(o)	mouth
orchi(o), orchid(o)	testis
-orexia	appetite, hunger
orth(o)	straight
-ory	pertaining to
-ose	sugar
-osis	condition (often an abnormal condition; sometimes, an increase), disease
osse(o)	bone or bony element
oste(o)	bone
-osmia	sense of smell
ot(o)	ear
-ous	pertaining to or characterized by
ovari(o)	ovary
ox(i)	oxygen
palat(o)	palate
pan-	all
pancreat(o)	pancreas
para-	near, beside, or abnormal
parasit(o)	parasite
par(o)	bearing offspring
-para	woman who has given birth
parathyroid(o)	parathyroid gland
patell(o)	patella
path(o), -pathy	disease
ped(o)	child (sometimes, foot)
pelv(i)	pelvis
pen(o)	penis
-penia	deficiency
-pepsia	digestion
per-	through or by
peri-	around
pericardi(o)	pericardium
perine(o)	perineum
periton(o)	peritoneum
-pexy	surgical fixation
phag(o)	eat, ingest
-phagia, -phagic, -phagy	eating, swallowing

Word Part	Meaning
phalang(o)	phalanx (bones of fingers or toes)
pharmac(o), pharmaceut(i)	drugs or medicine
pharyng(o)	pharynx
phas(o), -phasia	speech
phil(o)	attraction
phleb(o)	vein
-phobia	abnormal fear
phon(o)	voice
-phoresis	transmission
phot(o)	light
phren(o)	mind or diaphragm
-phylaxis	protection
-physis	growth
pil(o)	hair
pituitar(o)	pituitary gland
-plasma	substance of cells
plas(o), -plasia	formation, development
plast(o)	repair
-plasty	surgical repair
pleg(o), -plegia	paralysis
pleur(o)	pleura
-pnea	breathing
pneum(o)	lungs or air
pneumon(o)	lungs
pod(o)	foot
-poiesis	production
-poietin	that which causes production
poly-	many
post-	after, behind
poster(o)	back, behind
pre-	before in time or in place
presby(o)	old or old age
primi-	first
pro-	before in time or place; favoring, supporting
proct(o)	anus, rectum
prostat(o)	prostate
prote(o), protein(o)	protein
proxim(o)	near
pseudo-, pseud(o)	false
psych(o)	mind
-ptosis	prolapse (sagging or drooping)
-ptysis	spitting
pub(o)	pubis
pulm(o), pulmon(o)	lung
py(o)	pus
pyel(o)	renal pelvis
pylor(o)	pylorus
pyr(o)	fire
quad-, quadri-	four
rach(i), rachi(o)	vertebral or spinal column, spine (backbone)
radi(o)	radiant energy (sometimes, radius)
rect(o)	rectum
ren(o)	kidney
retin(o)	retina
retro-	behind, backward
rheumat(o)	rheumatism
rhin(o)	nose

Word Part	Meaning	Word Part	Meaning
rhythm(o), rrhythm(o)	rhythm	tert(i)	third
rhytid(o)	wrinkle	test(o), testicul(o)	testicle
-rrhage, -rrhagia	excessive bleeding or hemorrhage	tetra-	four
-rrhaphy	suture (uniting a wound by stitches)	therapeut(o), -therapy	treatment
-rrhea	flow or discharge	therm(o)	heat
-rrhexis	rupture	thorac(o)	thorax (chest)
sacr(o)	sacrum	thromb(o)	thrombus; clot
salping(o)	fallopian or uterine tube or auditory tube	thym(o)	thymus
		thyr(o), thyroid(o)	thyroid gland
-sarcoma	malignant tumor from connective tissue	tibi(o)	tibia
		-tic	pertaining to
scapul(o)	scapula (shoulder blade)	tom(o)	to cut
schis(o), schiz(o), schist(o), -schisis	split, cleft	-tome	an instrument used for cutting
scler(o)	hard	-tomy	incision (cutting into tissue)
-sclerosis	hardening	ton(o)	tone or tension
scop(o)	to examine, to view	tonsill(o)	tonsil
-scope	instrument used for viewing	top(o)	place or position
-scopy	visual examination	tox(o), toxic(o)	poison
scrot(o)	scrotum	trache(o)	trachea
seb(o)	sebum	trans-	across
secundi-	second	tri-	three
semi-	half, partly	trich(o)	hair
semin(o)	semen	-tripsy	surgical crushing
seps(o), sept(i)	infection	trop(o)	to stimulate
sept(o)	infection; septum	-tropic	stimulating
sial(o)	saliva; salivary glands	-tropin	that which stimulates
sialaden(o)	salivary glands	troph(o), -trophic, -trophy	nutrition
sigmoid(o)	sigmoid colon		
sin(o), sinus(o)	sinus	tympan(o)	eardrum
som(a), somat(o)	body	uln(o)	ulna (a forearm bone)
son(o)	sound	ultra-	excessive
-spasm	twitching, cramp	umbilic(o)	umbilicus
sperm(o), spermat(o)	spermatozoa	ungu(o)	nail
		uni-	one
spin(o)	spine	ur(o)	urinary tract, urine
spir(o)	to breathe (sometimes, spiral)	ureter(o)	ureter
splen(o)	spleen	urethr(o)	urethra
spondyl(o)	vertebrae	-uria	urine or urination
-stalsis	contraction	urin(o)	urine
staphyl(o)	grapelike cluster; uvula	uter(o)	uterus
-stasis	stopping, controlling	uvul(o)	uvula
-stenosis	narrowing; stricture	vag(o)	vagus nerve
stern(o)	sternum (breast bone)	vagin(o)	vagina
steth(o)	chest	valv(o), valvul(o)	valve
stomat(o)	mouth	varic(o)	twisted and swollen
-stomy	formation of an opening	vas(o)	vessel; ductus deferens
strept(o)	twisted	vascul(o)	vessel
sub-	beneath, under	ven(i), ven(o)	vein
super-	above, beyond, excessive	ventr(o)	belly
super(o)	superior (uppermost or above)	ventricul(o)	ventricle
supra-	above, beyond	venul(o)	venule
sym-, syn-	joined, together	vertebr(o)	vertebra
synov(o), synovi(o)	synovial membrane	vesic(o)	bladder or blister
tachy-	fast	vir(o), virus(o)	virus
tars(o)	ankle (sometimes, edge of eyelid)	viscer(o)	viscera
tel(e)	distant, far	vulv(o)	vulva
ten(o), tend(o), tendin(o)	tendon	xanth(o)	yellow
		xer(o)	dry
		-y	state or condition

B. English Words and Corresponding Word Parts

Meaning	Word Part
abdomen	abdomin(o)
abdominal wall	lapar(o)
able to	-able, -ible
abnormal	para-
abnormal softening	-malacia
above	epi-, super-, super(o), supra-
acid	acid(o)
across	trans-
adenoids	adenoid(o)
adrenaline	adrenalin(o)
adrenals	adren(o), adrenal(o)
after	post-
again	ana-
against	anti-, contra-
aged	ger(a), ger(o), geront(o)
air	pneum(o)
air sac	alveol(o)
albumin	albumin(o)
alkaline	alkal(o)
all	pan-
alveolus	alveol(o)
amnion	amni(o)
aneurysm	aneurysm(o)
ankle bone	tars(o)
anterior	anter(o)
anus	an(o)
anus and rectum	proct(o)
aorta	aort(o)
apex	apic(o)
appendix	append(o), appendic(o)
appetite	-orexia
arachnoid	arachn(o)
armpit	axill(o)
arms and legs	acr(o)
around	circum-, peri-
arteriole	arteriol(o)
artery	arter(o), arteri(o)
articulation	arthr(o), articul(o)
atrium	atri(o)
attraction	phil(o)
away from	ab-, ecto-, ex-, exo-, extra-
axilla	axill(o)
back	dors(o), poster(o)
backward	retr(o)
bacteria	bacter(i), bacteri(o)
bad	dys-, mal-
basic	alkal(o)
bearing offspring	par(o)
before	ante-, pre-, pro-
beginning	gen(o), -genic, -genesis, -genous
behind	poster(o), post-, retr(o)
belly side	ventr(o)
belonging to or pertaining to	-an, -ile
below normal	hypo-
below or beneath	hypo-, infer(o), infra-, sub-
beside	para-
between	inter-
beyond	super-, super(o), supra-

Meaning	Word Part
bile	bil(i), chol(e)
binding	-desis
birth	nat(o)
birth (give birth)	par(o)
woman who has given birth	-para
black	melan(o)
bladder	cyst(o), vesic(o)
bleeding, excessive	-rrhage, -rrhagia
blister	vesic(o)
blood	hem(a), hem(o), hemat(o), -emia
blood condition	-emia
blue	cyan(o)
body	som(a), somat(o)
bone	oste(o), osse(o)
bone marrow	myel(o)
bony element	osse(o)
brain	cerebr(o), encephal(o)
break	-clasia
breast	mamm(o), mast(o)
breast bone	stern(o)
breathe, breathing	-pnea, spir(o)
bronchi	bronch(o), bronchi(o)
bronchiole	bronchiol(o)
bursa	burs(o)
by	per-
calcaneus	calcane(o)
calcium	calc(i)
calculus	lith(o), -lith
cancer	cancer(o), carcin(o)
capable of	-able, -ible
carbon dioxide	-capnia
carpus	carp(o)
cartilage	chondr(o)
(to) cause an action or the result of an action	-ate
cause harm, injury, or pain	noc(i)
(that which) causes	-ant
cecum	cec(o)
cell	cyt(o), -cyte
cell, little	cellul(o)
cell substance	-plasma
cerebellum	cerebell(o)
cerebrum	cerebr(o)
cervix uteri	cervic(o)
change	meta-
characterized by	-ous
cheek	bucc(o)
chemical	chem(o)
chest	steth(o), thorac(o)
child	ped(o)
chorion	chori(o)
choroid	choroid(o)
clavicle	clavicul(o)
cleft	-schisis, schis(o), schist(o), schiz(o)
clot (thrombus)	thromb(o)
cluster	staphyl(o)

Meaning	Word Part
coagulation	coagul(o)
coal	anthrac(o)
coccyx	coccyg(o)
cochlea	cochle(o)
cold	cry(o)
collarbone	clavicul(o)
colon	col(o), colon(o)
color	chrom(o)
common bile duct	choledoch(o)
compartment	cellul(o)
condition	-ia, -iasis, -ism, -osis, -y
condition of the blood	-emia
conjunctiva	conjunctiv(o)
constant	home(o)
contraction	-stalsis
controlling	-stasis
cornea	corne(o), kerat(o)
cortex	cortic(o)
costae	cost(o)
cramp	-spasm
cranium	crani(o)
crown	coron(o)
cut (to cut)	tom(o)
incision or cutting	-tomy
instrument used to cut	-tome
cyst	cyst(o)
dead or death	necr(o)
decreased or deficient	-penia
destruction	lys(o)
that which destroys	-lysin
process of destroying	-lysis
capable of destroying	-lytic
development	plas(o), -plasia
diaphragm	phren(o)
difficult	dys-
digestion	-pepsia
digit	dactyl(o)
dilation	-ectasia, -ectasis
discharge	-rrhea
disease	nos(o), path(o), -osis, -pathy
dissolving	lys(o)
distant	dist(o), tel(e)
diverticula	diverticul(o)
dorsal	dors(o)
double	dipl(o), diplo-
down	de-
drooping	-ptosis
drugs	pharmac(o), pharmaceut(i)
dry	xer(o)
ductus deferens (vas deferens)	vas(o)
duodenum	duoden(o)
dust	coni(o)
dwarf	dwarf(o)

Meaning	Word Part
ear	aur(o), auricul(o), ot(o)
eardrum	myring(o), tympan(o)
ear wax	cerumin(o)
eat	phag(o)
eating	-phagia, -phagic, -phagy
edge of eyelid	tars(o)
egg (ovum)	o(o)
elderly	ger(a), ger(o), geront(o)
electricity	electr(o)
embolus	embol(o)
embryonic form	-blast, blast(o)
emitting or reflecting light	fluor(o)
endocardium	endocardi(o)
enlargement	-megaly
enzyme	-ase
epididymis	epididym(o)
epiglottis	epiglott(o)
equal	is(o)
erythema	erythemat(o)
esophagus	esophag(o)
examine	scop(o)
instrument used	-scope
process of examining	-scopy
excessive	ana-, hyper-, super-, ultra-
excessive preoccupation	-mania
excision	-ectomy
extremities	acr(o)
eye	ocul(o), ophthalm(o)
eyelid	blephar(o)
fallopian tube	salping(o)
false	pseudo-, pseud(o)
far	dist(o), tel(e)
fascia	fasci(o)
fast	tachy-
fat	adip(o), lip(o)
favoring	pro-
fear (abnormal)	-phobia
feeling	esthesi(o), -esthesia
female	gynec(o)
femur	femor(o)
fetus	fet(o)
few	olig(o)
fiber, fibrous	fibr(o)
fibrin	fibrin(o)
fibula	fibul(o)
fingers or toes	dactyl(o)
fire	pyr(o)
first	primi-
fish	ichthy(o)
flow	-rrhea
follicle	follicul(o)
foot	ped(o), pod(o)
for	pro-
form	morph(o)
forming	-genesis
formation	plas(o), -plasia
formation of an opening	-stomy

Meaning	Word Part
four	quad-, quadri-, tetra-
from	de-
front	anter(o)
fungus	fung(i), myc(o)
fusion	-desis
gall	bil(i), chol(e)
gallbladder	cholecyst(o)
genitals	genit(o), gon(o)
germ layer	-derm
gland	aden(o)
glans penis	balan(o)
glomerulus	glomerul(o)
glucose	gluc(o)
gonads (ovaries and testes)	gonad(o)
good	eu-
green	chlor(o)
growth	-physis
gums	gingiv(o)
hair	pil(o), trich(o)
half	hemi-, semi-
hand	chir(o)
hard	kerat(o), scler(o)
hardening	scler(o), -sclerosis
head	cephal(o)
hearing	acoust(o), audi(o)
heart	cardi(o)
heat	therm(o)
heel bone	calcane(o)
hemoglobin	hemoglobin(o)
hemorrhage	-rrhage, -rrhagia
hernia	-cele, herni(o)
hidden	crypt(o)
horny	kerat(o)
humerus	humer(o)
hunger	-orexia
hypophysis	hypophys(o), pituitar(o)
ileum	ile(o)
ilium	ili(o)
immature form	blast(o), -blast
immune, immunity	immun(o)
imperfect	atel(o)
incision	tom(o), -tomy
instrument used	-tome
incomplete	atel(o)
increase	-osis
individual	idio-
infection	seps(o), sept(i), sept(o)
inferior	infer(o)
inflammation	-itis
ingest	phag(o)
inside	en-, end-, endo-, in-
insulin	insulin(o)
intestine	enter(o), intestin(o)
iodine	iod(o)
iris	ir(o), irid(o)
ischium	ischi(o)
jejunum	jejun(o)
joined together	syn-, sym-
joint	arthr(o), articul(o)
ketone bodies	ket(o), keton(o)

Meaning	Word Part
kidney	nephr(o), ren(o)
killing	-cidal
kneecap	patell(o)
knowledge	log(o)
large	gigant(o), macr(o), megal(o), mega-, -megaly
large intestine	col(o), colon(o)
larynx	laryng(o)
life	bi(o)
light	phot(o)
lip	cheil(o)
lipid	lip(o)
liver	hepat(o)
living	bi(o)
lobe	lob(o)
location	top(o)
lower back	lumb(o)
lowermost	infer(o)
lung	pneum(o), pneumon(o), pulm(o), pulmon(o)
lymph	lymph(o)
lymph node	lymphaden(o)
lymph vessel	lymphangi(o)
lymphatics	lymph(o), lymphat(o)
male	andr(o)
mandible	mandibul(o)
many	multi-, poly-
masculine	andr(o)
maxilla	maxill(o)
measure	metr(o)
instrument used	-meter
process	-metry
mechanical	mechan(o)
mediastinum	mediastin(o)
medicine	-iatrics, -iatry, pharmac(o), pharmaceut(i)
membrane	-eum, -ium
meninges	mening(i), mening(o)
metacarpal (hand bone)	metacarp(o)
metatarsal (foot bone)	metatars(o)
middle	mid-, medi(o), meso-
midwife	obstetr(o)
milk	lact(o)
mind	ment(o), phren(o), psych(o)
month	men(o)
more than normal	hyper-
mouth	or(o), stomat(o)
movement	kinesi(o), -kinesia
mucus	muc(o)
muscle	muscul(o), my(o)
myocardium	myocardi(o)
nail	onych(o), ungu(o)
narrowing	-stenosis
nature	physi(o)
near	para-, proxim(o)
neck	cervic(o)
nerve	neur(o), nerv(o)
neuroglia	gli(o)
new	neo-

Meaning	Word Part
new opening	-stomy
next (as in a series)	meta-
night	noct(i), nyct(o)
no	a-, an-
none	nulli-
normal	norm(o), eu-
nose	nas(o), rhin(o)
not	a-, an-, in-
nucleus	kary(o), nucle(o)
nutrition	-trophic, troph(o), -trophy
old	ger(a), ger(o), geront(o), presby(o)
old age	presby(o)
on	epi-
one	uni-, mon(o)
one hundred, one-hundredth	centi-
one tenth (1/10)	deci-
one thousandth	milli-
one who	-er, -ist
one who studies	-logist
one who suffers	-iac
one with excessive preoccupation	-maniac
organs of reproduction	genit(o), gon(o)
origin	gen(o), -gen, -genic, -genesis, -genous
out	ecto-, ex-, exo-, extra-
outside	ecto-, exo-, extra-
outward	exo-
ovary	oophor(o)
ovum (egg)	o(o)
oxygen	ox(i)
pain	-algia, -dynia
palate	palat(o)
pancreas	pancreat(o)
paralysis	pleg(o), -plegia
parasite	parasit(o)
parathyroid gland	parathyroid(o)
partly	semi-
patella (kneecap)	patell(o)
pelvis	pelv(i)
penis	pen(o)
pericardium	pericardi(o)
perineum	perine(o)
peritoneum	periton(o)
perspiration	hidr(o)
pertaining to	-ac, -al, -an, -ar, -ary, -eal, -ic, -ical, -ile, -ive, -ory, -ous, -tic
pertaining to the science or study of	-logic, -logical
phalanges	phalang(o)
pharynx	pharyng(o)
phrases	-lexia
physician or treatment	iatr(o)
pituitary gland	hypophys(o), pituitar (o)
place (position)	top(o)
pleura	pleur(o)
poison	tox(o), toxic(o)

Meaning	Word Part
potassium	kal(i)
practitioner	-iatrician
pregnancy	-cyesis
pregnant female	-gravida
preoccupation (excessive)	-mania
process	-ation
production	-poiesis
that which causes	-poietin
produced by or in	-genic
producing	-genesis
prolapse	-ptosis
prostate gland	prostat(o)
protection	-phylaxis
protein	prote(o), protein(o)
pubis	pub(o)
pus	py(o)
pylorus	pylor(o)
radiant energy	radi(o)
radius	radi(o)
(to) record	gram(o)
record (the record)	-gram
recording instrument	-graph
recording process	-graphy
rectum	rect(o)
red, redness	erythr(o), erythemat(o)
removal	-ectomy
renal pelvis	pyel(o)
repair	plast(o)
reproduction	gon(o)
resembling	-oid
retina	retin(o)
reversing	de-
rheumatism	rheumat(o)
rhythm	rhythm(o), rrhythm(o)
ribs	cost(o)
rupture	-rrhexis
sac, fluid-filled	cyst(o)
sacrum	sacr(o)
sag	-ptosis
saliva	sial(o)
salivary gland	sial(o), sialaden(o)
same	ipsi-
sameness	home(o)
scanty	olig(o)
scapula (shoulder blade)	scapul(o)
scrotum	scrot(o)
sebum	seb(o)
second	secundi-
secrete	crin(o), -crine
seizure	-lepsy, leps(o)
self	aut(o)
semen	semin(o)
sensation	esthesi(o)
sense of smell	-osmia
sensitivity to pain	algesi(o), -algesia, -esthesia

Meaning	Word Part
septum	sept(o)
shape	morph(o)
shoulder blade	scapul(o)
side	later(o)
sigmoid colon	sigmoid(o)
single	mon(o)
sinus	sin(o), sinus(o)
situated above	super(o), super-, supra-
situated below	infer(o), infra-
skin	cutane(o), derm(a), dermat(o), -derm
skull	crani(o)
slow	brady-
small	micr(o), -ole
small intestine	enter(o)
sodium	natr(o)
soft, softening	-malacia
sound	ech(o), son(o)
specialist	-logist
speech	phas(o), -phasia
sperm, spermatozoa	spermat(o), sperm(o)
spider	arachn(o)
spinal cord	myel(o)
spine	rach(i), rachi(o), spondyl(o), spin(o)
spitting	-ptysis
spleen	splen(o)
split	schis(o), schist(o), schiz(o), -schisis
starch	amyl(o)
state	-y
sternum (breast bone)	stern(o)
sticky substance	gli(o)
stiff	ankyl(o)
stimulate	trop(o)
stimulating	-tropic
that which stimulates	-tropin
stomach	gastr(o)
stone	lith(o), -lith
stopping	-stasis
straight	orth(o)
stretching	-ectasia, -ectasis
stricture	-stenosis
study or science of	-logy
stupor	narc(o)
sugar	glyc(o), glycos(o), -ose
sun	heli(o)
supporting	pro-
surgical crushing	-tripsy
surgical fixation	-pexy
surgical puncture	-centesis
surgical repair	-plasty
suture	-rrhaphy
swallowing	-phagia, -phagic, -phagy
sweat	hidr(o)
swelling	-edema
symptom	sympt(o)
synovial membrane	synov(o), synovi(o)
tail	caud(o)

Meaning	Word Part
tail bone	coccyg(o)
tarsals (ankle bones)	tars(o)
tear (crying)	dacry(o), lacrim(o)
teeth	dent(i), dent(o), odont(o)
tendon	ten(o), tend(o), tendin(o)
tension	ton(o)
testis, testicle	orchi(o), orchid(o), test(o)
theory	-ia, -ism
thirst	dips(o), -dipsia
three	tri-
throat	pharyng(o)
thrombus	thromb(o)
through	dia-, per-, trans-
thymus	thym(o)
thyroid gland	thyr(o), thryoid(o)
tibia	tibi(o)
tissue	hist(o)
toe	dactyl(o)
together	sym-, syn-
tone	ton(o)
tongue	gloss(o), lingu(o)
tonsil	tonsill(o)
toward	ad-
trachea	trache(o)
transmission	-phoresis
treatment	iatr(o), -iatry, therapeut(o), -therapy
tree	dendr(o)
tumor	onc(o), -oma
tumor, malignant	-sarcoma from connective tissue
turn	trop(o)
twice	di-
twisted	strept(o)
twisted and swollen	varic(o)
twitching	-spasm
two	bi-, di-
ulna	uln(o)
umbilicus	omphal(o), umbilic(o)
under	infra-, sub-
upon	epi-
upper arm bone	humer(o)
uppermost	super(o)
ureter	ureter(o)
urethra	urethr(o)
urinary tract	ur(o)
urination	-uria
urine	ur(o), -uria, urin(o)
uterine tissue	metr(o)
uterine tube	salping(o)
uterus	hyster(o), uter(o)
uvula	staphyl(o), uvul(o)
vagina	colp(o), vagin(o)
vagus nerve	vag(o)
valve	valv(o), valvul(o)
varicose vein	varic(o)
vein	phleb(o), ven(o), ven(i)
ventral	ventr(o)
ventricle	ventricul(o)
venule	venul(o)
vertebra	spondyl(o), vertebr(o)

Meaning	Word Part	Meaning	Word Part
vertebral column	rach(i), rachi(o), spondyl(o), spin(o)	water	hydr(o)
vessel	angi(o), vas(o), vascul(o)	weakness	-asthenia
view	scop(o)	white	alb(o), albin(o), leuk(o), leuc(o)
instrument used	-scope	windpipe	trache(o)
process of viewing	-scopy	within	intra-
virus	vir(o), virus(o)	without	a-, an-, ecto-, ex-, exo-, extra
viscera	viscer(o)	words	-lexia, log(o)
vision	opt(o), optic(o)	wrinkle	rhytid(o)
voice	phon(o)	wrist bone	carp(o)
vomiting	-emesis	yellow	xanth(o)
vulva	vulv(o)	yellow, fatty plaque	ather(o)

Appendix IV: Solutions to Review Exercises

Chapter 1

Exercise 1
1. ophthalm
2. nas, rhin
3. thorac
4. spondyl, vertebr
5. abdomin

Exercise 2
1. combining form
2. combining form
3. word root
4. combining form
5. word root
6. word root
7. combining form
8. word root

Exercise 3
1. prefix
2. suffix
3. prefix
4. suffix
5. combining form
6. suffix
7. prefix
8. combining form

Exercise 4
1. prefix
2. suffix
3. suffix
4. suffix
5. prefix
6. suffix
7. prefix
8. prefix

Exercise 5
1. otic
2. otitis
3. otology
4. otoplasty
5. otorrhea
6. ototomy

Exercise 6
1. tonsillitis
2. uremia
3. cardioaortitis
4. urogenital
5. enteritis
6. enterocyst

Exercise 7
1. periappendicitis
2. unilateral
3. antiseptic
4. anemia

Exercise 8
1. acidosis
2. acromegaly
3. antiemesis
4. bronchoscopy
5. dysphagia
6. hypothyroidism
7. leukocytosis
8. malabsorption
9. myometrium
10. thrombophlebitis

Exercise 9
1. Alzheimer disease
2. Beckman thermometer

3. cesarean section
4. Foley catheter
5. Holter monitor

Exercise 10
1. A
2. A
3. B
4. B
5. A
6. A
7. B
8. A

Exercise 11
1. capsules
2. cataracts
3. calculi
4. cortices
5. diagnoses
6. meninges
7. neuroses
8. protozoa
9. vertices
10. viruses

Exercise 12
1. appendix
2. fungus
3. larynx
4. prognosis
5. sarcoma
6. spermatozoon
7. syndrome
8. thrombus

Exercise 13
1. six
2. long
3. sē
4. i in hī, e in sē, e in mē

Exercise 14
1. E
2. B
3. D
4. A
5. E
6. B
7. C
8. F

Exercise 15
1. to secrete
2. feeling or sensation
3. stomach
4. elderly
5. female
6. larynx
7. birth
8. new
9. straight
10. nose

Exercise 16
1. ped(o)
2. ot(o)
3. ophthalm(o)
4. ped(o)
5. cardi(o)
6. immun(o)
7. psych(o)

8. neur(o)
9. dermat(o)
10. ur(o)

Exercise 17

1. dermato/logic, dermato/logical; dermat(o), skin; -logic or -logical, pertaining to the study of
2. cardio/logic; cardi(o), heart; -logic, pertaining to the study of
3. cardi/ac; cardi, heart; -ac, pertaining to
4. gastr/ic; gastr, stomach; -ic, pertaining to
5. neuro/logic, neuro/log-ical; neur(o), nerve; -logic or -logical, pertaining to the study of
6. ophthalmo/logic, ophthalmo/logical; opthalm(o), eye; -logic or -logical, pertaining to the study of
7. ophthalm/ic; ophthalm, eye; -ic, pertaining to
8. ot/ic; ot, ear; -ic, pertaining to

9. ped/iatric; ped, child; -iatric, medical profession or treatment
10. patho/logic, patho/logical; path(o), disease; -logic or -logical, pertaining to the study of

Exercise 18

1. geriatrics
2. immunology
3. obstetrics
4. orthopedics
5. radiology

Exercise 19

1. obstetr/ics
2. endo/crino/logist
3. gyneco/logy
4. oto/laryngo/logist
5. ped/iatric(s)
6. patho/logist
7. an/esthesio/logy
8. neo/nato/logy

Exercise 20

1. rheumato/logist
2. immuno/logist
3. ortho/ped/ics
4. psych/iatry
5. neuro/surgery
6. uro/logist

Exercise 21

1. triage
2. epidemic
3. preventive
4. emergency
5. forensic

Exercise 22

1. cardiology
2. radiology
3. immunology
4. endocrinology
5. otolaryngology or rhinology
6. obstetrics
7. gastroenterology
8. urology
9. orthopedics
10. rheumatology

Exercise 23

1. E
2. A
3. B
4. C
5. D

Exercise 24

1. inpatients
2. outpatients
3. HIPAA

Exercise 25

1. chief complaint
2. diagnosis
3. family history
4. history and physical
5. history of present illness
6. health history
7. outpatient
8. physical examination
9. past medical history
10. review of systems
11. treatment
12. vital signs

Exercise 26

1. C
2. A
3. B
4. E
5. F
6. D

Exercise 27

1. generic
2. effects
3. Celebrex
4. pharmacist

Chapter 1 Self-Test

I.
1. A combining form is a word root with an attached vowel to which prefixes and suffixes can be added.
2. A prefix is placed before a word root to modify its meaning.
3. A suffix is attached to the end of a word or word part to modify its meaning.
4. A word root is the main body of a word.

II.
1. cardi/ac: cardi(o) is CF: -ac is S
2. gastr/ic: gastr(o) is CF; -ic is S
3. geronto/logy: geront(o) is CF; -logy is S
4. neuro/logy: neur(o) is CF; -logy is S
5. onco/logy: onc(o) is CF; -logy is S
6. ophthalmo/logical: ophthalm(o) is CF; -logical is S

7. ot/ic: ot(o) is CF; -ic is S
8. patho/logy: path(o) is CF; -logy is S
9. psych/iatry: psych(o) is CF; -iatry is S
10. uro/logic: ur(o) is CF; -ic is S

III.
1. atria
2. bullae
3. bursa
4. cervix
5. enchondroma
6. ganglia
7. index
8. microvilli
9. septa
10. syndromes

IV.
(No particular order)
1. anatomy
2. diagnostic test or procedure
3. pathology
4. surgery
5. therapy

V.
1. an-, without; esthesio, feeling or sensation; -logist, specialist
2. cardio, heart; -logy, specialty
3. dermato, skin; -logic, pertaining to the study of
4. gastr, stomach; -ic, pertaining to
5. ger, elderly or aged; -iatrics, medical profession
6. gyneco, female; -logy, study of
7. neo, new; nato, birth; -logist, specialist
8. neuro, nerve; -logy, study of
9. obstetr, midwife; -ic, pertaining to
10. ortho, straight; ped, child; -ist, specialist
11. ot, ear; -ic, pertaining to
12. onco, tumor; -logy, study of
13. ophthalmo, eye; -logic, pertaining to the study of

14. ped, child; -iatric, pertaining to profession or treatment
15. psych, mind; -iatry, medical profession

VI.
1. An anatomic pathologist is certified in the study of the effects of disease on the body's structure; a clinical pathologist is certified in the laboratory study of disease.
2. A clinical psychologist is not a physician (clinical psychology is a branch of psychology), whereas a psychiatrist is a medical doctor.
3. An internist is a medical specialist, whereas a physician intern is in postgraduate training before being licensed as a physician.
4. A primary health care provider sees patients in

his or her office and coordinates health care for individuals, often referring patients to specialists as needed; an emergency physician sees patients in the hospital emergency department.

5. Therapy means treatment, whereas triage is the sorting and prioritizing according to the patients' needs for care.

6. An anesthetic is a drug or agent that is capable of producing loss of feeling; anesthetics are given to a patient by an anesthesiologist or an anesthetist (nurse or other person trained in administered anesthetics).

VII.
1. cardiologist
2. obstetrician
3. anesthetist
4. neonatologist

5. gastroenterologist
6. radiologist
7. orthopedist
8. nerve cell
9. clinical pathologist
10. forensic

VIII.
1. internist
2. diagnosis
3. triage
4. cardiac
5. geriatrician
6. neonatal
7. endocrinology
8. pathology
9. neurosurgery
10. urology

IX.
cardiac, ophthalmic, psychiatry

X.
1. ACA
2. FDA
3. HPI
4. OTC
5. Pt
6. OB

7. DOB
8. Tx

XI.
1. anesthesiology
2. forensic
3. gastroenterology
4. orthopedics
5. pediatric
6. urological

XII.
1. skin
2. lungs
3. gerontologist
4. kidneys
5. ENT

XIII.
1. action
2. pharmacology
3. systemic
4. prescription
5. dose

XIV.
1. B
2. D
3. C
4. B
5. B

6. C
7. A
8. B
9. B
10. C
11. C
12. B
13. A
14. C
15. B
16. C
17. B
18. B
19. C
20. D

XV.
1. medical treatment performed mainly by manipulative and operative methods
2. treatment of disease using hormones
3. any disease of the nose
4. a physician specializing in the larynx
5. branch of cardiology specializing in children

Chapter 2

Exercise 1
1. C
2. A
3. B

Exercise 2
1. A
2. B
3. C
4. E
5. D

Exercise 3
1. E
2. D
3. F
4. G
5. A
6. C
7. B

Exercise 4
1. bacter(i), bacteri(o)
2. fung(i), myc(o)
3. staphyl(o)
4. sept(i), sept(o), seps(o)
5. strept(o)
6. vir(o), virus(o)

Exercise 5
1. bacilli
2. cocci
3. spirilla

Exercise 6
1-4 (No particular order): bacteria, fungi, protozoa, viruses

Exercise 7
1. weapons
2. Disease
3. bioterrorism
4. disseminated

Exercise 8
1. D
2. G
3. E
4. H
5. C
6. A
7. F
8. B

Exercise 9
1. append(o), appendic(o)
2. col(o), colon(o)
3. pod(o)
4. chir(o)
5. cephal(o)

6. or(o), stomat(o)
7. muscul(o), my(o)
8. nas(o), rhin(o)
9. cutane(o), derm(a), dermat(o)
10. hist(o)
11. tonsill(o)
12. trache(o)

Exercise 10
1. condition
2. inflammation
3. fear
4. prolapse
5. -mania
6. -oma
7. -pathy
8. -cele
9. -emia
10. -lith

Exercise 11
1. aden/itis: aden, gland; -itis, inflammation
2. appendic/itis: appendic, appendix; -itis, inflammation
3. cephal/ic: cephal, head; -ic, pertaining to

4. mast/itis: mast, breast; -itis, inflammation
5. muscul/ar: muscul, muscle; -ar, pertaining to
6. nas, nose; -al, pertaining to
7. neur/itis: neur, nerve; -itis, inflammation
8. ophthalm/itis: ophthalm, eye; -itis, inflammation
9. or/al: or, mouth; -al, pertaining to
10. oste/itis: oste, bone; -itis, inflammation
11. ot/itis: ot, ear; -itis, inflammation
12. tonsill/itis: tonsill, tonsil; -itis, inflammation

Exercise 12
1. carcin/oma: a cancerous tumor (or cancer)
2. dermat/itis: inflammation of the skin
3. ophthalmo/pathy: any disease of the eye
4. oto/pathy: a disease of the ear

Exercise 13
1. A
2. C
3. D
4. E
5. B
6. J
7. I
8. G
9. F
10. H

Exercise 14
1. blephar/al: blephar, eyelid; -al, pertaining to
2. cancer/ous: cancer, cancer; -ous, pertaining to
3. cerebr/al: cerebr, cerebrum; -al, pertaining to
4. mamm/ary: mamm, breast; -ary, pertaining to
5. trache/al: trache, trachea; -al, pertaining to

Exercise 15
1. lact/ase: the enzyme that breaks down lactose
2. lact/ose: main sugar found in milk
3. pyro/mania: disorder characterized by excessive preoccupation with fires
4. pyro/maniac: a person with a compulsion to set fires
5. neur/al: pertaining to a nerve

Exercise 16
1. B
2. D
3. H
4. J
5. E
6. A
7. I
8. G
9. C
10. F

Exercise 17
1. C
2. E
3. H
4. A
5. B
6. I
7. G
8. J
9. D
10. F

Exercise 18
1. microscope
2. hemolysin
3. hemolytic
4. ophthalmopathy
5. carcinogen
6. cephalometry
7. phagocyte
8. epilepsy

Exercise 19
1. white
2. green
3. blue
4. red
5. white
6. black
7. yellow

Exercise 20
1. xanthoderma
2. cyanosis
3. erythrocyte
4. albinism

Exercise 21
1. E
2. B
3. G
4. H
5. F
6. C
7. D
8. A

Exercise 22
1. -penia
2. -rrhea
3. -oid
4. -rrhexis
5. -spasm

Exercise 23
1. cardio/megaly: cardi(o), heart; -megaly, enlargement
2. my/algia: my(o), muscle; -algia, pain
3. ophthalm/algia: ophthalm(o), eye; -algia, pain
   ophthalmo/dynia: ophthalm(o), eye; -dynia, pain
4. ophthalmo/rrhagia: ophthalm(o), eye; -rrhagia, hemorrhage
5. ot/algia: ot(o), ear; -algia, pain
   ot/dynia: ot(o), ear; -dynia, pain

6. oto/rrhea: ot(o), ear; -rrhea, discharge

Exercise 24
1. pulse
2. respiration
3. auscultation
4. percussion
5. palpation
6. ambulation

Exercise 25
1. I
2. C
3. E
4. J
5. A
6. D
7. G
8. B
9. H
10. F

Exercise 26
1. E
2. A
3. B
4. D
5. E
6. F
7. C

Exercise 27
1. contrast
2. tomography
3. radioactive
4. resonance
5. sound

Exercise 28
1. temperature, pulse, respiration, and blood pressure
2. CT
3. No

Exercise 29
1. chem(o)
2. cry(o)
3. pharmac(o)
4. esthesi(o)
5. therm(o)
6. algesi(o)
7. narc(o)
8. therapeut(o)

Exercise 30
1. therapeutic
2. radiation
3. thermotherapy
4. cryotherapy

Exercise 31
1. G
2. A
3. F
4. H
5. I
6. J
7. B
8. D
9. C
10. E

Exercise 32
1. neur/ectomy
2. neuro/lysis
3. amnio/centesis
4. oto/plasty
5. ophthalmo/plasty
6. neuro/tripsy

Exercise 33
1. loosening, freeing, destroying
2. eye
3. suture
4. ear
5. brain
6. surgical repair
7. vessel
8. gland
9. incision
10. eyelid

Exercise 34
1. colono/scopy
2. append/ectomy
3. encephalo/tomy
4. osteo/tome
5. mammo/plasty
6. blepharo/plasty
7. chiro/plasty
8. angio/rrhaphy

Exercise 35
1. analgesic
2. anesthesia
3. neuromuscular
4. narcotic
5. radiopharmaceuticals
6. orally (*per os*)
7. water (*aqua*)
8. immediately (*statim*)
9. three times a day (*ter in die*)
10. every (*quaque*)

Chapter 2 Self-Test

I.
1. F
2. D
3. C
4. B
5. E
6. H
7. A
8. G

II.
1. E
2. C
3. B
4. D
5. A
6. F

III.
1. E
2. A
3. D
4. F
5. G
6. H
7. B
8. C

IV.
1. E
2. A
3. I
4. J
5. H
6. B
7. F
8. C
9. D
10. G

V.
1. symptom
2. chiroplasty
3. stasis
4. cardiomegaly
5. electrocardiogram
6. tracheostomy
7. adenectomy
8. ophthalmomalacia
9. otodynia
10. computed tomography
11. dermatitis
12. jaundice
13. appendicitis
14. encephalocele
15. phobia
16. biopsy
17. otopathy
18. histology
19. phagocyte
20. hemolyze
21. organic disease
22. nosocomial

VI.
(No particular order, one feature)
1. viruses: much smaller than bacteria; replicate only within a cell
2. bacteria: classified according to shape
3. fungi: absorb organic molecules from surroundings; may be parasitic
4. protozoa: only a few are pathogenic

VII.
1. amnio/centesis: amnion; surgical puncture
2. blepharo/plasty: eyelid; surgical repair
3. colo/scopy: colon; visual examination
4. echo/graphy: sound; process of recording
5. electro/cardio/graph: electricity; heart; instrument used to record
6. fluoro/scope: emitting or reflecting light; instrument used to view
7. oste/oid: bone; resembling
8. tomo/gram: to cut; a record

VIII.
1. hemorrhage
2. colectomy or colonectomy
3. ophthalmotomy
4. encephalotome
5. otoplasty
6. erythrocyte
7. disorder
8. carcinogen
9. ophthalmopathy
10. pyromania
11. neurotripsy
12. colopexy
13. angiorrhaphy
14. blepharedema
15. otoscopy
16. osteitis
17. myalgia
18. nasal
19. calculi
20. microscopy

IX.
1. medications used to treat malignant neoplasms
2. treatment using chemical agents
3. treatment of disease with medicine (drugs)
4. treatment of disease with heat

X.
1. palpation
2. percussion
3. auscultation

XI.
1. encephalocele
2. dermatitis
3. albinism
4. blepharoptosis

XII.
1. angio, vessel
2. blepharo, eyelid
3. chiro, hand
4. mammo, breast
5. ophthalmo, eye
6. oto, ear

XIII.
1. Mania is a disorder characterized by excessive preoccupation, whereas a phobia is a persistent, irrational fear of something.
2. Lactase is a type of enzyme that breaks down lactose, the major sugar found in milk.
3. Biopsy means the examination of tissue from the living body, whereas an autopsy is examination of the organs and tissues of a dead body.
4. An ophthalmoscope is the name of the instrument used in ophthalmoscopy, the examination of the interior of the eye.
5. Incision means cutting into, whereas excision means removal.
6. An electrocardiogram is the tracing obtained during electrocardiography, whereas electrocardiograph is the machine used.
7. An encephalotome is the name of the instrument used in encephalotomy, surgical incision of the brain.

XIV.
1. sound waves
2. pain
3. magnetic
4. nerve
5. ultrasound

XV.
1. twice per day
2. counter
3. abdomen
4. as needed
5. pressure

XVI.
cephalic, neurotripsy, ophthalmoplasty, cerebral, symptom

XVII.
1. BP
2. FEMA
3. HPF
4. MIS
5. NPO
6. Rx
7. SPECT
8. WMD
9. US
10. WHO

XVIII.
1. appendectomy
2. encephalotomy
3. calcipenia
4. neurolysis
5. sonography
6. virulence

XIX.
1. radiopharmaceuticals
2. antineoplastics
3. chemotherapy
4. analgesics
5. narcotic

XX.
1. E
2. D
3. A
4. C
5. C
6. B
7. A
8. C
9. D
10. E

XXI.
1. appendic/itis: inflammation of the appendix
2. blephar/itis: inflammation of the eyelid
3. chiro/spasm: cramping of the hand
4. encephal/itis: inflammation of the brain
5. leuko/cyte: white cell (white blood cell)
6. myo/cele: hernia of muscle
7. neuro/genic: originating in the nervous system
8. rhino/plasty: surgical repair of the nose
9. tracheo/scopy: visual examination of the trachea
10. xanth/ous: yellowish

Chapter 3

Exercise 1
(No particular order)
1. nucleus
2. cytoplasm
3. cell membrane

Exercise 2
organelles, cells, tissues, organs

Exercise 3
1. cell
2. tissue
3. organ
4. connective
5. epithelial
6. muscle
7. nervous
8. somatic
9. stem
10. congenital

Exercise 4
1. B
2. B
3. E
4. F
5. A
6. D
7. C
8. A

Exercise 5
1. bi/ped/al: bi-, two; ped, foot; -al, pertaining to
2. mono/vision: mon(o), one; vision, seeing
3. tri/plegia: tri-, three; -plegia, paralysis
4. super/vitamin/osis: super-, excessive; vitamin; -osis, condition

Exercise 6
1. A
2. E
3. G
4. F
5. B
6. H
7. D
8. C

Exercise 7
1. away from, toward
2. behind
3. inside
4. between
5. above
6. around
7. postnatal
8. extracellular
9. same
10. across

Exercise 8
1. anesthesia
2. anhydrous
3. aplastic
4. atraumatic
5. asymptomatic

Exercise 9
1. incompatible
2. indigestion
3. inattentive
4. incapable
5. inoperable

Exercise 10
1. A
2. F
3. A
4. B
5. D
6. B
7. G
8. E
9. E
10. C

Exercise 11
1. tachy(phasia)
2. mal(aise)
3. pre(cancerous)
4. macro(scopic)
5. eu(phoria)
6. post(anesthetic)
7. micr(otia)
8. dys(lexia)
9. contra(ceptive)
10. brady(phasia)

Exercise 12
1. mal/nutrition: mal-, poor; nutrition, nutrients
2. macro/cyte: macro-, large; -cyte, cell
3. mega/dose: mega-, large; dose
4. megalo/cyte: megalo-, large; -cyte, cell
5. micro/cyte: micro-, small; -cyte, cell

Exercise 13
1. frontal plane
2. transverse plane
3. sagittal plane

Exercise 14
1. front, anterior
2. tail or lower part of body, caudal (caudad)
3. head, cephalad
4. distant or far, distal
5. back side, dorsal
6. situated below, inferior
7. side or farther from midline, lateral
8. middle, medial or median
9. behind (toward the back), posterior
10. near, proximal
11. uppermost, superior
12. belly, ventral

Exercise 15
1. anterior
2. posterior
3. lateral

Exercise 16
1. posteroanterior
2. left lateral

Exercise 17
1. antero/medi/al: anter(o), front; medi, middle
2. antero/superior: anter(o), toward the front; superior, uppermost or above
3. cephal/ic: cephal(o), head
4. dorso/later/al: dors(o), behind or postero/lateral; poster(o), posterior; later, side
5. infero/median: infer(o), below; medi, middle

6. postero/extern/al: poster(o), posterior; extern, outer
7. postero/medi/al: poster(o), posterior; medi, middle
8. postero/superior: poster(o), toward the back; superior, uppermost or above
9. postero/intern/al: poster(o), posterior; intern, within
10. ventro/medi/an: ventr(o), bellyside; medi, middle

Exercise 18
1. supine
2. prone

Exercise 19
1. B
2. A
3. H
4. E
5. G
6. C
7. D
8. F

Exercise 20
1. RUQ
2. RLQ
3. LUQ
4. LLQ

Exercise 21
1. cranial
2. thoracic
3. abdominopelvic

Exercise 22
1. dactyl/itis: dactyl, finger or toe; -itis, inflammation
2. chiro/plasty: chir(o), hand; -plasty, surgical repair
3. omphal/ic: omphal, umbilicus; -ic, pertaining to
4. omphal/itis: omphal, umbilicus; -itis, inflammation

5. omphal/oma: omphal, umbilicus; -oma, tumor
6. omphalo/rrhagia: omphal(o), umbilicus; -rrhagia, hemorrhage
7. omphalo/rrhexis: omphal(o), umbilicus; -rrhexis, rupture
8. pelv/ic: pelv, pelvis; -ic, pertaining to
9. trans/thorac/ic: trans-, across (through); thorac, chest; -ic pertaining to
10. supra/thorac/ic: supra-, superior; thorac, chest; -ic pertaining to

Exercise 23
1. pyrogen
2. dysplasia
3. aplasia
4. hypoplasia
5. hyperplasia
6. anaplasia

Exercise 24
1. somatic
2. brain
3. somatopsychic
4. dehiscence
5. evisceration

Exercise 25
1. intra(cellular)
2. extra(cellular)
3. inter(stitial)

Exercise 26
1. F
2. A
3. B
4. D
5. G
6. C
7. E
8. F

Exercise 27
1. hyper/calc/emia: hyper-, greater than normal; calc, calcium; -emia, blood
2. hyper/kal/emia: hyper-, greater than normal; kal, potassium; -emia, blood
3. hyper/natr/emia: hyper-, greater than normal; natr, sodium; -emia, blood
4. hypo/calc/emia: hypo-, less than normal; calc, calcium; -emia, blood
5. hypo/kal/emia: hypo-, less than normal; kal, potassium; -emia, blood

6. hypo/natr/emia: hypo-, less than normal; natr, sodium; -emia, blood

Exercise 28
1. excessive loss of water from body tissue
2. swelling caused by excessive accumulation of fluid in the body tissues
3. molecules that conduct an electric charge
4. the regulation of water by the body
5. to redirect the flow of body fluid from one part of the body to another, or the device that is implanted to accomplish that purpose

Exercise 29
1. A
2. A
3. C
4. G
5. B
6. D
7. E
8. F

Exercise 30
1. F
2. C
3. B
4. G
5. A
6. E
7. D

Exercise 31
1. F
2. H
3. C
4. B
5. D
6. A
7. E
8. G

Exercise 32
1. hemato/log/ic: pertaining to hematology
2. hemato/poiesis: production of blood
3. hemato/poietic: pertaining to hematopoiesis

Exercise 33
1. anti/coagul/ant: anti-, against; coagul, coagulation; -ant, that which causes
2. coagul/ant: coagul, coagulation; -ant, that which causes

3. coagul/ate: coagul, coagulation; -ate, to cause a reaction
4. coagulo/pathy: coagul(o), coagulation; -pathy, disease

Exercise 34
1. fibrinolysis
2. coagulation
3. fibrin
4. fibrinolysin
5. fibrinogen

Exercise 35
(No particular order)
1. erythrocyte, red (blood) cell
2. leukocyte, white (blood) cell
3. thrombocyte, blood platelet

Exercise 36
(No particular order)
1. basophil
2. eosinophil
3. neutrophil
4. lymphocyte
5. monocyte

Exercise 37
1. erythro/cyt/ic: erythr(o), red; cyt, cell; -ic, pertaining to
2. erythro/poiesis: erythr(o), red; -poiesis, production
3. erythro/poietin: erythr(o), red; -poietin, that which causes production
4. karyo/megaly: kary(o), nucleus; -megaly, enlarged
5. nucle/oid: nucle, nucleus, -oid, resembling

Exercise 38
1. thrombo/cyto/penia: thromb(o), clot; cyt(o), cell; -penia, deficiency
2. thrombo/cyt/osis: thromb(o), clot; cyt, cell; -osis, increase
3. thrombo/lysis: thromb(o), thrombus; -lysis, destroying
4. thrombo/lytic: thromb(o), thrombus; -lytic, capable of destroying
5. thromb/osis: thromb(o), thrombus; -osis, abnormal condition

Exercise 39
1. thrombocyte
2. thrombus

3. clot
4. thrombolysis
5. hemolysis
6. thrombocytosis
7. anemia
8. fainting

Exercise 40
1. There is an increase in leukocytes in both, but in leukemia, leukocyte production is uncontrolled and many of the leukocytes are immature and nonfunctional.
2. Infection means the presence of living microorganisms within tissue, whereas inflammation is a protective response of body tissues to irritation or injury.

Exercise 41
1. hemoglobinopathy
2. hemolytic anemia
3. aplastic anemia

Exercise 42
1. macro/cyte: macr(o), large; -cyte, cell
2. megalo/cyte: megal(o), large; -cyte, cell
3. macro/cyt/osis: macr(o), large; -cyt, cell; -osis, abnormal increase
4. micro/cyte: micr(o), small; -cyte, cell
5. micro/cyt/osis: micr(o), small; -cyt, cell; -osis, abnormal increase

Exercise 43
1. hypo/chrom/ia: hypo-, less than normal; chrom, color; -ia, condition
2. hypo/chrom/ic: hypo-, less than normal; chrom, color; -ic, pertaining to
3. hyper/chrom/ic: hyper-, greater than normal; chrom, color; -ic, pertaining to

Exercise 44
1. agglutination
2. transfusion
3. autologous
4. homologous
5. clots (or coagulation)
6. hemostasis

Exercise 45
1. antigen
2. susceptible
3. immunoglobulin
4. interferon
5. Active
6. immunodeficiency

Exercise 46
1. E
2. F
3. C
4. A
5. D
6. B

Exercise 47
1. centimeter
2. deciliter
3. gram
4. kilogram
5. liter
6. microgram
7. milligram
8. milliliter
9. alert and oriented
10. blood pressure
11. chief complaint
12. date of birth
13. diagnosis
14. history
15. pulse
16. physical examination
17. respirations
18. range of motion
19. right upper quadrant
20. temperature

Exercise 48
1. b.i.d.
2. h
3. IV
4. min
5. p.o.
6. A&O
7. HEENT
8. L&W
9. WD/WN

Chapter 3 Self-Test

I.
1. J
2. C
3. F
4. B
5. G
6. A
7. E
8. D
9. I
10. H

II.
1. A
2. I
3. C
4. G
5. E
6. D
7. D
8. C
9. B
10. B
11. K

III.
1. A
2. C
3. B
4. C
5. B

IV.
1. A
2. C
3. D
4. B

V.
1. A
2. B
3. E
4. C
5. D
6. F

VI.
1. sagittal
2. transverse
3. frontal
4. superior
5. inferior
6. lateral

VII.
1. B
2. H
3. C
4. I
5. F
6. A
7. G
8. D
9. E

VIII.
1. hypertrophy
2. hyperplasia

IX.
1. extra
2. intra
3. inter

X.
(Any five; no particular order)
1-5. natural barriers (unbroken skin), complement, interferon, phagocytes, inflammation, mucus, cilia, normal flora, urination, chemicals in human tears, and acids of the stomach, vagina, and skin

XI.
1. cellul/ar: pertaining to or consisting of cells
2. coagul/ant: a substance that promotes coagulation
3. post/nas/al: post-, behind; nas(o), nose; -al, pertaining to
4. tachy/phas/ia: tachy-, fast; phas(o), speech; -ia, condition
5. trans/derm/al: trans-, across; derm(o), skin; -al, pertaining to

XII.
1. ante-, pre-: before
2. macro-, mega-: large
3. mono-, uni-: one
4. quad-, tetra-: four

XIII.
1. aplasia: lack of development of an organ or tissue
2. anaplasia: loss of differentiation of cells and their orientation, characteristic of tumors
3. dysplasia: abnormality in development (in anatomy, alteration in cell size, shape, and organization)
4. hyperplasia: abnormal increase in the number of normal cells
5. hypoplasia: underdevelopment of an organ or tissue

XIV.
1. mononeuropathy
2. triceps
3. fibrinogen
4. pandemic
5. polydactyly
6. circumduction
7. virulence
8. transdermal
9. mesoderm
10. symmetry
11. tissue
12. aplastic
13. front to back
14. farther from the origin
15. antibodies
16. inflammation
17. lying face downward
18. dermatosis
19. intracellular
20. diaphragm

XV.
1. abduction
2. polydactyly
3. hydrocephalus

XVI.
1. anesthesia
2. anhydrous
3. aplastic
4. asymptomatic
5. atraumatic

XVII.
1. allograft
2. electroencephalogram
3. microcyte
4. dysplasia
5. unilateral
6. hyponatremia
7. immunity
8. chirospasm
9. thrombolysis
10. thrombosis
11. dermatitis
12. abscess
13. supine
14. erythrocyte (or red blood cell)
15. suprathoracic
16. abdominopelvic
17. peritoneal
18. plantar
19. hematopoiesis
20. intracellular

XVIII.
1. An autologous tissue graft is transferred from one site to another site on the same body.
2. A homologous tissue graft is tissue removed from a donor and transplanted to a recipient of the same species.

XIX.

1. Afebrile means without fever; antifebrile means reducing fever or an agent that relieves or reduces fever.
2. Agglutination is a clumping together of cells as in testing blood. Coagulation is a complex chemical reaction in which a solid blood clot forms.
3. Erythropoiesis is production of erythrocytes. Erythropoietin is the substance that causes the bone marrow to produce erythrocytes.
4. Excretion is the body's way of eliminating wastes. Secretion is the process of discharging a chemical substance needed by the body into a cavity.
5. Inflammation is a normal response to injury or irritation. Infection is invasion of body tissue by pathogenic microorganisms.
6. Parietal peritoneum lines the walls of the abdominopelvic cavity; visceral peritoneum is reflected over the viscera
7. Plasma is the fluid part of blood. Interstitial fluid is not part of the blood and is located between cells in the body tissue.
8. Prone means lying face downward; supine means lying with the face upward.
9. Somatic cells are body cells in general; stem cells are undifferentiated cells that can give rise to other types of cells.

XX.

1. In postnatal, post- means after; in postnasal, post- means behind.
2. In supervitaminosis, super- means excessive; in suprarenal, supra- means above.
3. Both macro- and megalo- mean large, but when used together (as in describing erythrocytes), megalo- means larger than macro-.

XXI.

1. abduct
2. tachyphasia
3. anticoagulant
4. incompatible
5. ipsilateral
6. afebrile
7. hypochromic
8. hypoplasia
9. hyperkalemia
10. superior
11. extracellular
12. microcyte
13. postnatal
14. distal

XXII.

1. dehiscence
2. supratherapeutic
3. thrombocytopenia
4. anemia
5. thrombosis
6. immunodeficiency
7. hematologic
8. b.i.d.

XXIII.

1. hyponatremia
2. malaise
3. normocephalic
4. Hct
5. Hgb

6. pallor
7. bilaterally
8. dyspneic
9. edema
10. WNL

XXIV.

1. febrile
2. puncture
3. fever
4. antibiotic
5. distension

XXV.

1. A
2. E
3. B
4. F

XXVI.

abdomen, acrocyanosis, addiction, hydrocephalus, ipsilateral, toxicity

XXVII.

1. DNA
2. CBC
3. EEG
4. ROM
5. HCT or Hct
6. Hgb
7. WBC
8. RLQ
9. RPR
10. HIV

XXVIII.

1. anaphylaxis
2. anotia
3. exudate
4. chiroplasty
5. hyperpyrexia
6. immunocompromised
7. interstitial
8. parietal
9. staphylococcemia
10. omphalocele

XXIX.

1. vaccine/immunization
2. immunosuppressants
3. antipyretics

4. antihelmintics
5. antibacterials

XXX.

1. C
2. E
3. A
4. A
5. C
6. B
7. B
8. A
9. C
10. D
11. C
12. D
13. E
14. E

XXXI.

1. cephalo/centesis: surgical puncture of the skull (implied meaning)
2. dactyl/edema: swelling of the fingers or toes
3. dorso/dynia: pain of the back
4. erythr/oid: reddish in color; second meaning, pertaining to erthrocytes
5. extra/peritone/al: occurring or located outside the peritoneal cavity (implied meaning)
6. hemoglobino/meter: instrument used to measure hemoglobin
7. leuko/poiesis: production and development of leukocytes
8. ot/itis media: inflammation of the middle ear
9. peri/appendic/itis: inflammation of the tissue around the appendix
10. thromb/oid: clotlike, resembling a thrombus

Chapter 4

Exercise 1
1. cardiovascular
2. oxygen
3. dioxide
4. fluid

Exercise 2
1. B
2. A
3. D

4. C
5. E

Exercise 3
1. vessel
2. atrium
3. crown
4. mediastinum
5. septum; partition (sometimes, infection)

6. chest
7. valve
8. ventricle

Exercise 4
1. artery
2. arteriole
3. capillary
4. venule
5. vein

6. superior and inferior venae cavae

Exercise 5
1. E
2. D
3. B
4. A
5. C

Exercise 6
1. arteri/al: arteri, artery; -al, pertaining to
2. ven/ous: ven, vein; -ous, pertaining to
3. arterio/ven/ous: arteri(o), artery; ven, vein; -ous, pertaining to
4. atri/al: atri, atrium; -al, pertaining to
5. cardio/pulmon/ary: cardi(o), heart; pulmon, lungs; -ary, pertaining to
6. sept/al: sept, septum; -al, pertaining to
7. peri/cardi/al: peri-, around; cardi, heart; -al, pertaining to
8. endo/cardi/al: endo-, inside; cardi, heart; -al, pertaining to
9. myo/cardi/al: my(o), muscle; cardi, heart; -al, pertaining to
10. pulmon/ary: pulmon, lung; -ary, pertaining to
11. phlebo/tom/ist: phleb(o), vein; tom, to cut; -ist, one who
12. phlebo/tomy: phleb(o), vein; -tomy, incision
    veni/puncture: ven(i), vein; puncture

Exercise 7
1. myocardium
2. endocardium
3. pericardium
4. arteriovenous
5. endocardial
6. ventricular
7. septal
8. atrial

Exercise 8
1. aort/ic: aort, aorta; -ic, pertaining to
2. intra/aort/ic: intra-, within; aort, aorta; -ic, pertaining to
3. valv/al: valv, valve; -al, pertaining to valv/ar: valv, valve; -ar, pertaining to
4. valv/ate: valv, valve; -ate, the result of an action valvul/ar: valvul, valve; -ar, pertaining to

Exercise 9
1. venae cavae
2. atrium
3. right ventricle
4. lungs
5. left atrium
6. bicuspid (or mitral)
7. aorta
8. arterioles
9. capillaries
10. veins

Exercise 10
1. hypertension
2. bradycardia
3. diastole
4. systolic
5. Holter
6. lipids
7. lipoproteins

Exercise 11
1. echocardiography
2. aortography
3. arteriogram

Exercise 12
1. atrio/megaly: atri(o), atrium; -megaly, enlargement
2. cardio/myo/pathy: cardi(o), heart; my(o), muscle, -pathy, disease
3. endocard/itis: endocard, endocardium; -itis, inflammation
4. myocard/itis: myocard, myocardium; -itis, inflammation
5. pericard/itis: pericard, pericardium; -itis, inflammation

Exercise 13
1. atriomegaly
2. cyanosis
3. dysrhythmia
4. microcardia
5. anoxia

Exercise 14
1. increased pulse rate
2. low blood pressure
3. irregularity or loss of rhythm of the heart beat
4. the record produced in electrocardiography
5. enlargement of the heart

Exercise 15
1. cardiomegaly
2. fibrillation

3. asystole
4. infarct
5. ischemia
6. cardiovalvulitis
7. pericarditis
8. stenosis
9. endocarditis
10. shock

Exercise 16
1. aort/itis: aort, aorta; -itis, inflammation
2. aorto/sclerosis: aort(o), aorta; -sclerosis, hardening
3. aneurysm/al: aneurysm; -al, pertaining to
4. angio/card/itis: angi(o), vessel; card, heart; -itis, inflammation
5. arter/itis: arter, artery; -itis, inflammation
6. arterio/pathy: arteri(o), artery, -pathy, disease

Exercise 17
1. angiostenosis
2. aneurysmal
3. lymphangioma
4. arteriosclerosis
5. angiocarditis

Exercise 18
1. aneurysm
2. coronary
3. occlusion
4. thrombosis
5. atherosclerosis
6. aortosclerosis
7. stenosis

Exercise 19
1. B
2. C
3. D
4. A

Exercise 20
1. phlebo/plasty: phleb(o), vein; -plasty, surgical repair
2. pericardio/centesis: pericardi(o), pericardium; -centesis, surgical puncture
3. atrio/septo/plasty: atri(o), atrium; sept(o), septum; -plasty, surgical repair
4. angio/stomy: angi(o), vessel; -stomy, formation of a new opening
5. angio/tomy: angi(o), vessel; -tomy, incision

6. angi/ectomy: angi, vessel; -ectomy, excision
7. embol/ectomy: embol, embolus; -ectomy, excision

Exercise 21
1. D
2. B
3. F
4. A
5. C
6. E

Exercise 22
1. aden(o)
2. lymphaden(o)
3. lymphangi(o)
4. splen(o)
5. thym(o)
6. tonsill(o)

Exercise 23
1. lymphatic
2. lymph
3. veins
4. systemic
5. splenic
6. thymic
7. tonsillar

Exercise 24
1. lymphography
2. lymphadenography
3. biopsy

Exercise 25
1. D
2. B
3. A
4. E
5. C

Exercise 26
1. A
2. C
3. H
4. G
5. F
6. E

Exercise 27
1. thymic
2. lymphedema
3. splenorrhagia
4. tonsillectomy
5. lymphadenopathy

Exercise 28
1. antianginal
2. thrombolytics
3. hemostatics
4. anticoagulants
5. antihypertensives

Chapter 4 Self-Test

I.
1. lymphangi(o)
2. arter(o), arteri(o)
3. arteriol(o)
4. phlebo, ven(i), ven(o)
5. venul(o)

II.
1. tonsill(o)
2. lymphaden(o)
3. thym(o)
4. lymphangi(o)
5. splen(o)

III.
1. H
2. B
3. D
4. I
5. E
6. F
7. G
8. C
9. J
10. A

IV.
1. E
2. C
3. A
4. B
5. D

V.
(No particular order)
Maintains the internal fluid environment by returning proteins and tissue fluids to the blood; aids in the absorption of fats into the bloodstream; helps defend the body against micro-organisms and disease

VI.
1. adenoid/ectomy: excision of the adenoids
2. angio/graphy: radio-graphic visualization of the blood vessels
3. an/ox/ia: lack of oxygen in body tissues
4. atrio/megaly: enlargement of an atrium of the heart

5. cardio/vascul/ar: pertain-ing to the heart and blood vessels
6. echo/cardio/graphy: process of recording the heart using ultrasonic waves
7. end/arter/ectomy: excision of plaque from the inner wall of an artery
8. hemo/pericard/ium: blood within the pericar-dial space
9. phleb/ectomy: excision of a vein
10. thrombo/phleb/itis: inflammation of a vein accompanied by a blood clot

VII.
1. tachycardia
2. microcardia
3. hypertension
4. vasoconstriction

VIII.
1. lymphangitis
2. elephantiasis
3. lymphadenitis
4. aneurysm

IX.
1. thymoma
2. aortosclerosis
3. asystole
4. vasodilator
5. hypertension
6. tachycardia
7. lymphangitis
8. angiostenosis
9. tonsillectomy
10. splenorrhaphy

X.
1. myocardial infarction
2. atherosclerosis
3. coronary artery bypass
4. endocarditis
5. defibrillation
6. coronary thrombosis
7. atrial septal defect

8. rheumatic fever
9. peripheral artery disease
10. aneurysm

XI.
1. An embolus is one cause of a CVA (stroke).
2. Sometimes an intracoronary stent is placed in an artery as part of an angioplasty, any of several means of opening a vessel.

XII.
1. In systemic circulation, oxygenated blood is pumped from the heart to body tissues, then back to the heart. In pulmonary circulation, blood travels from the heart to the lungs to pick up oxygen and get rid of carbon dioxide.
2. An angiogram is the record produced in the process of angiography.

XIII.
1. C
2. B
3. D
4. E
5. F
6. A

XIV
1. aneurysm/ectomy: surgical excision of an aneurysm
2. epi/cardi/al: pertaining to the outer membrane of the heart; pericardial
3. lymph/angi/ectasia: dilation of (smaller) lymphatic vessels
4. pericardio/stomy: creation of an opening into the pericardium, usually for drainage
5. vascul/itis: inflammation of the blood vessels

XV.
1. asystole
2. arterial
3. tachycardic
4. cardiac
5. systolic
6. pulse

XVI.
1. ASHD
2. CPR
3. CVA
4. CABG
5. RA
6. HTN
7. LDH
8. PVC

XVII.
atherosclerosis, ischemia

XVIII.
1. angina pectoris
2. CAD
3. heart attack
4. HTN
5. hypercholesterolemia

XIX.
1. antihyperlipidemic
2. cardiomyopathy
3. lymphography
4. pericardium
5. thrombolytics
6. vasodilation

XX.
1. outer layer
2. cardiac tamponade
3. HTN
4. surgical puncture
5. atherosclerosis

XXI.
1. B
2. C
3. D
4. C
5. C
6. C
7. B
8. D
9. E
10. A

Chapter 5

Exercise 1
1. circulatory
2. oxygen
3. carbon
4. inspiration
5. expiration

Exercise 2
(no particular order)
1. nose
2. nasal cavity
3. sinuses

4. pharynx
5. larynx

Exercise 3
(no particular order)
1. trachea
2. bronchi

3. bronchioles
4. alveoli
5. lungs

Exercise 4
1. phren(o)
2. laryng(o)

3. pneum(o)
4. pharyng(o)
5. phas(o)
6. spir(o)

Exercise 5
1. oropharynx
2. larynx
3. bronchi
4. alveoli

Exercise 6
1. endo/nas/al: endo-, inside; nas, nose; -al, pertaining to
2. nas/al: nas, nose; -al, pertaining to
3. naso/lacrim/al: nas(o), nose; lacrim, tear; -al, pertaining to
4. or/al: or, mouth; -al, pertaining to
5. retro/nas/al: retr(o), behind; nas, nose; -al, pertaining to
6. supra/nas/al: supra-, above; nas, nose; -al, pertaining to

Exercise 7
1. in/spir/ation: process of breathing in
2. para/nas/al: pertaining to near the nose
3. pharyng/eal: pertaining to the pharynx
4. pulmon/ary: pertaining to the lungs
5. retro/nas/al: pertaining to behind the nose

Exercise 8
1. pharynx
2. septum
3. larynx
4. sinuses
5. epiglottis

Exercise 9
1. alveol/ar: alveol, alveoli; -ar, pertaining to
2. bronchi/al: bronchi, bronchi; -al, pertaining to
3. broncho/alveol/ar: bronch(o), bronchi; alveol, alveoli; -ar, pertaining to
4. endo/trache/al: endo-, inside; trache, trachea; -al, pertaining to
5. inter/alveol/ar: inter-, between; alveol, alveoli; -ar, pertaining to

6. trache/al: trache, trachea; -al, pertaining to

Exercise 10
1. extra/pleur/al: extra-, outside; pleur, pleura; -al, pertaining to
2. extra/pulmon/ary: extra-, outside; pulmon, lung; -ary, pertaining to
3. pleur/al: pleur, pleura; -al, pertaining to
4. pulmon/ic: pulmon, lung; -ic, pertaining to
5. sub/pulmon/ary: sub-, beneath; pulmon, lung; -ary, pertaining to

Exercise 11
1. alveoli
2. pleura
3. apex
4. lobes
5. diaphragm

Exercise 12
1. laryngo/graphy: laryng(o), larynx; -graphy, process of recording
2. laryngo/scope: laryng(o), larynx; -scope, instrument used for viewing
3. laryngo/scopy: laryng(o), larynx; -scopy, visual examination
4. mediastino/scope: mediastin(o), mediastinum; -scope, instrument used for viewing
5. mediastino/scopy: mediastin(o), mediastinum; -scopy, visual examination
6. tracheo/scopy: trache(o), trachea; -scopy, visual examination

Exercise 13
1. D
2. B
3. C
4. A
5. E

Exercise 14
1. oximeter
2. spirometry
3. bronchography
4. laryngoscopy
5. pharyngoscope

Exercise 15
1. anoxia
2. hypocapnia

3. dyspnea
4. apnea
5. alkalosis

Exercise 16
1. oxygen
2. hyperpnea
3. hyperventilation
4. hypercapnia
5. acidemia

Exercise 17
1. brady/pnea: slow breathing
2. eu/pnea: normal rate of breathing
3. hyp/ox/emia: decreased blood oxygen
4. ortho/pnea: breathing is difficult except in an upright position
5. phreno/plegia: paralysis of the diaphragm
6. tachy/pnea: greater than normal number of breaths per minute

Exercise 18
1. rhinorrhea
2. dysphasia
3. sinusitis
4. pharyngodynia
5. aphasia

Exercise 19
1. epiglott/itis: epiglott, epiglottis; -itis, inflammation
2. laryngo/pathy: laryng(o), larynx; -pathy, any disease of
3. laryngo/plegia: laryng(o), larynx; -plegia, paralysis
4. laryngo/spasm: laryng(o), larynx; -spasm, spasm

Exercise 20
1. D
2. A
3. B
4. C

Exercise 21
1. C
2. E
3. G
4. D
5. B
6. A
7. H
8. F

Exercise 22
1. G
2. E
3. A

4. D
5. F
6. B
7. C
8. H

Exercise 23
1. anthracosis
2. pneumoconiosis
3. atelectasis
4. hemoptysis

Exercise 24
1. emphysema
2. COPD (chronic obstructive pulmonary disease)
3. emphysema
4. cystic fibrosis

Exercise 25
1. increased pulse rate
2. increased respiratory rate
3. labored or difficult breathing
4. acute inflammation of the lungs and bronchi
5. a physician who specializes in the lungs and respiratory disorders

Exercise 26
1. bronchiolectasis
2. laryngotracheitis
3. bronchiolitis
4. trachealgia
5. bronchopulmonary

Exercise 27
1. laryngectomy
2. thoracocentesis
3. tracheoplasty
4. septoplasty
5. pneumonectomy

Exercise 28
1. asphyxia or asphyxiation
2. resuscitation
3. ventilator
4. tracheostomy
5. obstructive
6. transtracheal
7. orotracheal
8. lung
9. thoracostomy
10. lobectomy

Exercise 29
1. mucolytics
2. antiasthmatics
3. antihistamines
4. antitussives
5. bronchodilators

Chapter 5 Self-Test

I.
1. G
2. A
3. B
4. F
5. D
6. E
7. C

II.
1. A
2. G
3. D
4. B
5. C
6. E
7. F

III.
1. sin(o)
2. nas(o), rhin(o)
3. pharyng(o)
4. laryng(o)
5. trache(o)
6. bronch(o), bronchi(o)
7. phren(o)
8. alveol(o)
9. bronchiol(o)

IV.
nasal cavity 1; bronchi 5; larynx 3; pharynx 2; trachea 4; alveoli 7; bronchioles 6

V.
(No particular order)
1. provides oxygen and removes carbon dioxide
2. maintains acid–base balance
3. produces speech
4. facilitates smell
5. maintains body's heat and water balance

VI.
1. B
2. B
3. B
4. A
5. A
6. A
7. B

VII.
1. pneumothorax
2. hemothorax
3. bronchoscopy
4. thoracocentesis or thoracentesis

VIII.
1. eupnea
2. bradypnea
3. tachypnea
4. hyperpnea

IX.
1. pneumonitis
2. expectoration
3. apnea
4. exchange of CO_2 for O_2
5. parietal pleura
6. paroxysmal
7. orthopnea
8. alkalosis
9. spirometry
10. pulmonary edema

X.
1. thrombus
2. dysphonia
3. bronchoscopy
4. endonasal
5. pharyngitis
6. rhinolithiasis
7. alveolar
8. laryngography
9. rhinorrhagia
10. intranasal

XI.
1. Both have an abnormal respiration pattern of temporary absence of breathing.
2. They are both divisions of the pharynx.

XII.
1. Internal respiration is the delivery of oxygen to body cells with the removal of carbon dioxide, whereas external respiration is breathing (ventilation of the lungs).
2. Expiration is breathing out or letting out one's breath; inspiration is breathing in (drawing air into the lungs).
3. Pneumocentesis is surgical puncture of a lung to drain fluid that has accumulated in the lung itself; thoracentesis is surgical puncture of the chest wall and pleural space, either to obtain a specimen for biopsy or to treat pleural effusion.
4. The glottis is the vocal apparatus of the larynx; the epiglottis is a lidlike structure that closes off the glottis during swallowing.
5. Pneumothorax is air or gas in the pleural cavity; hemothorax is blood in the pleural cavity.

XIII.
1. tachypnea
2. bronchoconstriction
3. hypocapnia
4. exhalation

XIV.
1. COPD
2. bronchospasm
3. cannula
4. nebulizer
5. dyspnea
6. bronchodilation
7. paroxysmal
8. RPFT
9. hypoventilation
10. hypoxemia

XV.
1. malaise
2. pleural effusion
3. wheezes
4. crackles
5. pneumothorax
6. bronchitis
7. COLD
8. embolism
9. bronchodilator
10. expectorant

XVI.
1. shortness
2. hemoptysis
3. fluid
4. surgically removed
5. emphysema

XVII.
1. pharyngeal
2. laryngopathy
3. mesothelioma
4. parietal
5. spirometer
6. tracheostomy

XVIII.
laryngography, pneumonitis

XIX.
1. CPAP
2. TTO
3. URI
4. CPR
5. ECMO
6. RPFT

XX.
1. F
2. E
3. C
4. D
5. B
6. A

XXI.
1. C
2. B
3. C
4. A
5. E
6. A
7. B
8. D
9. B
10. C

XXII.
1. broncho/spiro/metry: the study of the ventilation of each lung separately
2. laryngo/stomy: surgical creation of an artificial opening into the larynx
3. pharyngo/plegia: paralysis of the muscles of the pharynx
4. pneumo/myc/osis: fungal disease of the lungs
5. sino/scopy: endoscopic examination of a paranasal sinus

Chapter 6

Exercise 1
(no particular order)
1. ingestion of food
2. digestion of food
3. absorption of nutrients
4. elimination of wastes

Exercise 2
(no particular order)
1. salivary glands
2. liver
3. gallbladder
4. pancreas

Exercise 3
1. starch
2. bile
3. sugar
4. milk
5. fats
6. protein
7. thirst
8. appetite
9. digestion
10. contraction

Exercise 4
1. H
2. I
3. J
4. G
5. B
6. F
7. E
8. D
9. C
10. A

Exercise 5
1. anus
2. gallbladder
3. common bile duct
4. large intestine; colon
5. duodenum
6. small intestine; intestines
7. esophagus
8. stomach
9. liver
10. ileum
11. jejunum
12. mouth
13. pancreas
14. rectum
15. salivary glands
16. mouth

Exercise 6
1. esophag/eal: esophag, esophagus; -eal, pertaining to
2. gastr/ic: gastr, stomach; -ic, pertaining to
3. oro/pharyng/eal: or(o), mouth; pharyng, pharynx; -eal, pertaining to
4. pharyng/eal: pharyng, pharynx; -eal, pertaining to

Exercise 7
1. enteritis
2. gastric
3. oropharyngeal
4. colonic
5. mucoid

Exercise 8
1. cheek
2. lip
3. stomach
4. gums
5. teeth
6. salivary gland
7. mouth
8. vagus nerve

Exercise 9
1. denti/lingual: dent, teeth; lingu(o), tongue; -al, pertaining to
2. gingiv/al: gingiv, gum; -al, pertaining to
3. glosso/pharyng/eal: gloss(o), tongue; pharyng, pharynx; -eal, pertaining to
4. inter/dent/al: inter-, between; dent, teeth; -al, pertaining to
5. maxill/ary: maxill, maxilla; -ary, pertaining to

Exercise 10
1. lingual
2. mandibular
3. periodontist
4. palatine
5. interdental

Exercise 11
1. mandible
2. maxilla
3. palate
4. gingivae
5. hypoglossal, sublingual
6. endodontium

Exercise 12
1. proct(o)
2. cec(o)
3. diverticul(o)
4. sigmoid(o)

Exercise 13
1. B
2. B
3. B
4. A
5. A
6. A
7. B

Exercise 14
1. duodenal
2. proctologist
3. retrocecal
4. ileal
5. pericolic

Exercise 15
1. cholecyst/ic: cholecyst, gallbladder; -ic, pertaining to

2. cholecysto/gastr/ic: cholecyst(o), gallbladder; gastr, stomach; -ic, pertaining to
3. choledoch/al: choledoch, common bile duct; -al, pertaining to
4. extra/hepat/ic: extra-, outside; hepat, liver; -ic, pertaining to
5. hepat/ic: hepat, liver; -ic, pertaining to
6. hepato/tox/ic: hepat(o), liver; tox, poison; -ic, pertaining to
7. pancreat/ic: pancreat, pancreas; -ic, pertaining to
8. supra/hepat/ic: supra-, above; hepat, liver; -ic, pertaining to

Exercise 16
1. cholecystogastric
2. hepatolytic
3. hypoglycemia
4. hyperglycemia
5. extrahepatic

Exercise 17
1. coloscopy
2. sialography
3. esophagogastroscopy
4. cholecystogram
5. fluoroscopy

Exercise 18
1. A
2. D
3. B
4. C
5. H
6. F
7. E
8. G

Exercise 19
1. anorexia
2. hyperemesis
3. eupepsia
4. exogenous
5. adipsia

Exercise 20
1. cheil/itis: cheil, lip; -itis, inflammation
2. gingiv/algia: gingiv, gum; -algia, pain
3. gingiv/itis: gingiv, gum; -itis, inflammation
4. gingivo/gloss/itis: gingiv(o), gum; gloss, tongue; -itis, inflammation

5. gingivo/stomat/itis: gingiv(o), gum; stomat, mouth; -itis, inflammation
6. gloss/itis: gloss, tongue; -itis, inflammation
7. glosso/pathy: gloss(o), tongue; -pathy, disease of
8. glosso/plegia: gloss(o), tongue; -plegia, paralysis

Exercise 21
1. cheil/osis: splitting of the lips and angles of the mouth
2. gingiv/algia: painful gums
3. end/odont/itis: inflammation of the endodontium
4. glosso/pyr/osis: sensation of pain, burning, and stinging of the tongue
5. pyo/rrhea: inflammation of the gingiva and the periodontal ligament
6. stomato/myc/osis: disease of the mouth caused by a fungus

Exercise 22
1. esophag/itis: esophag, esophagus; -itis, inflammation
2. esophago/dynia: esophag(o), esophagus; -dynia, pain
3. esophago/malacia: esophag(o), esophagus; -malacia, softening
4. gastr/ectasia: gastr, stomach; -ectasia, stretching
5. gastr/ic carcin/oma: gastr, stomach; -ic, pertaining to; carcin, cancer; -oma, tumor
6. gastro/malacia: gastr(o), stomach; -malacia, softening
7. gastro/megaly: gastr(o), stomach; -megaly, enlargement
8. gastro/pathy: gastr(o), stomach; -pathy, disease of

Exercise 23
1. gastralgia
2. gastropathy
3. gastroesophageal
4. esophagomalacia
5. esophagodynia, esophagalgia

Exercise 24
1. F
2. B
3. C
4. A
5. G
6. I
7. J
8. M
9. L
10. E
11. D
12. H
13. K

Exercise 25
1. enterostasis
2. appendicitis
3. gastroduodenitis
4. lipopenia

Exercise 26
1. gastroenteritis
2. dysentery
3. fistula
4. diverticulosis
5. fissure
6. irritable
7. hemorrhoids
8. impaction
9. intussusception
10. volvulus

Exercise 27
1. A
2. D
3. F
4. E
5. B
6. C
7. G
8. H

Exercise 28
1. hepatomegaly
2. cholestasis
3. hepatorenal
4. pancreatolysis
5. pancreatolith

Exercise 29
1. a physician specializing in diseases of the GI tract
2. inflammation of the colon
3. herniation of the stomach
4. a disease characterized by resistance to insulin or lack of insulin secretion

Exercise 30
1. cheilo/plasty: cheil(o), lip; -plasty, surgical repair
2. cheilo/rrhaphy: cheil(o), lip; -rrhaphy, suture
3. gloss/ectomy: gloss, tongue; -ectomy, excision
4. glosso/plasty: gloss(o), tongue; -plasty, surgical repair
5. glosso/rrhaphy: gloss(o), tongue; -rrhaphy, suture
6. stomato/plasty: stomat(o), mouth, -plasty, surgical repair
7. cheilo/stomato/plasty: cheil(o), lip; stomat(o), mouth; -plasty, surgical repair

Exercise 31
1. cheilo/rrhaphy: suture of the lip
2. cheilo/stomato/plasty: surgical repair of the lips and mouth
3. esophago/myo/tomy: incision into the esophageal muscle
4. esophago/stomy: formation of a new opening into the esophagus
5. gingiv/ectomy: excision of the gums
6. glosso/rrhaphy: suture of the tongue

7. jejuno/stomy: formation of a new opening into the jejunum
8. lip/ectomy: excision of subcutaneous fat
9. naso/gastr/ic: pertaining to the nose and stomach
10. stomato/plasty: surgical repair of the mouth

Exercise 32
1. esophago/gastro/plasty: esophag(o), esophagus; gastr(o), stomach; -plasty, surgical repair
2. gastro/pexy: gastr(o), stomach; -pexy, surgical fixation
3. gastro/rrhaphy: gastr(o), stomach; -rrhaphy, suture
4. pyloro/tomy: pylor(o), pylorus; -tomy, incision; my(o), muscle

Exercise 33
1. pylorotomy
2. gastropexy
3. jejunoileostomy
4. vagotomy
5. gastroduodenostomy

Exercise 34
1. ceco/ileo/stomy: cec(o), cecum; ile(o), ileum; -stomy, artificial opening
2. col/ectomy: col, large intestine; -ectomy, excision and hemi-, half
3. diverticul/ectomy: diverticul, diverticulum; -ectomy, excision
4. duodeno/tomy: duoden(o); -tomy, incision and -stomy, artificial opening
5. ileo/stomy: ile(o), ileum; -stomy, artificial opening
6. jejuno/tomy: jejun(o), jejunum; -tomy, incision

7. laparo/entero/stomy: lapar(o), abdominal wall; enter(o), small intestine; -stomy, artificial opening
8. palato/pharyngo/plasty: palat(o), palate; pharyng(o), pharynx (or throat); -plasty, surgical repair; uvulo/palato/pharyngo/plasty: uvul(o), uvula
9. procto/plasty: proct(o), anus and rectum; -plasty, surgical repair

Exercise 35
1. hemicolectomy
2. cecoileostomy
3. ileostomy
4. laparoenterostomy
5. diverticulectomy

Exercise 36
1. lithotripsy
2. pancreatotomy
3. pancreatolithectomy
4. hepatotomy
5. choledochostomy

Exercise 37
1. D
2. G
3. E
4. B
5. A
6. I
7. F
8. J
9. H
10. C

Exercise 38
1. antacids
2. antiemetics
3. antispasmodics
4. anorexiants
5. emetics

Chapter 6 Self-Test

I.
1. pharyng(o)
2. sial(o), sialaden(o)
3. hepat(o)
4. cholecyst(o)
5. duoden(o)
6. or(o), stomat(o)
7. esophag(o)
8. gastr(o)
9. pancreat(o)
10. jejun(o)
11. ile(o)
12. col(o), colon(o), or sigmoid(o)
13. an(o)

II.
1. C
2. B
3. D
4. A

III.
1. D
2. C
3. I
4. A
5. E
6. G
7. J
8. H
9. B
10. F

IV.
(No particular order)
1. carbohydrates: basic source of cell energy
2. fats: energy reserve, and help cushion and insulate vital organs
3. proteins: building material for development, growth, and maintenance of the body

V.

(No particular order)

1. liver = hepat(o)
2. gallbladder = cholecyst(o)
3. pancreas = pancreat(o)
4. salivary glands = sial(o) or sialaden(o)

VI.

1. cholecystogram
2. diverticulitis
3. lithotripsy
4. gastroscopy

VII.

1. ileo/cec/al: pertaining to the cecum and the ileum
2. choledocho/litho/tripsy: surgical crushing of a stone in the common bile duct
3. chole/stasis: interruption of the flow of bile
4. esophago/myo/tomy: incision (longitudinal) of the muscle of the esophagus to treat achalasia
5. gastro/duodeno/stomy: anastomosis of the stomach and duodenum

VIII.

1. gastroenterology
2. cholecystography
3. extracorporeal shock wave lithotripsy
4. anorexia nervosa
5. emaciation
6. colectomy
7. pyloric stenosis
8. hiatal hernia
9. lips and mouth
10. enterostasis

IX.

1. adipsia
2. gastropathy
3. amylase
4. hyperemesis
5. cholecystectomy
6. vagotomy
7. gastritis
8. pharyngeal
9. dyspepsia
10. duodenoscopy

X.

1. Ingestion is the way the body takes in nutrients and is the first stage of digestion. When nutrition is divided into four stages, digestion is the second stage.
2. Amylase is the enzyme that breaks down starch.

XI.

1. A fistula is an abnormal communication between two internal organs, or from an internal organ to the body surface. A fissure is a split or a crack.
2. Polydipsia is excessive thirst; polyphagia is excessive eating.
3. Gastralgia is a stomachache, which could be caused by gastritis, inflammation of the stomach.

XII.

1. eupepsia
2. hypoglycemia

XIII.

1. large intestine
2. abnormal new growth
3. gallbladder
4. abdominal wall
5. large intestine
6. abdomen
7. T
8. T
9. F
10. T
11. F
12. F

XIV.

1. stomach
2. liver
3. cholelithiasis
4. small intestine
5. diagnostic

XV.

1. gastrointestinal: pertaining to the organs of the GI tract

2. colitis: inflammation of the colon
3. colon: the large intestine, extending from the cecum to the rectum
4. diarrhea: frequent passage of loose watery stools
5. abdominal: pertaining to the abdomen
6. ulcerative colitis: a chronic, inflammatory disease of the large intestine and rectum
7. endoscopy: term is not always in reference to G.I., but as used here, the visualizing of the colon using a colonoscope
8. gastroenteritis: inflammation of the stomach and intestines
9. Crohn disease: a chronic inflammatory bowel disease, usually affecting the ileum, the colon, or another part of the G.I. tract
10. colorectal: pertaining to the colon and rectum
11. bowel sounds: sounds associated with movement of the intestinal contents through the G.I. tract
12. rectal: pertaining to the rectum
13. hepatosplenomegaly: enlargement of the liver and spleen
14. stool: feces
15. transverse colon: the portion of the colon that crosses the abdomen, between the ascending colon and the descending colon

XVI.

glossorrhaphy, nasogastric, varices

XVII.

1. AST
2. BMI
3. EGD
4. TMJ
5. HBV
6. UGI

XVIII.

1. emetic
2. palatopharyngoplasty
3. stomatomycosis
4. anastomosis
5. eructation
6. atresia

XIX.

1. C
2. E
3. F
4. B
5. D
6. A

XX.

1. C
2. E
3. B
4. A
5. C
6. B
7. D
8. C
9. C
10. C

XXI.

1. ceco/colo/stomy: surgical creation of an anastomosis between the cecum and the colon
2. esophago/gastr/ectomy: removal of the esophagus and stomach
3. hemi/gastr/ectomy: surgical removal of one half of the stomach
4. sialo/genous: producing saliva
5. sigmoido/sigmoido/stomy: surgical creation of an anastomosis of portions of the sigmoid colon

Chapter 7

Exercise 1

No particular order:

1. maintains homeostasis
2. filters the blood to remove wastes
3. maintains balance of water and other substances
4. maintains blood pH
5. excretes wastes via urine

Exercise 2

1. kidneys
2. ureters
3. urethra

Exercise 3

1. cyst(o)
2. vesic(o)
3. gon(o)
4. pyel(o)

5. ureter(o)
6. ur(o)
Exercise 4
1. cyst/ic: cyst, bladder, cyst, or fluid-filled sac; -ic, pertaining to
2. abdomino/cyst/ic: abdomin(o), abdomen; cyst, bladder, cyst, or fluid-filled sac; -ic, pertaining to
3. extra/cyst/ic: extra-, outside; cyst, bladder, cyst, or fluid-filled sac; -ic, pertaining to
4. inter/ren/al: inter-, between; ren, kidney; -al, pertaining to
5. genito/urin/ary: genit(o), organs of reproduction; urin(o), urine; -ary, pertaining to
6. recto/urethr/al: rect(o), rectum; urethr, urethra; -al, pertaining to
7. ren/al: ren, kidney; -al, pertaining to
8. supra/ren/al: supra-, above; ren, kidney; -al, pertaining to
9. ureter/al: ureter, ureter; -al, pertaining to
10. urethro/vagin/al: urethr(o), urethra; vagin, vagina; -al, pertaining to
Exercise 5
1. urethral
2. urinary
3. vesical
4. vesicoureteral
Exercise 6
1. pelvis
2. ureter
3. urethra
4. nephron
5. bladder

6. glomerulus
7. tubules
8. meatus
Exercise 7
(no particular order)
1. glomerular filtration
2. tubular reabsorption
3. tubular secretion
Exercise 8
1. sugar
2. sugar
3. ketone bodies
4. night
5. night
6. few or scanty
Exercise 9
1. albumin/uria: albumin, albumin; -uria, urine or urination
2. glycos/uria: glycos, sugar; -uria, urine or urination
3. hemat/uria: hemat, blood; -uria, urine or urination
4. keton/uria: keton, ketone bodies; -uria, urine or urination
5. protein/uria: protein, protein; -uria, urine or urination
Exercise 10
1. proteinuria
2. glycosuria
3. urinometer
4. pyuria
5. ketonuria
Exercise 11
1. cysto/metro/graphy: a urologic procedure that measures the amount of pressure on the bladder
2. nephro/stomy: surgical formation of a new opening into the renal pelvis
3. cysto/meter: an instrument used to measure aspects of the bladder

4. electro/myo/graphy: electric recording of muscular contraction
Exercise 12
1. C
2. E
3. A
4. F
5. D
6. B
Exercise 13
1. cystoscopy
2. cystourethroscopy or urethrocystoscopy
3. nephroscope
Exercise 14
1. F
2. C
3. A
4. D
5. G
6. E
7. J
8. I
9. B
10. H
Exercise 15
1. abnormal presence of sugar, especially glucose, in the urine
2. presence of protein in the urine
3. presence of blood in the urine
4. end products of lipid metabolism
5. complex disorder of carbohydrate, fat, and protein metabolism resulting from a deficiency or lack of insulin secretion by the pancreas or a resistance to insulin
Exercise 16
1. nephro/lysis: nephr(o), kidney; -lysis, loosening, freeing, or destroying

2. nephro/malacia; nephr(o), kidney; -malacia, abnormal softening
3. nephro/megaly: nephr(o), kidney; -megaly, enlargement
4. nephro/pathy: nephr(o), kidney; -pathy, any disease of
5. nephro/tox/ic: nephr(o), kidney; tox, poison; -ic, pertaining to
Exercise 17
1. hydronephrosis
2. nephromalacia
3. renovascular
4. nephropathy
5. nephromegaly
Exercise 18
1. hydroureter
2. cystocele
3. hyperplasia
4. nephrolithiasis
5. insipidus
6. hypospadias
7. epispadias
8. pyelonephritis
9. urethrostenosis
10. urethrorrhea
Exercise 19
1. transureteroureterostomy
2. lithotripsy
3. cystectomy
4. nephroureterectomy
5. lithotomy
Exercise 20
1. nephrectomy
2. ureterostomy
3. infection
4. pyelolithotomy
5. anticoagulant therapy
6. transurethral resection
Exercise 21
1. antispasmodics
2. antihypertensives
3. antidiuretics
4. antiinfectives

Chapter 7 Self-Test

I.
1. ren(o), nephr(o)
2. ureter(o)
3. cyst(o), vesic(o)
4. urethr(o)
II.
1. E
2. D
3. A

4. C
5. B
III.
(1 through 3, in no particular order)
filtering the blood; maintaining proper balance of water, salts, and acids; excreting waste products

IV.
1. F
2. F
3. T
4. F
5. F
6. F
7. F
8. T

V.
1. an/ur/ic: pertaining to absence of urine production or a urinary output of less than 100 mL per day
2. litho/tomy: the surgical excision of a calculus

3. noct/uria: excessive urination at night
4. olig/uria: a diminished capacity to form and pass urine—less than 500 mL per day
5. trans/urethral: through or across the wall of the urethra

VI.
1. nephrostomy
2. cystoscopy
3. urinometer
4. nephrotomogram

VII.
1. glomeruli
2. pyelolithotomy
3. nephromegaly
4. lithotripsy
5. intravenous urography
6. renal failure
7. incontinence
8. polyuria
9. endoscopy
10. uremia

VIII.
1. uropathy
2. interrenal
3. hematuria
4. urethrocele
5. glomerulonephritis
6. pyelitis
7. hemodialysis
8. extracystic
9. cystography
10. lithotripsy

IX.
1. All are structures pertaining to the entrance and exit of the renal arteries and renal veins. The hilum is the depression where the blood vessels, nerves, and lymphatic vessels enter or leave the kidney. Renal arteries carry blood to the kidneys, and renal veins carry blood away from the kidneys.
2. Kidneys produce renin, which assists in regulation of blood pressure.
3. Micturition and urination have the same meaning.
4. A urinometer is an instrument that measures specific gravity.

X.
1. In hypospadias, the urinary meatus is located on the underside of the penis, whereas in epispadias, the urinary meatus is located on the upper surface of the penis.
2. Tubular reabsorption means that some substances that the body conserves are reabsorbed into blood vessels surrounding the tubules, whereas tubular secretion is the way in which substances in the bloodstream are secreted into the tubules to be expelled in urine.
3. Anuria is more severe than oliguria. In anuria, less than 100 mL of urine per day is excreted. In oliguria, less than 500 mL of urine per day is excreted.
4. Diabetes insipidus is not related to diabetes mellitus but was so named because of the large quantity of urine excreted. Diabetes mellitus is true diabetes and results primarily from the deficiency or lack of insulin secretion by the pancreas or a resistance to insulin.
5. Hydroureter is caused by obstruction in the lower part of the ureter, whereas hydronephrosis is caused by obstruction in the upper part of the ureter.

XI.
1. polyuria
2. antidiuretic

XII.
1. glomerulus
2. proximal convoluted tube
3. Bowman capsule
4. distal convoluted tubule
5. collecting duct

XIII.
1. C
2. B
3. A
4. C
5. D

XIV.
1. B
2. E
3. A
4. C
5. E
6. D
7. C
8. B
9. A
10. C

XV.
1. painful
2. nocturia
3. UA

4. kidneys
5. BPH

XVI.
1. diuresis
2. lithotripsy
3. nephrolithiasis
4. pyelogram
5. ureteroplasty
6. uropathy

XVII.
1. B
2. A
3. C
4. D

XVIII.
1. a developmental defect in which the urethral orifice (opening) is too low, lying on the undersurface of the penis
2. narrowing of the urinary meatus
3. surgical repair of the urinary meatus

XIX.
hydronephrosis, gonorrhea

XX.
1. BUN
2. EMG
3. ESWL
4. ARF
5. VCUG

XXI.
1. cysto/rrhagia: hemorrhage from the bladder
2. keton/emia: the presence of ketones in the blood
3. nephro/toxic: toxic or destructive to a kidney
4. perineo/cele: a hernia in the perineal area
5. uro/genit/al: pertaining to the urinary and reproductive systems; genitourinary

Chapter 8

Exercise 1
1. offspring
2. genitalia
3. gonad
4. external
5. minora

Exercise 2
1. D
2. C
3. B
4. E
5. A

Exercise 3
1. vagina
2. organs of reproduction
3. uterus
4. month
5. measure or uterine tissue
6. ovum
7. ovary
8. ovary
9. uterus
10. vagina
11. perine(o)
12. cervic(o)
13. salping(o)
14. vulv(o)

Exercise 4
1. colpo/cyst/itis: colp(o), vagina; cyst, bladder; -itis, inflammation
2. ovari/an: ovari, ovary; -an, pertaining to
3. uter/ine: uter, uterus; -ine (understood to be pertaining to)

4. vagin/al: vagin, vagina; -al, pertaining to

Exercise 5

1. cervical
2. ovarian
3. intrauterine
4. perimetrium
5. myometrium
6. endometrium

Exercise 6

1. puberty
2. menstruation
3. menarche
4. climacteric

Exercise 7

1. menstruation
2. follicle-stimulating hormone
3. luteinizing hormone
4. ovulation
5. estrogen
6. progesterone

Exercise 8

1. speculum
2. cytology
3. dysplasia
4. gonadotropin
5. colposcopy
6. hysteroscopy
7. hysterosalpingography
8. laparoscopy

Exercise 9

1. E
2. B
3. D
4. A
5. C

Exercise 10

1. a/meno/rrhea: a-, without; men(o), month; -rrhea, discharge
2. dys/meno/rrhea: dys-, difficult or painful; men(o), month; -rrhea, discharge
3. meno/rrhagia: men(o), month; -rrhagia, hemorrhage
4. meno/rrhea: men(o), month; -rrhea, discharge
5. metro/rrhagia: metr(o), uterine tissue; -rrhagia, hemorrhage

Exercise 11

1. oophor/algia: oophor, ovary; -algia, pain
2. oophor/itis: oophor, ovary; -itis, inflammation

3. oophoro/pathy: oophor(o), ovary; -pathy, disease
4. oophoro/salping/itis: oophor(o), ovary; salping, uterine tube; -itis, inflammation
5. salping/itis: salping, uterine tube; -itis, inflammation
6. salpingo/cele: salping(o), uterine tube; -cele, herniation

Exercise 12

1. premenstrual
2. ovulation
3. anovulation
4. ovarian
5. pelvic
6. prolapse
7. retroversion
8. leiomyoma
9. fistula
10. cystocele

Exercise 13

1. colpo/plasty: colp(o), vagina; -plasty, surgical repair
2. colpo/rrhaphy: colp(o), vagina; -rrhaphy, suture
3. hyster/ectomy: hyster, uterus; -ectomy, excision
4. hystero/pexy: hyster(o), uterus; -pexy, surgical fixation
5. oophor/ectomy: oophor, ovary; -ectomy, excision
6. oophoro/hyster/ectomy: oophor(o), ovary; hyster, uterus; -ectomy, excision
7. oophoro/pexy: oophor(o), ovary; -pexy, surgical fixation
8. oophoro/salping/ectomy: oophor(o), ovary; salping, uterine tube; -ectomy, excision
9. ovari/an cyst/ectomy: ovari, ovary, -an, pertaining to; cyst, cyst; -ectomy, excision
10. hyster/ectomy: hyster, uterus; -ectomy, excision
11. salpingo/pexy: salping(o), uterine tube; -pexy, surgical fixation
12. salpingo/rrhaphy: salping(o), uterine tube; -rrhaphy, suture

13. vagin/ectomy: vagin, vagina; -ectomy, excision
14. vulv/ectomy: vulv, vulva; -ectomy, excision

Exercise 14

1. hormone
2. vulvectomy
3. oophoropexy
4. hysterectomy
5. laparohysterectomy
6. salpingectomy
7. ligation
8. salpingostomy
9. curettage
10. cryotherapy or cryosurgery

Exercise 15

1. colporrhaphy
2. salpingopexy
3. oophorohysterectomy
4. hysteropexy
5. laparoscope

Exercise 16

1. pertaining to the period of life after normal cessation of menstruation
2. removal of both ovaries and uterine tubes
3. examination of the external and internal female genitalia
4. herniation of the urinary bladder through the wall of the vagina

Exercise 17

1. glans penis
2. epididymis
3. testicle
4. rectum
5. scrotum
6. semen
7. urethra
8. vessel, vas deferens

Exercise 18

1. pen/ile: pen, penis, -ile, pertaining to
2. prostat/ic: prostat, prostate, -ic, pertaining to
3. scrot/al: scrot, scrotum; -al, pertaining to
4. spermat/ic: spermat, spermatozoa, -ic, pertaining to
5. testicul/ar: testicul, testicle; -ar, pertaining to

Exercise 19

1. spermatogenesis
2. testicle

3. seminiferous
4. testosterone
5. luteinizing

Exercise 20

1. C
2. A
3. B
4. D

Exercise 21

1. olig(o)
2. crypt(o)
3. varic(o)

Exercise 22

1. uro/logy
2. oligo/sperm/ia
3. crypt/orchid/ism
4. epididym/itis
5. hydro/cele

Exercise 23

1. torsion
2. varicocele
3. phimosis
4. balanitis
5. hyperplasia

Exercise 24

1. a/zoo/sperm/ia: condition of the absence of living sperm
2. orchid/algia: testicular pain
3. prostat/itis: inflammation of the prostate gland
4. an/orch/ism: condition of absence of the testis
5. hyper/trophy: enlargement in size

Exercise 25

1. A
2. G
3. D
4. E
5. C
6. F
7. B
8. H

Exercise 26

1. orchiotomy
2. vasostomy
3. transurethral
4. prostatectomy

Exercise 27

1. amni(o)
2. chori(o)
3. fet(o)
4. gonad(o)
5. ov(o)
6. spermat(o)

Exercise 28
1. gonad
2. gamete
3. zygote
4. ovulation
5. conception
6. implantation
7. fetus
8. chorion
9. spermatoblast
10. progesterone

Exercise 29
1. E
2. B
3. A
4. D
5. C

Exercise 30
1. postcoital
2. abstinence
3. intrauterine
4. contraceptive

Exercise 31
1. vasectomy
2. ligation
3. fertilization
4. contraception

Exercise 32
1. -cyesis
2. -gravida
3. -tropin
4. -para

Exercise 33
1. nulli/para: nulli-, none; -para, woman who has given birth
2. quadri/para: quadri-, four; -para, woman who has given birth
3. secundi/para: secundi-, second; -para, woman who has given birth
4. tri/para: tri-, three; -para, woman who has given birth; terti/para: terti-, third; -para, woman who has given birth

Exercise 34
1. D
2. F
3. G
4. E
5. A
6. B
7. I
8. H
9. J
10. C

Exercise 35
1. post/nat/al: pertaining to after birth
2. amnio/rrhexis: rupture of the amnion (inner fetal membrane)

3. primi/gravida: a female during her first pregnancy
4. ante/partum: before childbirth
5. neo/nato/logist: a physician who specializes in the care of newborn infants

Exercise 36
1. pregnancy
2. pelvimetry
3. amniocentesis
4. chorionic
5. fetoscope

Exercise 37
1. E
2. A
3. C
4. D
5. B

Exercise 38
1. C
2. E
3. A
4. B
5. D

Exercise 39
1. D
2. A
3. E
4. B
5. C

Exercise 40
1. laparotomy
2. amniorrhexis
3. cervical
4. laparorrhaphy

Exercise 41
1. D
2. C
3. B
4. A

Exercise 42
1. penile discharge
2. cocci in pair that are located inside and outside a cell
3. gonorrhea
4. *Neisseria gonorrhoeae*
5. penicillin or another antibiotic if patient is allergic to penicillin

Exercise 43
1. A
2. D
3. C
4. E
5. B

Exercise 44
1. antiandrogens
2. inhibitors
3. stimulants
4. uterine
5. antiretrovirals
6. tocolytics

Chapter 8 Self-Test

I.
1. oophor(o)
2. salping(o)
3. hyster(o)
4. cervic(o)
5. colp(o)

II.
1. vas(o)
2. urethr(o)
3. pen(o)
4. prostat(o)
5. epididym(o)
6. orchi(o)
7. scrot(o)

III.
1. umbilical cord
2. chorion
3. amnion
4. placenta
5. amniotic fluid
6. uterus

IV.
1. A
2. B
3. C

V.
1. A
2. B
3. C
4. A
5. D
6. F
7. E

VI.
1. D
2. C
3. A
4. B
5. E

VII.
1. E
2. D
3. A
4. B
5. C

VIII.
1. amniocentesis
2. vasectomy
3. sonogram

4. cystocele
5. fetoscope

IX.
1. anteversion
2. retroversion
3. anteflexion
4. retroflexion

X.
1. endo/metr/ium: lining of the uterus
2. erythro/blast/osis: a condition of embryonic forms of erythrocytes
3. hystero/scope: an endoscope used to visually examine the cervix and uterine cavity
4. laparo/rrhaphy: suture of the abdominal wall
5. neo/nato/logy: a specialty that cares for newborns
6. oophor/ectomy: surgical removal of one or both ovaries

7. protein/uria: protein in the urine
8. salping/itis: inflammation of a uterine tube
9. spermato/genesis: development or production of sperm
10. vaso/vaso/stomy: restoring the cut ends of the vas deferens

XI.
1. HCG
2. pelvimetry
3. dystocia
4. Down syndrome
5. gestational
6. cephalic
7. IUD
8. G_2P_2
9. genital warts
10. candidiasis
11. dysmenorrhea
12. speculum
13. laparoscopy

14. oophoritis
15. menarche
16. hysteropexy
17. leukorrhea
18. endometriosis
19. colpoplasty
20. anorchidism
21. sterility
22. prepuce
23. cryptorchidism
24. testicular torsion
25. orchialgia

XII.
1. ovarian
2. ovulation
3. estrogen
4. uterine
5. menstruation (or menses)

XIII.
1. neonate
2. multipara
3. spermatoblast
4. implantation
5. amniotomy
6. prostatectomy
7. hysterectomy
8. menorrhagia
9. salpingocele
10. episiotomy
11. vasotomy
12. cervicitis
13. vulvovaginitis
14. oligospermia
15. chancre
16. amniochorial or amniochorionic
17. fetal
18. ovulation
19. salpingopexy
20. colposcopy

XIV.
1. The ovaries and testes are gonads.
2. They are three types of uterine tissue; endometrium, the lining; myometrium, muscular tissue; perimetrium, the outermost tissue.
3. Menarche is the first occurrence of menstruation.
4. Spermatogenesis is the production of sperm, which are produced in the seminiferous tubules.

5. Prostate-specific antigen is a protein that may be present at high levels in the blood in men with prostatic carcinoma.
6. Both are extraembryonic membranes.
7. Both mean a female who has produced one viable offspring.

XV.
1. A chancre is the primary lesion of syphilis. A genital wart is the lesion of condyloma acuminatum.
2. A contraceptive patch is a skin patch that releases hormones and prevents conception during intercourse. A postcoital contraceptive is a pill that is taken after unprotected intercourse and blocks or terminates pregnancy.
3. Ovarian cysts may or may not be cancerous; ovarian cancer is a malignant neoplasm of the ovaries.
4. A urethrovaginal fistula occurs between the urethra and the vagina; a vesicovaginal fistula occurs between the bladder and the vagina.
5. A vasectomy, done for sterilization, is bilateral separation of the ends of the vas deferens. A vasovasostomy is a surgical procedure to reestablish function of the vas deferens on both sides, in a male who formerly has undergone a vasectomy.

XVI.
1. retroversion
1. aspermatogenesis
2. postpartum
3. postnatal

XVII.
1. C
2. A
3. D
4. E
5. B

XVIII.
1. D
2. H
3. G
4. F
5. B

XIX.
1. CPD
2. HCG or hCG
3. PVP
4. TUNA
5. HIV
6. HBV

XX.
1. OB
2. four times
3. after birth
4. dystocia
5. antenatal

XXI.
1. anorchidism
2. azoospermia
3. cauterization
4. epididymis
5. luteinizing
6. neurosyphilis
7. oophoralgia
8. parturition
9. spermatozoa
10. vesicovaginal

XXII.
1. pelvic: pertaining to the pelvis; or pelvic pressure: increased tightness within the pelvis
2. gravida 6: six pregnancies
3. para 5: five viable births
4. abortus 1: one abortion
5. postectopic pregnancy: the time after an abnormal pregnancy in which the embryo implants outside the uterine cavity
6. vaginal hysterectomy: removal of the uterus through the vagina
7. bilateral oophorosalpingectomy: removal of both ovaries and their accompanying uterine tubes
8. carcinoma of the cervix: cancer of the uterine cervix
9. benign prostatic hyperplasia: nonmalignant enlargement of the prostate

10. vagina: the canal which receives the penis during copulation; birth canal
11. cystocele: herniation of the urinary bladder through the vaginal wall
12. rectocele: herniation of the rectum through the vaginal wall
13. vaginal prolapse: loss of support that holds the vagina in place, allowing it to sag
14. perineoplasty: surgical repair of the perineum
15. colpoplexy: surgical fixation of the vagina

XXIII.
amniocentesis, contraceptive, menarche

XXIV.
1. C
2. E
3. E
4. C
5. D
6. A
7. B
8. D
9. D
10. B
11. C
12. B
13. D
14. C
15. C

XXV.
1. balano/plasty: plastic surgery of the glans penis
2. epididymo/orch/itis: inflammation of the epididymis and the testicle
3. feto/scopy: directly observing the fetus in utero, using a fetoscope introduced through a small incision in the abdomen
4. leio/myo/fibr/oma: a benign uterine leiomyoma with fibrous connective tissue
5. oo/sperm: a fertilized ovum; the cell resulting from the union of the sperm and ovum after fertilization

Chapter 9

Exercise 1

1. C
2. B
3. A

Exercise 2

1. myelo/blast: myel(o), bone marrow; -blast, embryonic form; -cyte, cell
2. osteo/blast: oste(o), bone; -blast, embryonic form
3. osteo/cyte: oste(o), bone; -cyte, cell
4. osteo/genesis: oste(o), bone; -genesis, producing or forming

Exe.rcise 3

1. marrow
2. epiphyses
3. periosteum
4. bone
5. musculoskeletal
6. ossification

Exercise 4

1. skeleton
2. skeletal
3. axial
4. appendicular

Exercise 5

1. sternum
2. cranium
3. cost(o)
4. spine
5. stern(o)

Exercise 6

1. cervical
2. thoracic
3. lumbar
4. sacral
5. coccygeal

Exercise 7

1. cost/al: cost, rib; -al, pertaining to
2. infra/cost/al: infra-, beneath; cost, rib; -al, pertaining to
3. infra/stern/al: infra-, beneath; stern, breast-bone; -al, pertaining to
4. intra/stern/al: intra-, within; stern, breastbone; -al, pertaining to
5. retro/stern/al: retro-, behind; stern, breastbone; -al, pertaining to
6. stern/al: stern, breast-bone; -al, pertaining to
7. sterno/cost/al: stern(o), breastbone; cost, rib; -al, pertaining to
8. supra/cost/al: supra-above; cost, rib; -al, pertaining to
9. supra/stern/al: supra-above; stern, breastbone; -al, pertaining to
10. thoraco/lumb/ar: thorac(o), thorax; lumb, lumbar; -ar, pertaining to
11. vertebro/cost/al: vertebr(o), vertebra; cost, rib; -al, pertaining to
12. vertebro/stern/al: vertebr(o), vertebra; stern, breastbone; -al, pertaining to

Exercise 8

1. thoracolumbar
2. cranial
3. supracostal
4. infrasternal
5. intervertebral

Exercise 9

1. tars(o)
2. fibul(o)
3. clavicul(o)
4. phalang(o)
5. calcane(o)
6. patell(o)
7. tibi(o)
8. scapul(o)
9. femor(o)
10. humer(o)
11. carp(o)

Exercise 10

1. costo/clavicul/ar: cost(o), rib; clavicul, clavicle, -ar, pertaining to
2. humer/al: humer, upper arm bone; -al, pertaining to
3. humero/radi/al: humer(o), humerus; radi, radius; -al, pertaining to
4. humero/scapul/ar: humer(o), humerus; scapul, scapula; -ar, pertaining to
5. humero/uln/ar: humer(o), humerus; uln, ulna; -ar, pertaining to

6. infra/clavicul/ar: infra-, under; clavicul, clavicle; -ar, pertaining to
7. infra/scapul/ar: infra-, under; scapul, scapula; -ar, pertaining
8. inter/scapul/ar: inter-, between; scapul, scapula; -ar, pertaining
9. scapul/ar: scapul, scapula; -ar, pertaining
10. scapulo/clavicul/ar: scapul(o), scapula; clavicul, clavicle; -ar, pertaining to
11. sterno/clavicul/ar: stern(o), breastbone; clavicul, clavicle; -ar, pertaining to
12. ulno/radi/al: uln(o), ulna; radi, radius; -al, pertaining to

Exercise 11

1. ilio/pub/ic: ili(o), ilium; pub, pubis; -ic, pertaining to
2. ischio/coccyg/eal: ischi(o), ischium; coccyg, coccyx; -eal, pertaining to
3. ischio/pub/ic: ischi(o), ischium; pub, pubis; -ic, pertaining to
4. sub/pub/ic: sub-, below; pub, pubis; -ic, pertaining to
5. supra/pub/ic: supra-, above; pub, pubis; -ic, pertaining to

Exercise 12

1. (No particular order) ilium, ischium, and pubis
2. (No particular order) ulna and radius
3. wrist
4. scapula

Exercise 13

1. carpo/phalang/eal: pertaining to the carpus and the phalanges
2. humero/scapul/ar: pertaining to the humerus (upper arm bone) and the scapula (shoulder blade)
3. inter/pub/ic: pertaining to between the pubic bones

4. ulno/radi/al: pertaining to the radius and ulna (lateral and medial forearm bones)
5. meta/carp/al: pertaining to the bones of the palm

Exercise 14

1. scapuloclavicular
2. carpophalangeal
3. ischiopubic
4. iliofemoral
5. sternoclavicular

Exercise 15

1. calcaneo/fibul/ar: calcane(o), calcaneus; fibul, fibula; -ar, pertaining to
2. calcaneo/tibi/al: calcane(o), calcaneus; tibi, tibia; -al, pertaining to
3. ilio/femor/al: ili(o), ilium; femor, femur; -al, pertaining to
4. infra/patell/ar: infra-, beneath; patell, patella; -ar, pertaining to
5. ischio/femor/al: ischi(o), ischium; femor, femur; -al, pertaining to
6. patello/femor/al: patell(o), patella; femor, femur; -al, pertaining to
7. pubo/femor/al: pub(o), pubis; femor, femur; -al, pertaining to

Exercise 16

1. C
2. A
3. B
4. D
5. E

Exercise 17

1. connective
2. articulation
3. synovial
4. joint
5. bursae
6. tendons
7. ligament
8. perichondrium

Exercise 18

(no particular order)

1. cardiac muscle (myocardium): located in the heart; involuntary.
2. skeletal muscle: functions in movement of the body; voluntary.

3. visceral muscle: located in the walls of blood vessels and organs; involuntary.

Exercise 19
1. B
2. A
3. E
4. F
5. H

Exercise 20
1. densitometry
2. electromyography
3. motion
4. erythrocyte
5. rheumatoid
6. joint
7. arthroscope
8. arthrocentesis

Exercise 21
1. arthrography
2. calciuria
3. intraarticular
4. electromyogram

Exercise 22
1. E
2. B
3. D
4. A
5. C

Exercise 23
1. E
2. C
3. B
4. F
5. G
6. D
7. A

Exercise 24
1. arthro/chondr/itis: arthr(o), joint; chondr, cartilage; -itis, inflammation
2. burs/itis: burs, bursa; -itis, inflammation
3. calcane/itis: calcane, heel bone; -itis, inflammation
4. calcaneo/dynia: calcane(o), heel bone; -dynia, pain
5. chondr/algia: chondr, cartilage; -algia and -dynia, pain
6. chondr/itis: chondr, cartilage; -itis, inflammation
7. chondro/pathy: chondr(o), cartilage; -pathy, disease

8. ischi/algia, ischio/dynia: ischi, ischium; -algia and –dynia, pain
9. rachi/algia, rachio/dynia: rachi or rachi(o), spine; -algia and –dynia, pain
10. sacro/dynia: sacr(o), sacrum; -dynia, pain
11. spondyl/algia: spondyl, vertebra; -algia, pain
12. stern/algia: stern, sternum; -algia, pain
13. synov/itis: synov, synovial membrane; -itis, inflammation
14. ten/algia, teno/dynia: ten or ten(o), tendon; -algia, -dynia, pain
15. tendin/itis: tendin, tendon; -itis, inflammation
16. tibi/algia: tibi, tibia; -algia, pain

Exercise 25
1. tendin/itis: inflammation of a tendon
2. spondyl/algia: pain in a vertebra
3. arthro/chondr/itis: inflammation of an articular cartilage
4. calcaneo/dynia: pain in the heel
5. tarso/ptosis: prolapse of the tarsus; flatfoot

Exercise 26
1. osteitis
2. chondrosarcoma
3. osteomyelitis
4. myocellulitis
5. leukemia

Exercise 27
1. cranio/cele: hernial protrusion of the brain through a defect in the skull
2. syn/dactyl/ism: condition of fused digits
3. osteo/sclerosis: abnormal hardness of bone
4. osteo/penia: decreased bone mass
5. rachi/schisis: fissure (split) of one or more vertebrae

Exercise 28
1. ankyl/osing spondyl/itis: ankyl, stiff; spondyl, spine; -itis, inflammation

2. ankyl/osis: ankyl, stiff; -osis, condition
3. arthr/algia: arthr, joint; -algia, pain
4. arthro/pathy: arthr(o), joint, -pathy, disease
5. arthro/sclerosis: arthr(o), joint; -sclerosis, hardening
6. dors/algia: dors, back; -algia, pain
7. osteo/arthro/pathy: oste(o), bones; arthr(o), joint; -pathy, disease
8. poly/arthr/itis: poly-, many; arthr, joint; -itis, inflammation
9. spondyl/arthr/itis: spondyl, vertebrae; arthr, joint; -itis, inflammation
10. spondylo/arthro/pathy: spondyl(o), vertebrae; arthr(o), joint; -pathy, disease

Exercise 29
1. a fracture in which the bone is broken into two pieces, but does not protrude through the skin
2. the smaller bone of the lower leg
3. joint pain
4. examination of the interior of a joint with an endoscope

Exercise 30
1. carpal
2. bursitis
3. arthrochondritis
4. temporomandibular
5. tarsoptosis
6. tumor
7. osteomalacia
8. bifida
9. osteoarthritis
10. myasthenia

Exercise 31
1. dorsalgia
2. ankylosis
3. myofibrosis
4. polymyalgia
5. spondylarthropathy

Exercise 32
1. B
2. C
3. A

Exercise 33
1. burs/ectomy: burs, bursa; -ectomy, excision
2. carp/ectomy: carp, carpus; -ectomy, excision
3. coccyg/ectomy: coccyg, coccyx; -ectomy, excision
4. cost/ectomy: cost, vertebra; -ectomy, excision
5. crani/ectomy: crani, skull; -ectomy, excision
6. cranio/plasty: crani(o), skull; -plasty, surgical repair
7. cranio/tomy: crani(o), cranium; -tomy, incision
8. myo/plasty: my(o), muscle, -plasty, surgical repair
9. myo/rrhaphy: my(o), muscle; -rrhaphy, suture
10. oste/ectomy: oste, bone; -ectomy, excision
11. osteo/plasty: oste(o), bone; -plasty, surgical repair
12. phalang/ectomy: phlang, finger or toe; -ectomy, excision
13. sterno/tomy: stern(o), sternum; -tomy, incision
14. tendo/plasty: tend(o), tendon; -plasty, surgical repair
15. teno/myo/plasty: ten(o), tendon; my(o), muscle; -plasty, surgical repair
16. teno/rrhaphy: ten(o), tendon; -rrhaphy, suture
17. teno/tomy: ten(o), tendon; -tomy, incision
18. vertebr/ectomy: vertebr, vertebra; -ectomy, excision

Exercise 34
1. arthroclasia
2. costectomy
3. arthrotomy
4. myelosuppression
5. antiinflammatories
6. chondrectomy
7. cranioplasty
8. myorrhaphy

Exercise 35
1. cranio/tomy: surgical incision into the skull

2. myo/rrhaphy: suture of a muscle
3. teno/myo/plasty: repair of a tendon and muscle

4. spondylo/syn/desis: spinal fusion
5. fasci/ectomy: excision of fascia

Exercise 36
1. antirheumatic
2. anti-osteoporotics

3. antiinflammatories
4. analgesics

Chapter 9 Self-Test

I.
1. cranium, crani(o)
2. clavicle, clavicul(o)
3. sternum, stern(o)
4. ribs (costae), cost(o)
5. vertebra, vertebr(o), spondyl(o)
6. scapula, scapul(o)
7. humerus, humer(o)
8. radius, radi(o)
9. ulna, uln(o)
10. carpus, carp(o)
11. metacarpals, metacarp(o)
12. phalanges, phalang(o)
13. ilium, ili(o)
14. ischium, ischi(o)
15. pubis, pub(o)
16. femur, femor(o)

II.
1. B
2. A
3. C
4. D

III.
1. electromyography
2. arthroscopy

IV.
1. G
2. B
3. E
4. D
5. A
6. C
7. F

V.
1. J
2. H
3. A
4. D
5. I
6. G
7. C
8. F
9. B
10. E

VI.
1. J
2. D
3. H
4. I
5. F
6. E

7. B
8. G
9. C
10. A

VII.
1. carpo/phalang/eal: pertaining to the wrist and fingers
2. chondro/sarcoma: malignant tumor derived from cartilage
3. osteo/lysis: destruction of bone
4. osteo/arthro/pathy: any disease affecting bones and joints
5. scapulo/clavicul/ar: pertaining to the shoulder blade and collarbone

VIII.
1. cervical
2. thoracic
3. lumbar
4. sacral
5. coccygeal

IX.
(No particular order)
support for the body, protection of soft body parts, movement, blood cell formation, and storage

X.
(No particular order)
skeletal: control movement of bones; visceral: contraction of organs and blood vessels; cardiac: contraction of the heart

XI.
1. sternoschisis
2. ulnoradial
3. arthropathy
4. electromyogram
5. decalcification
6. polydactylism
7. bone marrow
8. arthroscopy
9. tarsoptosis
10. osteoporosis

XII.
1. reduction
2. intercostal

3. osteoarthritis
4. coccygectomy
5. myocele
6. osteitis
7. scoliosis
8. myofascial
9. articular
10. arthrocentesis

XIII.
1. Myeloblasts are embryonic cells that will become myelocytes, which are precursors of granulocytic leukocytes.
2. Both terms mean pertaining to the sternum and vertebrae.

XIV.
1. The diaphysis is the long shaft of the long bone, whereas the epiphysis is one of the expanded ends.
2. Ligaments connect bones or cartilage; tendons attach the muscles to the bones.

XV.
1. suprasternal
2. adductor

XVI.
1. D
2. C
3. G
4. E
5. F
6. A
7. B

XVII.
1. burso/pathy: any disease of a bursa
2. musculo/tendin/ous: pertaining to the muscle and the tendon
3. osteo/chondr/al: pertaining to bone and cartilage
4. supra/patell/ar: pertaining to a location above the kneecap
5. teno/synov/itis: inflammation of the tendon and synovial membrane (joint lining)

XVIII.
1. rheumatoid
2. arthroplasty
3. osteoarthritis
4. extremity
5. ambulate

XIX.
1. ALL
2. CPK
3. ROM
4. MTP
5. EMG
6. DJD

XX.
femoral, iliofemoral

XXI.
1. RA
2. joint
3. extremities
4. bone
5. wrist

XXII.
1. arthroclasia
2. bisphosphonates
3. chondrosarcoma
4. myasthenia
5. rachischisis
6. sternocostal

XXIII.
1. comminuted proximal left femur fracture: fracture of the left thigh bone resulting in many bone fragments
2. herniated disk: rupture of the cartilage surrounding an intervertebral disk
3. arthralgia: painful conditions of the joints
4. spinal laminectomy: surgical removal of the bony arches of one or more vertebrae
5. right knee arthroscopy: examination of the interior of the right knee with an arthroscope
6. osteoporosis: abnormal loss of bone density and deterioration of the bone with increased fracture risk

XIV.
1. E
2. C

3. B
4. A
5. A

6. C
7. A
8. B

9. D
10. A

Chapter 10

Exercise 1
1. (No particular order) stimulates movement; senses changes both within and outside the body; provides us with thought, learning, and memory; maintains homeostasis with the help of the hormonal system
2. sensory, integrative, motor
3. (No particular order) central nervous system, peripheral nervous system

Exercise 2
1. nerv(o), neur(o)
2. gli(o)
3. dendr(o)

Exercise 3
1. sensory
2. brain
3. neurons, neuroglia
4. axon, dendrites
5. acetylcholine
6. reflex
7. neurons

Exercise 4
1. spider or arachnoid
2. cerebellum
3. cerebrum
4. meninges
5. spinal cord

Exercise 5
1. cerebro/spin/al: pertaining to the cerebrum and the spinal cord
2. cranio/cerebr/al: pertaining to the skull and the cerebrum
3. mening/eal: pertaining to the meninges

4. neuro/muscul/ar: pertaining to the nerves and muscles
5. sub/dural: beneath the dura mater

Exercise 6
1. peripheral
2. somatic
3. receptors
4. acetylcholine
5. epinephrine

Exercise 7
1. B
2. E
3. A
4. D
5. C

Exercise 8
1. alges/ia: algesi, pain; -ia, pertaining to (one "i" is omitted to facilitate pronunciation)
2. dys/kines/ia: dys-, bad or difficult; -kinesia, movement
3. neur/algia: neur, nerve; -algia, pain
4. par/esthesia: para-, abnormal; -esthesia, feeling (the "a" is omitted to facilitate pronunciation)
5. poly/neuro/pathy: poly-, many; neur(o), nerve; -pathy, disease
6. pseud/esthesia: pseudo-false; esthesi, feeling or sensation; -ia, condition (one "i" is omitted)

Exercise 9
1. cephalalgia
2. photophobia

3. polyneuritis
4. hyperalgesia
5. dyslexia

Exercise 10
1. A
2. D
3. C
4. B

Exercise 11
1. di/plegia: di-, two; -plegia, paralysis
2. hemi/plegia: hemi-, half; -plegia, paralysis
3. mono/plegia: mono-, one; -plegia, paralysis
4. quadri/plegia: quadri-, four; -plegia, paralysis

Exercise 12
1. cerebell/itis: inflammation of the cerebellum
2. encephalo/mening/itis: inflammation of the meninges and brain
3. hemi/plegia: paralysis of half of the body (one side only)
4. meningo/myelo/cele: an abnormal protrusion of the meninges and spinal cord
5. ventricul/itis: inflammation of a ventricle of the brain

Exercise 13
1. cephalgia
2. dyskinesia
3. dyslexia
4. narcolepsy

Exercise 14
1. bradykinesia
2. narcolepsy
3. intracranial

4. glioma
5. amyotrophic

Exercise 15
1. B
2. B
3. A
4. C

Exercise 16
1. pseudomania
2. psychosis
3. neurasthenia
4. pyrophobia
5. hyperkinesia

Exercise 17
1. shunt
2. aneurysmectomy
3. craniectomy
4. neurorrhaphy
5. neurotripsy

Exercise 18
1. neuro/lysis: release of a nerve sheath, disintegration of a nerve; loosening of adhesions
2. psycho/therapy: treatment of disorders of the mind by psychologic means
3. vago/tomy: severing branches of the vagus nerve
4. trans/cutane/ous: through the skin

Exercise 19
1. B
2. C
3. A

Exercise 20
1. neuroleptics
2. anticonvulsants
3. analgesics
4. anxiolytics
5. cholinesterase

Chapter 10 Self-Test

I.
1. dura mater
2. arachnoid
3. pia mater

II.
1. cerebellum
2. spinal cord
3. cerebrum

4. diencephalon
5. brain stem

III
1. poly/neur/algia: pain of several nerves simultaneously
2. aneurysm/ectomy: excision of an aneurysm

3. neuro/genic: originating in the nervous system
4. cranio/tomy: incision into the cranium
5. sub/dur/al: pertaining to the area under the dura mater

IV.
1. meningocele
2. ventriculoperitoneal
3. paraplegia

V.
1. A
2. B
3. A

VI.
1. dura mater
2. Alzheimer disease
3. paraplegia
4. cerebrovascular accident
5. myelogram
6. claustrophobia
7. meningocele
8. deep tendon reflex
9. bulimia
10. hypalgesia

VII.
1. meninges
2. cerebrum
3. cerebrospinal
4. neuron
5. neuroglia
6. axon
7. dendrite

VIII.
1. electroencephalogram
2. antidepressant
3. pseudomania
4. encephalomyelitis
5. agoraphobia
6. semiconscious
7. myelography
8. electroencephalography
9. neurolysis
10. narcolepsy

IX.
1. Both are types of cells of the nervous system.
2. Both are cytoplasmic projections of a neuron.
3. Both are meningeal membranes.

X.
1. The central nervous system, composed of the brain and spinal cord, is the control center of the body, whereas the peripheral nervous system is composed of the various nerve processes that connect the brain and spinal cord with receptors, muscles, and glands.
2. The somatic tissues are the skin and muscles involved in conscious activities; the autonomic tissues are the visceral organs, which function without conscious thought.

XI.
1. DTs
2. CSF
3. ALS
4. Ach
5. IAD

XII.
1. G
2. F
3. C
4. A
5. B
6. J
7. D

XIII.
acetylcholine, cerebral, neurectomy, occipital

XIV.
1. dysphasia
2. hyperkinesias
3. Alzheimer disease
4. anorexia
5. multiple sclerosis

XV.
1. algesia
2. aneurysmectomy
3. efferent
4. cholinesterase
5. cerebrotomy
6. psychotherapy

XVI.
1. ischemic
2. transient
3. speech
4. CVA
5. within
6. embolus

XVII.
1. B

2. C
3. D
4. E
5. F
6. G
7. A

XVIII.
1. E
2. C
3. D
4. C
5. B
6. A
7. B
8. E
9. C
10. D

XIX.
1. arachn/itis: inflammation of the arachnoid membrane
2. cardio/phobia: abnormal fear of heart disease
3. cerebro/cerebell/ar: pertaining to the cerebrum and the cerebellum
4. encephalo/malacia: softening of the brain
5. meningo/encephalo/myel/itis: inflammation of the meninges, brain, and spinal cord

Chapter 11

Exercise 1
1. peripheral
2. receptors
3. (no particular order) eyes, ears, skin, mouth, nose

Exercise 2
1. H
2. E
3. I
4. C
5. F
6. B
7. A
8. G
9. D
10. J

Exercise 3
1. conjunctiva
2. tear
3. cornea
4. iris
5. cornea, hard, horny

6. tear
7. vision
8. retina

Exercise 4
1. choroid(o), choroid
2. conjunctiv(o), conjunctiva
3. corne(o), corna
4. irid(o), iris
5. lacrim(o), tear
6. ocul(o), eyes; opt(o), eyes or sight
7. pupill(o), pupil
8. retin(o), retina

Exercise 5
1. B
2. D
3. C
4. E
5. A
6. F

Exercise 6
1. A
2. B
3. D
4. C

Exercise 7
1. retinopathy
2. ptosis
3. nyctalopia
4. conjunctivitis
5. glaucoma
6. blepharitis
7. ambylopia
8. photophobia
9. hordeolum or stye
10. achromatopsia

Exercise 8
1. accommodation
2. glaucoma
3. tonometry
4. visual field
5. nyctalopia

Exercise 9
1. E
2. F
3. C
4. D
5. A

Exercise 10
1. acoust(o); sound
2. audi(o); hearing
3. audi(o); hearing
4. aur(o), auricul(o), ot(o); ear
5. cochle(o); cochlea

Exercise 11
1. B
2. E
3. C
4. A
5. F
6. D

Exercise 12
1. tympanostomy
2. otoplasty
3. cochlear, cochlea

Exercise 13
1. photoreceptors
2. thermoreceptors
3. nociceptors
4. mechanoreceptors

Exercise 14
1. B
2. C
3. A
4. D

Exercise 15
1. ceruminolytics
2. pupil(s)
3. mydriatics
4. antiglaucoma
5. cycloplegics

Chapter 11 Self-Test

I.
1. D
2. F
3. A
4. C
5. E
6. B

II.
1. eyes
2. achromatopsia
3. tonometry
4. cochlea
5. eustachian
6. audiologist
7. media
8. skin
9. tongue
10. stapes

III.
1. They have the same meaning.
2. They are both brought about by a change in the lens of the eye.

IV.
1. myopia
2. cochlear

V.
1. iris
2. achromatic vision
3. intraocular pressure
4. ptosis
5. opening of the eustachian tube
6. semicircular canals
7. presbyopia
8. mydriatic

VI.
1. cerumen
2. hyperopia
3. anosmia
4. olfactory
5. nociceptor
6. mechanoreceptor
7. cryoextraction
8. blepharedema
9. blepharoptosis
10. anotia

VII.
1. pupil
2. iris
3. sclera
4. lacrimal duct
5. nasolacrimal dut

VIII.
1. Anosmia is impairment or absence of smell, whereas hyperosmia is increased sensitivity to smells or odors.
2. There is a weakness in distinguishing red from green in daltonism, whereas achromatic vision is total color blindness.

IX.
auricular, fluorescein angiography, vitreous humor

X.
1. ectropion
2. LASIK
3. mydriatic
4. otalgia

5. ceruminolytics
6. eustachian

XI.
1. C
2. B
3. E
4. C
5. D
6. C
7. C
8. A
9. C
10. A

XII.
1. ear pain
2. hearing
3. eardrum
4. middle ear
5. dizziness

XIII.
1. ALD
2. OU
3. IOL
4. AS
5. OS
6. AD

XIV.
1. B
2. D
3. C
4. A

XV.
1. diabetic retinopathy: abnormality of the lens caused by diabetes mellitus

2. nyctalopia: night blindness or poor vision in dim light
3. Meniere disease: chronic disease of the inner ear with hearing loss, tinnitus, and vertigo
4. tinnitus: noise or ringing in the ears
5. lacrimation: excessive secretion of tears or crying
6. ophthalmoscopic: pertaining to the eyes
7. sclera: white opaque, tough outer layer of the eye
8. iris: colored portion of the eye, which controls the pupil
9. ophthalmic: pertaining to the eye
10. ophthalmologist: eye specialist

XVI.
1. presence of calculi in the lacrimal sac or duct
2. outside the eye
3. inflammation of the iris
4. inflammation of the cornea
5. paralysis of the pupil

Chapter 12

Exercise 1
1. (no particular order)
   pituitary, adrenals, gonads, thyroid, pancreas, parathyroids, and pineal gland

Exercise 2
1. nervous
2. pituitary or hypophysis
3. gland
4. hormones

Exercise 3
1. B
2. E
3. H
4. K
5. D
6. I
7. I
8. G

9. F
10. A
11. A
12. C
13. J
14. L

Exercise 4
1. (no particular order)
   ADH and oxytocin

2. (no particular order)
   STH, MSH, TSH, PRL, FSH, LH, ACTH

Exercise 5
1. adeno/hypo/physis: gland portion (anterior) of the hypophysis (growth below the brain) or pituitary gland

2. neuro/hypo/physis: nerve portion (posterior) of the hypophysis (growth below the brain) or pituitary gland
3. hypo/thalamus: portion of the lower part of the brain (beneath the thalamus)
4. exo/crine: to secrete outside; the glands with ducts—different from endocrine
5. homeo/stasis: controlling the sameness, maintaining a balance

Exercise 6
1. somatotropin
2. melanocyte
3. euthyroid
4. androgenic
5. tropic

Exercise 7
1. lacto/genic: inducing the secretion of milk
2. ad/ren/al: pertaining to toward the kidney, the gland situated atop each kidney
3. retro/mamm/ary: pertaining to behind the breasts
4. lact/ation: (process of) milk production
5. adreno/cortico/tropic: stimulating the adrenal cortex

Exercise 8
1. D
2. D
3. A
4. D
5. D
6. C
7. D
8. D
9. D
10. B
11. E
12. D

Exercise 9
1. adrenals
2. kidneys
3. ovaries or testes
4. ovaries or testes
5. female breasts
6. thyroid

Exercise 10
1. D
2. C
3. B
4. E
5. A

Exercise 11
1. hyperthyroidism
2. hypoglycemia
3. ketonuria
4. glycosuria
5. mammography

Exercise 12
1. hyper/pituitar/ism: hyper-, greater than normal; pituitar, pituitary; -ism, condition
2. hypo/pituitar/ism: hypo-, below normal; pituitar, pituitary; -ism, condition
3. poly/dipsia: poly-, many; -dipsia, thirst
4. poly/uria: poly-, many; -uria, urination

Exercise 13
1. hyper/parathyroid/ism: hyper-, greater than normal; parathyroid, parathyroid; -ism, condition
2. hypo/parathyroid/ism: hypo-, below normal; parathyroid, parathyroid; -ism, condition
3. pituitar/y hypo/gonad/ism: pituitar, pituitary; -y, condition; hypo-, below normal; gonad, gonad; -ism, condition
4. hypo/gonad/ism: hypo-, below normal; gonad, gonad; -ism, condition

Exercise 14
1. adeno/carcin/oma: malignant tumor of a gland
2. poly/dipsia: excessive thirst
3. hypo/pituitar/ism: decreased activity of the pituitary gland

Exercise 15
1. hyperglycemia
2. polyphagia
3. polyuria
4. antidiuretic
5. glycosuria

Exercise 16
1. pancreatitis
2. mastodynia
3. mastocarcinoma
4. hyperadrenalism
5. hyperinsulinism

Exercise 17
1. D
2. F
3. C
4. H
5. I
6. J
7. E
8. B
9. A
10. G

Exercise 18
1. lumpectomy
2. thyroidectomy
3. mammoplasty
4. adrenalectomy
5. mastopexy
6. mastectomy

Exercise 19
1. antithyroid
2. antihyperglycemic
3. corticosteroids
4. hormone
5. hypothyroidism

Chapter 12 Self-Test

I.
(No particular order) pituitary, adrenals, gonads, pineal gland, thyroid, pancreas, parathyroids

II.
(No particular order) nervous system stimulates endocrine glands by nerve impulses; endocrine glands release hormones

III.
1. C
2. B
3. B
4. A
5. D

IV.
1. D
2. D
3. A
4. D
5. D
6. C
7. D
8. D
9. D
10. B
11. E
12. D
13. E

V.
1. B
2. F
3. C
4. E
5. G
6. A
7. D

VI.
1. adreno/cortic/al: pertaining to the adrenal cortex (outer portion)
2. endo/crine: to secrete internally (into the blood or lymph)
3. hyper/calc/emia: greater than normal amounts of calcium in the blood
4. mast/ectomy: surgical excision of one or both breasts
5. somato/tropin: growth hormone; agent that influences body growth

VII.
1. hypophysectomy
2. mammogram

VIII.
1. sweat gland
2. androgens
3. mammography
4. Cushing syndrome
5. acromegaly
6. diabetes insipidus
7. myxedema
8. pancreas
9. glycosylated hemoglobin
10. goiter

IX.
1. antidiuretic
2. hypopituitarism

X.
1. epinephrine
2. hypothyroidism
3. hirsutism
4. gonad
5. hyperglycemia

6. prolactin
7. pituitary or hypophysis
8. androgenic (or masculinizing)
9. homeostasis
10. glycosuria

XI.
1. Adrenal gland and suprarenal gland are synonyms; both refer to the flattened body above each kidney that secretes hormones.
2. The pituitary is the master gland and, via TSH, the thyroid gland is one of its target organs.
3. Insulin is one type of glucose-lowering agent, a substance that brings about a reduction in the blood glucose level.

XII.
1. An endocrine gland is ductless and secretes hormones into the bloodstream. An exocrine gland secretes its substances through ducts opening on an internal or external surface of the body.
2. Follicle-stimulating hormone is secreted by the pituitary gland and stimulates ovarian follicles to produce estrogen, a female sex hormone responsible for secondary sex characteristics and for preparing a suitable environment for a developing embryo.
3. Type 1 diabetes mellitus is an autoimmune process in which affected persons are dependent on insulin to prevent ketosis; individuals with type 2 diabetes mellitus are usually not dependent on insulin, and the disease is often controlled by diet and exercise and sometimes oral glucose-lowering agents.

XIII.
1. atriopeptin
2. fibrocystic
3. glycosylated
4. cachexia
5. myxedema
6. thyrotropin

XIV.
adenohypophysis, homeostasis, thyrotropin

XV.
1. ADH
2. FSH
3. PTH
4. STH
5. TCT

XVI.
1. polydipsia, polyuria (excessive urination) and chronic UTIs (urinary tract infections)
2. mastectomy
3. Both are high—she has hypercholesterolemia and hyperlipidemia.

4. Nonhealing leg ulcers and poorly healing skin wounds—both due to diabetes, which affects the blood vessels, causing slow healing
5. retinopathy (diseased eyes), neuropathy (diseased nerves), and nephropathy (diseased kidneys)
6. HbA_{1c} 9%, the amount of hemoglobin A_{1c} in the blood, provides an accurate long-term index of the patient's average blood glucose level

XVII.
1. B
2. A
3. C
4. D

XVIII.
1. excessive development of the male mammary glands, frequently secondary to increased estrogen levels; may occur in healthy adolescents
2. excision of both breasts
3. the circular pigmented area around the nipple
4. the arrest of bleeding
5. the mass of fat cells in the area of the axilla
6. to approximate is to bring close together; to reapproximate is to bring close together again, as in suturing together the edges of the skin after surgery

XIX.
1. exophthalmos
2. iodine
3. surgical repair
4. Type 2 diabetes mellitus
5. hormone

XX.
1. C
2. C
3. E
4. C
5. C
6. A
7. B
8. D
9. B
10. C

XXI.
1. para/thyro/tropic: stimulating the growth or activity of the parathyroid glands
2. endo/crino/pathy: a disease involving an endocrine gland or a dysfunction that decreases its secretion or response to a hormone
3. lactos/uria: lactose in the urine, a condition that may occur in late pregnancy or during lactation
4. pituitar/ism: any condition caused by a failure or defect of the pituitary gland
5. thyro/genic: originating in the thyroid gland

Chapter 13

Exercise 1
1. D vitamin synthesis
2. Elimination of wastes through perspiration
3. Regulation of body temperature through perspiration
4. Makes information about the environment available to the brain
5. Acts as barrier to pathogens

Exercise 2
1. A
2. F
3. G
4. B
5. A
6. D
7. C
8. E
9. C
10. D

Exercise 3
1. kerato/genesis: formation of keratin, a horny material

2. sub/cutane/ous: pertaining to beneath the skin
3. ecto/derm: outside (outermost) germ layer
4. dermato/logist: specialist in treatment of the skin
5. endo/derm: innermost germ layer

Exercise 4
1. dermis and epidermis (no particular order)
2. ectoderm
3. sebum
4. sudoriferous gland
5. ungual

Exercise 5
1. biopsy
2. needle
3. skin (or allergy)
4. sweat

Exercise 6
1. A
2. E
3. H
4. D
5. G
6. B
7. C
8. F

Exercise 7
1. albinism
2. cyanosis
3. ichthyosis
4. scleroderma
5. xerosis

Exercise 8
1. A
2. E
3. B
4. C
5. F
6. D

Exercise 9
1. A
2. D
3. C
4. E
5. B
6. F

Exercise 10
1. petechiae
2. nevus

3. keratosis
4. lipoma
5. Kaposi

Exercise 11
1. cysts
2. wheals
3. keloid
4. urticaria
5. laceration

Exercise 12
1. dermis
2. wound or laceration
3. contusion
4. frostbite

Exercise 13
1. follicul/itis: follicul, follicle; -itis, inflammation; cellul/itis: cellul, little cell or compartment; -itis, inflammation

2. hidr/aden/itis: hidr, perspiration; aden, gland; -itis, inflammation
3. leuko/derma: leuk(o), white; derma, skin
4. onycho/lysis: onych(o), nail; -lysis, loosening, freeing, or destroying
5. onycho/malacia: onych(o), nail; -malacia, softening
6. onycho/pathy: onych(o), nail; -pathy, disease
7. onych/osis: onych, nail; -osis, condition
8. onycho/myc/osis: onych(o), nail; myc, fungus; -osis, condition
9. tricho/pathy: trich(o), hair; -pathy, disease

10. trich/osis: trich, hair; -osis, condition (meaning is implied)

Exercise 14
1. C
2. D
3. A
4. B

Exercise 15
1. C
2. D
3. B
4. A

Exercise 16
1. rubefacients
2. pediculicides
3. transdermal
4. astringents
5. keratolytics
6. antipruritics
7. antiseborrheic
8. anesthetics

Chapter 13 Self-Test

I.
1. superficial partial-thickness (first degree)
2. deep partial-thickness (second degree)
3. full-thickness (third degree)
4. epidermis
5. dermis
6. subcutaneous fat

II.
(Any 5, no particular order) external body covering; acts as a barrier to microorganisms; helps regulate body temperature; provides information about the environment; helps eliminate wastes; synthesizes vitamin D

III.
(No particular order) hair protects the scalp, eyes, nostrils, and ears; nails protect the fingers and toes, and fingernails help us pick up small things; sebaceous glands produce sebum to keep hair and skin soft and inhibit bacterial growth; sweat glands eliminate waste and help regulate body temperature

IV.
1. A
2. G
3. C

4. D
5. H
6. F
7. E
8. B

V.
1. excoriation
2. petechiae
3. papules

VI.
1. electro/lysis: destruction by electricity
2. ichthy/osis: a condition in which the skin is dry, resembling scales
3. kerato/genesis: the formation of horny tissue (keratin)
4. melano/cyte: a cell capable of producing melanin
5. sclero/derma: hardening and thickening of the skin

VII.
1. allergy testing
2. cryosurgery
3. débridement
4. axillary
5. seborrheic dermatitis
6. sweat test
7. scleroderma
8. decubitus ulcer
9. deep partial thickness
10. necrotic

VIII.
1. keratin
2. dermis
3. sebum
4. sudoriferous
5. sweating (perspiration)

IX.
1. furuncle
2. scabies
3. laceration
4. albinism
5. contusion
6. onychopathy
7. alopecia
8. ichthyosis
9. thermoplegia
10. folliculitis

X.
1. Both are layers of the skin.
2. A curet is the instrument used in curettage.

XI.
1. A cyst is filled with fluid or a semisolid material; a nodule is solid.
2. A topical drug is applied directly to and exerts effects on the skin; a transdermal drug is delivered as a skin patch and is absorbed into the circulatory system.

XII.
ectoderm, hidradenitis, onychectomy

XIII.
1. AIDS
2. Bx or bx
3. HSV
4. ung
5. TBSA

XIV.
1. the removal of foreign material or dead and damaged tissue
2. abundant flushing of the open wound
3. VAC means vacuum-assisted closure. It is used to remove drainage and speed wound healing, using tubes and a pump to draw off fluids from the wound.
4. incision and drainage

XV.
1. B
2. F
3. D
4. E
5. C
6. A
7. G

XVI.
1. bulla
2. dehiscence
3. electrodessication
4. furuncle
5. rhytidoplasty
6. suppurative

XVII.
1. shingles
2. wheals
3. fever blisters
4. fungus
5. urticaria
XVIII.
1. C
2. B
3. E
4. A
5. D

XIX.
1. E
2. C
3. D
4. D
5. C
6. D
7. B
8. D
9. A
10. C

XX.
1. an/hidr/osis: inadequate (literal translation: lack of) perspiration
2. dermato/graph/ia: a skin condition characterized by wheals that develop from tracing on the skin with the fingernail or a blunt instrument

3. hyper/kerat/osis: overgrowth of the cornified epithelial layer of the skin
4. onycho/dys/trophy: a condition of malformed or discolored fingernails or toenails
5. tricho/phag/ia: the habit of eating hair

Chapter 14

Exercise 1
1. undifferentiated (or immature)
2. carcinogenesis
3. neoplasm
4. carcinogens
5. heart
6. cancer
7. cervical
Exercise 2
1. B
2. B
3. A
4. B
5. A
Exercise 3
(No particular order)
1. direct extension to neighboring tissue
2. permeation along lymph vessels and nodes
3. embolism via blood vessels

4. invasion of body cavity (diffusion)
Exercise 4
1. benign
2. cancerous (malignant)
3. grade
4. staging
Exercise 5
1. exfoliative
2. thyroid
3. radioisotope
4. biopsy
5. radioimmunoassay
6. imaging
7. emission
8. mammography
9. markers
10. biopsy
Exercise 6
1. C
2. D
3. J
4. G

5. F
6. A
7. D
8. H
9. J
10. E
11. G
12. G
13. I
14. G
15. H
16. B
17. B
Exercise 7
1. asymmetry
2. border
3. color
4. diameter
5. evolution (or elevation)
Exercise 8
1. remission
2. excision (biopsy)

3. resection
4. debulking
5. mastectomy
6. lumpectomy
7. cauterization
8. radiosensitive
9. fractionation
10. brachytherapy
11. pheresis or apheresis
12. immunotherapy
Exercise 9
(No particular order)
1. surgical excision
2. radiation therapy
3. systemic or biological therapy
Exercise 10
1. chemotherapy
2. papilloma
3. immunosuppressants
4. radiopharmaceuticals

Chapter 14 Self-Test

I.
1. B
2. A
3. A
4. B
5. A
6. B
7. A
8. B
II.
1. A
2. A
3. A
4. G
5. G
6. J
7. J
8. H

9. H
10. H
11. H
12. F
13. I
14. B
15. D
16. D
III.
1. asymmetry
2. border
3. color
4. diameter
5. evolution, elevation
IV.
(no particular order)
5. direct extension to neighboring tissue

6. permeation along lymph vessels and nodes
7. embolism via blood vessels
8. invasion of body cavity (diffusion)
V.
1. surgical excision
2. radiation therapy
3. systemic or biological therapy
VI.
1. differentiation
2. tumor marker tests
3. cancer staging
4. tumor grading system
5. radioimmunoassay
6. gamma knife radiation
7. SPECT

8. malignant melanoma
9. stereotactic mammography
10. sentinel lymph node biopsy
11. PSA
12. N
13. second
14. anaplasia
15. apheresis
VII.
1. fractionation
2. radiosensitive
3. remission
4. resection
5. brachytherapy
6. carcinogenesis
7. mastectomy

8. debulking
9. chemotherapy
10. radioresistant

VIII.
1. carcinoma
2. metastasis
3. remission
4. chemotherapy
5. neoplasm

IX.
1. T
2. F
3. F

4. T
5. F

X.
1. anaplasia
2. cauterization
3. metastasize
4. oncology
5. radiopharmaceutical
6. stereotactic

XI.
radioimmunoassay, remission, cytopathology

XII.
1. DNA
2. LINAC
3. BPH
4. PSA
5. RAIU
6. RIA

XIII.
1. A
2. C
3. B

XIV.
1. D
2. B
3. E
4. E
5. E
6. D
7. A
8. B
9. B
10. C

Self Test

I.
1. obstetrician
2. neonatologist
3. radiologist
4. nerve cell
5. clinical pathologist
6. symptom
7. chiroplasty
8. electrocardiogram
9. iatrogenic
10. analgesic
11. macroscopic
12. intramuscular
13. syndrome
14. between
15. thrombopenia
16. myocardial infarction
17. atherosclerosis
18. coronary thrombosis
19. atrial septal defect
20. rheumatic fever
21. pneumonitis
22. expectorate
23. parietal pleura
24. bronchodilators
25. orthopnea
26. pancreatography
27. extracorporeal shock wave lithotripsy
28. anorexia nervosa
29. emaciation
30. colectomy
31. intravenous urography
32. renal failure
33. vesicoureteral
34. polyuria
35. endoscopy tube
36. dysmenorrhea
37. endometriosis
38. anorchidism
39. dystocia
40. genital warts
41. sternoschisis
42. ulnoradial
43. arthropathy
44. electromyogram
45. polydactylism
46. central nervous system
47. paraplegia
48. meningocele
49. echoencephalography
50. Alzheimer disease
51. iris
52. achromatic vision
53. ptosis
54. semicircular canals
55. mydriatic
56. pancreas
57. goiter
58. mammography
59. diabetes insipidus
60. Cushing syndrome
61. débridement
62. seborrheic dermatitis
63. scleroderma
64. deep partial-thickness
65. necrosis
66. differentiation
67. radioimmunoassay
68. SPECT
69. second
70. sentinel lymph node biopsy

Bibliography/Illustration and Table Credits

Bibliography

American Cancer Society: *Cancer facts and figures 2016,* Atlanta, 2016, American Cancer Society.

Applegate EJ: *The anatomy and physiology learning system: textbook,* ed 4, Philadelphia, 2011, Saunders.

Ball JW, Dains JE, Flynn JA, Solomon BS, Stewart RW: *Seidel's guide to physical examination,* ed 8, St Louis, 2015, Mosby.

Bedolla M: *Essential Spanish for health care,* New York, 1997, Living Language.

Bonewit-West K: *Clinical procedures for medical assistants,* ed 9, Philadelphia, 2014, Saunders.

Centers for Disease Control and Prevention (website): www.cdc.gov. Accessed March 31, 2017.

Dorland's illustrated medical dictionary, ed 32, Philadelphia, 2011, Saunders.

Federal Bureau of Investigation: *Weapons of mass destruction* (website): http://www.fbi. gov/about-us/investigate/terrorism/wmd. Accessed March 31, 2017.

Ignatavicius DD, Workman MI: *Medical-surgical nursing: patient-centered collaborative care,* ed 8, Philadelphia, 2016, Saunders.

Joyce EV, Villanueva ME: *Say it in Spanish: a guide for health care professionals,* ed 3 Philadelphia, 2004, Saunders.

Lewis SM, Dirksen SR, Heitkemper MM, Bucher L: *Medical-surgical nursing, assessment and management of clinical problems,* ed 10, St Louis, 2017, Mosby.

Mosby's dictionary of medicine, nursing, and health professions, ed 9, St Louis, 2013, Mosby.

Spies SC: Planning for WMD terrorism response: factors to consider, *Journal of the American Society of Professional Emergency Planners* 7:1-15, 2000.

Taber's cyclopedic medical dictionary, ed 22, Philadelphia, 2013, FA Davis.

Velasquez M: *Velasquez Spanish and English dictionary,* El Monte, CA, 2006, Academic Learning Company.

Illustration and Table Credits

1001nights/E+/gettyimages.com **Unnumbered 1-9**

7activestudio/ iStock/Getty Images Plus /gettyimages.com **Unnumbered 7-2, Unnumbered 12-2**

aabejon/ iStock /Getty Images Plus/gettyimages.com **Unnumbered 6-11**

Abrahams PH, Boon J, Spratt JD: *McMinn's clinical atlas of human anatomy,* ed 6, St Louis, 2008, Mosby. Figures **3-3** (face), **3-24** (Photo), **9-5,** and **Unnumbered 9-4**

Abrahams PH, Spratt JD, Loukas M, van Schoor A-N, Hutchings RT: *McMinn and Abrahams' clinical atlas of human anatomy,* ed 7, St Louis, 2014, Mosby. **Unnumbered 1-3** (Exercise 1); Figures **9-8A** and **9-9**

Adam A, Dixon AK, Grainger RG, Allison DJ: *Grainger and Allison's Diagnostic Radiology,* ed 5, 2008, Churchill Livingstone. Figure **2-38B**

Albert RK, Spiro SG, Jett JR: *Clinical respiratory medicine,* ed 2, Philadelphia, 2004, Mosby. Figure **5-29A**

AlexRaths/ iStock / Getty Images Plus /gettyimages.com **Unnumbered 12-1**

alvarez/E+/gettyimages.com **Unnumbered 14-5**

Andregric/ iStock /Getty Images Plus/gettyimages.com Figure **9-8B**

andresr/E+/gettyimages.com **Unnumbered 10-1**

annedde/E+/gettyimages.com **Unnumbered 8-3**

Antonio_Diaz/ iStock / Getty Images Plus/gettyimages.com. Figure **3-36** photo inset: (right)

anyaivanova/ iStock /Getty Images Plus /gettyimages.com **Unnumbered 1-1, Unnumbered 2-1**

Applegate E: *The Anatomy and Physiology Learning System,* ed 4, 2011, Saunders/Elsevier. Figures **3-42, 3-49** and **4-30A**

asiseeit/E+/gettyimages.com **Unnumbered 10-12**

Aspinall RJ, Taylor-Robinson SD: *Mosby's Color Atlas and Text of Gastroenterology and Liver Disease,* London, 2002, Mosby, Ltd. Figure **6-9B&C, 6-10B**

Athanasoulis CA et al: *Interventional radiology,* Philadelphia, 1982, Saunders. Figure **7-28, A and B**

Aunt_Spray/ iStock /Getty Images Plus/gettyimages.com Figure **2-4A**

Ball JW, Dains JE, Flynn JA, Solomon BS and Stewart Rosalyn: *Seidel's guide to physical examination,* ed 8, St. Louis, 2015, Mosby. Figures **2-21, 2-31, 3-8 B** and **C, 3-20A, 5-6, 8-44A,** and **11-7; Unnumbered 8-6E**

Ballinger PW, Frank ED: *Merrill's atlas of radiographic positions and radiologic procedures,* vol 1, ed 9, St Louis, 1999, Mosby. Figure **2-35A**

Ballinger PW, Frank ED: *Merrill's atlas of radiographic positions and radiologic procedures,* ed 10, St Louis, 2003, Mosby. Figure **2-40, 9-32, 12-12C** (modified)

Baloncici/ iStock / Getty Images Plus /gettyimages.com Figure **10-27**

baona/ iStock / Getty Images Plus /gettyimages.com **Unnumbered 9-12**

baranozdemir/ iStock /Getty Images Plus/gettyimages.com **Unnumbered 7-10**

Barkauskas VH, Bauman LC, Darling-Fisher CS: *Health & physical assessment,* ed 3, St Louis, 2002, Mosby, Inc. Figures **3-30, 9-22A**

Barrett JP, Herndon DN: *Color atlas of burn care,* Philadelphia, 2001, Saunders. Figure **13-25D**

Beare PG, Myers JL: *Adult health nursing,* ed 3, 1998, Mosby. Figures **6-30, 12-25**

Behrman R, Kliegman R, Jenson HB: *Nelson's textbook of pediatrics,* ed 17, Philadelphia, 2004, Saunders. Figures **4-32** and **9-39; Unnumbered 4-8**

Belchetz PE, Hammond P: *Mosby's color atlas and text of diabetes and endocrinology,* London, 2003, Mosby. Figure **7-6B** and **12-21**

Bernstein E: *Laser treatment of tattoos.* J Clin Dermatol 24 (1): 2005, p. 43. Figure **13-34D**

Black JM, Hawks JH, Keene AM:*Medical-surgical nursing: clinical management for continuity of care,* ed 6, Philadelphia, 2001, Saunders. Figure **5-26** and **Unnumbered 10-3**

Black JM and Hawks JH: *Medical-surgical nursing: clinical management for positive outcomes,* ed 7, Philadelphia, 2005, Saunders. Figures **2-39, 9-23B,** and **12-24; Unnumbered 9-6** and **12-13**

Black JM, Hawks JH: *Medical-surgical nursing,* ed 8, 2009, Saunders. Figures **8-8** and **14-16**

blueringmedia/ iStock / Getty Images Plus/gettyimages.com Figure **10-8A; Unnumbered 14-2**

Bodansky HJ: *Pocket picture guide to diabetes,* London, 1989, Gower Medical Publishing. Figure **12-3** (Photomicrograph)

Bonewit-West K: *Clinical procedures for medical assistants,* ed 8, Philadelphia, 2012, Saunders. Figure **8-41**

Bonewit-West K: *Clinical procedures for medical assistants,* ed 9, Philadelphia, 2015, Saunders. Figures **2-30A, 7-6C**

Bontrager KL, Lampignano J: *Textbook of radiographic positioning and related anatomy,* ed 6, St Louis, 2005, Mosby. Figure **7-11** and **Unnumbered 7-5D**

Bork K, Brauninger W: *Skin diseases in clinical practice,* ed 2, 1999, Saunders. Figure **13-20**

bowdenimages/ iStock / Getty Images Plus /gettyimages.com **Unnumbered 11-3**

Boyle AC, Shipley M: *A colour atlas of rheumatology,* ed 3, London, 1993, Mosby-Year Book Europe Limited. Figure **9-34A**

Braunwald: *Heart disease: a textbook of cardiovascular medicine,* ed 6, Philadelphia, 2001, Saunders. Figure **4-15**

Brunzel NA: *Fundamentals of urine & body fluid analysis,* ed 2, St Louis, 2004, Saunders. Figure **7-7**

bulentgultek/DigitalVision Vectors/gettyimages.com **Unnumbered 1-4**

Callen JP, Greer KE, Hood AF, et al: *Color atlas of dermatology,* Philadelphia, 1992, Saunders. Figure **6-15**

Callen JP, Greer KE, Paller AS, Swinyer LJ: *Color atlas of dermatology,* ed 2, Philadelphia, 2000, Saunders. Figures **13-16, 13-21AB, 13-30,** and **13-31**

Canale ST: *Operative orthopaedics,* ed 9, St Louis, 1998, Mosby. Figure **9-27**

Canale ST, Beaty JH: *Campbell's Operative Orthopaedics,* ed 12, St. Louis, 2013, Mosby. Figure **9-31**

Canby C: *Problem based anatomy,* St. Louis, 2007, WB Saunders. Figure **8-16B**

Carlson K, Eisenstat S: *Primary care of women,* 1995, Mosby. Figure **6-12** and **Unnumbered 6-5A**

CarpathianPrice/iStock/Getty Images Plus/gettyimages.com **Unnumbered 8-2**

CasarsaGuru/E+/gettyimages.com **Unnumbered 14-1**

Cathy Yeulet/ Hemera / Getty Images Plus/ gettyimages.com Figure **8-35B**

Centers for Disease Control and Prevention, Atlanta, Georgia. Figures **2-10B, 2-11,** and **2-12**

choja/E+/gettyimages.com. Figure **4-10F**

Christian PE, Waterstram-Rich KM: *Nuclear Medicine and PET/CT*, 7e, 2012, Mosby. Figures **14-7** and **14-8**

Clark DA: *Atlas of neonatology*, 2000, Saunders. Figures **2-15** and **6-16; Unnumbered 2-5**

claudiodivizia/iStock/Getty Images Plus/gettyimages.com. Figure **3-40A**

Conlon CP, Snydman DR: *Mosby's color atlas and text of infectious diseases, 2000*, Mosby Ltd. Figure **13-32**

Copyright Dennis Kunkel Microscopy, Inc., 1994. Figure **3-41A**

© Drägerwerk AG & Co. KGaA, Lübeck, All rights reserved. No portion hereof may be reproduced, saved or stored in a data processing system, electronically or mechanically copied or otherwise recorded by any other means without our express prior written permission. Figure **5-29B**

© Joint Commission Resources. Oakbrook Terrace, IL: Joint Commission on Accreditation of Healthcare Organizations, 2016. Reprinted with permission. **Table 1-7**

Cotran RS, Kumar V, Collins T: *Robbin's pathologic basis of disease*, ed 7, Philadelphia, 2004, Saunders. Figure **8-56**

Courtesy Baxter Healthcare Corporation. Figure **7-23A**

Courtesy Biomet Orthopedics. Figure **9-45A**

Courtesy Cory J Bosanko, OD, FAAO. Eye Centers of Tennessee, Crossville, Tenn. Figure **11-6**

Courtesy Department of Neurological Surgery, Vanderbilt University Medical Center, Nashville, Tennessee. Figure **10-30A** and **14-14**

Courtesy Department of Pathology, Duke University Medical Center, Durham, North Carolina. Figure **7-16**

Courtesy Dr. Christine L. Williams, New York Medical College. Figure **3-5 A** and **Unnumbered 3-15**

Courtesy Dr. Dwight Parkinson, Departments of Surgery and of Human Anatomy and Cell Science, University of Manitoba, Winnipeg, Manitoba, Canada. Figure **10-19**

Courtesy Dr. Ellen Wald, Children's Hospital of Pittsburgh. Figure **8-27**

Courtesy Ellen Wald, MD, University of Wisconsin Children's Hospital. Figures **2-8A**

Courtesy Dr. M. McKenzie, Toronto, Canada. Figure **13-15**

Courtesy Dr. Jeffrey P. Callen. Figure **13-8**

Courtesy Ellen Peterson, University of California-Irvine. Figure **8-52C**

Courtesy Hannah Kruse, St. Paul, Missouri. Figure **2-24A**

Courtesy Janet Jones. Figure **5-27D**

Courtesy Joseph Imbriglia, MD, Allegheny General Hospital, Pittsburgh, Pa. Figure **3-5B**

Courtesy Ophthalmic Photography at the University of Michigan, WK Kellogg Eye Center, Ann Arbor, Mich. Figure **11-11**

Courtesy Peggy Leonard Zimmerman. Figure **1-2**

Courtesy Pilonidal Support Alliance, Long Beach, California. www.pilonidal.org Figure **13-9B**

Courtesy PresMark Publishing Co. www.presmark.com. Figure **5-15B**

Courtesy Professor A. Jackson, Department of Diagnostic Radiology, University of Manchester. Figure **2-41A**

Courtesy S. Ishihara, Washington University Department of Ophthalmology. Figure **11-4**

Courtesy the Royal College of Obstetricians and Gynaecologists. Figure **8-11B**

Courtesy Zimmer, Inc., Warsaw, Indiana. Figure **9-44**

Curry RA, Tempkin BB: *Sonography: introduction to normal structure and function*, St. Louis, 2004, Saunders. Figure **8-45A**

Custer RP: An atlas of the blood and bone marrow, ed 2, Philadelphia, 1974, Saunders. Figure **3-44**

Dalrymple NC, Leyendecker JR, Oliphant M: *Problem Solving in Abdominal Imaging*, 2009, Mosby. Figure **8-9**

Damjanov I, Linder J: *Anderson's pathology*, ed 10, St Louis, 1996, Mosby. Figure **6-20**

Damjanov I, Linder J: *Pathology: A color atlas*, 2000, St. Louis, Mosby. Figure **3-40B, 6-25B, 6-28B,** and **6-29; Unnumbered 6-5B**

Damjanov I, *Pathology for the health professions*, ed 5, Philadelphia, 2017, Saunders. Figure **2-24B, 6-24, 6-27, 7-15, 7-22,** and **14-3; Unnumbered 12-10**

Damjanov I, *Pathology for the health professions*, ed 5, Philadelphia, 2017, Saunders. Courtesy of the late Dr. Warren Lang, Jefferson Medical College, Philadelphia, PA. Figure **8-7B**

DaveAlan/ iStock /Getty Images Plus/gettyimages.com Figure **1-16A**

dblight/E+/gettyimages.com. Figure **10-12A**

dimdimich/ iStock /Getty Images Plus/gettyimages.com Figure **9-14B**

Dimedrol68/ iStock / Getty Images Plus/gettyimages.com. Figure **3-20B**

Dorland's illustrated medical dictionary, ed 32, Philadelphia, 2011, Saunders. Figure **3-39**

DragonImages/ iStock /Getty Images Plus/gettyimages.com **Unnumbered 5-1**

Drake R, Vogl W, Mitchell AWM: *Gray's anatomy for students*, ed 3, New York, 2015, Churchill Livingstone. Figures **4-31, 5-9B,** and **8-7C**

Draper BK, Robbins JR, Stricklin GP: Bullous Sweet's syndrome in congenital neutropenia: Association with pegfilgrastim. J Am Acad Dermatol, Elsevier, May, 2005. Figure **13-11E**

drbimages/ iStock / Getty Images Plus /gettyimages.com **Unnumbered 6-7, Unnumbered 12-16**

drbimages/E+/gettyimages.com **Unnumbered 2-10, Unnumbered 7-8, Unnumbered 10-10**

Earis JE, Pearson MG: *Respiratory medicine*, London, 1995, Times Mirror International Publishers. Figure **5-16**

EHStock/ iStock /Getty Images Plus/gettyimages.com **Unnumbered 6-3**

Elkin MK, Perry AG, Potter PA: *Nursing interventions & clinical skills*, ed 3, St. Louis, 2003, Mosby. Figure **6-35**

emreogan/ iStock /Getty Images Plus/gettyimages.com **Unnumbered 5-12**

Eraxion/iStock/Getty Images Plus/gettyimages.com Figure **8-25B; Unnumbered 6-2, Unnumbered 9-2, Unnumbered 11-2**

Evans A et al: *Atlas of breast disease management*, Philadelphia, 1998, Saunders. Figure **12-19B**

Falcone T, Goldberg JM: *Basic, Advanced, and Robotic Laparoscopic Surgery*, Philadelphia, 2010, Saunders/Elsevier. Figures **1-12, 6-37, 8-10B, 8-19, 8-22,** and **8-38**

FangXiaNuo/ iStock / Getty Images Plus /gettyimages.com **Unnumbered 10-14**

FangXiaNuo/E+/gettyimages.com. **Unnumbered 4-15**

FatCamera/E+/gettyimages.com **Unnumbered 1-7** (career photo)

ferlistockphoto/ iStock / Getty Images Plus/gettyimages.com. Figure **3-36** photo inset (left)

Finkbeiner WE, Ursell PC, Davis RL: Autopsy pathology: a manual and atlas, ed 2, Philadelphia 2009, Saunders. Figure **13-24B**

Firstsignal/iStock/Getty Images Plus/gettyimages.com **Unnumbered 13-2**

Fletcher CDM: *Diagnostic histopathology of tumors*, ed 3, London, 2007, ChurchillLivingstone. Figure **12-22**

Forbes BA, Sahm DF, Weissfeld AS: *Bailey & Scott's diagnostic microbiology*, ed 12, St Louis, 2007, Mosby. Figures **8-51B** and **8-52B**

francesco_de_napoli/ iStock / Getty Images Plus/gettyimages.com **Unnumbered 3-19**

franciscodiazpagador/ iStock / Getty Images Plus /gettyimages.com Figure **10-21**

Frank ED, Long BW, and Smith BJ: *Merrill's atlas of radiographic positioning and procedures*, ed 11, St. Louis, 2008, Mosby. Figure **3-19**

Frank ED, Long BW, Smith BJ: *Merrill's atlas of radiographic positions and radiologic procedures*, ed 12, St Louis, 2012, Mosby. Figures **12-12B** and **14-11**

freemixer/E+/gettyimages.com **Unnumbered 4-1**

Fuller JK: *Surgical Technology: principles and practice*, ed 6, 2013, Saunders. Figures **2-44, 3-47,** and **9-26B**

Gartner LP, Hiatt JL: *Color Textbook of Histology*, ed 3, Philadelphia, 2007, Saunders. Figure **3-4**

Geber86/ iStock / Getty Images Plus /gettyimages.com **Unnumbered 9-14**

giannonip/ iStock /Getty Images Plus/gettyimages.com Figure **2-41B**

Gitlan N, Strauss RM: *Atlas of Clinical Hepatology*, Philadelphia, 1995,WB Saunders. Figure **6-17**

GlobalStock/E+/gettyimages.com **Unnumbered 5-10**

Goering R, Dockrell H, Zuckerman M, Roitt I, Chiodini PL: *Mim's medical microbiology*, ed 5, St. Louis, 2013, Saunders. Figures **2-5AB** and **2-7AB**

Goldman L, Bennett JC: *Cecil Textbook of Medicine*, ed 21, Philadelphia, 2000, Saunders. Figure **13-12C**

Goldman L and Schafer AI: *Goldman's Cecil Medicine*, ed 24, Philadelphia, 2012, Saunders. Figure **14-10A**

Goldstein BJ, Goldstein AO: *Practical dermatology*, ed 2, St Louis, 1997, Mosby. Figures **2-25** and **4-34; Unnumbered 4-7**

grandriver/ iStock /Getty Images Plus/gettyimages.com **Unnumbered 7-12**

Greer I, Cameron I, Kitchner H, Prentice A: *Mosby's color atlas and text of obstetrics and gynecology*, London, 2001, Mosby Ltd. Figure **3-2B**

Gruber RP, Peck GC: *Rhinoplasty: state of the art*, St Louis, 1993, Mosby. Figure **2-46**

Habif TP, Campbell JL, Chapman MS et al: *Skin disease: diagnosis and treatment*, ed 3, Philadelphia, 1996, Saunders. Figure **13-29**

Habif TP: *Clinical dermatology: A color guide to diagnosis and therapy*, ed 6, 2016, Mosby. Figure **13-6, 13-12B**

Hagen-Ansert SL: *Textbook of Diagnostic Ultrasonography*, ed 5, St Louis, 2001, Mosby. Figure **4-14B**

Hagen-Ansert S: *Textbook of Diagnostic Ultrasonography*, ed 6, 2006, St. Louis, Mosby. Figure **2-42**

Hardy M, Snaith B: *Musculoskeletal Trauma*, London, 2011, Churchill-Livingstone. Figure **13-24A**

Harkreader H, Hogan MA, Thobaben M: *Fundamentals of nursing*, ed 3, St Louis, 2007, Saunders. Figures **3-21D, 5-30, 5-33** and **7-8A, 11-18**

Hart CA, Broadhead RL: *Color atlas of pediatric infectious diseases*, London, 1992, Mosby-Wolfe. Figure **3-37** and **Unnumbered 3-16**

Herlihy B: *The human body in health and illness*, ed 3, 2007, St. Louis, Saunders. Figure **12-10**

Herlihy B: *The human body in health and illness*, ed 5, Philadelphia, 2014, Saunders. **Unnumbered 3-13**

Hockenberry MJ, Wilson D: *Wong's essentials of pediatric nursing*, ed 9, 2013, Mosby. Figure **8-48**

Hockenberry MJ, Wilson D: Wong's nursing care of infants and children, ed 10, St Louis, 2015, Mosby. Figures **9-7B** and **13-33A**

Hoffman AV, Pettit JE: *Color atlas of clinical hematology*, ed 4, Philadelphia, 2009, Mosby. Figure **2-16**

Hordinsky MK, Sawaya ME, Scher RK: *Atlas of hair and nails*, 2000, Churchill Livingstone. Figure **12-19A**

huronphoto/E+/gettyimages.com **Unnumbered 9-10**

Ignatavicius DD, Workman ML, Mishler MA: *Medical-surgical nursing across the health care continuum*, ed 3, Philadelphia, 1999, Saunders. Figures **12-17** and **13-28**

Ignatavicius DD, Workman ML: *Medical-surgical Nursing: Critical thinking for collaborative care*, ed 5, Philadelphia, 2006, Saunders. Figures **5-14, 8-20, 10-30B, 13-19A; Unnumbered 13-6**

Ignatavicius MS. Workman MI: *Medical-surgical nursing: patient-centered collaborative care*, ed 7, 2013, Philadelphia, Saunders. Figure **10-31**

Ignatavicius MS, Workman MI: *Medical-surgical nursing: patient-centered collaborative care*, ed 8, Philadelphia, 2016, Saunders. **Table 11-2;** Figures **2-32A, 3-32, 5-3, 9-45B,** and **13-25C; Unnumbered 3-12**

ilbusca/E+/gettyimages.com Figure **11-5**

Imagesbybarbara/E+/gettyimages.com Figure **11-17A**

Ingalls AJ, Salerno MC: *Maternal and child health nursing,* ed 6, St Louis, 1987, Mosby. Figure **5-24**

Jacob S: *Atlas of human anatomy,* Philadelphia, 2002, Churchill Livingstone. Figure **3-23**

Jacob S: *Human anatomy: A clinically-orientated approach,* St Louis, 2008, Churchill-Livingstone. Figures **4-6A** and **7-2A**

James SR, Nelson K, and Ashwill J: *Nursing Care of Children: principles and practice,* ed 4, St. Louis, 2013, Saunders. Figure **2-1**

James WD: *Andrews' Diseases of the skin,* 2011, Elsevier. Figure **13-14**

James WD, Berger T, Elston T: *Andrews' Diseases of the skin: Clinical Dermatology,* 2016, Elsevier. Figure **13-27**

jaqy/ iStock /Getty Images Plus/gettyimages.com Figure **2-24C**

jarabee123/ iStock / Getty Images Plus /gettyimages.com Figure **13-9A**

jarenwicklund/ iStock / Getty Images Plus/gettyimages.com Figure **10-20**

jarun011/ iStock /Getty Images Plus /gettyimages.com Figure **14-6; Unnumbered 3-2**

Jarvis C: *Physical examination and health assessment,* ed 7, Philadelphia, 2016, Saunders. Figures **8-26, 9-20ABCDE, 9-22B, 10-10C**

jeffbergen/E+/gettyimages.com Figure **11-8**

JohnnyGreig/ iStock / Getty Images Plus /gettyimages.com **Unnumbered 13-3**

Juanmonino/ iStock / Getty Images Plus /gettyimages.com **Unnumbered 11-10, Unnumbered 13-13**

Juanmonino/E+/gettyimages.com **Unnumbered 5-8**

kali9/ iStock / Getty Images Plus /gettyimages.com **Unnumbered 12-12, Unnumbered 13-1**

kali9/E+/gettyimages.com Figure **13-34B; Unnumbered 7-3**

Kamal A, Brockelhurst JC: *Color atlas of geriatric medicine,* ed 2, St Louis, 1991, Mosby. Figures **2-23** and **9-30**

KatarzynaBialasiewicz/ iStock / Getty Images Plus /gettyimages.com Figure **12-23**

Keohane E, Smith L, Walenga J: *Rodak's Hematology: clinical principles and applications,* ed 5, St. Louis, 2015, Saunders. Figures **3-41B, 3-46B,** and **9-24B**

Kowalczyk N, Mace JD: *Radiographic Pathology for Technologists,* ed 5, 2009, Mosby. Figure **4-20B** and **Unnumbered 4-9**

KozyrevAnton/ iStock /Getty Images Plus/gettyimages.com Figure **9-42A**

Kumar P, Clark M: *Kumar & Clark's Clinical Medicine,* ed 9, Edinburgh, 2017, Elsevier. Figure **13-23**

Kumar V, Abbas AK, Aster J: *Robbins and Cotran Pathologic basis of disease,* ed 9, Philadelphia, 2015, Saunders. Figures **5-20** and **9-35**

Kumar V, Abbas AK, Aster J: *Robbins' Basic pathology,* ed 9, Philadelphia, 2013, Saunders. Figure **2-19**

kzenon/ iStock /Getty Images Plus/gettyimages.com **Unnumbered 9-1**

Ladida/E+/gettyimages.com **Unnumbered 2-12**

lawcain/ iStock /Getty Images Plus/gettyimages.com Figure **9-8C**

Lemmi FO, Lemmi CAE: *Physical assessment findings* CD-ROM, Philadelphia, 2000, Saunders. Figures **5-17A, 8-52A, 8-54, 8-55, 9-38A, 11-15,** and **13-12F; Unnumbered 13-5**

Lewis S, Heitkemper MM, Dirksen SR: *Medical-surgical nursing, assessment and management of clinical problems,* ed 6, St Louis, 2004, Mosby. Figures **7-10**

Lewis SM, Heitkemper MM, Dirksen SR, O'Brien PG, Bucher L: *Medical-surgical nursing: assessment and management of clinical problems,* ed 7, St Louis, 2007, Mosby. Figures **3-26** and **4-23A**

Lewis S, Dirksen SR, Heitkemper MM, Bucher L, Camera IM: *Medical-surgical nursing, assessment and management of clinical problems,* ed 8, St Louis, 2011, Mosby. Figure **7-29**

Lewis SL, Bucher L, Heitkemper MM, Dirksen SR, : *Medical-surgical nursing, assessment and management of clinical problems,* ed 9, St Louis, 2014, Mosby. **Table 10-1** (modified) and Figure **13-25 E**

Lewis SL, Bucher L, Heitkemper MM, Harding MM, Kwong J, Roberts D: *Medical-surgical nursing, assessment and management of clinical problems,* ed 10, St Louis, 2017, Mosby. Figures **9-21, 10-10AB**

Liebert PS: *Color atlas of pediatric surgery,* ed 2, Philadelphia, 1995, Saunders. Figures **9-37AB**

lirtlon/ iStock /Getty Images Plus/gettyimages.com Figure **2-4B**

lisafx/ iStock /Getty Images Plus/gettyimages.com **Unnumbered 5-3**

Long BW, Rollins JH, Smith BJ: *Merrill's atlas of radiographic positioning procedures,* ed 13, St. Louis, 2016, Mosby. Figure **2-33B, 2-36, 2-37, 2-43, 4-14A, 6-11, 9-4, 9-12, 9-13, 9-43, 12-12A** and **14-13**

lovro77/ iStock /Getty Images Plus/gettyimages.com **Unnumbered 7-1**

luckyraccoon/ iStock / Getty Images Plus/gettyimages.com **Unnumbered 3-8**

Mahan LK, Escott-Stump S: *Krause's food and nutrition therapy,* ed 12, Philadelphia, 2008, Saunders. Figure **6-28A**

Male D, Brostoff J, Roth D, and Roitt I: *Immunology,* ed 8, 2013, Mosby. Figure **3-48A** and **B**

Mark Kostich/ iStock / Getty Images Plus /gettyimages.com Figure **10-28**

Marks JG Jr, Miller JJ: *Lookingbill and Marks' principles of dermatology,* ed 4, Philadelphia, 2006, Saunders. Figures **13-11G, 13-21C**

Mason, RJ et al: *Murray and Nadel's Textbook of Respiratory Medicine,* ed 4, Philadelphia, 2005, Saunders. Figure **5-21**

Matteson PS: *Women's health during the childbearing years: a community-based approach,* St Louis, 2001, Mosby. Figure **9-7A**

Mehmet Hilmi Barcin/ iStock /Getty Images Plus/gettyimages.com Figure **1-16B**

Mendeloff AI, Smith DE, eds: Acromegaly, diabetes, hypermetabolism, proteinuria and heart failure. *Clin Pathol Conf Am J Med* 20:133, 1956. Figure **12-16**

Miles DA, Van Dis ML, Williamson GF, Jensen CW: *Radiographic Imaging for the Dental Team,* 4e, 2009, Saunders. Figure **2-35B**

Miller MD, Howard RF, Plancher KD: *Surgical Atlas of Sports Medicine,* 2003, Philadelphia, Saunders. Figure **9-26A**

Monahan FD, Neighbors M: *Medical-surgical nursing: foundations for clinical practice,* ed 2, Philadelphia, 1998, Saunders. Figures **5-13** and **13-5**

Monahan FD, Sands JK, Neighbors, M, Marek JF, Green CH: *Phipps' medical-surgical nursing: health and illness perspectives,* ed 8, St Louis, 2007, Mosby. Figures **3-15** and **10-29; Unnumbered 10-7**

Monkey Business Images Ltd/Monkey Business / Getty Images Plus/gettyimages.com. **Unnumbered 4-11**

monkeybusinessimages/ iStock / Getty Images Plus /gettyimages.com Figure **8-35A; Unnumbered 3-1, Unnumbered 3-17** patient photo, and **Unnumbered 3-18, Unnumbered 4-3, Unnumbered 8-1, Unnumbered 13-11**

Moore KL, Persaud TVN, Torchia MG: *The developing human,* ed 10, Philadelphia, 2017, Saunders. Figure **8-43**

MorePixels/ iStock /Getty Images Plus /gettyimages.com Figure **1-10**

Morse S, Moreland A, Holmes K, eds: *Atlas of sexually transmitted diseases and AIDS,* ed 2, London, 1996, Mosby-Wolfe. Figure **8-51A**

Morse SA, Ballard RC, Holmes KK, Moreland AA, eds: *Atlas of sexually transmitted diseases and AIDS,* ed 3, London, 2003, Mosby. Figure **2-6F**

Mourad LA: *Orthopedic disorders,* St Louis, 1991, Mosby. Figure **9-23A**

Murray PR, Rosenthal KS, Kobayashi GS, Pfaller MA: *Medical microbiology,* ed 3, St Louis, 1994, Mosby. Figure **2-6B**

Murray PR, Rosenthal KS, Pfaller MA: *Medical microbiology,* ed 8, Philadelphia, 2016, Saunders. Figure **8-57**

Murray SS, McKinney ES: *Foundations of maternal–newborn nursing,* ed 4, Philadelphia, 2006, WB Saunders. Figure **8-40**

Mutlu Kurtbas/E+/gettyimages.com **Unnumbered 1-2**

neicebird/ iStock /Getty Images Plus/gettyimages.com **Unnumbered 6-1**

Neustockimages/ iStock /Getty Images Plus /gettyimages.com Figure **1-9**

Neustockimages/E+/gettyimages.com **Unnumbered 14-7**

nicolas_/ iStock /Getty Images Plus/gettyimages.com. Figure **2-20**

nicomenijes/gettyimages.com Figure **1-1**

Noble J, ed: *Textbook of primary care medicine,* St Louis, 1996, Mosby. Figure **8-53**

Noble J and Greene HL: *Textbook of primary care medicine,* St Louis, ed 3, Mosby, 2001. Figures **13-11ABCDF, 13-12ADE, 13-19B, 14-10B** and **Unnumbered 13-7**

nyul/ iStock /Getty Images Plus/gettyimages.com **Unnumbered 1-5** (patient photo within Figure 1-15),

Obstetrics and Gynecology Clinics of North America, 2005, Invasive Antenatal Interventions in Complicated Multiple Pregnancies. Figure **8-34**

Osborn AG: *Diagnostic neuroradiology,* St Louis, 1994, Mosby. Figure **10-22**

Pagana KD, Pagana TJ: *Mosby's diagnostic and laboratory test reference,* ed 7, St. Louis, 2004, Mosby. Figure **14-5**

Palay DA, Krachmer JH, editors: *Ophthalmology for the primary care physician,* ed 2, St Louis, 2005, Mosby. Figures **2-18, 2-32B, 11-2B; Unnumbered 2-8**

Patton KT, Thibodeau GA: *Anatomy & physiology,* ed 8, St Louis, 2013, Mosby/Elsevier. Figures **10-3A, 11-22B; Unnumbered 3-7**

Patton KT, Thibodeau GA: *Anatomy & physiology,* ed 9, St Louis, 2016, Mosby/Elsevier. Figures **1-11A, 4-21, 10-12B** (modified), **11-22A, 12-2** (modified), and **13-2.**

Patton KT, Thibodeau GA: *The human body in health & disease,* ed 6, St. Louis, 2014. Figures **3-16, 3-34,** and **8-49**

Patton KT, Thibodeau GA: *The human body in health & disease,* ed 7, St. Louis, 2018, Elsevier/Mosby. Figures **8-6B** and **C, 8-24B,** and **8-32**

Patton KT, Thibodeau GA: *Structure and Function of the Body,* ed 15, St. Louis, 2016, Elsevier/Mosby. Figure **6-14**

PavlovskiJenya/ iStock / Getty Images Plus /gettyimages.com Figure **12-20**

Perkin GD et al: *Atlas of clinical neurology,* ed 3, Philadelphia, 2011 Saunders. Figure **10-18**

Perry AG, Potter PA, Elkin MK, *Nursing interventions and clinical skills,* ed 6, St Louis, 2016, Mosby. Figure **5-32**

Perry AG, Potter PA, Ostendorf W: *Clinical nursing skills and techniques,* ed 9, St. Louis, 2018, Mosby. Figure **2-27A**

Phipps WJ, Monahan FD, Sands JK, Neighbors M, Marek JF and Green-Nigro CJ: *Phipps' Medical Surgical Nursing,* ed 8, St. Louis, 2007, Mosby. Figure **2-33A**

Photo Researchers, Inc. All Rights Reserved. Figure **5-15A**

Photodisc CD: *Health and medicine 2,* vol. 40, Getty Images, Inc., Seattle, WA. Figure **1-7**

pidjoe/E+/gettyimages.com **Unnumbered 8-12**

Polaski AL, Tatro SE: *Luckmann's core principles and practice of medical-surgical nursing,* Philadelphia, 1996, Saunders. Figures **8-12, 10-11**

Potter PA, Perry AG: *Basic nursing,* ed 7, St Louis, 2011, Mosby. Figure **5-5**

Potter PA, Perry AG, Stockert P, Hall A: *Fundamentals of Nursing,* ed 8, St. Louis, 2013, Mosby-Elsevier. Figures **2-28B&C, 4-10E,** and **5-27C**

Potter PA, Perry AG, Stockert P, Hall A: Fundamentals of Nursing, ed 9, St. Louis, 2017, Mosby. Figure **2-27B, 2-28A&D, 2-29C,** and **5-27AB; Unnumbered 2-4C**

Price S, Wilson L: *Pathophysiology: clinical concepts of disease processes,* ed 6, St Louis, 2003, Mosby. Figure **7-12**

Proctor DB, et al: *Kinn's The Medical Assistant,* ed.13, 2017, Saunders/Elsevier. Figure **4-12**

Rakel RE: *Textbook of family medicine,* ed 7, Philadelphia, 2007, Saunders. Figure **14-10D**

Rakel RE, Rakel DP: *Textbook of family medicine,* ed 8, Philadelphia 2012, Saunders. Figure **11-14**

real444/E+/gettyimages.com **Unnumbered 11-8**

Regezi JA, Sciubba JJ, Jordan RC: *Oral pathology: clinical pathologic correlations,* ed 6, Philadelphia, 2012, Saunders. Figure **2-8B**

Roberts J, Hedges J: *Clinical procedures in emergency medicine,* ed 5, Philadelphia, 2010, Saunders. Figure **6-13**

Rodak BF, Carr JH: *Clinical hematology atlas*, ed 5, St Louis, 2017, Saunders. Figure **3-46A**

Rodak BF: *Hematology: Clinical Principles and Applications, ed* 2, St. Louis, 2002, Saunders. Figures **2-10A** and **3-31**

Rumack CM, Wilson SR, Charboneau JW, and Levine D: *Diagnostic Ultrasound,* ed 4, 2011, Mosby. Figure **8-45B** and **Unnumbered 8-7C**

scanrail/iStock/Getty Images Plus/gettyimages.com **Unnumbered 2-2**

Schoenwolf GC, Bleyl SB, Brauer PR, Francis-West PH: *Larsen's Human Embryology,* ed 4, London, 2008, Churchill Livingstone. Figure **8-33**

Sean_Warren/E+/gettyimages.com Figure **1-16C**

Seidel HM, Ball JW, Dains JE, Benedict GW: *Mosby's guide to physical examination*, ed 5, St Louis, 2003, Mosby. Figures **1-13, 2-14AB, 2-29A; Unnumbered 2-4A**

Seidel HM, Ball, JW, Dains JE, Benedict GW: *Mosby's guide to physical examination*, ed 6, St Louis, 2006, Mosby. Figure **5-17B**

SensorSpot/E+/gettyimages.com **Unnumbered 4-13, Unnumbered 6-9, Unnumbered 8-10, Unnumbered 12-18** and **Unnumbered 12-20**

SensorSpot/Vetta/gettyimages.com **Unnumbered 8-14**

shawshot/ iStock / Getty Images Plus/ gettyimages.com Figure **8-37**

Shiland BJ: *Mastering Healthcare Terminology,* ed 5, St. Louis, 2016, Mosby. Figure **11-12**

shmuel/E+/gettyimages.com Figure **8-44B**

Snopek AM: *Fundamentals of special radiographic procedures,* 5e, St Louis, 2006, Saunders. Figure **4-11** and **4-29BC**

Snowleopard1/E+/gettyimages.com **Unnumbered 2-3,** Figures **14-12** and **14-15**

Sorrentino S, Remmert L: *Mosby's Textbook for Nursing Assistants,* ed 9, St Louis, 2017, Mosby. Figure **7-8B**

Sorrentino SA: *Mosby's textbook for nursing assistants,* ed 5, St. Louis, 2000, Mosby. Figure **4-10D**

Steve Debenport/E+/gettyimages.com **Unnumbered 14-3**

stevecoleimages/ iStock / Getty Images Plus /gettyimages.com **Unnumbered 13-9**

Stevens A, Lowe JS, Scott I: *Core Pathology,* ed 3, St Louis, 2009, Mosby. Figure **9-2**

Stone DR, Gorbach SL: *Atlas of infectious diseases,* Philadelphia, 2000, Saunders. Figures **4-33, 9-42B** and **Unnumbered 4-6**

Svane G, Potchen EJ, Sierra A, Azavedo E: *Screening mammography, breast cancer diagnosis in asymptomatic women,* St. Louis, 1993, Mosby. **Unnumbered 12-14**

Swartz MH: *Textbook of physical diagnosis: history and examination,* ed 7, Philadelphia, 2015, Saunders. Figures **2-32C, 5-12, 9-41, 11-19, 11-21, 12-11B** and **13-18**

Symonds EM, MacPherson MBA: *Color atlas of obstetrics and gynecology,* London, 1994, Mosby-Wolfe. Figure **8-11A**

Talbot LA, Myers-Marquardt M: *Pocket guide to critical care assessment,* ed 3, St Louis, 1997, Mosby. Figure **5-8**

Tassii/E+/gettyimages.com **Unnumbered 9-3**

tdhster/iStock/Getty Images Plus/gettyimages.com **Unnumbered 10-2**

Thibodeau GA, Patton KT: *Anatomy & physiology,* ed 3, St Louis, 1996. Figure **9-17**

Thibodeau GA, Patton KT: *Anatomy & Physiology,* ed 6, St. Louis, 2007, Mosby. Figure **5-23**

Thibodeau GA, Patton KT: *The human body in health & disease,* ed 5, St. Louis, 2010, Elsevier/Mosby. Figures **9-1, 10-25, 11-20** and **12-14; Unnumbered 11-5**

Thompson JM, Wilson SF: *Health assessment for nursing practice,* St Louis, 1996, Mosby. Figure **3-22**

Tille PM: *Bailey & Scott's diagnostic microbiology,* ed 14, St Louis, 2017, Mosby. Figure **2-6D**

TommL/E+/gettyimages.com Figure **2-38A**

Topol E: *Textbook of interventional cardiology,* 1990, Saunders. Figure **4-29A**

Townsend C, Beauchamp RD, Evers BM, Mattox K: *Sabiston textbook of surgery,* ed 18, Philadelphia, 2008, Saunders. Figure **14-10C**

vgajic/E+/gettyimages.com Figure **1-8**

Vidic B, Suarez FR: *Photographic atlas of the human body*, St Louis, 1984, Mosby. Figure **5-2**

vuk8691/ iStock /Getty Images Plus/gettyimages.com **Unnumbered 12-11**

Walter JB: *An introduction to the principles of disease,* ed 2, Philadelphia, 1982, Saunders. Figure **9-33**

Waterstram-Rich KM, Gilmore D: *Nuclear Medicine and PET/CT,* 8e, 2017, Mosby. Figures **14-9ABC**

Weston WL, Lane AT, Morelli JG: *Color textbook of pediatric dermatology,* ed 4, St Louis, 2007, Mosby. Figures **2-17, 13-17** and **Unnumbered 2-6**

White GM, Cox NH: *Diseases of the skin: A color atlas and text,* ed 2, St. Louis, 2006, Mosby. Figures **2-9** and **13-13**

WILLSIE/ iStock /Getty Images Plus/gettyimages.com Figure **9-11B**

Wilson SF, Giddens JF: *Health assessment for nursing practice,* ed 3, St Louis, 2005, Elsevier. Figure **13-7**

Wilson SF, Giddens JF: *Health Assessment for Nursing Practice,* ed 5, St. Louis, 2013, Mosby. Figures **2-29B, 5-19** and **Unnumbered 2-4B**

Wilson SF, Giddens JF: *Health assessment for nursing practice,* ed 6, St. Louis, 2017, Mosby. Figures **3-12, 3-14, 9-16, 12-11A**

Wilson SF, Thompson JM: *Respiratory disorders,* St Louis, 1990, Mosby. Figure **5-7**

WiroKlyngz/ iStock / Getty Images Plus/gettyimages.com. Figure **3-36** photo inset: (center)

yodiyim/iStock/Getty Images Plus/gettyimages.com **Unnumbered 5-2**

Young AP, Proctor DB: *Kinn's the medical assistant: an applied learning approach,* ed 13, Saunders, 2017. Figure **3-10**

Zacarian SA: *Cryosurgery,* St Louis, 1985, Mosby. Figure **2-13**

Zakus S: *Mosby's clinical skills for medical assistants,* 2001, Mosby. Figures **2-2, 7-6A** and **Unnumbered 7-5C**

zimmytws/ iStock /Getty Images Plus/gettyimages.com Figure **1-14**

Zitelli BJ, Davis HW: *Atlas of pediatric physical diagnosis,* ed 3, St Louis, 1997, Mosby. Figures **9-36, 9-38B** and **Unnumbered 10-6**

Zitelli & Davis: *Atlas of pediatric physical diagnosis,* ed 4, Philadelphia, 2002, Mosby. Figure **3-29** and **3-45**

Zitelli BM, McIntire SC, Nowalk AJ: *Zitelli and Davis' Atlas of pediatric physical diagnosis,* ed 6, Philadelphia, 2012, Saunders. Figures **2-22, 6-21, 6-36, 7-20AB, 8-28, 9-38C, 11-10, 12-15,** and **12-18; Unnumbered 2-7, Unnumbered 11-1**

Index/Glossary

Page numbers followed by the letter *f* refer to figures; those followed by the letter *t* refer to tables.

680

amnion (**am**-nē-on) the thin membrane that lines the chorion and contains the fetus and the amniotic fluid around it. 72, 371

amniorrhexis (am-nē-ō-**rek**-sis) rupture of the amnion. 378

amniotomy (am-nē-**ot**-uh-mē) deliberate rupture of the fetal membranes to induce labor. 386

amputation (am-pū-**tā**-shun) the removal of a limb or other appendage or outgrowth. 585

amylase (**am**-uh-lās) an enzyme that breaks down starch. 254

amylolysis (am-uh-**lol**-uh-sis) the breaking down of starch, or its conversion to sugar. 254

analeptic (an-uh-**lep**-tik) invigorating or a drug that acts as a central nervous system stimulant. 93

analgesic (an-ul-**jē**-zik) relieving pain; a medication that relieves pain. 76
opioid a., pain relievers for severe pain that act on the central nervous system (CNS). 491
narcotic a., drug that relieves pain, can cause numbness and induce a state of unconsciousness. 491
nonnarcotic a., a class of substances that relieve pain and have little to no potential for abuse. 491

anaphylactic reaction (an-uh-fuh-**lak**-tik rē-**ak**-shun) acute allergic response after exposure to an antigen. 140

anaphylaxis (an-uh-fuh-**lak**-sis) a manifestation of immediate hypersensitivity in which exposure of a sensitized individual to a specific antigen or hapten results in urticaria, pruritus, and angioedema, followed by vascular collapse and shock and often accompanied by life-threatening respiratory distress; a general term originally applied to the situation in which exposure to a toxin resulted not in development of immunity (prophylaxis) but in hypersensitivity. 140

anaplasia (an-uh-**plā**-zhuh) a loss of differentiation of cells and of their orientation to one another and to their axial framework and blood vessels, a characteristic of tumor tissue. 116, 602

anastomose (uh-**nas**-tuh-mōs) to create a connection between two formerly separate structures. 285, 285*f*

anastomosis (uh-nas-tuh-**mō**-sis) an opening created by surgical, traumatic, or pathologic means between two normally distinct organs or spaces; a communication between two vessels by collateral channels. 285
gastroduodenal a., surgical connection of the stomach and duodenum after removal of a portion of either of the two structures. 285
gastrojejunal a., a surgical procedure in which the stomach is directly attached to the jejunum. 285

anatomic (an-uh-**tom**-ik) pertaining to anatomy or to the structure of the body. 100
a. pathologist, a physician specializing in the study of the effects of disease on the structure of the body. 15
a. plane, points of reference by which imaginary dissecting lines are drawn through the body to describe locations. 102
a. position, the position in which the body is erect, facing forward with the arms at the sides and the palms toward the front. 102,102*f*

anatomy (uh-**nat**-uh-mē) the science of the structure of living organisms. 22, 102

androgen (**an**-drō-jun) any substance that possesses masculinizing activities, such as the testicular hormone, testosterone. 537, 550*f*

andropathy (an-**drop**-uh-thē) any disease peculiar to the male sex. 550

anemia (uh-**nē**-mē-uh) a condition in which the blood is deficient in red blood cells, hemoglobin, or both. 132, 132*t*
sickle cell a., a genetically caused defect of hemoglobin synthesis, occurring almost exclusively in black individuals, characterized by the presence of sickle-shaped erythrocytes in the blood and homozygosity for S hemoglobin. Signs and symptoms include arthralgia, acute abdominal pain, and leg ulcerations. 136

anesthesia (an-es-**thē**-zhuh) having no feeling or sensation. 76, 76*f*
epidural a., regional anesthesia produced by injection into the epidural space. 490
nerve block a., a loss of sensation in a region of the body, produced by injecting a local anesthetic along the course of a nerve or nerves. 489

anesthesiologist (an-us-thē-zē-**ol**-uh-jist) a physician who specializes in the administration of anesthetics during surgery. 17

anesthesiology (an-us-thē-zē-**ol**-uh-jē) the branch of medicine that studies anesthesia and anesthetics. 17

anesthetic (an-us-**thet**-ik) pertaining to or producing anesthesia; an agent that produces anesthesia. 17, 76
general a., induction of a state of unconsciousness with the absence of pain sensation over the entire body.. 27. 76*f*
local anesthetic, loss of feeling in a restricted area of the body. 27, 76*f*
topical a., a local anesthetic applied directly to the area to be anesthetized. 287

anesthetist (uh-**nes**-thuh-tist) a nurse or technician trained to administer anesthetics. 17

aneurysm (**an**-ū-riz-um) a sac formed by localized dilation of an artery or vein, or of the heart. 183, 183*f*, 472, 472*f*

aneurysmectomy (an-ū-riz-**mek**-tuh-mē) surgical removal of the sac of an aneurysm. 488

angiectomy (an-jē-**ek**-tuh-mē) removal or resection of a vessel. 189

angina pectoris (an-**jī**-nuh **pek**-tuh-ris) severe pain and constriction about the heart caused by an insufficient supply of blood to the heart itself. 112, 181

angiocardiography (an-jē-ō-kahr-dē-**og**-ruh-fē) radiography of the heart and major vessels after injection of a radiopaque contrast medium into a blood vessel or one of the cardiac chambers. 178

angiocarditis (an-jē-ō-kahr-**dī**-tus) inflammation of the heart and great blood vessels. 184

angiography (an-jē-**og**-ruh-fē) radiographic visualization of vessels of the body. 178
coronary a., radiographic visualization of coronary vessels of the heart. 178
digital subtraction a., radiographic visualization that provides computer-enhanced radiographic images of blood vessels filled with contrast material. 178
fluorescein a., a procedure that uses fluorescein and rapid serial photography to study blood movement through vessels of the eye. 510
pulmonary a., the radiographic examination of the blood vessels of the lungs. 219
renal a., the process of producing a radiograph of the renal arteries. 316

angioma (an-jē-**ō**-muh) a tumor whose cells tend to form blood or lymph vessels. 47, 47*f*, 183

angioplasty (**an**-jē-ō-plas-tē) surgical repair of the blood vessels. 73
balloon a., a method of dilating or opening an obstructed blood vessel by threading a small, balloon-tipped catheter into the vessel, inflating the balloon, and compressing arteriosclerotic lesions against the walls of the vessel. 188, 188*f*
excimer laser coronary a., the opening of an occluded artery with laser energy delivered through a fiberoptic probe. 187
laser-assisted a., the opening of an occluded artery with laser energy delivered through a fiberoptic probe. 187
percutaneous transluminal coronary a., compression of fatty deposits of plaque in a coronary artery by an inflated balloon on the end of a catheter; balloon catheter dilation. 188
percutaneous transluminal renal a., enlargement of the lumen of a renal artery via an incision of the skin overlying the artery. 328

angiorrhaphy (an-jē-**or**-uh-fē) suture of a vessel or vessels. 73

angiostenosis (an-jē-ō-stuh-**nō**-sis) narrowing of the caliber of a vessel. 183

angiostomy (an-jē-**os**-tuh-mē) surgical formation of a new opening into a blood vessel. 189

angiotomy (an-jē-**ot**-uh-mē) incision or severing of a blood or lymph vessel. 189

ankylosing spondylitis (ang-kuh-**lō**-sing spon-duh-**lī**-tis) inflammation of the spine marked by stiffening of the spinal joints and ligaments so that movement becomes increasingly painful and difficult. It is a form of rheumatoid arthritis that affects the spine, and affects the male sex almost exclusively. 441

ankylosis (ang-kuh-**lō**-sis) immobility of a joint. 441

anomaly (uh-**nom**-uh-lē) marked deviation from the normal standard, especially as a result of congenital defects. 39

anorchidism (an-**or**-ki-diz-um) absence of testes. 368

anorchism (an-**or**-kiz-um) congenital absence of the testis, either unilaterally or bilaterally. 368

anorexia (an-ō-**rek**-sē-uh) lack or loss of appetite for food. 269
a. nervosa, a mental disorder occurring predominantly in female individuals, having onset usually in adolescence, and characterized by refusal to maintain a normal minimal body weight; intense fear of becoming obese that is undiminished by weight loss; disturbance of body image resulting in a feeling of being fat even when extremely emaciated; and amenorrhea (in the female sex). 485, 485

anorexiant (an-ō-**rek**-sē-unt) causing anorexia or loss of appetite. 283, 290

anosmia (an-**oz**-mē-uh) absence of the sense of smell. 520

anotia (an-**ō**-shuh) congenital absence of one or both ears. 116, 516

anovulation (an-ov-ū-**lā**-shun) absence of ovulation. 352

anoxia (uh-**nok**-se-uh) a total lack of oxygen; often used interchangeably with *hypoxia* to mean a reduced supply of oxygen to the tissues. 181, 220

antacid (ant-**as**-id) 1. counteracting acidity; 2. a substance that counteracts or neutralizes acidity, usually of the stomach. 290

anteflexion (an-tē-**flek**-shun) 1. forward curvature of an organ or part; 2. the forward curvature of the uterus. 355, 355*f*

antemortem (an-tē-**mor**-tum) before death. 96

antenatal (an-tē-**nā**-tul) occurring or formed before birth; prenatal. 379

antepartum (an-tē-**pahr**-tum) in obstetrics, before the onset of labor, with reference to the mother. 379

anterior chamber (an-**tēr**-ē-ur **chām**-bur) the part of the anterior cavity of the eye in front of the iris. 505

anteversion (an-tē-**vur**-zhun) the forward tipping or tilting of an organ; displacement in which the uterus is tipped forward but is not bent at an angle. 355, 355*f*

anthracosis (an-thruh-**kō**-sis) a usually asymptomatic form of pneumoconiosis caused by deposition of coal dust in the lungs. 230

antiaggregants (an-tē-**ag**-ruh-gunts) medications that act against the amassing together of platelets. 197

antiandrogens (an-tē-**an**-druh-junz) drugs that block the effect of androgens. 391

antianginal drugs (an-tē-an-jī-nul drugz) medications used in the treatment of angina pectoris. 196

antianxiety drug (an-tē-ang-**zī**-uh-tē drug) a medication that reduces anxiety. 491, 492

antiarrhythmic (an-tē-uh-**rith**-mik) preventing or alleviating cardiac arrhythmia; an agent that prevents or alleviates arrhythmia (antiarrhythmic drug). 196

antiarthritic (an-tē-ahr-**thrit**-ik) an agent that alleviates arthritis; alleviating arthritis. 447

antiasthmatic (an-tē-az-**mat**-ik) alleviating asthma; a drug that alleviates asthma. 238

antibacterials (an-tē-bak-**tēr**-ē-ulz) antimicrobial treatments used in the treatment or prevention of bacterial infections. 143, 587, 588

antibiotic (an-tē-bī-**ot**-ik) destructive of life; a chemical substance that inhibits the growth of or kills other microorganisms. 115, 143, 586
a. sensitivity test, a laboratory method of determining the susceptibility of organisms to therapy with antibiotics. 43*f*, 312

antibody (**an**-ti-bod-ē) an immunoglobulin that interacts only with the antigen that induced its synthesis or with an antigen closely related to it. 139, 140, 140*f*

anticoagulant (an-tē-kō-**ag**-ū-lunt) preventing blood clotting; any substance that prevents blood clotting. 127, 142, 196

anticonvulsant (an-tĕ-kun-**vul**-sunt) preventing or relieving convulsions; an agent that prevents or relieves convulsions. 491

antidepressant (an-tĕ-dĕ-**pres**-unt) preventing or relieving depression; an agent that is used to treat the symptoms of depression. 491

antidiabetics (an-tĕ-dī-uh-**bet**-iks) drugs used to treat diabetes mellitus by lowering the blood glucose level. 290

antidiarrheal (an-tĕ-dī-uh-**rē**-ul) counteracting diarrhea; an agent that is effective in combating diarrhea. 290

antidiuretics (an-tĕ-dī-ū-**ret**-iks) agents or drugs that control the body's water balance by reducing urination. 308, 330, 535, 535f

antiemetic (an-tĕ-uh-**met**-ik) preventing or alleviating nausea and vomiting; an agent that prevents or alleviates nausea and vomiting. 290

antifebrile (an-tĕ-**feb**-ril) relieving or reducing fever; an agent that relieves or reduces fever. 115

antiflatulents (an-tĕ-**flat**-ū-lunts) drugs used the alleviation or prevention of excessive intestinal gas. 290

antifungals (an-tĕ-**fung**-gulz) medications that limit or prevent the growth of fungal organisms. 143, 587, 588

antigen (**an**-ti-jun) any substance that is capable, under appropriate conditions, of inducing a specific immune response and of reacting with the products of that response. 139

prostate-specific a. (PSA), a protein produced by the prostate that may be elevated in patients with cancer or other disease of the prostate. 365

antiglaucoma drugs (an-tĕ-glaw-**kō**-muh drugz) medicines that are used to prevent or alleviate glaucoma. 521

antigout agents (an-tĕ-**gout** ā-junts) medications that work to either correct overproduction or underexcretion of uric acid. 448

antihelmintics (an-tĕ-hel-**min**-tiks) drugs used to treat infections with parasitic worms. 143

antihistamine (an-tĕ-**his**-tuh-mĕn) a drug that counteracts the action of histamine. 141, 142, 238, 588

antihyperglycemic agent (an-tĕ-hī-pur-glī-**sē**-mik ā-junt) medication that lowers blood glucose levels. 556

antihyperlipidemics (an-tĕ-hī-pur-lip-i-**dē**-miks) agents that reduce lipid levels in the blood. 196-197

antihypertensive (an-tĕ-hī-pur-**ten**-siv) counteracting high blood pressure; an agent that reduces high blood pressure. 196, 330

anti-infective (an-tĕ-in-**fek**-tiv) capable of killing or preventing the multiplication of infectious agents; an agent that so acts. 115, 143, 330, 588

antiinflammatory (an-tĕ-in-**flam**-uh-tor-ē) counteracting or suppressing inflammation; an agent that counteracts or suppresses the inflammatory process. 115, 142, 448, 491, 588

antimicrobial (an-tĕ-mī-**krō**-bē-ul) killing microorganisms or suppressing their multiplication or growth; an agent that kills microorganisms or suppresses their multiplication or growth. 115, 143, 584

antimigraine drugs (an-tĕ-**mī**-grān drugz) medications used to reduce the effects or intensity of migraine headaches. 491

antineoplastic (an-tĕ-nē-ō-**plas**-tik) inhibiting or preventing the development of neoplasms; checking the maturation and proliferation of malignant cells; an agent having such properties. 76, 142, 615

antinuclear antibody (ANA) **test** (an-tĕ-**nōō**-klē-ur **an**-ti-bod-ē test) a blood test used primarily to help diagnose systemic lupus erythematosus, although a positive result may also indicate other autoimmune diseases. 430

anti-osteoporotics (an-tĕ-os-tē-ō-puh-**rot**-iks) drugs used to treat osteoporosis. 448

antiparkinsonian agents (an-tĕ-pahr-kin-**sō**-nē-un ā-junts) drugs that attempt to replace dopamine and treat or halt the symptoms of Parkinson disease. 491

antiperspirant (an-tĕ-**pur**-spur-unt) inhibiting or preventing perspiration; an agent that inhibits or prevents perspiration. 101

antiplatelet drugs class of pharmaceuticals that decrease platelet aggregation and inhibit thrombus formation. 197

antiprotozoals (an-tĕ-prō-tuh-**zō**-ulz) medications used to treat parasitic protozoal infections. 143

antipruritic (an-tĕ-prōō-**rit**-ik) relieving or preventing itching; an agent that relieves or prevents itching. 586, 588

antipsoriatics (an-tĕ-sor-ē-**at**-iks) drugs that prevent or counter psoriasis. 588

antipsychotic (an-tĕ-sī-**kot**-ik) drugs that are effective in the treatment of psychosis. 492

antipyretic (an-tĕ-pī-**ret**-ik) relieving or reducing fever; an agent that relieves or reduces fever. 115, 142

antiretrovirals (an-tĕ-ret-rō-**vī**-rulz) medications for the treatment of infection by retroviruses, primarily HIV. 391

antiseborrheic drugs (an-tĕ-seb-ō-**rē**-ik drugz) medications that are effective in treating seborrheic dermatitis, dandruff. 588

antiseptic (an-ti-**sep**-tik) pertaining to asepsis; a substance that inhibits the growth and development of microorganisms without necessarily killing them. 70, 587

antisocial (an-tĕ-**sō**-shul) acting against the rights of others. 478

antispasmodic (an-tĕ-spaz-**mod**-ik) relieving spasm, usually of smooth muscle; an agent that relieves muscle spasms. 290, 330

antithyroid drug (an-tĕ-**thī**-roid drug) medication that counteracts the functioning of the thyroid. 554, 556

antituberculars (an-tĕ-tōō-**bur**-kū-lurz) drugs that are used to treat tuberculosis. 143

antitussive (an-tĕ-**tus**-iv) relieving or preventing cough; an agent that relieves or prevents cough. 238

antivirals (an-tĕ-**vī**-rulz) drugs used to treat viral infections. 143, 587, 588

anuria (an-**ū**-rē-uh) complete suppression of urinary secretion by the kidneys. 317

anus (**ā**-nus) the distal or terminal opening of the alimentary canal. 257

anxiolytics (ang-zē-ō-**lit**-iks) medication or other interventions that inhibits anxiety. 492

aorta (ā-**or**-tuh) the main trunk from which the systemic arterial system proceeds. 167, 172f

coarctation of the a., a localized malformation of the aorta that causes narrowing of the lumen of the vessel. 179

aortic (ā-**or**-tik) of or pertaining to the aorta. 172

a. insufficiency (AI), aortic regurgitation. 183

a. regurgitation, blood flow from the aorta back into the left ventricle during diastole. 183

a. stenosis, a narrowing or stricture of the aortic valve. 183

a. valve, a valve in the heart between the left ventricle and the aorta. 168

aortitis (ā-or-**tī**-tis) inflammation of the aorta. 184

aortogram (ā-**or**-tō-gram) the radiographic record resulting from aortography. 177

aortography (ā-or-**tog**-ruh-fē) radiography of the aorta after the injection of an opaque medium. 177

aortosclerosis (ā-or-tō-skluh-**rō**-sis) abnormal hardening of the aorta. 184

aphagia (uh-**fā**-juh) refusal or loss of the ability to swallow. 270

aphasia (uh-**fā**-zhuh) defect or loss of the power of expression by speech, writing, or signs, or of comprehending spoken or written language, because of injury or disease of the brain. 224, 476

apheresis (af-uh-**rē**-sis) withdrawal of blood from a donor's body, removal of one or more components from the blood, and transfusion of the remaining blood back to the circulation; pheresis. 614

aphonia (ā-**fō**-nē-uh) loss of voice. 224

aplasia (uh-**plā**-zhuh) lack of development of an organ or tissue. 116, 117t, 228

apnea (**ap**-nē-uh) cessation of breathing. 220

sleep a., transient periods of cessation of breathing during sleep. 220, 471

appendectomy (ap-en-**dek**-tuh-mē) surgical removal of the vermiform appendix. 286, 287f

appendicitis (uh-pen-di-**sī**-tis) inflammation of the vermiform appendix. 275, 275f, 287f

appendix (uh-**pen**-diks) an accessory part attached to a main structure.

vermiform a., a wormlike process extending from the cecum. 262

approximate (uh-**prok**-si-māt) (verb) to bring close together. 74

apraxia (uh-**prak**-sē-uh) neurological disorder characterized by the inability to perform purposeful movement that the person is physically able and willing to do. 480

arachnoid (uh-**rak**-noid) resembling a spider's web; the middle of the three meninges. 466

arachnophobia (uh-rak-nō-**fō**-bē-uh) abnormal fear of spiders. 485

areola (uh-**rē**-ō-luh) a circular area of a different color, surrounding a central point. 539, 539f

aromatase inhibitors (uh-**rō**-muh-tās in-**hib**-i-turz) medications that block aromatase, which turns the hormone androgen into small amounts of estrogen in the body. 391

arrhythmia (uh-**rith**-mē-uh) any variation from the normal rhythm of the heartbeat. 179-180

arteriogram (ahr-**tēr**-ē-ō-gram) a radiograph of an artery after injection of a radiopaque medium. 177, 177f

renal a., a radiographic record of the renal arteries. 316, 316f

arteriograph (ahr-**tēr**-ē-ō-graf) an image produced by arteriography. 177

arteriography (ahr-tēr-ē-**og**-ruh-fē) radiography of arteries after injection of radiopaque material into the bloodstream. 177

arteriole (ahr-**tēr**-ē-ōl) a minute arterial branch, especially one just proximal to a capillary. 165

arteriopathy (ahr-tēr-ē-**op**-uh-thē) any arterial disease. 184

arteriosclerosis (ahr-tēr-ē-ō-skluh-**rō**-sis) a group of diseases characterized by thickening and loss of elasticity of arterial walls. 175, 183

arteritis (ahr-tuh-**rī**-tis) inflammation of an artery. 184

artery (**ahr**-tuh-rē) a vessel through which the blood passes away from the heart to the various parts of the body. 164, 164f

pulmonary a., either of the arteries supplying blood to the lungs. 166, 168

renal a., one of two arteries that carries blood to the kidneys. 304, 305f

arthralgia (ahr-**thral**-juh) pain in a joint. 441

arthrectomy (ahr-**threk**-tuh-mē) the excision of a joint. 446

arthritis (ahr-**thrī**-tis) inflammation of joints. 441

rheumatoid a., a chronic systemic disease primarily of the joints, marked by inflammatory changes in the synovial membranes and articular structures and by muscle atrophy and bone loss. In late stages, deformity and ankylosis develop. 442, 442f

arthrocentesis (ahr-thrō-sen-**tē**-sis) puncture and aspiration of a joint. 430

arthrochondritis (ahr-thrō-kon-**drī**-tis) inflammation of the cartilage of a joint. 436

arthroclasia (ahr-thrō-**klā**-zhuh) the surgical breaking down of an ankylosis to secure free movement. 446

arthrodesis (ahr-thrō-**dē**-sis) the surgical fixation of a joint. 446

arthrodynia (ahr-thrō-**din**-ē-uh) pain in a joint. 441

arthrogram (**ahr**-thrō-gram) a radiographic record after introduction of opaque contrast material into a joint. 430

arthrography (ahr-**throg**-ruh-fē) radiography of a joint after injection of opaque contrast material. 430

arthrolysis (ahr-**throl**-i-sis) destruction of a joint; the operative loosening of adhesions in an ankylosed joint. 446

arthropathy (ahr-**throp**-uh-thē) any joint disease. 441

cardioplegia (kahr-dē-ō-**plē**-juh) arrest of myocardial contraction, as may be induced in performance of surgery on the heart. 186

cardioplegic solutions (kahr-dē-ō-**plē**-jik suh-**loo**-shunz) drugs that are used to stop myocardial contractions so that surgery can be performed on the heart. 186

cardiopulmonary (kahr-dē-ō-**pool**-muh-nar-ē) pertaining to the heart and lungs. 171

   c. bypass, a procedure used in heart surgery in which the blood is diverted from the heart and lungs by means of a pump oxygenator and returned directly to the aorta. 186, 187f

   c. resuscitation (CPR), the reestablishing of heart and lung action as indicated for cardiac arrest or apparent sudden death. 185-186, 234

cardiovalvulitis (kahr-dē-ō-val-vū-**lī**-tis) inflammation of the valves of the heart. 182

cardiovascular (kahr-dē-ō-**vas**-kū-lur) pertaining to the heart and blood vessels. 123, 163

cardioversion (**kahr**-dē-ō-vur-zhun) the restoration of normal heart rhythm by electric shock. 186

cardioverter (**kahr**-dē-ō-vur-tur) a device that delivers a direct-current shock to restore normal heart rhythm. 186, 187f

caries (**kar**-ēz) decay or death of bone or teeth. 270

carpals (**kahr**-pulz) the bones of the wrist. 418

carpectomy (kahr-**pek**-tuh-mē) surgical removal of the wrist bones. 447

carpoptosis (kahr-pop-**tō**-sis) wristdrop. 476

carpus (**kahr**-pus) the wrist; the joint between the arm and the hand. 418

cartilage (**kahr**-ti-luj) fibrous connective tissue present in adults and forming most of the temporary skeleton in the embryo. 422

cast (kast) a solid reproduction of an enclosed space such as a hollow organ; a rigid dressing, molded to the body while pliable, and hardening as it dries, to give firm support. 444

cataract (**kat**-uh-rakt) an opacity of the eye, or in the lens or capsule, that impairs vision or causes blindness. 511, 511f

cathartic (kuh-**thahr**-tik) a substance which causes cleansing or purging of the body, especially the bowels. 290

catheter (**kath**-uh-tur) a flexible tube passed through body channels for withdrawal from or introduction of fluids into a body cavity. 64

   c. dilation, increasing the diameter of a vessel, such as a ureter or the urethra, by introducing a catheter slightly larger than the vessel. 328, 328f

   Foley c., an indwelling catheter that has a balloon filled with air or liquid to train it in place in the bladder. 313, 313f

   indwelling c., a urethral catheter that is held in position in the urethra. 313, 313f

catheterization (kath-uh-tur-i-**zā**-shun) passage of a tubular, flexible instrument into a body channel or cavity for withdrawal or introduction of fluids into a body cavity. 64, 64f, 314f

   suprapubic c., introduction of a catheter through the skin about one inch above the symphysis pubis to drain urine from the urinary bladder. 314, 314f

   ureteral c., insertion of a catheter into the ureter. 314, 314f

   urethral c., insertion of a catheter through the urethra into the urinary bladder. 314, 314f

   urinary c., passage of a catheter through the urethra into the bladder. 313, 314f

catheterize (**kath**-uh-ter-īz) to introduce a catheter within a body cavity. 64

caudad, caudal (**kaw**-dad, **kaw**-dul) pertaining to a tail or tail-like appendage; denoting a position more toward the tail. 103

cauterization (kaw-tur-i-**zā**-shun) destruction of tissue with a hot or cold instrument, electric current, caustic substance, or other agent. 360

cauterize (**kaw**-tur-īz) to perform cauterization. 360

cavity (**kav**-i-tē) a hollow space within a larger structure.

   abdominopelvic c., the body cavity that is formed by the abdominal and pelvic cavities. 111, 111f

   cranial c., the cavity of the skull containing the brain and other tissues. 110, 111f, 111t

   dorsal c., the posterior body cavity that is divided into the cranial and the spinal cavities. 110, 111f, 111t

   medullary c., the space in the diaphysis of a long bone; marrow cavity. 409, 409f

   oral c., the space within the mouth, containing the tongue and teeth. 257

   pericardial c., the space between the visceral pericardium and the parietal pericardium. 168, 169f

   pleural c., the space within the thorax that contains the lungs. 215

   ventral c., the anterior body cavity that is subdivided into the thoracic and the abdominopelvic cavity. 111, 111f, 111t

cecoileostomy (sē-kō-il-ē-**os**-tuh-mē) a surgical procedure that creates an anastomosis between the cecum and the colon. 287

cecum (**sē**-kum) the first part of the large intestine, extending from the ileum to the colon. 262, 263f

cellulitis (sel-ū-**lī**-tis) an acute, spreading, edematous, suppurative inflammation of the deep subcutaneous tissue and sometimes muscle, which may be associated with abscess formation. 583, 583f

Celsius (**sel**-sē-us) a temperature scale in which 0 is the freezing point of water and 100 is the boiling point of water at sea level. 94

centigrade (**sen**-ti-grād) consisting of or having steps or degrees. 94, 94f

centimeter (**sen**-ti-mē-tur) a unit of length equal to one hundredth of a meter. 93

cephalalgia, cephalgia (sef-uh-**lal**-juh, suh-**fal**-juh), headache. 474

cephalometer (sef-uh-**lom**-uh-tur) an instrument for measuring the head, or also for positioning the head in radiography. 4, 54

cephalometry (sef-uh-**lom**-uh-trē) measurement of the dimensions of the head. 54, 54f

cephalopelvic disproportion (CPD) (sef-uh-lō-**pel**-vik dis-prō-**por**-shun) an unusually large fetal head in proportion to the maternal pelvis. 381

cerebellitis (ser-uh-bel-**ī**-tis) inflammation of the cerebellum. 478

cerebellum (ser-uh-**bel**-um) a large, dorsally projecting part of the hindbrain that is concerned with the coordination of movements. It consists of a median lobe and two lateral lobes. 467, 467f

cerebral (suh-**rē**-brul, **ser**-uh-brul) pertaining to the cerebrum. 52, 467

   c. aneurysm, a thin sac filled with blood, formed by dilatation of the walls of an artery in the brain. 472, 472f, 476

   c. angiography, radiography of the cerebral blood vessels. 472

   c. hemisphere, either half of the cerebrum. 467

   c. hemorrhage, the rupture of a blood vessel, usually an artery, within the brain. 476

cerebrospinal fluid (CSF) (ser-uh-brō-**spī**-nul **floo**-id) the fluid that bathes the cerebrum and the spinal cord. 466

cerebrotomy (ser-uh-**brot**-uh-mē) incision of the brain. 74, 488

cerebrovascular (sur-uh-brō-**vas**-kū-lur) pertaining to the blood vessels of the cerebrum.

   c. accident (CVA), a condition involving the blood vessels of the brain, generally associated with ischemic or hemorrhagic lesions. 184, 476, 477f

cerebrum (**ser**-uh-brum, suh-**rē**-brum) the main portion of the brain, occupying the upper part of the skull. 467, 467f

cerumen (suh-**roo**-mun) the waxlike secretion found within the external meatus of the ear; earwax. 514

ceruminolytics (suh-roo-mi-nō-**lit**-iks) medications that dissolve or loosen earwax to allow for its removal. 521

cervical (**sur**-vi-kul) pertaining to the neck or the cervix.

   c. cancer, cancer of the uterine cervix. 349, 349f

   c. cap, a contraceptive device that consists of a cap that fits directly over the cervix to prevent sperm from entering the cervical canal. 374

   c. dilation, the diameter of the opening of the cervix during labor. 378, 378f

   c. polyp, an outgrowth of epithelial tissue of the cervix uteri. 356

cervicitis (sur-vi-**sī**-tis) inflammation of the cervix. 356

cervicocolpitis (sur-vi-kō-kol-**pī**-tis) inflammation of the cervix and the vagina. 346

cervix (Cx) (**sur**-viks) neck; a constricted portion of an organ. 346

   c. uteri, the narrow lower end of the uterus. 346

cesarean section (CS or C-section) (suh-**zar**-ē-un **sek**-shun) incision through the abdominal and uterine walls for delivery of a fetus. 379, 379f

chancre (**shang**-kur) the primary sore of syphilis; a painless, eroded papule occurring at the site of entry of the infection. 387, 387f

chancroid (**shang**-kroid) a nonsyphilitic sexually transmitted disease caused by *Haemophilus ducreyi*. 388

cheilitis (kī-**lī**-tis) inflammation of the lip. 270

cheiloplasty (kī-lō-plas-tē) surgical repair of a defect in the lip. 282

cheilorrhaphy (kī-**lor**-uh-fē) suturing of the lip; surgical repair of a congenitally cleft lip. 282

cheilosis (kī-**lō**-sis) splitting and scaling of the lips and angles of the mouth, a characteristic of riboflavin deficiency. 270

cheilostomatoplasty (kī-lō-stō-**mat**-ō-plas-tē) plastic surgery of the lips and mouth. 282

chemical addiction (kem-i-kul uh-**dik**-shun) a compulsive need for a certain drug, or drawing toward a habit-forming drug. 97

chemoreceptor (kē-mō-rē-**sep**-tur) a nerve ending that detects chemical stimuli, found in the nose and on the tongue. 520

chemotherapeutic (kē-mō-ther-uh-**pū**-tik) using cytoxic agents to treat cancer. 142, 615

chemotherapy (kē-mō-**ther**-uh-pē) treatment of disease by chemical agents. 76

chiroplasty (kī-rō-plas-tē) surgical repair of the hand. 72, 115

chiropody (kī-**rop**-uh-dē) podiatry. 114

chirospasm (kī-rō-spaz-um) cramping of the hand; writer's cramp. 114

chlamydia (kluh-**mid**-ē-uh) a member of bacteria of the phylum *Chlamydiae*, which multiply only within an appropriate host. 322, 350

chlamydiosis (kluh-mid-ē-ō-sis) any infection caused by species of *Chlamydia*. 388

cholangiography (kō-lan-jē-**og**-ruh-fē) radiography of the biliary ducts after the use of a contrast medium. 267, 267f

cholangitis (kō-lan-**jī**-tis) inflammation of a bile duct. 280

cholecystectomy (kō-luh-sis-**tek**-tuh-mē) surgical removal of the gallbladder.

   laparoscopic c., removal of the gallbladder through small incisions in the abdominal wall. 288

cholecystitis (kō-luh-sis-**tī**-tis) inflammation of the gallbladder. 281

cholecystogram (kō-luh-**sis**-tō-gram) a radiograph of the gallbladder. 267

cholecystography (kō-luh-sis-**tog**-ruh-fē) x-ray examination of the gallbladder after the bile is rendered radiopaque. 267, 267f

cholecystotomy (kō-luh-sis-**tot**-uh-mē) surgical incision of the gallbladder. 289

choledochitis (kō-luh-dō-**kī**-tis) inflammation of the common bile duct. 281

choledochojejunostomy (kō-led-uh-kō-juh-**joo**-**nos**-tuh-mē) surgical anastomosis of the common bile duct and the jejunum. 289

choledocholithiasis (kō-led-uh-kō-li-**thī**-uh-sis) the presence of calculi in the common bile duct. 281

choledocholithotripsy (kō-led-uh-kō-**lith**-ō-trip-sē) the crushing of a gallstone within the common bile duct. 289

choledochostomy (kō-led-uh-**kos**-tuh-mē) surgical formation of an opening into the common bile duct and drainage by catheter or T-tube. 289

cholelithiasis (kō-luh-li-**thī**-uh-sis) the presence of gallstones. 281, 281f

cholestasis (kō-luh-**stā**-sis) suppression of bile flow. 280

cholesteatoma (kō-luh-sē-uh-**tō**-muh) a cystic mass composed of epithelial cells and cholesterol that is found in the middle ear. 517

cholesterol (kuh-**les**-tur-ol) a compound that is widely distributed in animal tissues. It is normally found in bile and is the principal constituent of most gallstones. An increased blood level of cholesterol in most individuals constitutes an increased risk for development of coronary heart disease. 175

cholinergic (kō-lin-**ur**-jik) parasympathomimetic (activated or transmitted by acetylcholine). 470

cholinesterase inhibitors (kō-lin-**es**-tur-ās in-**hib**-i-turz) drugs that penetrate the blood brain barrier and enhance cholinergic transmission in the brain. 492

chondral (**kon**-drul) pertaining to cartilage. 422

chondralgia (kon-**dral**-juh) pain in a cartilage; chondrodynia. 436

chondrectomy (kon-**drek**-tuh-mē) surgical removal of a cartilage. 446

chondritis (kon-**drī**-tis) inflammation of the cartilage. 436

chondrodynia (kon-drō-**din**-ē-uh) pain that originates in cartilage. 436

chondroid (**kon**-droid) resembling cartilage. 422

chondroma (kon-**drō**-muh) a benign tumor of mature cartilage. 438

chondropathy (kon-**drop**-uh-thē) any disease of the cartilage. 436

chondroplasty (**kon**-drō-plas-te) surgical repair of the cartilage. 446

chondrosarcoma (kon-drō-sahr-**kō**-muh) a malignant tumor derived from cartilage cells or their precursors. 438

chorion (**kor**-ē-on) the outermost fetal membrane, which forms the fetal part of the placenta. 371

chorionic (kor-ē-**on**-ik) pertaining to the chorion. 350
  c. villi, vascular projections on the surface of the chorion that infiltrate the maternal blood sinuses of the endometrium and help form the placenta. 380
  c. villus sampling, the sampling of placental tissues for prenatal diagnosis of potential genetic defects. 380, 381*f*

choroid (**kor**-oid) a vascular layer of tissue between the retina and the sclera. 505

chronic (**kron**-ik) showing little change or slow progression over a long period. 38
  c. obstructive pulmonary disease (COPD), any disorder marked by persistent obstruction of bronchial air flow; same as chronic obstructive lung disease (COLD). 231, 231*f*

chyme (kīm) the semifluid, homogeneous material produced by gastric digestion of food. 255

ciliary body (**sil**-ē-ar-ē **bod**-ē) the thickened part of the eye that joins the iris with the anterior portion of the choroid. 505

circulation (sur-kū-**lā**-shun) movement of an object or substance through a circular course so that it returns to its starting place.
  pulmonary c., the blood flow through the network of vessels between the heart and the lungs. 165, 166*f*
  systemic c., the general blood circulation of the body, not including the lungs. 165, 166*f*

circumcision (sur-kum-**sizh**-un) surgical removal of all or part of the foreskin. 97, 369

circumduction (sur-kum-**duk**-shun) the active or passive circular movement of a limb or the eye. 96, 96*f*, 427

cirrhosis (si-**rō**-sis) a chronic liver disease characterized by marked degeneration of liver cells with eventual increased resistance to flow of blood through the liver. 280, 280*f*

cisterna chyli (sis-**tur**-nuh **kī**-lī) a dilated portion of the thoracic duct that receives lymph from several lymph-collecting vessels. 190

claustrophobia (klaws-trō-**fō**-bē-uh) morbid fear of closed places. 485

clavicle (**klav**-i-kul) the collarbone; an elongated curved bone, connecting the breastbone to a scapula. 417, 418*f*

cleft lip (kleft lip) opening or split in the upper lip. 272, 272*f*, 385

cleft palate (kleft **pal**-ut) opening or split in the roof of the mouth (palate). 272, 385

climacteric (klī-**mak**-tur-ik) the syndrome of endocrine, somatic, and psychic changes that occur at the termination of the reproductive period in the female sex; menopause. 347

clinical depression (**klin**-i-kul di-**presh**-un) a mood disturbance characterized by exaggerated feelings of sadness, despair, and discouragement. 486

clinical psychologist (**klin**-i-kul sī-**kol**-uh-jist) a psychologist who uses psychological knowledge and techniques in the treatment of people who have emotional difficulties. 19

clinical psychology (**klin**-i-kul sī-**kol**-uh-jē) the use of psychologic knowledge and techniques in the treatment of emotional difficulties. 19

clitoris (**klit**-uh-ris) a small erectile body in the female homologous to the male glans penis. 342

coagulant (kō-**ag**-ū-lunt) promoting, accelerating, or making possible the coagulation of blood; an agent that promotes or accelerates the coagulation of blood. 127

coagulate (kō-**ag**-ū-lāt) to become clotted or to cause clotting. 127

coagulation (kō-ag-ū-**lā**-shun) formation of a clot. 127, 127*f*

coagulopathy (kō-ag-ū-**lop**-uh-thē) any disorder of blood coagulation. 127

cocci (**kok**-sī) spheric bacteria; plural of coccus. 42, 43*f*

coccygectomy (kok-si-**jek**-tuh-mē) excision of the coccyx. 447

coccyx (**kok**-siks) the tailbone, the small bone that forms the caudal extremity of the vertebral column. 414

cochlea (**kok**-lē-uh) anything of a spiral form; a spirally wound tube, resembling a snail shell, which forms part of the inner ear. 514

coitus (**kō**-i-tus) sexual union between male and female during which the penis is inserted into the vagina. 362
  c. interruptus, withdrawal of the penis from the vagina before ejaculation. 373

colectomy (kō-**lek**-tuh-mē) removal of part of the large intestine. 73, 287

colic (**kol**-ik) painful spasm of a hollow or tubular soft organ; pertaining to the large intestine. 257

colitis (kō-**lī**-tis) inflammation of the large intestine. 276

colon (**kō**-lun) the part of the large intestine extending from the cecum to the rectum. 257, 263*f*
  ascending c., the portion of the colon that rises on the right side of the abdomen from the cecum to the transverse colon. 263*f*
  descending c., the portion of the colon on the left side of the abdomen that extends from the transverse colon to the sigmoid colon. 263*f*
  sigmoid c., the S-shaped part of the colon. 262, 263*f*
  transverse c., the part of the colon that runs transversely across the upper part of the abdomen. 263*f*

colonoscope (kō-**lon**-ō-skōp) a flexible endoscope that permits visual examination of the colon; coloscope. 266, 266*f*

colonoscopy (kō-lun-**os**-kuh-pē) examination by means of the colonoscope. 73, 266, 266*f*

colopexy (**kō**-lō-pek-sē) surgical fixation or suspension of the colon. 73

color vision deficiencies (**kul**-ur **vizh**-un dē-**fish**-un-sēz) any of several abnormal conditions characterized by inability to distinguish colors. 511

colorrhaphy (kō-**lor**-uh-fē) suture of the colon. 73

coloscope (**kol**-ō-skōp) colonoscope. 73

coloscopy (kō-**los**-kuh-pē) examination of the colon by means of an elongated flexible endoscope; same as colonoscopy. 73, 266, 266*f*

colostomy (kuh-**los**-tuh-mē) surgical formation of a new opening from the large intestine to the surface of the body. 286, 286*f*

colostrum (kuh-**los**-trum) the thin, milky fluid secreted by the mammary gland the first few days before or after birth. 539

colpectomy (kol-**pek**-tuh-mē) excision of the vagina. 358

colpitis (kol-**pī**-tis) inflammation of the vagina; vaginitis. 352

colpocystitis (kōl-pō-sis-**tī**-tis) inflammation of the vagina and of the bladder. 346

colpodynia (kol-pō-**din**-ē-uh) vaginal pain. 356

colpohysterectomy (kol-pō-his-tur-**ek**-tuh-mē) surgical removal of the uterus by way of the vagina. 358

colpoplasty (**kol**-pō-plas-tē) plastic surgery of the vagina. 358

colporrhaphy (kol-**por**-uh-fē) suture of the vagina. 358

colposcope (**kol**-pō-skōp) an instrument for examining the vagina and cervix. 350

colposcopy (kol-**pos**-kuh-pē) examination of the vagina and cervix using a colposcope. 350, 350*f*

coma (**kō**-muh) a profound unconsciousness from which the patient cannot be aroused. 470, 475

complement (**kom**-pluh-munt) proteins in the blood that play a vital role in the body's immune defenses. 139

compulsion (kom-**pul**-shun) a persistent and irresistible impulse; a compulsive act or ritual. 484

conception (kun-**sep**-shun) the onset of pregnancy, marked by implantation of the blastocyst in the endometrium. 371

concussion (kun-**kush**-un) an injury resulting from impact with an object; loss of function associated with a blow or fall. 474
  cerebral c., loss of consciousness caused by a blow to the head. 475

condom (**kon**-dum) (male condom) thin sheath (usually latex) worn over the penis to collect semen to prevent impregnation or infection; (female condom) thin sheath (usually latex) worn in the vagina to collect semen. 374*t*

condyloma acuminatum (kon-duh-**lō**-muh uh-kū-mi-**nāt**-um) a papilloma usually occurring on the mucous membrane or skin of the external genitals or in the perianal region, caused by an infectious virus; venereal wart. 390, 390*f*

congenital (kun-**jen**-i-tul) present at or existing from the time of birth. 39

conjoined twins (kun-**joind** twinz) identical twins that are joined in utero. 385

conjunctiva (kun-**junk**-ti-vuh) the thin membrane lining the eyelids and covering the exposed whites of the eyes. 505

conjunctivitis (kun-junk-ti-**vī**-tis) inflammation of the conjunctiva, the membrane that lines the eyelids and covers the exposed surface of the sclera. 511

contagious (kun-**tā**-jus) capable of being transmitted from one individual to another. 40

contraception (kon-truh-**sep**-shun) prevention of conception or impregnation. 373

contraceptive (kon-truh-**sep**-tiv) anything used to diminish likelihood of or to prevent impregnation. 101, 373
  c. patch, skin patch that releases hormones that prevent pregnancy. 374*t*
  injectable c., progestin that is administered intramuscularly to prevent ovulation. 374*t*
  oral c., a hormonal compound taken orally that blocks ovulation. 374*t*
  postcoital c., pill that must be taken within 72 hours after unprotected intercourse, which blocks or terminates pregnancy in first days after intercourse. 373

contralateral (kon-truh-**lat**-ur-ul) associated with a particular part on an opposite side. 98, 98*f*

contusion (kun-**tōō**-zhun) a bruise; an injury of a part without a break in the skin. 474, 580, 580*f*

convulsion (kun-**vul**-shun) a violent involuntary contraction or series of contractions of the involuntary muscles; seizure. 480

copulation (kop-ū-**lā**-shun) sexual intercourse; coitus. 362

corium (**kor**-ē-um) alternative for dermis. 568

corn (korn) a hardening and thickening of the skin of the toes, caused by pressure. 434, 577

cornea (**kor**-nē-uh) the transparent structure forming the anterior part of the fibrous tunic of the eye. 505

coronary (**kor**-uh-nar-ē) encircling in the manner of a crown. This term is applied to vessels and ligaments, but especially to the heart's arteries. 168
  c. angiogram, a radiograph of the coronary blood vessels filled with a contrast medium. 178
  c. angiography, radiographic examination of the blood vessels. 178

coronary (*Continued*)

c. arteriography, radiographic examination of the coronary arteries. 177

c. artery, one of a pair of arteries that branch from the aorta, which supply blood to the heart. 169*f*

c. artery bypass, open heart surgery in which a prosthesis or a section of a blood vessel is grafted onto one of the coronary arteries. 186-187, 187*f*

c. artery bypass graft (CABG), a section of vein or other conduit grafted between the aorta and a coronary artery distal to an obstruction. 186-187, 187*f*

c. artery disease (CAD), myocardial damage caused by insufficient blood supply; also called *coronary heart disease (CHD)*. 184

c. occlusion, complete obstruction of an artery of the heart, usually from progressive atherosclerosis. 184

c. thrombosis, development of an obstructive thrombus in a coronary artery. 184

percutaneous c. intervention, the management of coronary artery occlusion by any of various catheter-based procedures. 187

coronavirus (kuh-**rō**-nuh-**vī**-rus) any virus belonging to the family Coronaviridae, which causes respiratory disease and possibly gastroenteritis in humans. 226

corpus luteum (**kor**-pus **loo**-tē-um) a yellow mass in the ovary formed by an ovarian follicle that has matured and discharged its ovum. 347

corpuscle (**kor**-pus-ul) any small mass or body. 127

cortex (**kor**-teks) the outer layer of an organ. 538

cerebral c., the convoluted layer of gray matter covering each cerebral hemisphere. 467, 467*f*

corticosteroids (kor-ti-kō-**ster**-oidz) cortisone-like medicines used to provide relief or inflamed areas of the body. 142, 556, 588

cortisone (**kor**-ti-sōn) a natural glucocorticoid secreted by the adrenal cortex. 538

coryza (kō-**rī**-zuh) an acute condition of the nasal mucous membrane with a profuse discharge from the nostrils. 224

costa (**kos**-tuh) rib. 414

costectomy (kos-**tek**-tuh-mē) removal of a rib. 447

counterirritants (coun-tur-**ir**-i-tunts) a general term for a substance which creates irritation or mild inflammation in one location with the goal of lessening discomfort and/or inflammation in another location. 588

crackles (**krak**-ulz) abnormal nonmusical sounds heard on auscultation, primarily during inhalation. 217

craniectomy (krā-nē-**ek**-tuh-mē) excision of a segment of the skull. 447, 447*f*, 488*t*

craniocele (**krā**-nē-ō-sēl) protrusion of the brain through a defect in the skull. 440

cranioplasty (**krā**-nē-ō-plas-tē) plastic surgery of the skull. 447, 488*t*

craniotome (**krā**-nē-ō-tōm) an instrument used in craniotomy. 447, 447*f*

craniotomy (krā-nē-**ot**-uh-mē) cutting into the skull. 447, 447*f*, 488*t*

cranium (**krā**-nē-um) the skull; the skeleton of the head. 412, 466

creatine (**krē**-uh-tin) an important nitrogenous compound produced by metabolic activity in the body.

c. kinase (CK) test, a blood test used to detect damage to the heart muscle. 175

c. phosphokinase (CPK), creatine kinase, an enzyme in muscle, brain, and other tissue. 430

creatinine (krē-**at**-i-nin) a substance formed from the metabolism of creatine. 310

c. clearance, the rate at which creatinine is cleared from the blood by the kidneys. 312

cretinism (**krē**-tin-iz-um) a condition caused by congenital lack of thyroid secretion, marked by arrested physical and mental development. 548, 548*f*

croup (**kroop**) a condition resulting from acute obstruction of the upper airway caused by allergy, foreign body, infection, or new growth, occurring chiefly in infants and children, and characterized by resonant barking cough and hoarseness. 225

crust (krust) an outer layer of solid matter formed by the drying of a secretion. 577

cryoextraction (krī-ō-ek-**strak**-shun) removal of tissue, such as a cataract, using an extremely cold probe. 513

cryosurgery (krī-ō-**sur**-jur-ē) destruction of tissue by application of extreme cold. 359, 585

ophthalmic c., the use of extreme cold to remove a cataract or to cause the edges of a detached retina to heal. 513

cryotherapy (krī-ō-**ther**-uh-pē) treatment of tissue using cold temperatures. 343, 585

cryptorchidism (krip-**tor**-ki-diz-um) a developmental defect in which the testes remain in the abdominal cavity; undescended testes. 366, 366*f*

curet (kū-**ret**) a spoon-shaped instrument for removing material from a surface. 343, 570, 570*f*

curettage (kū-ruh-**tahzh**) scraping of a cavity for removal of a growth or other material; curettement. 570, 570*f*

cuspids (**kus**-pid) canine teeth. 258

cyanosis (sī-uh-**nō**-sis) blueness of the skin and mucous membranes. 55, 55*f*, 572

cycloplegics (sī-klō-**plē**-jiks) agents that cause paralysis of the ciliary muscle of the eye, allowing vision problems to be measured. 521

cyst (sist) any sac that contains a fluid, either normal or abnormal, and is lined by epithelium. 573

ovarian c., a globular sac that develops in or on the ovary. 353, 353*f*, 358*f*

pilonidal c., congenital cysts in the sacrococcygeal area.. 573, 573*f*

sebaceous c., abnormal sac of sebum from the sebaceous follicles. 573, 573*f*

cystectomy (sis-**tek**-tuh-mē) excision of a cyst; excision or resection of the urinary bladder. 327

ovarian c., removal of an ovarian cyst. 358, 358*f*

cystic (**sis**-tik) pertaining to a cyst; pertaining to the urinary bladder or to the gallbladder. 306

c. fibrosis, an inherited disease of exocrine glands that affects the pancreas, the respiratory system, and the sweat glands. 231-232, 232*f*, 571

cystitis (sis-**tī**-tis) inflammation of the bladder. 323

cystocele (**sis**-tō-sēl) herniation of the urinary bladder into the vagina. 323, 323*f*, 357, 357*f*

cystography (sis-**tog**-ruh-fē) radiography of the bladder after injection of the organ with an opaque solution. 315

cystolith (**sis**-tō-lith) a calculus within the bladder. 324

cystolithiasis (sis-tō-li-**thī**-uh-sis) the presence of a stone in the urinary bladder. 324

cystolithotomy (sis-tō-li-**thot**-uh-mē) the removal of a calculus by incision of the bladder. 327

cystometer (sis-**tom**-uh-tur) an instrument for measuring the neuromuscular mechanism of the bladder. 314

cystometrography (sis-tō-muh-**trog**-ruh-fē) the graphic recording of the pressure exerted at varying degrees of filling of the urinary bladder. 314

cystoplasty (**sis**-tō-plas-tē) plastic surgery of the bladder. 329

cystoscope (**sis**-tō-skōp) an instrument used for visual examination of the bladder. 316, 317*f*

cystoscopy (sis-**tos**-kuh-pē) visual examination of the urinary tract with an instrument inserted through the urethra. 316

cystostomy (sis-**tos**-tuh-mē) formation of an opening into the urinary bladder. 329

cystotomy (sis-**tot**-uh-mē) incision of the bladder. 329

suprapubic c., incision of the skin above the urinary bladder to removal a stone. 329

cystourethritis (sis-tō-ū-rē-**thrī**-tis) inflammation of the bladder and urethra. 324

cystourethrography (sis-tō-ū-ruh-**throg**-ruh-fē) x-ray examination of the urinary bladder and the urethra. 315

cystourethroscopy (sis-tō-ū-rē-**thros**-kuh-pē) visual examination of the urinary bladder and the urethra. 316

cytology (sī-**tol**-uh-jē) study of cells. 71, 349

cytopathology (sī-tō-puh-**thol**-uh-jē) a branch of pathology that studies and diagnoses diseases on the cellular level. 605

cytotoxic agents (sī-tō-**tok**-sik **ā**-junts) immunosuppressive drugs. 71, 142, 615

cytotoxicity (sī-tō-tok-**sis**-i-tē) having a deleterious effect on cells. 141

cytotoxin (sī-tō-tok-sin) a toxin or antibody that has specific toxic action on cells of special organs. 141

dacryocystitis (dak-rē-ō-sis-**tī**-tis) inflammation of the lacrimal sac. 512

dactylitis (dak-tuh-**lī**-tis) inflammation of a finger or toe. 115

dactylogram (dak-**til**-ō-gram) a fingerprint taken for purposes of identification. 114

dactylography (dak-tuh-**log**-ruh-fē) the study of fingerprints. 114

dactylospasm (dak-tuh-**lō**-spaz-um) cramping or twitching of the fingers or toes. 114

daltonism (**dawl**-tun-iz-um) a weakness in perceiving colors distinctly. 506, 507*f*

deafness (**def**-nis) a condition characterized by a loss of hearing that makes it impossible for an individual to understand speech through hearing alone. 516

débride (dā-**brēd**) to remove foreign material and contaminated or devitalized tissue by sharp dissection. 585

débridement (dā-brēd-**maw**) the removal of foreign material and necrotized or contaminated tissue from or adjacent to an infected or traumatic lesion until surrounding healthy tissue is exposed. 585

debulking (dē-**bulk**-ing) surgical removal of as much of the mass of a tumor as possible to increase the chance that chemotherapy or radiation therapy will kill more tumor cells. 611

decalcification (dē-kal-si-fi-**kā**-shun) the loss of calcium from bone. 436

decongestants (dē-kun-**jes**-tunts) agents that reduces congestion or swelling. 238

defecate (**def**-uh-kāt) to evacuate feces from the rectum. 276

defecation (def-uh-**kā**-shun) the evacuation of fecal material from the rectum. 263

defect (**dē**-fekt) an imperfection, failure, or absence.

atrial septal d., a congenital heart defect in which there is an opening between the atria. 179

ventricular septal d., the most common congenital cardiac anomaly, characterized by one or more abnormal openings in the septum separating the ventricles. 179, 179*f*

defibrillation (dē-fib-ri-**lā**-shun) termination of fibrillation, usually by electroshock. 180

defibrillator (dē-**fib**-ri-lā-tur) an apparatus used to stop fibrillation by application of brief electroshock to the heart, directly or through electrodes placed on the chest wall. 180, 180*f*

dehiscence (dē-**his**-uns) a splitting open. 117, 117*f*, 584

dehydration (dē-hī-**drā**-shun) removal of water from a substance; the condition that results from excessive loss of body water. 120

dementia (duh-**men**-shuh) loss of intellectual function caused by organic brain disease. 482

dendrite (**den**-drīt) one of the threadlike extensions of a neuron's cytoplasm. 464, 464*f*

dentalgia (den-**tal**-juh) toothache. 270

dentilingual (den-ti-**ling**-wul) pertaining to the teeth and tongue. 259

denture (**den**-chur) a complement of teeth, either natural or artificial; ordinarily used to designate artificial replacement for the natural teeth. 258

dermabrasion (dur-muh-**brā**-zhun) a surgical procedure that uses an abrasive disk or other mechanical method to plane the skin. 586

dermatitis (dur-muh-**tī**-tis) inflammation of the skin. 49, 49*f*, 119, 575

contact d., acute or chronic dermatitis caused by materials or substances coming in contact with the skin. 575, 575*f*

seborrheic d., a common chronic inflammatory skin disease characterized by greasy scales and yellowish crusts. 576

dermatologist (dur-muh-**tol**-uh-jist) a specialist in skin diseases. 566

dermatology (dur-muh-**tol**-uh-jē) the study of the skin and skin diseases. 566

dermatome (**dur**-muh-tōm) an instrument for cutting thin skin slices for skin grafts; the area of skin supplied with afferent nerve fibers by a single posterior spinal root. 568, 568*f*

duct (dukt) a passage with well-defined walls.
ejaculatory d., the passage formed by the junction of the duct of the seminal vesicles and ductus deferens through which semen enters the urethra. 361
nasolacrimal d., a tubular passage that carries tears from the eye to the nose. 213, 505

ductus (duk-tus) a general term for a passage with well-defined walls; a duct.
d. deferens, the excretory duct of the testis; vas deferens. 361

duodenitis (dōō-od-uh-**nī**-tis) inflammation of the duodenum. 276

duodenoscope (dōō-ō-**dē**-nō-skōp) an endoscope for examination of the duodenum. 266

duodenoscopy (dōō-ō-duh-**nos**-kuh-pē) endoscopic examination of the duodenum. 266

duodenostomy (dōō-ō-duh-**nos**-tuh-mē) formation of a new opening into the duodenum. 287

duodenotomy (dōō-ō-duh-**not**-uh-mē) incision into the duodenum. 287

duodenum (dōō-ō-**dē**-num, dōō-**od**-uh-num) the part of the small intestine that connects with the stomach. 260*f*, 261

Dupuytren contracture (dū-pwē-**trah** kun-**trak**-chur) contracture of the palmar fascia causing the ring and little fingers to bend into the palm so that they cannot be extended. 435, 435*f*

dura mater (doo-ruh **mā**-tur) the outermost and toughest of the three membranes of the brain and spinal cord. 466

dwarfism (**dworf**-iz-um) a disease in which the person is much smaller than the normal size of humans. The condition is caused by insufficient growth hormone in childhood. 547, 547*f*

dysarthria (dis-**ahr**-thrē-uh) a speech disorder consisting of imperfect articulation caused by loss of muscular control after damage to the nervous system. 476

dyscrasia (dis-**krā**-zhuh) an abnormal state or condition. 135

dysentery (**dis**-un-ter-ē) any of a number of disorders marked by inflammation of the intestine, especially the large intestine, with abdominal pain and frequent stools. 275

dyskinesia (dis-ki-**nē**-zhuh) difficulty in performing voluntary movement, which is characterized by involuntary muscle movement, including tics. 473

dyslexia (dis-**lek**-sē-uh) inability to read, spell, and write words, despite the ability to see and recognize letters. 101, 473

dysmenorrhea (dis-men-uh-**rē**-uh) painful menstruation. 352

dyspepsia (dis-**pep**-sē-uh) poor digestion. 269

dysphagia (dis-**fā**-jē-uh) difficulty in swallowing. 269

dysphasia (dis-**fā**-zhuh) speech impairment. 224, 476

dysphonia (dis-**fō**-nē-uh) difficulty in speaking or weak voice. 224

dysphoria (dis-**for**-ē-uh) disquiet, restlessness, or malaise. 102

dysplasia (dis-**plā**-zhuh) abnormality of development; in pathology, alteration in size, shape, and organization of adult cells. 116, 349

dyspnea (disp-**nē**-uh) difficult breathing. 132, 220

dysrhythmia (dis-**rith**-mē-uh) disturbance of rhythm. 180

dystocia (dis-**tō**-shuh) abnormal or difficult labor. 383

dystrophy (**dis**-truh-fē) faulty nutrition. 54
m. dystrophy, a genetically determined myopathy characterized by atrophy and wasting away of muscles. 440

dysuria (dis-**ū**-rē-uh) difficult or painful urination. 317

ecchymosis (ek-i-**mō**-sis) a small hemorrhagic spot, larger than a petechia, in the skin or mucous membrane forming a nonelevated, rounded or irregular, blue or purplish patch. 577, 577*f*

echocardiogram (ek-ō-**kahr**-dē-ō-gram) the record produced by echocardiography. 176
transesophageal e. (TEE), an endoscopic/ultrasound test that provides ultrasonic imaging of the heart from a retrocardiac vantage point. 176

echocardiography (ek-ō-kahr-dē-**og**-ruh-fē) recording of the heart walls or internal structures of the heart and neighboring tissue by the echo obtained from beams of ultrasonic waves directed through the chest wall. 176, 176*f*
Doppler e., a technique in which ultrasonography is used to evaluate the direction and pattern of blood flow within the heart. 176, 176*f*

echoencephalogram (ek-ō-en-**sef**-uh-luh-gram) a recording produced by an echoencephalograph. 472

echoencephalography (ek-ō-en-sef-uh-**log**-ruh-fē) the use of ultrasound to study the brain. 472

echography (uh-**kog**-ruh-fē) a diagnostic aid in which ultrasonic waves are directed at the tissues. A record is made of the sound waves reflected back through the tissues to differentiate structures. 65

eclampsia (uh-**klamp**-sē-uh) convulsions occurring in a pregnant woman with hypertension, proteinuria, and/or edema. 382

ectoderm (**ek**-tō-durm) in embryology, the outermost layer of cells in the blastoderm. 569

ectropion (ek-**trō**-pē-on) a turning outward of the eyelid. 512

eczema (**ek**-zuh-muh) a dermatitis occurring as a reaction to many endogenous and exogenous agents, characterized in the acute stage by erythema, edema associated with a serous exudate oozing and vesiculation, and crusting and scaling. 577

edema (uh-**dē**-muh) an abnormal accumulation of fluid in intercellular spaces in the tissues. 58
pulmonary e., abnormal diffuse, extravascular accumulation of fluid in the pulmonary tissues. 230

effacement (uh-**fās**-munt) the taking up or obliteration of the cervix in labor in which it is so changed that only the thin external os remains. 378

effusion (uh-**fū**-zhun) the escape of fluid into a part or tissue; an effused material. 182
pleural e., presence of liquid in the pleural space. 182, 229, 229*f*

ejaculation (ē-jak-ū-**lā**-shun) a sudden act of expulsion, as of the semen. 361

electrocardiogram (ē-lek-trō-**kahr**-dē-ō-gram) a tracing produced by the electrical impulses of the heart. 61, 175*f*

electrocardiograph (ē-lek-trō-**kahr**-dē-ō-graf) an instrument used to record the electrical current produced by the heart contractions. 174

electrocardiography (ē-lek-trō-kahr-dē-**og**-ruh-fē) recording the electrical currents of the heart muscle. 61, 62*f*, 174

electrodessication (ē-lek-trō-des-i-**kā**-shun) dehydration of tissue by the use of a high-frequency electric current. 586

electroencephalogram (ē-lek-trō-en-**sef**-uh-lō-gram) a record produced by the electrical impulses of the brain. 118, 472

electroencephalograph (ē-lek-trō-en-**sef**-uh-lō-graf) a machine used to record the electrical impulses of the brain. 118, 472

electroencephalography (EEG) (ē-lek-trō-un-sef-uh-**log**-ruh-fē) the recording of the electrical currents of the brain by means of electrodes applied to the scalp or to the surface of the brain or placed within the substance of the brain. 118, 472, 472*f*

electrolysis (ē-lek-**trol**-uh-sis) destruction by passage of a galvanic electrical current, as in removal of excessive hair from the body. 587

electrolytes (ē-**lek**-trō-līts) substances that dissociate into ions when fused or in solution and thus becomes capable of conducting electricity. 122

electromyogram (ē-lek-trō-**mī**-ō-gram) the record obtained by electromyography. 428

electromyography (EMG) (ē-lek-trō-mī-**og**-ruh-fē) the recording and study of the intrinsic electrical properties of skeletal muscle. 315, 428, 429*f*

electrophoresis (ē-lek-trō-fuh-**rē**-sis) the movement of charged suspended particles through a liquid in response to changes in an electric field.
hemoglobin e., identification of different types of hemoglobin based on their differing electrophoretic mobilities. 135

electrophysiology studies (ē-lek-trō-fiz-ē-**ol**-uh-jē stud-ēz) evaluations of the mechanisms of production of electrical phenomena and the use of electrode catheters to study the effects of electricity on tissue, such as study of the heart rhythm. 178

elephantiasis (el-uh-fun-**tī**-uh-sis) a disease caused by a parasitic infestation and characterized by inflammation and obstruction of the lymphatics and increased size of nearby tissue. 58

elimination (ē-lim-i-**nā**-shun) 1. the act of expulsion or of extrusion, especially of expulsion from the body; 2. omission or exclusion, as in an elimination diet. 252

emaciation (ē-mā-shē-**ā**-shun) excessive leanness; a wasted condition of the body. 269

embolectomy (em-buh-**lek**-tuh-mē) surgical removal of an embolus from a blood vessel where it has lodged. 189

embolism (**em**-buh-liz-um) the sudden blocking of a vessel by a clot or foreign material brought to its site of lodgment by the bloodstream. 131

embolus (**em**-bō-lus) a clot or other plug brought by the bloodstream and forced into a smaller vessel where it lodges, thus obstructing circulation. 131
cerebral e., a mass of undissolved matter present in a blood vessel in the brain, blocking blood flow, and results in tissue ischemia distal to the blockage. 476
pulmonary e., the blockage of a pulmonary artery by an embolus. 230, 230*f*

embryo (**em**-brē-ō) derivatives of the fertilized ovum that eventually become the offspring. 371, 371*f*, 372*f*

emesis (**em**-uh-sis) vomiting; an act of vomiting. 58, 269

emetic (uh-**met**-ik) a medicine that induces vomiting. 290

emphysema (em-fuh-**sē**-muh) an accumulation of air in tissues or organs; pulmonary disease characterized by destruction of many of the alveolar walls. 231

empyema (em-pī-ē-muh) accumulation of pus in a cavity of the body. If used without a descriptive qualifier, it refers to thoracic empyema. 229

encephalitis (en-sef-uh-**lī**-tis) inflammation of the brain. 118, 479

encephalocele (en-**sef**-uh-lō-sēl) hernia of part of the brain and meninges through a skull defect. 48, 49*f*

encephalography (en-sef-uh-**log**-ruh-fē) radiography of the brain. 471

encephalomeningitis (en-sef-uh-lō-men-in-**jī**-tis) inflammation of the brain and its membranes. 479

encephalomyelitis (en-sef-uh-lō-mī-uh-**lī**-tis) inflammation of the brain and spinal cord. 479

encephalomyelopathy (en-sef-uh-lō-mī-uh-**lop**-uh-thē) a disease involving the brain and spinal cord. 475

encephalopathy (en-sef-uh-**lop**-uh-thē) any disease of the brain. 475

encephalotome (en-**sef**-uh-luh-tōm) an instrument for incision of the brain. 74

encephalotomy (en-sef-uh-**lot**-uh-mē) incision of the brain. 74

endarterectomy (end-ahr-tur-**ek**-tuh-mē) excision of the atheromatous inner wall of an artery. 189
carotid e., surgical excision of atheromatous segments of the inner walls of a carotid artery. 189

endocarditis (en-dō-kahr-**dī**-tis) inflammation of the inner lining of the heart. 178

endocardium (en-dō-**kahr**-dē-um) the membrane lining the inner surface of the heart. 168

endocrine (**en**-dō-krin, **en**-dō-krīn) secreting internally; applied to organs that secrete hormones into the bloodstream. 16

endocrinologist (en-dō-kri-**nol**-uh-jist) a physician who treats diseases arising from disordered internal secretions. 16

endocrinology (en-dō-kri-**nol**-uh-jē) the science that studies the endocrine glands and the hormones they produce. 16

endoderm (**en**-dō-durm) the innermost of the three primary germ layers of the embryo. 568

endodontics (en-dō-**don**-tiks) the branch of dentistry concerned with the cause, prevention, diagnosis, and treatment of conditions that affect the tooth pulp, root, and surrounding tissues. 259

endodontist (en-dō-**don**-tist) a dentist who specializes in prevention and treatment of conditions that affect the tooth pulp, root, and surrounding tissues. 259

endodontitis (en-dō-don-**tī**-tis) inflammation of the dental pulp. 270

endodontium (en-dō-**don**-shē-um) dental pulp. 259

endogastric (en-dō-**gas**-trik) pertaining to the interior of the stomach. 261

endometriosis (en-dō-mē-trē-ō-sis) ectopic endometrium located in various places, usually in the pelvic cavity. 355, 355*f*

endometritis (en-dō-mē-**trī**-tis) inflammation of the lining of the uterus. 355

endometrium (en-dō-**mē**-trē-um) the membrane that lines the cavity of the uterus. 346

endonasal (en-dō-**nā**-zul) within the nose. 213

endorphin (en-**dor**-fin) any of three amino acid residues that bind to opioid receptors in the brain and have potent analgesic activity. 465 **endoscope** (en-dō-skōp) an instrument for the examination of the interior of a hollow viscus. 63, 63*f*

endoscopic sphincterotomy (en-dō-**skop**-ik sfingk-tur-**ot**-uh-mē) incision of a constricting sphincter through an endoscope. 288

endoscopy (en-**dos**-kuh-pē) visual inspection of any cavity of the body by means of an endoscope. 63, 63*f*, 96

enteritis (en-ter-**ī**-tis) inflammation of the intestine, especially the small intestine. 257

enterostasis (en-ter-ō-**stā**-sis) the stopping of food in its passage through the intestine. 278

entropion (en-**trō**-pē-on) a rolling inward of the eyelid.. 512. 512*f*

enuresis (en-ū-**rē**-sis) involuntary discharge of urine after the age at which urinary control should have been achieved; often used with specific reference to involuntary discharge of urine occurring during sleep at night (bed-wetting). 318

enzyme (**en**-zīm) a protein molecule that catalyzes chemical reactions of other substances without itself being destroyed or altered. 47
angiotensin-converting e. inhibitors, antihypertensive medications that block the formation of angiotensin II. 51

eosinophil (ē-ō-**sin**-ō-fil) a granular leukocyte with a nucleus that usually has two lobes and cytoplasm containing coarse, round granules that are readily stained by eosin. 130

epicardium (ep-i-**kahr**-dē-um) the layer of serous pericardium on the surface of the heart. 168

epidemic (ep-i-**dem**-ik) occurring suddenly in numbers clearly in excess of normal expectancy. 21

epidemiologist (ep-i-dē-mē-**ol**-uh-jist) a physician or medical scientist who specializes in epidemic study. 21

epidemiology (ep-i-dē-mē-**ol**-uh-jē) 1. the study of the relationships of factors determining the frequency and distribution of diseases in the human community; 2. the field of medicine dealing with the determination of causes of localized outbreaks of infection or other disease of recognized cause. 21

epidermis (ep-i-**dur**-mis) the outermost, nonvascular layer in the skin. 96, 568, 568*f*

epididymis (ep-i-**did**-uh-mis) the elongated cordlike structure along the posterior border of the testis that provides for storage, transit, and maturation of spermatozoa and is continuous with the ductus deferens. 361

epididymitis (ep-i-did-uh-**mī**-tis) inflammation of the epididymis. 368

epiglottides (ep-i-**glot**-i-dēs) the plural of epiglottis. 214

epiglottis (ep-i-**glot**-is) the lidlike structure composed of cartilage that covers the larynx during swallowing; epiglottides (plural). 214

epiglottitis (ep-i-glo-**tī**-tis) inflammation of the epiglottis. 226

epilepsy (**ep**-i-lep-sē) a recurrent disorder of cerebral function characterized by sudden, brief attacks of altered consciousness, motor activity, or sensory phenomena. 54, 480

epinephrine (ep-i-**nef**-rin) a hormone secreted by the adrenal medulla. It is a potent stimulator of the sympathetic nervous system and a powerful vasopressor, increasing blood pressure and cardiac output. 465, 538

epiphysis (uh-**pif**-uh-sis) either end of a long bone. 409

episiotomy (uh-piz-ē-**ot**-uh-mē) surgical incision of the female perineum to enlarge her vaginal opening for delivery. 386

epispadias (ep-i-**spā**-dē-us) a developmental anomaly consisting of absence of the upper wall of the urethra. 323

epistaxis (ep-i-**stak**-sis) hemorrhage from the nose; nosebleed. 224

erectile dysfunction (uh-**rek**-tīl dis-**funk**-shun) inability of the male individual to achieve or maintain an erection. 366

erection (uh-**rek**-shun) the condition of being made rigid and elevated, especially that of the penis. 363

eructation (uh-ruk-**tā**-shun) the casting up of wind from the stomach through the mouth; belching. 269

erythema (er-uh-**thē**-muh) redness of the skin produced by congestion of the capillaries. 573

erythroblast (uh-**rith**-rō-blast) embryonic form of a red blood cell. 135

erythroblastosis fetalis (uh-rith-rō-blas-**tō**-sis fi-**ta**-lus) a type of hemolytic anemia of the fetus or newborn infant, caused by the transplacental transmission of maternally formed antibody. 135, 384

erythrocyte (uh-**rith**-rō-sīt) a red blood cell; mature form is a nonnucleated, biconcave disk. 55, 127, 136*f*
e. sedimentation rate (ESR), the rate at which red blood cells settle out in a tube of unclotted blood, expressed in millimeters per hour. 430

erythrocytopenia (uh-rith-rō-sī-tō-**pē**-nē-uh) a deficiency in the number of red blood cells; anemia. 132

erythrocytosis (uh-rith-rō-sī-**tō**-sis) an increase in the number of red blood cells. 132

erythropenia (uh-rith-rō-**pē**-nē-uh) a deficiency in the number of red blood cells. 132

erythropoiesis (uh-rith-rō-poi-ē-sis) the production of red blood cells. 130

erythropoietin (uh-rith-rō-**poi**-uh-tin) a hormone chiefly secreted by the kidney in the adult that acts on stem cells of the bone marrow to stimulate red blood cell production. 130, 306

escharotomy (es-kuh-**rot**-uh-mē) surgical incision of the constricting, damaged tissue of a burned area. 586

esophageal (uh-sof-uh-**jē**-ul) pertaining to the esophagus. 257
e. achalasia, an abnormal condition characterized by constriction of the lower portion of the esophagus because of the inability of a muscle to relax. 272
e. atresia, an abnormal esophagus that ends in a blind pouch or narrows to a thin cord and does not provide a continuous passage to the stomach. 272
e. varices, enlarged, swollen veins at the lower end of the esophagus that are susceptible to hemorrhage. 272

esophagectomy (uh-sof-uh-**jek**-tuh-mē) excision of all or part of the esophagus. 283

esophagitis (uh-sof-uh-**jī**-tis) inflammation of the esophagus. 274

esophagoduodenostomy (uh-sof-uh-gō-gas-trō-dōō-od-uh-nos-stuh-mē) surgical anastomosis between the esophagus and the duodenum. 285

esophagodynia (uh-sof-uh-gō-**din**-ē-uh) pain in the esophagus. 274

esophagogastroduodenoscopy (EGD) (uh-sof-uh-gō-gas-trō-dōō-od-uh-**nos**-kuh-pē) endoscopic examination of the esophagus, stomach, and duodenum. 266, 266*f*

esophagogastroplasty (uh-sof-uh-gō-**gas**-trō-plas-tē) plastic surgery of the esophagus and stomach. 286

esophagogastroscopy (uh-sof-uh-gō-gas-**tros**-kuh-pē) endoscopic examination of the esophagus and stomach. 266

esophagogastrostomy (uh-sof-uh-gō-gas-**tros**-tuh-mē) forming a new opening between the stomach and the esophagus. 285

esophagogram (uh-**sof**-uh-gō-gram) a radiograph of the esophagus. 267

esophagojejunostomy (uh-sof-uh-gō-juh-**jōō**-**nos**-tuh-mē) surgically creating a new opening between the esophagus and jejunum. 285

esophagomalacia (uh-sof-uh-gō-muh-**lā**-shuh) softening of the esophagus. 274

esophagomyotomy (uh-sof-uh-gō-mī-**ot**-uh-mē) incision through the muscular coat of the esophagus. 283

esophagoscopy (uh-sof-uh-**gos**-kuh-pē) examining the esophagus using an endoscope. 266

esophagostomy (uh-sof-uh-**gos**-tuh-mē) creation of an opening into the esophagus. 283

esophagram (uh-**sof**-uh-gram) a radiograph of the esophagus. 267

esophagus (uh-**sof**-uh-gus) a muscular canal extending from the throat to the stomach. 255

estrogen (**es**-truh-jun) the female sex hormones, including estradiol, and estrone; a generic term for estrus-producing compounds. Estrogens are responsible for female secondary sex characteristics. During the menstrual cycle, estrogens act on the female genitalia to produce a suitable environment for fertilization, implantation, and nutrition of the early embryo. 346, 538, 550*f*

eupepsia (ū-**pep**-sē-uh) normal digestion. 254

euphoria (ū-**for**-ē-uh) an exaggerated feeling of physical and mental well-being. 102

eupnea (yōōp-**nē**-uh) normal breathing. 223

eustachian tube (ū-**stā**-kē-un tōōb) the auditory tube, which extends from the middle ear to the pharynx. 214, 515

euthyroid (ū-**thī**-roid) normal thyroid function. 536

eversion (ē-**vur**-zhun) a turning inside-out; a turning outward, as of the sole of the foot or the eyelid. 427

evisceration (ē-vis-ur-**ā**-shun) removal of the viscera from the abdominal cavity; the protrusion of an internal organ through a wound or surgical incision. 117, 117*f*

Ewing sarcoma (ū-ing sahr-**kō**-muh) a highly malignant, metastatic tumor of bone. 438

excimer laser (ek-si-mur **lā**-zur) a laser whose beam, in the ultraviolet spectrum, breaks chemical bonds instead of generating heat to destroy tissue. 513

excision (ek-**sizh**-un) removal, as of an organ, by cutting. 72
surgical e., removal of a body part or tissue as a surgical procedure. 612

excoriation (eks-kō-rē-**ā**-shun) a skin injury caused by trauma, such as scratching, abrasion, or a chemical or thermal burn. 575, 576*f*

excretion (eks-**krē**-shun) the act, process, or function of excreting; material that is excreted. 124, 304

exfoliation (eks-fō-lē-**ā**-shun) a falling off in scales or layers. 572

exfoliative cytology (eks-**fō**-lē-uh-tiv sī-**tol**-uh-jē) the study of cells, their origin, structure, function, and pathology. 607

exhalation (eks-huh-**lā**-shun) expelling air from the lungs by breathing. 210

exophthalmos (ek-sof-**thal**-mos) abnormal protrusion of the eyeball. 544, 544*f*

expectorants (ek-**spek**-tuh-runts) drugs that increase bronchial secretion and enhance the expulsion of mucus. 238

expectorate (ek-**spek**-tuh-rāt) spitting or coughing up materials from the air passageways leading to the lungs. 231

expiration (ek-spi-**rā**-shun) the act of expelling air from the lungs or breathing out; death. 210

expulsion (ek-**spul**-shun) the act of expelling. 378, 378*f*

extension (ek-**sten**-shun) the movement by which the ends of a jointed part are pulled away from each other; a movement that brings the members of a limb into or toward a straight condition. 426, 426*f*

extensor (ek-**sten**-sor) any muscle that extends a joint. 426

extracorporeal (eks-truh-kor-**por**-ē-ul) situated or occurring outside the body. 186
e. membrane oxygenator (ECMO), a device that oxygenates a patient's blood outside the body and returns the blood to the patient's circulatory system. 236

extraocular (eks-truh-**ok**-ū-lur) outside the eye. 506

extremities (ek-**strem**-i-tēz) the upper or lower limbs; hands or feet. 114

exudate (eks-ū-dāt) fluid or other substances that have been slowly discharged from cells or blood vessels through small pores or breaks in the membrane. 124

fallopian tube (fuh-**lō**-pe-un tŏŏb) the duct that extends laterally from the fundal end of the uterus and terminates near the ovary; uterine tube. 344, 344*f*

family practice (**fam**-i-lē **prak**-tis) the medical specialty concerned with the planning and provision of the comprehensive primary health care of all family members, regardless of age or sex, on a continuing basis. 14

fascia (**fash**-ē-uh) a sheet or band of fibrous tissue that covers the muscles and various other organs of the body. 425

fasciectomy (fas-ē-**ek**-tuh-mē) excision of fascia. 445

fatigue (fuh-**tēg**) a state of increased discomfort and decreased efficiency resulting from prolonged or excessive exertion; loss of capacity to respond to stimulation. 101

febrile (**feb**-ril) pertaining to or characterized by fever. 115

feces (**fē**-sēz) the excrement discharged from the intestines. 253, 263

femur (**fē**-mur) the thigh; the thigh bone. 420

fetoscope (**fē**-tō-skōp) a specially designed stethoscope for listening to the fetal heartbeat; an endoscope for viewing the fetus in utero. 380, 381*f*

fetus (**fē**-tus) the unborn offspring in the postembryonic period, after major structures have been outlined—in humans from 7 to 8 weeks after fertilization until birth. 371

fibrillation (fib-ri-**lā**-shun) involuntary muscle contraction caused by spontaneous activation of single muscle cells or muscle fibers. 180
  atrial f., a cardiac arrhythmia characterized by disorganized electric activity in the atria. 180
  ventricular f., cardiac arrhythmia marked by rapid, uncoordinated, and ineffective contraction of the ventricles. 180

fibrin (**fī**-brin) an insoluble protein that forms long threads that compose blood clots. 127

fibrinogen (fī-**brin**-ō-jun) a protein in plasma that is essential for clotting of blood. 127

fibrinolysin (fī-bri-**nol**-uh-sin) a substance that dissolves fibrin clots and also breaks down certain coagulation factors. 127

fibrinolysis (fī-bri-**nol**-uh-sis) destruction of fibrin. 127

fibromyalgia (fī-brō-mī-**al**-juh) chronic pain in muscles and soft tissues surrounding joints. 443

fibrosarcoma (fī-brō-sahr-**kō**-muh) a malignant tumor composed of cells and fibers that produce collagen. 438

fibula (**fib**-ū-luh) the smaller of the two lower leg bones. 420

fimbria (**fim**-brē-uh) any structure that resembles a fringe or border, such as the long fringelike extension of a uterine tube that lies close to the ovary. 344

fissure (**fish**-ur) a split; a cleft or groove. 276, 276*f*, 574, 575*f*

fistula (**fis**-tū-luh) an abnormal communication between two internal organs, or from an internal organ to the body surface. 276, 356, 356*f*

fixation (fik-**sā**-shun) the act of holding, operating, or suturing in a fixed position; the use of a fixative to preserve, as a biological specimen; in psychoanalysis, an arrest at a particular stage of psychosexual development.
  external f., a method of stabilizing fractures by pins drilled into the bony parts through the overlying skin and held in a fixed position by a rigid connector. 444, 445*f*
  internal f., a method of stabilizing fractures using pins, rods, plates, screws, and/or other materials to immobilize a bone fracture. 444, 445*f*

flexion (**flek**-shun) the act of bending; being bent. 426

flexor (**flek**-sor) any muscle that flexes a joint. 426

fluid (**flŏŏ**-id) a substance, especially liquid, that is able to follow and adjust its shape to that of a container.
  extracellular f., the portion of body fluid outside cells and is made up of interstitial fluid and blood plasma. 120, 120*f*
  intercellular f., the fluid between and among cells. 119, 120*f*
  interstitial f., tissue fluid or fluid occupying spaces between tissue cells. 120, 120*f*
  intracellular f., the fluid that is located within cells. 119, 120*f*
  lacrimal f., tears that keep the eyeball moist. 505

fluoroscope (**floor**-ō-skōp) a device used in fluoroscopy for examining deep structures by means of x-rays. 66, 66*f*

fluoroscopy (floo-**ros**-kuh-pē) examination by means of a fluoroscope, a device that allows both structural and functional visualization of internal structures. 66, 66*f*

folliculitis (fuh-lik-ū-**lī**-tis) inflammation of a follicle or follicles; used ordinarily in reference to hair follicles but sometimes in relation to follicles of other kinds. 583

foramen magnum (fō-**rā**-mun **mag**-num) the opening in the occipital bone through which the spinal cord passes from the brain. 412, 467

fractionation (frak-shun-**ā**-shun) in radiology, a division of the total dose of radiation into smaller doses given at intervals. 613

fracture (fx) (**frak**-chur) a break or rupture in a bone; the breaking of a part, especially a bone. 432-433, 433*f*
  closed f., one that does not produce an open wound in the skin. 432, 433*f*
  comminuted f., one in which the bone is crushed or splintered. 433, 433*f*
  compound f., open fracture. 432, 433*f*
  compression f., a break in which bone surfaces are forced into each other. 432, 475*f*
  greenstick f., one in which only one side of a bone is broken. 433
  impacted f., one in which one fragment is firmly driven into the other. 433, 433*f*
  open f., one in which a wound through the overlying or adjacent soft tissues communicates with the site of the break. 432, 433*f*
  simple f., closed fracture. 432, 433*f*
  spiral f., a bone break that is spiral to the bone's long axis. 433
  transverse f., one at right angles to the axis of the bone. 433, 433*f*

frequency (**frē**-kwun-sē) the number of occurrences of a periodic or recurrent process per unit time. 317

friction rub (**frik**-shun rub) a dry grating sound heard with a stethoscope during auscultation. 216, 217*f*

frontal (**frun**-tul) pertaining to the forehead; denoting a plane that divides the body into anterior and posterior portions. 467*f*
  f. lobe, the largest of five lobes constituting each of the two cerebral hemispheres. 467, 467*f*
  f. plane, a flat surface that divides the body into front and back portions. 102

frostbite (**frost**-bīt) damage to tissues as the result of exposure to low environmental temperatures. 582

fundus (**fun**-dus) the bottom or base of anything. 260, 260*f*

fungus (**fun**-gus) a general term used to denote a group of microorganisms that includes mushrooms, yeasts, and molds; fungi (plural). 44

furuncle (**fū**-rung-kul) a painful nodule formed in the skin by circumscribed inflammation enclosing a core; a boil. 576

gamete (**gam**-ēt) a male or female reproductive cell; spermatozoon or ovum. 371

gamma knife procedure (**gam**-uh nīf prō-**sē**-jur) a method for destroying tumors with a focused beam of gamma radiation; gamma knife radiation. 489, 489*f*

gastralgia (gas-**tral**-juh) pain of the stomach; stomachache. 274

gastrectasia (gas-trek-**tā**-zhuh) stretching of the stomach. 274

gastrectomy (gas-**trek**-tuh-mē) removal of all or part of the stomach. 285, 285*f*

gastric (**gas**-trik) pertaining to the stomach. 257

gastrin (**gas**-trin) any of several hormones released from fibers in the vagus nerve and the pylorus that stimulate the flow of gastric juice. 542

gastritis (gas-**trī**-tis) inflammation of the stomach. 273

gastroduodenitis (gas-trō-dŏŏ-ō-duh-**nī**-tis) inflammation of the stomach and duodenum. 276

gastroduodenostomy (gas-trō-dŏŏ-ō-duh-**nos**-tuh-mē) formation of a new opening between the stomach and the duodenum. 285, 285*f*

gastroenteritis (gas-trō-en-tur-**ī**-tis) inflammation of the stomach and intestines. 275

gastroenterologist (gas-trō-en-tur-**ol**-uh-jist) a physician who specializes in the stomach and intestines and their diseases. 14

gastroenterology (gas-trō-en-tur-**ol**-uh-jē) the study of the stomach and intestines and associated diseases. 263

gastroenterostomy (gas-trō-en-tur-**os**-tuh-mē) surgical creation of an artificial passage between the stomach and intestines, usually the jejunum. 285, 285*f*

gastrointestinal (GI) (gas-trō-in-**tes**-ti-nul) pertaining to the stomach and the intestines. 252
  lower g. series, the use of a contrast agent, often barium sulfate, to make the lower digestive tract more distinct during radiographic examination; barium enema. 267
  upper g. series, the use of a contrast agent, often barium sulfate to make the upper digestive tract more distinct during a series of x-ray images; barium meal. 267

gastrojejunostomy (gas-trō-juh-jŏŏ-**nos**-tuh-mē) surgical creation of an anastomosis between the stomach and the jejunum; also, the anastomosis so established. 285, 285*f*

gastromalacia (gas-trō-muh-**lā**-shuh) abnormal softening of the stomach. 274

gastromegaly (gas-trō-**meg**-uh-lē) enlargement of the stomach. 274

gastropathy (gas-**trop**-uh-thē) any disease of the stomach. 274

gastropexy (**gas**-trō-pek-sē) surgical fixation of the stomach to the abdominal wall. 286

gastroplasty (**gas**-trō-plas-tē) plastic surgery of the stomach. 284

gastrorrhaphy (gas-**tror**-uh-fē) suture of the stomach. 286

gastroschisis (gas-**tros**-ki-sis) a birth defect in which the intestines protrude outside of the baby's body, through a hole beside the umbilicus. 385

gastroscope (**gas**-trō-skōp) instrument for viewing inside the stomach. 266

gastroscopy (gas-**tros**-kuh-pē) inspection of the interior of the stomach by means of the gastroscope. 266

gastrostomy (gas-**tros**-tuh-mē) surgical creation of an artificial opening in the stomach through the abdominal wall. 283

generic name (juh-**ner**-ik nām) the official established name of a drug that is used by every company. 26

genital (**jen**-i-tul) pertaining to the genitals. In its plural form, genitals refers to the reproductive organs. 342
  g. herpes, herpes genitalis; herpetic lesions on the male or female genitalia. 389, 390*f*
  g. warts, condyloma acuminatum; venereal warts; papillomas occurring on the genitalia, caused by an infectious virus. 390, 390*f*

genitalia (jen-i-**tā**-lē-uh) the reproductive organs. 342

genitourinary (GU) (jen-i-tō-**ū**-ri-nar-ē) pertaining to the genital and urinary organs; urogenital. 306, 342
  g. infection, invasion of the genitourinary tract by microorganisms. 322

geriatrician (jer-ē-uh-**trish**-un) a specialist in geriatrics. 17

geriatrics (jer-ē-**at**-riks) the branch of medicine that deals with problems and diseases of old age. 17

gerodontics (jer-ō-**don**-tiks) dentistry dealing with dental problems of older people. 259

gerodontist (jer-ō-**don**-tist) a dentist specializing in dental problems of older people. 259

gerontology (jer-on-**tol**-uh-jē) the branch of science that deals with the problems of aging in all of its aspects. 17

gestation (jes-**tā**-shun) the period from the fertilization of the ovum until birth in a viviparous animal. 376

gigantism (jī-**gan**-tiz-um) a condition in which a person reaches an abnormal stature, caused by excessive growth hormone during childhood. 547, 547*f*

gingiva (**jin**-ji-vuh) the gum; the mucous membrane with supporting and fibrous tissue that covers the tooth-bearing border of the jaw. 258
gingivalgia (jin-ji-**val**-juh) pain in the gums. 270
gingivectomy (jin-ji-**vek**-tuh-mē) cutting away part of the gums. 282
gingivitis (jin-ji-**vī**-tis) inflammation of the gum. 270
gingivoglossitis (jin-ji-vō-glos-**ī**-tis) inflammation of the gums and tongue. 270
gingivostomatitis (jin-ji-vō-stō-muh-**tī**-tis) inflammation of the gums and mouth. 270
gland (gland) an aggregation of cells that are specialized to secrete or excrete materials not related to their ordinary needs. 530, 531*f*
  adrenal g., a flattened body above either kidney that secretes steroid hormones, epinephrine, and norepinephrine. 531, 538*t*
  apocrine sweat g., one of several sweat glands that open into hair follicles rather than directly onto the surface of the skin. 569, 569*f*
  Bartholin g., one of two small mucous glands located in each lateral wall of the vestibule of the vagina, near the vaginal opening. 342
  bulbourethral g., one of two small glands located on each side of the prostate and secreting a fluid that helps make up seminal fluid. 361
  endocrine g., a gland that secretes hormones directly into the blood. 530, 530*f*
  exocrine g., any of the glands that discharge their secretions through ducts opening on internal or external surfaces of the body. 530, 530*f*
  lacrimal g., one of a pair of glands situated superiorly and laterally to the eye bulb. 505
  mammary g., the milk-secreting organ of female mammals. 538
  master g., the pituitary gland. 532, 532*f*, 533*f*, 540*t*
  parathyroid g., any one of four glands lying beside the thyroid gland that are responsible for secreting a hormone that regulates calcium and phosphorus in the body. 531, 531*f*
  paraurethral g., a gland of the female urethra, secreting a fluid that helps make up vaginal fluid. 342
  parotid g., the largest of the paired salivary glands, located in front of the ear. 260, 260*f*
  pineal g., the small, slightly flat, cone-shaped gland located under the cerebrum that secretes melatonin. 531
  pituitary g., the hypophysis, a small, oval, two-lobed body at the base of the brain that regulates other glands by secretion of hormones. 531, 532, 532*f*, 533*f*, 540*t*
  sebaceous g., a gland in the skin that secretes sebum, the oily material that keeps hair from becoming dry and forms a protective film on the skin. 569
  sublingual g., a salivary gland that lies under the tongue. 260, 260*f*
  submandibular g., one of a pair of salivary glands. 260, 260*f*
  sudoriferous g., sweat gland, a gland in the skin that is responsible for production of sweat. 569
  vestibular g., any one of four small glands, two on each side of the vaginal orifice. 342
glans penis (glanz **pē**-nis) the cap-shaped expansion at the end of the penis. 362
Glasgow coma scale (glas-gō **kō**-muh skāl) a quick standardized system for assessing the degree of impairment of consciousness. 470
glaucoma (glaw-, glou-**kō**-muh) a group of eye diseases characterized by an increase in intraocular pressure, which causes pathologic changes in the optic disk and typical defects in the field of vision. 511
glia cell (**glī**-uh sel) one of the cells that make up the supporting nerve of nervous tissue. 463
glioma (glī-**ō**-muh) a tumor composed of tissue that represents neuroglia. The term is sometimes extended to include all the primary intrinsic neoplasms of the brain and spinal cord. 479
glomerular (glō-**mer**-ū-lur) pertaining to the glomerulus.
  g. filtration, the renal process whereby fluid of the fluid is filtered across the capillaries of the glomerulus and into the urinary space of Bowman capsule. 307
  g. filtration rate (GFR), a kidney function value that can be determined from the amount of filtrate formed by the glomeruli of the kidney. 308, 308*f*
glomerulonephritis (glō-mer-ū-lō-nuh-**frī**-tis) a type of nephritis in which there is inflammation of the glomeruli. 319
glomerulopathy (glō-mer-ū-**lop**-uh-thē) any disease of the renal glomeruli. 319
glomerulus (glō-**mer**-ū-lus) a small cluster, as of blood vessels or nerve fibers; often used alone to designate one of the renal glomeruli, which act as filters. 292
glossectomy (glos-**ek**-tuh-mē) surgical removal of the tongue. 282
glossitis (glos-**ī**-tis) inflammation of the tongue. 270
glossopathy (glos-**op**-uh-thē) any disease of the tongue. 270
glossoplasty (glos-**ō**-plas-tē) plastic surgery of the tongue. 282
glossoplegia (glos-ō-**plē**-juh) paralysis of the tongue. 270
glossopyrosis (glos-ō-pī-**rō**-sis) pain, burning, itching, and stinging of the mucous membranes of the tongue without apparent lesions of the affected areas. 270
glossorrhaphy (glos-**or**-uh-fē) suture of the tongue. 282
glottis (**glot**-is) the vocal apparatus of the larynx. 214
glucagon (**gloo**-kuh-gon) hormone secreted by the alpha cells of the islets of Langerhans in response to hypoglycemia, acetylcholine, some amino acids, and growth hormone. 265, 541
glucocorticoid (gloo-kō-**kor**-ti-koid) any of a group of steroids produced by the adrenal cortex. 538
glucose (**gloo**-kōs) a sugar found in certain foodstuffs, especially fruit, and normal blood; dextrose. 254, 541
  g. lowering agent, a drug that lowers the blood glucose. 554
  g. tolerance test (GTT), a test of the body's ability to metabolize carbohydrates; involves administering a standard dose of glucose and measuring the blood and urine for glucose levels. 545

gluten (**gloo**-tun) a substance present in cereal grains, especially wheat, that can cause illness in people with celiac disease. 269
glycolysis (glī-**kol**-uh-sis) the enzymatic breakdown of glucose to simpler compounds. 253-254
glycosuria (glī-kō-**sū**-rē-uh) the presence of sugar in the urine. 311, 545
goiter (**goi**-tur) enlargement of the thyroid gland, causing a swelling in the front part of the neck. 544, 548
gonad (**gō**-nad) an organ that produces eggs or sperm; ovary or testis. 342, 353, 531
gonadotropic (gō-nuh-dō-**trō**-pik) capable of stimulating the ovaries or the testes. 536
  g. hormone, a general term that means a hormone that stimulates the gonads and includes follicle-stimulating hormone (FSH) and luteinizing hormone. 536
gonadotropin (gō-nuh-dō-**trō**-pin) a substance that stimulates the gonads, especially the hormone secreted by the pituitary gland that stimulates the ovaries or testes. 350, 536
  human chorionic g., a hormone present in the urine and many body fluids of pregnant female individuals that forms the basis of testing for pregnancy. 350, 380, 542
gonococcus (GC) (gon-ō-**kok**-us) an organism of the species Neisseria gonorrhoeae, the cause of gonorrhea. 387
gonorrhea (gon-ō-**rē**-uh) infection caused by Neisseria gonorrhoeae; transmitted sexually in most cases but also by contact with infected exudates in neonatal children at birth, or by infants in households with infected inhabitants. It is characterized by discharge and painful urination in male individuals and often is asymptomatic in female individuals. 322-323, 350, 387*f*
gout (gout) hereditary metabolic disease that is a form of acute arthritis and is marked by inflammation of the joints. Gout is characterized by hyperuricemia and deposits of urates in and around joints. Any joint may be affected, but gout usually begins in the knee or foot. 442
graafian follicle (**grah**-fē-un **fol**-i-kul) development of the primary oocyte in the ovary to the stage where the ovum is fully developed. 347
graft (graft) a tissue or organ taken from a site or a person and inserted into a new site or person, performed to repair a defect in structure; transplant.
  homologous g., a tissue removed from a donor for transplantation to a recipient of the same species. 138
grafting (**graft**-ing) transplantation.
  corneal g., transplantation of corneal tissue from one human eye to another. 513
gravid (**grav**-id) pregnant. 377
gravida (**grav**-i-duh) a pregnant woman. 377
gumma (**gum**-uh) a lesion in late stages of syphilis. 388
gynecologist (gī-nuh-**kol**-uh-jist) a physician who treats diseases of the female sex. 14
gynecology (gī-nuh-, jin-uh-**kol**-uh-jē) the branch of medicine that treats female diseases, especially those of the genital and urinary systems. 342
gynecomastia (gī-nuh-kō-**mas**-tē-uh) excessive development of the male mammary glands, sometimes even to the functional state. 550, 550*f*
halitosis (hal-i-**tō**-sis) offensive breath. 271
hallux valgus (**hal**-uks **val**-gus) angulation of the great toe away from the midline of the body, or toward the other toes. 434, 434*f*
hammertoe (**ham**-ur-tō) a toe with dorsal flexion of the first phalanx and plantar flexion of the second and third phalanges. 434, 434*f*
haversian canals (huh-**ver**-zhun kuh-**nalz**) the channels of compact bone that contain blood vessels, lymph vessels, and nerves. 409
headache (**hed**-āk) pain in the head. 474
  cluster h., a headache similar to migraine, recurring as often as two or three times a day over a period of weeks; then there may be absence of symptoms for weeks or months. 474, 474*f*
  migraine h., paroxysmal attacks of headache frequently unilateral, usually accompanied by disordered vision and gastrointestinal disturbances. 474, 474*f*
  muscle contraction h., result from the long-sustained contraction of skeletal muscles around the scalp, face, neck, and upper back; also called *tension headache*. 474, 474*f*
  tension h., a pain that affects the head as a result of overwork or emotional strain and involves tension in the muscles of the neck, face, and shoulder. 474
heart (hahrt) the muscular cone-shaped hollow organ that pumps blood throughout the body. 169*f*
  congestive h. failure, a condition characterized by weakness, breathlessness, and edema in lower portions of the body resulting from venous stasis and reduced outflow of blood. 182, 230
  h. block, impairment in conduction of an impulse in heart excitation. 180
  h. flutter, a type of irregular heart rhythm. 180
heat hydrotherapy (hēt hī-drō-**ther**-uh-pē) the use of warm water in the treatment of disease. 587
Heimlich maneuver (**hīm**-lik muh-**noo**-vur) an emerging procedure for dislodging a bolus of food or other obstruction from the trachea to prevent asphyxiation. 233, 233*f*
heliotherapy (hē-lē-ō-**ther**-uh-pē) treatment of disease by exposing the body to sunlight. 587
hemangioma (hē-man-jē-**ō**-muh) an extremely common benign tumor, occurring most commonly in infancy and childhood, made up of newly formed blood vessels and resulting from malformation of angioblastic tissue of fetal life. 183
hemapheresis (hē-muh-fuh-**rē**-sis) selective removal of certain components of the blood via a machine designed specifically for this purpose. 613
hematemesis (hē-muh-**tem**-uh-sis) vomiting of blood. 269
hematochezia (hē-muh-tō, hem-uh-tō-**kē**-zhuh) presence of blood in the feces. 268

hematocrit (hē-**mat**-uh-krit) a tube with graduated markings used to determine the volume of packed red cells in a blood specimen by centrifugation; by extension, the measurement obtained using this procedure or the corresponding measurements produced by automated blood cell counters. 128

hematology (hē-muh-**tol**-uh-jē) the study of blood and blood-forming tissues and their physiology and pathology. 51, 126

hematoma (hē-muh-**tō**-muh) any localized collection of blood, usually clotted, in an organ, tissue, or space. 125, 125f, 476, 476f
  epidural h., accumulation of blood in the epidural space. 476, 476f
  intracerebral h., accumulation of blood within the brain tissue. 476, 476f
  subdural h., accumulation of blood in the subdural space. 476, 476f

hematopoiesis (hē-muh-tō-poi-**ē**-sis) the formation and development of blood cells. 126

hematuria (hē-muh-, hem-uh-**tū**-rē-uh) the presence of blood in the urine. 311

hemicolectomy (hem-ē-kō-**lek**-tuh-mē) excision of approximately half of the colon. 93, 287

hemiplegia (hem-ē-**plē**-juh) paralysis of one side of the body. 477f, 478

hemodialysis (hē-mō-dī-**al**-uh-sis) the process of diffusing blood through a semipermeable membrane for the purpose of removing toxic materials and maintaining acid-base balance in cases of impaired kidney function. 324, 325f

hemoglobin (hē-mō-**glō**-bin) the oxygen-carrying red pigment of red blood cells. 135
  glycosylated h., a hemoglobin A molecule in which the concentration represents the average blood glucose level over the previous several weeks. 545

hemoglobinopathy (hē-mō-glō-bin-**op**-uh-thē) a hematologic disorder caused by genetically determined abnormal hemoglobin. 135

hemolysin (hē-**mol**-uh-sin) a substance that causes destruction of red blood cells. 131

hemolysis (hē-**mol**-uh-sis) destruction of red blood cells that results in the liberation of hemoglobin. 53, 131

hemolytic (hē-mō-**lit**-ik) pertaining to, characterized by, or producing hemolysis. 53
  h. disease of the newborn (HDN), hemolytic erythroblastosis fetalis. 135, 383

hemolyze (hē-mō-līz) to subject to or to undergo hemolysis. 53

hemopericardium (hē-mō-per-i-**kahr**-dē-um) an effusion of blood within the pericardium. 182

hemophilia (hē-mō-**fil**-ē-uh) a hereditary hemorrhagic disorder caused by deficiency of antihemophilic factor VIII or IX. 134

hemoptysis (hē-**mop**-ti-sis) the spitting of blood or blood-stained sputum. 231

hemorrhoid (**hem**-uh-roid) a varicose dilation of a vein of the anal canal inside or just outside the rectum that causes pain, itching, and bleeding. 276, 276f

hemorrhoidectomy (hem-uh-roid-**ek**-tuh-mē) excision of hemorrhoids. 287

hemostasis (hē-mō-**stā**-sis, hē-**mos**-tuh-sis) the checking of the flow of blood either by coagulation or surgical means; interruption of blood flow through any vessel or to any part of the body. 137

hemostatics (hē-mō-**stat**-iks) agents used to reduce bleeding by speeding up the clotting of blood or by the formation of an artificial clot. 197

hemothorax (hē-mō-**thor**-aks) a collection of blood in the chest cavity. 228, 229f

hepatectomy (hep-uh-**tek**-tuh-mē) excision of part of the liver. 289

hepatitis (hep-uh-**tī**-tis) inflammation of the liver. 138, 279
  viral h., hepatitis caused by a viral infection, such as hepatitis A virus (HAV), hepatitis B virus (HBV), or hepatitis C virus (HCV). 389

hepatoma (hep-uh-**tō**-muh) a tumor of the liver, especially hepatocellular carcinoma. 279

hepatomegaly (hep-uh-tō-**meg**-uh-lē) enlargement of the liver. 279

hepatopathy (hep-uh-**top**-uh-thē) any disease of the liver. 279

hepatosplenomegaly (hep-uh-tō-splē-nō-**meg**-uh-lē) enlargement of the liver and spleen. 279

hepatotomy (hep-uh-**tot**-uh-mē) surgical incision of the liver. 289

hermaphroditism (hur-**maf**-ruh-di-tiz-um) a rare condition resulting from a chromosomal abnormality in which both testicular and ovarian tissue exist in the same person. 366

hernia (**hur**-nē-uh) protrusion of an organ or part of it through an abnormal opening. 48
  hiatal h., protrusion of any structure through the esophageal hiatus of the diaphragm. 273, 273f

herniated disk (**hur**-nē-āt-ud disk) herniation of an intervertebral disk. 435, 435f

herniation (hur-nē-**ā**-shun) abnormal protrusion of an organ or other body structure through a defect or natural opening in a covering, membrane, muscle, or bone. 48

hernioplasty (**hur**-nē-ō-plas-tē) surgical repair of a hernia. 114

herpes (**hur**-pēz) a word that at one time was used to indicate any inflammatory skin disease marked by small vesicles in clusters and caused by a virus. Its use as a single word is imprecise but often refers to the condition of cold sores or fever blisters. 575
  h. genitalis, herpetic blisters on the male or female genitalia. 389-390, 390f
  h. simplex virus (HSV), herpes simplex virus 1 (HSV-1) or herpes simplex virus 2 (HSV-2). 224, 389, 575
  h. zoster, an acute infection caused by reactivation of the latent varicella zoster virus; shingles. 479, 479f, 575, 576

hesitancy (**hez**-uh-tun-sē) tending to hold back or delay momentarily. In urinary hesitancy there is decrease in the force of the stream, often with difficulty in beginning the flow. 317

hidradenitis (hī-drad-uh-**nī**-tis) inflammation of a sweat gland. 583

hilum (**hī**-lum) anatomic nomenclature for a depression or pit at the part of an organ where vessels and nerves enter. 215, 304

hirsutism (**hur**-sōōt-iz-um) abnormal hairiness, especially an adult male pattern of hair distribution in women. 550, 550f

histamine (**his**-tuh-mēn) a substance present in the body that has known pharmacologic action when released from injured cells. Histamine can also be produced synthetically. 141

histamine-2 receptor antagonists (**his**-tuh-mēn-2 rē-**sep**-tur an-**tag**-uh-nists) medications used to treat duodenal ulcers and prevent their return. 290

histocompatibility (his-tō-kum-pat-i-**bil**-i-tē) the ability of donor tissue to survive after a transplant, rather than being rejected by the immune system of the patient who receives the tissue. 585

histologist (his-**tol**-uh-jist) one who studies tissue. 61

histology (his-**tol**-uh-jē) study of the minute structure, composition, and function of tissues. 61

holistic health (hō-**lis**-tik helth) a concept that a concern for health requires a perception of the individual as an integrated system rather than one or more separate parts. 13f, 14

Holter monitor (**hōl**-tur **mon**-i-tur) a type of ambulatory ECG monitor. 175, 175f

homeostasis (hō-mē-ō-**stā**-sis) sameness or stability in the normal body state of an organism. 121

hordeolum (hor-**dē**-ō-lum) a localized, purulent, inflammatory staphylococcal infection of one or more sebaceous glands. 512

hormone (**hor**-mōn) a chemical substance produced in the body that has a specific effect on the activity of certain cells or organs. 530
  adrenocorticotropic h. (ACTH), the hormone secreted by the adenohypophysis that stimulates the adrenal cortex. 538
  anterior pituitary hormone, hormone secreted by the adenohypophysis. 533f, 534
  antidiuretic h., a hormone that decreases the production of urine. 308, 535
  follicle-stimulating h., a gonadotropin that stimulates the growth and maturation of the graafian follicles in the ovaries and stimulates spermatogenesis in the male. 347, 536
  growth h., a hormone secreted by the pituitary gland that stimulates growth. 537
  h. replacement therapy (HRT), a combination of estrogen and progesterone, an intervention for women who experience symptoms of menopause or those at high risk for osteoporosis (abnormal loss of bone density) and deterioration of bone tissue. 357
  interstitial cell–stimulating h., a hormone secreted by the pituitary gland that stimulates the production of testosterone by the interstitial cells of the testes. 536
  lactogenic h., one of the gonadotropic hormones produced by the anterior pituitary; stimulates and maintains secretion of milk in postpartum mammals. 538
  luteinizing h., a hormone secreted by the anterior pituitary gland that stimulates secretion of the sex hormones by the ovaries and testes. 347, 536
  melanocyte-stimulating h., a hormone secreted by the anterior pituitary gland that controls the intensity of pigmentation in pigmented cells. 537
  parathyroid h., a hormone secreted by the parathyroid glands. 542
  posterior pituitary h., hormone secreted by the posterior pituitary, either ADH or oxytocin. 532, 532f, 533f
  somatotropic h., somatotropin; growth hormone. 537
  thyroid-stimulating h., a substance secreted by the pituitary gland that controls the release of thyroid hormone. 536

humerus (**hū**-mur-us) the bone of the upper arm, extending from shoulder to elbow. 417

Huntington chorea (**hun**-ting-tun kuh-**rē**-uh) an autosomal dominant disease characterized by chronic, progressive, complex, jerky movements and mental deterioration terminating in dementia. 478

hydrocele (**hī**-drō-sēl) a circumscribed collection of fluid, especially pertaining to fluid collection in the scrotum. 367

hydrocelectomy (hī-drō-sē-**lek**-tuh-mē) excision of a hydrocele. 369

hydrocephalus, hydrocephaly (hī-drō-**sef**-uh-lus, hī-drō-**sef**-uh-lē) a condition characterized by abnormal accumulation of cerebrospinal fluid (CSF) within the skull with enlargement of the head, atrophy of the brain, mental retardation, and convulsions. 122, 122f, 480

hydronephrosis (hī-drō-nuh-**frō**-sis) distention of the kidney with urine, as a result of obstruction of the ureter. 321, 321f

hydrophobia (hī-drō-**fō**-bē-uh) rabies, a viral disease transmitted to a human by the bite of an infected animal. 479

hydrothorax (hī-drō-**thor**-aks) a collection of water fluid in the pleural cavity. 228

hydroureter (hī-drō-ū-**rē**-tur) abnormal distention of the ureter caused by obstruction from any cause. 321, 321f

hypalgesia (hī-pal-**jē**-zē-uh) decreased sensitivity to pain. 473

hyperacidity (hī-pur-uh-**sid**-i-tē) an excessive amount of acid. 284

hyperadrenalism (hī-pur-uh-**drē**-nul-iz-um) increased activity of the adrenal glands. 549

hyperalgesia (hī-pur-al-**jē**-zē-uh) extreme sensitivity to pain. 473

hyperalimentation (hī-pur-al-uh-men-**tā**-shun) the intravenous infusion of a hypertonic solution that contains sufficient nutrients to sustain life. 283

hypercalcemia (hī-pur-kal-**sē**-mē-uh) an increased level of calcium in the blood. 122, 549

hypercalciuria (hī-pur-kal-sē-**ū**-rē-uh) excessive calcium in the urine. 431

hypercapnia (hī-pur-**kap**-nē-uh) excessive carbon dioxide in the blood. 221

hypercholesterolemia (hī-pur-kō-les-tur-ol-**ē**-mē-uh) the most common inherited type of high fat or lipid levels in the blood. 175

hyperemesis (hī-pur-**em**-uh-sis) excessive vomiting. 269

hyperemia (hī-pur-**ē**-mē-uh) excessive blood flow to a part of the body. 125

hyperglycemia (hī-pur-glī-**sē**-mē-uh) an increased amount of sugar in the blood. 265, 320, 545

hyperinsulinism (hī-pur-**in**-suh-lin-iz-um) excessive secretion of insulin by the pancreas, resulting in an increased level of insulin in the blood and hypoglycemia. 552

hyperkalemia (hī-pur-kuh-**lē**-mē-uh) abnormally high concentration of potassium in the blood. 122

hyperkinesia, hyperkinesis (hī-pur-ki-**nē**-zhuh, hī-pur-ki-**nē**-sis) abnormally increased muscular function or activity. 484

hyperlipidemia (hī-pur-li-pi-**dē**-mē-uh) increased lipids in the blood. 175

hypernatremia (hī-pur-nuh-**trē**-mē-uh) a greater than normal concentration of sodium in the blood. 122

hyperopia (hī-pur-**ō**-pē-uh) an error of refraction in which rays of light entering the eye are brought to a focus behind the retina; also called *farsightedness*. 510, 510*f*

hyperosmia (hi-pur-**oz**-mē-uh) increased sensitivity of smell. 520

hyperoxemia (hī-pur-ok-**sē**-mē-uh) increased amount of oxygen in the blood. 235

hyperparathyroidism (hī-pur-par-uh-**thī**-roid-iz-um) increased secretion of hormone by the parathyroids. 549

hyperpituitarism (hī-pur-pi-**tōō**-i-tuh-riz-um) increased secretion by the pituitary gland. 547

hyperplasia (hī-pur-**plā**-zhuh) abnormal increase in the number of normal cells in a tissue. 116, 116*f*
  benign prostatic h., nonmalignant, noninflammatory enlargement of the prostate. 322, 322*f*, 367

hyperpnea (hī-pur-**nē**-uh, hī-purp-**nē**-uh) an abnormal increase in depth and rate of respiration. 221

hyperpyrexia (hī-pur-pī-**rek**-sē-uh) a highly increased body temperature of around 105 F or higher. 115

hypersecretion (hī-pur-sē-**krē**-shun) excessive secretion. 530

hypersensitivity (hī-pur-sen-si-**tiv**-i-tē) a state in which the body reacts with an exaggerated response to a foreign agent. 140

hypertension (hī-pur-**ten**-shun) increased blood pressure. 174
  renal h., hypertension resulting from renal artery stenosis or other kidney disorders. 322

hyperthermia (hī-pur-**thur**-mē-uh) greatly increased body temperature. 585

hyperthyroidism (hī-pur-**thī**-roid-iz-um) increased activity of the thyroid gland. 544, 548

hypertonicity (hī-pur-tō-**nis**-i-tē) the state of having increased tone. 424

hypertrophy (hī-**pur**-truh-fē) enlargement of an organ caused by an increase in the size of preexisting cells. 116, 116*f*

hyperventilation (hī-pur-ven-ti-**lā**-shun) abnormally increased pulmonary ventilation, resulting in greater than normal loss of carbon dioxide, which if prolonged may lead to alkalosis. 221

hypnotic (hip-**not**-ik) inducing sleep; pertaining to or of the nature of hypnotism; a drug that acts to induce sleep. 490

hypoadrenalism (hī-pō-uh-**drē**-nul-iz-um) decreased activity of the adrenal glands. 550

hypoalgesia (hī-pō-al-**jē**-zē-uh) decreased sensitivity to pain. 96, 473

hypocalcemia (hī-pō-kal-**sē**-mē-uh) decreased amount of calcium in the blood. 122, 549

hypocapnia (hī-pō-**kap**-nē-uh) deficiency of carbon dioxide in the blood resulting from hyperventilation and eventually leading to alkalosis. 221

hypochondria (hī-pō-**kon**-drē-uh) abnormal anxiety about one's health. 486

hypochondriac (hī-pō-**kon**-drē-ak) pertaining to the hypochondrium; a person who has morbid anxiety about his or her health but has no attributable cause. 110

hypochondriasis (hī-pō-kon-**drī**-uh-sis) a stomatoform disorder characterized by an interpretation of normal sensations as indications of serious problems. 486

hypochromia (hī-pō-**krō**-mē-uh) abnormal decrease in the hemoglobin content of the erythrocytes. 136

hypoglycemia (hī-pō-glī-**sē**-mē-uh) an abnormally low concentration of glucose in the blood. 265, 541, 552

hypogonadism (hī-pō-**gō**-nad-iz-um) decreased functional activity of the gonads with retardation of sexual development. 549
  pituitary h., a deficiency in the secretory activity of the ovary or testes caused by hyposecretion of pituitary hormones. 549

hypoinsulinism (hī-pō-in-su-lin-iz-um) deficient secretion of insulin by the pancreas. 550

hypokalemia (hī-pō-kuh-**lē**-mē-uh) abnormally low potassium concentration in the blood. 122

hyponatremia (hī-pō-nuh-**trē**-mē-uh) deficiency of sodium in the blood. 122

hypoparathyroidism (hī-pō-par-uh-**thī**-roid-iz-um) decreased secretion of hormone by the parathyroids. 549

hypophysectomy (hī-pof-uh-**sek**-tuh-mē) surgical removal or destruction of the pituitary. 554, 554*f*

hypophysis (hī-**pof**-uh-sis) the pituitary gland. 531

hypopituitarism (hī-pō-pi-**tōō**-i-tuh-riz-um) decreased activity of the pituitary gland. 547

hypoplasia (hī-pō-**plā**-zhuh) incomplete development or underdevelopment of an organ or tissue. 116

hypopnea (hī-**pop**-nē-uh) abnormal decrease in the depth and rate of breathing. 223

hyposecretion (hī-pō-suh-**krē**-shun) diminished secretion as of a gland. 550

hypospadias (hī-pō-**spā**-dē-us) a developmental anomaly in which the urethra opens inferior to its usual location. 323

hypotension (hī-pō-**ten**-shun) decreased blood pressure. 174

hypothalamus (hī-pō-**thal**-uh-mus) the part of the brain most concerned with moderating behavior related to internal physiologic states. 467, 467*f*, 533, 539*f*

hypothermia (hī-pō-**thur**-mē-uh) low body temperature. 584

hypothyroidism (hī-pō-**thī**-roid-iz-um) decreased activity of the thyroid gland. 93, 548

hypotonicity (hī-pō-tō-**nis**-i-tē) the state of being hypotonic. 424

hypoventilation (hī-pō-ven-ti-**lā**-shun) a state in which there is a reduced amount of air entering the pulmonary alveoli. 221

hypovolemia (hī-pō-vō-**lē**-mē-uh) decreased volume of circulating blood in the body. 182

hypoxemia (hī-pok-**sē**-mē-uh) deficient oxygen in the blood. 222

hypoxia (hī-**pok**-sē-uh) a condition of decreased oxygen. 220

hysterectomy (his-tur-**ek**-tuh-mē) removal of the uterus. 358
  abdominal h., removal of the uterus through an incision in the abdominal wall. 358
  radical h., removal of ovaries, fallopian tubes, lymph nodes, lymphatic channels as well as the uterus and cervix. 358
  vaginal h., a hysterectomy performed through the vagina. 358

hysteria (his-**ter**-ē-uh) a now obsolete term formerly used in psychiatry for a dramatic attack involving intense emotional display. 50

hysteropathy (his-tuh-**rop**-uh-thē) any uterine disease or disorder. 354

hysteropexy (**his**-tur-ō-pek-sē) surgical fixation of the uterus. 358

hysteroptosis (his-tur-op-**tō**-sis) falling or prolapse of the uterus. 354, 354*f*

hysterosalpingogram (his-tur-ō-sal-**ping**-gō-gram) the record produced by x-ray examination of the uterus and uterine tubes after the injection of opaque material. 350, 351*f*

hysterosalpingography (his-tur-ō-sal-ping-**gog**-ruh-fē) radiography of the uterus and uterine tubes after injection of opaque material. 350, 351*f*

hysteroscope (**his**-tur-ō-skōp) an endoscope used in direct visual examination of the uterus. 350, 351*f*

hysteroscopy (his-tur-**os**-kuh-pē) inspection of the interior of the uterus with an endoscope. 350, 351*f*

ichthyosis (ik-thē-**ō**-sis) any of several generalized skin disorders marked by dryness and scaliness, resembling fish skin. 572, 572*f*

ileitis (il-ē-**ī**-tis) inflammation of the ileum. 276

ileostomy (il-ē-**os**-tuh-mē) surgical creation of an opening into the ileum, usually by establishing a stoma on the abdominal wall. 287

ileum (**il**-ē-um) the distal portion of the small intestine, which extends from the jejunum to the cecum. 261

ilium (**il**-ē-um) the lateral flaring portion of the hip bone. 419

immunity (i-**mū**-ni-tē) being immune; security against a particular disease; nonsusceptibility to the invasive or pathogenic effects of certain antigens. 139, 140*f*

immunization (im-ū-ni-**zā**-shun) the induction of immunity. 139

immunocompromised (im-ū-nō-**kom**-pruh-mīzd) having the immune response attenuated by administration of immunosuppressive drugs, by irradiation, by malnutrition, or by some disease processes. 141

immunodeficiency (im-ū-nō-duh-**fish**-un-sē) a deficiency in immune response. 138

immunoglobulin (im-ū-nō-**glob**-ū-lin) a protein of animal origin that has known antibody activity. 139

immunologist (im-ū-**nol**-uh-jist) a person who makes a special study of immunology. 18

immunology (im-ū-**nol**-uh-jē) the branch of medical science concerned with the response of the organism to antigenic challenge, recognition of self from nonself, and all of the aspects of immune phenomena. 18

immunosuppressant, immunosuppressive (im-ū-nō-suh-**pres**-unt, im-ū-nō-suh-**pres**-iv) pertaining to or inducing immunosuppression., or an immunosuppressive agent. 141

immunotherapy (im-ū-nō-**ther**-uh-pē) the prevention of disease with substances that stimulate the immune response. 141

impaction (im-**pak**-shun) the condition of being firmly lodged or wedged. 278
  fecal i., a collection of puttylike or hardened feces in the rectum or sigmoid. 278

implant (**im**-plant) 1. an encapsulated radioactive substance embedded in tissue for therapy; 2. in surgery, material inserted or grafted into an organ or structure of the body.
  cochlear i., an electronic device that is surgically implanted in the cochlea of a deaf person to improve hearing. 518, 518*f*
  subdermal i., an implant that is placed in the dermis. 374*t*

implantation (im-plan-**tā**-shun) attachment of the fertilized egg to the epithelial lining of the uterus and its embedding in the compact layer of the endometrium. 371

impotence agents (**im**-puh-tuns **ā**-junts) drugs that treat erectile dysfunction by increasing blood flow to the the penis and causing an erection. 391

incision (in-**sizh**-un) a cut or wound produced by a sharp instrument; the act of cutting. 72
  i. and drainage (I&D), a surgical cut into a wound and drainage of pus, blood, or other fluid. 586

incisor (in-**sī**-zur) any of the four anterior teeth in either jaw. 258

incompatibility (in-kum-pat-i-**bil**-i-tē) the unsuitability of one thing to another. 585

incus (**ing**-kus) any of the three ossicles in the middle ear. 514

induration (in-dū-**rā**-shun) the quality of being or becoming hard; an abnormally hard spot. 571

infarct (**in**-fahrkt) an area of necrosis in a tissue caused by local ischemia resulting from obstruction of circulation to the area. 181

infarction (in-**fahrk**-shun) the formation of a localized area of necrosis caused by insufficient blood supply, produced by an occlusion.
  myocardial i., death of an area of the heart muscle, occurring as a result of oxygen deprivation. 181, 181*f*

infection (in-**fek**-shun) the invasion of the body by pathogenic microorganisms; a disease caused by the invasion of pathogenic microorganisms. 41

chlamydial i., the most common sexually transmitted disease (STD) in the United States. 322, 350

nonspecific genital i., a genital infection caused by various microorganisms that are not included in the usual types of genitourinary infections. 388

nosocomial i., hospital-acquired infection that was not present or incubating before the patient's admission and is acquired 72 hours or longer after admission. 39

infectious (in-**fek**-shus) capable of being transmitted; pertaining to a disease caused by a microorganism; producing infection. 41*t*

i. mononucleosis, an acute infectious disease that primarily affects lymphoid tissue. The cause of most cases of infectious mononucleosis is the Epstein-Barr virus. 133

inferior (in-**fēr**-ē-ur) situated below or directed downward; in anatomy it is used in reference to the lower surface of a structure or to the lower of two or more similar structures. 103, 104*f*

infertility (in-fur-**til**-i-tē) diminished or absent capacity to produce offspring. 372

inflammation (in-fluh-**mā**-shun) a localized protective response elicited by injury or destruction of tissues. 115

influenza (in-flōō-**en**-zuh) an acute viral infection involving the respiratory tract. 226

ingest (in-**jest**) taking food, medicine, etc., into the body by mouth. 54

ingestion (in-**jes**-chun) the act of taking food, medicines, etc., into the body by mouth. 252

inhalation (in-huh-**lā**-shun) drawing air or other substances into the nasal or oral respiratory route; any drug administered by the respiratory route. 210

inhale (in-**hāl**) to take into the lungs by breathing. 99

injection (in-**jek**-shun) the forcing of a liquid into a part; a substance that is injected. 98, 98*f*

collagen i., a reconstructive "plumping" technique in cosmetic surgery. 586, 586*f*

inotropes (**in**-ō-trōps) agents that alter the force of muscular contraction and change the force of cardiac contractions. 197

inspection (in-**spek**-shun) observation of a patient using the eyes. 61

inspiration (in-spi-**rā**-shun) the drawing of air into the lungs. 210

insula (**in**-suh-luh) a portion of the cerebral cortex. 467

insulin (**in**-suh-lin) a hormone secreted by the beta cells of the islets of Langerhans of the pancreas into the blood. 265, 541, 541*f*, 553

i. pump, a portable battery-operated instrument that delivers a measured amount of insulin through the abdominal wall. 553, 554*f*

intake and output (I&O) (**in**-tāk and **out**-poot) the measurement of the amount of fluid that is given to a patient, as well as the amount of fluid secreted in a specific time, usually 24 hours. 310

integument (in-**teg**-ū-munt) a covering or investment. 566

interferon (in-tur-**fēr**-on) any of a family of glycoproteins that exert nonspecific antiviral activity, have immunoregulatory functions, and can inhibit the growth of nonviral intracellular parasites. 139

internal os (in-**tur**-nul os) the internal opening of the cervical canal. 383

internist (in-**tur**-nist) a specialist in internal medicine. 14

interstitial (in-tur-**stish**-ul) pertaining to or situated between parts or in the interspaces of a tissue. 120

i. cells of Leydig, cells in the testes that are responsible for the production of testosterone. 362, 362*f*

intervertebral (in-tur-**vur**-tuh-brul) between two contiguous vertebrae. 414

i. disk, the layer of fibrocartilage between the bodies of adjoining vertebrae. 414

intrathecal (in-truh-**thē**-kul) within a sheath or within the spinal canal. 468

intrauterine (in-truh-**ū**-tur-in) within the uterus. 135

i. device (IUD), a contraceptive device inserted into the uterine cavity. 374, 374*f*

i. transfusion, the introduction of blood directly into the bloodstream of a fetus while the fetus is in the uterus. 135

intubation (in tōō-**bā**-shun) insertion of a tube into a body canal or organ.

endotracheal i., insertion of a tube into the trachea. 235

nasotracheal i., insertion of a tube through the nose into the trachea to serve as an airway. 235, 235*f*

orotracheal i., insertion of a tube through the mouth into the trachea to serve as an airway. 235, 235*f*

intussusception (in-tuh-suh-**sep**-shun) the prolapse of one part of the intestine into the lumen of an immediately joining part. 278

inversion (in-**vur**-zhun) a turning inward, inside-out, upside-down, or other reversal of the normal relation of a part. 426*f*, 427

in vitro (in vē-trō) in an artificial environment or within a test tube. 128

i. fertilization (IVF), a method of fertilizing human ova outside the body by exposing mature ovum to living sperm. 372

in vivo (in **vē**-vo) within the living body. 128

ipsilateral (ip-si-**lat**-ur-ul) situated on, pertaining to, or affecting the same side. 96, 98*f*

iridectomy (ir-i-**dek**-tuh-mē) surgical removal of part of the iris of the eye. 513

iris (**ī**-ris) the circular pigmented membrane behind the cornea. 504

ischemia (is-**kē**-mē-uh) deficiency of blood from functional constriction or actual obstruction of a blood vessel. 181

ischialgia (is-kē-**al**-juh) pain in the ischium. 436

ischiodynia (is-kē-ō-**din**-ē-uh) pain in the ischium. 436

ischium (**is**-kē-um) the inferior, dorsal portion of the hip bone. 419

islets of Langerhans (**ī**-lets ov **lahng**-uhr-hahnz) irregular microscopic structures scattered throughout the pancreas and constituting the endocrine portion. In humans they are composed of at least three types of cells that secrete insulin, glucagon, and somatostatin. 531

isograft (**ī**-sō-graft) surgical transplantation of tissue from identical twins. 138

jaundice (**jawn**-dis) yellowness of the skin, sclerae, and excretions because of increased bilirubin in the blood and deposition of bile pigments. 56, 56*f*, 279, 279*f*, 572

jejunoileostomy (juh-jōō-nō-il-ē-**os**-tuh-mē) formation of a new opening between the jejunum and the ileum. 285

jejunostomy (juh-jōō-**nos**-tuh-mē) surgical creation of a permanent opening between the jejunum and the surface of the abdominal wall; also the opening it creates. 283

jejunotomy (juh-jōō-**not**-uh-mē) surgical incision of the jejunum. 287

jejunum (juh-**jōō**-num) that portion of the small intestine that extends from the duodenum to the ileum. 261

joint (joint) the site of junction or union between two or more bones. 422

j. crepitus, a clicking sound often heard in movement of joints. 436

metatarsophalangeal j., any of the joints between the metatarsals and the bones of the toes. 422

synovial j., a general classification of joints that have a cavity between articulating bones and are freely movable. 422

temporomandibular j., one of a pair of joints connecting the mandible of the jaw to the temporal bone of the skull. 423

Kaposi sarcoma (**kah**-pō-shē sahr-**kō**-muh) a malignant neoplastic proliferation characterized by the development of bluish-red cutaneous nodules, usually on the lower extremities, that slowly increase in size and number and spread to more proximal sites. 389, 389*f*, 578

karyomegaly (kar-ē-ō-**meg**-uh-lē) abnormal enlargement of the cell nucleus. 130

Kegel exercises (**kā**-gul ek-**sur**-sīz-uz) exercises performed to strengthen the pubococcygeal muscle. 329

keloid (**kē**-loid) a sharply-elevated, irregularly-shaped, progressively-enlarging scar resulting from formation of excessive amounts of collagen in the dermis during connective tissue repair. 580, 580*f*

keratin (**ker**-uh-tin) a protein that forms the epidermis, hair, and all horny tissue. 567

keratogenesis (ker-uh-tō-**jen**-uh-sis) the formation of horny material. 567

keratolytics (ker-uh-tō-**lit**-iks) medications that remove warts and other lesions in which the epidermis produces excess skin. 588

keratoma (ker-uh-**tō**-muh) a horny tumor; a tumor composed of keratin. 577

keratometer (ker-uh-**tom**-uh-tur) measurement of the cornea. 509

keratosis (ker-uh-**tō**-sis) any horny growth; a condition of the skin characterized by the formation of horny growths or excessive development of the horny growth. 578

seborrheic k., a common benign, noninvasive tumor of the skin characterized by soft, crumbly plaques, varying in pigmentation and occurring most often on the face, trunk, and extremities usually in middle life. 578, 578*f*

ketoacidosis (kē-tō-as-i-**dō**-sis) acidosis accompanied by the accumulation of ketone bodies (ketosis) in the body tissues and fluids. 311

ketone (**kē**-tōn) a compound that is a normal end product of lipid metabolism. 311, 545

ketonuria (kē-tō-**nū**-rē-uh) excretion of ketones in the urine. 311, 545

kidney (**kid**-nē) either of the two bean-shaped organs in the lumbar region that filter the blood, excreting the waste products in the form of urine and regulating the concentration of certain ions in the extracellular fluid. 305*f*, 306, 319*f*

k. dialysis, removal of impurities or wastes from the blood of patients with renal failure or various toxic conditions. 324, 325*f*

kleptomania (klep-tō-**mā**-nē-uh) an uncontrollable impulse to steal objects unnecessary for personal use or monetary value. 486

kyphosis (kī-**fō**-sis) abnormally increased convexity in the curvature of the thoracic spine as viewed from the side; hunchback. 440, 440*f*

labia (**lā**-bē-uh) fleshy edges, usually designating the labia majora and labia minora. 342

l. majora, a pair of elongated folds running downward and backward from the mons pubis in the female. 342

l. minora, a small fold of skin located on each side between the labium majorus and the opening of the vagina. 342

labor (**lā**-bur) the function by which the product of conception is expelled from the uterus through the vagina to the outside world. 378

labyrinth (**lab**-uh-rinth) a complex structure in the inner ear that contains the organs of hearing and balance. 514

laceration (las-ur-**ā**-shun) the act of tearing; a torn, ragged wound. 580, 580*f*

lactase (**lak**-tās) an enzyme that breaks down lactose. A deficiency of this enzyme may result in symptoms of lactose intolerance. 51

lactation (lak-**tā**-shun) the secretion of milk or the period of milk secretion. 539

lactiferous (lak-**tif**-ur-us) producing or conveying milk. 539

lactogenesis (lak-tō-**jen**-uh-sis) the origin or formation of milk. 539

lactose (**lak**-tōs) the main sugar present in milk of mammals. 51

l. intolerance, a sensitivity disorder resulting in the inability to digest lactose from milk products. 51

laminectomy (lam-i-**nek**-tuh-mē) excision of the posterior arch of a vertebra. 446

laparocholecystotomy (lap-uh-rō-kō-luh-sis-**tot**-uh-mē) removal of the gallbladder by incision of the abdominal wall. 289

laparoenterostomy (lap-uh-rō-en-tur-**os**-tuh-mē) surgical creation of an artificial opening into the intestine through the abdominal wall. 287

laparohysterectomy (lap-uh-rō-his-tuh-**rek**-tuh-mē) laparoscopic fixation of the uterus. 358

laparorrhaphy (lap-uh-**ror**-uh-fē) suture of the abdominal wall. 386

laparoscope (**lap**-uh-rō-skōp) an endoscope used for examining the peritoneal cavity. 72, 350, 351*f*

laparoscopy (lap-uh-**ros**-kuh-pē) examination of the interior of the abdomen with a laparoscope. 72, 350, 351*f*

laparotomy (lap-uh-**rot**-uh-mē) surgical incision through the abdominal wall. 386

laryngalgia (lar-in-**gal**-juh) pain in the larynx. 224

laryngectomy (lar-in-**jek**-tuh-mē) excision of the larynx. 234, 234*f*

laryngitis (lar-in-**jī**-tis) inflammation of the voice box. 225

laryngography (lar-ing-**gog**-ruh-fē) radiography of the larynx after instillation of a radiopaque substance. 219

laryngopathy (lar-ing-**gop**-uh-thē) any disease of the larynx. 226

laryngopharynx (luh-ring-gō-**far**-inks) that portion of the pharynx below the upper edge of the epiglottis, opening into the larynx and esophagus. 213

laryngoplegia (luh-ring-gō-**plē**-juh) paralysis of the voice box. 226

laryngoscope (luh-**ring**-guh-skōp) instrument used for examination of the larynx. 219

laryngoscopy (lar-ing-**gos**-kuh-pē) examination of the larynx with a laryngoscope. 219

laryngospasm (luh-**ring**-gō-spaz-um) spasmodic closure of the larynx. 226

laryngotracheitis (luh-ring-gō-trā-kē-**ī**-tis) inflammation of the larynx and the trachea. 233

laryngotracheobronchitis (luh-ring-gō-trā-kē-ō-brong-**kī**-tis) inflammation of the larynx, trachea, and bronchi. 233

larynx (**lar**-inks) the organ of voice; the air passage between the lower pharynx and the trachea. 17, 213

laser (**lā**-zur) abbreviation for light amplification by stimulated emission of radiation.
l. treatment, therapeutic use of laser. 586
l. retinal photocoagulation, using laser to make pinpoint scars to stabilize a detached retina. 513

LASIK (**lā**-sik) acronym for laser-assisted in-situ keratomileusis, a retractive surgery on the cornea for correction of distant vision. 513

lavage (lah-**vahzh**) the irrigation or washing out of an organ; to wash out or irrigate. 284

leiomyoma (lī-ō-mī-**ō**-muh) a benign tumor derived from smooth muscle, most commonly of the uterus; also called *fibroid* and *fibroid tumor.* 356, 356*f*

lens (lenz) the crystalline structure of the eye that is responsible for refraction of light rays; a curved transparent piece of plastic or glass that is shaped to refract light in a specific way. 505
extraction of the l., removal of the lens of the eye to treat a cataract. 513

lesion (**lē**-zhun) any pathologic or traumatic discontinuity of tissue or loss of function of a part. 573
primary l., a sore or wound that is the initial reaction to injury or disease. 574, 574*f*
secondary l., changes in the appearance of a primary lesion resulting in a different-appearing lesion. 574, 575*f*

lethargy (**leth**-ur-jē) a lowered level of consciousness marked by listlessness, drowsiness, and lack of feeling or emotion. 101

leukapheresis (lōō-kuh-fuh-**rē**-sis) a type of apheresis in which the leukocytes are selectively removed. 615

leukemia (lōō-**kē**-mē-uh) a disease of the blood-forming organs characterized by a marked increase in the number of leukocytes, including young forms of leukocytes not usually seen in circulating blood. 133
lymphoblastic l., leukemia in which lymphoblasts are the predominant type of leukocyte. 439
lymphocytic l., leukemia in which lymphocytes are the predominant type of leukocyte. 439
myelocytic l., leukemia in which myelocytes are the predominant type of leukocyte. 439
myelogenous l., leukemia in which polymorphonuclear leukocytes are the predominant type of leukocyte. 439

leukocyte (**lōō**-kō-sīt) a white blood cell. 127, 127*f*

leukocytopenia (lōō-kō-sī-tō-**pē**-nē-uh) a deficiency in the number of white blood cells. 133

leukocytosis (lōō-kō-sī-**tō**-sis) a transient increase in the number of leukocytes in the blood. 133

leukoderma (lōō-kō-**der**-muh) localized loss of skin pigmentation. 583

leukopenia (lōō-kō-**pē**-nē-uh) a deficiency in the number of leukocytes in the blood. 133

leukoplakia (lōō-kō-**plā**-kē-uh) a white patch on a mucous membrane. 261, 261*f*

leukorrhea (lōō-kō-**rē**-uh) a white, viscid discharge from the vagina or uterine cavity. 356

ligament (**lig**-uh-munt) a band of fibrous tissue that connects bones or cartilages and supports and strengthens joints. 423

linear accelerator (**lin**-ē-ur ak-**sel**-ur-ā-tur) a device used by oncologists to deliver and target radiation therapy. 612, 612*f*

lipase (**lip**-ās, **lī**-pās) an enzyme that breaks down fats. 265

lipectomy (li-**pek**-tuh-mē) excision of a mass of subcutaneous adipose tissue. 284, 586

lipid (**lip**-id) a fat. 175, 254

lipoid (**lip**-oid) resembling fat. 254

lipolysis (li-**pol**-uh-sis) the dissolution of fat. 586

lipoma (lip-**ō**-muh) a tumor composed of fatty tissue. 577

lipopenia (lip-ō-**pē**-nē-uh) a deficiency of fats in the body. 279

lipoprotein (lip-ō, lī-pō-**prō**-tēn) any of the lipid-protein complexes in which lipids are transported in the blood. 175
high-density l., a plasma protein that contains approximately 50% lipoprotein along with cholesterol, triglycerides, and phospholipid and is associated with decreased cardiac risk profiles. 175
low-density l., a plasma protein containing relatively more cholesterol and triglycerides than protein. 175

liposuction (lip-ō-**suk**-shun) surgical removal of localized fat deposits using high-pressure vacuum, applied by means of a subdermal cannula. 284, 586, 586*f*

lithotomy (li-**thot**-uh-mē) incision of a duct or organ for removal of a calculus. 326

lithotripsy (**lith**-ō-trip-sē) the crushing of a calculus within the urinary system or gallbladder, followed at once by the washing out of the fragments. 288, 326, 326*f*
extracorporeal shock wave l., a procedure for treating gallstones and upper urinary tract stones. The patient is immersed in a large tub of water or placed in contact with a water cushion. A high-energy shock wave is focused on the stone, which disintegrates into particles small enough to be expelled. 288, 326, 326*f*
laser l., destruction of a calculus using laser. 288

lithotriptor (**lith**-ō-trip-tur) an instrument for crushing calculi. 288

lithotrite (**lith**-ō-trīt) an instrument for crushing a urinary calculus. 326

lobe (lōb) a roundish projection of any structure, such as brain, liver, or lung.
frontal l., the largest of the five lobes of each of the cerebral hemispheres. 467, 467*f*
occipital l., one of the five lobes of each cerebral hemisphere. 467, 467*f*
parietal l., a portion of each cerebral hemisphere that is covered by the parietal bone. 467, 467*f*

lobectomy (lō-**bek**-tuh-mē) excision of a lobe, as removal of a lobe of the lung, brain, or liver.
hepatic l., excision of a lobe of the liver. 289
pulmonary l., removal of a lobe of the lung. 236

lobule (**lob**-ūl) a small lobe. 539

local effect (**lō**-kul uh-**fekt**) the impact of a therapeutic agent on specific tissues rather than on the whole body. 26

lordosis (lor-**dō**-sis) the anterior concavity in the curvature of the lumbar and cervical spine as viewed from the side. The term is used to refer to abnormally increased curvature (swayback) and to the normal curvature (normal lordosis). 440

lumen (**lōō**-mun) the cavity or channel within a tube. 183

lumpectomy (lum-**pek**-tuh-mē) surgery to remove cancer or other abnormal tissue from the breast. 555

lunula (**lōō**-nū-luh) a small crescent- or moon-shaped area. 569

lupus erythematosus (LE) (**lōō**-pus er-uh-them-uh-**tō**-sis) a group of connective tissue disorders primarily affecting women with a spectrum of clinical forms in which cutaneous disease may occur with or without systemic involvement. 441, 441*f*
cutaneous l. e., a form of lupus erythematosus in which the skin may be the only organ involved, or it may precede the involvement of other systems. 441
discoid l. e. (DLE), a chronic form of cutaneous lupus erythematosus in which the skin lesions mimic those of the systemic form but systemic signs are rare, although multisystem manifestations may develop after many years. 441, 572
systemic l. e., a chronic inflammatory, collagen disease affecting many systems of the body. 441, 441*f*

lymph (limf) a transparent fluid found in lymphatic vessels consisting of a liquid portion and cells that are mostly lymphocytes. 123, 163, 190, 192*f*
l. node, any of the small knots of lymphatic tissue found at intervals along the course of the lymphatic vessels. 190

lymphadenectomy (lim-fad-uh-**nek**-tuh-mē) surgical excision of a lymph node or nodes. 195

lymphadenitis (lim-fad-uh-**nī**-tis) inflammation of a lymph node. 193, 193*f*

lymphadenopathy (lim-fad-uh-**nop**-uh-thē) any disease of the lymph nodes. 193

lymphangiography (lim-fan-jē-**og**-ruh-fē) radiography of the lymphatic vessels after the injection of contrast medium. 193

lymphangioma (lim-fan-jē-**ō**-muh) a tumor composed of newly formed lymph channels. 193

lymphangitis (lim-fan-**jī**-tis) inflammation of a lymphatic vessel. 194, 194*f*

lymphatics (lim-**fat**-iks) a system of vessels that collects tissue fluids from all parts of the body and returns the fluids to the blood circulation; lymphatic system. 190

lymphedema (lim-fuh-**dē**-muh) chronic edema of an extremity because of obstruction within the lymph vessels or the lymph nodes, resulting in accumulation of interstitial fluid. 58*f*, 194, 194*f*

lymphocyte (**lim**-fō-sīt) any of the mononuclear leukocytes found in the blood, lymph, and lymphoid tissues that are responsible for humoral and cellular immunity. 130

lymphogenous (lim-**foj**-uh-nus) producing lymph; produced from lymph or in the lymphatics. 190

lymphogram (**lim**-fō-gram) a radiograph of the lymphatic vessels and lymph nodes. 193

lymphography (lim-**fog**-ruh-fē) radiography of the lymphatic vessels and nodes after injection of radiopaque material. 193

lymphoma (lim-**fō**-muh) a lymphatic tumor; any neoplastic disorder of lymphoid tissue. 194

lymphostasis (lim-**fos**-tuh-sis) stoppage of lymph flow. 194

macrocyte (**mak**-rō-sīt) a very large cell, usually referring to a very large red blood cell. 102, 136

macrocytosis (mak-rō-sī-**tō**-sis) an increase in the number of large red blood cells. 136

macrophage (**mak**-rō-fāj) any of the mononuclear phagocytes found in the walls of blood vessels and in loose connective tissue. 139

macular degeneration (MD) (**mak**-ū-lur dē-jen-ur-ā-shun) a progressive deterioration of the macula lutea of the retina. 511, 511*f*

macule (**mak**-ūl) a discolored spot on the skin that is not elevated above the surface. 574, 574*f*

magnetic resonance imaging (MRI) (mag-**net**-ik rez-ō-nuns **im**-uh-jing) a noninvasive method of creating images of body parts based on the magnetic properties of chemical elements within the body. 68, 68f

malacia (muh-**lā**-shuh) a morbid softness or softening of a tissue or part. 58

malaise (ma-**lāz**) a general feeling of ill health. 101

malaria (muh-**lar**-ē-uh) an infectious disease mainly found in parts of Africa, Asia, Turkey, the West Indies, Central and South America, and Oceania, caused by intracellular protozoa of the genus *Plasmodium* and usually transmitted by the bites of infected mosquitoes. 45

malignant (muh-**lig**-nunt) tending to grow worse and threatening to result in death. 48

malleus (**mal**-ē-us) one of the three ossicles in the middle ear. 514

malnutrition (mal-nōō-**trish**-un) poor nutrition. 102, 269

malocclusion (mal-uh-**klōō**-zhun) improper position of the teeth resulting in the faulty meeting of the teeth or jaws. 271, 271f

mammalgia (muh-**mal**-juh) painful breast. 552

mammogram (**mam**-uh-gram) a radiograph of the breast. 545, 545f

mammography (muh-**mog**-ruh-fē) the use of x-ray examination to diagnose diseases of the breast. 545, 545f
  stereotactic m., biopsy using a computer and imaging to localize a target lesion, especially of the breast. 606, 606f

mammoplasty (**mam**-ō-plas-tē) surgical repair of the breast. 74, 555
  augmentation m., plastic surgery to increase the size of the female breast. 75f, 555
  reduction m., plastic surgery to reduce the size of the female breast. 555

mandible (**man**-di-bul) the bone of the lower jaw. 258

mania (**mā**-nē-uh) a phase of bipolar disorder characterized by expansiveness, elation, agitation, hyperexcitability, hyperactivity, and increased speed of thought and speech (flight of ideas); also called *manic syndrome;* as a combining form, it signifies obsessive preoccupation. 50, 486

mast cell stabilizers (mast sel **stā**-buh-lī-zurz) medications used to prevent or control certain allergic disorders. 238

mastalgia (mas-**tal**-juh) pain in the breast. 552

mastectomy (mas-**tek**-tuh-mē) surgical removal of a breast. 555, 555f
  simple m., removal of the breast, but not all the lymph nodes. 555, 555f

mastitis (mas-**tī**-tis) inflammation of the breast. 552

mastocarcinoma (mas-tō-kahr-si-**nō**-muh) carcinoma of the mammary gland. 552

mastodynia (mas-tō-**din**-ē-uh) painful breast. 552

mastoiditis (mas-toid-**ī**-tis) inflammation of the mastoid antrum and cells. 517

mastopexy (**mas**-tō-pek-sē) plastic surgery to correct a pendulous breast. 555

mastoptosis (mas-tō-**tō**-sis) sagging breasts. 555

maxilla (mak-**sil**-uh) the irregularly shaped bone that helps form the upper jaw. 248

mechanoreceptor (mek-uh-nō-re-**sep**-turz) a receptor that is excited by mechanical pressures or distortions, as those responding to sound, touch, and muscular contractions. 519

mediastinoscope (mē-dē-uh-**stī**-nō-skōp) an endoscope used to examine the mediastinum. 219

mediastinoscopy (mē-dē-as-ti-**nos**-kuh-pē) examination of the mediastinum using an endoscope inserted through an anterior midline incision just above the thoracic inlet. 219

mediastinum (mē-dē-uh-**stī**-num) a median partition; an area in the middle of the chest that contains the heart and its large vessels, trachea, esophagus, thymus, and lymph nodes. 168, 215

medicine (**med**-i-sin) a drug or remedy; the science of diagnosis and treatment of disease and the maintenance of health; the nonsurgical treatment of disease. 13
  emergency m., medical specialty that deals with acutely ill or injured patients who require immediate medical treatment. 21
  forensic m., a branch of medicine that deals with the application of medical knowledge to the purposes of law. 21
  internal m., the branch of medicine concerned with the study of the physiological and pathological characteristics of the internal organs and with the medical diagnosis and treatment. 14
  preventive m., the branch of medicine that aims at prevention of disease and promotion health. 21

medulla (muh-**dul**-uh) the innermost part of an organ or structure. 467, 538
  adrenal m., the inner portion of the adrenal gland, which secretes epinephrine. 538, 541

megadose (**meg**-uh-dōs) a dose that greatly exceeds the amount usually prescribed. 102

megalocyte (**meg**-uh-lō-sīt) an extremely large red blood cell. 102, 136

megalomania (meg-uh-lō-**mā**-nē-uh) a disordered mental state characterized by delusions of grandeur. 486

melanin (**mel**-uh-nin) the dark pigment of the skin, hair, eye, and certain tumors. 55, 537

melanocyte (**mel**-uh-nō-sīt, muh-**lan**-ō-sīt) a black cell; a cell that produces melanin. 578

melanoma (mel-uh-**nō**-muh) a tumor arising from the melanocytic system of the skin and other organs. When used alone the term refers to malignant melanoma. 48f, 578, 578f
  malignant m., a malignant neoplasm of melanocytes that occurs most often in the skin but may occur elsewhere. 48f, 578, 578f

melatonin (mel-uh-**tō**-nin) a hormone synthesized by the pineal gland, the secretion of which increases during exposure to light; in mammals it influences hormone production, and in many species it regulates seasonal changes, such as reproductive pattern and fur color. In humans it is implicated in the regulation of sleep, mood, puberty, and ovarian cycles. 540

membrane (**mem**-brān) a thin layer of tissue that covers a surface, lines a cavity, or divides a space or organ. 55
  extraembryonic m., the membranes external to the developing embryo; the amnion and chorion. 371

menarche (muh-**nahr**-kē) the beginning of menstrual function. 347

meninges (muh-**nin**-jēz) the three membranes covering the brain and the spinal cord: dura mater, arachnoid, and pia mater. 466, 466f

meningioma (muh-nin-jē-**ō**-muh) a benign, slow-growing tumor of the meninges. 479

meningitis (men-in-**jī**-tis) inflammation of the meninges, the membranes that cover the brain and the spinal cord. Meningitis is caused by a variety of infectious microorganisms. 479

meningocele (muh-**ning**-gō-sēl) a hernial protrusion of meninges through a defect in the skull or vertebral column. 478, 478f

meningomyelocele (muh-ning-gō-**mī**-uh-lō-sēl) hernial protrusion of the spinal cord and the meninges through a defect in the spine. 478

menopause (**men**-ō-pawz) that period in a woman's life when menstruation ceases. 347

menorrhagia (men-uh-**rā**-juh) abnormally profuse menstruation. 352

menorrhea (men-uh-**rē**-uh) menstruation; too profuse menstruation. 352

menses (**men**-sēz) menstruation, the monthly flow of blood from the female genital tract. 347

menstrual cycle (**men**-strōō-ul **sī**-kul) the recurring cycle of change in the endometrium in which part of it is shed, then regrows, proliferates, is maintained for several days, and is shed again at menstruation. 346

menstruation (men-strōō-**ā**-shun) the cyclic, physiologic discharge through the vagina of blood and mucosal tissues from the nonpregnant uterus. 347

mesoderm (**mez**-ō-durm) in embryology, the middle layer of cells in the blastoderm. 96, 568

mesothelioma (mē-zō-thē-lē-**ō**-muh) a tumor derived from mesothelial tissue. 230

metabolism (muh-**tab**-uh-liz-um) the sum of all the physical and chemical processes by which living organized substance is produced and maintained (anabolism), and also the transformation by which energy is made available for the uses of the organism (catabolism). 253

metacarpal (met-uh-**kahr**-pul) pertaining to the metacarpus, the part of the hand between the wrist and fingers; one of the bones of the metacarpus. 418

metastasis (muh-**tas**-tuh-sis) a growth of pathogenic microorganisms or of abnormal cells distant from the site primarily involved by the morbid process. 602, 602f

metastasize (muh-**tas**-tuh-sīz) to form new foci of disease in a distant part by metastasis. 604, 604f

metatarsal (met-uh-**tahr**-sul) pertaining to the metatarsus; a bone of the metatarsus. 420

method (**meth**-ud) a technique or procedure for producing a desired effect.
  basal body temperature method, a natural method of family planning that relies on identifying the fertile period of the menstrual cycle by the increased basal body temperature that occurs with ovulation. 374t
  calendar or rhythm m., a natural family planning method using fertility awareness and avoidance of coitus during that period. 374t
  natural family planning m., any of several methods of conception control that do not rely on a medication or a physical device in avoiding pregnancy. 374t
  symptothermal m., a method of family planning that incorporates awareness of ovulation and changes in basal body temperature. 374t

metritis (muh-**trī**-tis) inflammation of uterine tissue. 345

metrorrhagia (mē-trō-**rā**-juh) uterine bleeding, usually of normal amount, occurring at completely irregular intervals, the period of flow sometimes being prolonged. 352

microbe (**mī**-krōb) a minute living organism, such as a bacterium, protozoan, or fungus. 115

microbiology (mī-krō-bī-**ol**-uh-jē) the science that deals with the study of microorganisms. 40

microcardia (mī-krō-**kahr**-dē-uh) smallness of the heart. 180

microcyte (**mī**-krō-sīt) an abnormally small erythrocyte, five microns or less in diameter. 102, 136

microcytosis (mī-krō-sī-**tō**-sis) an increase in the number of undersized red blood cells. 136

microorganism (mī-krō-**or**-gan-iz-um) a minute living organism, usually microscopic; types include bacteria, rickettsiae, viruses, molds, yeasts, and protozoa. 40, 40f

microscope (**mī**-krō-skōp) an instrument for viewing small objects that must be magnified to be seen. 53, 53f

microscopy (mī-**kros**-kuh-pē) viewing things with a microscope. 53

microtia (mī-**krō**-shuh) severe hypoplasia or aplasia of the pinna of the ear with a blind or absent external auditory meatus. 100, 100f

micturition (mik-tū-**ri**-shun) urination. 308

midbrain (**mid**-brān) the part of the brain that connects the pons and the cerebellum with the hemispheres of the cerebrum; mesencephalon. 467

midsection (mid-**sek**-shun) a cut through the middle of an organ or part. 96

milligram (**mil**-i-gram) one thousandth of a gram. 94

milliliter (**mil**-i-lē-tur) a metric unit of measurement that is one thousandth of a liter. 93

mineralocorticoid (min-ur-ul-ō-**kor**-ti-koid) any of the group of corticosteroids, principally aldosterone, predominantly involved in the regulation of electrolyte and water balance in the body. 538, 538t

minerals (**min**-ur-ulz) solid inorganic substances that occur in nature. 77

miotics (mī-**ot**-iks) substances that causes constriction of the pupil of the eye. 521

mitral (**mī**-trul) pertaining to the mitral or bicuspid valve; shaped like a miter.
m. valve, a bicuspid valve situated between the left atrium and the left ventricle; bicuspid valve. 167, 170*f*
m. valve prolapse (MVP), protrusion of one or both cusps of the mitral valve back into the left atrium during ventricular contraction. 182

mittelschmerz (**mit**-ul-shmertz) pain associated with ovulation, usually occurring in the middle of the menstrual cycle. 352

molar (**mō**-lur) a posterior tooth that is used for grinding food and acts as a major jaw support in the dental arch. 258

Monilia (mō-**nil**-ē-uh) a genus of fungi. 371

moniliasis (mon-i-**lī**-uh-sis) candidiasis; any infection caused by a species of *Candida*, especially *Candida albicans*. 391

monocyte (**mon**-ō-sīt) an important type of leukocyte that is mononuclear. 94, 130

mononeuropathy (mon-ō-noo-**rop**-thē) any disease or disorder that affects a single nerve trunk. 93

monoplegia (mon-ō-**plē**-juh) paralysis of a limb. 478

monovision (**mon**-ō-vish-un) vision resulting from correction of one eye for near vision and the other eye for far vision, especially with contact lens. 95

mons pubis (monz **pū**-bis) the rounded fleshy prominence over the symphysis pubis. 342

mood stabilizers (mō͞od **stā**-bi-lī-zerz) drugs used to treat mood disorders. 492

mucoid (**mū**-koid) resembling mucus. 255

mucolytic (mū-kō-**lit**-ik) dissolving mucus; an agent that dissolves or destroys mucus. 238

mucosa (mū-**kō**-suh) mucous membrane. 255

mucous (**mū**-kus) pertaining or relating to or resembling mucus; mucoid; covered with mucus; secreting, producing, or containing mucus. 124, 255

mucus (**mū**-kus) the free slime of the mucous membranes, composed of secretion of the glands, various salts, desquamated cells, and leukocytes. 124

multicellular (mul-tē-**sel**-ū-lur) consisting of more than one cell. 93

multigravida (mul-tē-**grav**-i-duh) a female who has been pregnant more than once. 377

multipara (mul-**tip**-uh-ruh) a female who has produced more than one viable offspring. 377

multiple myeloma (**mul**-ti-pul mī-uh-**lō**-muh) a disseminated type of plasma cell dyscrasia characterized by multiple bone marrow tumors. 439

murmur (**mur**-mur) an auscultatory sound, particularly a periodic sound of short duration of cardiac or vascular origin. 179
heart m., an abnormal sound heard on auscultation of the heart, caused by altered blood flow into a chamber or through a valve. 179

muscle (**mus**-ul) an organ that produces movement of an animal by contraction. 424
arrector pili m., minute smooth muscle attached to the connective tissue sheath of the hair follicle, capable of causing the hair to stand erect. 569
m. relaxant, an agent that causes the muscles to relax. 449
perineal m., any of the muscles of the perineum. 315
skeletal m., striated muscles that are attached to bones and bring about voluntary movement. 424, 424*f*
visceral m., smooth involuntary muscle of the internal organs. 424, 424*f*

myalgia (mī-**al**-juh) pain in a muscle or muscles. 58, 432

myasthenia (mī-us-**thē**-ne-uh) muscle weakness. 443
m. gravis, a disease characterized by muscle weakness, caused by a functional abnormality. 443, 482

mycodermatitis (mī-kō-dur-muh-**tī**-tis) inflammation of the skin caused by a fungus. 576

mydriatic (mid-rē-**at**-ik) an ophthalmic agent that dilates the pupil. 509

myelin sheath (**mī**-uh-lin shēth) the sheath surrounding the axon of some (the myelinated) nerve cells. 464

myelitis (mī-uh-**lī**-tis) inflammation of the bone marrow; inflammation of the spinal cord. 438

myeloblast (**mī**-uh-lō-blast) embryonic form of blood cell found in the bone marrow. 410

myelocyte (**mī**-uh-lō-sīt) a cell found in the bone marrow. 410

myelogram (**mī**-uh-lō-gram) x-ray image of the spinal cord. 472

myelography (mī-uh-**log**-ruh-fē) radiography of the spinal cord after injection of a contrast medium into the subarachnoid space. 472

myelosuppression (mī-uh-lō-suh-**presh**-un) inhibition of bone marrow activity. 429

myelosuppressive (mī-uh-lō-suh-**pres**-iv) inhibiting bone marrow activity; an agent that inhibits bone marrow activity. 447

myoblast (**mī**-ō-blast) embryonic cell that becomes a cell of the muscle fiber. 424

myocarditis (mī-ō-kahr-**dī**-tis) inflammation of the heart muscle. 178

myocardium (mī-ō-**kahr**-dē-um) the middle and thickest layer of the heart wall, made up of cardiac muscle. 168, 424

myocele (**mī**-ō-sēl) hernia of the muscle. 443

myocellulitis (mī-ō-sel-ū-**lī**-tis) inflammation of cellular tissue and muscle. 438

myodynia (mī-ō-**din**-ē-uh) pain in a muscle. 432

myofibrosis (mī-ō-fī-**brō**-sis) replacement of muscle tissue by fibrous tissue. 443

myolysis (mī-**ol**-i-sis) destruction of muscle tissue. 443

myomalacia (mī-ō-muh-**lā**-shuh) morbid softening of muscle. 443

myometritis (mī-ō-muh-**trī**-tis) inflammation of the myometrium, the muscular substance of the uterus. 355

myometrium (mī-ō-**mē**-trē-um) the smooth muscle of the uterus. 346

myopathy (mī-**op**-uh-thē) any disease of muscle. 443

myopia (mī-ō-**pē**-uh) the error of refraction in which rays of light entering the eye are brought to a focus in front of the retina; also called *nearsightedness*. 510

myoplasty (**mī**-ō-plas-tē) surgical repair of a muscle. 447

myorrhaphy (mī-**or**-uh-fē) suture of divided muscle. 447

myringitis (mir-in-**jī**-tis) inflammation or infection of the tympanic membrane. 517

myxedema (mik-suh-**dē**-muh) a condition resulting from hypothyroidism characterized by dry, waxy swelling of the skin. 548

narcolepsy (**nahr**-kō-lep-sē) recurrent, uncontrollable brief episodes of sleep. 480

narcotic (nahr-**kot**-ik) pertaining to or producing narcosis, nonspecific and reversible depression of function of the central nervous system (CNS) marked by stupor or insensibility produced by drugs; an agent that produces insensibility or stupor, applied especially to the opioids. 76
n. drugs, analgesics that produce insensibility or stupor. 491

naris (**nā**-ris) either of the external orifices of the nose; nares (**nā**-rēz) (plural). 213

nasogastric (nā-zō-**gas**-trik) pertaining to the nose and stomach. 283
n. tube, any tube passed into the stomach through the nose. 283

nasolacrimal sac (na-zō-**lak**-ri-mul sak) a pouch that receives tears from the lacrimal duct, from which tears drain into the nasolacrimal duct. 505

nasopharyngitis (nā-zō-far-in-**jī**-tis) inflammation of the nasopharynx. 225

nasopharynx (nā-zō-**far**-inks) the upper part of the pharynx, continuous with the nasal passages. 213

nasoscope (**nā**-zō-skōp) instrument for examining inside the nose. 218

nebulizer (**neb**-ū-lī-zur) a device for creating and throwing an aerosol spray. 238

necrosis (nuh-**krō**-sis) death of tissue. 125, 583, 584*f*

neonate (**nē**-ō-nāt) a newborn child. 379

neonatologist (nē-ō-nā-**tol**-uh-jist) a physician who specializes in care of the newborn. 379

neonatology (nē-ō-nā-**tol**-uh-jē) the branch of medicine dealing with treatment of the newborn infant. 16, 379

neoplasm (**nē**-ō-plaz-um) a new or abnormal growth either benign or malignant. 48, 278*f*

nephrectomy (nuh-**frek**-tuh-mē) surgical excision of a kidney. 325, 325*f*
laparoscopic n., removal of a kidney through several small incisions in the abdominal wall. 326

nephritis (nuh-**frī**-tis) inflammation of the kidney. 319
interstitial n., inflammation of the interstitial tissue of the kidney, including the tubules. 319

nephrolith (**nef**-rō-lith) a kidney stone. 324

nephrolithiasis (nef-rō-li-**thī**-uh-sis) a condition marked by the presence of kidney stones. 324

nephrolithotomy (nef-rō-li-**thot**-uh-mē) removal of renal calculi by cutting into the kidney. 327

nephrolysis (nuh-**frol**-uh-sis) destruction of kidney tissue; freeing of a kidney from adhesions. 320

nephromalacia (nef-rō-muh-**lā**-shuh) softening of the kidney. 320

nephromegaly (nef-rō-**meg**-uh-lē) enlargement of the kidney. 320

nephron (**nef**-ron) the structural and functional unit of the kidney. 307, 307*f*

nephropathy (nuh-**frop**-uh-thē) any disease of the kidneys. 320
obstructive n., a kidney disease caused by obstruction of the urinary tract. 320, 320*f*

nephropexy (**nef**-rō-pek-sē) surgical fixation of a floating kidney. 329

nephroptosis (nef-rop-**tō**-sis, nef-rō-**tō**-sis) downward displacement of the kidney; floating kidney. 324

nephrosclerosis (nef-rō-skluh-**rō**-sis) hardening of the kidney caused by renovascular disease. 322

nephroscope (**nef**-rō-skōp) an instrument inserted into an incision in the renal pelvis for viewing the interior of the kidney. 316, 317*f*

nephroscopy (nuh-**fros**-kuh-pē) visualization of the kidney using a nephroscope. 316, 317*f*

nephrosonography (nef-rō-sō-**nog**-ruh-fē) ultrasonic scanning of the kidney. 316

nephrostomy (nuh-**fros**-tuh-mē) a surgical procedure in which a catheter is inserted directly into the renal pelvis to drain the kidney. 314
percutaneous n., placement of a catheter into the kidney through the skin, providing for diversion of the renal output, certain surgical procedures, including biopsies, and infusion of substances to dissolve calculi. 328, 328*f*

nephrotomogram (nef-rō-**tō**-mō-gram) a sectional radiograph of the kidney obtained by nephrotomography. 316, 316*f*

nephrotomography (nef-rō-tō-**mog**-ruh-fē) radiologic visualization of the kidney by tomography after intravenous introduction of contrast medium. 316, 316*f*

nephroureterectomy (nef-rō-ū-rē-tur-**ek**-tuh-mē) excision of a kidney and all or part of the ureter. 326

neuralgia (noo-**ral**-juh) pain of a nerve. 473

neurasthenia (noor-us-**thē**-nē-uh) a nervous condition characterized by chronic weakness, easy fatigability, and sometimes exhaustion. 487

neurectomy (noo-**rek**-tuh-mē) excision of a part of a nerve. 489

neuritis (noo-**rī**-tis) inflammation of a nerve. 49

neuroglia (noo-**rog**-lē-uh) the supporting structure of nervous tissue. 463

neurohypophysis (noor-ō-hī-**pof**-uh-sis) the posterior lobe of the pituitary gland. 533, 539*f*

neuroleptics (noor-ō-**lep**-tiks) drugs that depress nerve function; a major tranquilizer. 492

neurologist (noo-**rol**-uh-jist) a specialist in the treatment of nervous diseases. 19

neurology (noo-**rol**-uh-jē) the branch of medicine that deals with the study of the nervous system. 14, 19

neurolysis (noo-**rol**-i-sis) release of a nerve sheath by cutting it longitudinally; operative breaking up of perineural adhesions; relief of tension on a nerve; exhaustion of nervous energy; destruction of nerve tissue. 72, 489

neuroma (noo-**rō**-muh) a tumor made up of nerve cells and nerve fibers. 480
  Morton n., a neuroma resulting from compression of a branch of the plantar nerve by the metatarsal heads. 435
neuromuscular blocking drugs (noor-ō-**mus**-kū-lur **blok**-ing drugz) a group of drugs that prevents motor nerve endings from exciting skeletal muscle, thus causing paralysis of the affected area. 76, 449
neuron (**noor**-on) any of the conducting cells of the nervous system. 18, 19, 19*f*, 463, 464*f*
  motor n., one of various efferent nerve cells that transmit impulses from either the brain or spinal cord. 465
  sensory n., an afferent nerve cell conveying sensory impulses. 465
neuropathy (noo-**rop**-uh-thē) inflammation or degeneration of the peripheral nerves. 519
  obstructive n., pathological change in the peripheral nervous system due to an obstruction. 320
  peripheral n., disease of the peripheral nerves, most commonly those of the extremities. 476
neuroplasty (**noor**-ō-plas-tē) plastic repair of a nerve. 489
neurorrhaphy (noo-**ror**-uh-fē) suturing of a cut nerve. 489
neurosurgeon (**noor**-ō-sur-jun) a surgeon who specializes in work on the nervous system. 19
neurosurgery (noor-ō-**sur**-jur-ē) surgery of the nervous system. 19
neurosyphilis (noor-ō-**sif**-i-lis) the central nervous system (CNS) manifestations of syphilis. 388
neurotripsy (**noor**-ō-trip-sē) surgical crushing of a nerve. 489
neutrophil (**noo**-trō-fil) a granular leukocyte having a nucleus with three to five lobes and cytoplasm containing fine inconspicuous granules. 130
nevus (**nē**-vus) any congenital lesion of the skin; a birthmark. 577
nitroglycerin (nī-trō-**glis**-ur-in) a drug used chiefly in the prophylaxis and treatment of angina pectoris, administered sublingually. 196
nociceptor (nō-si-**sep**-tur) a receptor for pain caused by injury to body tissues. 519
nocturia (nok-**tū**-rē-uh) excessive urination at night. 318
node (nōd) a small mass of tissue as a swelling, knot, or protuberance, either normal or abnormal.
  atrioventricular node, specialized heart muscle fibers that receive impulses from the sinoatrial node and transmit them to the bundle of His. 171
  axillary n., one of the lymph glands in the axilla. 190
  cervical lymph n., any of a cluster of lymph nodes located in the neck. 190
  inguinal n., any of the nodes in the upper femoral triangle of the thigh. 190
  lymph n., one of the many small oval structures that filter the lymph and fight infection, and in which lymphocytes, monocytes, and plasma cells are formed. 49*f*
  n. of Ranvier, one of several constrictions in the myelin sheath of a nerve fiber. 464, 464*f*
  sinoatrial n., a knot of modified cardiac tissue that acts as a natural pacemaker of the heart. 170
nodule (**nod**-ūl) a small node that is solid and can be detected by touch. 573
nonsteroidal antiinflammatory drugs (non-ster-**oid**-ul an-tē-in-**flam**-uh-tor-ē drugz) medications used to treat inflammation. 77, 142, 448, 491
norepinephrine (nor-ep-i-**nef**-rin) one of the naturally occurring catecholamines; a neurohormone and a major neurotransmitter. It is also secreted by the adrenal medulla and is released predominantly in response to hypotension and stress. 538
normocyte (**nor**-mō-sīt) a normal-sized red blood cell. 136
nuclear medicine imaging (**noo**-klē-ur med-i-sin **im**-uh-jing) a medical specialty involving using radioactive substances in the diagnosis and treatment of disease. 266
nucleoid (**noo**-klē-oid) resembling a nucleus. 130
nullipara (nuh-**lip**-uh-ruh) a female individual who has never borne a child. 93, 378
nutrition (**noo**-trish-un) the sum of the processes involved in taking in nutrients and assimilating and using them; nutriment. 252
  total parenteral n., the intravenous administration of the total nutrient requirements of a patient with gastrointestinal dysfunction. 283
nyctalopia (nik-tuh-**lō**-pē-uh) poor vision at night or in dim light. 511
nycturia (nik-**tū**-rē-ul) frequent urination during the night, especially the passage of more urine at night than during the day. 318
obesity (ō-**bēs**-i-tē) an increase in body weight beyond the limitation of skeletal and physical requirements, as the result of an excessive accumulation of fat in the body. 269
  endogenous o., obesity resulting from the dysfunction of the endocrine or metabolic function. 269
  exogenous o., obesity caused by a caloric intake greater than needed. 269
obsession (ob-**sesh**-un) a recurrent, persistent thought, image, or impulse that is unwanted and comes involuntarily. 484
obstetrician (ob-stuh-**tri**-shun) a physician who specializes in the treatment of pregnancy, labor, and delivery. 376
obstetrics (ob-**stet**-riks) a branch of surgery that deals with the management of pregnancy and delivery. 16, 376
ointment (**oint**-munt) a medication that contains fat and is of such consistency that it melts when applied to the skin. 587
olfaction (ol-**fak**-shun) the sense of smell; the act of smelling. 213, 520
oligospermia (ol-i-gō-**spur**-mē-uh) deficiency in the number of spermatozoa in the semen. 368
oliguria (ol-i-**gū**-rē-uh) excretion of a diminished amount of urine in relation to the fluid intake, usually defined as less than 500 mL per 24 hours. 317
omphalitis (om-fuh-**lī**-tis) inflammation of the navel. 115
omphalocele (**om**-fuh-lō-sēl) hernia of the navel. 114, 114*f*

omphaloma (om-fuh-lō-**lō**-muh) tumor of the navel. 115
omphalorrhagia (om-fuh-lō-**rā**-juh) hemorrhage from the umbilicus. 115
omphalorrhexis (om-fuh-lō-**rek**-sis) rupture of the umbilicus. 115
omphalus (**om**-fuh-lus) the navel. 114
oncologist (ong-**kol**-uh-jist) a specialist in the study and treatment of tumors. 70
  radiation o., oncologist who specializes in radiation therapy. 18, 70
oncology (ong-**kol**-uh-jē) study of tumors. 18, 70
  radiation o., the medical specialty that treats cancer with ionizing radiation. 18, 70
onychectomy (on-i-**kek**-tuh-mē) excision of a nail or nail bed; removal of the claws of an animal. 585
onycholysis (on-i-**kol**-i-sis) detachment of the nail from the nail bed. 583, 583*f*
onychomalacia (on-i-kō-muh-**lā**-shuh) softening of the nails. 583
onychomycosis (on-i-kō-mī-**kō**-sis) a disease of the nails caused by a fungus. 583, 583*f*
onychopathy (on-i-**kop**-uh-thē) any disease of the nails. 583
onychophagia (on-i-kō-**fā**-juh) habit of biting the nails. 570
onychophagist (on-i-**kof**-uh-jist) one who has the habit of nail biting. 570
onychosis (on-i-**kō**-sis) a condition of atrophy or dystrophy of the nails. 583
ooblast (**ō**-ō-blast) an embryonic egg. 372
oogenesis (ō-ō-**jen**-uh-sis) the origin and formation of eggs in the female sex. 348
oophoralgia (ō-ō-ur-**al**-juh) ovarian pain. 353
oophorectomy (ō-of-uh-**rek**-tuh-mē) the removal of an ovary or ovaries. 358
  laparoscopic o., removal of the ovaries using a laparoscope and making small incisions in the abdominal wall. 358
oophoritis (ō-of-uh-**rī**-tis) inflammation of an ovary. 353
oophorohysterectomy (ō-of-uh-rō-his-tur-**ek**-tuh-mē) removal of the uterus, ovaries, and uterine tubes. 358
oophoropathy (ō-of-uh-**rop**-uh-thē) any disease of the ovaries. 353
oophoropexy (ō-**of**-uh-rō-pek-sē) surgical fixation of the ovary. 358
oophorosalpingectomy (ō-of-uh-rō-sal-pin-**jek**-tuh-mē) surgical removal of an ovary and uterine tube. 358
oophorosalpingitis (ō-of-uh-rō-sal-pin-**jī**-tis) inflammation of an ovary and uterine tube. 353
ophthalmalgia (of-thul-**mal**-juh) pain in the eye. 58
ophthalmitis (of-thul-**mī**-tis) inflammation of the eye. 49
ophthalmodynia (of-thal-mō-**din**-ē-uh) pain in the eye. 58
ophthalmologist (of-thul-**mol**-uh-jist) a physician who specializes in the diagnosis and treatment of eye disease. 58
ophthalmology (of-thul-**mol**-uh-jē) the study of the eye and its diseases. 17, 17*f*
ophthalmomalacia (of-thal-mō-muh-**lā**-shuh) abnormal softness of the eye. 58
ophthalmometer (of-thul-**mom**-uh-tur) an instrument for measuring the eye. 509
ophthalmopathy (of-thul-**mop**-uh-thē) any disease of the eye. 50
ophthalmoplasty (of-**thal**-mō-plas-tē) plastic surgery of the eye or its appendages. 72
ophthalmorrhagia (of-thal-mō-**rā**-juh) hemorrhage from the eye. 58
ophthalmoscope (of-**thal**-mō-skōp) an instrument used to examine the interior of the eye. 62, 63*f*, 508
ophthalmoscopy (of-thul-**mos**-kuh-pē) examination of the eye using an ophthalmoscope. 508
ophthalmotomy (of-thul-**mot**-uh-mē) incision of the eyeball. 72
opioid antagonists (ō-pē-oid an-**tag**-uh-nists) receptor antagonists that act to block the receptor, preventing the body from responding to opioids and endorphins. 27
optic (**op**-tik) pertaining to the eyes or to sight.
  o. disc, the small blind spot on the surface of the retina. 506
  o. nerve, one of a pair of nerves that transmit visual impulses. 506
optometrist (op-**tom**-uh-trist) a specialist in optometry. 508
orchialgia (or-kē-**al**-juh) pain in a testis. 368
orchidalgia (or-ki-**dal**-juh) pain in a testis. 368
orchiditis (or-ki-**dī**-tis) inflammation of a testicle. 368
orchidopexy (**or**-ki-dō-pek-sē) orchiopexy. 368
orchiectomy (or-kē-**ek**-tuh-mē) excision of one or both testes. 368
orchiepididymitis (or-kē-ep-i-did-i-**mī**-tis) inflammation of a testicle and an epididymis. 368
orchiopathy (or-kē-**op**-uh-thē) any disease of the testes. 366
orchiopexy (or-kē-ō-pek-sē) surgical fixation of an undescended testis in the scrotum. 369
orchioplasty (**or**-kē-ō-plas-tē) plastic surgery of a testis. 368
orchiorrhaphy (or-kē-**or**-uh-fē) orchiopexy or suturing a testicle for fixation purposes. 368
orchiotomy (or-kē-**ot**-uh-mē) incision and drainage of a testis. 368
orchitis (or-**kī**-tis) inflammation of a testis. This is not a common disorder, but it can occur in a variety of infectious diseases. 368
oropharynx (or-ō-**far**-inks) that part of the pharynx between the soft palate and the upper edge of the epiglottis. 213
orthodontics (or-thō-**don**-tiks) the branch of dentistry concerned with irregularities of teeth and malocclusions and associated facial problems. 259
orthodontist (or-thō-**don**-tist) a dentist who specializes in orthodontics. 259
orthopedic (or-thō-**pē**-dik) pertaining to the correction of deformities of the musculoskeletal system. 444
  o. surgeon, a surgeon who specializes in orthopedics. 20
orthopedics (or-thō-**pē**-diks) that branch of surgery specially concerned with the preservation and restoration of the function of the skeletal system, its articulations, and associated structures. 20, 21*f*
orthopedist (or-thō-**pē**-dist) an orthopedic surgeon. 20, 21*f*, 444
orthopnea (or-thop-**nē**-uh) a condition in which breathing is possible only when the person is in an upright position. 222

ossicle (**os**-i-kul) a small bone, such as the malleus, the incus, or the stapes of the middle ear. 514, 514*f*

ossification (os-i-fi-**kā**-shun) the development of bone. 410

ostealgia (os-tē-**al**-juh) any pain associated with an abnormal condition within a bone. 438

ostectomy, osteectomy (os-**tek**-tuh-mē, os-tē-**ek**-tuh-mē) excision of a bone or a portion of a bone. 447

osteitis (os-tē-**ī**-tis) inflammation of a bone. 49
    o. deformans, a disease of bone marked by repeated episodes of increased bone resorption followed by excessive attempts at repair, resulting in weakened deformed bones of increased mass; also called *Paget disease*. 436

osteoarthritis (os-tē-ō-ahr-**thrī**-tis) degenerative joint disease characterized by degeneration of the articular cartilage, hypertrophy of bone at the margins, and changes in the synovial membrane. 442

osteoarthropathy (os-tē-ō-ahr-**throp**-uh-thē) any disease of the bones and joints. 441

osteoblast (**os**-tē-ō-blast) embryonic form of a bone cell. 410

osteochondritis (os-tē-ō-kon-**drī**-tis) inflammation of the bone and cartilage. 436

osteochondroma (os-tē-ō-kon-**drō**-muh) a benign tumor of bone and cartilage. 438

osteocyte (**os**-tē-ō-sīt) a cell that makes up the bone matrix. 410

osteodynia (os-tē-ō-**din**-ē-uh) pain in the bone. 438

osteogenesis (os-tē-ō-**jen**-uh-sis) the formation of bone. 410

osteoid (**os**-tē-oid) resembling bone. 58

osteolysis (os-tē-**ol**-uh-sis) destruction of the bone. 436

osteomalacia (os-tē-ō-muh-**lā**-shuh) a skeletal disorder characterized by a disturbance in bone metabolism. 436

osteomyelitis (os-tē-ō-mī-uh-**lī**-tis) inflammation of the bone and bone marrow caused by a pyogenic organism. 438

osteopenia (os-tē-ō-**pē**-nē-uh) reduced bone mass caused by insufficient bone synthesis to keep pace with normal bone destruction. 437

osteoplasty (**os**-tē-ō-plas-tē) plastic surgery of the bones. 447

osteoporosis (os-tē-ō-puh-**rō**-sis) reduction in the amount of bone mass, leading to fractures after minimal trauma. 436, 437*f*

osteosarcoma (os-tē-ō-sahr-**kō**-muh) a malignant primary neoplasm of bone composed of a malignant connective tissue stroma with evidence of malignant, osteoid, bone, or cartilage formation. 438

osteosclerosis (os-tē-ō-skluh-**rō**-sis) the hardening or abnormal density of bone. 436

osteotome (**os**-tē-ō-tōm) an instrument used to cut bone. 447

osteotomy (os-tē-**ot**-uh-mē) the surgical cutting of a bone. 74

otalgia (ō-**tal**-juh) pain in the ear; earache. 58, 517

otitis (ō-**tī**-tis) inflammation of the ear. 517
    o. externa, inflammation or infection of the external canal or the auricle of the external ear. 517
    o. interna, inflammation or dysfunction of the canals of the inner ear, resulting in vertigo. 517
    o. media, inflammation of the middle ear. 517

otodynia (ō-tō-**din**-ē-uh) pain in the ear; earache. 58

otolaryngologist (ō-tō-lar-ing-**gol**-uh-jist) a physician who specializes in otolaryngology. 17

otolaryngology (ō-tō-lar-ing-**gol**-uh-jē) that branch of medicine concerned with medical and surgical treatment of the head and neck, including the ears, nose, and throat. 17

otologist (ō-**tol**-uh-jist) a physician trained in the diagnosis and treatment of disease and disorders of the ear. 17

otology (ō-**tol**-uh-jē) the study of the ear, including the diagnosis and treatment of its diseases and disorders. 17

otomycosis (ō-tō-mī-**kō**-sis) a lesion of the external ear caused by a fungus infection. 517

otopathy (ō-**top**-uh-thē) any disease of the ear. 50

otoplasty (ō-tō-plas-tē) plastic surgery of the ear. 73, 518

otorrhea (ō-tō-**rē**-uh) discharge from the ear. 58, 517

otosclerosis (ō-tō-skluh-**rō**-sis) a pathologic condition of the ear in which there is formation of spongy bone and that usually results in hearing loss. 517

otoscope (ō-tō-skōp) an instrument for viewing inside the ear. 515

otoscopic examination (ō-tō-**skōp**-ik eg-zam-i-**nā**-shun) use of an otoscope to examine the ear. 515

otoscopy (ō-**tos**-kuh-pē) viewing the inside of the ear using an otoscope. 60, 60*f*, 515

oval window (ō-vul **win**-dō) an aperture in the wall of the middle ear, leading to the inner ear. 515

ovary (**ō**-vuh-rē) the female gonad; either of the paired female organs in which eggs are formed. 343

ovulation (ov-ū-**lā**-shun) the discharge of an egg from a vesicular follicle of the ovary. 347, 348*f*, 371
    o. method, a natural method of family planning that uses observation of changes in the character and quantity of cervical mucusa to determine the time of ovulation. 374*t*
    o. stimulants, (ov-ū-**lā**-shun stim-**ū**-lunts) drugs that stimulate ovulation. 391

ovum (**ō**-vum) an egg; the female reproductive germ cell; ova (plural). 343, 371

oxygenation (ok-si-juh-**nā**-shun) the act, process, or result of adding oxygen. 236

oxytocics (ok-sē-**tō**-siks) drugs that hasten or facilitate childbirth by stimulating uterine contractions. 392

oxytocin (ok-sē-**tō**-sin) a pituitary hormone that stimulates uterine contractions and milk ejection. 386, 535

palate (**pal**-ut) the roof of the mouth, which separates the nasal and oral cavities. 213

palatitis (pal-uh-**tī**-tis) inflammation of the palate. 225

palatoplasty (**pal**-uh-tō-plas-tē) plastic reconstruction of the palate. 236

pallor (**pal**-ur) paleness or absence of skin coloration. 132

palpation (pal-**pā**-shun) the act of feeling with the hand; the application of the fingers with light pressure to the surface of the body for the purpose of determining the consistency of the parts beneath in physical diagnosis. 61

palpitation (pal-pi-**tā**-shun) a subjective sensation of an unduly rapid or irregular heartbeat. 180

palsy (**pawl**-zē) paralysis.
    Bell p., unilateral facial paralysis of sudden onset caused by facial nerve lesion and resulting in characteristic facial distortion. 477, 477*f*
    cerebral p., a brain disorder characterized by paralysis and lack of muscle coordination. 478, 478*f*

pancreas (**pan**-krē-us) a large, elongated gland situated transversely behind the stomach, between the spleen and the duodenum. The external secretion of the pancreas contains a variety of digestive enzymes. An internal secretion, insulin, is concerned with the regulation of carbohydrate metabolism. Glucagon is also produced by the pancreas. 264*f*, 531

pancreatectomy (pan-krē-uh-**tek**-tuh-mē) excision of the pancreas. 289

pancreatitis (pan-krē-uh-**tī**-tis) inflammation of the pancreas. 281, 550

pancreatoduodenostomy (pan-krē-uh-tō-dōō-ō-duh-**nos**-tuh-mē) surgical anastomosis of a pancreatic duct, cyst, or fistula to the duodenum. 554

pancreatography (pan-krē-uh-**tog**-ruh-fē) x-ray examination of the pancreas, performed during surgery by injecting contrast medium into the pancreatic duct. 267

pancreatolith (pan-krē-**at**-ō-lith) a pancreatic stone. 281

pancreatolithectomy (pan-krē-uh-tō-li-**thek**-tuh-mē) surgical excision of pancreatic calculi. 289

pancreatolithiasis (pan-krē-uh-tō-li-**thī**-uh-sis) presence of pancreatic stones. 281

pancreatolysis (pan-krē-uh-**tol**-i-sis) destruction of pancreatic tissue. 281

pancreatotomy (pan-krē-uh-**tot**-uh-mē) incision of the pancreas. 289

pandemic (pan-**dem**-ik) a widespread epidemic of a disease. 93

panic attack (**pan**-ik uh-**tak**) an episode of acute anxiety that occurs unpredictably with numerous symptoms including chest pain or palpitations. 485

Papanicolaou or **Pap smear** (pap-uh-**nik**-ō-lā-ōō, pap smēr) collection of material from areas of the body that shed cells, especially the cervix and the vagina, followed by microscopic study of the cells for diagnosing cancer. 349, 349*f*

Papanicolaou test (pap-uh-**nik**-ō-lā-ōō test) a smear method of examining stained exfoliative cells. 349

papule (**pap**-ūl) a red, elevated, solid, and circumscribed area of the skin. 512
    abdominal p., abdominocentesis. 574, 574*f*

paralysis (puh-**ral**-i-sis) the loss of muscle function, sensation, or both. 477

paracentesis (par-uh-sun-**tē**-sis) a procedure in which fluid is withdrawn from a body cavity. 113
    abdominal p., removal of excess fluid from the peritoneal cavity. 113

paramedic (par-uh-**med**-ik) a person who acts as an assistant to a physician or in place of a physician until a physician is available. 96

paranoia (par-uh-**noi**-uh) a condition characterized by an elaborate, overly suspicious system of thinking. 487

paranormal (par-uh-**nor**-mul) beyond normal or natural. 96

paraphilia (par-uh-**fil**-ē-uh) a psychosexual disorder characterized by recurrent intense sexual disorders. 486

paraplegia (par-uh-**plē**-juh) paralysis of the legs and lower part of the body, often caused by disease or injury to the spine. 477, 477*f*

parasympathetic (par-uh-sim-puh-**thet**-ik) referring to the nerves that are part of the autonomic system and work against the sympathetic nerves. 470

parathormone (PTH) (par-uh-**thor**-mōn) parathyroid hormone. 542

parathyroidectomy (par-uh-thī-roid-**ek**-tuh-mē) removal of one or more of the parathyroid glands. 554

parenteral (puh-**ren**-tur-ul) injection into the body, not through the alimentary canal. 283

paresthesia (par-es-**thē**-zhuh) an abnormal touch sensation, such as burning or prickling, often in the absence of an external stimulus. 473

parity (**par**-i-tē) the classification of a woman by the number of live-born children and stillbirths she has delivered at more than 20 weeks of gestation. 377

parotitis (par-ō-**tī**-tis) inflammation of the parotid gland. 261
    epidemic p., mumps. 272

paroxysmal (par-ok-**siz**-mul) occurring in sudden, periodic attacks or recurrence of symptoms of a disease. 228

parturition (pahr-tū-**ri**-shun) childbirth. 376

patella (puh-**tel**-uh) the kneecap, a lens-shaped bone situated in front of the knee. 420

patellar response (puh-**tel**-ur rē-**spons**) a deep tendon reflex elicited by a sharp tap on the tendon just distal to the patella. 465

patent (**pā**-tunt) open, unobstructed, or not closed.
    p. ductus arteriosus (PDA), an abnormal opening between the pulmonary artery and the aorta. 179

pathogen (**path**-ō-jun) any disease-producing agent or microorganism. 40

pathogenicity (path-ō-juh-**nis**-i-tē) the ability of a pathogenic agent to produce a disease. 40

pathologist (puh-**thol**-uh-jist) a physician who specializes in the study of the essential nature of disease. 15
    clinical p., a physician specialized in the branch of pathology that is applied to the solution of clinical problems, especially the use of laboratory methods in clinical diagnosis. 15
    surgical p., a physician specialized in the study of disease processes that are surgically accessible for diagnosis or treatment. 15

pathology (puh-**thol**-uh-jē) the study of the changes caused by disease in the structure or functions of the body. 15, 22
anatomical p., study of the effects of disease on the body's structure. 15
clinical p., the study of disease by the use of laboratory tests and methods. 15
pediatrician (pē-dē-uh-**tri**-shun) a physician who specializes in the treatment of children's diseases. 16, 16*f*
pediatrics (pē-dē-**at**-riks) the branch of medicine that is devoted to the study of children's diseases. 16
pediculicides (puh-**dik**-ū-li-sīdz) substances used to treat lice. 588
pediculosis (puh-dik-ū-**lō**-sis) infestation with lice of the family Pediculidae. 572
pedodontics (pē-dō-**don**-tiks) the branch of dentistry that deals with the teeth and mouth conditions of children. 259
pedodontist (pē-dō-**don**-tist) a dentist who specializes in the teeth and mouth conditions of children. 259
pelvic (**pel**-vik) pertaining to the pelvis. 111
p. exenteration, the surgical removal of all reproductive organs and their lymph nodes, as well as most pelvic organs. 360
p. girdle, a bony ring formed by the hip bones, the sacrum, and the coccyx. 417
pelvimetry (pel-**vim**-uh-trē) the measurement of the dimensions and capacity of the pelvis. 381
pelvis (**pel**-vis) the lower portion of the trunk. The word also means any basin-like structure. 111, 410*f*
renal p., in the kidney, the funnel-shaped structure at the upper end of the ureter. 308
penile (**pē**-nīl) pertaining to or affecting the penis. 362
p. prosthesis, a device that can be surgically implanted in the penis to treat erectile dysfunction. 369, 369*f*
penis (**pē**-nis) the male organ of urination and copulation. 362
pepsin (**pep**-sin) any of several enzymes of gastric juice that break down proteins. 542
percussion (pur-**kuh**-shun) the act of striking a part with short, sharp blows as an aid in diagnosing the condition of the underlying parts by the sound obtained. 61
pericardiocentesis (per-ē-kahr-dē-ō-sen-**tē**-sis) surgical puncture of the pericardial cavity for the aspiration of fluid. 189
pericarditis (per-i-kahr-**dī**-tis) inflammation of the pericardium. 178
pericardium (per-i-**kahr**-dē-um) the sac enclosing the heart and the roots of the great vessels. 168
parietal p., the outer layer of the double membrane that surrounds the heart. 168
visceral p., the surface of the pericardial membrane that is in direct contact with the heart. 168, 169*f*
perichondrium (per-i-**kon**-drē-um) the layer of fibrous connective tissue that invests all cartilage except the articular cartilage of synovial joints. 422
pericolitis (per-ē-kō-**lī**-tis) inflammation of the connective tissue around the colon. 96
perimetrium (per-i-**mē**-trē-um) the serous coat of the uterus. 346
perineum (per-i-**nē**-um) the pelvic floor and the associated structures occupying the pelvic outlet; it is bounded anteriorly by the pubic symphysis, laterally by the ischial tuberosities, and posteriorly by the coccyx; the region between the thighs, bounded in the male sex by the scrotum and anus and in the female sex by the vulva and anus. 315, 342
periodontics (per-ē-ō-**don**-tiks) the branch of dentistry that deals with the study and treatment of the periodontium. 259
periodontist (per-ē-ō-**don**-tist) a dentist who specializes in periodontics. 259
periodontitis (per-ē-ō-don-**tī**-tis) inflammation of the periodontium, caused by residual food, bacteria, and tartar that collect in the spaces between the gum and the lower part of the tooth crown. 271
periodontium (per-ē-ō-**don**-shē-um) the tissues investing and supporting the teeth. 259
periosteum (per-ē-**os**-tē-um) a tough fibrous membrane that surrounds a bone. 409
peristalsis (per-i-**stawl**-sis) movement by which the alimentary canal propels its contents. It consists of a wave of contraction passing along the tube for variable distances. 252
peritoneal dialysis (per-i-tō-**nē**-uhl dī-**al**-uh-sis) dialysis in which the lining of the peritoneal cavity is used as the dialysis membrane. 325
peritoneum (per-i-tō-**nē**-um) the serous membrane that lines the walls of the abdominal and pelvic cavities and invests the internal organs in those cavities. 51, 112*f*
parietal p., the peritoneum that lines the abdominal and pelvic walls and the undersurface of the diaphragm. 112
visceral p., a continuation of the parietal peritoneum reflected at various places over the viscera. 112
perspiration (pur-spi-**rā**-shun) sweating; sweat. 124, 569
perspire (pur-**spīr**) to sweat or excrete sweat. 96
pertussis (pur-**tus**-is) an acute, highly contagious infection of the respiratory tract, most frequently affecting young children, usually caused by *Bordetella pertussis*. 225
petechia (puh-**tē**-kē-uh) a pinpoint, nonraised, perfectly round, purplish red spot caused by intradermal or submucous hemorrhage. 577, 577*f*
phagocyte (**fā**-gō-sīt) any cell that ingests something else. The term usually refers to polymorphonuclear leukocytes, macrophages, and monocytes. 54
phagocytosis (fā-gō-sī-**tō**-sis) the engulfing of microorganisms, other cells, and foreign particles by phagocytes. 139
phalangectomy (fal-un-**jek**-tuh-mē) excision of a finger or toe. 447
phalanges (fuh-**lan**-jēz) bones of the fingers or toes. 418
pharmaceutic (fahr-muh-**soo**-tik) relating to medicinal drugs, or a medicinal drug. 25

pharmaceutical (fahr-muh-**soo**-ti-kul) pertaining to pharmacy or to drugs; medicinal drug. 25, 67
pharmaceutics (fahr-muh-**soo**-tiks) the science of preparing, using, or dispensing medicines. 25
pharmacist (**fahr**-muh-sist) one who is licensed to prepare, sell, or dispense drugs and compounds and to make up prescriptions. 27
pharmacokinetics (fahr-muh-kō-ki-**net**-iks) the study of the body's absorption, distribution, metabolism, and excretion of drugs. 26
pharmacology (fahr-muh-**kol**-uh-jē) the study of drugs and their origin, properties, and effects on living systems. 25
pharmacotherapy (fahr-muh-kō-**ther**-uh-pē) treatment of disease with medicines. 75
pharmacy (**fahr**-muh-sē) the science of preparing, compounding, and dispensing medicines; a place where drugs and medicinal supplies are prepared, compounded, and dispensed. 27
pharyngalgia (far-in-**gal**-juh) pain in the pharynx. 225
pharyngitis (far-in-**jī**-tis) inflammation of the throat. 224
streptococcal p., pharyngitis caused by streptococci; strep throat. 43
pharyngodynia (fuh-ring-gō-**din**-ē-uh) pain in the throat; sore throat. 225
pharyngomycosis (fuh-ring-gō-mī-**kō**-sis) any fungal infection of the pharynx. 225
pharyngopathy (far-ing-**gop**-uh-thē) any disease of the pharynx. 225
pharyngoscope (fuh-**ring**-gō-skōp) an instrument for examining the throat. 218
pharynx (**far**-inks) the throat; the cavity behind the nasal cavities, mouth, and larynx, communicating with them and with the esophagus. 213, 252
phimosis (fī-**mō**-sis) constriction of the preputial orifice so that the prepuce cannot be retracted back over the glans. 367
phlebectomy (fluh-**bek**-tuh-mē) removal of a vein or a segment of a vein. 189
phlebitis (fluh-**bī**-tis) inflammation of a vein. 185
phleboplasty (**fleb**-ō-plas-tē) plastic repair of a vein. 189
phlebostasis (fluh-**bos**-tuh-sis) controlling the flow of blood in a vein. 185
phlebotomist (fluh-**bot**-uh-mist) one who practices phlebotomy. 171
phlebotomy (fluh-**bot**-uh-mē) incision of a vein, as for the letting of blood; needle puncture of a vein for the drawing of blood; venipuncture. 171
phlegm (flem) abnormally thick mucus secreted by the mucosa of the respiratory passages during certain infectious processes. 218
phobia (**fō**-bē-uh) a persistent, irrational, intense abnormal fear or dread. 49, 485
phobophobia (fō-bō-**fō**-bē-uh) irrational fear of acquiring a phobia. 485
photodermatitis (fō-tō-dur-muh-**tī**-tis) an abnormal skin reaction produced by light. 576
photophobia (fō-tō-**fō**-bē-uh) abnormal sensitivity to light, especially of the eyes. 511
photoreceptor (fō-tō-rē-**sep**-tur) a nerve ending that detects light, found in the human eye. 519
phrenitis (fruh-**nī**-tis) inflammation of the diaphragm. 222
phrenodynia (fren-ō-**din**-ē-uh) pain in the diaphragm. 222
phrenoplegia (fren-ō-**plē**-juh) paralysis of the diaphragm. 222
phrenoptosis (fren-op-**tō**-sis, fren-ō-**tō**-sis) downward displacement of the diaphragm. 222
physician (fi-**zish**-un) an authorized practitioner of medicine, as one graduated from a college of medicine or osteopathy and licensed by the appropriate board; one who practices medicine as distinct from surgery. 14
emergency p., a physician who deals with acutely ill or injured patients requiring immediate medical treatment. 21
pia mater (**pī**-uh, **pē**-uh **mā**-tur) the innermost of the three meninges covering the brain and the spinal cord. 466
pituitary (pi-**too**-i-tar-tē) the hypophysis, a small oval two-lobed body at the base of the brain. It regulates other glands by secretion of hormones. 531, 531*f*, 533, 533*f*
p. cachexia, a profound and marked state of constitutional disorder with general ill health caused by hypopituitarism. 548
placenta (pluh-**sen**-tuh) an organ characteristic of true mammals during pregnancy, joining mother and offspring. 371, 371*f*
p. previa, a placenta that develops in the lower uterine segment, in the zone of dilatation, so that it covers or adjoins the internal os. 383, 383*f*
placental stage (pluh-**sen**-tul stāj) the third stage in childbirth, which extends from the expulsion of the child until the placenta is expelled. 378, 378*f*
plane (plān) a flat surface determined by the position of three points in space; a specified level; to rub away or abrade; a superficial incision in the wall of a cavity or between layers of tissue. 102
anatomic p., any of several longitudinal sections used in the study of anatomy. 102, 103*f*
body p., an imaginary flat surface used to identify the position of the body. 102
coronal p., the body plane that divides the body into front and back portions; frontal plane. 102, 103*f*
frontal p., the body plane that divides the body into front and back portions. 102, 103*f*
midsagittal p. the plane vertically dividing the body through the midline into right and left halves. 102
sagittal p., the body plane that divides the body into left and right sides. 102, 103*f*
transverse p., the body plane that divides the body into upper and lower portions. 102, 103*f*
plaque (plak) any patch or flat area; a superficial, solid, elevated skin lesion equal to or greater than 1.0 cm (0.5 cm according to some authorities) in diameter; a patch of atherosclerosis. 574, 574*f*
plasma (**plaz**-muh) the fluid portion of the blood. 120
p. cell, a cell found in the bone marrow, connective tissue, and sometimes the blood. 191

shunt (shunt) to turn to one side, divert, or bypass; a passage or anastomosis between two natural channels, especially between blood vessels. 122, 186, 488
  ventriculoperitoneal s., a surgically-created passageway consisting of plastic tubing and one-way valves between a cerebral ventricle and the peritoneum for the draining of excess cerebrospinal fluid (CSF) in hydrocephalus. 488, 488*f*

sialadenitis (sī-ul-ad-uh-**nī**-tis) inflammation of a salivary gland. 281

sialography (sī-uh-**log**-ruh-fē) radiographic demonstration of the salivary glands after injection of radiopaque substances. 267

sialolithiasis (sī-al-ō-li-**thī**-uh-sis) a condition characterized by the presence of stones in the salivary ducts or glands. 281

sigmoidoscope (sig-**moi**-dō-skōp) a rigid or flexible endoscope with appropriate illumination for examining the sigmoid colon. 266

sigmoidoscopy (sig-moi-**dos**-kuh-pē) inspection of the sigmoid colon through a sigmoidoscope. 266

sign (sīn) an indication of the existence of something as opposed to the subjective sensations (symptoms) of the patient. 56

silicosis (sil-i-**kō**-sis) pneumoconiosis caused by inhalation of the dust of stone, sand, or flint containing silicon dioxide with formation of generalized nodular fibrotic changes in both lungs. 231

sinus (**sī**-nus) a recess, cavity, or channel. 213
  paranasal s., one of several cavities that communicate with the nasal cavity and are lined with a mucous membrane. 213, 213*f*

sinusitis (sī-nus-**ī**-tis) inflammation of a sinus. 224, 224*f*

skeleton (**skel**-uh-tun) the hard framework of the animal body. 411
  appendicular s., the bones of the upper and lower limbs. 411, 412*f*, 417
  axial s., the bones of the cranium, vertebral column, ribs, and sternum. 411, 412*f*

skin (skin) the tough, supple membrane that covers the entire surface of the body.
  accessory s. structure, any of the hair, nails, sebaceous, or sweat glands that are embedded in the dermis. 568
  s. flap, a layer of skin, usually separated by dissection from a deeper layer of tissue. 585, 585*f*
  s. infection, any of various infections caused by specific types of bacteria, viruses, and fungi. 576, 576*f*

slit-lamp examination (slit lamp eg-zam-i-**nā**-shun) examining the various layers of the eye with a bright light usually after the pupils have been dilated. 509, 509*f*

smoking cessation drugs (**smōk**-ing suh-**sā**-shun drugz) medicines that help people stop smoking cigarettes or using other forms of tobacco. 239

Snellen chart (**snel**-un chahrt) one of several charts used in testing visual acuity. 484*f*, 508, 509*f*

somatic (sō-**mat**-ik) pertaining to the body.
  s. cell, all of the body cells that have the diploid number of chromosomes. 90
  s. death, absence of electrical activity of the brain for a specified period of time under rigidly defined circumstances. 118

somatotropin (sō-muh-tō-trō-pin) growth hormone. 537

somesthetic (sō-mes-**thet**-ik) pertaining to body feeling or sensation. 118

sonography (suh-**nog**-ruh-fē) the process of using sound waves bouncing off body tissue to form a picture of an internal organ; ultrasonography. 68

spasm (**spaz**-um) a sudden, violent, involuntary contraction of a muscle or a group of muscles, attended with pain and interference with function, producing involuntary movement and distortion; a sudden but transitory constriction of a passage, canal, or orifice. 58

specific gravity (spuh-**sif**-ik **grav**-i-tē) the ratio of the density of a substance to the density of another substance accepted as a standard, water often being the standard for liquids or solids. 310

specimen (**spes**-i-mun) a small sample intended to show the nature of the whole.
  catheterized urine s., a sample of urine obtained by catheterization. 312
  clean-catch s., a urine sample that is as free of bacterial contamination as possible without the use of a catheter. 312
  shaved s., a sample of tissue for microscopic study that is collected using a razor blade from a superficial lesion. 570
  voided specimen, a sample of urine for examination that has been obtained by voiding. 312

speculum (**spek**-ū-lum) an instrument used to examine a body orifice or cavity.
  vaginal s., an instrument used to hold open the vaginal opening for inspection of the vaginal cavity. 348, 349*f*

spermatoblast (**spur**-muh-tō-blast) embryonic form of a sperm. 372

spermatocele (**spur**-muh-tō-sēl) a swelling of the epididymis or of the rete testis containing spermatozoa. 367, 367*f*

spermatogenesis (spur-muh-tō-**jen**-uh-sis) the process of formation of sperm. 368

spermatozoon (spur-muh-tō-**zō**-on) a mature male sperm cell, which serves to fertilize the ovum; spermatozoa (plural). 363, 363*f*, 371

sphincter (**sfingk**-tur) a ringlike band of muscle fibers that constricts a passage or closes a natural opening. 260
  anal s., internal and external muscles of the anus. 276, 276*f*

spina bifida (**spī**-nuh **bif**-i-duh) a developmental abnormality marked by defective closure of the bony encasement of the spinal cord. 439, 439*f*

spinal (**spī**-nul) pertaining to the vertebral column. 414
  s. cord, a long, nearly cylindric structure located in the vertebral canal, and part of the central nervous system (CNS). 468, 468*f*
  s. fluid, the fluid that flows through and protects the brain and spinal cord; cerebrospinal fluid (CSF). 468

spirilla (spī-**ril**-uh) spiral-shaped bacteria that have polar flagella for motility. 42

spirochetes (**spī**-rō-kēts) tiny spiral bacteria with motility based on axial filaments; includes the organism that causes syphilis. 42, 387

spirometer (spī-**rom**-uh-tur) the instrument used in spirometry. 218, 218*f*
  incentive s., an instrument used to encourage voluntary deep breathing by providing visual feedback about inspiratory volume. 237, 237*f*

spirometry (spī-**rom**-uh-trē) a measurement of the breathing capacity of the lungs. 218, 218*f*

spleen (splēn) a large, glandlike organ situated in the upper left part of the abdominal cavity that destroys erythrocytes at the end of their usefulness and serves as a blood reservoir. 191

splenectomy (splē-**nek**-tuh-mē) removal of the spleen. 195

splenomegaly (splē-nō-**meg**-uh-lē) enlargement of the spleen. 194

splenopathy (splē-**nop**-uh-thē) any disease of the spleen. 194

splenopexy (**splē**-nō-pek-sē) surgical fixation of the spleen. 195

splenoptosis (splē-nop-**tō**-sis, splē-nō-**tō**-sis) downward displacement of the spleen. 194

splenorrhagia (splē-nō-**rā**-juh) hemorrhage from the spleen. 194

splenorrhaphy (splē-**nor**-uh-fē) suture of the spleen. 195

splint (splint) to fasten; an appliance used to hold in position a displaced or movable part. 444

spondylalgia (spon-duh-**lal**-juh) a painful vertebra. 436

spondylarthritis (spon-dul-ahr-**thrī**-tis) inflammation of joints between vertebrae. 441

spondylarthropathy (spon-duh-lō-ahr-**throp**-uh-thē) any disease of the joints and spine. 441

spondylosyndesis (spon-duh-lō-sin-**dē**-sis) surgical immobilization or ankylosis of the spine; spinal fusion. 445

sprain (sprān) a joint injury in which some of the fibers of a supporting ligament are ruptured but the continuity of the ligament remains intact. 432

sputum (**spū**-tum) material ejected from the trachea, bronchi, and lungs through the mouth. 218

stapes (**stā**-pēz) one of the three ossicles in the middle ear, resembling a tiny stirrup. 514, 514*f*

staphylococcemia (staf-uh-lō-kok-**sē**-mē-uh) a condition in which staphylococci are present in the blood; septicemia caused by staphylococci. 131

staphylococci (staf-uh-lō-**kok**-sī) plural of staphylococcus. *Staphylococcus* is a genus of gram-positive bacteria consisting of cocci, usually unencapsulated, 0.5 to 1.5 microns in diameter. The organisms occur singly, in pairs, and in irregular clusters. 43

stasis (**stā**-sis) a stoppage or diminution of the flow of blood or other body fluid in any part; a state of equilibrium among opposing forces. 58, 58*f*

stem cell (stem sel) cell that has the ability to divide without limit and give rise to specialized cells. 90
  stem cell transplantation, bone marrow transplant that infuses healthy stem cells into the body to replace damaged or diseased bone marrow. 614

stenosis (stuh-**nō**-sis) narrowing or stricture of a duct or canal. 182
  renal artery s., partial or complete blocking of one or both renal arteries. 322
  valvular s., a narrowing or stricture of any of the heart valves. 182

stent (stent) a mold or slender rodlike or threadlike device used to provide support for tubular structures or to maintain their patency. 188, 188*f*
  intracoronary s., a stent used to provide support for a coronary artery. 188

stereotactic radiosurgery (ster-ē-ō-**tak**-tik rā-dē-ō-**sur**-jur-ē) a method of treating tumors by ionizing radiation rather than surgical incision. 489, 613, 613*f*

stereotaxis (ster-ē-ō-**tak**-sis) a type of surgery or radiotherapy characterized by computerized positioning to locate the site. 488*t*, 489

sternalgia (stur-**nal**-juh) pain in the breastbone. 436

sternoschisis (stur-**nos**-ki-sis) congenital fissure of the sternum. 440

sternotomy (stur-**not**-uh-mē) incision of the sternum. 447

sternum (**stur**-num) the breastbone, a plate of bone forming the middle anterior wall of the thorax. 414

steroid (**ster**-oid) any of a large number of hormonal substances with a similar basic chemical structure, produced mainly in the adrenal cortex and gonads. 531

stethoscope (**steth**-ō-skōp) an instrument by which various internal sounds of the body are conveyed to the ear of the listener. 60, 60*f*

stillbirth (**stil**-birth) the delivery of a dead child; fetal death. 383

stimulants (**stim**-ū-lunts) substances that raise the levels of physiological or nervous activity of the body. 492

stoma (**stō**-muh) any minute pore, orifice, or opening on a free surface; the opening established in the abdominal wall by colostomy, ileostomy, etc. 73, 73*f*

stomatitis (stō-muh-**tī**-tis) inflammation of the mouth. 270

stomatodynia (stō-muh-tō-**din**-ē-uh) painful mouth. 270

stomatomycosis (stō-muh-tō-mī-**kō**-sis) a mouth disease caused by a fungus. 270

stomatoplasty (**stō**-muh-tō-plas-tē) surgical repair of the mouth. 282

strabismus (struh-**biz**-mus) an abnormal condition in which the visual axes of the eyes are not directed at the same point. 511, 511*f*

strain (strān) an overstretching or overexertion of some part of the musculature. 432

streptococcemia (strep-tō-kok-**sē**-mē-uh) the presence of streptococci in the blood. 131

streptococci (strep-tō-**kok**-sī) plural of *Streptococcus*, a genus of gram-positive cocci occurring in pairs or chains. 43

stress test (stres test) a method of evaluating cardiovascular fitness. While exercising, the person is subjected to steadily increasing levels of work, and the amount of oxygen consumed and an electrocardiogram are monitored. 176-177
  thallium s. t., a stress test that measures the response to thallium. 177
  treadmill s. t., a stress test that measures the response to exercise. 176-177

stricture (**strik**-chur) decrease in the caliber of a canal, duct, or other passage. 183

stridor (**strī**-dur) a harsh, high-pitched respiratory sound such as the inspiratory sound often heard in acute laryngeal obstruction. 217

stroke (strōk) a sudden and severe attack; cerebrovascular accident (CVA). 184, 184*f*, 476, 477*f*

embolic s., stroke that occurs when a blood clot or other embolus reaches an artery in the brain, lodges there, and blocks the flow of blood. 184*f*, 476, 477*f*

hemorrhagic s., stroke caused by cerebrovascular hemorrhage. 184*f*, 476, 477*f*

ischemic s., stroke resulting from inadequate blood flow to the brain caused by partial or complete occlusion of a cerebral artery. 476

thrombotic s., a stroke syndrome caused by cerebral thrombosis. 184*f*, 476, 477*f*

stupor (**stoo** -pur) a state of unresponsiveness in which the individual seems unaware of the surroundings. 470

subdural (sub-**doo**-rul) between the dura mater and the arachnoid. 467

s. space, the space between the dura mater and the arachnoid. 467

superficial (soo-pur-**fish**-ul) situated on or near the surface. 96, 106

superior (soo-**pēr**-ē-ur) situated above, or directed upward. 103, 104*f*

supersensitivity (soo-pur-sen-si-**tiv**-i-tē) excessive sensitivity, as that following damage of a nerve supply to a body part. 93

supervitaminosis (soo-pur-vī-tuh-min-**ō**-sis) a condition resulting from excessive ingestion (swallowing or taking by mouth) of vitamins. 95

supination (soo-pi-**nā**-shun) the act of assuming the supine position, or the state of being supine. Applied to the hand, the act of turning the palm forward or upward. 107, 107*f*

supine (**soo**-pīn, soo-**pīn**) lying with the face upward. 107

suppuration (sup-ū-**rā**-shun) forming pus; the act of discharging pus. 576

surgery (**sur**-jur-ē) the branch of medicine that treats diseases, injuries, and deformities by manual or operative methods; the place in a hospital where surgery is performed. 20, 22

plastic s., surgery that is concerned with restoration, reconstruction, correction, or improvement in the shape and appearance of body structures. 20

robotic s. the application of robotics in surgery. 20*f*

stereotactic s., any of several surgical techniques to treat specific tiny areas of pathological tissue in deep-seated structures of the central nervous system (CNS) using heat, cold, radiation, and ultrasound. 489

susceptibility (suh-sep-ti-**bil**-i-tē) a state of vulnerability, readily affected or acted on, such as a diminished immunity to infection. 139

suture (**soo**-chur) the act of uniting a wound by stitches; a type of joint in which the opposed surfaces are closely united, as in the skull; material used in closing a surgical or traumatic wound with stitches; a stitch or stitches made to secure the edges of a wound. 73

suturing (**soo**-chur-ing) bringing together edges of a wound using sterile suture material and a needle. 584

symmetry (**sim**-uh-trē) correspondence of parts on opposite sides of a dividing line. 96

sympathectomy (sim-puh-**thek**-tuh-mē) transection, resection, or other interruption of some portion of the sympathetic nervous pathways. 490

sympathetic (sim-puh-**thet**-ik) a sympathetic nerve or the sympathetic nervous system; pertaining to sympathy. 469

symptom (**simp**-tum) any subjective evidence of disease or of a patient's condition. 56

synapse (**sin**-aps) the junction between two neurons. 465

synaptic bulb (si-**nap**-tik bulb) the end of an axon where a neurotransmitter is released to either enhance or inhibit the transmission of an impulse. 465

syncope (**sing**-kuh-pē) a temporary loss of consciousness because of generalized cerebral ischemia; a faint. 132

syndactylism, syndactyly (sin-**dak**-tuh-liz-um, sin-**dak**-tuh-lē) a congenital anomaly characterized by the fusion of the fingers or toes. 96, 440, 440*f*

syndrome (**sin**-drŏm) a set of symptoms that occur together and collectively characterize or indicate a particular disease or abnormal condition. 96, 97

acquired immunodeficiency s. (AIDS), an epidemic, transmissible retroviral disease caused by infection with human immunodeficiency virus (HIV), manifested in severe cases as profound depression of cell-mediated immunity. 141, 389

adrenogenital s., adrenal virilism. 549

carpal tunnel s. (CTS), a complex of symptoms resulting from compression of the median nerve in the carpal tunnel. 434

chronic fatigue s., a condition characterized by disabling fatigue, accompanied by many symptoms, including muscle pain, multijoint pain, unrefreshing sleep, and malaise. 443

Cushing s., a group of signs and symptoms associated with hypersecretion of the glucocorticoids by the adrenal cortex. 549, 549*f*

Down s., chromosome disorder characterized by a small flattened skull, short, flat-bridge nose, epicanthal fold, short phalanges, widened spaces between the first and second digits of hands and feet, and moderate to severe mental retardation. Also called *trisomy 21* and *nondisjunction*; formerly called *mongolism*. 383, 383*f*

fetal alcohol s., a congenital syndrome caused by excessive consumption of alcohol by the mother during pregnancy. 385

fibromyalgia s., a form of nonarticular rheumatism characterized by musculoskeletal pain, stiffness, spasm, fatigue, and severe sleep disturbance. 443

hepatorenal s., functional renal failure, without pathologic renal changes, associated with cirrhosis and ascites or with obstructive jaundice. 279

malabsorption s., a complex of signs and symptoms resulting from disorders in the intestinal absorption of nutrients, characterized by anorexia, weight loss, abdominal bloating, muscle cramps, bone pain, and an abnormal amount of fat in the feces. 269

syndrome (*Continued*)

nephrotic syndrome, a clinical classification that includes all diseases of the kidney characterized by chronic loss of protein in the urine and subsequent depletion of body protein. 319

polycystic ovary s., a clinical symptom complex associated with polycystic ovaries. 353

premenstrual s., a condition that occurs several days before the onset of menstruation, characterized by one or more of the following: irritability, emotional tension, anxiety, depression, headache, breast tenderness, and water retention. 352

Sjögren s., a symptom complex of unknown cause, usually occurring in middle-aged or older women, marked by keratoconjunctivitis, xerostomia, and the presence of a connective tissue disease, usually rheumatoid arthritis but sometimes systemic lupus erythematosus, scleroderma, or polymyositis. 441

tarsal tunnel s., an abnormal condition caused by compression of a nerve and characterized by pain and numbness in the sole of the foot. 434

toxic shock s. (TSS), a severe infection with *Staphylococcus aureus* characterized by high fever of sudden onset, vomiting, diarrhea, and myalgia, followed by hypotension and, in severe cases, shock. The syndrome affects almost exclusively menstruating women using tampons, although a few women who do not use tampons and a few male individuals have been affected. 353

synovitis (si-nō-**vī**-tis) inflammation of a synovial membrane. 436

syphilis (**sif**-i-lis) a sexually transmitted disease caused by *Treponema pallidum* that is characterized by lesions that may involve any organ or tissue. 350, 387, 387*f*

congenital s., syphilis acquired in utero and manifested by any of several characteristic malformations and by neurologic changes and active mucocutaneous syphilis at the time of birth or shortly afterward. 388

system (**sis**-tum) a collection of parts, that unified, make a whole.

afferent s. division of the nervous system that conducts or conveys toward a center. 463, 469

autonomic nervous s., the part of the nervous system related to involuntary body functions. 463*f*, 469, 469*f*

body s., several organs of the body that work together to accomplish a set of functions. 91, 92*t*

cardiovascular s., body system consisting of the heart and blood vessels. 92*t*, 163

central nervous s. (CNS), the control center of the body, composed of the brain and the spinal cord. 462, 462*f*, 463*f*

circulatory s., the network of channels through which the fluids of the body circulate, composed of the cardiovascular system and the lymphatic system. 163

digestive s., the organs, structures, and accessory glands of the gastrointestinal tube through which food passes. 92*t*, 252

efferent s., division of the nervous system that conveys away from a center. 463, 469

endocrine s., the network of ductless glands and other structures that elaborate and secrete hormones into the bloodstream. 92*t*, 530

integumentary s., the skin and its appendages, hair, nails, sweat and sebaceous glands. 92*t*, 567

lymphatic s., a complex network of capillaries, vessels, ducts, nodes, and organs that help protect and maintain the internal fluid environment of the body by conveying lymph and producing various blood cells. 92*t*, 163, 190

motor s., the portion of the peripheral nervous system that carries impulses to the somatic and autonomic tissues; the efferent system. 469

musculoskeletal s., all of the muscles, bones, joints, and related structures that function in the movement of body parts and organs. 408

nervous s., the intricate network of structures that activates, coordinates, and controls all the functions of the body. 92*t*, 462

peripheral nervous s., the various nerve processes that connect the brain and the spinal cord with receptors, muscles, and glands. 462, 462*f*, 463*f*, 469

reproductive s., the male and female gonads, associated ducts and glands, and external genitalia that function in the procreation of offspring. 92*t*, 342

respiratory s., the complex of organs and structures that performs the pulmonary ventilation of the body and exchange of oxygen and carbon dioxide between the air and blood circulating through the lungs. 92*t*, 210

sensory s., the portion of the peripheral nervous system that carries impulses to the central nervous system (CNS) from the visceral and somatic tissues; the afferent system. 463, 469

urinary s., all organs and ducts involved in the secretion and elimination of urine. 92*t*, 304

systemic (sis-**tem**-ik) affecting the body generally; supplying those parts of the body that receive blood through the aorta.. 26, 131

systole (**sis**-tō-lē) the contraction or period of contraction of the heart, especially of the ventricles. 174

systolic pressure (sis-**tol**-ik **presh**-ur) blood pressure measured at the height of ventricular contraction. 174

tachycardia (tak-i-**kahr**-dē-uh) fast heartbeat; fast pulse. 101*f*, 132, 175, 220

paroxysmal atrial t., palpitations and a racing heartbeat that occur and stop suddenly. 180

tachyphasia (tak-ē-**fā**-zhuh) fast speech. 101

tachypnea (tak-ip-**nē**-uh, tak-ē-**ne**-uh) rapid breathing. 223

target organ (**tahr**-gut **or**-gun) the organ or structure toward which the effects of a drug or hormone are primarily directed. 530, 530*f*

tarsals (**tahr**-sulz) the bones of the ankle. 420

tarsoptosis (tahr-sop-**tō**-sis) falling of the tarsals; fallfoot; fallen arch. 434

tarsus (**tahr**-sus) the seven bones composing the articulation between the foot and the leg; also the cartilaginous plates of the eyelids. 420

taste buds (tāst budz) any of the many peripheral taste organs distributed over the tongue, epiglottis, and the roof of the mouth. 520, 520*f*

tattoo removal (ta-tōō ri-mōō-vul) multiple treatments, either dermabrasion or laser removal of a tattoo. 586

tearing (tēr-ing) watering of the eye, usually caused by excessive tear production. 505

telecardiogram (tel-uh-kahr-dē-ō-gram) a heart tracing that registers distant from the patient by means of electrical sending of the signal. 112

telecardiography (tel-uh-kahr-dē-og-ruh-fē) the process of recording the heart that registers distant from the patient by means of electric sending of the signal. 175

temporal lobe (tem-puh-rul lōb) the lateral region of the cerebrum. 467, 467f

tenalgia (tē-nal-juh) pain in a tendon. 436

tendinitis (ten-di-nī-tis) inflammation of tendons and tendon-muscle attachments. 436

tendon (ten-dun) a fibrous cord by which a muscle is attached. 423, 423f

tendonitis (ten-duh-nī-tis) tendinitis; inflammation of a tendon. 436

tendoplasty (ten-dō-plas-tē) surgical repair of a tendon. 447

tenodynia (ten-ō-din-ē-uh) pain of a tendon. 436

tenomyoplasty (ten-ō-mī-ō-plas-tē) surgical repair of a tendon and muscle. 447

tenorrhaphy (tuh-nor-uh-fē) union of a divided tendon by a suture. 447

tenotomy (tuh-not-uh-mē) cutting of a tendon. 447

tertipara (tur-tip-uh-ruh) a woman who has had three pregnancies that resulted in viable offspring; tripara. 378

testalgia (tes-tal-juh) testicular pain. 368

testicular torsion (tes-tik-ū-lur tor-shun) axial rotation of the spermatic cord cutting off blood supply to the testicle. 367

testis (tes-tis) the male gonad; either of the egg-shaped glands located in the scrotum, in which sperm are formed. 361, 362f, 367f

testosterone (tes-tos-tuh-rōn) a hormone secreted by the testes that brings about induction and maintenance of male secondary sex characteristics. 362, 537

tetanus (tet-uh-nus) an acute, often fatal, infectious disease caused by the anaerobic bacillus *Clostridium tetani*, which usually enters the body through a contaminated puncture wound. 479

tetany (tet-uh-nē) a nervous condition characterized by intermittent or continuous tonic muscle contractions involving the extremities. 432

tetraiodothyronine (tet-ruh-ī-ō-dō-thī-rō-nēn) thyroxine, a thyroid hormone. 536

tetralogy (te-tral-uh-jē) any group of four related factors.
  t. of Fallot, a combination of congenital cardiac defects consisting of pulmonary stenosis, right ventricular hypertrophy, and interventricular septal and aortic defects. 93, 179

thalamus (thal-uh-mus) the largest subdivision of the diencephalon. 467

therapeutic angiogenesis (ther-uh-pū-tik an-jē-ō-jen-uh-sis) treatment of ischemic organs or tissues; for example, puncturing an ischemic heart to stimulate the creation of new blood vessels. 188

therapy (ther-uh-pē) treatment of disease. 22

thermometer (thur-mom-uh-tur) an instrument for determining temperatures. 59
  axillary t., a thermometer placed in the armpit to record the temperature. 59, 60f
  oral t., a clinical thermometer that is usually placed under the tongue. 59, 60f
  rectal t., a clinical thermometer that is inserted in the rectum. 59, 60f
  tympanic t., a thermometer designed to measure temperature electronically at the tympanic membrane. 59, 60f

thermoplegia (thur-mō-plē-juh) heatstroke or sunstroke. 584

thermoreceptor (thur-mō-rē-sep-tur) a nerve ending, usually in the skin, that is sensitive to a change in temperature. 519

thermotherapy (thur-mō-ther-uh-pē) treatment of disease by the application of heat. 70

thoracentesis (thor-uh-sen-tē-sis) surgical puncture of the chest wall into the parietal cavity for aspiration of fluids. 236, 236f

thoracic (thuh-ras-ik) pertaining to the chest. 108, 414, 415f
  t. duct, the common trunk of many lymphatic vessels in the body. 191f

thoracocentesis (thor-uh-kō-sen-tē-sis) surgical puncture of the chest wall for the aspiration of fluid. 236

thoracodynia (thor-uh-kō-din-ē-uh) pain in the chest. 112

thoracoplasty (thor-uh-kō-plas-tē) surgical removal of ribs, allowing the chest wall to collapse a diseased lung. 236

thoracostomy (thor-uh-kos-tuh-mē) surgical opening in the wall of the chest. 236, 236f

thoracotomy (thor-uh-kot-uh-mē) surgical incision of the wall of the chest. 108

thorax (thor-aks) chest; the part of the body that is encased by the ribs and extends from the neck to the respiratory diaphragm. 108, 414

thrombectomy (throm-bek-tuh-mē) surgical removal of a blood clot. 131

thrombocyte (throm-bō-sīt) a blood platelet. 129

thrombocytopenia (throm-bō-sī-tō-pē-nē-uh) a decrease in the number of platelets in circulating blood. 131

thrombocytosis (throm-bō-sī-tō-sis) an increase in the number of platelets in the peripheral blood. 131

thrombogenesis (throm-bō-jen-uh-sis) origin of a blood clot; clot formation. 131

thrombolymphangitis (thromb-bō-lim-fan-jī-tis) inflammation of a lymph vessel caused by a blood clot. 194

thrombolysis (throm-bol-i-sis) dissolution of a blood clot. 131
  intravascular t., use of a thrombolytic agent delivered via a catheter to dissolve an internal blood clot. 189

thrombolytic (throm-bō-lit-ik) dissolving or breaking up a blood clot; an agent that dissolves or breaks up a blood clot. 131, 197, 490

thrombolytics (throm-bō-lit-iks) drugs that are capable of dissolving a blood clot. 197, 490

thrombopenia (throm-bō-pē-nē-uh) a deficiency in the number of platelets in circulating blood. 131

thrombophlebitis (throm-bō-fluh-bī-tis) inflammation of a vein caused by a blood clot. 185

thromboplastin (throm-bō-plas-tin) coagulation factor III. 128
  partial t. time, a test for detecting coagulation defects. 128

thrombosis (throm-bō-sis) the presence of a blood clot. 131
  intravascular t., blood clot within a blood vessel. 184-185, 189
  renal vein t., a blood clot in a renal vein. 322
  venous t., an abnormal condition in which a clot forms in a vein; phlebothrombosis. 185

thrombus (throm-bus) an aggregation of blood factors, primarily platelets and fibrin with entrapment of cellular elements, frequently causing vascular obstruction at the point of its formation; thrombi (plural). 127, 131

thymectomy (thī-mek-tuh-mē) excision of the thymus gland. 195

thymoma (thī-mō-muh) tumor derived from elements of the thymus. 194

thymopathy (thī-mop-uh-thē) any disease of the thymus. 194

thymosin (thī-mō-sin) a substance secreted by thymic epithelial cells that maintains immune system functions and can restore T-cell function in thymectomized animals. 542

thymus (thī-mus) a glandlike body in the anterior mediastinal cavity that usually reaches its maximum development during childhood and then undergoes involution. 191, 542

thyrocalcitonin (TCT) (thī-rō-kal-si-tō-nin) calcitonin; a hormone produced by the thyroid gland that is concerned with the homeostasis of the blood calcium level. 536

thyroid (thī-roid) the thyroid gland, a highly vascular organ at the front of the neck; pertaining to the thyroid gland. 531, 544f
  thyroid drugs, medications that are used to supplement natural thyroid hormones. 556

thyroid drugs (thī-roid drugz) medications that are used to supplement natural thyroid hormones. 556

thyroidectomy (thī-roid-ek-tuh-mē) surgical removal of the thyroid gland. 554

thyroiditis (thī-roid-ī-tis) inflammation of the thyroid gland. 548

thyropathy (thī-rop-uh-thē) any disease of the thyroid gland. 548

thyrotoxicosis (thī-rō-tok-si-kō-sis) a morbid condition caused by excessive thyroid secretion; symptoms are sweating, weight loss, tachycardia, and nervousness. 548

thyrotropin (TSH) (thī-rot-ruh-pin) a hormone of the anterior pituitary that stimulates the thyroid. 536

thyroxine (T₄) (thī-rok-sin) an iodine-containing hormone secreted by the thyroid gland. Its chief function is to increase cell metabolism. 536

tibia (tib-ē-uh) the inner and larger bone of the leg below the knee. 420

tibialgia (tib-ē-al-juh) pain of the tibia. 436

tinea (tin-ē-uh) any of various skin disorders popularly called *ringworm.* 577, 577f

tinnitus (tin-i-tus, ti-nī-tus) a noise in the ears, such as ringing, buzzing, or roaring. 132, 517

tissue (tish-ōō) an aggregation of similarly specialized cells united in the performance of a particular function. 91
  connective t., tissue that binds together and provides support for various structures. 422
  epithelial t., tissue that forms the covering of body surfaces. 91
  hypoxic t., a decreased amount of oxygen within the tissue. 583
  muscle t., tissue that produces movement. 91
  nervous t., tissue that coordinates and controls many body activities, found in the brain, spinal cord, and nerves. 91
  subcutaneous adipose t., fat deposits beneath the skin. 568, 568f

tocolytics (tō-kō-lit-ics) labor suppressants; medications used to suppress premature labor. 392

tomogram (tō-mō-gram) a radiogram produced by the process of tomography. 67

tomography (tō-mog-ruh-fē) the recording of internal body images at a predetermined plane by means of the tomograph.
  computed axial t., former name of computed tomography. 65
  computed t. (CT), a radiologic technique in which transmission patterns are recorded by electronic detectors and stored in a computer, which then reconstructs a view of internal structures of the body. 67, 67f
  positron emission t., a computerized radiographic technique that uses radioactive substances to examine the metabolic activity of various body structures. 67, 67f

tonometer (tō-nom-uh-tur) an instrument used in measuring tension or pressure, especially intraocular pressure. 509, 509f

tonometry (tō-nom-uh-trē) the measuring of intraocular pressure by determining the resistance of the eyeball to indentation by an applied force. 509, 509f

tonsil (ton-sil) a small, rounded mass of tissue, especially of lymphoid tissue; generally used alone to designate the palatine tonsil. 192
  lingual t., one of the small, rounded masses of tissue near tongue. 192
  palatine t., one of the small, rounded masses of tissue near palate. 192
  pharyngeal t., one of the small, rounded masses of tissue near pharynx. 192

tonsillectomy (ton-si-lek-tuh-mē) excision of the tonsils. 195

tonsillitis (ton-si-lī-tis) inflammation of the tonsils, especially the palatine tonsils. 49

tonsilloadenoidectomy (ton-si-lō-ad-uh-noid-ek-tuh-mē) excision of lymphoid tissue from the throat and nasopharynx (tonsils and adenoids). 195

topical (top-i-kul) pertaining to a particular surface area, as a topical anti-infective applied to a certain area of the skin and affecting only the area to which it is applied. 287
  t. medication, any drug that is applied to the skin or a mucous membrane. 587, 589

tourniquet (toor-ni-kut) a device applied around an extremity to control the circulation and prevent the flow of blood to or from the distal area. 185

toxemia (tok-**sē**-mē-uh) the condition resulting from the spread of bacterial products (toxins) by the bloodstream. 132

toxic (**tok**-sik) poisonous; pertaining to poisoning. 69

t. dose (TD), the amount of a substance that may be expected to produce a toxic effect. 70

toxicity (tok-**sis**-i-tē) the quality of being poisonous, especially the degree of virulence of a toxic microbe or of a poison. 141

toxicologist (tok-si-**kol**-uh-jist) one who specializes in the study of poisons. 70

toxicology (tok-si-**kol**-uh-jē) the science that deals with poisons. 70

toxin (**tok**-sin) a substance produced by certain animals, some higher plants, and pathogenic bacteria that is highly poisonous for other living organisms. 70

toxoid (**tok**-soid) a toxin treated in a way that destroys its deleterious properties without destroying its ability to stimulate antibody production. 140

trabeculae (truh-**bek**-ū-lē) plural of trabecula, a supporting or anchoring strand of connective tissue, such as one extending from a capsule into the substance of the enclosed organ. 409

trachea (**trā**-kē-uh) the windpipe. 211*f*, 212

trachealgia (trā-kē-**al**-juh) pain in the trachea. 233

tracheomalacia (trā-kē-ō-muh-**lā**-shuh) softening of the windpipe. 233

tracheitis (trā-kē-**ī**-tus) inflammation of the trachea. 233

tracheoplasty (**trā**-kē-ō-plas-tē) plastic surgery of the windpipe. 236

tracheoscopy (trā-kē-**os**-kuh-pē) examination of the interior of the windpipe. 219

tracheostenosis (trā-kē-ō-stuh-**nō**-sis) narrowing or contraction of the trachea. 233

tracheostomy (trā-kē-**os**-tuh-mē) surgical formation of a new opening into the windpipe from the neck. 234

t. tube, tube through which transtracheal oxygen is delivered. 235, 235*f*

tracheotomy (trā-kē-**ot**-uh-mē) surgically cutting into the windpipe. 74, 234

traction (**trak**-shun) the act of drawing or exerting a pulling force. 444

trade name (trād nām) drug name under which a company usually trademarks a generic drug. 26

tranquilizer (**trang**-kwi-līz-ur) a drug with a calming, soothing effect. 491

transcutaneous electrical nerve stimulation (TENS) (trans-kū-**tā**-nē-us ē-**lek**-tri-kul nurv stim-ū-**lā**-shun) a method for relief of pain by placement of electrodes over the painful site and delivery of small amounts of electrical current. 490, 490*f*, 587

transdermal drug delivery (trans-**dur**-mul drug dē-**liv**-ur-ē) a method of applying a drug to unbroken skin. 587

transfusion (trans-**fū**-zhun) the introduction of whole blood or blood components directly into the bloodstream of a person. 137

blood t., the introduction of whole blood or a component to replace blood that is lost. 137

t. reaction, an adverse reaction to blood received in a transfusion. 138

transient ischemic attack (**tran**-shent, **tran**-sē-unt is-kē-mik uh-**tak**) a brief attack (from a few minutes to an hour) of cerebral dysfunction of vascular origin, with no persistent neurologic deficit. 476

transplant ([noun] **trans**-plant) an organ or tissue used for grafting; the process of removing and grafting such an organ or tissue; ([verb] trans-**plant**) to transfer tissue from one part to another. 141

autologous t., surgical transplantation of any tissue from one part of the body to another location in the same individual. 447

bone marrow t., the transfer of bone marrow to stimulate production of bone marrow. 447, 614

corneal t., grafting of corneal tissue from one human eye to another. 513

intraocular lens t., insertion of a plastic artificial lens, generally after cataract removal. 513

renal t., replacement of a diseased kidney with a healthy one from a donor. 325, 325*f*

transthoracic (trans-thuh-**ras**-ik) through the chest cavity or across the chest wall. 115

transtracheal (trans-**trā**-kē-ul) through the wall of the trachea.

t. oxygen (TTO), the administration of oxygen via a low-flow catheter inserted directly into the trachea. 234, 234*f*

transureteroureterostomy (trans-ū-rē-tur-ō-ū-rē-tur-**os**-tuh-mē) surgical connection of one ureter to another. 327, 327*f*

transurethral (trans-ū-**rē**-thrul) performed through the urethra. 329

t. microwave thermotherapy (TUMT), destruction of prostatic tissue using microwave energy, performed through the urethra. 369

t. needle ablation (TUNA), destruction of prostatic tissue using low level radiofrequency energy, performed through the urethra. 369

t. resection (TUR), the surgical removal of a structure, performed through the urethra. 329

t. resection of the prostate (TURP), resection of the prostate by means of a cystoscope passed through the urethra. 329, 329*f*, 369

trauma (**traw**-muh) an injury or wound, whether physical or psychic. 38

tremor (**trem**-ur) an involuntary quivering or trembling. 481

triage (trē-**ahzh**, **trē**-ahzh) the sorting and prioritizing of patients for treatment. 21

triceps (**trī**-seps) a muscle that has three heads at its origin. 93, 95*f*

Trichomonas (trik-ō-**mō**-nus) a genus of parasitic flagellated protozoa. 349-350

trichomoniasis (trik-ō-mō-**nī**-uh-sis) infection with *Trichomonas*, a genus of parasitic protozoa found in the intestinal and genitourinary tracts. 45, 45*f*, 390

trichopathy (tri-**kop**-uh-thē) any disease of the hair. 583

trichosis (tri-**kō**-sis) any disease or abnormal growth of the hair; growth of hair in an unusual place. 583

triglyceride (trī-**glis**-ur-īd) a neutral fat synthesized from carbohydrates for storage in animal adipose cells. 175

triiodothyronine (T₃) (trī-ī-ō-dō-**thī**-rō-nēn) one of the thyroid hormones. 536

trimester (trī-**mes**-tur) a period of 3 months. 376

tripara (**trip**-uh-ruh) a female who has borne three children. 378

triplegia (trī-**plē**-juh) paralysis on one side of the body and, in addition, paralysis of an arm or a leg on the opposite side. 95

trocar (**trō**-kahr) surgical instrument with a three-sided cutting point enclosed in a tube for inserting in a body cavity. 72

tubal ligation (**tōō**-bul lī-**gā**-shun) cauterization or tying off of the uterine tubes to prevent passage of eggs and thus prevent pregnancy. 359, 359*f*, 375

t. l. reversal, reconnection of the fallopian tubes that have been previously blocked to prevent conception. 375

tubercle (**tōō**-bur-kul) any of the small, rounded, granulomatous lesions produced by infection with *Mycobacterium tuberculosis;* it is the characteristic lesion of tuberculosis. A nodule, or small eminence, such as a rough, rounded eminence on a bone. 231

tuberculosis (TB) (tōō-bur-kū-**lō**-sis) an infectious bacterial disease caused by species of *Mycobacterium* that is chronic in nature and commonly affects the lungs. 231

tubular reabsorption (**tōō**-bū-lur rē-ab-**sorp**-shun) conservation of certain substances, including much of the water, as fluid passes through the renal tubules. 307, 308*f*

tubule (**tōō**-būl) a small tube. 307

distal t., the portion of the nephron lying between the descending loop of Henle and the collecting duct in the kidney. 307

proximal t., the portion of the nephron between the glomerulus and the loop of Henle. 307

seminiferous t., one of several small channels of the testes in which spermatozoa develop. 362

tumor (**tōō**-mur) a new growth of tissue in which cell multiplication is uncontrolled; neoplasm. 48

benign t., a localized tumor that has a fibrous capsule and is not malignant. 48, 48*f*

fibrogenic t., a tumor composed of fibrous tissue. 438

localized t., a new tumor in which the cancer has not metastasized. 605

malignant t., a malignant neoplasm that characteristically invades surrounding tissue and metastasizes to distant parts if treatment does not intervene. 48, 48*f*, 602

primary t., the original cancerous tumor from which cancer may spread. 600

t. marker test, procedure in which certain substances are found at higher than normal levels in the blood, urine, or body tissue of some people with cancer. 606

t. grade, grading system depending on the amount of abnormality. 604

Wilms tumor, a malignant neoplasm of the kidney occurring in young children. 318

tuning fork test (**tōō**n-ing fork test) a screening procedure of hearing in which a small metal instrument consisting of a stem and two prongs produce a constant pitch when either prong is struck, and used by physicians to test air and bone conduction. 516, 517*f*

tympanic membrane (tim-**pan**-ik **mem**-brān) the thin membranous partition between the external acoustic meatus and the tympanic cavity. 514

tympanostomy (tim-puh-**nos**-tuh-mē) surgical incision of the eardrum performed to relieve pressure and release pus or fluid from the middle ear. 518, 518*f*

ulcer (**ul**-sur) a local defect or excavation of the surface of an organ or tissue, produced by sloughing of necrotic inflammatory tissue. 574, 575*f*

decubitus u., a sore in the skin over a bony prominence that results from ischemic hypoxia of the tissues caused by prolonged pressure; pressure ulcer. 579, 579*f*

ulna (**ul**-nuh) the inner and larger bone of the forearm. 418

ultrasonography (ul-truh-suh-**nog**-ruh-fē) the visualization of deep structures of the body by recording the reflections of pulses of ultrasonic waves directed into the tissues. 68

ultrasound (**ul**-truh-sound) mechanical radiant energy with a frequency greater than 20,000 cycles per second; ultrasonography. 68, 381*f*

ultraviolet (UV) (ul-truh-**vī**-uh-lut) beyond the violet end of the spectrum. 93, 571

umbilical region (um-**bil**-i-kul rē-jun) abdominal region in the area of the umbilicus. 110

umbilicus (um-**bil**-i-kus) the navel. 114

undifferentiated cells (un-dif-ur-**en**-she-āt-ud selz) biological cells that can differentiate into specialized cells and can divide to produce more stem cells. 600

urea (ū-**rē**-uh) the chief nitrogenous constituent of urine and the major nitrogenous end product of protein metabolism. 310

uremia (ū-**rē**-mē-uh) an accumulation of toxic products in the blood caused by inadequate functioning of the kidneys. 318

ureter (ū-**rē**-tur, **ū**-ruh-tur) the tubular organ through which urine passes from the kidney to the bladder. 304

ureteral dysfunction (ū-**rē**-tur-ul dis-**funk**-shun) a disturbance of a ureter that may be caused by mechanical irritation of a stone. 324

ureterectomy (ū-rē-tur-**ek**-tuh-mē) surgical removal of all or a part of a ureter. 328

ureteritis (ū-rē-tur-**ī**-tis) inflammation of a ureter. 324

ureterocele (ū-**rē**-tur-o-sēl) hernia of the ureter. 324

ureterocystoneostomy (ū-rē-tur-ō-sis-tō-nē-**os**-tuh-mē) surgical transplantation of the ureter to a different site of attachment to the bladder. 328

ureterocystostomy (ū-rē-tur-ō-sis-**tos**-tuh-mē) surgical transplantation of a ureter to a different site in the bladder; ureteroneocystostomy. 328

ureterolith (ū-**rē**-tur-ō-lith) a stone that is lodged or has formed in the ureter. 324

ureterolithiasis (ū-rē-tur-ō-li-**thī**-uh-sis) formation of stones in a ureter. 324

ureterolithotomy (ū-rē-tur-ō-li-**thot**-uh-mē) the removal of a calculus from the ureter by incision. 324

ureteropathy (ū-rē-tur-**op**-uh-thē) any disease of the ureter. 324

ureteroplasty (ū-**rē**-tur-ō-plas-tē) surgical repair of the ureter. 329

ureteropyelonephritis (ū-rē-tur-ō-pī-uh-lō-nuh-**frī**-tis) inflammation of the ureter, renal pelvis, and the kidney. 324

Pronunciation Guide

Pronunciation of medical terms is located in an alphabetical list at the end of each chapter.

Phonetic spelling with few marks is used for simplicity.

There are three basic rules:

1. The syllable that gets the greatest stress is **bold**faced. Single syllable words have no stress mark.
2. Long vowels are marked with a straight line above them.
3. Short vowels are unmarked.

See to the right for consonant sounds, and individual and combined vowel sounds.

Vowels

ā	m*a*te	a	b*a*t
ē	b*ea*m	e	m*e*t
ī	b*i*te	i	b*i*t
ō	h*o*me	o	g*o*t
ū	f*ue*l	u	b*u*t
uh	sof*a*	aw	*a*ll
oi	b*oi*l	ou	f*ow*l
ōō	b*oo*m	oo	b*oo*k

Consonants

b	*b*ook	m	*m*ouse	ch	*ch*in
d	*d*og	n	*n*ew	ks	si*x*
f	*f*og	p	*p*ark	kw	*qu*ote
g	*g*et	r	*r*at	ng	si*ng*
h	*h*eat	s	*s*igh	sh	*sh*ould
j	*j*ewel, *g*em	t	*t*in	th	*th*in, *th*an
k	*c*art, pi*ck*	w	*w*ood	zh	mea*s*ure
l	*l*ook	z	*s*ize, pha*s*e		